Comprehensive PEDIATRIC Ophthalmology

Comprehensive PEDIATRIC Ophthalmology

PK Mukherjee
MS
Consultant and Counselor
Former Dean, Professor and Head
Department of Ophthalmology
Pt Jawahar Lal Nehru Memorial Medical College
Raipur, Chhattisgarh, India

JAYPEE

JAYPEE BROTHERS MEDICAL PUBLISHERS
The Health Sciences Publisher
New Delhi | London

Jaypee Brothers Medical Publishers (P) Ltd

Headquarters
Jaypee Brothers Medical Publishers (P) Ltd
EMCA House, 23/23-B
Ansari Road, Daryaganj
New Delhi 110 002, India
Landline: +91-11-23272143, +91-11-23272703
+91-11-23282021, +91-11-23245672
Email: jaypee@jaypeebrothers.com

Corporate Office
Jaypee Brothers Medical Publishers (P) Ltd
4838/24, Ansari Road, Daryaganj
New Delhi 110 002, India
Phone: +91-11-43574357
Fax: +91-11-43574314
Email: jaypee@jaypeebrothers.com

Overseas Office
JP Medical Ltd.
83, Victoria Street, London
SW1H 0HW (UK)
Phone: +44 20 3170 8910
Fax: +44 (0)20 3008 6180
Email: info@jpmedpub.com

Website: www.jaypeebrothers.com
Website: www.jaypeedigital.com

Comprehensive Pediatric Ophthalmology

First Edition: **2025**

ISBN: 978-93-6616-156-3

Printed at: Samrat Offset Pvt. Ltd.

Dedicated to

My family and friends

Contributors

Jaya Lalwani MD
Professor and Head
Department of Anesthesia
Pt Jawahar Lal Nehru Memorial Medical College
Raipur, Chhattisgarh, India

PK Mukherjee MS
Consultant and Counselor
Former Dean, Professor and Head
Department of Ophthalmology
Pt Jawahar Lal Nehru Memorial Medical College
Raipur, Chhattisgarh, India

Preface

Currently, the world has a staggering population of 8.2 billion people. In spite of all efforts, it is increasing and may reach a stage beyond a manageable number. The condition is worse in the underdeveloped world. India is in an unenviable first place among all with its population of 1.44 billion, out of which 24% are in the pediatric age group, requiring special attention. In India, the number of totally blind persons stands at about three hundred thousand; 50% of them have nonretrieval vision, many of which could have been prevented and cured if proper steps had been taken at the appropriate time.

As against this, an unsurmountable number of 9.3 million children are referred to as visually handicapped; the majority of them are manageable with present-day advanced technology that includes prophylaxes, medical management and high-grade surgery. The percentage of children with subnormal vision varies from place to place and the methodology used to record them. Surprisingly, it is less in preschool children, most of which are congenital anomalies amounting to 1 in 14 as compared to 1 in 4 in school-going children, mostly with errors of refraction and amblyopia. The childhood visual handicap leaves the subjects in a state of underprivilege both socially and economically.

Such a massive problem requires proper planning and management by especially trained persons who have ventured in this field. That requires a large number of ophthalmologists, most of them working as general ophthalmologists dealing with neonatal disorders to advanced retinal morbidity without being proficient in a particular subspecialty. They deal with pediatric ophthalmology in the same way as they would deal with adult persons.

Pediatric ophthalmology heads the list of such faculties that have assumed a status of a superspecialty. This resulted in the establishment of separate departments for pediatric ophthalmology in most of the medical colleges to create a large army of pediatric ophthalmologists; naturally, the books available on eye disorders have small chapters on pediatric ophthalmology which are not sufficient to deal with ever-increasing superspecialization in pediatric ophthalmology. There is a paucity of books in this field. The present work does not claim to answer all the requirements. The present work can be taken as a handy, quick way to answer many day-to-day ocular problems in children and adolescents, who comprise one-fourth of all ophthalmic cases. The book deals with usual ocular problems besides a special chapter on genetics and ocular anesthesia. The book avoids details of therapeutic and surgical procedures for which the readers may refer to larger books. The present book may at the most be considered as a handbook to meet day-to-day requirements.

PK Mukherjee

Acknowledgments

The most difficult part of writing a book is to acknowledge the contribution of many friends, fellows, and well-wishers. The list runs in hundreds. At the top of the list is Dr Jaya Lalwani, Professor of Anesthesia at Pt Jawahar Lal Nehru Memorial Medical College, Raipur, Chhattisgarh, India. She, in spite of her heavy schedule, has kindly written the much-needed chapter on anesthesia in pediatric ophthalmology. I am indebted to her, and I am also thankful to Dr Dilip Lalwani, Consultant in Ophthalmology, for his suggestions and supply of clinical pictures. Padma Shri Dr AK Dabke was kind enough to go through the chapter on genetics.

I express my heartfelt gratitude to Dr SL Adile, Former Director, Medical Education, Government of Chhattisgarh; Dr AK Chandrakar, Vice Chancellor, Ayush University of Medical Science, Raipur; Dr Somen Misra, Professor and Head of the Department of Ophthalmology, AIIMS, Raipur; Dr ML Garg, Dean, Government Medical College, Kanker; Dr Nidhi Pandey, Director, Regional Institute of Ophthalmology Medical College, Raipur; and Dr Santosh Patel, Professor, Department of Ophthalmology, Pt Jawahar Lal Nehru Memorial Medical College, for their unending help in writing the book. I am thankful to Dr Anand Deshpande, Professor and Head of Department, Bhilai Medical College, and Dr LC Madaria, former Professor and Head of Department, Government Medical College, for the clinical pictures contributed.

I am thankful to Dr Madan Deshpande, Bilaspur; Dr Yamini of the Regional Institute of Ophthalmology at Pt Jawahar Lal Nehru Memorial Medical College; and Dr Richa Chatterjee, Dr Biplab Chatterjee, and Dr Satish Batalia for providing me with clinical pictures. I am indebted to Dr Santosh G Honavar for permission to use photographs of retinoblastoma, published in IJO and other publications. I extend my gratitude to various editors of IJO who have permitted me to use material from the journal from time to time.

I am intensely grateful to Shri Jitendar P Vij (Group Chairman) of M/s Jaypee Brothers Medical Publishers (P) Ltd, New Delhi, India for his help in getting this work published. I am also immensely thankful to Mr Ankit Vij (Managing Director), Mr MS Mani (Group President), Ms Pooja Bhandari [Director—Production (Books and Journals)], Ms Sunita Katla (Executive Assistant to Group Chairman and Publishing Manager), Mr Ashwani Kumar Singh [Senior Manager—Production (Books and Journals)], Ms Neha Verma (Cover Designer), Somoshri Banerji (Development Editor) and others, without whose involvement this work would not have been possible.

I am very thankful to Sri Anil Kumar Prasad, my computer assistant, who had immense patience in typing, retyping, correcting the manuscript, drawing the pictures, and making the charts and tables. Without his efforts, this book would not have been possible.

I am thankful to all the persons who have permitted me to use their clinical pictures in the book.

Lastly, I am thankful to my wife, Protima Mukherjee, who has been the driving force behind writing this book and other books published earlier. Without her forbearance, it would not have been possible to complete the project. I appreciate the tolerance of my daughters and sons-in-law, for whom I could not spare much time during this project.

Contents

CHAPTER

1 Embryology

The eyes start developing at an early stage of embryogenesis. The presence of future eyes becomes obvious 2 weeks after conception, i.e., at the 2.00 mm stage of the embryo. The ocular structures are part of the central nervous system; the development of the eye is closely associated with the development of the brain. The eyeball and the optic nerve are out pouching of the developing central nervous system. The central nervous system itself develops from the neural groove, which gives rise to a neural tube that occupies a dorsal position in the growing embryo; the eyes develop from the cephalic end of the neural tube, to which are added cells from the surface ectoderm and mesoderm **(Figs. 1.1 and 1.2)**.

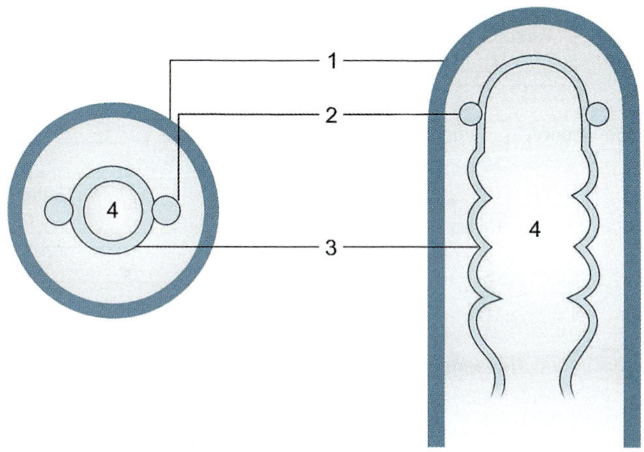

Fig. 1.1: Early evidence of embryonic eye. (1) Surface ectoderm; (2) Embryonic plate; (3) Neuroectoderm; (4) Neural tube.

Involvement of surface ectoderm, mesoderm, and neural ectoderm is an intricate process; failure at any stage of this process will lead to congenital malformation of not only the eye and its adnexa but also the developing central nervous system; thus, developmental anomalies can be ocular in isolation, oculocerebral, or cerebral.

The surface ectoderm is the outermost layer of the developing eye, the neural ectoderm is the innermost, and the mesoderm is insinuating in between.

The chart that follows shows different structures that arise from different layers **(Flowchart 1.1)**.

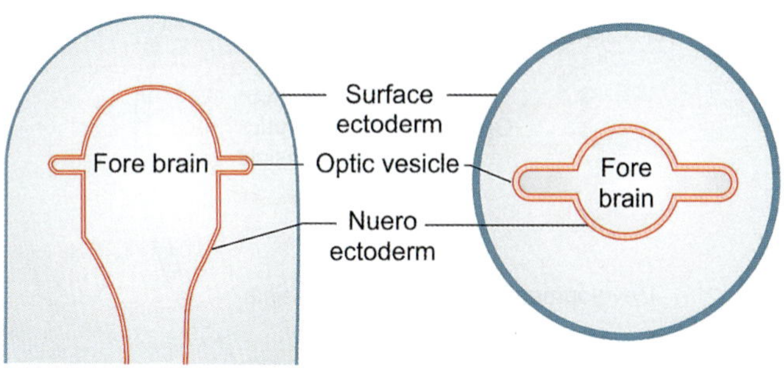

Fig. 1.2: Early evidence of optic vesicle.

> *Structures that have multiple origin*
> - *Lids:* Surface ectoderm and mesoderm
> - *Vitreous:* Neuroectoderm, mesoderm, and surface ectoderm
> - *Bruch's membrane:* Neuroectoderm and mesoderm

Two weeks after conception, at the 2.5 mm stage, the neuroectoderm exhibits the first evidence of future eyeballs and optic nerves, as the embryonic plate sees **(Figs. 1.1 and 1.2)**. The embryonic plate gets converted into the neural crest (ridge), neural tube (cylinder), and optic vesicle successively. At about 4 weeks, i.e., the 9.00 mm stage, the anterior part of the neural tube closes fully; at this point, the neuroectoderm grows toward the surface ectoderm. The neuroectoderm toward the surface is transformed into a shallow spherical structure and is called the primary optic vesicle, from which will develop two layers of the future retina. The tubular structure joining the optic vesicle to the forebrain is called the optic stalk, from which will develop the optic nerve.

The optic vesicle grows toward the surface ectoderm till it comes into contact with the surface ectoderm. The contact of the optic vesicle with the surface ectoderm triggers thickening in the surface at the spot where the two meet. This thickened surface is called the lens placode,

Flowchart 1.1: Structures arising from different layers of the embryo.

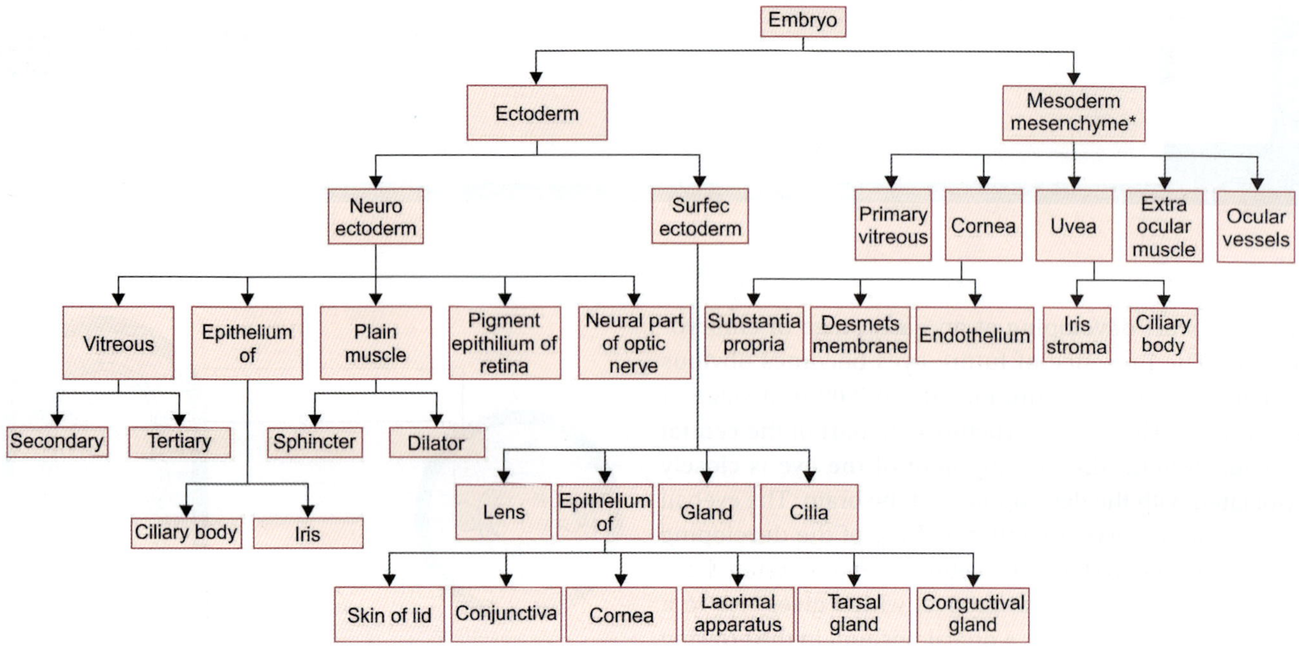

*Mesenchyme is embryonic mesoderm from which arise connective tissue, blood vessel, blood and lymphatic.

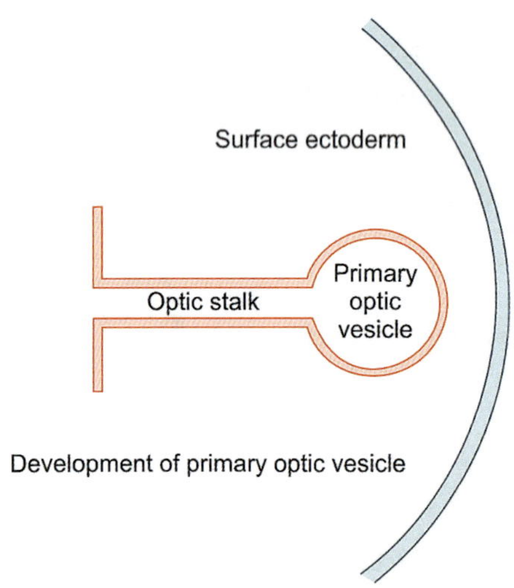

Fig. 1.3: Development of primary optic vesicle.

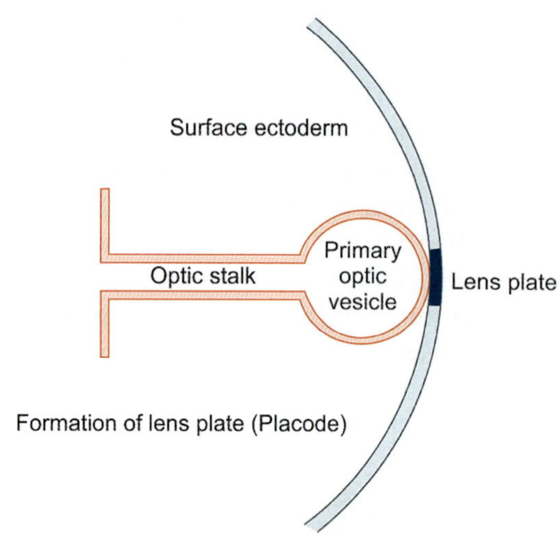

Fig. 1.4: Formation of lens plate (placode).

the precursor of the lens **(Figs. 1.3 and 1.4)**. Simultaneously with the formation of the lens placode, changes are initiated at the vertex of the optic vesicle. The apex of the vesicle develops a saucer-like depression that gradually sinks backward **(Fig. 1.5)** to form a two-layered cup called the optic cup **(Figs. 1.6 and 1.7)**. The development of the two layers of the optic cup is not uniform and equal throughout the circumference; it is slower at the ventral surface, giving rise to a groove at the lower part, to an extent ending from the rim of the cup to the forebrain in the optic stalk. The fault is called by various names, i.e., the optic fissure, fetal fissure, choroidal fissure, or embryonal fissure **(Figs. 1.8 and 1.9)**. The outer layer of the cup gives rise to the retinal pigment layer; from the inner layer, develop the remaining retinal layers. The two layers are approximated, but there is a potential space in between the two. The choroidal fissure is the space through which the mesoderm will enter the future eyeball.

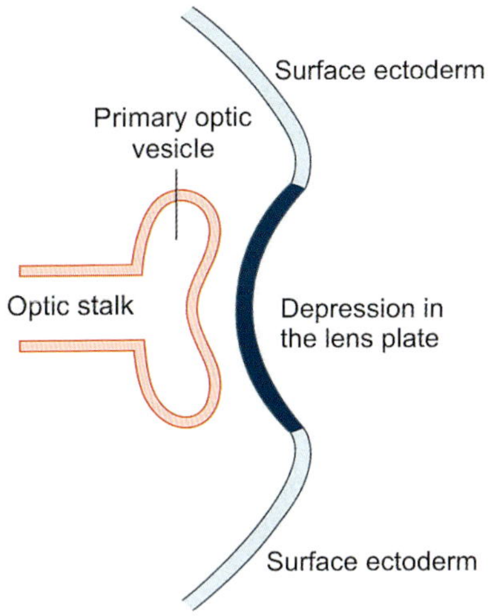

Fig. 1.5: Formation of lens vesicle (early stage).

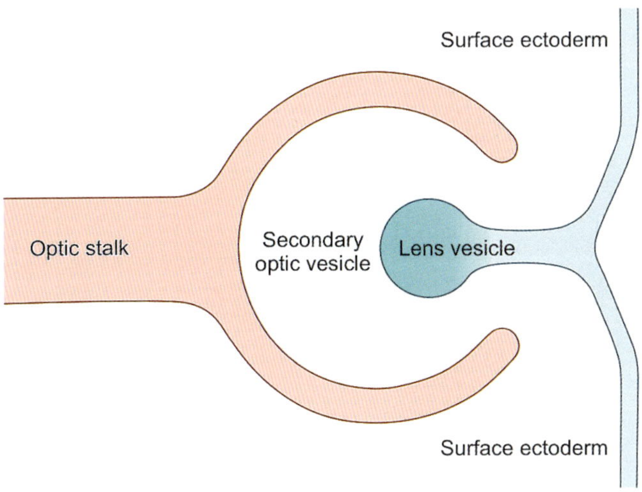

Fig. 1.6: Formation of secondary optic vesicle.

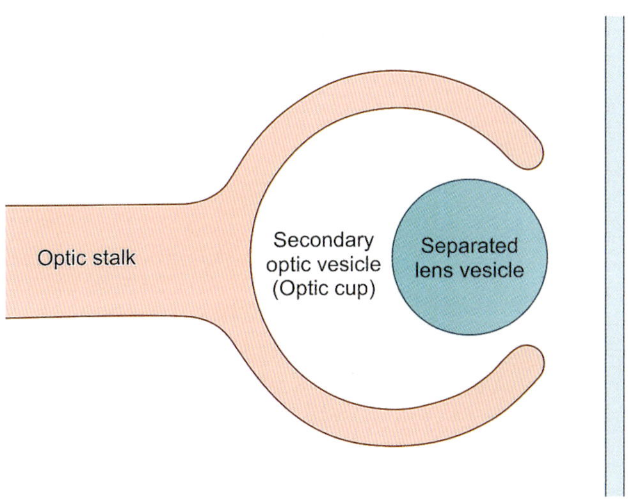

Fig. 1.7: Formation of lens vesicle.

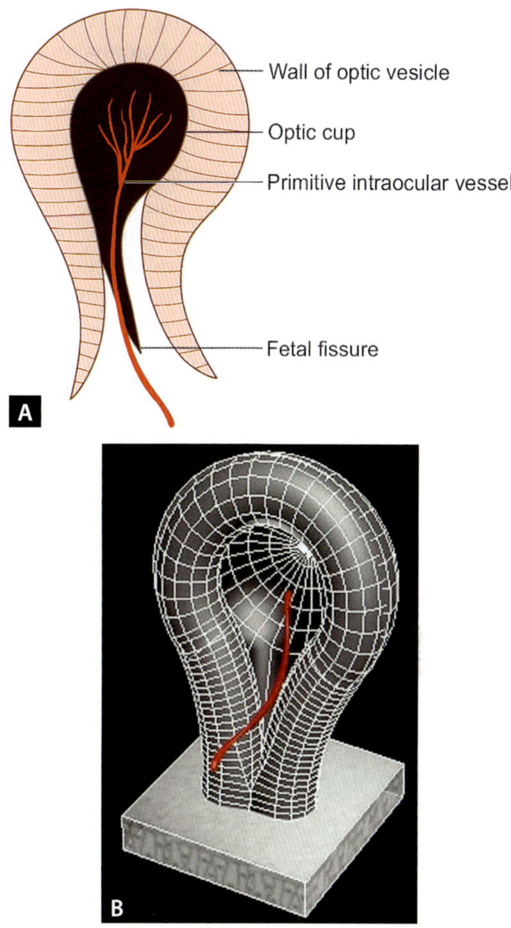

Figs. 1.8A and B: Development of fetal fissure and entry of mesodermal tissue.

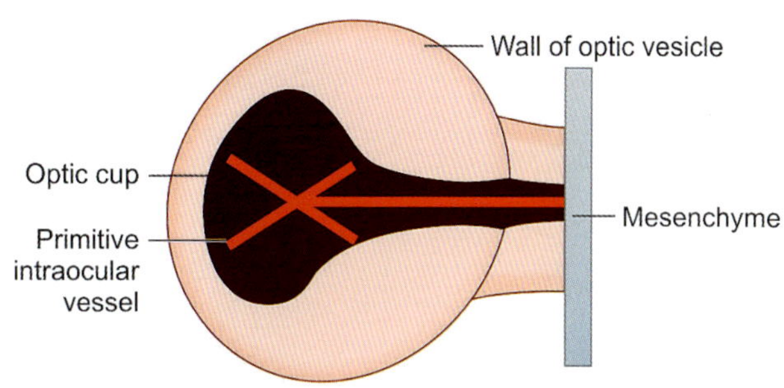

Fig. 1.9: Optic vesicle, optic cup, primitive intraocular blood vessel, and paraxial mesenchyme.

SUGGESTED READING

1. Banu Mathy SP, Natchair G. Anatomy of the eye, 2nd edition. Madurai: Arvind Eye Hospital; 1998.
2. Barber AN. Embryology of the Human Eye. St. Louis: Mosby; 1955.

3. Demston AKO, Murry PI. Embryology. In: Demston AKO, Murry PI (Eds). Oxford handbook of ophthalmology. New Delhi: Oxford University Press; 2006.
4. Duke Elder S, Cook C. Embryology in the System of Ophthalmology, Volume 3, part 1, System of Ophthalmology, 1st edition. London: Henry Kimpton; 1963.
5. Hamming N, Apple D. Anatomy and embryology of the eye in principles and practices of ophthalmology. In: Peyman GA, Saunder DR, Goldberg MF (Eds). Pediatric dermatology, 1st Indian Edition. New Delhi: JP Brother; 1981.
6. Keeny AH. Embryology. In: Keeny AH (Ed). Modern Ophthalmology, Volume 1. London: Butterworth's; 1963.
7. Kozart DM. Embryology of the Human Eye. In: Schcie HG, Albert DM (Eds). The Text Book of Ophthalmology, 9th edition. London: WB Saunders Company; 1977.
8. Mahesh KS. Neuroophthalmology, 4th edition. Madurai: Arvind Eye Hospital; 2007.
9. Mann Ida. Development of the Human Eye, 3rd edition. London: British Medical Association; 1964.
10. Nema HV. Congenital anomalies of the eye and its adnexa. In: Nema HV. Anatomy of the Eye and its Adnexa, 2nd edition. New Delhi: JP Brother; 1991.
11. Riordan-Eva P. Chapter 1: Anatomy & Embryology of the Eye. In: Vaughan D, A. Taylor A, Riordan-Eva P (Eds). General Ophthalmology, 15th edition. Stamford, Connecticut: Appleton & Lange; 1999.

CHAPTER

2 Development of Specific Structures of Eye

DEVELOPMENT OF LIDS, LACRIMAL APPARATUS, AND CONJUNCTIVA

LIDS

The upper and lower lids develop from two separate sources; the upper lid develops from the frontonasal process in two parts, i.e., a large later part and a smaller medial part that fuse to form the upper lid. A fault in their fusion results in coloboma of upper lid that may just be a notch or large enough to expose the cornea. The lower lid develops from a single maxillary process. The lids develop partly from ectoderm and partly from mesoderm. The skin on the outer surface and the conjunctiva on the inner surface are ectodermal, the main bulk of the lids are mesodermal. To begin with the lid are just mesenchymal buds, one above and one below the developing globe, they creep in front of the cornea from canthus to canthus and are fused, initially there is no interpalpebral fissure in between them, till fifth month, there after the lids start separating from the middle, spreading on either side, this gives rise to the interpalpebral fissure that is fully developed and functional at birth. The tarsal plates and the muscles are mesodermal. The tarsal glands, and sweat glands develop from the ectodermal cells of the lids along with lashes.

LACRIMAL SYSTEM

The lacrimal system consists of two parts, i.e., the lacrimal gland and lacrimal passages. The former is divisible in ectodermal glands and mesodermal connective tissue.

Lacrimal Glands

The glands, develop as solid cords from the superior temporal aspect of upper conjunctival fornix and grow toward the fossa for lacrimal gland in the orbit, the cords get ramified and canalized, surrounded by mesoderm. Lacrimal glands start developing by the end of second month of gestation, they are not fully developed at birth, it takes about 3 years to be fully developed. The lacrimal gland do not start secreting tears before 4 weeks postnatal hence there is no watering in infants eyes. The discharge in infants is only conjunctival secretion. Each lacrimal gland develops as a solid epithelial bud from superior temporal conjunctival epithelium of the fornix, the buds are initially without lumen, it takes about 3 months of embryogenesis for them to get canalized and form acini. The orbital condenses round the acini to complete the development. By this time developing levator insinuates itself in the substance of the gland to divide it in two parts, i.e., orbital and palpebral parts.

> Lacrimal ectoderm is only epithelial tissue in orbit; that is liable to develop malignancy.

Lacrimal Passage

The lacrimal passage is intimately related to development of frontal and maxillary processes of the face, the two bony processes form a groove in between. The groove is later converted in to bony nasolacrimal duct. The surface ectoderm finds its way in the canal from above and below, to completely line the bony canal; they meet in the middle, thus forming the nasolacrimal duct, the upper end grows up and is dilated to be converted in to the lacrimal sac, the canaliculi sprout from the later aspect of the sac to end in for mining the puncta.

The development of the lacrimal gland. The lacrimal glands are ectodermal in origin; surrounded by mesoderm. The ectodermal part comes from conjunctiva; and the mesodermal part from orbit.

Lacrimal Drainage

> The lacrimal drainage system is fully developed at birth in contrast to gland that takes 3 years postnatal to be developed.

The sac begins as a solid cord of epithelium between the lateral nasal process and maxillary process. The upper part distends to form the sac. The solid cord extending down gets canalized to form nasolacrimal duct. The canalization starts both at the upper and lower ends simultaneously to meet in the middle, just before birth. The puncta, the canaliculi, and the nasolacrimal duct should be patent and functional at birth. Sometimes some solid epithelial debris may be left in the nasolacrimal duct causing congenital obstruction of nasolacrimal duct.

CONJUNCTIVA

The conjunctiva too has dual development, i.e., mesoderm and ectodermal. It is intimately associated with development of the lids. The fused upper and lower lids create a pouch in front of the developing globe, called the conjunctival sac, from the wall of the sac will develop the conjunctival epithelium and its glands, the rest of conjunctiva is mesodermal. The plica semilunaris and caruncle share the developmental process of both lids and conjunctiva.

DEVELOPMENT OF CORNEA, SCLERA, AND EXTRAOCULAR MUSCLE

CORNEA

The development cornea involves both ectoderm and mesoderm. The corneal epithelium is ectodermal in nature, the rest of the cornea is mesodermal. During early days of development, the vortex of the optic vesicle touches the inner surface of the surface ectoderm, this initiates thickening of the surface epithelium to form the lens placode that separates from the surface ectoderm and passes in the optic vesicle to develop as lens. The void in the surface ectoderm is bridged and becomes the epithelium of cornea. The space between the developing corneal epithelium and the lens vesicle is filled by mesoderm. The mesoderm is divided in two parts, from the anterior will develop the stroma of cornea and corneal endothelium, from the remaining will develop the stroma of the iris. In the space between the endothelium of lens will develop the future anterior chamber. The invading mesoderm gives rise to Bowman's membrane, stroma, Descemet's membrane, and endothelium. The Descemet's membrane develops independently while Bowman's membrane is the condensation from the stroma under the corneal epithelium.

SCLERA

The sclera is entirely mesodermal in development. It develops from the paraxial mesoderm that condenses round the optic cup. The sclera gets well differentiated by 5th month, initially the future limbus is far posteriorly placed than in actual life, and it is nearer to the developing equator, an area where the recti are attached. By 12th week the condensing mesoderm encircles the optic nerve and the lamina develops, the recti become evident and the Tenon's capsule develops. The sclera develops by 16th week. The sclera has no role in determining the size of the globe that is influenced by developing retina, in contrast to this the size of sclera definitely influences growth of orbit. At birth the sclera is so thin and translucent that the underlying uvea imparts it a blue tinge, the sclera gradually thickens and turns opaque white.

EXTRAOCULAR MUSCLES

All the striated muscle develop from paramedian mesoderm; the extraocular muscles are no exception. The extraocular muscles to begin with arise from a common mesodermal mass at the back of optic cup, that later differentiates in three definite parts; from each will develop muscles specifically marked to be supplied by designated cranial nerve. The levator, superior rectus, medial rectus, inferior rectus, and inferior oblique develop from largest common mesodermal mass to be supplied by third nerve. The superior oblique develops from a separate smaller mass to be supplied by fourth nerve the lateral rectus develops from another small mass to be supplied by sixth nerve. Development of levator overlaps development of superior rectus, this common embryogenesis results in levator getting its nerve supply from a twig of third nerve that passes through the mass of superior rectus, hence both are involved in common congenital anomalies, dystrophies, and degenerations. It is worth noting that the first mass gives rise to four extraocular muscles, i.e., three recti and one oblique to be supplied by single cranial nerve, the mass that gives rise to later rectus and superior oblique are smaller, in spite of smaller mass the muscles arising from them have individual single nerve supply. The recti develop earlier than the oblique as embryo genesis of recti are simpler than oblique; congenital anomalies of recti are less common than oblique. The orbicularis oculi develops from mesoderm of the lid by 12th week of gestation, it is part of mesenchyme of second pharyngeal arch. Embryogenesis of extraocular muscles are closely related to cranial mesoderm and migrating neural crest cells. The Tenon's capsule, parts of ligaments of extraocular muscles, and orbital fat develop along with extraocular muscles.

DEVELOPMENT OF ORBIT

The bones and periosteum of the orbit are mesodermal in origin. They develop from the mesodermal mass around the developing eye ball. The different walls develop from different mesodermal masses. The lateral wall and the floor develop from maxillary mesoderm, the medial develops from the later nasal process. The development of the roof is more complex, it develops from the mesodermal cover of the fore brain. Till 28th week, the orbital rim and equator of the globe are in the same plane, there after the orbital bones start growing faster than the globe, the rim ending in a more anterior position than the globe. The size of the growing orbit is far less than a developed orbit, the orbital walls are almost snug with the globe. At birth the orbital rim is almost circular. The diameter of the orbit at birth is relatively large when compared to face, intraorbital distance in a new born is 16 mm that increases to 25–28 mm in adults.

DEVELOPMENT OF ANTERIOR CHAMBER

The anterior chamber is a space between cornea on one side and iris pupil and lens on the other side, bordered by angle of anterior chamber and trabecular meshwork. The developing anterior chamber becomes evident at 20 mm stage as a cleavage in the paraxial mesoderm between the corneal endothelium and the iris stroma. The sequence of development is as follows:

Once lens placode separates from the surface ectoderm, it gets converted to lens vesicle, the mesoderm from the edge of the optic cup grows in the space between the surface ectoderm and lens vesicle. The mesoderm that fills the gap divides in to two parts, from the anterior part develops cornea except its epithelium, from the posterior part develop the stroma of iris. The anterior chamber starts as a chink in the mesoderm and spreads up to the angle. As the anterior chamber develops the space cleared of mesoderm is filled by aqueous. In early fetal life the anterior chamber and its angle are very narrow, till the enhanced growth of the anterior segment pushes the corneal scleral angle forward, complete differentiation of angle structures take place only after birth. The anterior chamber is fully developed at birth but shallow. The canal of Schlemm is formed by fourth month as venous channel from the margin of optic cup. The angle is formed still 2 months later.

DEVELOPMENT OF THE LENS

The development of lens has two parts, i.e., lens vesicle and lens proper.

The development of the lens goes through the following phases:

Surface ectoderm—Lens placode—Lens vesicle—
Primary lens fibers—Cortex—Nucleus

Lens Vesicle

It has been noted earlier **(Figs. 1.5 to 1.7)** that once the lens placode has formed it bows backwards as a cup that deepens to form lens vesicle. Initially it is open towards the exterior till its lips close. The vesicle is lined by single layer of surface ectoderm. After sometimes it detaches from the surface ectoderm as a hollow sphere and migrates in the optic cup. The gap in the surface ectoderm left by the lens vesicle closes to give rise to corneal epithelium **(Fig. 2.1)**.

The wall toward the surface ectoderm forms the lens epithelium. The cells of the posterior wall do not divide, they only elongate to form columnar epithelium **(Fig. 2.2)**.

- Surface ectoderm, will give rise to epithelium of cornea.
- Space where mesenchymal will give rise to remaining layers of cornea.
- Cuboidal cells of anterior wall.
- Remaining part of lens vesicle.

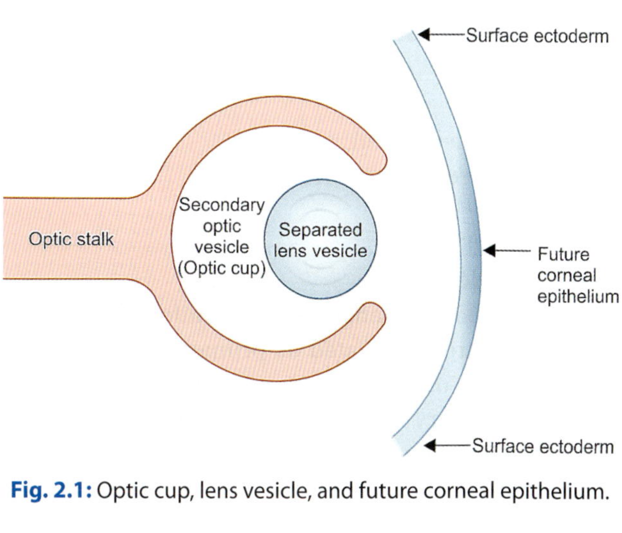

Fig. 2.1: Optic cup, lens vesicle, and future corneal epithelium.

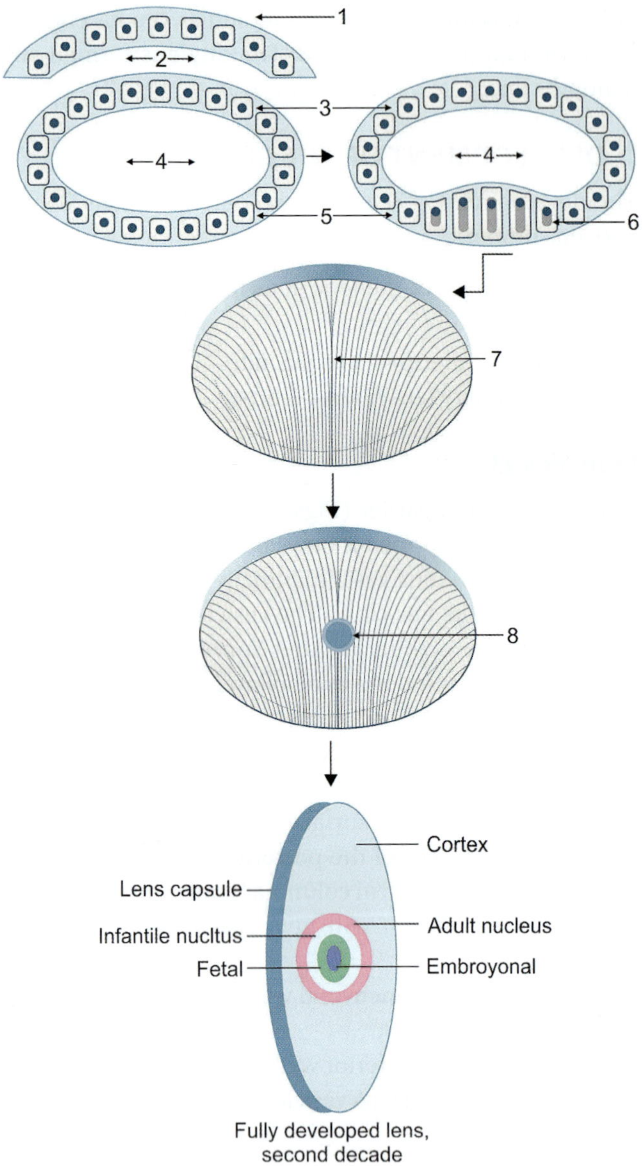

Fig. 2.2: Stages of development of lens.

- Cells of posterior wall.
- Columnar cells of posterior wall.
- Developing cortex.
- Embryonal nucleus.
- Fully developed lens.

They increase in length, spread uniformly to fill the cavity. They are designated as primary lens fibers and are precursor of embryonic nucleus; in contrast to this the secondary lens fibers arise from the equatorial cells of the anterior epithelium and keep on multiplying throughout the life. The secondary lens fibers are laid down concentric with each other. The inner layers get squeezed and pushed toward the center to give rise to various nuclei, that are named as—fetal, infantile, and adult. The fetal nucleus develops between third and eighth week, infantile nucleus starts developing in the last week of gestation and grows till puberty. The adult nucleus develops after puberty and keeps growing throughout the life. The fibers laid over the adult nucleolus become cortex that is responsible for majority of lenticular mass.

Thus the developing lens has:

- Single layered anterior wall.
- From the posterior develop the columnar cells.
- From the equator develop various nuclei; the equatorial cells are in fact the migrated anterior cells.
- Fibers laid over the nuclei will form the cortex.
- The anterior and posterior walls combine to form the anterior and posterior lens capsule, respectively.
- They are in fact the basement membrane of the lens epithelium.

Lens is virtually a mass of epithelium wrapped in capsule.

Suspensory ligament develops from tertiary vitreous. The suspensory ligaments are well developed by fourth month of gestation (See development of vitreous).

DEVELOPMENT OF VITREOUS

The vitreous has dual origin spread over three stages, i.e., primary, secondary, and tertiary. The primary vitreous is mesenchymal in origin. The rest are neuroectodermal. The primary is first to appear only to disappear by the time the secondary vitreous is fully developed. The primary vitreous contains hyaloid vasculature that is converted to tunica vasculosa lentis (TVL), the sole source of blood supply to the developing lens. The primary vitreous is pushed toward the developing lens. The Cloquet's canal develops in primary vitreous. The Cloquet's as hyaloid canal which is infect and empty space in the middle of the developing vitreous, it is a perivascular sheath that surround the developing hyaloid vasculature.

The secondary vitreous is avascular. It forms the main bulk of adult vitreous. The secondary vitreous is neuro-ectodermal in origin, derived from the inner surface of optic cup, the base of the adult vitreous is the thickened part of the secondary vitreous.

The tertiary vitreous is not true vitreous, it in fact is the suspensory ligament of the adult lens. It develops from the neuroectoderm of the ciliary body.

DEVELOPMENT OF UVEA

The three components that are collectively called uvea; are iris, ciliary body, and choroid. They not only differ in tissue but also in embryogenesis, the iris and ciliary body contain both muscle and blood vessels. The choroid is devoid of musculature, it is vascular, with plenty of pigments, which are present in iris and ciliary body in less quantity.

The iris and ciliary body have dual origin, i.e., neuroectoderm and mesoderm, the choroid minus the Bruch's membrane is mesodermal. The Bruch's membrane is partly neuroectodermal and partly mesodermal. The surface ectoderm has no role in development of uvea. The structures in uvea that are ectodermal are: epithelium of ciliary body, pigment epithelium of iris, sphincters of iris, and iris melanocytes. From the mesoderm develops the stroma.

IRIS

The stroma of the iris is mesenchymal, while the pigment epithelium, the sphincter and dilators are neuroectodermal in nature. The stroma develops behind the surface ectoderm, in front of anterior lens capsule. Over the stroma develops the two epithelial layers which are ectodermal, the anterior epithelial layer is continuous with outer layer of the optic cup, and is anterior extension of pigment epithelium of the retina. The posterior layer of the epithelium is derived from inner layer of the optic cup and represents the sensory retina; from the anterior tip of the pigment epithelium develop the splinter and dilator muscle of iris. The iris is fully pigmented at birth but lighter in color than adult, paucity of pigment makes it lighter, excess makes it dark, absence of pigment results in albinism.

FORMATION OF PUPIL

The pupil is a dynamic structure without tissue. Earlier it has been noted that a membrane of mesodermal origin stretches across the lip of the optic cup, which later; atrophies and disappears. The membrane besides mesoderm also contains part of tunica vasculosa lentis. Which gradually atrophy and disappear leaving the anterior lens capsule clear, with a circular aperture, bordered by pigmented fringe. This clear space is the pupil. A remnant of the mesodermal membrane attached to the iris collaret is called persistent pupillary membrane.

CILIARY BODY

Embryo genetically the ciliary muscles and it is epithelium have different origins, the muscles are mesodermal, the epithelia are neuroectodermal. The undifferentiated ciliary muscle become evident by third month of gestation and then differentiate in longitudinal, oblique, and circular muscles. The ciliary epithelium is neuroectodermal, it develops from the lip of the optic cup, with pigmented outer layer and nonpigmented inner layer. The ciliary processes, about 70–75 in number develop from the ciliary epithelium.

CHOROID

The choroid that constitute the largest volume of the uvea structurally differs from iris and ciliary body, it lacks epithelium, stroma, and muscle, and it is luxuriant in blood vessels of three sizes, with plenty of pigment and connective tissue. It has a special noncellular tissue called Bruch's membrane, the Bruch's membrane is partly ectodermal and partly mesodermal, it is avascular. The choroidal vessels develop in three stages according to their caliber. The choriocapillaries that are thinnest develop first. In the 3rd month develop; the venae verticosae and their tributaries. In the last phase the branches from short ciliary vessels develop.

UVEAL CIRCULATION

The earliest presence of uveal circulation becomes evident at the posterior aspect of developing optic vesicle. It begins with primitive internal carotid giving off two branches—the dorsal and ventral ophthalmic arteries respectively, from one of them, i.e., the dorsal ophthalmic which is fore runners of posterior ciliary arteries develops single hyaloid artery, that gives rise to central retinal artery, main hyaloid artery, and vasa hyaloidia propria. The anterior uveal circulation develops from the anterior ciliary system of circulation; through the muscular branches of the ophthalmic artery.

UVEAL MELANOCYTES AND BRUCH'S MEMBRANE

The melanocytes of uvea develop from the neural crest by fifth month of gestation. The Bruch's membrane is secreted by the outer wall of the optic cup. By the time the Bruch's membrane is formed rudimentary vertex veins also start developing at different quarters of the globe.

DEVELOPMENT OF RETINA AND MACULA

Retina

The retina proper is neuroectodermal; the retinal vessels are mesenchymal and part of hyaloid system of vasculature. The retina develops from two walls of the optic cup. The inner wall gives rise to neural retina. From the outer wall develops the pigment epithelium of not only the retina but also pigment epithelium of ciliary body and iris. The neurosensory retina develops in three layers, from the first layer that is outermost layer of inner wall of the optic cup develop the rods and cones, from the next layer develop the bipolar cells and the ganglion cells from the third layer develop the nerve fiber layer.

Macula

Macula being a part of retina shares a common embryogenesis with retina, i.e., it is neuroectodermal in nature, develops from the inner layer of optic cup; with following differences:

- Initially the part of retina where future macula will develop grows faster than rest of the retina up to third month.
- Then it goes in a phase of retardation, while rest of surrounding retina grows in usual pace, for next 5 months.
- This is followed by an acceleration in growth macula keeping in pace with rest of retina.
- At 6 months it is thicker than surrounding retina.
- By seventh month it starts thinning, this happens due to spreading out of ganglion cells from the center of developing macula.
- The fovea at birth has only one layer each of ganglion cells and outer nuclear layer.
- Macula is not fully developed at birth.
- It continues to grow up to 4 months postnatal.

DEVELOPMENT OF INTRAOCULAR VASCULATURE (UVEO-RETINAL)

Embryogenesis of intraocular vasculature consists of development of retinal, hyaloid, and uveal system (*See* **Flowchart 2.1** in the following text).

Development of retinal circulation is not well understood. The commonly accepted view is that it develops from the posterior aspect of hyaloid artery as central retinal artery which bifurcates in to nasal and temporal branches, the hyaloid artery ahead of the bifurcation atrophies, the central retinal arteries keep growing in to superior and inferior branches.

Flowchart 2.1: Flowchart showing development of hyaloid system and tunica vasculosa lentis.

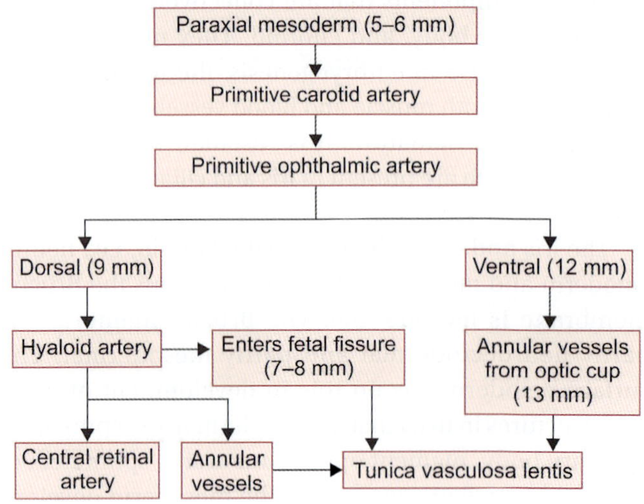

The intraocular vessel system is mesodermal in origin and enter the optic stalk and vesicle via the foetal fissure. The system develops from two sources i.e. the embryonic dorsal and ventral ophthalmic arteries which are branches of internal carotid. The intraocular vessels develop partly from each.

All the three systems of intraocular vasculature cannot be separated from each other in toto.

At places they overlap, i.e., the retinal system is offshoot of hyaloid system, while from the termination of hyaloid system develops the posterior part of tunica vasculosa lentis, the lateral parts of tunica gets twigs from anterior uveal system.

> The intraocular vessels not only supply nutrition to the eye but also act as stimulus for its development.

HYALOID SYSTEM

The system consist of:

- Hyaloid artery
- Tunica vasculosa lentis
- Vessels of persistent pupillary membrane

Development of hyaloid artery is shown in **Figure 2.3**.

The hyaloid artery is the only source of blood supply to the developing lens. It is a branch of dorsal ophthalmic artery, it enters the developing eye through the fetal fissure, once it gets in the developing eye it traverses through the vitreous in the Cloquet canal to reach the posterior surface of the developing lens, thus it stretches from the developing optic nerve head to the lens. The hyaloid system is divided in two parts. From the first (anterior) part; develop the vessels of iris and pupillary membrane. The second (posterior) part gives rise to hyaloid artery, hyaloidia propria, and tunica vasculosa lentis **(Fig. 2.4)**.

The following **Flowchart 2.2** depicts distribution of hyaloid system.

From the base of the main hyaloid artery springs the central retinal artery. The terminal end of hyaloid artery

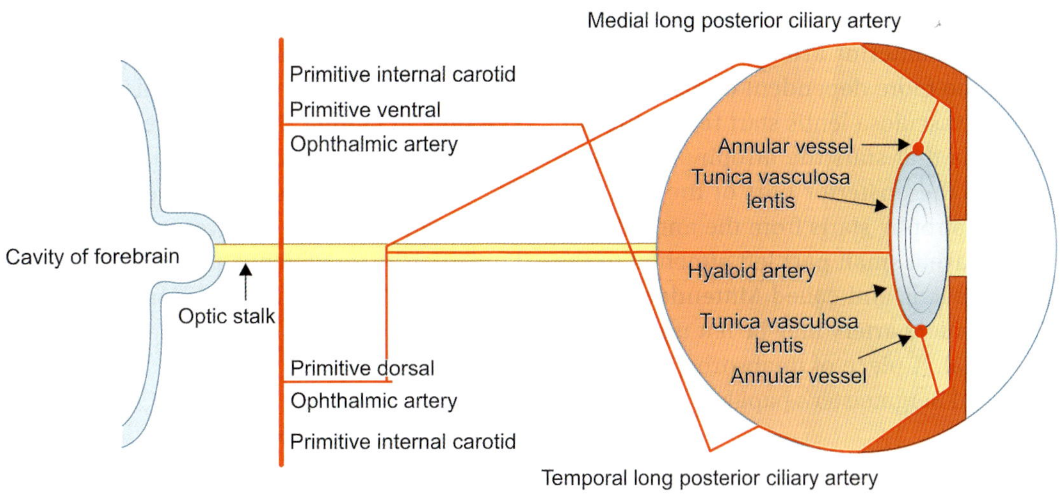

Fig. 2.3: Development of uveal and hyaloid blood vessels.

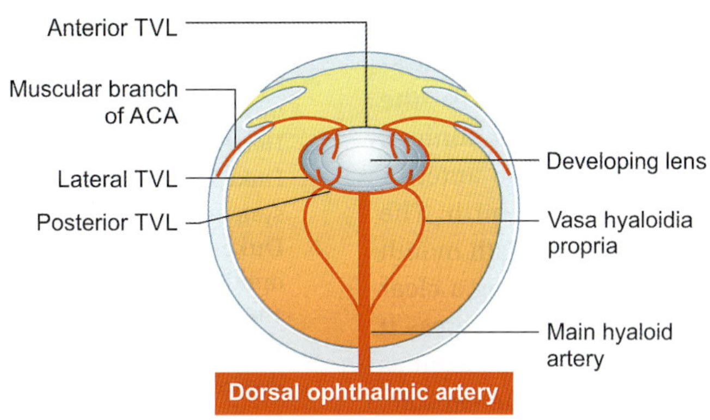

Fig. 2.4: Development of tunica vasculosa lentis. (ACA: anterior ciliary artery; TVL: tunica vasculosa lentis)

Flowchart 2.2: Branches of hyaloid system.

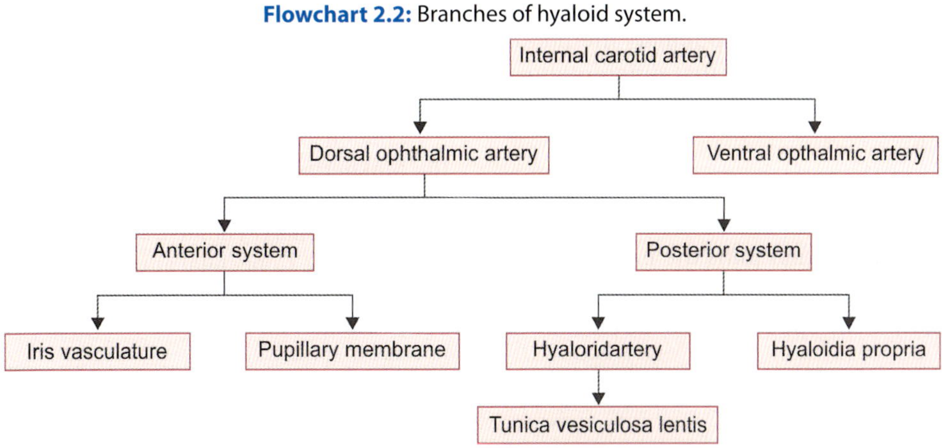

sprouts small twigs before reaching the posterior surface of the lens, the small twigs join to form posterior part of tunica vasculosa lentis, which is junction of two separate vascular systems, i.e., intra- and extraocular. Once it has reached the posterior surface of the lens, it is joined by vessels from anterior uveal vascular system through the muscular branches of anterior arteries. Once the lens has developed and no more dependent on tunica for its nutrition the tunica vasculosa lentis start regressing and atrophy, the impetus that stars the atrophy is not well elucidated, at birth the posterior part of the tunica is fully regressed. The atrophy starts from the anterior end may occasionally leave a small part left attached to the posterior pole of the lens and called Mittendorf's spot. A bit of atrophied hyaloid artery may be left unabsorbed in the Cloquet's canal. A piece of unabsorbed vessel on the optic disc is called Bergmeister's papilla.

FORMATION OF TUNICA VASCULOSA LENTIS

Tunica vasculosa lentis is a fibrovascular envelop that covers the developing lens from all sides, it is also a junction where the two systems of circulation, i.e., intra- and extraocular meet. The tunic has three parts—the posterior, lateral, and anterior. The posterior tunic is the earliest to atrophy, followed by later; the anterior is the last to disappear, leaving no trace at birth. The anterior tunica vasculosa lentis atrophies by sixth month of gestation, beginning from the center, leaving a clear and bright anterior lens capsule, if it fails to regress it may get attached to the lens capsule and be mistaken as posterior synechiae, or leave an opacity on the capsule, rarely it may get attached to cornea and mistaken as iridocorneal dysgenesis. The membrane develops from the mesenchymal tissue, anterior to the iris, posterior to the cornea. The typical persistent pupillary membrane is attached to the collaret of the iris that differentiates it from posterior synechiae. The peripheral thick part arises from the iris stroma.

DEVELOPMENT OF OPTIC NERVE

The optic stalk is a conduit that joins the fore brain and the optic cup, it is the fore runner of future optic nerve, at the inferior surface of the optic stalk lies the fetal fissure extending from the optic vesicle to the fore brain, through the stalk pass the retinal nerve fibers and the retinal vasculature. By third month the mesoderm along with fine capillaries enter the optic nerve from bellow. The outer covering of the optic nerve, i.e., the dura, arachnoid, and pia develop between third and seventh month, the lamina develops still later. The myelination starts at about seventh month, from the cephalic end and grow toward the globe, stopping at lamina. The optic nerve fibers develop from retinal fiber layers, grow back to reach the brain through the optic stalk, the neural tissues are neuroectodermal, the covering tissues and vessels are mesodermal. The lamina cribrosa which is in fact part of sclera becomes evident by fifth month of gestation, gets fibrous tissue from choroid and sheaths of optic nerve till eighth month of gestation.

SUGGESTED READING

1. Banumathy SP. Natchair Geeta anatomy of the eye, 2nd edition. Madurai: Arvind eye hospital; 1998.
2. Demston AKO, Murry PI. Embryology in Oxford Hand Book of Ophthalmology. New Delhi: Oxford University Press; 2006.
3. Duke Elder S, Cook C, Embryology in system of ophthalmology, volume 3, part 1, 1st edition. London: Henry Kimpton; 1963.
4. Duke Elder S, Wyber KC. Anatomy of the visual system in system of ophthalmology. London: Henry Kimpton; 1961.
5. Duke Elder S. Congenital deformities in system of ophthalmology, volume 3, part 2. London: Henry Kimpton; 1964.
6. Hamming ND, Apple D. Anatomy and embryology of the eye in principle and practice or ophthalmology, volume 1. In: Peyman GA, Saunder DR, GoldBerg (Eds). New Delhi: JP Brothers; 1981.
7. Keeny AH. Embryology in modern ophthalmology, volume 1. London: Butter Worths; 1963.
8. Mahesh KS. Neuro ophthalmology, 4th edition, Madurai: Arvind eye hospital; 2007.
9. Mann Ida. Development of human eye, 3rd edition. London: British medical Association; 1964.
10. Mukherjee PK. Outline of development of the eye in pediatric ophthalmology, 1st edition. New Delhi: New age international (P) limited; 2005.
11. Nema HV. Congenital anomalies of eye and its adnexa in anatomy of the eye and its adnexa, 2nd edition. New Delhi: JP Brother; 1991.

CHAPTER 3

Congenital Anomalies of Eyes and Adnexa

Congenital anomalies of ocular interest are not uncommon; they may be uni- or binocular; when bilateral, they are generally symmetric; they may be apparent at birth or discovered later; they may be symptomatic or asymptomatic.

The congenital anomalies of the eye and adnexa can be put into the following groups:

- Ocular
- Adnexal
- Combination of the above
- Associated with cranial deformity
- Associated with anomalies of the central nervous system (CNS)
- Associated with congenital anomalies of other organs

CAUSES OF CONGENITAL ANOMALIES OF EYES

The causes of congenital anomalies can be put into two broad groups, i.e.,

1. Nongenetic
2. Genetic

NONGENETIC CAUSES

Nongenetic causes are as follows:

Aftermath of maternal infection: The common maternal infections that cause congenital ocular anomalies are predominantly viruses like rubella, herpes simplex, varicella zoster, cytomegalovirus, Epstein–Barr virus, and Zika virus. The most common bacterial maternal infection to cause congenital anomalies is syphilis. Parasitic maternal infections, too, have been thought to cause congenital anomalies, the most common being toxoplasmosis.

- Drugs and toxins
- Trauma
- Maternal diabetes
- Teratogenicity

Genetic

All types of genetic variation can cause congenital anomalies of the eyes and adnexa.

The common examples are: Anophthalmos and its variations, aniridia, albinism, ectopia lentis, neurofibromatosis, and other hamartomas.

CLASSIFICATION OF CONGENITAL OCULAR ANOMALIES

There is no single classification that can cover all the aspects of ocular congenital anomalies. One of the practical classifications based on topography is shown in **Flowchart 3.1**.

The other topographical classification can be as mentioned in **Flowchart 3.2**.

CONGENITAL ANOMALIES OF LIDS

The anomalies are as follows:

Muscles:

- *Levator:* Ptosis, lid retraction, cryptophthalmos
- *Muller's:* Horner's syndrome
- *Orbicularis:* Bell's palsy

Lid margin:

- Coloboma, distichiasis, and ankyloblepharon
- Epicanthus
- Microblepharon
- Epiblepharon
- Euryblepharon

Congenital anomalies of the lid are generally bilateral and may or may not be symmetric, concurrent, isolated, or associated with other craniofacial congenital anomalies.

Flowchart 3.1: Classification of congenital anomalies of ocular and nonocular structures.

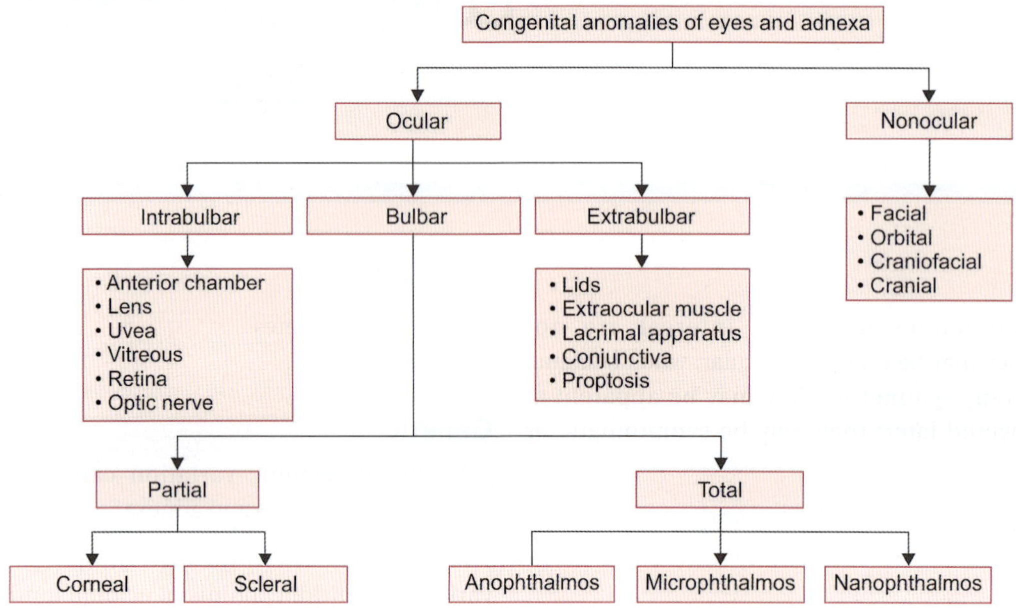

Flowchart 3.2: Other possible classifications of congenital anomalies of the eyes.

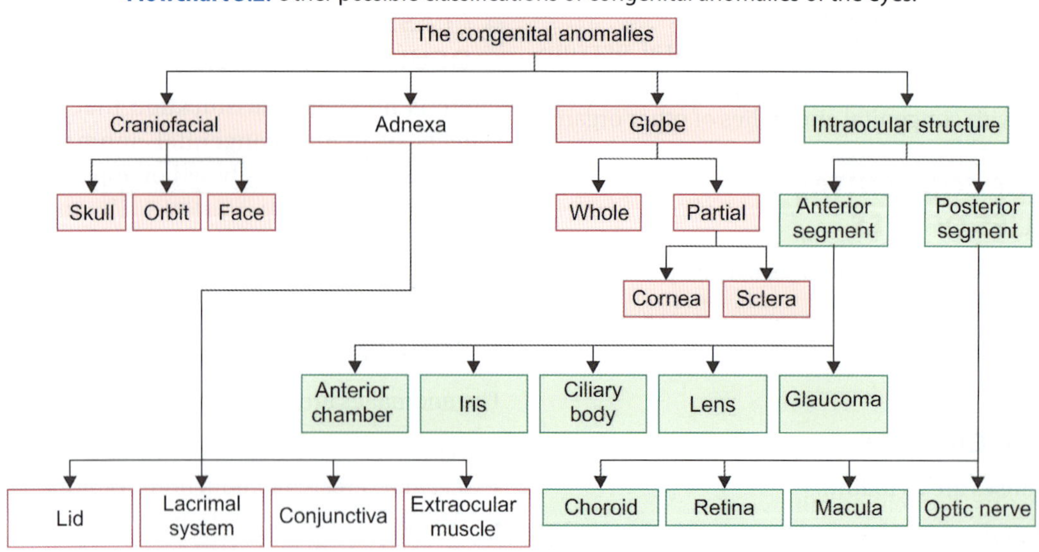

CONGENITAL ANOMALIES OF THE LACRIMAL SYSTEM

The lacrimal system for clinical purposes is divided into two parts, i.e., the lacrimal gland and the lacrimal drainage system.

Congenital Anomalies of Lacrimal Gland

Congenital anomalies of the lacrimal gland are rare.

Absence of the lacrimal gland (rare).

This is the least common congenital anomaly of the lacrimal gland. The development of the lacrimal gland solely depends on the development of the conjunctiva. The lacrimal gland develops from the conjunctiva of the upper fornix. It is only natural that if the fornix/conjunctiva is absent developmentally, the lacrimal gland will not develop. It should be noted that the lacrimal gland is present and functioning in anophthalmos where conjunctiva is present; the gland is absent in cryptophthalmos because conjunctiva is absent in this condition.

Aberrant Lacrimal Gland

Aberrant lacrimal glands are not accessory lacrimal glands. They are rare and mistaken for dermoids, epidermoids, or dermolipomas. Their development is similar to that of the usual lacrimal gland. They develop as epithelial cords from developing conjunctiva generally in the upper fornix. Incidentally, they have been reported from the iris and ciliary body as well. The exact cause of the phenomenon is not understood.

Alacrima

Absence of tears in the presence of lacrimal glands is called alacrima (extremely rare). It is a total or partial absence of tears. It is a generally bilateral condition and is noticed during the early months by parents, who complain that the child has red eyes with mucus discharge and that there is no watering from the eyes. On examination, both basic and reflex tearing are absent. The exact cause is not known. The most widely accepted theory is lack of communication between the lacrimal nucleus and the neural communication of the gland. This theory gets credence because the condition is invariably associated with anomalies of the sixth and seventh nerves and autonomic dysfunction known as Riley Day syndrome.

Riley Day Syndrome

This is a rare disease seen in some Jewish children. This is also called familial dysautonomia. It is an autosomal recessive disorder and bilateral; there is no lacrimal secretion. It has both ocular and systemic features.

The ocular features are: Diminished or absent tearing; both reflex and basic. The cornea has hypoesthesia, leading to recurrent keratitis, corneal opacity, and vascularization. The pupils are hypersensitive to pilocarpine. It constricts promptly to even 0.25% pilocarpine, which has no effect on a normal pupil.

Systemic manifestations are varied; they include increased vasomotor instability, episodes of hypertension, abnormal sweating, a lack of cutaneous sensation, and tendon reflex recurrent fever.

The cause is attributed to a lack of an enzyme that interferes with the production of noradrenaline and adrenaline from dopamine. The condition should be differentiated from other causes of cloudy corneas in infants. There is no known treatment.

Congenital Sinus of the Lacrimal Gland (Rare)

The congenital sinus of the lacrimal gland is rare and unilateral. The genesis of the malady is not well established. It may open just above the lateral canthus, in the fornix, or on the superior lateral aspect of the tarsal conjunctiva. It is a source of water. Excision of the tract is the preferred treatment.

In this anomaly, an epithelial-lined tract from the lacrimal gland opens on the skin surface. Most probably, this is one of the misdirected lacrimal ducts that, instead of opening in the fornix, opens on the skin at the outer canthus. It looks like a translucent depression, sometimes surrounded by a tuft of hair. A fine probe can be passed. It can also be visualized following the injection of radioactive, opaque dye. Whenever the gland is activated, tears dribble out of the opening, especially during eating. It becomes a constant source of infection in the gland.

Treatment is isolating the tract fully and removing it in toto with the proper closure of the gland end of the sinus; otherwise, recurrence is common.

Anomalies of the Lacrimal Drainage Passage

Anomalies of the lacrimal drainage passage can be:

- Puncta and canaliculi
- *Lacrimal sac:*
  - Congenital mucocele
  - Congenital fistula
  - Nasolacrimal duct. Obstruction

Anomalies of Puncta and Canaliculi

They are rare. The puncta may be absent or pinpointed. The canaliculi are either ectatic or absent. Both cause epiphora.

Anomalies of the Lacrimal Sac

Congenital mucocele: Congenital mucocele of the sac occurs when the nasolacrimal duct and canaliculi have not developed. It presents as a tense, subcutaneous, bluish, and diffuse swelling between the nose and medial canthus **(Fig. 3.1)**.

The swelling is non reducible; the condition is often mistaken as hemangioma or meningocele. The condition waxes and wanes in size or may all together disappear, with the spontaneous opening of the nasolacrimal duct. The mucocele transilluminates with a narrow transilluminator.

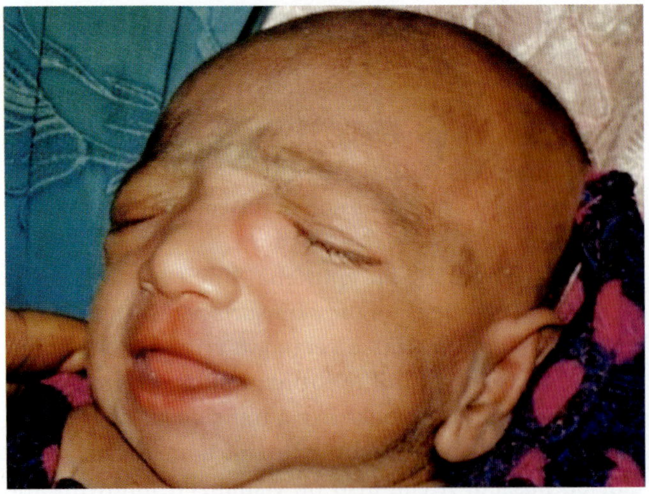

Fig. 3.1: Congenital mucocele of the lacrimal sac.
Courtesy: Dr Preeti Gupta.

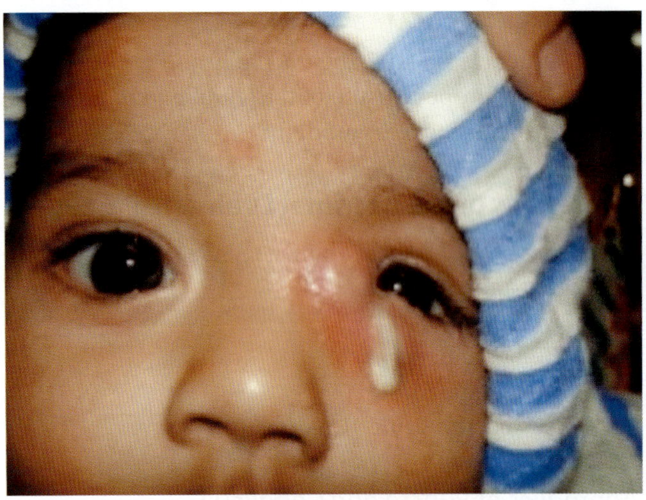

Fig. 3.2: Fistula developing in the congenital mucocele of the sac.
Courtesy: Dr Preeti Gupta.

USG helps in differentiating it from hemangioma and meningocele. It may get infected.

Congenital fistula: In this rare condition, there is a fistula on the lower end of the sac below the medial canthus, which generally arises from the sac but may arise from the common canaliculus. The opening goes unnoticed unless the tear production starts, with trickling tears from the opening. Histologically, the tract has a similar appearance with canaliculus **(Fig. 3.2)**.

Congenital anomalies of nasolacrimal duct: These are commonly referred to as congenital dacryocystitis. This is a misnomer that should better be replaced by the term congenital nasolacrimal duct obstruction with or without infection. The inflammation of the sac is not present at birth. Infection is superimposed.

The nasolacrimal duct obstruction is the most common congenital anomaly of the eye and adnexa. It is seen in 6–7% of all full-term babies. The incident is more premature, and unilateral involvement is more common.

The nasolacrimal duct developed as a soiled cord between the lacrimal bone and maxillary process to get canalized before birth. The canalization starts at the superior end. At birth, the whole of the canal should be canalized. Occasionally, some membranes or epithelial debris are left in the canal, which causes obstruction to the canal. The most common site of obstruction is at the level of the Hasner valve.

Ninety percent of babies with nasolacrimal duct block will have a functional canal following spontaneous clearing of the block by the first month. Only ducts that do not open up by the third week develop symptoms.

Clinical features of congenital nasolacrimal duct obstruction: The most common presenting feature is constant epiphora. Mild conjunctival congestion and mucopurulent discharges are frequent accompaniments. In a fortnight, the sac gets distended. Pressure on the sac causes purulent discharge from one or both the puncta. The explanation for delayed infection is the nonproduction of tears by the lacrimal gland before 3 weeks. There is no watering of the eyes before 3 weeks, even when the infant cries.

Once an infection has set in, there is no chance of the duct opening automatically. No amount of antibiotics will ameliorate the condition. The only remedy to disrupt the obstruction is either indirectly or directly. The indirect procedure is to press the distended sac firmly to expel the fluid downward, forcing the obstructing debris down. This is achieved by applying pressure over the sac in such a way that the contents do not regurgitate in the conjunctival sac but are forced down. The pressure should be directed posteriorly. Any amount of massaging the skin parallel to the nose bridge will be futile. The expression of the sac is carried out five to six times a day. In 2–3 days, the regurgitation will become negative, but epiphora will persist. Each expression is followed by the instillation of broad-spectrum antibiotic-soluble drops. The procedure may have to be continued for 10–15 days.

The direct method consists of repeated syringing of the nasolacrimal duct. If this fails, the next alternative is nasolacrimal duct probing under general anesthesia.

If all these minor efforts fail, the only way left is to do a dacryocystorhinostomy, either external or endonasal. Ballooning or intubations of the nasolacrimal duct too have poor success.

Laser disruption of the obstruction via the endonasal root, too, has been tried with unequal success.

Differential diagnosis of congenital nasolacrimal duct obstruction: The condition should be differentiated from all the conditions that cause watering from the eyes in a neonate.

They are as follows:

- *Infection*
  - Conjunctiva—ophthalmia neonatorum **(Fig. 3.3)**
  - Cornea: Keratitis (rare)
- *Trauma:*
  - Birth trauma
  - Chemical (iatrogenic)
- *Congenital anomalies:*
  - Congenital glaucoma **(Fig. 3.4)**
  - Congenital proptosis
  - Large coloboma of the lid

Crocodile Tear

This is a paradoxical tearing due to the misdirection of the seventh nerve through the sphenopalatine ganglion. It is generally unilateral. The symptoms are typical and diagnostic. There is watering from one eye during mastication. Its acquired form is more common, which develops following facial palsy in adults. No effective treatment is available.

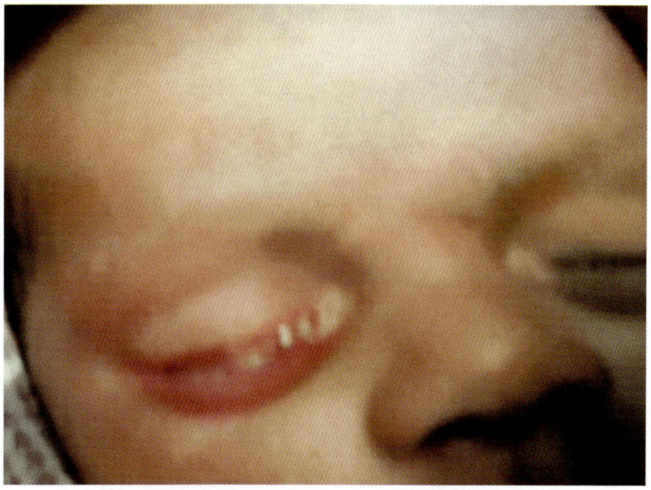

Fig. 3.3: Ophthalmia neonatorum.
Courtesy: Dr Preeti Gupta.

CONGENITAL ANOMALIES OF CONJUNCTIVA

In spite of the large size of the conjunctiva, congenital anomalies of the conjunctiva are less frequent, less conspicuous, and non-vision-threatening. Congenital anomalies of the conjunctiva are generally associated with deformities of the lid.

The congenital anomalies of conjunctiva are:

- Epitarsus
- Dermoid
- Dermolipoma
- Telangiectasia
- Lymphangiomas
- Melanosis

Epitarsus

Epitarsus is an infrequent anomaly in the form of an additional layer of conjunctiva over the tarsus, attached on either side, forming a pouch that opens on the lid margin, with hardly any clinical importance except recurrent conjunctivitis.

Dermoids

Dermoids are common congenital anomalies of the conjunctiva **(Fig. 3.5)**.

They are choristomas in nature.

> Choristomas are normal tissue in an abnormal place. They are tissues derived from the germinal cell layer. They are foreign to a particular site. They are classified as per tissue of origin.

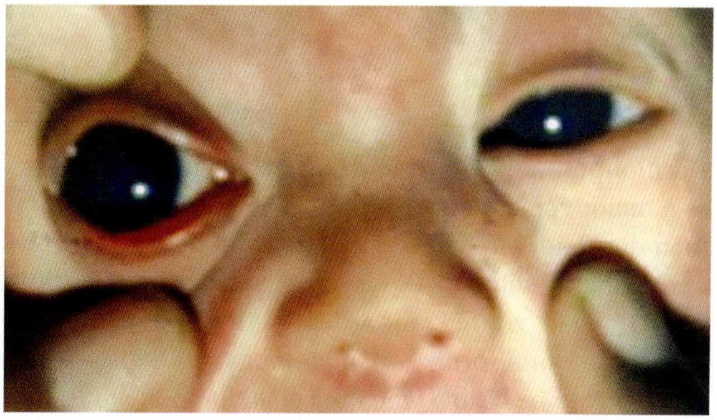

Fig. 3.4: Congenital glaucoma.
Courtesy: Dr Somen Misra.

Besides the conjunctiva and orbit, they are seen in the skin, oral cavity, and even internal organs.

The most common site for them to grow in the eye is the limbus **(Figs. 3.6 to 3.9)**.

Conjunctival Dermoid

Most of them are located at the inferior temporal limbus; they may rarely develop away from the limbus, even on the caruncle. There, sizes range from pinhead to as large as the cornea. They may be corneoscleral.

Protruding through the interpalpebral fissure, associated with or without coloboma in the lower lid, dermoids rarely grow inward. The dermoids are sporadic, present at birth, and may be small enough to be missed. After birth, they grow steadily but slowly to reach maximum size at puberty. At puberty, they may show a spurt in growth; once the maximum size has been reached, the growth stops. The dermoids are not known to turn malignant; they do not get infected nor do they rupture.

The dermoid contains both ectodermal and mesodermal tissues. The first gives rise to hair, sebaceous glands, smooth muscle, and nerve twigs. The mesoderm gives rise to blood vessels and cartilage.

The dermoids are dome-shaped growths sitting astride the limbus. They are dirty gray in color with a rough, slightly pigmented surface. A few hairs may be found growing on the apex of the growth. The dermoids are nonblinding and may cause diminished vision by way of irregular astigmatism. Limbal dermoids are a constant feature of Goldenhar syndrome.

Treatment-wise, all dermoids do not need treatment. The only treatment is surgical removal for cosmetic reasons, with the drawback of residual corneal opacity and uncorrectable irregular astigmatism. The dermoids do not recur after removal.

Dermolipoma

Dermolipoma, like dermoids, are choristomas, with fat as a major constituent. They are congenital, less frequent than dermoid, rarely diagnosed at birth, become obvious in childhood, the growth when fully developed is visible, as yellowish white, smooth growth from under the superotemporal fornix, or small, not visible on primary gaze, only to be visible when the child looks down and in. They too are nonblinding, without a chance of turning malignant, and soft in consistency. The conjunctiva

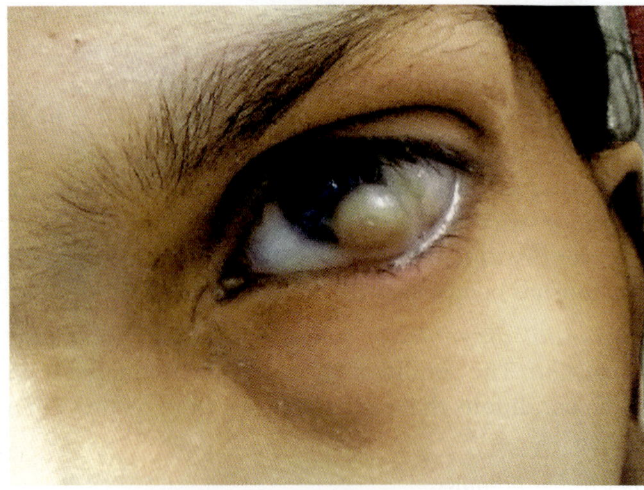

Fig. 3.5: Dermoids of the limbus.

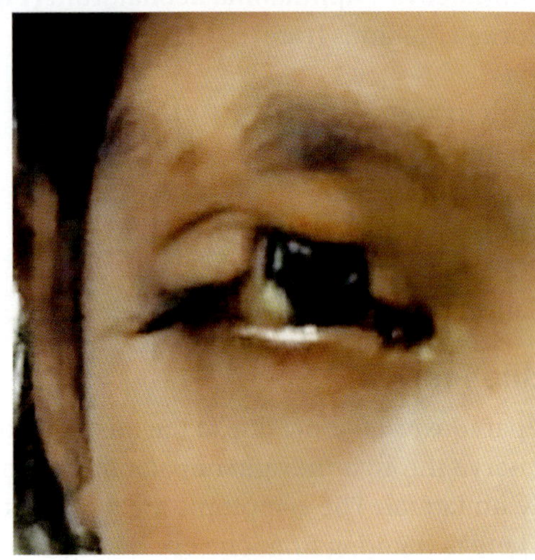

Fig. 3.6: Dermoid at limbus with full-thickness coloboma upper lid.

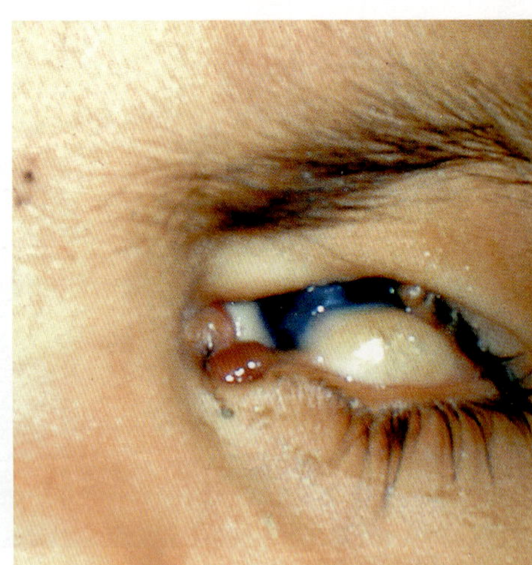

Fig. 3.7: Dermoid at the limbus with shallow coloboma lower lid.

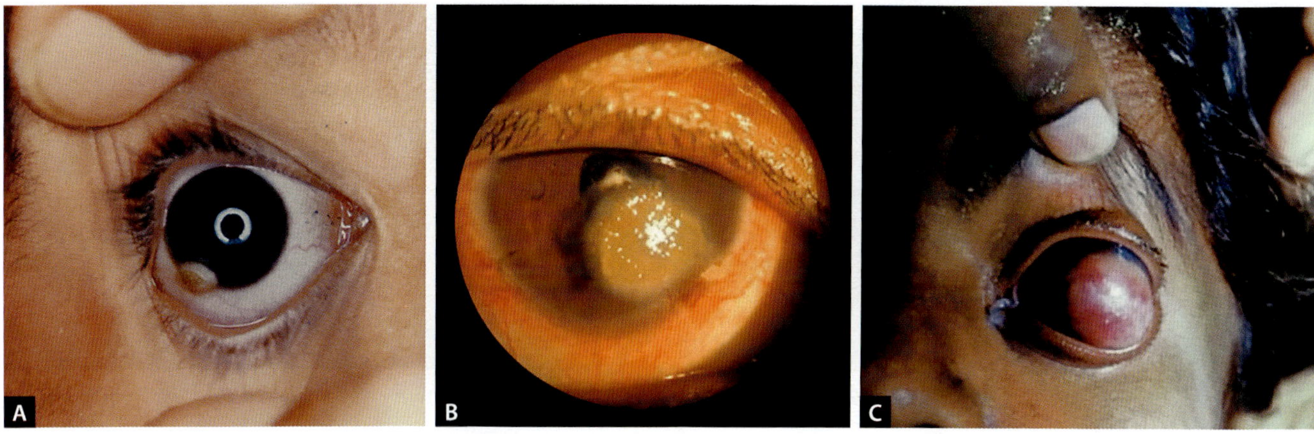

Figs. 3.8A to C: Dermoids of various sizes and sites.
Courtesy: (A and C) Dr Somen Misra; (B) Dr Nupur Chakrawarty.

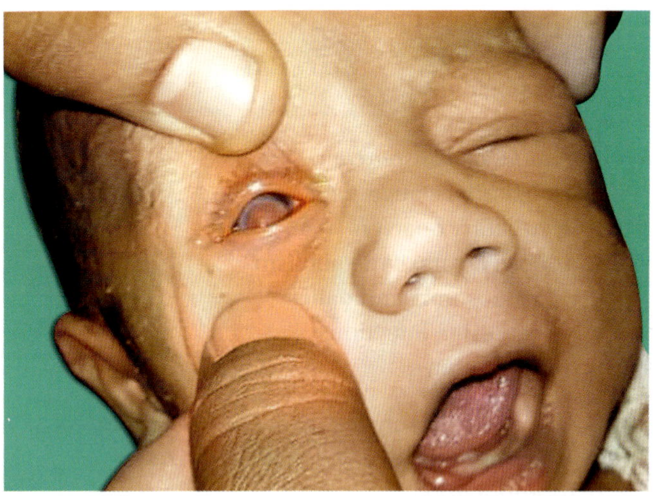

Fig. 3.9: Central corneal dermoid in a newborn.

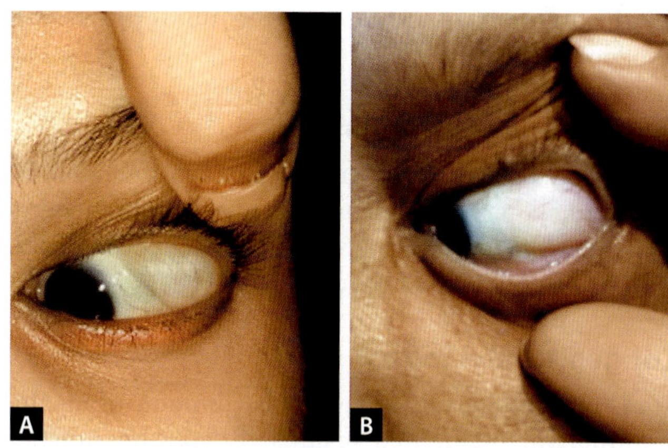

Figs. 3.10A and B: Dermolipomas noticed since childhood.

can be moved over the growth; they have a tendency to grow back in the orbit. There is no specific treatment **(Figs. 3.10A and B)**.

Congenital Telangiectasia

Congenital telangiectasia is a hereditary, congenital condition of autosomal recessive trait, present either at birth or discovered at puberty, with either ocular involvement or systemic features of cutaneous telangiectasia, epistaxis, or hematuria. The ocular findings consist of conjunctival and/or retinal telangiectasia. The conjunctival lesion can present as a small bunch of vessels arising from a common point in star fashion or as a bunch of dilated vessels in the lower bulbar conjunctiva or fornix **(Fig. 3.11)**.

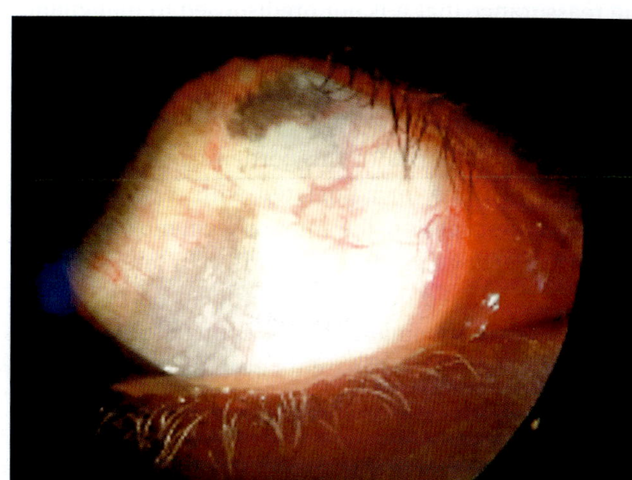

Fig. 3.11: Congenital telangiectasia.

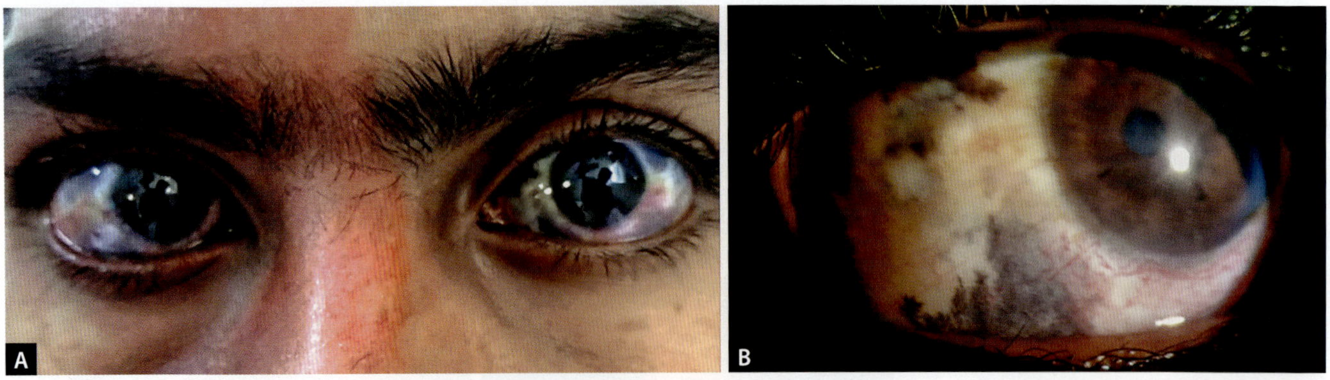

Figs. 3.12A and B: Congenital melanosis of conjunctiva.

The vessels have a tendency to bleed even with slight trauma, and the conjunctival lesions do not interfere with vision. This is in contrast to retinal lesions, which are invariably associated with visual symptoms. The small conjunctival lesions may be obliterated with cryoapplication.

Congenital Lymphedema

Congenital lymphedema is rarer than the above conditions, may be hereditary, and generally manifest in childhood as a solid mass in the conjunctiva that may spill over the lid. There is no specific treatment.

Congenital Melanosis

Congenital melanosis is the most common of all the conjunctival pigmented lesions. It may be present at birth or develop later. Usually, it does not grow or spread and does not require any treatment except for the reassurance that it is not predisposed to malignancy (**Figs. 3.12A and B**).

CONGENITAL ANOMALIES OF CORNEA

Congenital anomalies of the cornea can be localized to the cornea only or associated with a wider ocular deformity, dysgenesis of the anterior segment, or systemic anomalies. They can be unilateral or bilateral; when bilateral, they need not be symmetric and may be mild enough to be symptomless or gross enough to be detected on diffuse light even by parents even at birth. Many of them have genetic predispositions.

Isolated corneal anomalies can be:

- *Anomaly of size:*
  - Microcornea
  - Megalocornea
  - Buphthalmos
- *Anomaly of curvature:*
  - Keratoconus
  - Keratoglobus
  - Cornea plana
- *Anomalies of transparency:*
  - Congenital glaucoma
  - Hereditary opacity
  - Inborn errors of metabolism
  - Chromosomal anomalies
  - Intrauterine infection
  - Birth trauma

The conditions are acronymed as S T U M P E D (Basak SK).

S—*S*clerocornea and other anomalies of size
T—*T*ears and trauma
U—*U*lcers
M—*M*etabolic
P—*P*eters' anomaly and other mesodermal dysgenesis syndromes
E—*E*dema
D—*D*ermoids and dystrophies

Microcornea

Microcornea is a common congenital anomaly of the cornea. In its milder form, it may be missed in casual examination; its presence is obvious in severe form. It may be an isolated feature or associated with more serious anomalies such as microphthalmos and coloboma of the uvea. It may be sporadic or may have a genetic background. It may be seen in many members of the family; it is generally bilateral. An eye with microcornea may be otherwise normal with normal vision.

A cornea smaller than 10 mm in diameter qualifies to be called a microcornea. The corneal curvature is generally flatter, making the eye hypermetropic **(Fig. 3.13)**, and it may be predisposed to narrow-angle glaucoma.

Other anomalies associated with microcornea are: Microphthalmos, narrow interpalpable fissure, anterior insertion of recti, nanophthalmos, early development of cataracts, and amblyopia. The treatment consists of correction of existing errors in refraction to salvage as much vision as possible, prevention of glaucoma, and management of amblyopia. Unilateral microphthalmos may be hidden by a suitable prosthesis for cosmetic reasons.

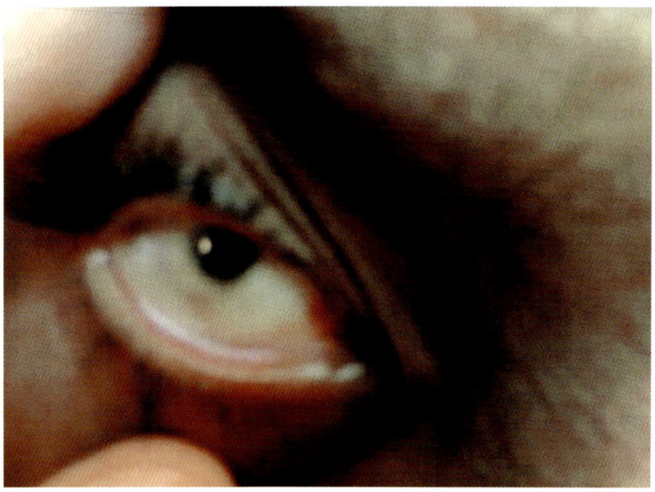

Fig. 3.13: Microcornea in microphthalmos.
Courtesy: Professor ML Garg.

Megalocornea

A cornea larger than 13 mm in diameter is called a megalocornea. It may occasionally be as large as 16 mm. Megalocornea is present at birth and its size does not change with age; the corneal curvature is more than normal, resulting in myopic astigmatism with the rule. It is bilateral and symmetric. The cornea is transparent; the anterior chamber is deep without iridodonesis; and the angle is wide without dysgenesis. It is more frequent in boys. The condition should be differentiated from congenital glaucoma, a blinding condition, and benign keratoglobus. Most of the cases do not require much treatment except correction of the error of refraction.

Common differences between megalocornea keratoglobus and buphthalmos are highlighted in **Table 3.1**.

Keratoglobus

Keratoglobus is a bilateral, rare, nonprogressive condition with increased corneal curvature and normal diameter. The corneal thickness is uniformly less than normal. It is almost symptomless, as noticed on routine examinations.

TABLE 3.1: Difference between megalocornea keratoglobus and buphthalmos.

Clinical feature	*Megalocornea*	*Keratoglobus*	*Buphthalmos*
Laterality	Bilateral	Bilateral—65%	Unilateral—35%
Sex	More common in boys	Equal in both sexes	More common in boys
Progress	Stationary	Stationary	Progressive
Vision	Variable	Variable	Poor
Refraction	Astigmatism with rule	Irregular myopic astigmatism	Astigmatism against the rule
Transparency cornea	Clear	Clear	Cloudy
Descemet's membrane	Normal	Normal	Ruptured
Lacrimation	Nil	Nil	Prominent feature
Photophobia	Absent	Absent	Prominent
Angle of AC	Normal	Normal	Malformed
Tension	Normal	Normal	Raised
Corneal diameter	>13 mm	11–12 mm	13–16 mm
Corneal curvature	Normal	Increased	Increased
Corneal thickness	Uniform	Thin	Thin
Genetics	X-linked	Autosomal recessive	Autosomal recessive

It should be differentiated from buphthalmos, early keratoconus, and megalocornea.

Cornea Plana

Cornea plana is a rare congenital disorder of the globe where there is a reduction in corneal and scleral curvature with a shallow anterior chamber. The cornea is reduced in all dimensions. It gives the impression of mild ptosis and enophthalmos. Flat corneas cause curvature and hypermetropia. No specific treatment is required except correction of the error of refraction.

Keratoconus

Keratoconus is a noninfective, nontraumatic, progressive condition of uncertain origin; it may be congenital. The proponents of this theory consider it to be a congenital defect of mesodermal tissue. The mucopolysaccharides and collagen in corneal stroma too have been blamed. Some studies have come out with the theory that it is a dystrophy, hence congenital, not manifesting at birth. Others postulate that it is degeneration, hence acquired. Still others consider it to be due to a not yet identified chemical, probably an enzyme that damages the corneal stroma by a radical-induced oxidative process. Due to its varied presentation, it is often missed in the milder early stages. A fully developed disorder is difficult to miss. The condition makes its presence felt at about 4–5 years of age, generally in one eye; the other eye may follow or may remain unaffected. Bilateral involvement is less common; when present, the disorder is not symmetric. The most common mode of presentation is painless, gradual, diminished distant vision in a noncongested eye. There is no lacrimation either. The other, supposed to be a normal eye too, may have diminished distant vision to a lesser degree; the most common error of refraction is compound myopic astigmatism, with the spherical component showing a gradual increase. The condition is progressive, often self-arresting; the progress stops by the second decade with either no sequel or minimal scarring. Initially, the vision is well corrected by either spectacles, suitable contact lenses, or both.

Keratoconus has worldwide distribution; it is more common among dark races. It is more common among boys. There is no genetic predisposition. It has been found among the siblings; the siblings may not have a fully developed picture; in them, it may manifest as progressive compound myopic astigmatism without other features of keratoconus.

There are two patterns of progress for the disorder:

1. Progresses relentlessly up to the third decade and then stops
2. Progresses for the first few years, then slows or may stop progressing

There is a spurt in increment in puberty. The sudden and fast increase in corneal stretching may cause rupture in Descemet's membrane, leading to the accumulation of fluid in the stroma, causing edema with a loss of transparency, then turning translucent, followed by total opacification. By this time, the fluid percolates through Bowman's membrane to reach the epithelium, producing edema, throwing the epithelium into painful bullae, causing hydrops of the cornea. (See below.)

Other less common symptoms of keratoconus are: Diplopia, polyopia, haloes, glare, and redness. Watering and photophobia are features of hydrops of the cornea.

Keratoconus can be divided in various ways. They are:

- Clinical
- Keratometry
- Tomography
- In-grades
    - Suspect
    - Forme fruste (subclinical)
    - Incipient
    - *Developed:* Mild, moderate, or severe
- *Depending on:*
    - Steepness of the cornea (keratometry)
    - Thickness of the cornea (pachymetry)
    - Shape of cone:
        - *Nipple:* Central, with a diameter of 5 mm or less
        - *Oval:* Inferonasal, >5 mm
        - *Globus:* Covering more than 75% of the cornea

Suspect: A boy between 10 and 15 years old with a history of a frequent increase in the myopic power of lenses, generally in both eyes, with similar history in at least one parent and siblings, a history of atopia, and a spring cataract. The vision was not corrected to 6/6 with the best correction. The eye is free of other morbidities.

Forme fruste: Forme fruste or subclinical keratoconus in an eye with clinical features of keratoconus in the other eye that looks normal with a slit lamp and Placido disc. But topography shows increased steepening, an asymmetric bow-tie appearance, and a skewed radial axis. These eyes may not progress or pass into fully developed keratoconus; the eyes have subnormal vision that can be corrected fully.

Incipient keratoconus: The incipient stage is a stage more advanced than forme fruste; some authors deny its relevance. All children with too frequent and ever-increasing spectacle and compound myopic astigmatism should be suspected of having keratoconus unless proved otherwise. The most useful investigation is video keratography, which picks up subtle findings and records progress.

Developed keratoconus: A fully developed keratoconus is not difficult to discern even by simple oblique illumination in a youth in the second decade, probably with a positive family history, complaining of relentless progress in myopic power and nonimprovement of vision with glasses or contact lenses.

On examination, the child is found to have the following features in various combinations:

- Both eyes may be involved.
- There is neither redness nor watering.
- The eyes may be straight or may squint, with subnormal, noncorrectable vision.
- On oblique illumination, the cornea shows a distinct conical bulge, and the apex of the cone is decentered down and in.
- As the patient looks down, the apex of the cone bisects the lower lid. This is called Munson's sign.
- The anterior chamber is uniformly deep, without iridodonesis.
- On slit-lamp examination, the central part of the cornea is thin, with normal thickness on the periphery.
- Positive Rizzuti sign
  Rizzuti sign: If a narrow beam of bright light, i.e., from a slit lamp, is thrown on the temporal limbus of an eye with normal corneal curvature, the nasal limbus lights up as a bright crescent. In the case of keratoconus, the beam of light assumes a triangular configuration with the apex away from the limbus; the distance of the apex from the limbus denotes the depth of the anterior chamber and the angle between the two limbs shows the steepness of the cornea **(Fig. 3.14)**.
- *Vogt's line:* These are linier opacities at the level of stroma, they disappear under pressure only to re appear as the pressure is removed.
- *Fleischer's ring:* The ring develops at the base of the cone due to deposition of iron; the exact source of iron is not clear.

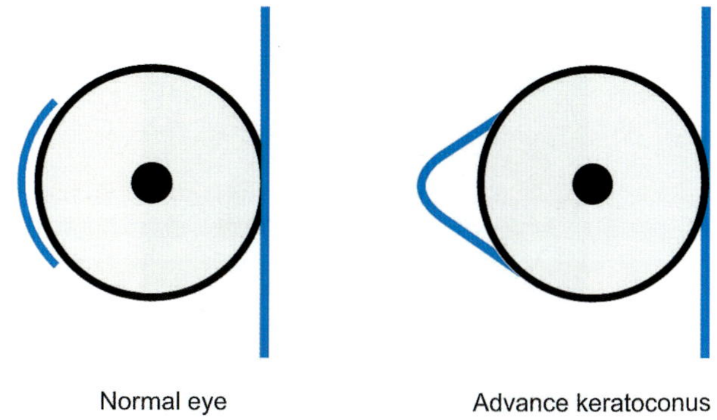

Fig. 3.14: Positive Rizzuti sign.

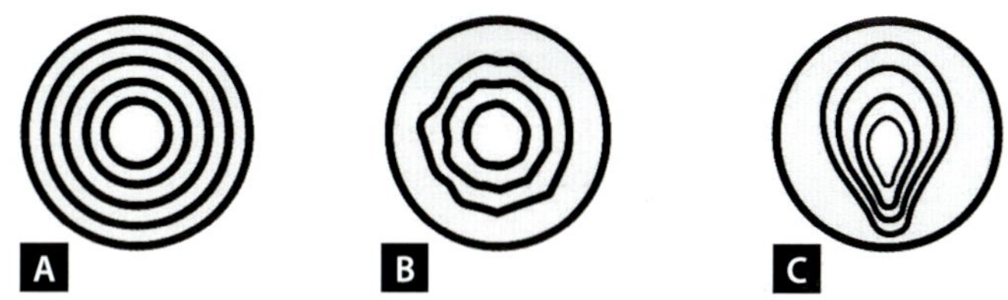

Figs. 3.15A to C: Types of mires in normal cornea and keratoconus. (A) Normal eye with regular mires; (B) Keratoconus with irregular mires; (C) Advance keraoconus egg-shaped mires.

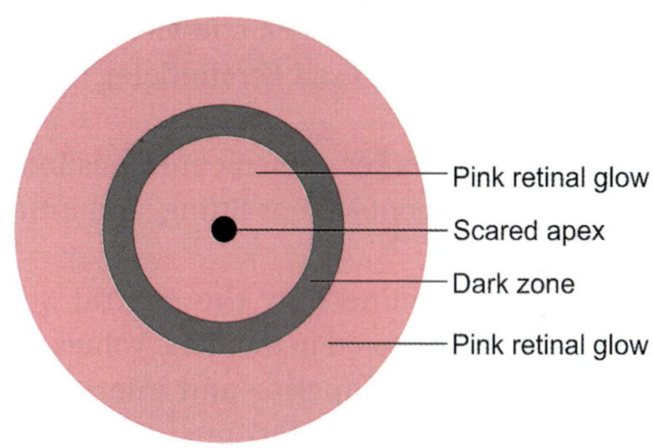

Fig. 3.16: Features of distant direct ophthalmoscopy in keratoconus.

- On retroillumination, a black spot stands out against pink glow. This represents the scarred apex of the cone.
- Retinoscopy reveals compound myopic or irregular myopic astigmatism.
- Placidoscope shows irregular mires, egg-shaped mires, and compression of mires **(Figs. 3.15A to C)**.
- Distant direct ophthalmoscopy gives a specific pattern of a central black dot surrounded by a pink glow, encircled by a dark zone with a pink peripheral glow. The dot in the center represents scarred apex, while the dark ring represents the base of the cone **(Fig. 3.16)**.
- *Keratometry:* The principle of a keratometer is as simple as the principle of Purkinje image formation,

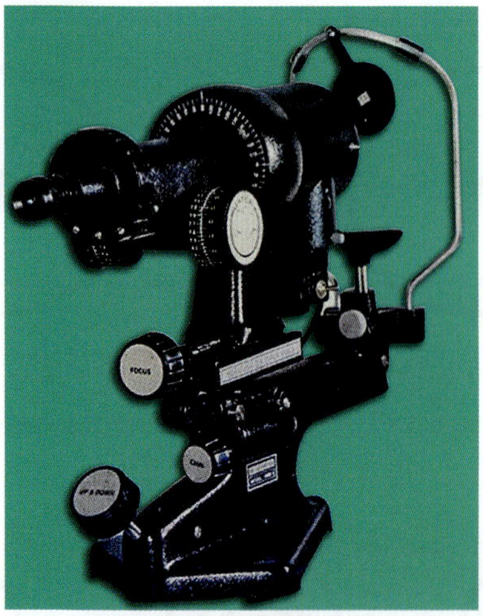

Fig. 3.17: B & L model keratometer.
Courtesy: Appasamy Association.

which is based on the principle of image formation by a convex mirror. The anterior corneal surface acts as a convex mirror. The size of the image depends on the curvature of the cornea. The image is smaller when the curvature is greater, and vice versa. Photograph of a commonly used keratometer is shown in **Figure 3.17**.

The various uses of a keratometer are measurement of corneal astigmatism, contact lens fitting, and intraocular lens (IOL) calculation.

Keratometers examine only the central 3 mm of cornea. The results are noted in diopters. Values > 47.20D or asymmetry between superior and inferior dioptric values are suggestive of keratoconus; values between 47.20D and 48D are considered mild; values between 48D and 53D are taken as moderate; and values >53D are called advanced keratoconus.

- *Pachymeter:* Pachymeters are a group of instruments that can be either optical or ultrasonic. The optical pachymeter measures the thickness of an optical section of the cornea. The ultrasonic pachymeter uses an ultrasonic probe to measure the thickness, which is measured via contact between the ultrasonic probe and the cornea.

  This measures the thickness of the cornea. Reading of 500 μm is considered mild, 300–500 moderate, and <300 microadvanced.
- *Photokeratoscopy* (video keratography, tomography): It gives a three-dimensional image of elevation and depression on both surfaces in color code. Blue is designated cool; it represents flattening. Orange and red mean steep and are called hot.
- *Anterior segment optical coherence tomography (OCT):* Analogous to ultrasonography, it uses light in place of sonic waves thus giving a high-resolution image of the cornea, anterior chamber, and iris.

Complications of Kertoconus

- Most of the keratoconus have few complications, i.e., permanent reduction in vision, uncorrectable myopic astigmatism, intolerance to contact lenses, and amblyopia.
- The majority of keratoconus stops progressing by the third decade; by this time, the patient gets adjusted to contact lenses.
- The only serious complication is the development of hydrops.

The hydrops develop suddenly at puberty. Mostly in girls, there is a sudden increase in the size of the cone with an abrupt change in curvature; there is stretching of all the layers of the cornea, which is most marked in Descemet's membrane. This is followed by the imbibement of fluid in the stroma. The water-laden stroma passes the fluid to the epithelium, throwing it into the bullae, which causes pain, lacrimation, photophobia, and redness. The cornea turns opaque. Hydrops is a self-healing disorder; it takes 3–4 months for Descemet's membrane to get repaired, even without treatment. The purpose of treatment is to alleviate the pain and watering by way of oral analgesics and local hyperosmolar solutions like 5% NaCl and ophthalmic-grade glycerine, along with local broad-spectrum antibiotic drops by day and ointment at night.

Differential diagnoses include all conditions with increased corneal curvature, i.e., megalocornea, keratoglobus, keratobuphthalmos, and central Descemetocele.

Ocular disorders frequently associated with keratoconus are: Ectopia lentis, aniridia, congenital cataract, retinitis pigmentosa, Leber's congenital amaurosis, floppy eye syndrome, and spring catarrh. Spring catarrh has been often blamed for aggravated keratoconus; one unsubstantiated theory of the worsening of keratoconus in spring catarrh is constant rubbing of the eyes.

Systemic disorders associated are:

- Systemic allergy, atopia, eczema, hay fever, and asthma
- *Syndromes:* Apert syndrome, Down syndrome, Marfan syndrome, Ehlers–Danlos syndrome (EDS), and Crouzon syndrome

Management

Management depends on the severity of the case; it ranges from simple spectacles in the mildest case to specialized surgery in the most advanced case.

The following is the most frequent protocol:

- *Mild:* Spectacle, soft toric contact lens. Both require frequent changes.
- *Moderate:* Rigid gas-permeable lens or scleral lens
- *Severe:*
  - Intact endothelium—deep anterior lamellar keratoplasty (DALK)
  - Damaged. Endothelium full-thickness keratoplasty
  - *Other methods:* Intracorneal segment (intact), superficial keratectomy, excimer laser phototherapeutic keratectomy, Bowman's layer transplant, phakic IOL, and corneal collagen cross-linking (CXL).

Corneal collagen cross linking: This is one of the most effective nonsurgical, nonoptical methods of management of keratoconus, suitable for moderately severe cases in patients between 16 and 40 years with corneas with a thickness not <400 μm and keratometry readings <60D. The procedure is done under topical anesthesia. The corneal epithelium is removed and riboflavin drops are instilled, one drop every 5 minutes six times. The cornea is exposed to ultraviolet A (365 nm) for 30 minutes. The eye is bandaged for a day or two.

The combination of riboflavin and photosensitization by ultraviolet brings about biomechanical changes in the corneal matrix, raising the corneal strength by 300%.

Ancillary methods in management

- *Antioxidants:* These are administered on the presumption that radicals are due to their oxidative properties that harm the corneal collagen, which is prevented by antioxidants.
- Antihistamines
- Mast cell stabilizers
- Cyclosporine drop
- Steroid drops
- Nonsteroidal anti-inflammatory drug (NSAID) drops
- Hyperosmotic drops
- Lubricants
- Dark glasses

Posterior Keratoconus

The condition is far less common than keratoconus. In this condition, there is steepening of the endothelium due to a defect in Descemet's membrane to which the iris gets attached, giving the appearance of Peter's anomaly and leaving an intact epithelium. It generally progresses unilaterally and may be associated with the anterior lenticonus.

CONGENITAL CAUSES OF CORNEAL HAZE

Corneas at birth are mildly hazy and pass off within a few hours to a day or two; thereafter, the corneas are transparent and bright. On some occasions, this does not happen, and the corneas are left permanently hazy or frankly opaque at birth. The opacity may be generalized or localized, central or peripheral, or vascularized. Anterior segment dysgenesis is a common accompaniment.

CONGENITAL ANOMALIES OF GLOBE

The globe develops in two parts, i.e., the cornea and sclera, along with the recti muscles. Out of all the tissues that constitute the globe, only the corneal epithelium develops from the surface ectoderm.

Congenital anomalies of the globe vary from a minor degree of microphthalmos to a severe anomaly of anophthalmos, where the eyeball is absent along with the optic nerve and extraocular muscles.

Congenital anomalies around the globe can occur in the following conditions:

- Fault in the development of the primary optic vesicle: Anophthalmos
- Failure of the optic cup to develop and differentiate: Uveal anomalies, retinal and macular anomalies, colobomatous cystic eyeball
- Failure of the eyeball to grow: Nanophthalmos

Anophthalmos

Anophthalmos is the extreme form of congenital anomaly of the eye, with a normal orbit, lids, and conjunctiva without trace of structures that constitute the eye, i.e., the cornea, sclera, muscles, vessels, nerves, and the eyeball with its contents. Such complete pictures are rare. Clinically, an eye with an absence of too much tissue is taken as an anophthalmos. In fact, such cases may be cases of extreme degrees of microphthalmos. They can be unilateral or bilateral; when unilateral, the ipsilateral orbit is smaller than its counterpart.

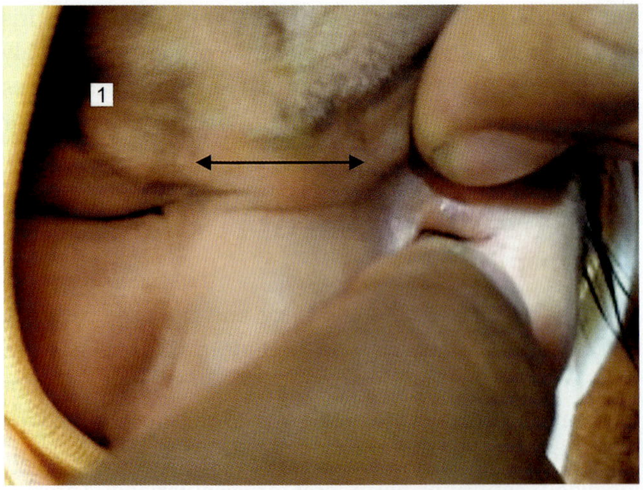

Fig. 3.18: Severe bilateral microphthalmos.
Courtesy: Dr Nupur Chakrawarti.

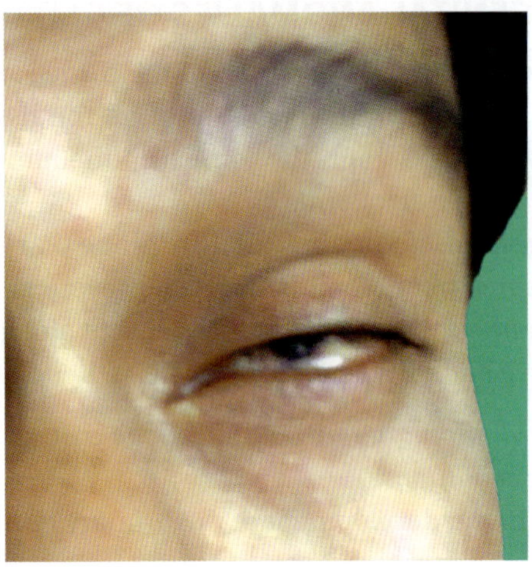

Fig. 3.19: Microphthalmos.
Courtesy: Dr Nupur Chakrawarti.

In both instances, the interpalpebral fissures are narrowed to a slit. The condition is not to be confused with acquired postinfection, post-traumatic enophthalmos, or congenital Horner's syndrome, where the eyeball is pulled back.

Microphthalmos

These are eyes with a size smaller than expected at the normal stage of development **(Figs. 3.18 and 3.19)**.

They can be unilateral or bilateral; later, they are more common. When bilateral, they are not mirror images of each other. In unilateral cases, the other eye is variably normal or may have defects independent of the microphthalmic eye **(Fig. 3.20)**.

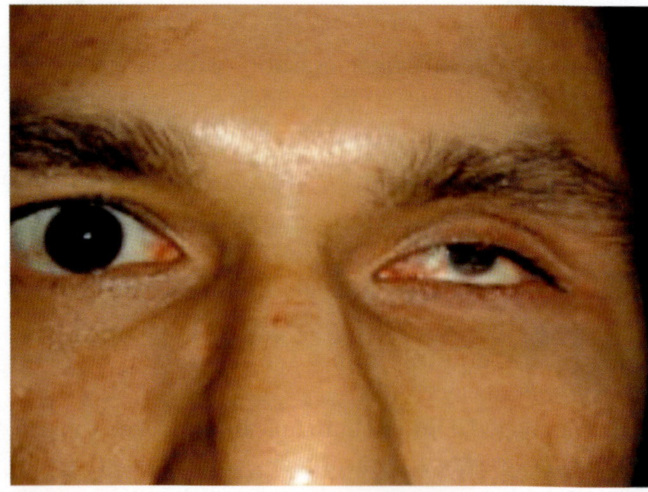

Fig. 3.20: Left eye microphthalmos.

Flowchart 3.3: Classification of microphthalmos.

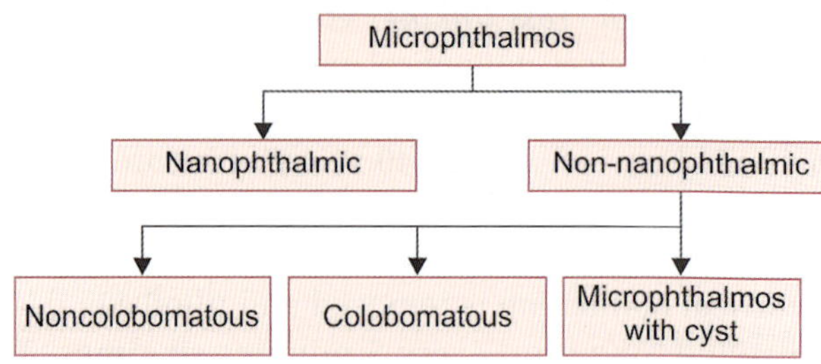

Flowchart 3.3 is a commonly used classification of microphthalmos.

The condition can be genetic or sporadic. It may be seen in otherwise normal children or in children with multiple anomalies. The orbit on the side of the microphthalmos is smaller than its counterpart. The interpalpebral fissure is narrow, giving the impression of ptosis. The movements are normal; generally, the vision is subnormal. It may even be absent and the eyes suffer from various types of errors of refraction.

Clinically, microphthalmos has been divided into two broad groups, i.e., nanophthalmic and non-nanophthalmic. The latter is divided into colobomatous and microphthalmos with cysts **(Flowchart 3.3)**.

Nanophthalmos

It is also referred to as pure or true microphthalmos and is considered a phenotype of microphthalmos **(Fig. 3.21)**. It is rare and often missed. The eye is fully developed anatomically and in function, baring its overall dimension, which is two-thirds of normal volume. The axial

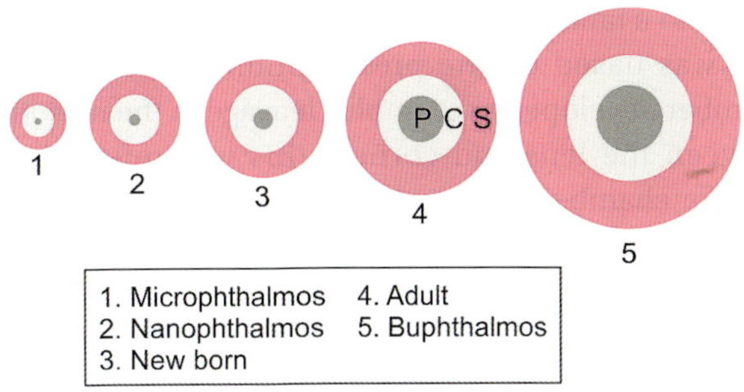

Fig. 3.21: Relative size of the sclera, cornea, and pupil in various congenital anomalies of the globe. (C: cornea; P: pupil; S: sclera)

length of a new-born eye should be 16.5 mm at birth and grow to 24 mm by the third year; in the case of nanophthalmos, this postnatal growth is absent, leaving a dwarfed eye.

This retardation starts in the embryo after the fetal fissure has closed without any tissue incarcerated in it; thus, there is no coloboma in the nanophthalmic eye.

Nanophthalmos is mostly a genetic disorder; it can be both autosomal dominant and recessive; rarely, it is sporadic. It is a bilateral condition that is invariably identical, seen equally among boys and girls and generally detected in primary school. The child may not complain, but the teacher notices that the child has a visual handicap; the child may squint due to high hypermetropia, which is axial, generally without astigmatism. The position of the globe in the orbit is normal, and the movements are normal with good accommodation and convergence matching with age and error of refraction. There is no ptosis or proptosis. The corneal diameter is less but not as small as what is called the microcornea; the cornea is flatter, adding to the hypermetropia to some extent. The anterior chamber is shallow with an occludable angle that predisposes the eye to narrow-angle glaucoma in adulthood. Some of the eyes are predisposed to wide-angle glaucoma as well. The pupil is small and central, with a brisk light reflex. The refraction may be as high as +10–15D. Requiring the child thick glasses for distant vision may require near addition.

The old dictum says that phakic patients with aphakic glasses is a nanophthalmic patient.

The lens is in a normal position with normal shape, size, curvature, and transparency; this makes the lens too big for the eye, predisposing it to lens-induced glaucoma. Amblyopia is a hindrance to full correction of vision that should get priority in management.

The next problem that requires attention is glaucoma, which could be narrow angle, wide angle, lens-induced, aphakic, or even malignant. It is better to give medical treatment a try for glaucoma because surgery is always fraught with intractable complications like uveal effusion syndrome* and malignant glaucoma†. Such calamities can occur even following a penetrating wound or the repair of a corneal or corneoscleral wound in a nanophthalmic eye. Thus, management is: Correction of the error of refraction, correction of near vision if needed, management of amblyopia, treatment of glaucoma medically, and if medical treatment fails, restoration to surgery with precaution.

Colobomatous Microphthalmos (Microphthalmos with Intraocular Coloboma)

These are small eyes with coloboma of the retina and uvea. They are more common than simple colobomas of the uvea that may be present in eyes with normal dimensions. The eyes are smaller in all dimensions, set deep in the orbit that gives an impression of enophthalmos, the cornea is small with <10 mm diameter, the anterior chamber is shallow, and the pupil may be normal or distorted due to the coloboma of the iris that may be a small notch at the lower pupillary margin or extend up to the limbus and beyond. The condition is associated with a fault in the fetal fissure; hence, the colobomas are at 6 o'clock. It is common for the retina to be involved with the coloboma of the choroid; the colobomas of the uvea and retina may be independent of each other. The vision varies from normal to severe loss depending on the extent of the coloboma, flattening of the cornea, and short anteroposterior length. The eyes are hypermetropic with an occludable angle. Peripheral lenticular opacity behind the coloboma is common.

Congenital conditions associated with noncolobomatous microphthalmos are:

- Anterior segment dysgenesis
- Persistent hyperplastic primary vitreous (PHPV)

**Uveal effusion syndrome:* It is an idiopathic exudative detachment of the choroid and ciliary body along with the retina. It is supposed to be due to obstructed blood flow from the posterior segment due to thickened sclera that throttles the venae vorticosae.

†*Malignant glaucoma:* It is also known as ciliary block glaucoma and aqueous misdirection glaucoma. It is seen in phakic, aphakic, and pseudophakic eyes. The most common phakic cause is filtering operations in narrow-angle glaucoma and angle closure glaucoma; this makes the nanophthalmic eye vulnerable to the disorder. (For details, see the chapter on glaucoma.)

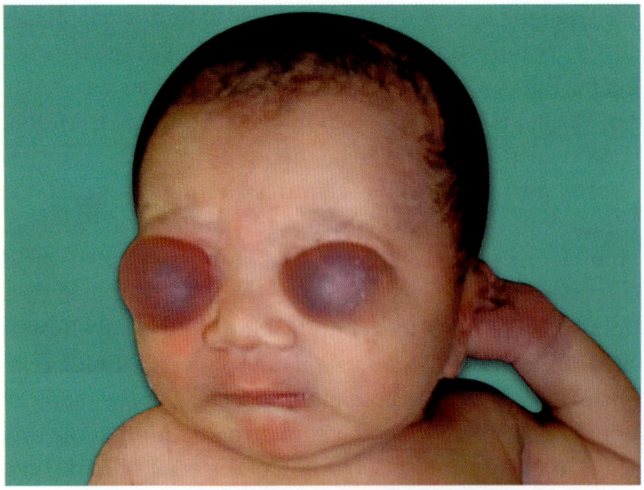

Fig. 3.22: Bilateral cryptophthalmos.
Courtesy: Dr M Minocha.

- Retinal dysplasia
- Cataract
- Glaucoma

The microphthalmic eyes with the above anomalies are called complicated microphthalmos.

Microphthalmos with Cyst

Normally, during development, the retina and vitreous do not protrude through the fetal fissure. In rare instances, they may get incarcerated in the closing fetal fissure or may protrude through the fissure and convert into a cyst below the eye **(Fig. 3.22)**.

Three things can happen following incarceration or protrusion:

1. The eye is either of normal size or minimally microphthalmic, with a small cyst on the inferior surface.
2. The formed eye has a fairly large cyst.
3. The eye is rudimentary, and the cyst is large enough to push the rudimentary eye back and up. The lower lid is stretched over the protruding cyst; the cyst behind the lid is covered by conjunctiva.

CONGENITAL ANOMALIES OF ANTERIOR CHAMBER

All the structures except the lens are related to the anterior chamber, i.e., the cornea, iris, and iridocorneal junction. The angle of the anterior chamber may be involved in various congenital anomalies of the anterior chamber, singly or in combination. Such anomalies have been designated in various ways. Initially, they were thought to be due to a fault in the formation of the anterior chamber. This was based on the presumption that the anterior chamber developed as a simple cleavage in the mesoderm between the lens and cornea; this was referred to as anterior chamber cleavage syndrome.

Later, they were separated into the following groups:

- Ectodermal dysgenesis
- Mesodermal dysgenesis
- Combination of the two

The common congenital anomalies involving the anterior chamber are:

- Posterior embryotoxon
- Axenfeld syndrome
- Reiger's anomaly and Reiger's syndrome
- Peter's anomaly and Peter's syndrome
- Trabecular dysgenesis

Posterior Embryotoxon

Posterior embryotoxon is the mildest congenital anomaly in the anterior chamber. It has no clinical significance, is without symptoms, does not involve vision, does not progress, and has no complications. The only blemish that can be attributed to it is cosmetic. It is more common in persons with raised lipids. In about 10% of cases, mostly in the third decade, it can be seen as an arcus without raised lipid.

The pathogenesis is said to lie in the terminal Descemet's membrane; the membrane develops a split on the periphery, followed by thickening of Schwalbe's line, which is moved anteriorly by 1 mm. The arcus need not be complete; it is often fragmented. The condition needs to be differentiated from arcus juveniles, which develop at the termination of Bowman's membrane.

The rest of the cornea, anterior chamber, iris, and angle of the anterior chamber are normal; the anomaly per se does not cause any errors in refraction. It does not require any treatment.

Axenfeld Syndrome

This is bilateral mesodermal dysgenesis of the anterior chamber with a prominent and anteriorly placed Schwalbe's line, to which are attached a few strands of iris. The iris attachments are patchy, not encircling the whole interior side of the angle. Except for attachment to Schwalbe's line, the iris does not show any change; the pupil is central, circular, and brisk. The iris attachment should be differentiated from goniosynechiae and peripheral anterior synechiae; the rest of the cornea is normal. The condition does not interfere with vision; unless glaucoma develops, glaucoma is seen in 50% of eyes; glaucoma develops in the fourth to fifth decade due to changes in angle, which are difficult to treat medically. Surgical treatment is also not very satisfactory; neither is laser.

Reiger's syndrome and Axenfeld syndrome may coexist, making the conditions worse, and are commonly known as Axenfeld–Reiger syndrome.

Reiger's Anomaly

This may be considered to be an advanced stage of Axenfeld syndrome. It is better referred to as iridocorneal dysgenesis with a clear anterior chamber angle. Unlike Axenfeld syndrome, where the iris does not show any change, Reiger's syndrome has a moth-eaten appearance to the iris. The iris is hypoplastic with multiple partial or full-thickness defects leading to polycoria, pseudocornea, slit-like pupils, corectopia, and irregular pupils. The defects in the iris can be trance-illuminated. Though the angle is not directly involved, it can be involved in extensive iridocorneal adhesions causing glaucoma, which is common. Other findings reported are cloudy corneas and lenticular opacity secondary to glaucoma, persistent hyaloid vessels, and the absence of retinal and choroidal pigment epithelium. All cases of Reiger's anomaly should be kept under observation for the rise of intraocular tension; once glaucoma develops, it is difficult to manage.

Reiger's Syndrome

The syndrome has many systemic anomalies, besides those of Reiger's anomaly, related to teeth and the maxilla. The systemic anomalies are microdontia, hypodontia, and hypoplasia of the maxilla.

Peter's Anomally

Peter's anomaly is the severest form of mesodermal dysgenesis of the anterior chamber; it is the rarest of all the dysgenesis of the anterior chamber, involving the posterior stroma, Descemet's membrane, and endothelium in a leucomatous lesion. In contrast to other dysgenesis where the corneal lesions are confined to the periphery, Peter's anomaly involves the central cornea, leaving the periphery mostly clear. Glaucoma is of varied nature and severity.

It can be either sporadic or autosomal recessive. It is bilateral, without sex predilection, present at birth, and difficult to treat.

As per severity and corneal involvement, the condition has been put into the following grades:

- Combination of Axenfeld syndrome and Reiger's anomaly, to which is added an endothelial defect in front of the pupil. The corneal defect is a facet in Descemet's membrane; the endothelium is absent over the facet, and strands of iris are attached to the periphery of the facet. Absence of endothelium causes edema of the stroma, which in turn leaves a generalized haze in the cornea. The anterior chamber is irregular in depth, absent from the center, and is slit-like in the periphery. The lens is not involved.
- Absence of features of Axenfeld and Reiger's anomaly, central corneal adhesion involving the posterior stroma, Descemet's membrane, and endothelium.
- Consists of clinical features above with adhesion of the anterior lens capsule to the facet
- The addition of systemic anomalies is called Peter's syndrome.

The summary of various mesodermal dysgenesis of anterior chamber is given in **Table 3.2**.

Trabecular Dysgeneses

The trabecular meshwork develops from mesoderm, which also gives out buds for blood vessels at the rim of the optic cup. The developing tissues are liable for congenital anomalies, i.e., mesodermal and iridocorneal dysgenesis.

TABLE 3.2: Summary of various mesodermal dysgenesis of anterior chamber.

Anomaly	*Clinical features*
Posterior embryotoxon	Prominent, centrally shifted, Schwalbe's line, good vision, no glaucoma
Reiger's anomaly	Prominent Schwalbe's line, to which strands of peripheral iris are attached, variable vision, glaucoma developing in adolescence or in fourth decade
Reiger's syndrome	Above features with skeletal deformity
Peter's anomaly: • *Type 1:* Combination of Axenfeld and Reiger's anomaly with central corneal facet to which are attached strands of iris, no lenticular adhesion to cornea, poor vision, glaucoma • *Type 2:* Incomplete separation from cornea, corneal opacity • *Type 3:* Above features with adhesion of anterior lens capsule to the corneal facet. Poor vision, glaucoma, short stature, cleft lip, mental retardation	

The first gives rise to primary congenital glaucoma. (See childhood glaucoma, where the rest of the ocular structure is developmentally normal.)

Trabecular dysgenesis is present at birth and mild enough to be missed on casual observation. All the eyes with trabecular dysgenesis may not have raised intraocular pressure; the hallmark of congenital glaucoma, i.e., the rise of pressure, manifests soon after birth.

The exact mechanism of the anomaly's development is not well elucidated. The dispute revolves around two factors, i.e., is it an anatomical maldevelopment or aberration of growth that fails to keep pace with the growth of the eye?

There are no skeletal deformities associated with trabecular dysgenesis; the only common feature between trabecular and mesodermal dysgenesis is glaucoma, and it is after math.

It is more common among boys, involvement of both eyes is more common, and uniocular cases are most probably not true trabecular dysgenesis.

On gonioscopy, the angle is wide, yet the trabecular meshwork is not visualized. It is plastered with a thin membrane of doubtful origin, eponymed as Barkan's membrane, which prevents aqueous to reach Schlemm's canal, causing a rise in intraocular pressure, terminating in intractable glaucoma.

Trabecular dysgenesis may be confused with iridocorneal endothelial dysgenesis, which is present at birth, initially asymptomatic, up to the end of the first decade, to manifest in adulthood, is generally unilateral with a distorted pupil, and is in tractable glaucoma.

CONGENITAL ANOMALIES OF THE LENS

The lens starts developing at the very early stage of gestation and continues to grow throughout gestation, resulting in numerous congenital anomalies.

The common congenital anomalies are:

- *Morphological:*
  - Microspherophakia
  - Microphakia
  - Coloboma of the lens
  - Lenticonus
  - Lenti globus
  - Umbilication
- *Topographical:* Ectopia lentis
- *Anomalies of transparency:* Congenital cataract

The congenital anomalies of the lens can be:

- Confined to the lens only, i.e., congenital cataract, simple ectopia lenticonus, coloboma, and anomalies of shape and size
- Associated with congenital anomalies of other structures, i.e., the coloboma lens associated with coloboma of the ciliary body; ectopia lentis et pupillae; displacement of the lens associated with a slit-like pupil
- Associated with systemic anomalies: Marfan syndrome, Marchesani syndrome, homocystinuria, etc.

Anomalies of Size and Shape

Microspherophakia

The normal lens is almost spherical until the middle of development, after which it flattens and becomes disc-shaped. If the flattening and increase in diameter are arrested, the lens remains spherical and small. This happens due to the arrest of growth between the fifth and sixth months of gestation. It is not clear if a lens can be small, not spherical, and vice versa. Most probably, all small lenses are spherical.

Microspherophakia can be:

- *Primary microspherophakia:* Familial; there can be only microspherophakia without any systemic disorder.
- *Associated microspherophakia:* Along with multiple systemic anomalies, i.e.,
  - Lowe syndrome*
  - Peter's anomaly
  - Weill–Marchesani syndrome
  - Hyperlysinemia
  - Apert syndrome†
  - Rarely congenital rubella, megalocornea, and ectopia lentis

---

**Lowe syndrome* is associated with congenital cataracts of various grades, diminished vision, and renal problems developing in the first year of life, along with CNS damage leading to mental retardation. It is an X-linked disorder. Management of renal disorders should get priority over ocular disorders.

†*Apert syndrome* is a congenital disorder with variable heredity; it includes ocular and craniofacial deformities. The ocular features are cataracts, either primary or secondary, and craniofacial anomalies, i.e., craniosynostosis, proptosis, squint, papilledema, and optic atrophy.

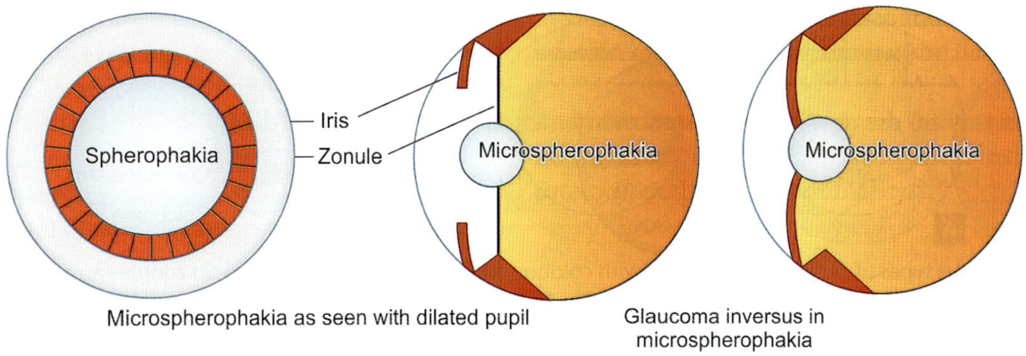

Fig. 3.23: Anterior and lateral views of spherophakia with a dilated and constricted pupil.

Microspherophakia is generally bilateral, with reduced equatorial diameter and increased anteropost-erior thickness of the lens to 5.00 mm in contrast to 3.4–4.5 mm in adults. The diameter ranges between 6.75 and 7.00 mm in contrast to 9 mm in adults. The lenticular mass is reduced from 7.5 to 80%. There is diminished distant vision due to lenticular myopia that may be as high as –20D. In an undilated pupil, there may be mild iridodonesis. When dilating the pupil, the lens looks like an oil drop in the center of the dilated pupil.

Intact zonules are visible on slit-lamp examination. Real trouble starts when the pupil is constricted; the small spherical lens acts as a ball in the socket and produces pupillary block glaucoma, and this is called glaucoma inversus. Generally, mydriasis is known to cause glaucoma, which is relieved by miosis, but here is a condition where miosis causes glaucoma, which is relieved by mydriasis **(Fig. 3.23)**.

Management: If there is no glaucoma inversus, all that is required is to correct myopia by the appropriate method

- Prophylactic laser iridotomy or surgical iridectomy may circumviate possibility of inverse glaucoma.

  The next alternative is to keep the pupil mildly diluted and observe for any rise in tension.

> The condition is not to be confused with aniridia, where the zonules are visible due to the absence of an iris with a normal lens diameter.

- Microphakia (*see* above)
- *Coloboma of the lens:* This is a deformity of the lens at the equator of the lower pole without loss of substance; it can be a notch or a wider flatting of circumference **(Figs. 3.24A to C)**.

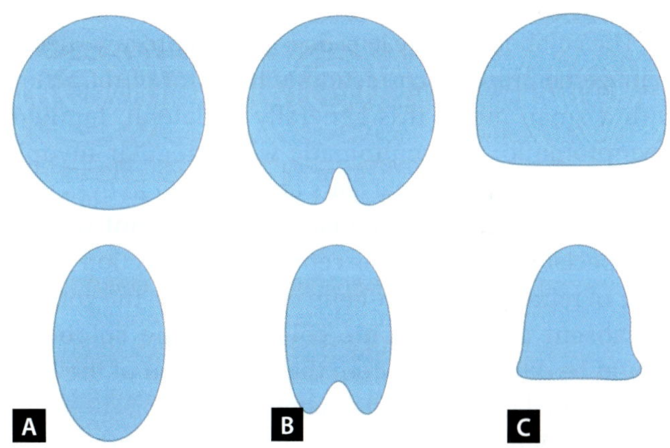

Figs. 3.24A to C: Congenital coloboma of lens—anteroposterior and lateral views: (A) Lens without coloboma; (B) Lens with notch coloboma; (C) Lens with a flat coloboma.

Congenital coloboma does not occur without coloboma of the ciliary body because the mechanism of coloboma does not lie in the lens but in the zonule.

Isolated iris or choroidal colobomas do not result in colobomas of the lens. Notch coloboma is less common than flattening of the circumference, which is always present at the lower circumferences of the lens. The flattened equator is thicker than the rest of the lens and rounded, resulting in irregular myopic astigmatism.

The lens adjacent to the coloboma may have opacity. The opacity spares the embryonal and fetal nuclei. Age-related cataracts are known to develop in the colobomatous lens early. Giant retinal tears are more common with the coloboma of the lens. The coloboma is not visible with an undilated pupil; it becomes obvious only with wide mydriasis. On slit-lamp examination, the zonules are absent adjacent to the coloboma. The coloboma should be differentiated from the subluxation of the lens; a subluxated lens retains its smooth curvature

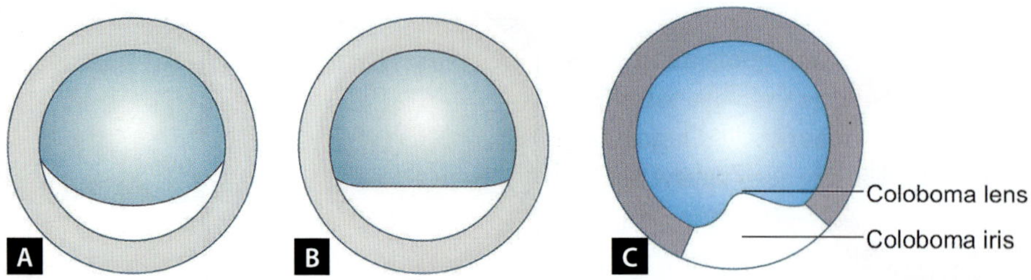

Figs. 3.25A to C: Various types of coloboma of the lens with coloboma of the iris, and ciliary body: No zonules are present at the sight of coloboma. (A) The lens subluxated up, showing a round border; (B) A large coloboma lens showing a straight border; (C) Coloboma lens with coloboma iris.

while the surface of the coloboma is flat or concave **(Figs. 3.25A to C)**.

The coloboma of the lens does not require any special management except correction of the error of refraction with a small pupil. It is generally unilateral, familial, asymptomatic, or symptomatic with irregular myopic astigmatism. Giant retinal tears are common in eyes with coloboma of the lens. The condition does not require any special management, except for the correction of the error of refraction. On slit-lamp examination, the zonules are absent adjacent to the coloboma. The coloboma should be differentiated from the subluxation of the lens. A subluxated lens retains its smooth curve.

- *Lenticonus:* This is an abnormal bulge of the capsule along with the cortex in the central part of the lens. Lenticonus can be either anterior lenticonus or posterior lenticonus. In both conditions, the lens capsule bulges outside the lens in the former, in the aqueous, and later, in the vitreous, in the anteroposterior axis of the lens.
    - *Anterior lenticonus:* It is rarely isolated; most of the time, it is associated with Alport syndrome* and is bilateral. In oblique illumination, the deformity looks like a translucent bulge at the anterior pole of the lens. The bulge may get opacified later. The patients have diminished distant vision due to curvature-lenticular myopia, which is worsened by miosis **(Fig. 3.26)**. On silt-lamp examination, the area looks like an oil drop. On reflected light, it may look darker than the rest of the retinoscopy glow and give scissor movement; the fundus looks distorted. The condition does not require any treatment except the correction of lenticular myopia. The other alternative is clear lens extraction with IOL.

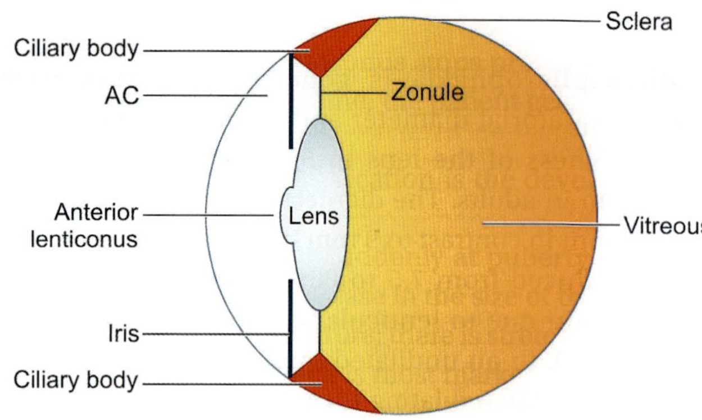

Fig. 3.26: Anterior lenticonus.

    - *Posterior lenticonus:* Posterior lenticonus is more common than anterior lenticonus. The patient reports earlier because the defect is at the nodal point, causing disproportionate loss of vision **(Fig. 3.27)**. It is generally unilateral; it can occur alone or with Lowe syndrome.† The condition becomes obvious only under slit-lamp examination or during retinoscopy. It is seen as a circular bulge in the posterior pole, like an oil drop. As long as the bulge is not opacified, it gives a translucent appearance. If the cortex herniates in the bulges,

**Alport syndrome:* The ocular features of Alport syndrome, besides anterior lenticonus, are corneal opacities, posterior polymorphous corneal dystrophy, central perimacular and peripheral fleck retinopathies, temporal retinal thinning, and, rarely, macular holes. It is generally associated with renal disorders and defective hearing. Also known as oculocerebral renal syndrome due to the dominant involvement of the brain and kidney besides the eyes, it is a sex-linked recessive disorder seen mostly in boys. It may be detected at birth due to the presence of dense bilateral congenital cataracts and glaucoma, and it may have corneal keloid. The central nervous manifestations are seizures and mental retardation. The child may survive until adulthood and die of renal failure.

†*Lowe syndrome* is a multisystem disorder affecting the nervous system and kidneys, along with ocular features.

it invariably gets opaque and looks like a posterior polar cataract. The bulge can be seen in the USG and CT. The management is similar to that of the anterior lenticonus. Posterior lenticonus requires PCIOL more often than anterior lenticonus.

- *Lentiglobus:* It is a larger form of anterior lenticonus. The diagnosis is made on a slit-lamp examination, and ultrasonography authors believe that a lenticonus is about 2–2.5 mm at its base and a lentiglobus is larger. The most probable etiology is congenital fault in the anterior lens capsules.
- *Umbilication of lens:* This is seen on both capsules. It is a depression in the capsules. It is again not clear whether it is a separate anomaly or a forme fruste of membranous cataract. The umbilication may just be a small depression on the anterior capsule or may be a large crater on both surfaces, giving a dumb-bell-like appearance on the narrow beam of the slit lamp.

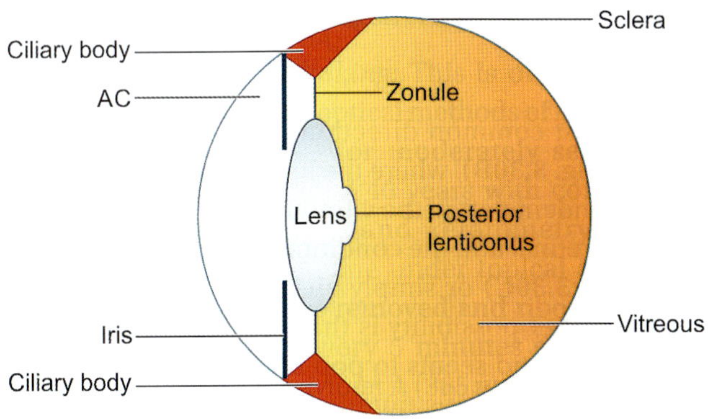

Fig. 3.27: Posterior lenticonus.

Ectopia Lentis (Lenticular Dystopia)

The normal lens is suspended and centered behind the normal pupil, in front of the vitreous, by the zonules. The zonules not only keep the lens in place but also maintain its shape. The line joining the anterior and posterior poles of the lens passes through the center of the normal pupil. Even on the widest dilatation of the pupil, no aphakic area is visible in the pupillary area, as shown in **Figure 3.28**.

Any shift from this normal position is called ectopia lentis. The lens gets shifted from its usual position due to the absence of at least 50% of the zonules in a segment. The lens moves away from the area of the absent zonule; that is, if the zonules are absent in the lower parts, the lens will shift up and vice versa **(Fig. 3.29)**.

The ectopia can be congenital or acquired, unilateral or bilateral; when bilateral, it need not be symmetric. Congenital ectopia is more commonly bilateral. The congenital ectopia is noticed in childhood and is generally nonprogressive. It may or may not be associated with systemic anomalies. Ectopia lentis has a strong genetic background and may be associated with other ocular anomalies without systemic manifestation.

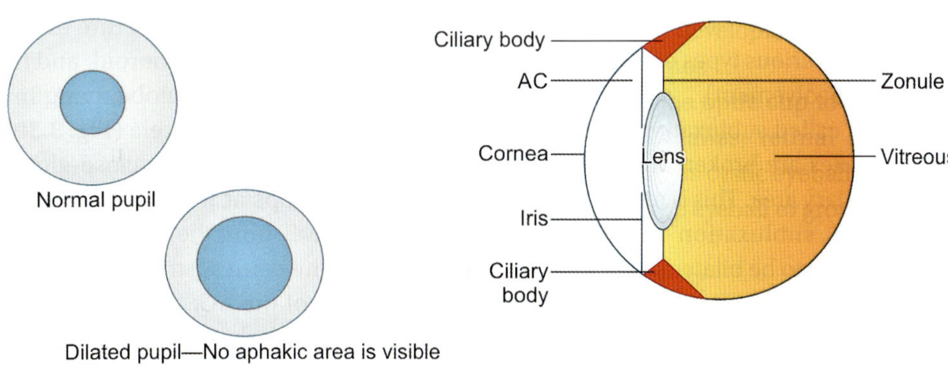

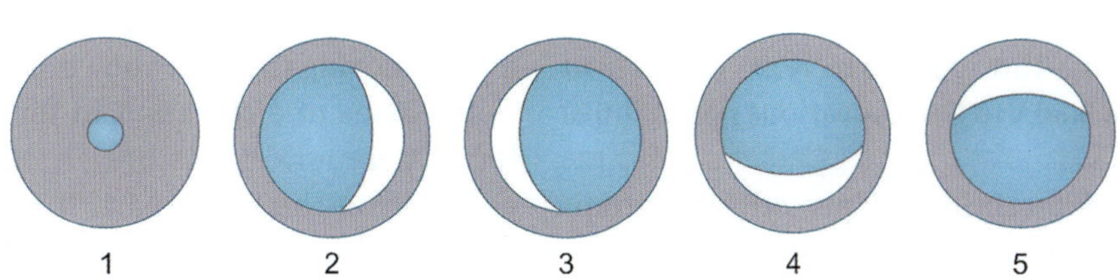

Fig. 3.28: Normal position of lens in normal and dilated pupil. (1) Undilated pupil—no dislocation visible; (2) Subluxated medially; (3) Subluxated laterally; (4) Subluxated upward; (5) Subluxated downward.

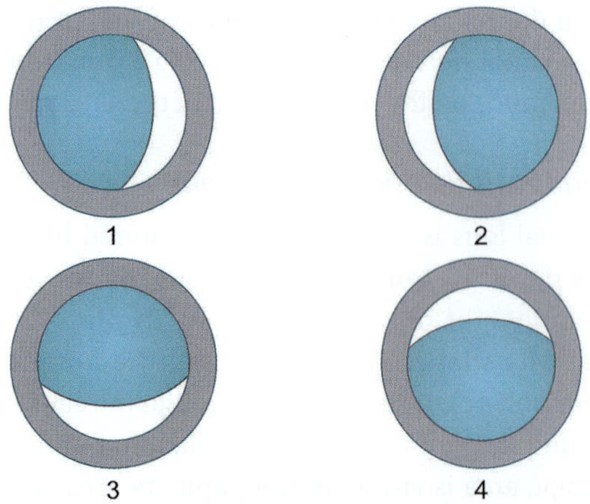

Fig. 3.29: Various possibility shift of ectopic lens. (1) Subluxated medially; (2) Subluxated laterally; (3) Subluxated upward; (4) Subluxated downward.

Causes of acquired ectopia lentis (in all ages):

- Trauma
- Idiopathic
- Long-standing anterior uveitis
- Syphilis
- High myopia
- Buphthalmos
- Hypermature cataract
- Pseudoexfoliation syndrome

Topographical classification of ectopia lentis

Topographically, ectopia lentis is of two types:

1. Partial
2. Complete

Flowchart 3.4 shows the various types of ectopia lentis (Without or with systemic involvement).

Partial ectopia lentis is called subluxation of the lens; here, almost half the zonules are broken and the lens is partially visible in the pupillary area. This is more common than the second type, i.e., subluxation with systemic syndromes. This is more likely to be bilateral.

Complete ectopia lentis is also called a luxated or dislocated lens. It characteristics are as follows: All the zonules are broken, and the lens is not visible in the pupillary area. The pupillary area looks like a pupil in aphakia following intracapsular lens extraction **(Fig. 3.30C)**. **Figures 3.30A to G** show various possibilities for dislocated lenses.

The lens can be either dislocated posteriorly, entrapped in the pupil, or dislocated in the anterior chamber. **Figures 3.30B to G** show various possible positions of dislocated lens.

Flowchart 3.4: Types of ectopia lentis (without or with systemic involvement).

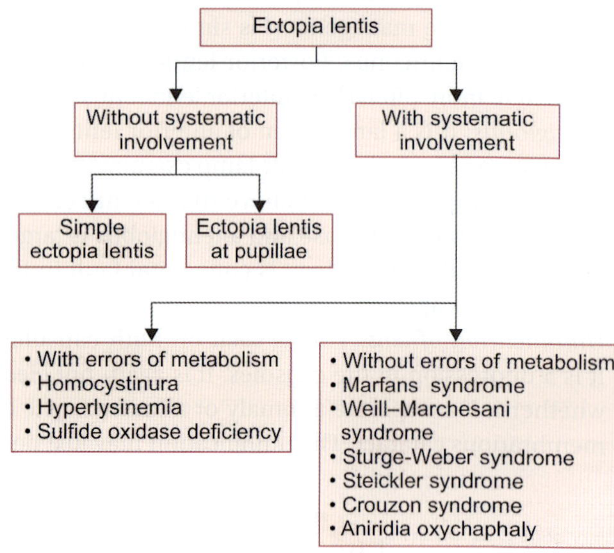

The most common direction of dislocation is in the vitreous **(Fig. 3.30B)**, where the lens generally sinks at the most dependent part of the vitreous; rarely it may get fixed under the retina, and the condition is called ectopia lentis fixate **(Fig. 3.30C)** or simply an immoveable dislocated lens. The other possibility is that the lens bobbles in the fluid vitreous and seems to pop up in the pupillary area. This condition is lentis nutans **(Fig. 3.30D)**. This lens is capable of migrating in the anterior chamber **(Fig. 3.30E)** or getting entrapped in the pupil **(Fig. 3.30F)**.

In cases of trauma with rupture of sclera, the lens may pass under the retina and choroid, and the dislocated lens may extrude outside the globe, lying in subconjunctival space. This is called phacocele **(Fig. 3.30G)**. This happens commonly following a blunt close-globe injury. The rent generally develops at the upper part of the globe, a few millimeters away from the limbus. The eyeball is soft with flattening of the cornea, striations in the cornea, resulting in shallowing of the AC. Vitreous may find access to the anterior chamber through the pupil. The management of phacocele is to incise the conjunctiva, and gradually easing the lens out through the incision, close the sclera after removing the uvea and vitreous entrapped.

In cases of dislocation in the anterior chamber, the lens is generally visible in the anterior chamber, generally at the lower part. It may be clear or opaque. The anterior chamber is deep, and some fluid vitreous may be present in the anterior chamber. The pupil is jet black, as seen following intracapsular lens extraction.

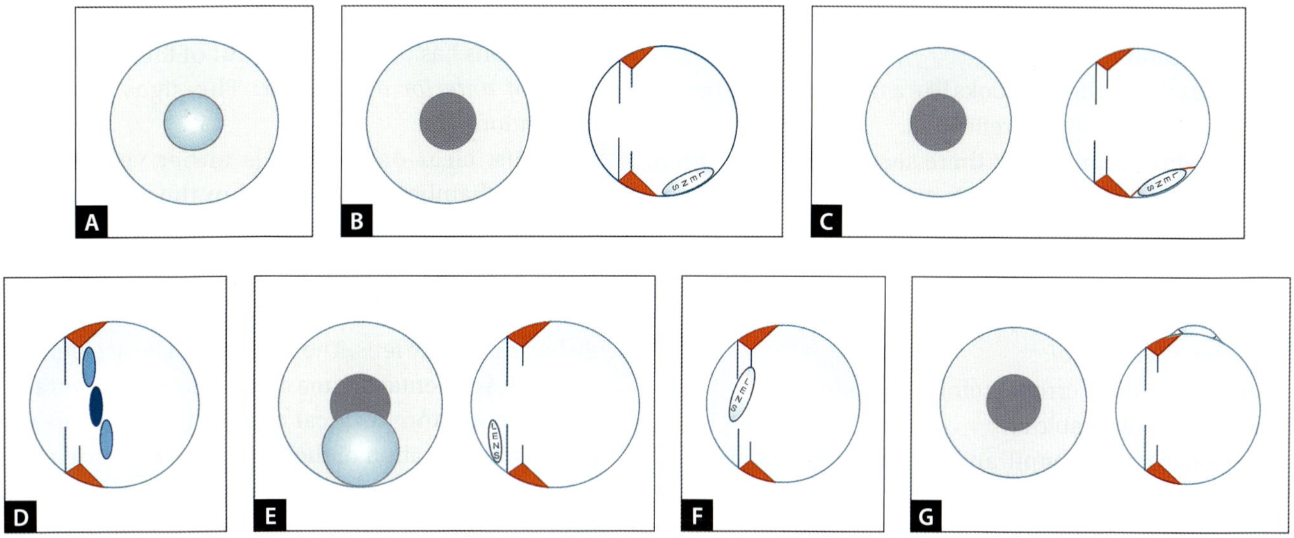

Figs. 3.30A to G: Various types of dislocated lens. (A) Lens in normal position; (B) Lens dislocated in vitreous; (C) Dislocated lens, trapped under retina—lentis fixate; (D) Lentis nutans wandering lens; (E) Lens dislocated in anterior chamber; (F) Lens entrapped in pupil; (G) Phacocele—lens extruded outside.

The lens may touch the endothelium of the cornea, resulting in decompensation; rarely, it may have raised intraocular pressure. The management is lensectomy with anterior vitrectomy and treating the eye as an aphakic eye.

There are two situations where a dislocated lens is not visible, either by an indirect ophthalmoscope or by ultrasonography:

1. The lens has been extruded out of a globe (phacocele)
2. The lens has been absorbed (less common)

Clinical features of subluxated lens (Ectopia lentis): Congenital developmental or acquired ectopia lentis shares common clinical features. *Symptoms are as follows:*

- *No symptoms:* Milder form, where the edge of the subluxated lens remains behind the iris with a normal pupil
- *Diminished distant vision:* Due to irregular lenticular astigmatism
- Uniocular subluxations may go unnoticed.
- The edge of the dislocated lens passes through the normal-sized pupil, causing partial aphakic and partial phakic pupils. The phakic part is generally myopic, while the aphakic part is hypermetropic and amblyopic.
- *Sudden improvement of vision:* Sudden improvement of vision: In cases of long-standing mature cataracts getting subluxated or dislocated, causing a clear aphakic pupil, the patient is able to see through the aphakic area, which has better vision than before. (This does not happen in children.)
- *Pain redness:* The ectopic eye may develop pain and redness in the following conditions:
    - Glaucoma is secondary to the entrapment of the lens in the pupil.
    - Glaucoma inversus
    - Decompensation of the cornea due to the lens in AC rubbing against the corneal endothelium
- Squint
- Nystagmus
- Symptoms of systemic disorder

Signs of ectopia lentis (subluxation) of all types:

- The eyes may look normal externally, but only close scrutiny may show signs of ectopia. The eyes with prominent ectopia on oblique illumination show a localized area of tremulousness over the defective zonule with an irregular depth of AC over the phakic area and deep over the aphakic area.
- Uniformly deep AC occurs when the dislocation of the lens is in the vitreous. The pupil looks as if an intracapsular lens extraction has been done.
- The lens may be visible in the anterior chamber, with a deep anterior chamber.
- *Retinoscopy:* The types of movements in ectopia lentis are:
    1. Phakic area, when clear, gives myopic astigmatic refraction.

2. The aphakic area gives simple high hypermetropic refraction.
3. The edge of the lens looks like a thin, black crescent due to total internal reflection.

- On fundus examination, there seem to be two optic discs present in the same eye, one large seen through the phakic (myopic) area and the other small seen through the aphakic (hypermetropic) area.

Management of simple ectopia lentis
Management consists of:

- Correction of the error of refraction optically.
  The options available are:
  - Constrict the pupil and give myopic astigmatic correction either in spectacle or in contact lens
  - Dilate the pupil and give aphakic correction with near addition
  - Lensectomy, vitrectomy with sclera suspended PC IOL or AC IOL (no more in vogue)
- Prevention of glaucoma by:
  - Local beta blockers/carbonic anhydrase inhibitors
  - Laser iridotomy in cases of pupillary block

Signs of dislocated lens:
The signs depend on the position of the dislocated lens.

- *Signs of posterior dislocations:* In cases of posterior dislocation, the signs and symptoms of aphakia are present as they happen following intracapsular lens extraction without any mark of incision.

  They are: Deep AC, tremulous iris without iridectomy, jet black pupil vitreous may protrude through the pupil, the floating lens may be seen moving up and down behind the iris, and the vision is reduced to counting fingers, which in uncomplicated dislocation may improve with +10 DSph.

  The dislocated lens is visible following wide mydriasis, lying at the bottom of the vitreous; the lens may be transparent or may have various degrees of opacity. In the case of a transparent lens, the retinal vessels underneath are visible. The cataractous lens blocks the retinal vessels.

  The differential diagnoses of the posterior dislocation of the lens are: Retinal detachment, localized choroidal effusion, peripheral retinal granuloma, and parasitic cyst.

  There are the following possibilities if the dislocated lens is not visible in the vitreous, even with an indirect ophthalmoscope and USG:
  - The lens has been absorbed completely.
  - The lens has been excreted out of the sclera.
- *Signs of anterior dislocation:* The signs of anterior dislocations are:
  The lens, clear or opaque, is either visible in the anterior chamber or entrapped in the pupillary area. Anterior dislocation causes the deepest AC.

Causes of dislocation of the lens (in all ages):

- *Trauma:* This is the most common cause of posterior dislocation of the lens. The trauma can be accidental or surgical. Accidental trauma can be blunt or penetrating. A very common surgical method associated with posterior dislocation of the lens used to be attempted: Intracapsular lens extraction. Fortunately, this does not happen anymore; however, the lens can be dislocated during small-incision extracapsular cataract extraction or during capsulorhexis.
- *Congenital*: Any of the congenital causes of subluxation may end in dislocation.
- Hypermatured cataract
- Syphilis
- Annular intercalary staphylomas
- Buphthalmos
- Spontaneous

Management of dislocated lens:

- A lens in AC or an incarcerated pupil is an emergency. This lens should be removed by A limbal incision and, if necessary, a vitrectomy should be performed.
- Lenses caught in the pupil may be pushed back by applying gentle pressure to the cornea and pupil constricted with 4% pilocarpine. However, these do not succeed always. In such an event, the lens is better removed.
- *Lens in the vitreous:*
  - It need not be tempered if asymptomatic.
  - A symptomatic dislocated lens is best removed by total vitrectomy.
  - In the case of phacocele, the conjunctiva over the extruded lens is incised, and the lens is eased out gently. The incarcerated uvea and vitreo are managed as per practice.

Complications of dislocated lens:

- *Anterior dislocation:* Pupillary block, trabecular block, uveitis, and corneal decompensation
- *Posterior dislocation:* Uveitis, secondary glaucoma, tractional retinal detachment

Specific types of ectopia lentis: Specific types of ectopia lentis can be without or with systemic involvement.

- *Ectopia lentis without systemic involvement*
    - *Familial ectopia lentis:* This is also called simple ectopia lentis. It runs in families, the displacement is generally bilaterally symmetrical, upward it is more common in males, and the association of myopia is frequent. Though there are no obvious systemic involvements, they are considered to be forme fruste of Marfan syndrome.
    - *Ectopia lentis with ectopic pupil* **(Figs. 3.31A and B)**: This is a condition of ectopia of the lens with a shifted pupil, or corectopia (ectopia pupil). This condition involves the pupil and lens without any systemic involvement. The pupil is shifted away from its normal position, i.e., corectopic, and the lens is subluxated. The cause of the combination is not well understood. The corectopic pupil may be circular or slit-like. The direction of the lenticular shift is opposite to the shift of the pupil. The condition is generally associated with early cataracts, secondary glaucoma, and retinal detachment.

    Management of ectopia lentis et ectopia pupillae
    - Asymptomatic cases need no treatment.
    - Due to the shift of the pupil, there may be diminished distance as well as near-vision.

    Various options available to improve the vision are:
    Mydriasis: This may cause a dislocated lens to migrate in the AC, accompanied by complications of the lens in the AC.

    Surgical enlargement of the pupil by sphinctero-tomy or LASER iridoplasty.

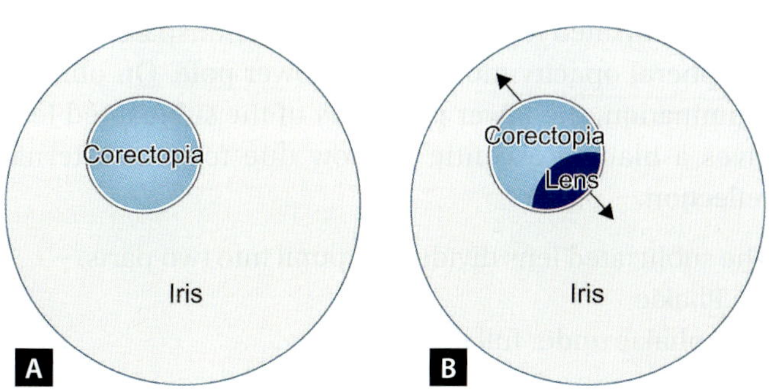

Figs. 3.31A and B: Ectopic lentis et corectopia. (A) Corectopia without involving the lens; (B) Ectopic lentis et corectopia. The small pupil shifted up and the lens shifted down.

- *Ectopia lentis with systemic involvement:* Ectopia lentis, with systemic involvement, is divided into two classes:
    1. Without an error of metabolism, they are:
        - Marfan syndrome
        - Weill–Marchesani syndrome
        - EDS
        - Sturge–Weber syndrome
        - Stickler syndrome
        - Crouzon syndrome
        - Oxycephaly
        - Aniridia
    2. With an error in metabolism, they are:
        - Homocystinuria
        - Hyperlysinemia
        - Sulfide oxidase deficiency

Marfan syndrome: This is the most common and important form of ectopia lentis the world over, with extensive systemic involvement due to multiple congenital anomalies. The ocular findings are bilateral and almost symmetrical. The exact cause is not known, but the most widely accepted view is that it is mesodermal dysplasia. It has a strong heredity; it is an autosomal dominant disorder that may be present not only in siblings but also in preceding and following generations. When present in the family, all the affected members may not have all the classical features. It is seen in all races and in both sexes, with boys outnumbering girls; the condition is present at birth but diagnosed in childhood. There are no biochemical changes.

It has three sets of components, all of which may not be present at the same time. However, the presence of any one set of components makes it mandatory for other systems to be examined and investigated for congenital anomalies.

The components are:
- Ocular
- Skeletal
- Cardiac

A child with Marfan syndrome may present with symptoms pertaining to systemic defects and, on examination, found to have ocular features and vice versa. The internist pays more attention to the skeletal and cardiac defects; the skeletal defects are benign, but the cardiac defects may be fatal. The physicians decide Marfan syndrome as per Ghent diagnostic criteria, which in turn depend on major and minor criteria in two organs and a

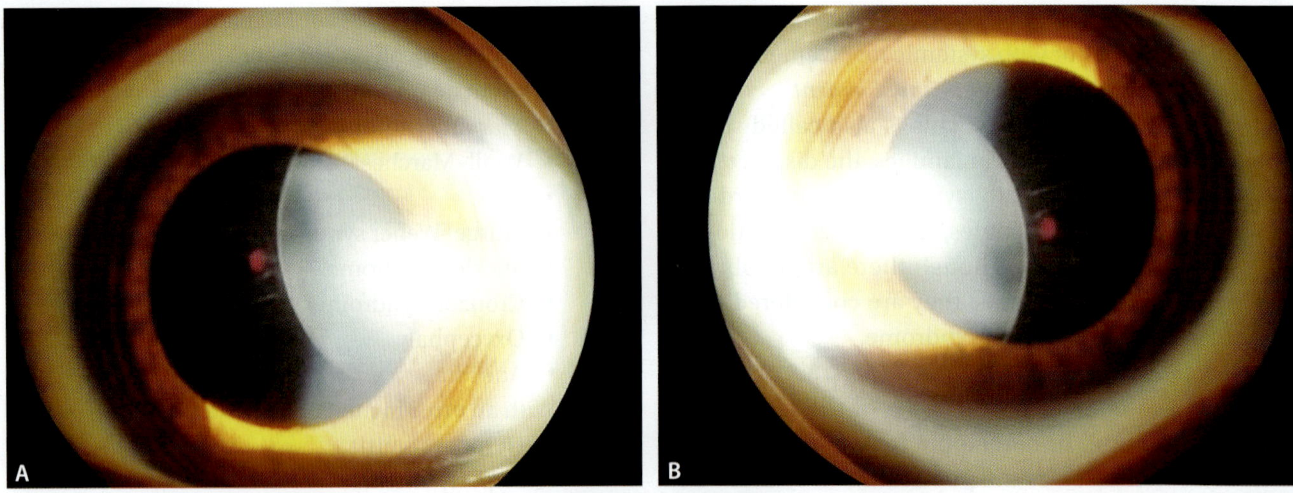

Figs. 3.32A and B: Bilateral subluxation of lens up and out.

minor criterion in the third organ. The major criteria have more clinical features than the minor criteria (see below).

The most striking features are skeletal changes. The most spectacular ocular finding is in the lens. The lenticular changes are bilateral, symmetric, and nonprogressive.

The ocular features are:

- Diminished distant vision
- Uniocular diplopia may become polyopia if both eyes are open.
- Retained accommodation until the lens is dislocated
- Bilateral symmetric upward subluxation of the lens
- Early onset of cataracts
- Less common ocular features are:
    - Microspherophakia
    - Glaucoma
    - Angle anomaly
    - Pupillary block
    - Hypoplasia of the dilator muscles
    - Peripheral retinal degeneration
    - Rhegmatogenous retinal detachment
    - Megalocornea
    - Uveal coloboma
    - Amblyopia
    - Squint

The ocular signs are:

Lens: The most common finding is subluxation of the lens; both lenses are subluxated, and the most common form of subluxation is up and out **(Figs. 3.32A and B)**.

The subluxated lenses are mirror images of each other **(Fig. 3.33)**.

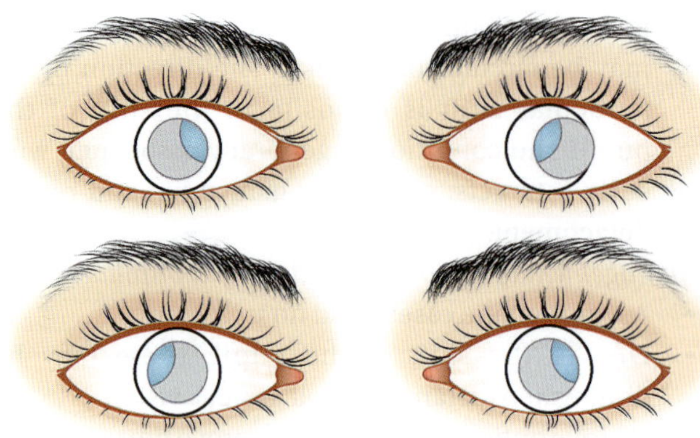

Fig. 3.33: Mirror image of the ectopia lens in Marfan syndrome.

The subluxated lenses remain clear until the development of the usual age-related cataract. Age-related cataracts develop early in subluxated lenses. The clear subluxated lens may have central transparency with peripheral opacity mostly at the lower pole. On oblique illumination, the lower periphery of the subluxated lens gives a black crescentic shadow due to total internal reflection.

The subluxated lens divides the pupil into two parts.

1. Phakic
2. Aphakic under full mydriatic

Retinoscopy: Retinoscopy done under full mydriasis gives two types of refraction.

Myopic astigmatism through a subluxated lens.

Simple hypermetropic refraction through the aphakic part. If the eye has axial myopia, which is common with Marfan syndrome, the hypermetropic refraction will be less than +10D. In cases of posterior dislocation, the whole of the pupil will give aphakic refraction.

Slit-lamp examination: The zonules that are not visible even with full mydriasis in the normal eye become visible in Marfan syndrome. Some of them may be totally absent or broken; on rare occasions, the anterior vitreous may bulge in the pupillary area **(Fig. 3.34)**.

Anterior chamber: The anterior chamber has irregular depth, deep over aphakia, and shallow over dislocation.

Iris: The iris is hypoplastic, so the pupil is small and resistant to mydriasis. The iris may show transillumination. The iris over the aphakic area may show tremulousness.

Ciliary body: As the ciliary body is not affected, the accommodation may be retained.

Fundus: Fundus can be seen through a dilated pupil, showing duplication of the disc—one smaller seen through the aphakia and the other large seen through the subluxated lens.

Other ocular changes: The following are some of the ocular changes seen in Marfan syndrome: They are not very constant and may be found in various combinations. Flattened cornea, retinal detachment, axial myopia, myopic fundus changes, angle anomalies, glaucoma, either due to an angle anomaly or due to a lens entrapped in the pupil, early cataract, scleral thinning, and spherophakia.

The eyes may be orthophoric or show various types of tropia. Nystagmus is rare.

The non-ocular features can be divided into two broad groups, i.e., facial and axial. The facial features are: Distinct, like dolichocephaly (long, narrow skull), enophthalmos, micrognathia (small jaw), flat cheek bones, a high, arched palate, and crowding of teeth.

The skeletal features are: Tall, lanky, stooping stature; a span of outstretched hands that is more than the height of the patient; scoliosis and kyphosis; a barrel-shaped chest; arachnodactyly; hyperexpandable joints; scanty subcutaneous fat; and a tendency for hernias.

The skeletal feature almost always attracts the attention of the parents, who think that the child is too thin for this age and consult a pediatrician, who is invariably the first to come to the diagnosis of Marfan syndrome and finds that the child is lanky with slender limbs and a long spidery figure (arachnodactyly). The fingers are too long for the circumference of the wrist. There are about 10 wrist and thumb signs; all are not present in all cases. The two common signs that are invariably present are the Murdoch wrist sign and the Steinberg thumb sign.

If a normal child clasps his forearm with the opposite hand just above the wrist, none of his fingertips reaches the tip of the thumb. If the tips of the thumb and finger overlap each other, the Murdoch sign is positive **(Figs. 3.35 and 3.36)**.

Similarly, if the child flexes his fingers over the flexed thumb across the palm, the tip of the thumb just reaches the ulnar border of the palm. If the tip of the flexed thumb

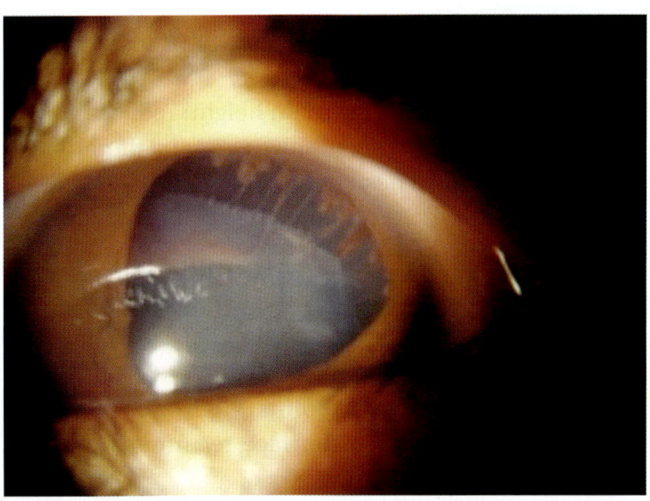

Fig. 3.34: Photograph showing zonule in subluxated lens. *Courtesy:* Dr Santosh Patel.

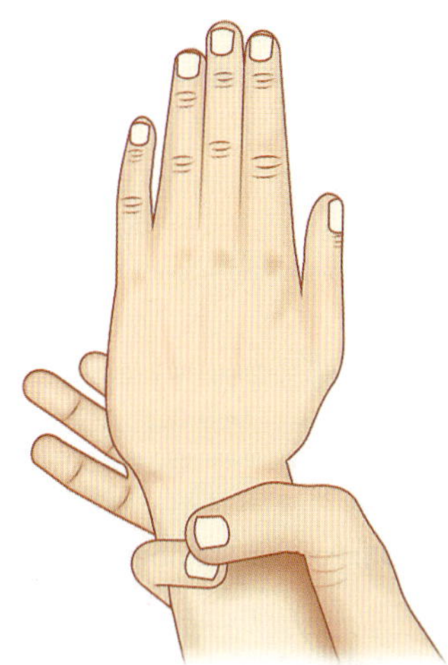

Fig. 3.35: Positive Murdoch sign.

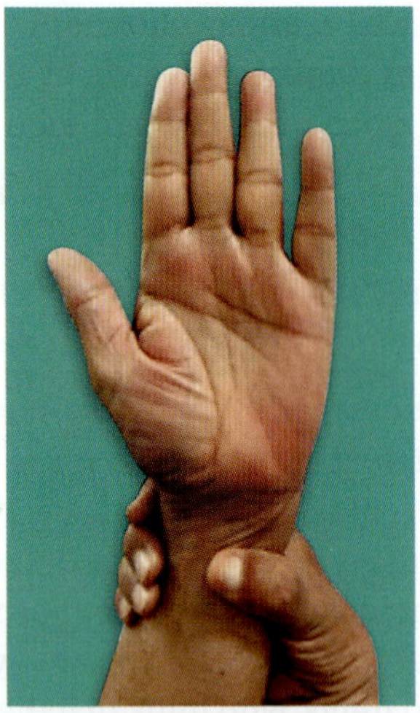

Fig. 3.36: Negative Murdoch sign.

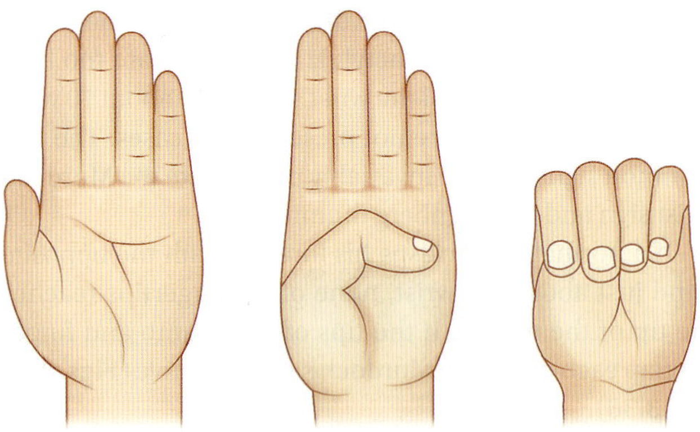

Fig. 3.37: Negative Steinberg sign.

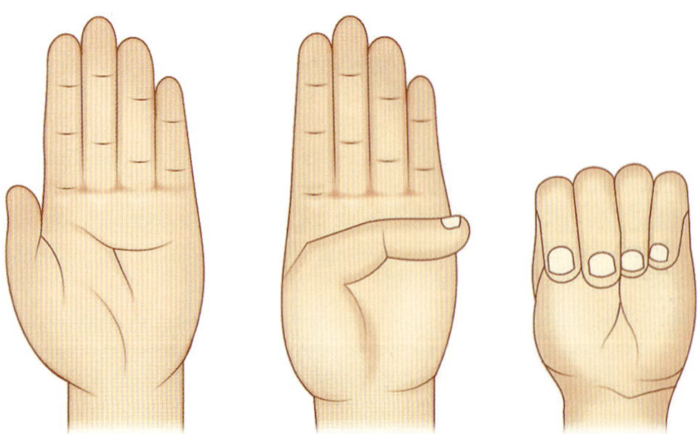

Fig. 3.38: Positive Steinberg sign.

is protruding beyond the ulnar border, the Steinberg sign is positive **(Figs. 3.37 and 3.38)**. Both signs are due to extralong fingers.

The ocular and skeletal signs are not fatal; they are visual and cosmetic. Long, slender arms and a lanky gait cause embracement in a growing child. To this is added the diminishment of distant vision. In contrast to these, cardiovascular changes are potentially fatal and may cause sudden death. The clinical features of the cardiac components of Marfan syndrome are: Breathlessness, palpitation, unexplained tiredness, and failure to gain weight. The cardiac features are put under the following headings:

- *Disorder of large vessels:* Aortic regurgitation, dilatation of the aortic ring, dissecting aneurysm of the aorta, aneurysm of the ascending and descending aorta, rupture of the aneurysm is invariably the cause of sudden death.
- *Disorder of the heart:* Persistent foramen ovale, dilatation of the aortic ring, mitral valve prolapse

Diagnosis:

- Diagnosis of a full-blown case is not difficult with skeletal and ocular changes.
- Patients with minimal findings require a complete ocular and physical examination, including family history suggesting Marfan syndrome and a history of unexplained sudden death in a young adult in the family.
- There is no biochemical test that may confirm the diagnosis, in contrast to homocystinuria, which closely resembles Marfan syndrome.

The most widely used criteria are Ghent's nosological criteria, which divide the condition into two major and one minor criteria.

The major criteria consist of:

- *Ocular:* Ectopia lentis
- *Skeletal:* Arm span more than height; reduced upper-to-lower segment ratio; positive wrist and thumb signs; scoliosis; pigeon chest; funnel chest
- *Cardiovascular:* Aortic aneurysm, aortic dilatation, dissecting aneurysm

The minor criteria consist of:

- *Ocular:* Ectopia lentis, flat cornea, axial myopia, more than 3D
- *Skeletal:* Hyperflexible joints, high-arched palate, crowded teeth, long and thin face, recurrent dislocation of joints, inguinal hernia
- *Cardiovascular:* Mitral valve prolapse, widened aortic ring, descending aneurysm.

To confirm the diagnosis, the patient should have:

- Two major criteria in two organs with at least one minor criterion in the third organ
- One major criterion is involvement in one organ and involvement in another organ with mutations in the *FBN1-1* gene.

Differential diagnosis

Differential diagnoses consist of the following:

- Familial ectopia lentis
- Ectopia lentis et pupillae
- Homocystinuria
- Weill-Marchesani syndrome
- Sulfide oxidase deficiency
- Hyperlysinemia
- EDS*
- Stickler syndrome†
- Brittle cornea syndrome‡

Treatment of Marfan syndrome

Being a genetic, congenital, and multiple organ disorder, there is no curative or preventive treatment. The management is aimed at prolonging the life span, preventing crippling disabilities, and salvaging as much vision as possible. Systemic management is best left to pediatricians and physicians.

The ocular disorders are managed by:

- Improving vision of axial myopia and aphakia following refraction
- Constricting the pupil and correcting index myopia
- Dilating pupil and correct aphakia
- Removal of the dislocated lens
- Prophylactic beta-blockers for glaucoma
- Surgical management of glaucoma
- Management of squints and amblyopia
- Counseling
- Rehabilitation by low-vision aid

> The patients have normal intelligence and no biochemical changes in the blood.

Weill-Marchesani syndrome: This condition is less common than Marfan syndrome. There are some similarities between Marfan and Weill-Marchesani syndromes: Both have bilateral subluxation of lenses, both are mesodermal dysgenesis without any biochemical change or lowered intelligence, both have cardiac anomalies, and both syndromes have three components of ocular, skeletal, and cardiac involvement.

- The ocular components of Weill-Marchesani syndrome are: Bilateral, symmetrical inferior subluxation of the lens with loss of accommodation. The lens is generally microspherophakia, with a tendency to move forward and either get incarcerated in the pupil, causing pupillary block, or dislocate in the anterior chamber. The anterior chamber is generally shallow.

  Glaucoma is due to multiple factors acting individually or in combination. They are pupillary block due to spherophakia, glaucoma inversus due to miosis, and trabecular obstruction by the iris.
- The skeletal changes consist of: Short stubby stature, muscular body with spade-like hands, brachycephaly, without kyphosis, scoliosis, or arachnodactyly.
- The cardiac anomalies are variable.

Management

The first and foremost part of management is the prevention of pupillary block glaucoma and glaucoma inversus by laser iridotomy or surgical iridectomy. If the lens is subluxated down, it will constrict the pupil and

---

**Ehlers-Danlos syndrome*: This is a rare genetic, multisystemic disorder of connective tissue with multiple ocular involvements. It occurs in structures rich in connective tissue, i.e., sclera, cornea, extraocular muscles, and zonules.

The ocular features are: Lax lids; the upper lid can be pulled down up to the chin with or without ptosis, various forms of squint (70%), mild proptosis, axial myopia, myopic and macular degeneration, angioid streak, and ectopia lentis. Due to the high collagen content, corneal involvements are frequent, which include a thin cornea, a brittle cornea, the keratoconus, and the keratoglobus. Due to the same reason, scleral disorders are also common; they are blue sclera, posterior, and equatorial staphylomas. Congenital and developmental glaucoma. The coats of the eyeball are predisposed to rupture, even with a trivial blunt injury.

The main systemic involvements are: Hypermotile joints, extreme stretch ability of the skin, frequent subcutaneous hemorrhages, kyphoscoliosis, and vascular anomalies.

†*Stickler syndrome* is hereditary, congenital, and progressive with oculopathy—poor vision, giant tear, vitreoretinal degeneration, rhegmatogenous retinal detachment, congenital myopia, and ectopia lentis. Connective tissues all over the body are involved, resulting in joint problems and poor hearing.

‡*Brittle cornea syndrome*: Congenital progressive bilateral autosomal recessive, extreme thinning of the cornea, fragile corneal thickness <400 μm, spontaneous perforation of the cornea, high myopia, posterior staphylomas, and squint.

provide aphakic correction. If the lens is behind the pupil, mid-dilate the pupil and provide myopic correction. A completely dislocated lens in the vitreous is best left as such if there is no symptom. A symptomatic lens from the vitreous may be removed along with a complete vitrectomy, and an anterior dislocated lens should be removed by a limbal incision, as this is more likely to cause corneal decompensation.

Homocystinuria: The existence of this condition was not known until the early sixties of the last century. Patients were put in the category of incomplete Marfan syndrome with mental retardation; however, it was realized that it was an error in the metabolism of the amino acid methionine. The fault lies in cystathionine beta synthase, which leads to the accumulation of homocysteine and methionine in the body. The level of homocysteine is high in both blood and urine. In this condition, homocysteine is excreted in urine. Mental retardation is seen in all patients. The condition is congenital, yet the infants appear healthy. The syndrome, too, has three components: Ocular, skeletal, and systemic.

- *The ocular involvements* have many similarities to the ocular features of Marfan syndrome. It consists of bilateral subluxations of the lens. About 50% of cases develop ectopic lenses by the end of the first decade of life. It is presumed that about 90% people with homocystinuria do develop subluxation of the lens sometimes or other. The zonules are broken and can be seen matted on the lens surface. The lens may cause pupillary block, get incarcerated in the pupil, get dislocated in the AC, or fall in the vitreous with the usual complications.
- *The skeletal features* are also akin to Marfan syndrome and may be called Marfanoid habitus with malar flush, knock-knee, and osteoporosis. Pathological fractures are common. Arachnodactyly is less common. The patients have thin, light-colored hair.
- *The systemic features* are more pronounced than those of Marfan syndrome. In contrast to Marfan syndrome, which has loose joints, patients with homocystinuria have tight joints. The systemic features are hematological, hepatological, and neurological. The neurological features are mental retardation and seizures. The hematological conditions are blood clotting disorders and premature atherosclerosis. The patients have high anesthetic complications that can prove fatal.

The presence of homocysteine in urine is detected by a sodium nitroprusside test. The test is simple, but one of the reagents is sodium cyanide. It has to be done with proper precaution under supervision. The test consists of adding 2 mL of 5% sodium cyanide to 5 mL of freshly collected urine. After 10 minutes, 4 drops of sodium nitroprusside are added to this mixture. A bright red color develops in the presence of homocysteine in urine; the test is not specific, and cysteine also gives a positive nitroprusside result. The presence of homocysteine should be confirmed by amino acid analysis and enzyme assays in the blood.

Management

The first step is to reduce serum homocysteine by administering vitamin B6 (pyridoxine) in large doses and restricting methionine in the diet. Those who do not respond to the B6 and low-methionine diets are treated with betaine (trimethylglycine). It is postulated that these two steps taken by children with homocystinuria delay or decrease the chance of ectopia lentis. The medical treatment has to be taken for the rest of your life.

> In view of the high risk of general anesthesia, all children with ectopia lentis should be tested for homocystinuria prior to surgery to avoid complications of anesthesia.

The summary of three main congenital causes of ectopia lentis is depicted in **Table 3.3**.

CONGENITAL ANOMALIES OF UVEA

Congenital anomalies of the uvea consist of congenital anomalies of the iris, ciliary body, and choroid.

Congenital Anomalies of Iris

Out of the three parts of the uvea, the iris has the maximum number of congenital anomalies. Iris is partly ectodermal and partly mesodermal in origin; hence, it is involved not only in anomalies of the uvea but also in those of the cornea.

Common congenital anomalies of the iris are:

- Aniridia
- Persistent pupillary membrane
- Coloboma
- Deformity of the pupil
- Iridocorneal dysgenesis
- Pigmentary anomalies

Aniridia

The term aniridia is a misnomer; logically, the term should mean total absence of iris in the eye, but that is not true with

TABLE 3.3: Congenital causes of ectopia lentis.

Features	*Marfan syndrome*	*Homocystinuria*	*Weill–Marchesani syndrome*
Genetics	Autosomal dominant	Autosomal recessive	Variable
Ocular features			
Lens	• Subluxate up and out • Nonprogressive • May dislocate • May become opaque	• Subluxate down • Tendency to dislocate	• Microspherophakia • Tendency to dislocate
Anterior chamber	• Normal • Irregular—shallow over phakic area; deep over aphakic area	Normal	Normal or iris bombe with constricted pupil
Iris	• Hypoplastic • Poorly developed dilator • Iridodonesis	Iridodonesis	Iridodonesis
Pupil	• Miotic • Difficult to dilate	Normal	Normal
Angle	Abnormal	Normal	Normal
Glaucoma	• Due to mesodermal dysgenesis of angle • Lens entrap in pupil	Nil	Glaucoma inversus
Accommodation	Fairly good	Poor to absent	May be lost
Refraction	• Overall—myopia • Index myopia in phakic area • Hypermetropia in aphakic area	Nonspecific	Lenticular myopia
Skeletal changes			
Height	Tall, lanky, slender	Tall, slender, lanky	Short, stubby
Limbs	• Long, thin • Length of outstretched arms more than height	Nonspecific	Short, stubby
Finger	• Arachnodactyly • Positive Murdoch and Steinberg sign	Arachnodactyly	• Short spade like palm • Short thick finger
Joints	Loose, hyperextensible	Hyper extensible	Stiff
Skull	Dolichocephaly/Normal	Dolichocephaly/Normal	Brachycephaly
Spine	• Scoliosis • Kyphosis	Scoliosis	Normal
Chest	• Long • Slender • Pigeon chest	Long Slender	Short wide
Palate	High arched	Normal	Normal
Subcutaneous tissue	Poorly developed	Poorly developed	Well formed
Cardiovascular changes			
Heart	• Aortic valve dilatation • Mitral valve prolapse	Variable	Variable
Large vessels	• Aneurysm of aortic arch • Aneurysm of descending aorta	Nil	Nil
Thromboembolic phenomena	Nil	Common	Nil
Anesthetic risk	Guarded	High	Guarded
Other changes			
Intelligence	Normal	Low	Normal
Life expectancy	Normal	Low	Normal
Biochemical test	Nil	Sodium nitroprusside, cyanide test positive	Nil

clinical aniridia. Clinically, an eye is said to have aniridia if no iris is visible on oblique illumination but shreds of iris are visible on gonioscopy, some with free ends floating in the aqueous and some plastered against the trabecular meshwork, impeding the free flow of the aqueous.

Aniridia is rare, bilateral, mostly hereditary, and rarely sporadic, equally distributed among boys and girls, and may run in families.

Other ocular structures involved are:

Cornea, angle, lens, macula, and optic nerve. The cornea shows a uniform haze or may be clear. The corneal changes are attributed to stem cell anomalies. Micropannus is common; anterior chamber is deep, without a line of demarcation between the anterior and posterior chambers. The lens is in place, may be clear, and have scattered opacities. The zonules are normal and visible; however, luxation of the lens is frequent.

Glaucoma develops slowly in the second decade, is intractable, and does not respond to usual medical or surgical treatment. Aqueous suppressant drugs are administered to keep aqueous production low. Prophylactic goniotomy before a set of glaucoma is claimed to work. The other parts to be involved are the macula and optic nerve, both of which are hypoplastic; the cause of hypoplasia is not known.

The first symptom to attract the attention of parents is intolerance to light; this is not true photophobia but is brought about by the absence of the iris. As the child grows, it is found that the child has uncorrectable vision.

The probable causes of diminished vision are: Corneal opacity, macular and optic nerve hypoplasia, error of refraction, amblyopia, nystagmus, and glaucoma.

Sporadic cases may harbor Wilms' tumor, making it mandatory for all children with aniridia to undergo abdominal ultrasonography.

The overall prognosis is poor.

Persistent Pupillary Membrane

It is not a true congenital anomaly of the iris; it is a failure of the anterior part of the tunica vasculosa lentis to disappear either at birth or within a few months. More than 50% of children are born with a minor degree of the disorder that disappears by the end of the first year. In rare instances, it remains unabsorbed, and the patient may not be aware of its presence unless told on routine examination.

The condition may be unilateral or bilateral; it need not be symmetric when bilateral. It may just be a fine strand of iris tissue visible only on a slit lamp under high power and bright light; it may be extensive enough to spread all over the anterior surface of the iris, including the pupil. The strands are attached to the iris collarettes and may be mistaken for posterior synechiae, which arise at the pupillary border of the posterior surface of the iris. The persistent pupillary membrane consists of mesodermal tissue and obliterated blood vessels. The free end of the strand may float in the aqueous solution and get attached to the anterior lens capsule **(Figs. 3.39A to D)**.

They do not hamper vision or pupillary reaction and do not require treatment.

Congenital Coloboma of Iris

Congenital coloboma of the iris cannot be discussed separately from the coloboma of the ciliary body and

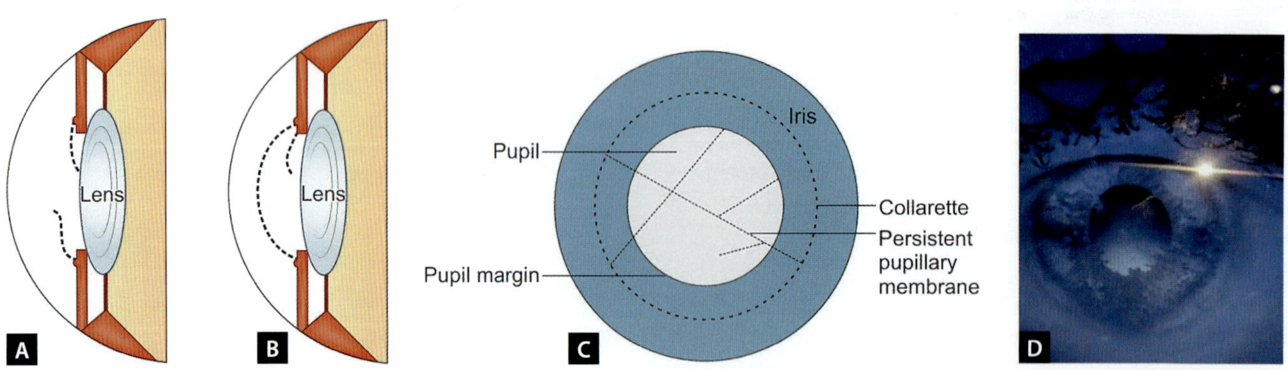

Figs. 3.39A to D: Various possibilities of persistent pupillary membrane. (A to C) Various types of persistent pupillary membrane; (D) Extensive persistent pupillary membrane.
Courtesy: (D) Dr SC Batalia.

the choroid. The coloboma of these structures have been reported in isolation as well. Colobomas of the uvea are found even in apparently normal eyes or with microphthalmos. Their presence in microphthalmic eyes is common.

Congenital anomalies of the uvea can be broadly divided into two groups, i.e., colobomatous and non-colobomatous. The colobomatous anomalies involve all three parts of the uvea: Iris, ciliary body, and choroid; the noncolobomatous anomalies are confined to the iris and choroid.

Isolated colobomas of the iris are most common among uveal colobomas. The usual shape of the iris coloboma is like a keyhole, which is narrow at the lower part; if the width of the coloboma at the upper part is as wide as the pupil, the coloboma assumes the shape of an inverted U or a hairpin **(Fig. 3.40)**. A wide and extensive pan-uveal coloboma gives a white reflex on retinoscopy **(Figs. 3.41A to D)**.

The acquired coloboma of iris should be differentiated from congenital coloboma.

The characteristics of acquired coloboma are shown in **Figure 3.42**.

Characteristics of the acquired coloboma of the iris are:
- There is a history of trauma, whether surgical or accidental.
- They can be anywhere on the iris.
- Their edges are sharp.
- There is no pigmentary border.
- They do not react independently to light or accommodation.

The longer the unfused area of the fetal fissure, the larger will be the coloboma. Minimal failure will result in a

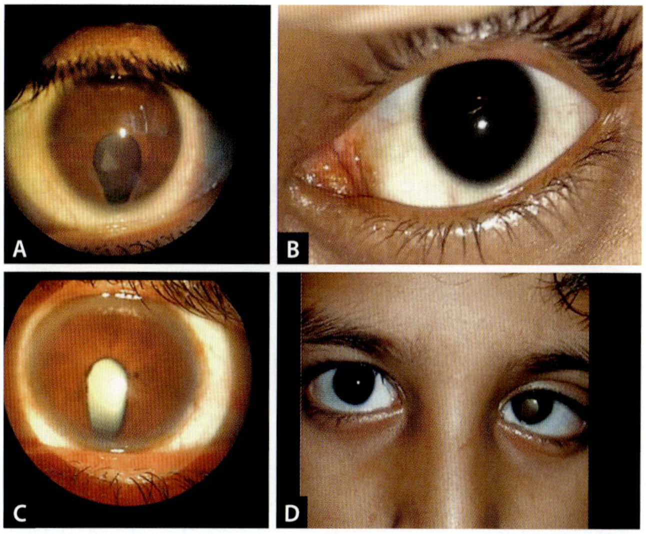

Figs. 3.41A to D: Coloboma of the iris. (A and B) A typical congenital iris colobomas; (C) Typical iris coloboma with congenital cataracts; (D) Bilateral congenial coloboma of the iris with retrolental white reflex.

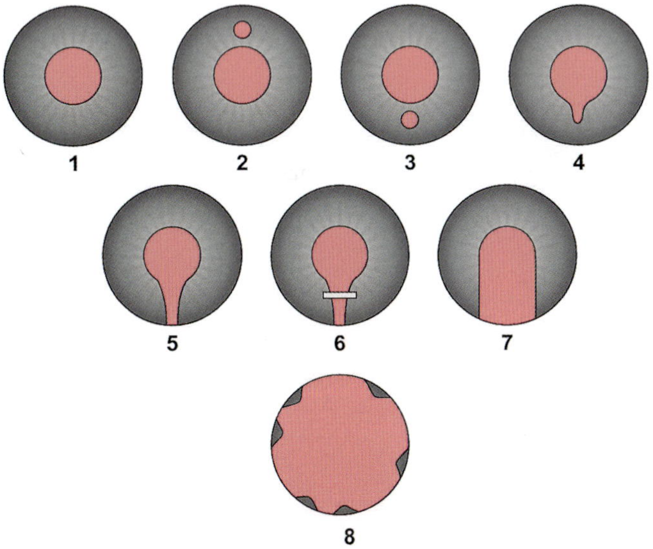

Fig. 3.40: Various types of congenital iris coloboma. (1) Iris without coloboma; (2) Atypical coloboma; (3) Partial typical coloboma; (4) Notch coloboma; (5) Key whole coloboma; (6) Bridge coloboma; (7) Hairpin coloboma; (8) Aniridia.

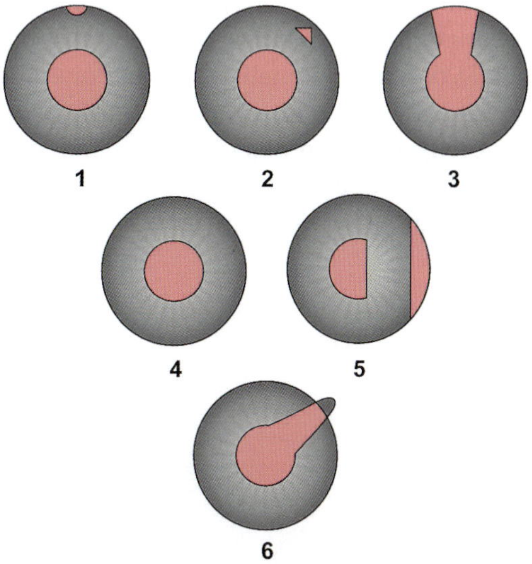

Fig. 3.42: Various types of acquired iris coloboma. (1) Peripheral basal iridectomy; (2) Button hole iridectomy; (3) Broad-based iridectomy; (4) Iridotomy; (5) Irido dialysis; (6) Iris prolapse at limbus.

notch coloboma at the pupillary margin, and an extensive area of nonfusion will result in a pan-uveal coloboma extending from the pupillary margin to the optic disc. As the fetal fissure is situated at the inferior aspect of the optic cup and stalk, it is natural that all congenital uveal colobomas develop at the lower aspect of the globe and are called typical coloboma. A typical congenital coloboma is extremely rare, with an unexplained mechanism of their production.

Coloboma of Ciliary Body

Isolated colobomas of the ciliary body are least frequent; ciliary colobomas are best visualized with an indirect ophthalmoscope and are delineated in ultrasonography and OCT. Ciliary body colobomas are associated with colobomas of the lens that may subluxate up; this happens due to the absence of zonules in the coloboma. The sclera over the ciliary coloboma looks like a translucent subconjunctival streak **(Fig. 3.43)**.

Coloboma of Choroid

Congenital colobomas of the choroid are the largest coloboma; they share the same etiology of faulty closure of the fetal fissure and are hence located at the 6 o'clock position. They are generally continuous with the coloboma of the iris and ciliary body; in rare instances, a choroidal coloboma may develop between the ciliary body and disc at 6 o'clock meridian without touching each other; such colobomas are generally vertically oval **(Fig. 3.44)**.

The congenital colobomas are generally bilateral; occasionally, they are too small and too peripheral, only to be seen by an indirect ophthalmoscope. Large colobomas give a white reflex on retinoscopy. The choroidal colobomas are parabolic in shape, with a rounded head toward the disc and an open, wide lower base toward the ciliary body. A large coloboma reaches up to the lower border of the disc, rarely including it. A still wider coloboma may reach up to the macula.

All choroidal colobomas are in fact retinochoroidal in nature. The retina is absent over the choroidal colobomas, the sclera is visible between the edges of the colobomas, and the edges of the colobomas are generally clear-cut or may be irregular with clumps of pigment similar to the edges of healed choroiditis, resembling miniature ora. The retinal vessels are not affected by coloboma; they travel across the floor of the coloboma without changing course. The floor of the coloboma is mildly depressed; it may be part of ectasia that may be large enough to become a cystic eyeball. The semblance of the edge of the large choroidal coloboma to the peripheral retina makes it vulnerable to rhegmatogenous retinal detachment and subretinal neovascularization. Large colobomas are associated with diminished vision; the colobomas produce corresponding negative scotomas.

Children with uveal coloboma have varied vision, ranging from normal to perception of light, depending on the position and extent of coloboma. Errors of refraction are common. Squints are frequent in unilateral cases. Amblyopia is common with large congenital colobomas.

> All the colobomas of the uvea, irrespective of the part of the uvea involved, have one common etiology, i.e., failure of the fetal fissure to close.

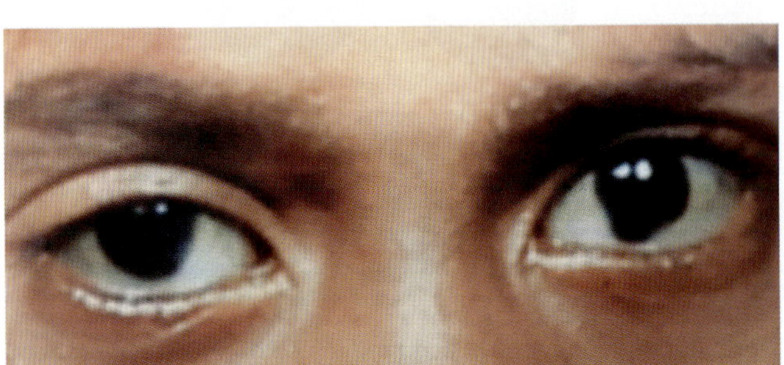

Fig. 3.43: Photograph showing bilateral iridociliary coloboma in microphthalmos.

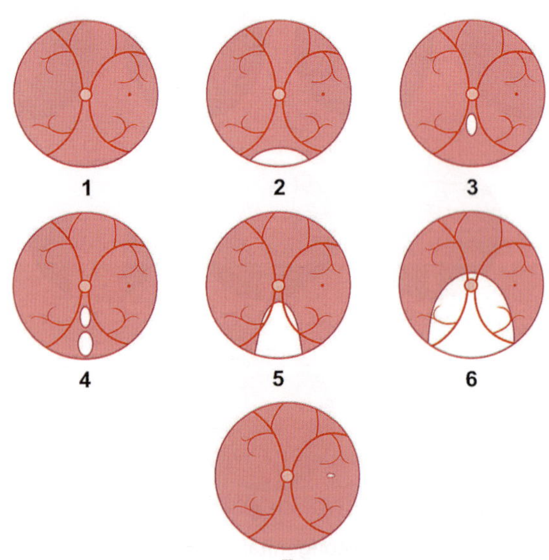

Fig. 3.44: Congenital coloboma of the choroid. (1) No coloboma; (2 to 6) Various types of choroidal coloboma; (3) Macular coloboma.

Flowchart 3.5 depicts various types of congenital coloboma of the eye.

Congenital Anomalies of the Pupil

The congenital anomalies of the pupil can be one of the following:

- *Size:*
    - Different: Anisocoria
    - Small: Microcoria
- *Number:*
    - Polycoria
    - Pseudocoria
- *Position:* Corectopia
- *Shape:* Dyscoria and coloboma of the iris

Anisocoria: The term denotes the different sizes of pupils in two eyes. Even under physiological conditions, the pupils are not equal in size and position; the difference is so small that it requires close scrutiny to find out the difference. A difference of 2 mm between the sizes of the pupils in two eyes is clinically considered to be anisocoria. One of the causes is congenital Horner's syndrome, which itself is rare; the unaffected side is smaller. This is in contrast to yet another rare cause, i.e., congenital third nerve palsy, where the pupil on the affected side is large. A birth injury may also cause anisocoria. The common acquired causes of anisocoria are unilateral instillations of miotic/mydriatic, head injury, or trauma to the iris.

Flowchart 3.5: Types of congenital coloboma.

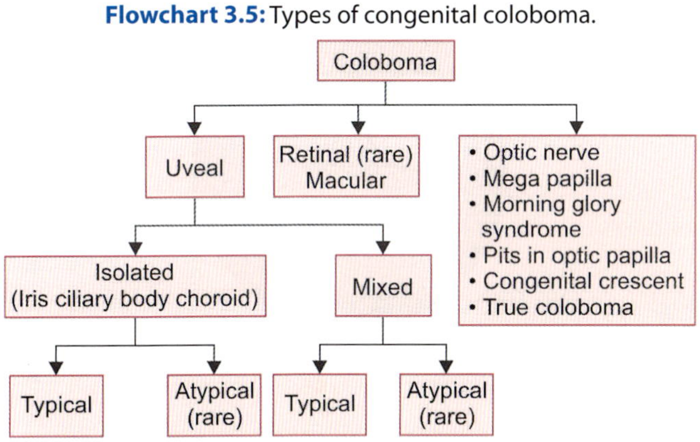

The various combinations can be **(Fig. 3.45):**

- One pupil is normal; the other is either dilated or constricted.
- One pupil is constricted, the other dilated.
- Both are constricted and unequal.
- Both are unequally dilated.

Anisocoria alone has no clinical significance and does not require any treatment.

> The pupil that dilated more in dim light is affected pupil.

Microcoria: The pupil of a newborn is smaller than the pupil after a few days. Both pupils of the newborn are of the same size and react to bright light. The condition is said to be microcoria if it remains <2 mm in size after a month. Such pupils seldom reach adult size and remain small throughout their lives. The most probable cause is the maldevelopment of the sphincters of the pupil. Microcoria have no clinical significance. It should be differentiated from the acquired cause of microcoria.

Polycoria: More than one pupil in an eye is called polycoria. It can be either a true polycoria that is rare or a pseudopolycoria. A true polycoria has its own pigmented margin and independent constrictors and dilators, each pupil reacting separately to light. The exact mode of their occurrence is not known **(Fig. 3.46)**.

Most probably, there is maldevelopment of smooth muscles.

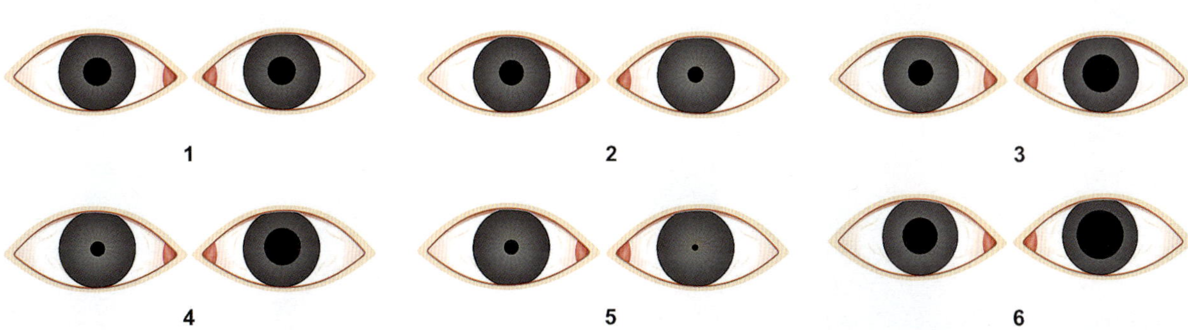

Fig. 3.45: Anisocoria of different grades. (1) Normal: Both pupils are of equal size; (2) The right pupil is normal, the left is constricted; (3) Right pupil normal, left dilated; (4) Right pupil constricted, left dilated; (5) Both pupils were constricted, left more than right; (6) Both pupils dilated, left more than right.

Pseudopolycoria: Pseudopolycoria is more common than true polycoria. It is always acquired, more likely to be unilateral, and more frequent than congenital. The main difference between the two is the presence of a sphincter in true polycoria. In eyes with pseudopolycoria, the pupil is not capable of reacting independently and lacks a dark pupillary border. The pupil in pseudopolycoria does not participate in pupillary constriction, but its borders show movement when the original one reacts. The congenital pseudopolycoria is supposed to be a modified iris coloboma; the congenital pseudopolycoria does not require any treatment unless it is associated with other anomalies of the iris.

Causes of pseudopolycoria (at all ages)

- Congenital
  - Simple
  - Associated with:
    - Mesodermal dysgenesis
    - Iridocorneal endothelial dysgenesis
- Trauma
  - Surgical
    - Iridectomy
    - Iridotomy
  - Accidental
    - Iridodialysis
    - Penetrating injury
- Postinflammatory
- Essential iris atrophy
- Iridoschisis

Corectopia (Ectopia pupillae): It is a congenital shift of a pupil from its usual position in the central iris. It is always single and is sometimes associated with ectopia lentis **(Fig. 3.47)**. The ectopic pupil acts like any physiological pupil, i.e., reacts to light and accommodation **(Fig. 3.48)**.

Dyscorea: This is a state of distorted pupil. The most common cause is coloboma of the iris; it may be a notch coloboma at the lower border of the pupil or a typical coloboma of the iris. A classical dyscoria is a pupil that has a shape different than a circle without a persistent pupillary membrane, or coloboma. It is shaped as a vertical spindle

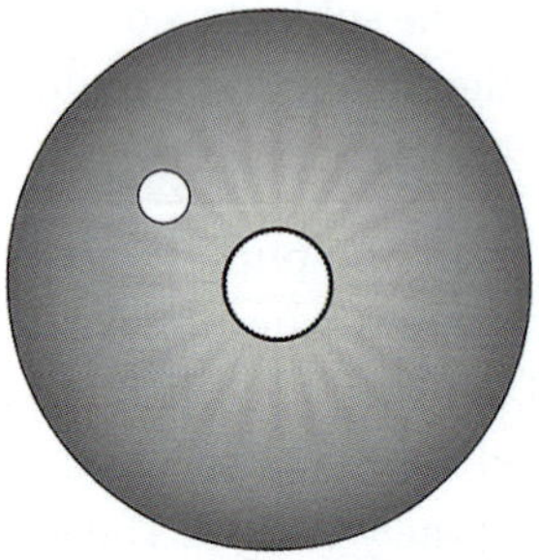

Fig. 3.46: Congenital true polycoria.

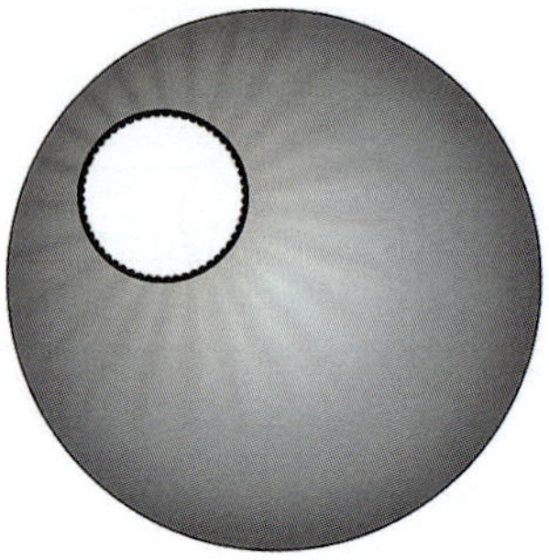

Fig. 3.47: Corectopia (ectopia pupillae).

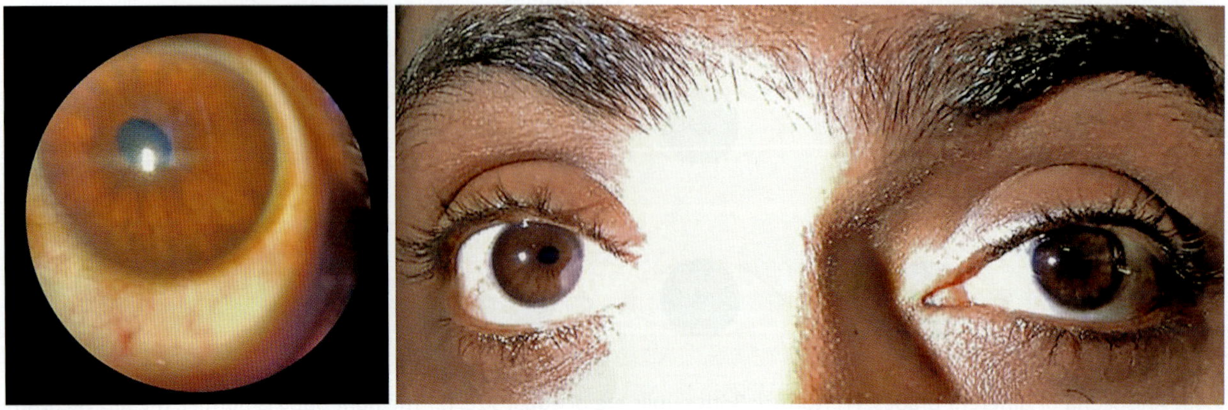

Fig. 3.48: Corectopia.
Courtesy: Dr Nupur Chakrawarty.

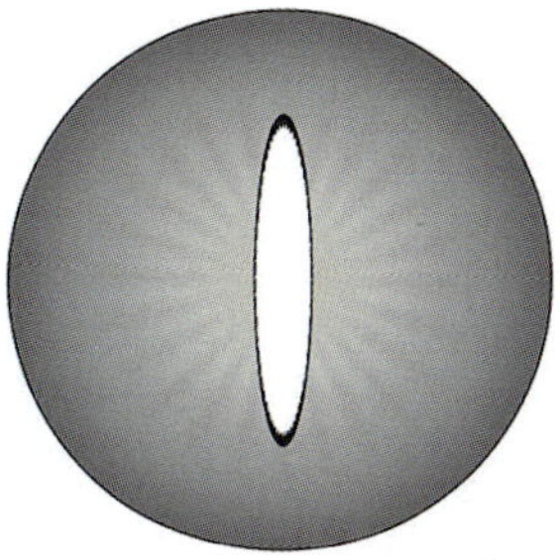

Fig. 3.49: Dyscoria in bright light.

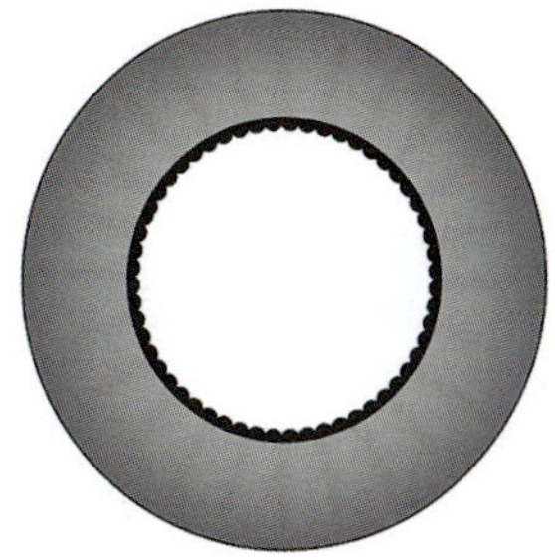

Fig. 3.50: Dyscoria in dim light.

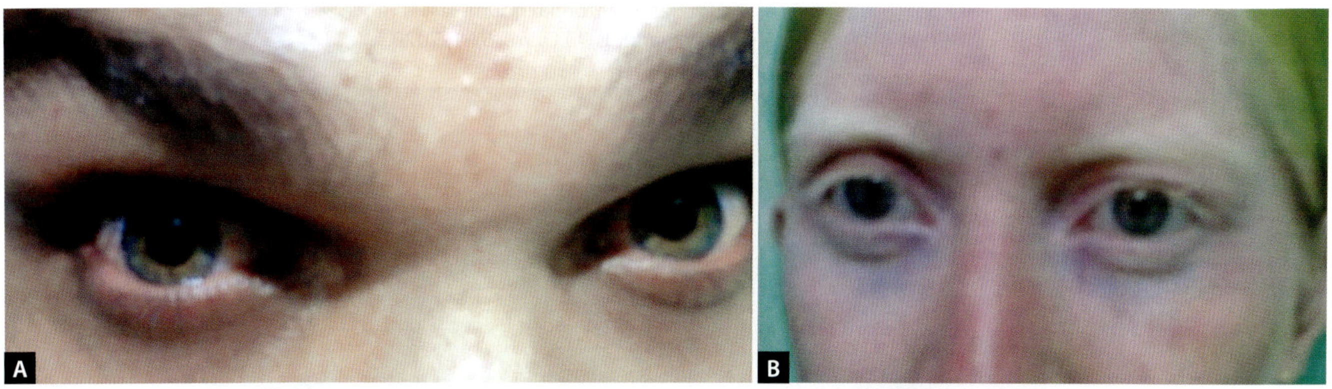

Figs. 3.51A and B: Isochromatic iris (A) in a normal boy and (B) in an albino.

in the presence of bright light that goes back to a circular shape as the light is removed; it is bilateral **(Figs. 3.49 and 3.50)**. The cause of the condition is not known. It has no clinical significance.

Pigmentary Anomalies of Uvea

Congenital pigmentary anomalies of the uvea are best seen in the iris. They are:

- Heterochromia
- Albinism

Heterochromia of the Iris

Heterochromia denotes a difference in color of the iris, either in one or both eyes. The color of the iris is a genetically determined factor. A uniformly light iris is not heterochromic; it may be called isochromia **(Figs. 3.51A and B)**.

Both iris are equally light colored; hence, they are not called heterochromic.

Heterochromia of iris can be: One eye has normal color; the other is either hypopigmented or hyperpigmented.

The two eyes have different colors.

One eye has a sectarian color difference.

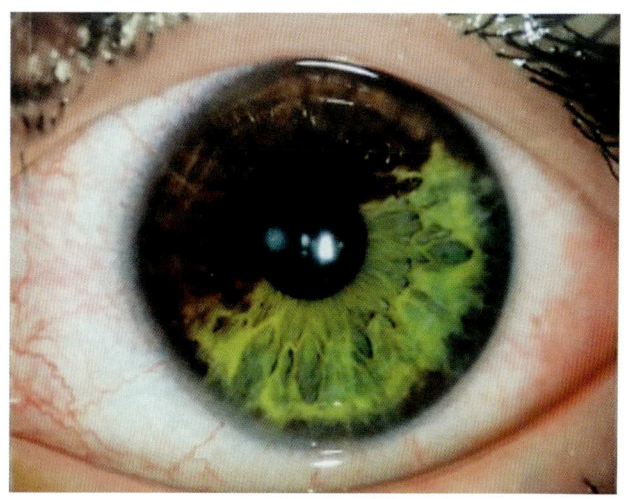

Fig. 3.52: Heterochromia iridis.

Courtesy: Shiva Sankar T, Honaver S (Eds). I.J.O. 2020; 68-3-2020.

This is called heterochromia iridis **(Fig. 3.52)**.

Eye with lighter colour is abnormal.

Heterochromia of iris: It has been noted earlier that the color of the iris is genetically determined; it can be dark or light colored, almost bordering blue. Normally, the colors

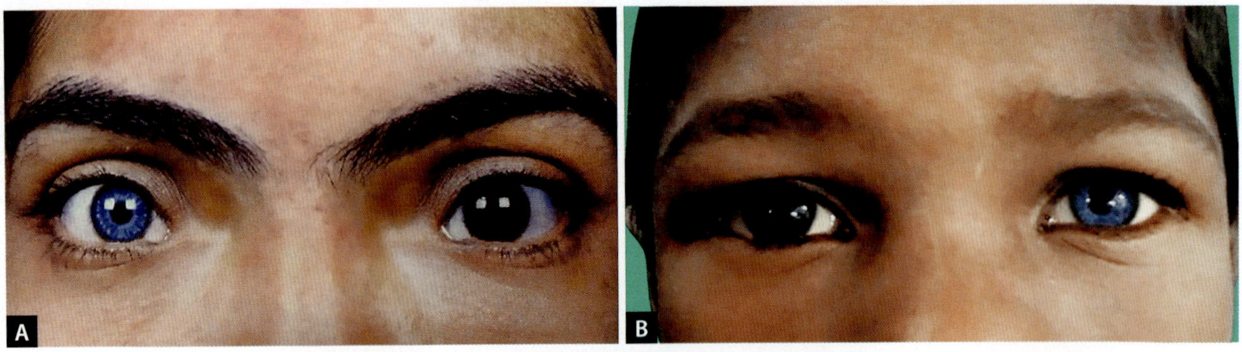

Figs. 3.53A and B: Heterochromia iridum.
Courtesy: Dr Santosh G Honavar (Eds) I.J.O. Vol. 67-1, 2020.

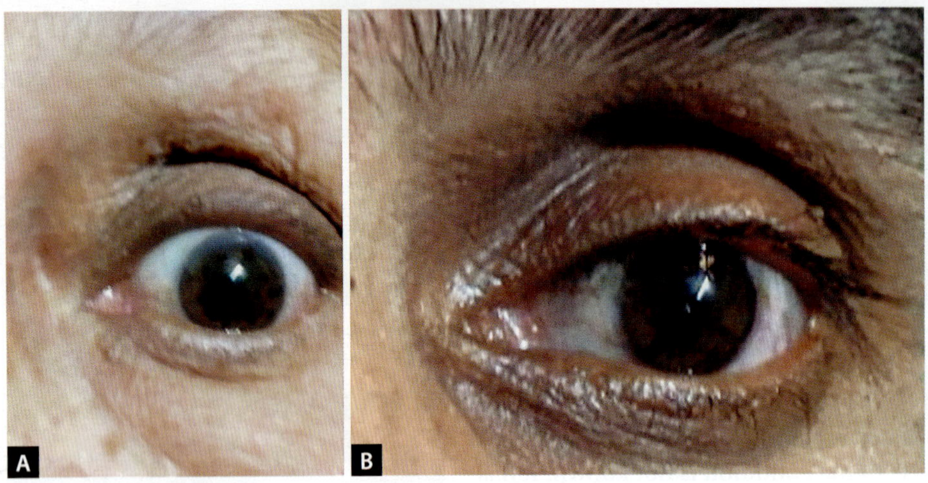

Figs. 3.54A and B: Iris freckle.

of the two eyes are the same. A deference in color, either between the two eyes or in one, could be heterochromia iris.

The differences can be as follows:

- One eye is of normal color; the other is of a different color. It could be heterochromia iridum **(Figs. 3.53A and B)**.

Congenital heterochromia of iris does not require any treatment.

Other causes of heterochromia of the iris at all ages

Heterochromia of the iris can be congenital or acquired. They are:

- Waardenburg syndrome*
- Trauma, accidental, or surgical
- Postinflammatory
- Iris freckle **(Figs. 3.54A and B)**
- Melanoma iris
- Ectropion of iris
- Drugs
- Fuchs' heterochromic iridocyclitis†
- Hemifacial atrophy
- Siderosis
- Chalcosis

Albinism (Achromasia)

Albinism is not a true congenital anomaly of the tissues of the body. It is a derangement of an enzyme tyrosine that is responsible for the manufacture of melanin, a pigment

Waardenburg syndrome is an infrequent congenital, genetic, multisystemic disorder including ocular involvement. The ocular signs include hypertelorism, synophrys (eyebrows joining in the midline), and heterochromia. Systemic manifestations are many; some prominent among them are light-colored skin and hair, white forelock, various degrees of hearing loss, and cleft lip.

†*Fuchs' heterochromic iridocyclitis* is a unilateral condition of low-grade anterior uveitis with heterochromia. The exact cause is not known; the condition predisposes to early age-related cataracts and glaucoma. There is no specific treatment; mild steroid drops may be sufficient; the patient should be under regular observation.

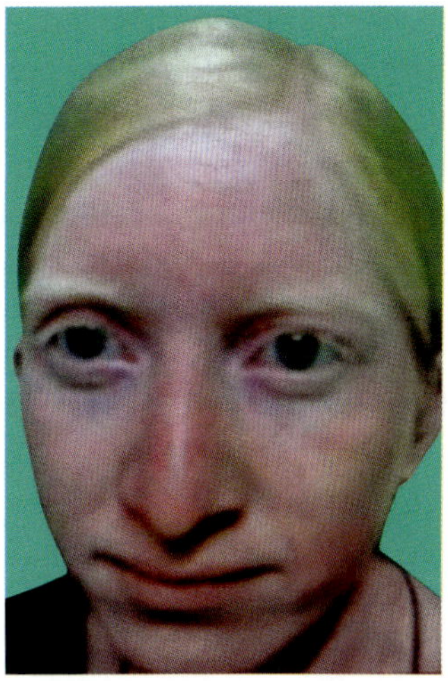

Fig. 3.55: Oculocutaneous albinism.

that imparts color to skin, hair, lashes, uvea, and retina. It is a genetically determined metabolic disorder present at birth due to the total or partial absence of melanin. In albinism, the enzyme tyrosinase is not converted to DOPA, the precursor of melanin.

Albinism has been classified variously, the most common used being oculocutaneous **(Fig. 3.55)**, cutaneous/ocular, and systemic.

Oculocutaneous Albinism

Out of the two forms, this condition is more common. It is easy to diagnose due to the obvious pale skin and hair, pink pupil, light-colored iris that is almost white, uncontrollable movement of the eyes, diminished vision, and glare. 80–90% of all albinos belong to this category. It is equally distributed among the two sexes in all races; in white races, the diagnosis may be missed due to a milder difference in natural skin color and albinotic paleness. In darker races, it is a curiosity that may turn into a social stigma. Oculocutaneous albinism is divided into two classes on the basis of biochemical tests. They are: Tyrosinase is positive (incomplete) and tyrosinase is negative (complete).

Tyrosine positive is the milder of the two, is autosomal recessive, and is considered to be an incomplete form. The other, called complete, shows maximum involvement of all pigmented tissues, with a complete absence of pigment in the eyes and skin. If both parents have oculocutaneous albinism, one positive and the other negative, their children will have normal eyes and skin, as the children are heterozygous for both types.

Ocular Albinism

This is the milder of the two, with only ocular involvement. The affected males have normal skin and hair; the carrier women may show no ocular involvement. The ocular structures involved are the uvea and retinal pigment epithelium. Involvement of the iris is first to draw attention; the pupil does not look pink as in the oculocutaneous variety. The pupil in oculocutaneous albinism is not really as red as it is considered to be; it is the reflected light that, in the absence of retinal and uveal pigment, looks red.

Some carriers have transillumination of the iris. The carriers have good vision; the retinal and choroidal vessels stand out against the pale background. Due to peripheral retinal lesions, the patients have poor scotopic vision. The albinotic fundus may show a hypoplastic macula. The eyes with a hypoplastic macula have marked nystagmus, squints, uncorrectable errors of refraction, and congenital color effects. The decussation of fibers at the chiasma is invariably faulty, leading to a corresponding field defect.

Achromatopsia

Achromatopsia is not a maldevelopment of the eyes. The eyes are structurally normal with subnormal vision and its sequel. It is a rare condition present at birth and is an autosomal recessive disorder. It is a state of complete absence of color sense; the fault lies in the cones resulting in gross subnormal vision and sensory nystagmus, which is a constant feature. The children do not have photophobia or glare, yet they like to keep their eyes closed for a long time, allowing the rods to be in a state of prolonged adaptation time, helping to have some peripheral vision. The fundus looks normal, and the diagnosis is confirmed by an electroretinogram. There is no specific treatment; all that is done is to salvage as much vision as possible by providing extradark glasses with the required power and suitable low vision correction.

Noncolobomatous Congenital Anomalies of UVEA

Three rare conditions that come under this category are:

1. Choroideremia
2. Choroidal sclerosis
3. Gyrate atrophy

The last is not found in children. The conditions are congenital in origin, manifesting in the second decade only to progress to near blindness. The first two cause diminished night vision that needs to be differentiated from two more common causes of night blindness, i.e., vitamin A deficiency and retinitis pigmentosa. Other symptoms common among them are loss of central vision and field of vision; both conditions are progressive. It may lead to a state of legal blindness.*

Choroideremia

The main symptom that brings the child for consultation is diminished night vision in the second decade. It is bilateral, progressive, X-linked, and far more severe among boys than in girls. In females, the condition is stationary. The females are carriers. The males become totally blind in about 10 years.

The fundus changes become obvious in puberty as salt-pepper fundus, degeneration of the retinal pigment epithelium, and progressive atrophy of the choroid leaving sclerosed vessels exposing the sclera. Initially,the disc and retina are normal, but ultimately they get atrophied. Electroretinogram shows changes in both rods and cones. The two conditions that need to be differentiated are xerophthalmia, which does not have fundus changes and shows dramatic improvement following administration of vitamin A in therapeutic doses, and the other condition is retinitis pigmentosa, which has a classical picture and does not respond to a large dose of vitamin A.

Choroidal Sclerosis

This condition is seen in two forms: Juvenile and adult. The first involves central vision, mostly starting around 15 years of age; it starts as a patch of central choroiditis. There is no night blindness in juvenile form. The second has a predominant peripheral defect, resulting in night blindness and a constricted field.

Gyrate Atrophy

This is a combined uveoretinal inherited dystrophy brought on by a defect in protein metabolism caused by a deficiency of the enzyme ornithine aminotransferase. There is progressive myopia and loss of peripheral vision developing in childhood. It is diagnosed by a typical fundus picture of circular patches of chorioretinal atrophy scattered all over the periphery. The circular patches join each other to form a ring all round the periphery, sparing the macula. The patches on the periphery are the cause of night blindness and peripheral constriction of field. There is no specific treatment; administration of vitamin B6 in large doses is claimed to be beneficial. This most probably acts on blood ornithine.

CONGENITAL ANOMALIES OF OPTIC NERVE

The two mechanisms responsible for congenital anomalies of the optic nerve head are faulty closure of embryonal fissures and faults in the absorption of arteries:

- Faulty closure of the embryonal fissure causes:
  - True coloboma
  - Megalopapilla
  - Morning glory syndrome
  - Congenital crescent
  - Congenital pit
- Fault in the absorption of hyaloid arteries causes Bergmeister papilla.
- Miscellaneous congenital anomalies of optic nerve are:
  - Opaque nerve fiber
  - Pseudoneuritis
  - Hypoplasia
  - Drusen of the optic nerve

Congenital anomalies of the optic nerve vary in appearance and clinical features; they may be as mild and benign as a speck of an opaque nerve fiber or tilled disc to as serious as the total absence of the disc. The anomaly may be localized to the nerve only or may be part of more extensive anomalies with changes in the uveoretinal complex. Congenital anomalies of the optic nerve are often associated with cranial or craniofacial anomalies. The symptoms may be influenced by its association with retinal disorders.

Isolated anomalies of the disc have diminished, uncorrectable vision, specific field changes, sluggish pupils [relative afferent pupillary defect (RAPD)], absent light reflex, and poor color vision. The symptoms may be associated with nonspecific symptoms and signs of an error of refraction, squint, amblyopia, or nystagmus.

**Legal blindness:* A person is considered legally blind if he/she has central visual acuity of 20/200 or worse in the better eye with best correction or if he/she has visual field restriction where the widest diameter is 20° or less in the better-seeing eye.

Most of the congenital anomalies of the optic nerve located in the disc are:

- Aplasia of the disc
- Hypoplasia of the disc
- Oblique, tilted disc (dysversion)
- Coloboma of the disc (pseudoglaucomatous disc)

- Pit of the disc.
- Opaque nerve fiber
- Pseudopapilledema (pseudoneuritis)
- Drusen of the optic nerve
- Morning glory syndrome
- Megalopapilla
- Congenital optic atrophy
- Bergmeister papilla
- Glial veil on disc
- Loop of blood vessels on the disc
- Pigment on the disc

Aplasia of the optic disc: This is the rarest and most severe form of congenital anomaly of the disc, where all the elements of the nerve, i.e., the nerve fibers, its covering, and blood vessels, are absent, as are the retinal elements. The posterior scleral foramen is bridged by the choroid. There is no vision; it is unilateral and may be associated with microphthalmos. The eyes show large esotropia, uveal coloboma, and hypoplasia of the iris and nystagmus.

Hypoplasia of the disc: This is one of the more common anomalies of the disc. With varied presentation, which may be uniocular or binocular, clinical presentation need not be the same in two eyes when bilateral. Incidences of unilateral cases are more common. The typical hypoplastic disc is generally small; the small size is attributed to the smaller number of axons in the nerve. The color of the disc ranges from normal pink to pale. The border is not sharp. It is surrounded by a hypopigmented ring. The vessels arise from the center of the disc and branch in a normal fashion. The condition may be associated with other anomalies, like aniridia and hypoplasia of the fovea. Gross reduction of vision is the rule; paradoxically, some eyes have near-normal vision with poor color sense. The small disc is reflected as a small blind spot. Nerve fiber defects may be present. The child is generally brought for consultation due to diminished vision, squints, or nystagmus; the eyes are often hypermetropic. There is no specific treatment. Vision, whenever present, should be corrected to the best level.

Dysversion of the disc (congenital crescent, Fuchs' coloboma): The anomaly is frequent and may go unnoticed if unilateral with fairly good vision. It is found in 3% of eyes, out of which 80% are bilateral. The crescent may be the only anomaly present or be associated with anomalies of the skull and face like Crouzon syndrome, Apert syndrome, hypertelorism, and other craniofacial dysostoses. The eye may squint. The cause of diminished vision is generally an error of refraction, which is frequently myopic astigmatism. The disc is vertically oval, with a crescent at the lower part and blurring at the upper pole of the disc, which may be mistaken for the beginning of papilledema. A combination of crescent and blurring results in field changes that may be confused with chiasmal lesions. The differentiating point is that a chiasmal lesion respects the midline, which the ocular lesions lack.

Congenital coloboma of the disc: Isolated coloboma of the disc is far less common than uveoretinal although all of them share a common etiology, i.e., incomplete closure of the embryonic fissure. That is why optic nerve colobomas are frequently associated with retinouveal coloboma. The coloboma of the optic nerve is often associated with multiple systemic disorders, like trisomy. It often exists with retrobulbar cysts and peripapillary scleral staphyloma. It is bilateral in 60% of cases and frequently hereditary. Occasionally, a band of uveal tissue bridges the coloboma, dividing the coloboma into two parts and giving the impression of two discs. The posterior scleral foramen is enlarged with normal blood vessels; the color of the disc, not involved in coloboma, is pale and may be mistaken for glaucomatous.

Symptoms depend on the extent of coloboma and associated local and systemic conditions. The most common symptom is diminished vision, which may range between just perception of light and loss of only a few lines on the Snellen chart, along with the usual conditions of amblyopia, squint, and nystagmus.

Morning glory syndrome: This is a rare unilateral congenital anomaly of the disc, thought to be a variant of congenital coloboma of the disc. The posterior scleral foramen may be enlarged with enlarged papilla and cup; the disc tissue outside the cup has the appearance of a pale rim from which the retinal vessels sprout instead of arising from the center. The blood vessels radiate from the rim in a cartwheel fashion. The rim is elevated than the rest of the surrounding retina. The excavation sometimes contains remnants of hyaloid blood vessels; the rim is surrounded by a ring of uveoretinal tissue. The condition is prone to rhegmatogenous retinal detachment in later life; a lesion may be large enough to cause a white reflex in the pupillary area.

> *Disc changes that may present as white reflexes in the pupillary area:*
> - Large, opaque fiber
> - Large chorioretinal coloboma
> - Morning glory syndrome
> - Coloboma of the optic nerve
> - Persistent hyperplastic primary vitreous

Congenital pit of the optic nerve head: This condition was thought to be rare, as most of them were diagnosed with central serous chorioretinopathy, which was in fact a sequel to the condition and not vice versa. The condition is mostly unilateral; when bilateral, one eye is more affected, the disc with the disorder is larger, equal among boys and girls, and sporadic. It has been reported in siblings.

The condition is present at birth without symptoms and becomes symptomatic by the second or third decade. The exact cause is not known, but the common assumptions are that it is a variant of atypical coloboma of the uvea or retina. The second theory is that it is backward herniation of neuroectodermal tissue during the closure of a fetal fissure through the lamina.

It may be asymptomatic throughout life and/or discovered on routine fundus examinations and passed as a large, nonglaucomatous disc of no significance. The patient seeks ophthalmic consultation in the late third decade for uncorrectable central vision and metamorphopsia. On examination, the disc may look slightly enlarged, with a bluish depression on the floor of the lamina that is more prominent than normal. The depressions vary in number from single to four or five, mostly on the temporal half; the size varies between one tenth of the disc and half of the disc. The depth of the pit ranges between ½ and 5D. The disc vessels not only traverse over the pit; they may dip in larger pits. Most of the pits are gray; they may be yellow or even olive green, or black.

The loss of central vision and distortion of vision are explained by the presence of accumulation of sub- or inter-retinal fluid. The nature of the fluid is debatable, i.e., vitreous or cerebrospinal fluid (CSF); accumulation of fluid is called optic disc pit maculopathy, and it has the shape of a pear with its narrow end toward the disc. The maculopathy is best visualized and assessed by indirect ophthalmoscope, +90D, and OCT. Most of the eyes turn out to be hypermetropic.

A differential diagnosis consists of the following:

- Small coloboma of the disc
- Berlins edema
- Central serous retinopathy
- Cystoids cause macular edema
- Subretinal neovascularization

There is no specific treatment. Various modes of management, like vitrectomy, laser, and gas tamponade, have been tried without much help.

Megalopapilla

These are rare cases of unusually large congenital discs, without any symptom or complication. The exact cause of the anomaly is obscure and may be a variant of the morning glory symptom. The cup is proportionately large, giving the false impression of a glaucomatous disc.

Myelinated Nerve Fiber (Medullated Nerve Fiber, Opaque Nerve Fiber)

Myelination of the optic nerve is not an uncommon fundus finding; it is innocuous and symptomless. Hence, neither the child nor the parents are aware of its existence. It is discovered on routine fundus examinations. It is worth noting that all nerves in the body are myelinated; the myelin protects and insulates the nerves and helps in the conduction of impulses. Loss of myelin in any nerve causes a conduction defect, which applies to the optic nerve as well.

Myelination of the optic nerve starts at the lateral geniculate of the body and travels down toward the disc, only to stop at the lamina by the seventh month of gestation, leaving the disc nonmyelinated. If the process of myelination overshoots its limit, it progresses forward to spill over the retina in a specific pattern. Normal retinal fibers are nonmyelinated; hence, they are not visible under white light. Once they get myelinated, they become visible as white, fluffy patches.

The opaque nerve fibers start at the edge of the disc, is flame shaped with apex away from the disc. The medullated fibers are visible at birth or may take a few weeks to be visible. Generally, there is a single patch in the supratemporal quadrant of the disc; in rare instances, the process can encircle the whole periphery. The patches grow along the course of the retinal vessels; they are white in color with a crenated border which is fluffy in texture. The vessels are obscured by the myelination or may dip in the substance, only to emerge at some distance. The patch may be as small as a speck or large enough to reach as far as the retinal periphery; rarely does a patch touch the disc margin and develop away from it as an isolated island, and it is mistaken for a large patch of exudate.

The myelinated nerve fibers do not produce a visual defect; they cause a field defect as negative scotomas corresponding to the patch, the most common being an irregular enlargement of the blind spot. The condition is benign, not warranting treatment. Small patches are known to fade without treatment. Large patches may produce a white reflex on retinoscopy.

Pseudoneuritis (Pseudopapilledema)

It is a common, symptomless, nonprogressive, bilateral congenital anomaly of the optic disc that may be misdiagnosed as early optic disc swelling, exposing the child to a battery of unnecessary, costly investigations.

The condition may be considered to be the reverse of the coloboma of the disc, where the posterior scleral foramen is too large for the normally present number of nerve fibers in the disc; in contrast to this, the posterior scleral foramen is too small to accommodate the normal number of nerve fibers in pseudoneuritis. The fibers heap up and spill out, giving the appearance of swollen papillas. That may be confused with either neuritis or early papilledema. The condition being none of the two, the first is an inflammatory process and the latter gives to a rise in intracranial pressure, while pseudoneuritis is a congenital anomaly of the posterior scleral foramen with normal intracranial pressure and noninflammatory. The condition is revealed during routine fundus examinations. The first question to be put to the child is about his vision; a normal vision excludes neuritis in the vast majority of cases. The absence of neurological deficiencies excludes papilledema.

The eye is generally hypermetropic of moderate power and may have astigmatism; the media is clear without cells in front of the disc. The disc is smaller than normal with a smudged border; the cup is absent, without peripapillary edema and splinter hemorrhage or exudate. The swelling is less than 3D; the color of the disc is mildly hyperemic. The vessels are of normal caliber and tortuosity; the retina does not have exudates or hemorrhages. The central and peripheral fields are normal, color sense is not changed, and the retina has shot silk appearance. Differential diagnosis consists of early papilledema, optic neuritis, drusen of the disc, small opaque nerve fibers, glial proliferation, and glial vessels on the disc. The condition does not require any specific treatment.

Drusen of Optic Disc

Drusen of the optic disc is a benign, nonvision-threatening, nonfatal condition that masquerades as two serious conditions, i.e., optic neuritis and papilledema, exposing the child to unnecessarily costly investigations. Though the condition may be obvious at birth, it is not considered to be a true congenital malady. When it is not detected at birth, it will not be diagnosed in the next 8–10 years. The drusen is invariably bilateral but not always symmetric; when unilateral on first examination, there is a good percentage of children who will get the other eye involved in the next one decade. It has a strong predisposition to positive family history, so much so that it is mandatory to examine the fundus of both parents. A large percentage of at least one may be found to harbor unrecognized drusen. The siblings too may share the same malady; it is an autosomal dominant trait. The presence of drusen in any of the family members almost excludes the possibility of papilledema in a suspected child.

Drusen is not a tumor. It is the accumulation of a proteinaceous, calcified material of unknown origin along with immature neuroglia in the substance of the nerve. It does not get vascularized. It starts in the substance of the nerve away from the lamina, gradually shifting toward the lamina. The growth is not visible on ophthalmoscopy unless it reaches the lamina; when it does, it becomes an oval growth of variable sizes ranging between 1 mm × 4 mm in diameter and half of this in depth. The drusen, due to its high calcium content, is well delineated on X-rays. It is also visible on ultrasonography in both A and B modes, OCT, and fundus fluorescein angiography (FFA). On FFA, drusen gives autofluorescence and OCT can be supplemented with FFA.

As the drusen reaches the lamina, it pushes the lamina forward, obliterating the cup and initiating a state resembling a swollen disc, along with anomalous blood vessels without peripapillary or parapapillary hemorrhage or exudate.

The drusen is symptomless and noticed on routine fundus examinations; the presence of a swollen disc rings concern for the physician, who, out of apprehension, orders a battery of investigations, all of which turn out to be negative. This impasse could be avoided if the fundi of parents are scrutinized. If any of them reveal

TABLE 3.4: Difference between drusen, papilledema, and papillitis.

Drusen	*Papilledema*	*Papillite*
Developmental	Acquired	Acquired
Not related to intracranial pressure	Solely dependent on intracranial pressure	There is no relation to raised intracranial pressure
Not related to the closure of cranial sutures.	Does not develop till the cranial sutures are open	Not related to the closure of cranial sutures
Present at birth but may manifest in the second decade	Acquired	Acquired
Bilateral	Bilateral	Generally unilateral
Strong family history	There is no family history	There is no family history
Vision is not effected	Vision not effected	Vision reduced
Nonsystemic	Prominent systemic features	There are no systemic features
Initially minimal disc edema	Variable disc edema	Mild disc edema
Gray-colored disc	Hyperemic disc	Hyperemic disc
Variable disc change	Enlarged blind spot	Field normal or may show nerve fiber defect

drusen, no further investigation is required. The only positive finding may be a slight loss of peripheral field on the auto perimeter. In adults, the disc that has drusen since childhood becomes gray. A long-standing drusen in an adult may protrude in the vitreous like a small mulberry; drusen in children does not show a tendency to bleeding. The adult may suffer not only bleeding but also choroidal neovascularization. **Table 3.4** shows difference among the above three conditions.

Differential diagnosis: The differential diagnosis consists of many disorders; common among them are pseudoneuritis, optic neuritis, impending papilledema, hypoplasia of the disc, glial proliferation, and Bergmeister papilla.

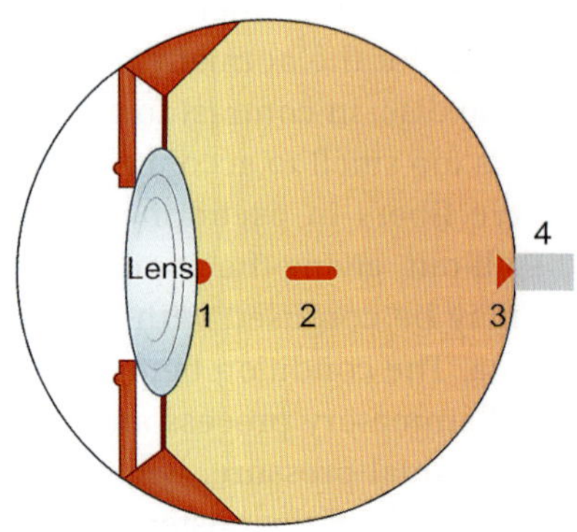

Fig. 3.56: Various congenital anomalies of the hyaloid artery. (1) Mittendorf's dot; (2) Piece of hyaloid artery in the vitreous; (3) Bergmeister papilla; (4) Optic nerve.

Glial Proliferation (Glial Veil)

These are rare, asymptomatic, nonprogressive anomalies of the hyaloid vasculature on the disc. They are considered to be milder form of Bergmeister papilla, discovered on routine fundus examinations. The veil differs from Bergmeister papilla in appearance. The glial proliferations are membranous, covering the surface of the disc, or may be localized on the temporal disc. The Bergmeister papillas protrude in the vitreous **(Fig. 3.56)** which shows various types of congenital anomalies of hyaloid vessels.

Bergmeister Papilla

Bergmeister papilla is not an anomaly of the optic disc; it is a failure of the hyaloid vessels to regress by the time of birth. The natural history of regression of the hyaloid artery is as follows.

During the early weeks of the development of the eye, the hyaloid artery runs through the middle of the developing vitreous between the disc and the posterior surface of the lens and forms the posterior part of the tunica vasculosa lentis that supplies blood to the developing lens. As the lens grows, its nutrition is taken over by aqueous, replacing the hyaloid system. The hyaloid artery atrophies and regresses; the regression starts from the lenticular end and should completely disappear at birth, leaving a potential canal in its place. The potential tract is not visible by any optical device and is called the Cloquet canal. During its regression, bits of the hyaloid artery may be left unabsorbed in pieces in three forms—a small bit attached to the posterior pole of the lens, called Mittendorf's dot; a piece left in the colloquist canal in the mid-vesicles; and a piece attached to the optic disc, called the Bergmeister papilla. The remnants are symptomless and were discovered on retinoscopy and ophthalmoscopy, requiring no treatment.

CONGENITAL ANOMALIES OF MACULA

Dysplasia

Dysplasia of the macula is rare, commonly associated with other congenital anomalies, i.e., microphthalmos, medullated nerve fiber, aniridia, and coloboma of the disc. Unilateral myopia is a common feature with dysplasia of macula.

Hypoplasia

Hypoplasia of the macula is also rare; it is probably a milder form of aplasia of the macula. In this case, the macula stops differentiating at a particular stage of growth, between the sixth and eighth weeks of gestation.

Coloboma

Coloboma of the macula differs from the coloboma of the uvea and retina in the sense that the uveoretinal colobomas are due to the failure of the closure of the embryonic fissure. Macular coloboma lacks such a simple explanation; the cause of macular coloboma is not clear to the extent that there is a school that thinks that these are in fact secondary to effect of intrauterine infection and have blamed toxoplasma as the most probable cause. Others consider them to be atypical colobomas. To understand the etiology of congenital anomalies of macula, it is better to recapitulate physiology and natural history of the development of macula. Macula is packed with cones with exceptionally few rods; hence, it is associated with photopic central vision, color vision, and contrast sensitivity. It has no role in scotopic vision.

The development of the macula differs from the rest of the retina in various ways due to some inherent differences. From the rest of the retina, the differences are as follows:

- Until 3 months of gestation, the growth of the macula does not differ from the rest of the retina.
- Between 3 and 8 months, there is a period of retardation in differentiation.
- After 8 months, the differentiation picks up and continues till birth.
- The central area continues to grow up to the fourth month after birth.
- The macula gets its blood supply from the choriocapillaries.
- The retinal vessels do not transverse into the avascular zone of the macula.
- The factors responsible for congenital anomalies can be activated during any stage of development.
- The embryogenesis of macular colobomas is independent of the closure of the fetal fissure.
- The coloboma of the macula may be considered an atypical coloboma of the fundus.

The macular colobomas are genetic and can be either autosomal dominant or recessive, bilateral and not always symmetric, with profound loss of vision, nystagmus, and squint. They are a common cause of esotropia in children. When children with coloboma of macula grow, they are found to be severe color deficient. Clinically, there are two types of macular coloboma, i.e., pigmented and nonpigmented. The first consists of a mass of pigment on the macular area, through which the retinal vessels traverse; the underlying choroidal vessels are visible. The bare sclera shines through. The sclera does not show any excavation. In the other type, there is no heaping of pigment; the vessels stop at the border of the patch. The sclera underneath is bare and excavated.

The size of the coloboma varies; it may occasionally be as large as the disc, and its shape varies from a circular to a horizontal ellipse. In congenital macular coloboma, the borders are irregular with clumps of pigment, are nonprogressive, and are visible with a direct ophthalmoscope **(Fig. 3.57)**.

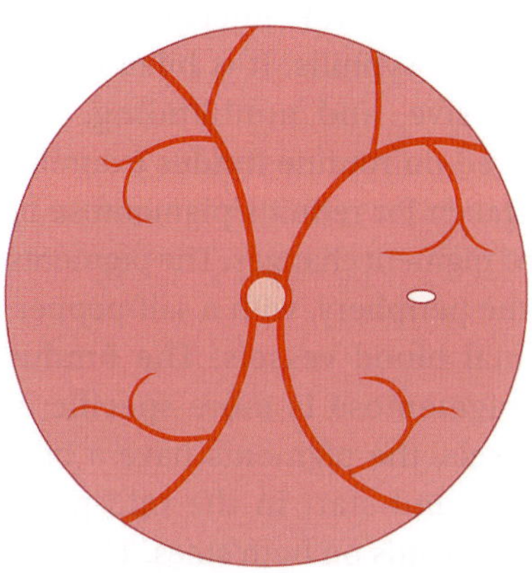

Fig. 3.57: A macular coloboma.

A large macular coloboma may give a white reflex on retinoscopy. There is no treatment. The child may be brought up with a visual handicap.

CONGENITAL ANOMALIES OF RETINA

Earlier, it was noted that the retina develops from both the layers of the optic cup and lies in proximity to the choroid, optic nerve, and vitreous. From the outer layer develops the layer of retinal pigment epithelium. The remaining layers, i.e., the nuclear, plexiform, and ganglion cells that constitute the neural component of the retina, develop from the inner layer; hence, congenital anomalies can be precipitated by maldevelopment of any or both layers to which can be added the choroid, blood vessels, vitreous, and optic nerves in various combinations. The clinical picture depends on the position, extent, and involvement of nonretinal tissues. The anomalies can be central or peripheral, and unilateral or bilateral, and they are equally distributed among boys and girls. Some of the anomalies are obvious at birth, while others are found later on routine examination.

The anomalies have been categorized in various ways:

1. Origin: Outer wall or inner wall
2. Position: Central/peripheral
3. Simple/composite
4. Ophthalmoscopic appearance
5. Tissues involved

The most effective would be a combination of 3 and 5 from the above list.

The following are some of congenital anomalies of retina:

- *Congenital embryonic pigmentary retinopathy (CEPR):* It is not an anatomical maldevelopment. It is an after-effect of an intrauterine infection, mostly by rubella, influenza, and syphilis. It is bilateral, symptomless, nonprogressive, and nonblinding. The condition is discovered on routine fundus examinations and is often mistaken for retinitis pigmentosa because of its associated pigment changes. The pigments of CEPR are seen on the periphery, with a salt-pepper appearance and normal blood vessels. The fundus picture in retinitis pigmentosa is more specific; with narrow blood vessels, the pigments have a bone corpuscle appearance and start in the mid-periphery like a band that expands on both sides. The most important symptom is relentless night blindness.
- *Congenital retinal dysplasia:* It is a bilateral non-progressive disease caused following viral infection. Some drugs if consumed during pregnancy may cause congenital retinal dysplasia, and even vitamin A deficiency in the mother too has been blamed for the defect. It can be genetic as well. The common features of the conditions are retinal folds and formation of rosettes.
- *Congenital retinal fold:* This is yet another congenital disorder that causes a white reflex in the pupil. It is due to the proliferation of neural tissue in the optic vesicle that may be an isolated disorder or associated with persistent primary hyperplastic vitreous. Occasionally, the bands may extend from ciliary processes to the disc.
- *Congenital rosette formation:* There are two forms, i.e., a common variety seen in microphthalmic eyes and a less frequent variety in nonmicrophthalmic eyes. This occurs when the growth of neural elements exceeds normal limits. They are also often mistaken for retinoblastoma even on histopathological examination due to their striking resemblance to rosettes of retinoblastoma. There are clumps of tissue buried in the retina or protruding in the vitreous.
- *Congenital gliosis:* This is a rare disorder that is often mistaken for retinoblastoma due to excessive glial proliferation.
- *Congenital retinal detachment:* This condition too gives a white pupillary glow, generally seen in the microphthalmic eye, secondary to the unequal growth of two layers of the optic cup.
- *Congenital retinoschisis:* Retinoschisis is split in the sensory retina at the level of the outer plexiform layer. The condition runs in families, is present at birth, and is diagnosed only when the child presents with uncorrectable diminished vision and is initially mistaken for retinal detachment.

CONGENITAL ANOMALIES OF VITREOUS

The most common congenital anomaly is persistent primary vitreous.

Persistent hyperplastic primary vitreous is one of the important congenital anomalies of the eyes that masquerade as one of the fatal ocular pediatric conditions, i.e., retinoblastoma. To understand its genesis, it is better to go through the development of the vitreous again.

The development of the vitreous is a complex process that involves both the ectoderm and the mesoderm. Initially, it was thought that the development of the vitreous was solely ectodermal; then the theory of mesodermal origin was put forward. Later, it was realized that the vitreous has a dual origin consisting of the ectoderm and mesoderm. The former consists both types of ectoderm, i.e., surface and neuroectoderm that participate in the development of the vitreous. The vitreous develops in three stages: Primary, secondary, and tertiary. The first two are involved in the development of the vitreous. The last is not really part of the vitreous; it is in fact a lenticular zonule. The primary vitreous is the initial stage that is ultimately replaced by the secondary vitreous.

The primary vitreous has multiple sources of origin:

- Mesenchymal cells and fibroblasts from the rim of the optic cup
- Mesenchymal cells from the hyaloid vasculature
- Cells from the embryonic lens
- Cells from the inner layer of the optic cup

Initially, it is the primary vitreous that fills the retrolental space from the posterior lens capsule to the optic disc. The primary vitreous gradually atrophies to be replaced by the secondary vitreous, which is clinically known as the vitreous gel, after birth. After the primary vitreous disappears, all that is left of it is the Cloquet canal, which has no clinical significance. The secondary vitreous starts developing in the second month of gestation and is fully developed at birth; it consists of vitreous gel and hyalocytes. The two important functions of the vitreous are optical and mechanical, by which it keeps the retina snug with the choroid. The vitreous is prone to proliferation, which causes the formation of bands.

Persistent hyperplastic primary vitreous is seen in full-term neonates, generally unilateral, without any systemic involvement. The pathogenesis of PHPV is the nonregression of the primary vitreous and its conversion into a proliferative mass. Clinically, PHPV is divided into two types, i.e., the more common anterior and less common posterior types.

Anterior persistent hyperplastic primary vitreous: This condition is seen in the microphthalmic eye of a newborn. In 90% of cases, it is unilateral. The cause of microphthalmos is not well understood, i.e., is it the cause or effect of the anomaly? The common hypothesis is that the absorption of primary vitreous acts as an impetus for further development of the eye; if that does not happen, the growth of the eye stops. The microphthalmos may be severe enough to be detected by the mother or may be so minimal that it requires a close look to detect it. In a full-blown case of PHPV, the eye is smaller in all dimensions with features of a microphthalmic eye, i.e., a small cornea, a shallow AC small pupil with or without an iris coloboma, the iris stroma is vascularized, the vessels may cross the pupil or may course over the lens, with marked retrolental features, better seen following mydriasis. The findings are as follows: The ciliary processes are elongated enough to be seen behind the lens. The ciliary processes are found to be anchored to the white mass that is proliferating in the primary vitreous. As the proliferating primary vitreous contracts, it pulls the ciliary process centrally. There are two things that happen due to the pull: The first is rent in the posterior lens capsule, with aqueous seeping in the cortex, causing the lens to swell; pushing the iris forward, obliterating angle, causing secondary glaucoma. This has a paradoxical effect on the size of the eye. An eye that was microphthalmic is converted to a buphthalmic eye; recurrent hemorrhage and posterior synechiae make the glaucoma worse. The eye that was blind without pain becomes a painful blind eye. The other effect of the pull on the proliferating band is traction retinal detachment, which enhances the white reflex in the pupillary area.

Natural history of persistent hyperplastic primary vitreous: Microphthalmos → Primary hyperplastic vitreous → Proliferation → Retrobulbar white mass → Elongation of ciliary process → Rent in posterior lens capsules → Cataract → Swollen lens → Secondary angle closure glaucoma → Buphthalmos → Blindness

The other situation that worsens the condition is tractional retinal detachment.

Posterior persistent hyperplastic primary vitreous: The condition is less frequent than its anterior counterpart; it is also unilateral and seen in full-term neonates. The difference between the two lies in their location. The posterior variety is placed deep in the vitreous near the disc, either as an opaque, dense membrane or as a nonopaque retinal fold that extends toward either the periphery or the posterior surface of the lens, the first situation causing traction detachment and the second, complicated cataract. The opaque membrane can cause a white reflex in the pupillary area. Some authors think that it is a variant of morning glory syndrome.

Flowchart 3.6: Development of the ocular vasculature.

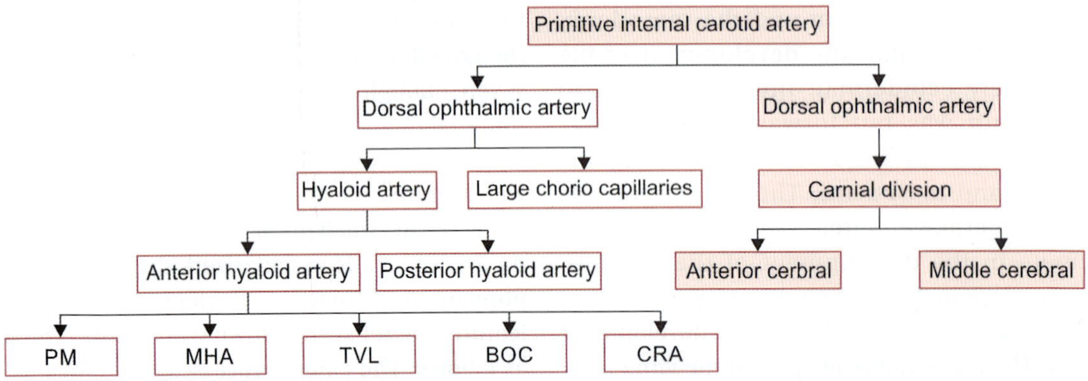

(BOC: branch to optic cup; CRA: central retinal artery; MHA: main hyaloid artery; PM: pupillary membrane; TVL: tunica vasculosa lentis)

The congenital anomalies of the retina can be divided into two broad groups that are retinouveal and vascular. To understand congenital vascular anomalies of retina, it is better to recapitulate the embryogenesis of blood supply of retina which comes from the internal carotid system while the adnexa is mainly supplied by the external carotid system.

The intraocular vasculature is divided into:

- Hyaloid system
- Retinal system
- Uveal system

Fully developed vitreous and lens are avascular; during embryogenesis, they are dependent on vessels developing from the internal carotid, such as the hyaloid artery, and the tunica vasculosa lentis, which is one of the terminal branches of the hyaloid artery. The tunica vasculosa lentis and hyaloid systems disappear before birth.

DEVELOPMENT OF HYALOID SYSTEM OF BLOOD VESSELS

In short, the development of the hyaloid system of blood vessels is as follows: Primitive dorsal and ventral ophthalmic arteries branch from the developing internal carotid artery; they are the main source of blood supply to the eye and its adnexa. The hyaloid system develops from this complex. The developing hyaloid artery, after sprouting from the dorsal ophthalmic artery, gets into the eye through the fetal fissure in the cephalic end to take up a central position in the substance of the developing optic nerve when the fetal fissure closes. A part of the hyaloid artery growing in the optic nerve becomes the central retinal artery, and the remaining part continues to form the posterior part of the tunica vasculosa lentis. The developing hyaloid artery is the main source of blood supply to the retina until the hyaloid artery regresses. Regression of the hyaloid artery acts as a stimulus for retinal angiogenesis.

Flowchart 3.6 partially outlines the development of the ocular vasculature.

DEVELOPMENT OF RETINOUVEAL VASCULATURE

The fully developed retina has two sources of blood supply: Retinal and choriocapillaries, which have independent embryogenesis with a common origin from primitive internal carotid arteries. The choroid supplies the outer retina and the inner layers, depending on the retinal vasculature. The developing retina is avascular until 4 months of gestation; at this stage, the hyaloid artery, a branch of the dorsal ophthalmic artery, reaches the embryonic fissure. In the embryonic fissure, the hyaloid does not give off any branches; it branches only upon reaching the optic vesicle, a branch that continues to become the main hyaloid artery that reaches the back of the developing lens to form the posterior part of the tunica vasculosa lentis. When the hyaloid artery is growing, a bullous structure made of solid endothelial cells appears at the optic nerve, at the base of the hyaloid artery.

This is the primitive central retinal artery. By the sixth month of gestation, the central retinal artery starts canalization and bifurcation in two branches, i.e., the nasal and temporal branches. The branches are without pericytes, which will appear only after 2 weeks postnatal. Retinal vessels assume adult dimensions by the fifth month postnatal. Vegetative endothelial growth factors play an important role in the development of superficial retinal vessels. Each of the temporal and nasal branches will branch to form superior and inferior retinal arteries; on the temporal side, they will arch over the macula, not reaching the avascular zone. Thus, the macula is devoid of retinal blood; it gets blood supply from the underlying choriocapillaries. The temporal and nasal branches do not grow at the same pace; the nasal branches reach the ora at birth, while the temporal branches grow at a slower pace and fail to reach the ora serrata, which is a contributing factor to the development of retinopathy in prematurity.

Like hyaloid and retinal vasculature, the uveal vasculature also develops from the primitive internal carotid artery. It has been noted that the primitive internal carotid artery gives rise to dorsal and ventral branches. The dorsal is chiefly used to supply the superficial retinal layers and form the tunica vascular lentis; it also gives rise to the common temporal ciliary artery running on the temporal side of the optic stalk and cup. From the ventral branch arises the ciliary artery on the nasal side; these two are the precursors of posterior ciliary arteries. The short posterior ciliary arteries come from the dorsal ophthalmic artery via a plexus of capillaries around the optic cup.

Congenital anomalies of the sclera: It has been seen earlier that the sclera is essentially mesodermal in origin. It develops from condensed mesoderm around the optic cup. The sclera develops in two parts, i.e., the anterior and posterior sclera. The anterior component develops earlier than the posterior component. The developing recti are closely related to the development of the anterior sclera. The developing recti grow backward from their insertion. The eyeball is mostly sclera. The cornea contributes only the anterior 1/6th of the surface. The shape and size of the eyeball depend on the retina. The congenital anomalies of the sclera can be localized to the sclera only or be associated with congenital anomalies of the uvea and retina.

The isolated anomalies are:

- Congenital staphylomas:
  - Equatorial
  - Posterior
- Sclerocornea
- Intrascleral nerve loop
- Blue sclera

Equatorial staphylomas: It is estimated that about 6% of normal eyes have asymptomatic equatorial congenital scleral staphylomas hidden under the recti, becoming apparent during strabismus or retinal surgery and mistaken as postinflammatory. Rarely, they may be visible between the recti under oblique illumination **(Fig. 3.58)**.

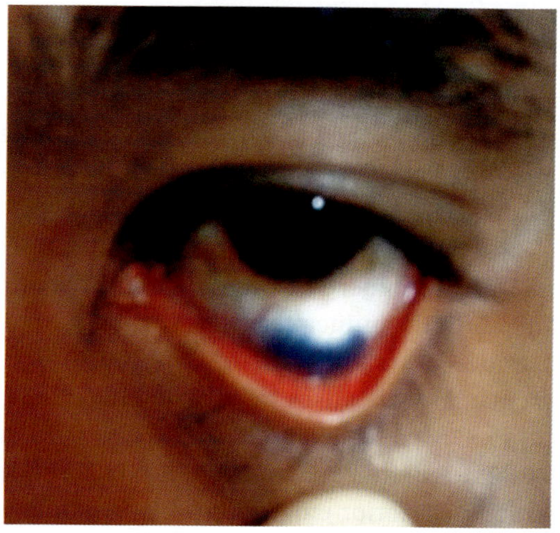

Fig. 3.58: Congenital staphylomas of the sclera.

Posterior staphylomas: These are exclusively seen in congenital axial myopia, round the posterior pole; they most probably develop during embryogenesis and increase as myopia increases. A difference in myopic refraction in the same meridian should raise suspicion, which is confirmed by wide-field OCT, indirect ophthalmoscopy, and ultrasonography.

Sclerocornea: This is a rare mesodermal dysgenesis that can be sporadic or hereditary. The sclera creeps over the cornea, obliterating the corneoscleral sulcus. There is no difference between the curvature of the cornea and the sclera. The cornea is invariably vascularized. The condition is generally partial, leaving a clear cornea in the center and there are some reports of sclerocornea totalis. The condition is nonprogressive and can be associated with microcornea and corneal plana. The anterior chamber is shallow, with an occludable angle, glaucoma, and cataracts.

Intrascleral nerve loop (Axenfeld nerve loop): This is a minor, often missed or ignored congenital anomaly of unknown origin. It develops when one of the branches of the long ciliary nerve changes its course and, instead of being intraocular, emerges on the surface of the sclera under the conjunctiva as a white nodule about 1 mm in diameter, generally on the nasal side, a little away from the limbus, not requiring any treatment.

Blue sclera: At birth, the sclera is thin, almost translucent; this is attributed to the lower number of scleral fibers in the neonatal sclera. The dark choroid imparts it a blue tinge that is referred to as the blue sclera. As the child grows, more opaque fibers are added to the still-developing sclera; by 1 year, the sclera gets its marble white color. In rare instances, this does not happen, and the sclera remains thin and blue. The blue tinge, per se, does not have any clinical significance unless it is accompanied by yet another systemic disorder, i.e., osteogenesis imperfecta (OI) that causes multiple fractures and bony deformities. Occasionally, the cornea is also thin, making it vulnerable to rupture even by trivial injury. Keratoconus, keratoglobus, posterior embryotoxon, and glaucoma are common in the blue sclera.

CONGENITAL ANOMALIES OF THE ORBIT

The congenital anomalies of the orbit can be due to any or many of the following:

- Isolated or associated with other anomalies
- Fault in the bones of the orbit
- Fault in the contents of the orbit
- Faults in the surrounding structures

Isolated Congenital Anomalies of the Orbit

They are hypertelorism, vertical displacement of orbit, and shallow orbit.

Hypertelorism is a congenital increase in intraorbital distance; it can be familial without any clinical significance. Otherwise, congenital hypertelorism gives an impression of a pseudodivergent squint. It may be associated with the vertical displacement of one of the orbits. The cause of hypertelorism is said to be abnormal growth of the bones of the forehead and base of the skull. It is not to be confused with the more common conditions of telecanthus, which is increased intracanthal distance with normal intraorbital and interpupillary distance, and epicanthus, which is an extra fold of skin between the medial canthus and nose. Hypertelorism is a constant feature of Waardenburg syndrome.

Shallow orbit: Congenital shallow orbits are seen in some congenital anomalies of the base of the skull due to premature fusion of bones, mainly in Crouzon and Apert syndromes.

As the development of the orbit is intimately related to the development of the skull and face, the congenital anomalies of the two are also closely associated; hence, cranial and craniofacial dysostosis are being discussed under congenital anomalies of the orbit.

The common cranial deformities with ocular involvement are given in **Table 3.5**.

CRANIOFACIAL DYSOSTOSES

Some of the common craniofacial and ophthalmic interests are:

- Oxycephaly (tower skull)
- Crouzon syndrome
- Apert syndrome
- Mandibulofacial dysostosis
    - Treacher–Collins syndrome
    - Goldenhar syndrome
    - Waardenburg syndrome

Microencephaly is a rare congenital developmental defect of the skull due to a small brain **(Fig. 3.59)**.

TABLE 3.5: Common cranial deformities with ocular involvement.

Nomenclature	***Features***
Scaphocephaly (Dolichocephaly)	Elongated, narrow skull
Brachycephaly	Short, wide skull
Plagiocephaly	Orbital asymmetry, flattened forehead, continued growth of contralateral side of skull, orbit on the affected side is shifted down and out trigonocephaly triangular deformity of anterior cranial fossa, hyper telorism
Acrocephaly	Tower skull due to multiple suture closures

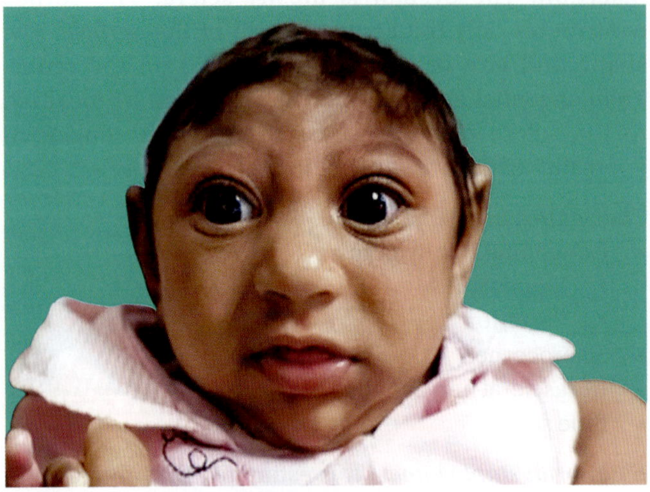

Fig. 3.59: Microencephaly.

TABLE 3.6: Clinical features of various craniofacial anomalies.

Condition	*Ocular feature*	*Systemic feature*
Oxycephaly	Bilateral shallow orbit, proptosis, ptosis, squint, papilledema, optic atrophy, exposure keratitis, nystagmus, cataract	Present at birth: Fusion of coronary and lambdoidal sutures of the skull
Crouzon syndrome	Shallow orbit, bilateral proptosis downward slant of the outer canthus, proptosis, frog-like face, bilateral divergent squint nystagmus, exposure keratitis	Present at birth, common in boys, dolichocephaly, underdeveloped maxilla, diminished hearing, and mental retardation
Apert syndrome	Hypertelorism, shallow orbit, mongoloid slant of the interpalpebral fissure, squint, optic atrophy, astigmatism, and amblyopia	May be familial, low-set ears, tower skull with syndactyly, underdeveloped maxilla, high-arched palate, prominent forehead, and cardiac malformation
Mandibulofacial dysostoses		
• Treacher–Collins syndrome	Bilaterally symmetrical, normal eyeball, good vision, coloboma of the lower lid	Hypoplasia of the facial bones abnormal hair line, deformity of the external ear, loss of hearing, sinus between the ear and mouth
• Franceschetti syndrome	Loss of lashes poorly developed lower tarsus, squint, and astigmatism	Same as above (some authors do not differentiate between (Treacher–Collins and Franceschetti syndromes)
• Goldenhar syndrome	Coloboma upper lid, microphthalmos, hypoesthesia of cornea nasolacrimal duct defect, squint, epibulbar dermoids	Congenital, sporadic, more common in boys besides oculoauriculovertebral anomalies; the child may have cardiac, renal, and CNS anomaly. The auricular changes consist of preauricular appendages, distorted meatus, distorted pinna, and absent auditory canal. The vertebral changes are hemi vertebra occipitalization of vertebra and fusion of cervical vertebra Cardiac changes are varied
• Waardenburg syndrome	Hypertelorism, epicanthus, lateral shift of puncta, heterochromia iridis, joined eyebrows, blepharophimosis	Familial, white forelock deafness, mutism vitiligo
• Hypertelorism	Bilateral symmetric broad nose bridge. Distance between two orbits increased, puncta are displaced outward, ptosis epicanthus inversus, squint, pseudosquint amblyopia	Familial

Clinical Featured of Common Craniofacial Dysostoses

Clinical features of common craniofacial dysostoses are given in **Table 3.6**.

CONGENITAL ANOMALIES OF EXTRAOCULAR MUSCLE

The congenital anomalies of extraocular muscles can be broadly divided into the following groups:

- Ptosis and its variants
- Retraction syndromes
- Superior oblique sheath syndrome
- Double elevator palsy
- Strabismus fixus

Except for simple ptosis, all congenital anomalies of extraocular muscles are associated with ocular deviation, which may be frank tropia or phoria. Converting to tropia, the congenital deviations may be secondary to single or multiple defects.

Probable Causes of Congenital Anomalies of Extraocular Muscles

The causes are as follows:

- Absence of muscle
- Hypoplasia of the muscle
- Abnormal insertion of muscle
- Abnormal adhesion between the affected muscle and adjacent structures
- Aberrant innervations of the muscle

- Congenital fibrosis of the muscle
- Abnormal fascial sheath
- Extra muscle
- Abnormal origin of muscle
- The last two are extremely rare

The congenital anomalies of extraocular muscles may involve a single muscle, as in Brown's syndrome, or more than one, as in Duane's retraction syndrome and double elevator palsy. They are generally uniocular, maybe obvious at birth, or may take some months or years to become apparent. The most common symptom that brings the child for consultation is a squint, which may be associated with abnormal head posture. They generally have binocular, single vision.

Duane's Retraction Syndrome

This is the most common congenital anomaly of extraocular muscles, with an array of presentations that have been reported by three different persons, independently and separately at different times, each putting emphasis on a group of features that were later put together to constitute the syndrome in its present form. The persons were Duane, Stilling, and Turk; hence, the syndrome has been eponymed variously in different combinations. However, it is more popularly referred to as Duane's retraction syndrome because retraction of the globe is a constant feature in all variations.

Variable duction defect with narrowing of palpebral aperture and retraction of globe in an attempt to adduct **(Figs. 3.60 to 3.64)**.

The incident may be as high as 4–5% among all cases of squint, without any racial predilection. Most of the time, the condition is sporadic but may show autosomal dominance. It is more common among girls. The left eye

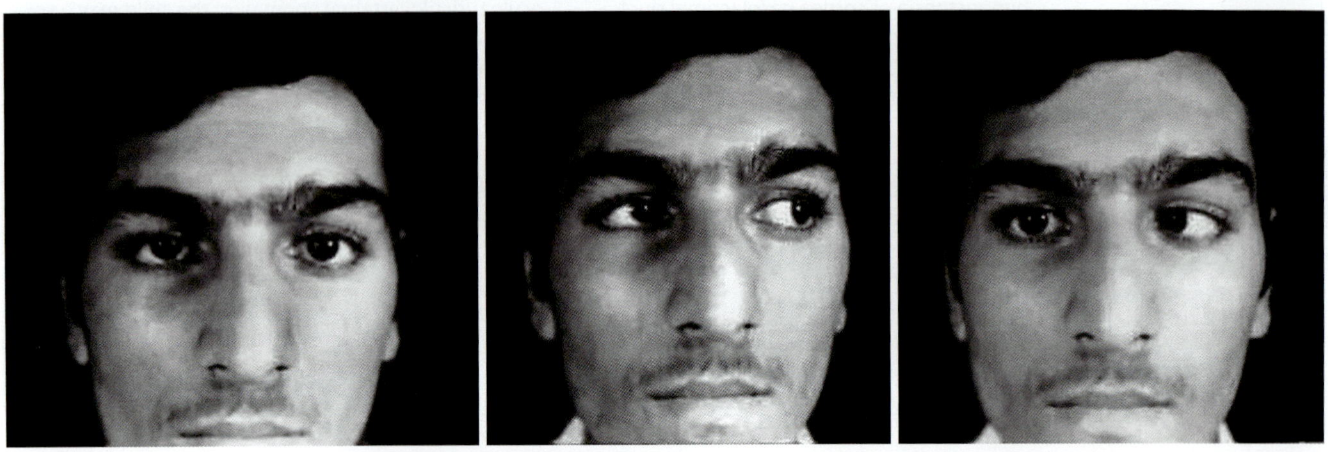

Fig. 3.60: Duane's retraction syndrome, right eye, no abduction of the right eye.

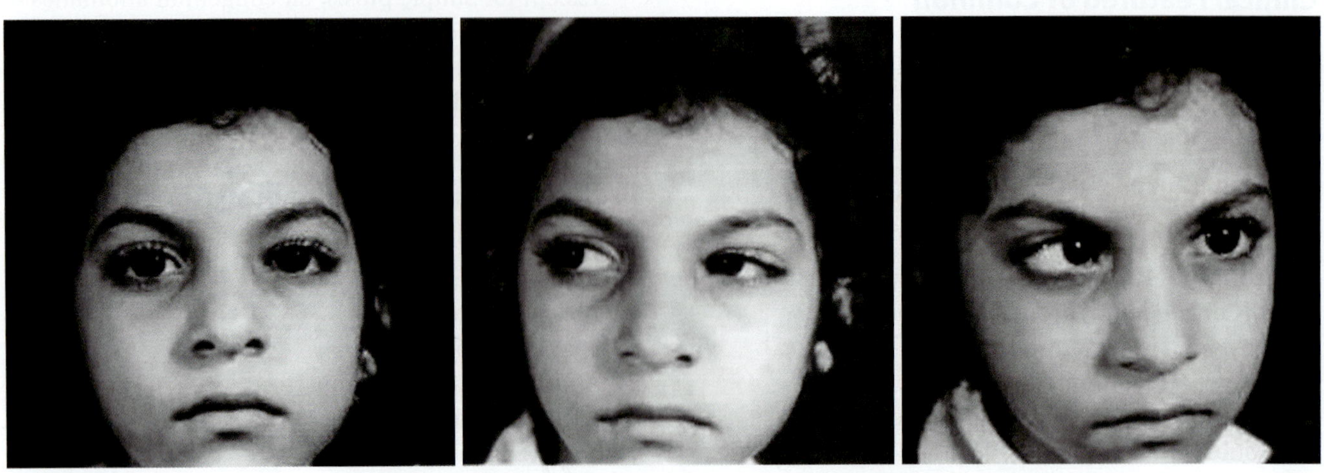

Fig. 3.61: Duane's retraction syndrome, left eye, narrowing of left eye in adduction.

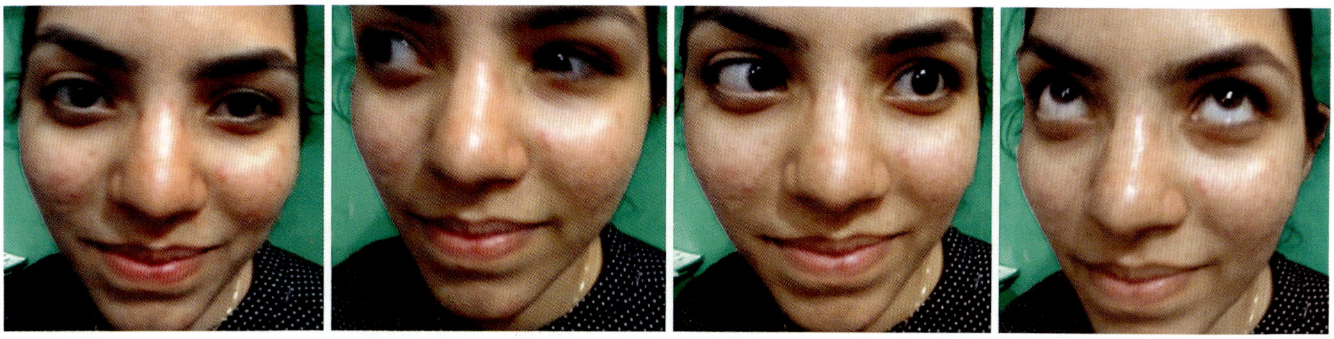

Fig. 3.62: Duane's retraction syndrome, left eye.

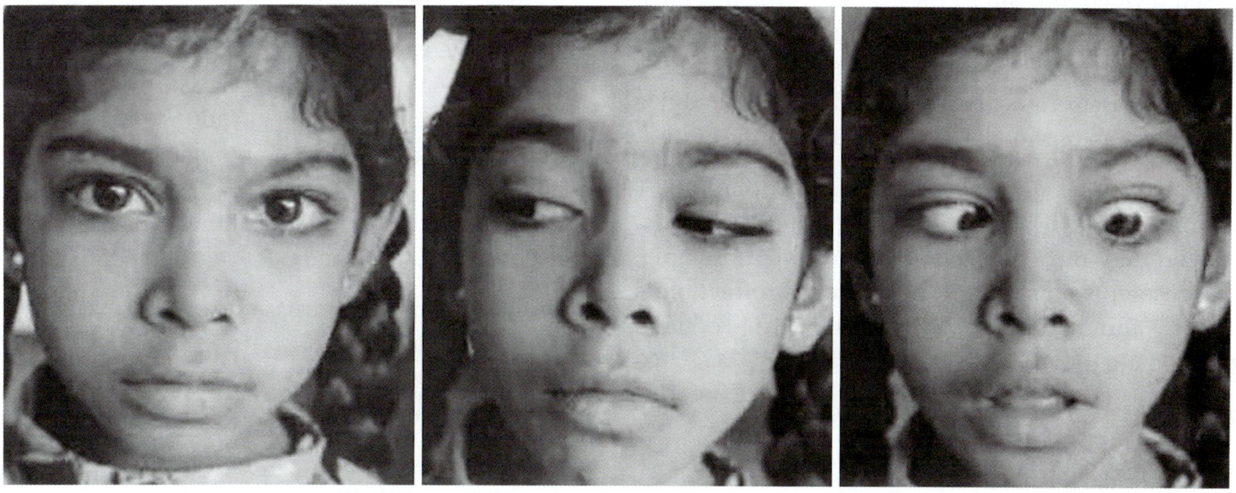

Fig. 3.63: Duane's retraction syndrome shows down shoot left eye.

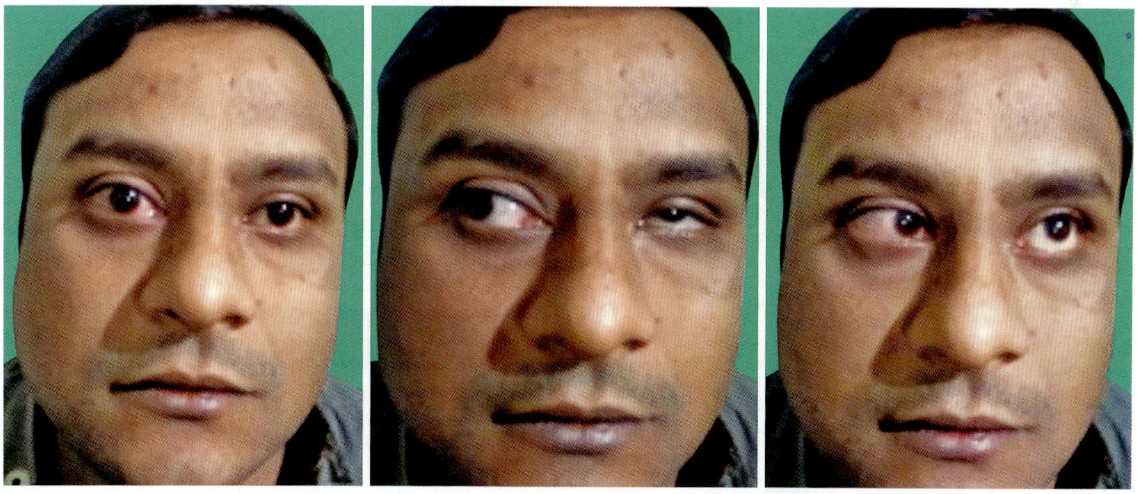

Fig. 3.64: Duane's retraction syndrome, left eye.

is more often involved; bilateral involvement too has been reported. The condition may be mistaken for congenital lateral rectus palsy.

The syndrome is present at birth but not noticed till 3 or 4 years of age, when the parents become aware of squints and a narrowing of the interpalpebral aperture on some gazes. The condition takes another 2–3 years to be fully developed; thereafter, it becomes stationary; there is no diplopia. No acquired form has been reported.

The child is brought for examination for any or many of the following:
- Routine checkup and found to have the condition
- Bizarre movement of the lids
- Squint
- Diminished vision
- Abnormal head posture

Depending on clinical presentation, the condition has been divided into three types: Type 1, which is most common, amounting to 85% of all cases **(Fig. 3.65)**. Type 2 comprises 12%, and the remaining belongs to type 3. A separate category may be added to the above where there is an upshoot of the eye on horizontal gaze.

The common types of deviations are: Esotropia in 65% and exotropia in 15%. The remaining are orthophoric. AV deviations, too, have been reported. Amblyopia, when present, is anisometric. The error of refraction is moderate and mostly hypermetropic with reduced accommodation.

Clinical features of the three types are as follows:
- *Type 1:*
  - Abnormal head posture
  - Orthophoria or esotropia in the primary gaze
  - Absent or reduced abduction
  - Narrowing of the palpebral fissure in adduction
  - Retraction of the globe in adduction

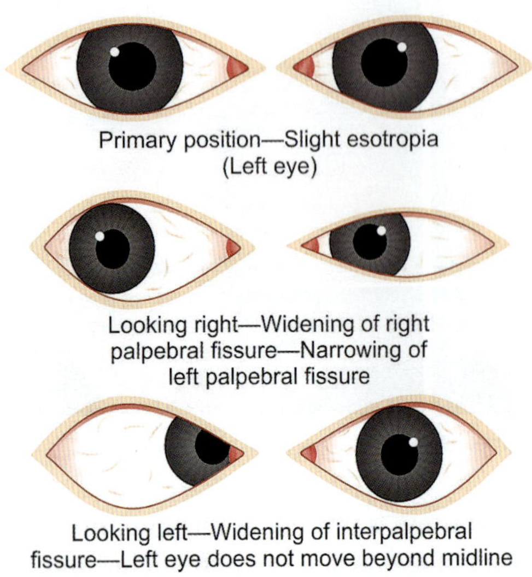

Fig. 3.65: Type one Duane's retraction syndrome involving left eye.

  - Widening of the palpebral fissure on abduction
  - Up- or downshoot of globe in adduction.
  - EMG shows abnormal innervations of the lateral rectus.
- *Type 2:*
  - Mostly exotropic
  - Slightly reduced abduction
  - Absent adduction
  - Narrowing of the palpebral fissure on adduction
  - Retraction of the globe on adduction
- *Type 3:*
  - Orthophoria
  - Reduced adduction
  - Reduced abduction
  - Narrowing of the palpebral fissure on adduction
  - Retraction of the globe on adduction

Table 3.7 is a comparison among types 1, 2, 3 as given by Huber (1974).

Ahluwalia (2017) modified Huber's classification into three groups, i.e., A, B, and C.

Accordingly, in primary gazes, the affected eye in:
- Type A is esotropic
- Type B is exotropic
- Type C is straight

Bilateral duane's retraction syndrome: It is estimated that some children with Duane's retraction syndrome have bilateral involvement, not always symmetric or equally severe in two eyes. The bilateral cases have been divided into following types, i.e., with or without fusion and with an AV pattern.

Differential diagnosis: Differential diagnosis consists of the following conditions:
- Congenital lateral rectus pals
- Infantile esotropia
- Medial rectus muscle entrapment

TABLE 3.7: Comparison among three types of Duane's retraction syndrome.

Type	*Frequency*	*Primary gaze*	*Primary feature*	*Globe retraction*
1	85%	Eso/Ortho	Reduced abduction	Mild
2	14%	Eso/Ortho	Reduced abduction	Sever
3	1%	Eso/Ortho	Both abduction and adduction are reduced	Moderate

(Eso: esotropia; Ortho: orthophoria)

- Moebius syndrome
- Strabismus fixus
- Congenital fibrosis syndrome
- Nystagmus blocking syndrome

Congenital lateral rectus palsy: Is an infrequent, self-limiting condition that resolves automatically in a month or two, leaving no aftereffects, most probably due to delayed myelination, birth trauma, or raised intracranial pressure.

Infantile esotropia

Medial rectus entrapment: It is never congenital. It may develop any time after birth and may be a part of battered baby syndrome, child abuse, sports injuries, or road traffic accidents. It is more common in the second decade.

Moebius syndrome: It is a congenital, bilateral, polyneuronal anomaly with multiple skeletal anomalies. The infant is brought with complaints of an inability to suckle, an expressionless face, and a peculiar cry. On examination, the child has a round expressionless face due to absent nasolabial fold and orbicularis under action; the above features are attributed to bilateral upper motor seventh nerve involvement. The eyes cannot be moved beyond midline, the eyes show esotropia of variable degrees, the eyes may be fixed in adduction due to absent or poor action of the sixth nerve, esotropia when present is large, the child may cross fixate, occasionally the child may have gaze palsy, forced duction is positive, and the medial rectus may be inserted nearer to the limbus. The AV pattern is common. The next cranial nerve to be involved is the twelfth, resulting in difficulty in suckling, bleat-like cry; the tip of the tongue shows evidence of atrophy. Other cranial nerves may be involved.

Multiple skeletal defects are not uncommon with Moebius syndrome. They are: Congenital anomalies of the digits, club feet, and abnormal gait. Mental retardation is common.The condition should be differentiated from strabismus fixus. There is no specific treatment; each problem requires different management.

Strabismus fixus: This is rarer than Moebius syndrome; it is congenital, without neurological defect, and presents with large-angle bilateral esotropia; rarely, there may be exotropia. The cause is attributed to congenital fibrosis of the medial rectus.

Congenital fibrosis syndrome: This is yet another rare, congenital, bilateral, restrictive, polygenic squint. The probable fault being in the third nerve nucleus, that is, hypoplastic. On the basis of genetics, it has been divided into two types, i.e., autosomal dominant and recessive. The first is referred to as classical; it consists of bilateral mild-to-moderate ptosis and a third nerve under action without pupillary involvement. The eyes cannot be elevated above the horizontal midline. The other type comprises large exotropia, with a gross restriction of both vertical and horizontal movements.

Nystagmus blocking syndrome: It is a form of infantile esotropia developed to dampen nystagmus. The mechanism of the phenomenon is based on the presumption that nystagmus can be reduced by convergence, which leads to sustained esotropia with secondary changes in the medial rectus. It should be differentiated from the bilateral sixth nerve under action and cross-fixation.

Conditions that mimic Duane's retraction syndrome:

- *Medial orbital fracture:* This is associated with diplopia that is absent in Duane's retractions syndrome.
- *Vertical retraction syndrome:* Globe retraction and narrowing of palpebral fissure on vertical movement of eye

Less common features associated with Duane's retraction syndrome: The conditions belong to four categories, i.e., ocular, auricular, skeletal, and neural.

Ocular: Ptosis, jaw winking, epibulbar dermoids, dysplasia of the iris, pupillary anomaly, heterochromia of the iris, uveal coloboma, cataract, microphthalmos, morning glory syndrome, error of refraction, amblyopia, nystagmus

Auricular: Deformity of the external ear; sensory neural deafness.

Skeletal: Deformity of limbs, cleft palate, deformity of face, vertebral anomaly, spina bifida, phocomelia

Neural: Anomalies of cranial nerves three, four, and six in different combinations.

Syndromes associated with Duane's retraction syndrome are: Goldenhar, Klippel–Feil (Okihiro), Duane-radial ray, renal ocular syndrome.

Goldenhar syndrome is a congenital multisystemic anomaly consisting of ocular and nonocular features.

The ocular features are Duane's retraction syndrome and limbal dermoids. The nonocular features consist of facial anomalies, which are a deformed ear, nose, soft palate, lip, and mandible on one side. The condition is due to faulty development of the first and second branchial arches.

Klippel-Feil (Okihiro) syndrome is a prominent disorder of cervical vertebrae, along with Duane's retraction syndrome. It is composed of fusion of cervical vertebrae leading to a short neck, a low hairline, and diminished neck movement.

Duane-radial ray syndrome affects not only movement of the eyes and retraction of the globe but also deformity in the arms and hands.

Etiology of duane's retraction syndrome: The exact cause is not well understood; the causes are multifactorial. One common factor agreed upon by all is that it is a congenital anomaly that begins during early embryogenesis and may not only be confined to extraocular muscles but also their nerve supply. There may be some genetic factors involved. The most widely accepted theory is "miss wiring of two horizontal muscles", i.e., innervations of the lateral rectus by an anomalous branch of the lower division of the third nerve that causes involuntary contraction of both the horizontally acting muscles simultaneously, leading to retraction of the globe, which in turn results in a narrowing of the palpebral fissure.

Other possibilities are: Absence of the third nerve nucleus and hypoplasia of the sixth nerve trunk.

Less accepted theories are: Rigid lateral rectus, abnormal attachment of lateral rectus, rigid medial rectus acting as a band, and abnormal adhesion of medial rectus at its origin.

Treatment of Duane's retraction syndrome: There is no specific treatment for the anomaly; all cases do not require treatment. Treatment is indicated only in cases of gross head turns. Correction of head turn, changes in palpebral fissure, and squint should be preceded by correction of the error of refraction and management of amblyopia. Recession of the medial rectus may reduce retraction; prisms have been tried to minimize head turn without a uniform result. The standard procedure followed for type 1 Duane's syndrome is unilateral or bilateral recession of the medial rectus. Resection of the lateral rectus is better avoided because it rarely increases abduction and worsens retraction.

Brown Syndrome (Superior Oblique Tendon Sheath Syndrome)

Brown syndrome is almost as common a cause of retraction tropia as Duane's retraction syndrome. It is mostly congenital in children and may be acquired in the second decade secondary to craniofacial trauma and inflammation. When congenital retraction is discovered in infancy or childhood, the child is not aware of the condition. Abnormal head posture is the main feature that brings the child for consultation; observant parents may become aware of squints and bizarre movements of the lid. It is unilateral in 90% of cases. Bilaterality adds difficulty to otherwise easy diagnoses; it is a little more common in girls and is more frequent in the right eye. There may be a positive family history, and many of the siblings may show various degrees of the disorder that may be obvious in old family group photographs **(Fig. 3.66)**.

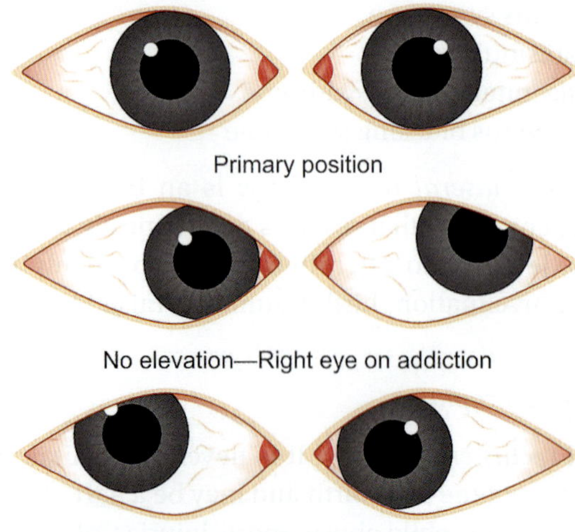

Fig. 3.66: Brown's syndrome—right eye

The commonly accepted theory of the condition is that the superior oblique loses its smoothness as it passes over the trochlea, most commonly due to congenital short and tight superior oblique tendon sheath and less commonly due to thickening of the muscle.

Abnormal head postures, i.e., chin up and head tilt, in isolation or in combination, are the most common features for consultation. The child may occasionally complain of diplopia; diminished vision and amblyopia are common. On examination, most of the affected eyes are orthophoric in the primary position; otherwise, they may be hypertrophic to various degrees, and an AV pattern may be present. Most diagnostic features are reduced or absent elevation in adduction. The eye cannot be elevated beyond midline in adduction. Elevation improves as the eye abducts so much so that it starts elevating in primary gaze; the elevation is maximum in abduction. Retraction of the globe and downshoot may be present in adduction. The forced duction test is positive. There is no overaction of the ipsilateral superior oblique. Occasionally, the condition is bilateral. Depending on severity, the condition has been divided into three categories, i.e., mild, moderate, and severe:

Mild: Orthophoria in primary gaze, no downshoot in adduction

Moderate: Orthophoria in primary gaze, downshoot on adduction

Severe: Hypotropia in primary gaze, downshoot in adduction, and chin up

Binocular singles are present in the primary and lower gazes.

Differential diagnosis: Diagnosis is not difficult in a child with an elevated chin, restricted elevation in adduction, and a positive family history.

However, the following conditions should be kept in mind:

- *Inferior oblique palsy:* Negative forced duction test
- *Double elevator palsy:* Reducedelevation on adduction and abduction
- *Blow-out fracture of orbit:* Positivehistory of injury to orbit, evidence of fracture on CT.
- *Congenital fibrosis syndrome:* Positive forced duction test in all fields

Management of Brown syndrome: The condition is self-limiting in many cases; hence, it is better to observe the child till the end of the first decade unless the child has prominent hypotropia in the primary gaze and marked chin elevation. Correction of errors in refraction and management of amblyopia should get priority over all other modes of treatment. The surgical procedures used are to weaken the superior oblique by tenotomy.

Double Elevator Palsy (Monocular Elevation Deficiency)

This is an infrequent, unilateral congenital anomaly of elevation in all positions due to underaction or absence of elevation. The disorders follow involvement of the elevators of the eye, i.e., the superior rectus and inferior obliques, in combination or isolation **(Figs. 3.67A and B)**.

The most probable cause is hypoplasia of the nucleus of the third nerve concerned with elevation. The eye is hypotrophic in the primary gaze with true or pseudoptosis, retaining Bell's phenomenon. The hypodeviation may occasionally be latent. Chin is raised, amblyopia is common, and elevation of the chin and hypertropia reduce the chance of amblyopia.

There are three possible types of the condition:

1. Prominent inferior rectus with normal superior rectus
2. Reduced elevation, negative forced duction test, diminished superior rectus action
3. Combination of the above two

Differential diagnosis consists of:

- Brown syndrome
- Abnormal insertion of the superior and/or inferior rectus
- Congenital fibrosis of the inferior rectus
- Blow-out fracture

Double Depressor Palsy

This is far less common than double elevator palsy; it may be considered the reverse of monocular elevation palsy. It is due to the underaction of the inferior rectus and superior oblique. The eye is hypertrophic in its primary position.

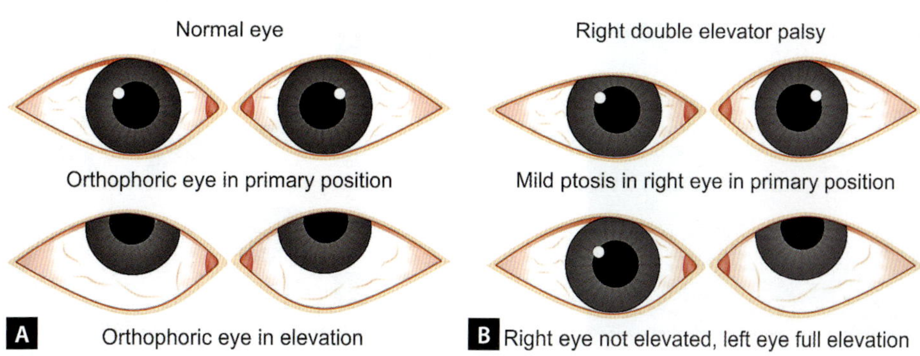

Figs. 3.67A and B: (A) Normal eye without elevation palsy; (B) Right double elevation palsy.

Strabismus Surso-Adductorius

It is generally bilateral and symmetric, causing marked elevation when the eye is adducted. It is common in horizontal squints: Esotropia (70%) and exotropia (30%). There is no vertical deviation in the primary position. Hypertropia develops when the eye looks to the other side, i.e., right hypertropia on the left gaze and vice versa. V pattern is common. It is commonly confused with dissociated vertical deviation (DVD). There are two clinical types: Primary and secondary. The primary is bilateral without head tilt; the cause of the condition is not known. Secondary types are unilateral, secondary to superior oblique palsy. The treatment is surgical.

The two conditions that are not really congenital but mimic strabismus surso-adductorius are inferior oblique overaction (IOOA) and DVD.

Inferior oblique overaction: This is the elevation of the affected eye when adducted. It is more commonly unilateral; it is generally seen in horizontal squints in children. It has been put into two groups, i.e., primary and secondary. The primary often involves both eyes, the cause of which is obscure and is seen in 70% congenital esotropia and the remaining 30% in accommodative esotropia. The secondary type is unilateral and secondary to superior oblique palsy. The characteristic of the primary type is excess elevation of the adducted eye; the condition may have minimal vertical deviation in the primary gaze with moderate head tilt. The secondary type is characterized by elevation on adduction; hypertropia of the affected eye is a rule. The child has an abnormal head posture with positive Bielschowsky test **(Fig. 3.68)**.

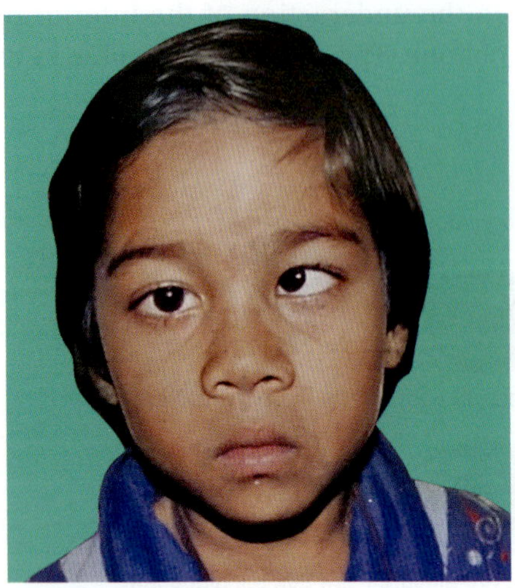

Fig. 3.68: Inferior oblique overaction.
Courtesy: Dr Somen Misra.

Dissociated vertical divergence: This phenomenon is generally associated with infantile esotropia but can happen in the straight eye as well. It was discovered during the first 3 years. The cause is not well understood. It is presumed to be a disorder of supranuclear innervations of the ocular muscles. The child may look normal with a tendency to the malady when tired or daydreaming. The drifts may be frequent or only once or twice a day; the amount of drifts may change even every hour; they are unmasked by a simple cover test **(Figs. 3.69A and B)**.

The eye under cover deviates up for some duration and spontaneously drifts to a normal position or even lower. Faulty enervation of one eye allows it to move independently without voluntarily exerting effort.

The condition is thought to be cortical suppression. There is no diplopia; the presence of diplopia indicates the absence of suppression. The divergence is due to asymmetries in bilateral cases. The up movement is generally associated with esotropia. Nystagmus is common.

Congenital Vertical Fibrosis

This is a rare familial condition. The most common form is vertical squint. The eyes are fixed permanently in the downgaze with an elevated chin. There may be associated ptosis, and the most common muscle involved is the inferior rectos.

Adherence Syndrome

This is a rare congenital anomaly of two adjacent muscles, i.e., lateral rectus and inferior oblique, or superior rectus

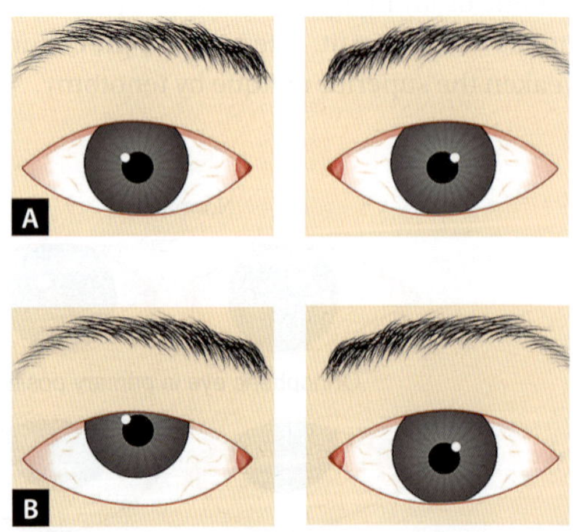

Figs. 3.69A and B: Cover test in DVD. (A) Normal eye, no deviation under cover; (B) Up drifts under cover in DVD. (DVD: dissociated vertical divergence)

and superior oblique. The adherence is nonspecific, and in spite of the involvement of obliques, the clinical presentation is that of the involved horizontal rectus.

List of congenital vertical strabismus:

- IOOA
- DVD
- Double elevator palsy
- Double depressor palsy
- Brown syndrome
- Congenital fibrosis syndrome
- Adherence syndrome

SUMMARY OF EMBRYOLOGY OF THE EYE AND ITS ADNEXA

Table 3.8 depicts origin of various parts of eye and its adnexa.

CLINICAL PROBLEMS OF CONGENITAL ANOMALIES OF EYES AND ITS ADNEXA

The common problems that parents bring the child for consultation are:

- Cosmetic **(Figs. 3.70 and 3.71)**
- Diminished vision
- Amblyopia
- Nystagmus
- White reflex in the pupil **(Fig. 3.72)**
- Large cornea with watering **(Fig. 3.73)**

TABLE 3.8: Origin of various parts of eye and its adnexa.

Tissue	*Part developed*
Surface ectoderm	• Lens • Epithelium of: Cornea, conjunctiva, lacrimal gland, lacrimal passages, and part of the vitreous
Neural ectoderm	• Part of the vitreous • Epithelium of the iris, ciliary body, and retina • Sphincter and dilator of the pupil • Neural component of the optic nerve
Mesoderm	• Sclera, choroid, orbit, extraocular and lid muscles • Hyaloid vessels, optic nerve sheath, and vessels
Combined	• Lacrimal gland • Cornea • Iris • Vitreous • Bruch membrane

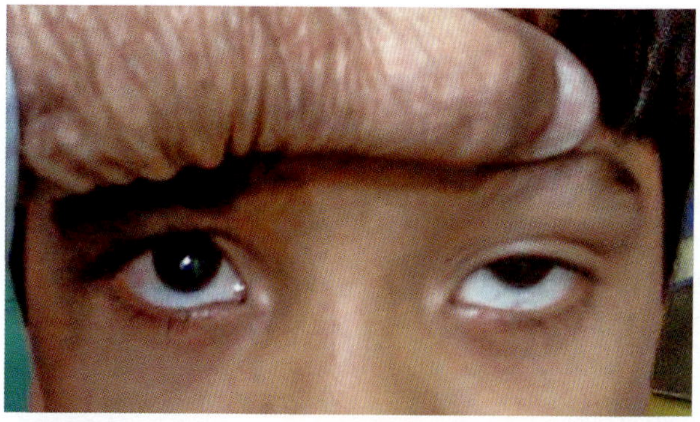

Fig. 3.70: Cosmetic defect due to congenital anomaly: Congenital ptosis.

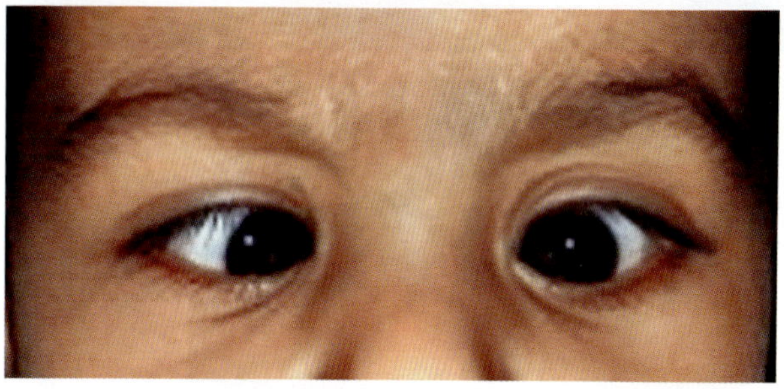

Fig. 3.71: Cosmetic defect due to congenital anomaly: Pseudosquint.

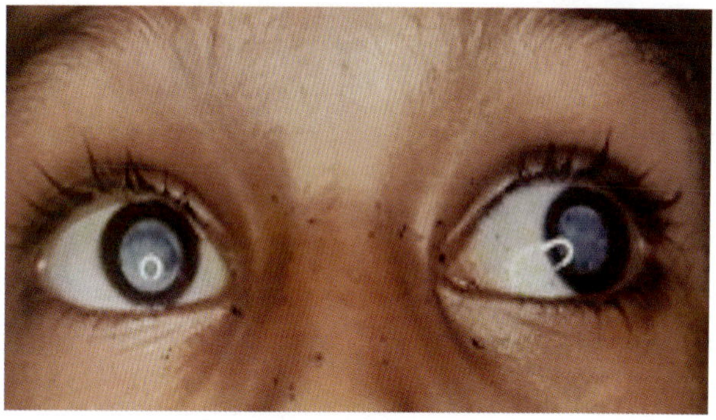

Fig. 3.72: Congenital cataract.
Courtesy: Dr Somen Misra.

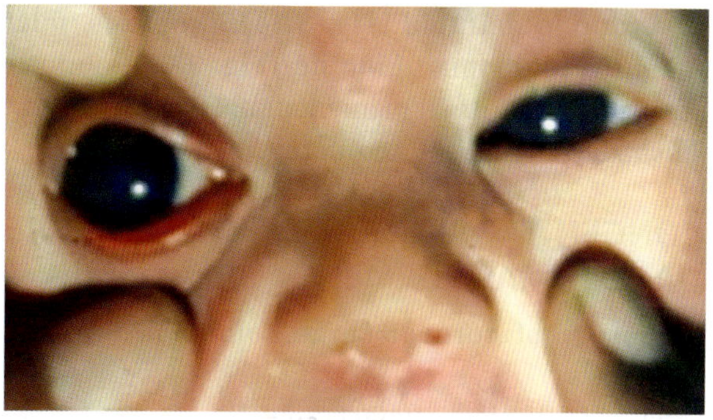

Fig. 3.73: Buphthalmos.
Courtesy: Dr Somen Misra.

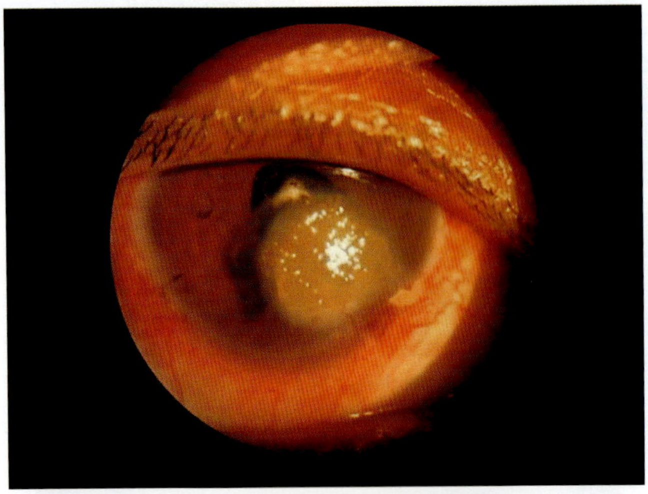

Fig. 3.74: Corneal opacity (dermoid).

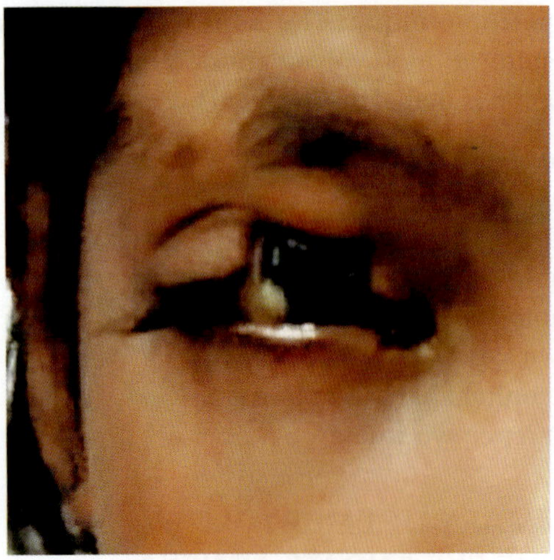

Fig. 3.75: Large coloboma of the lid.
Courtesy: Dr Nupur Chakarwarty.

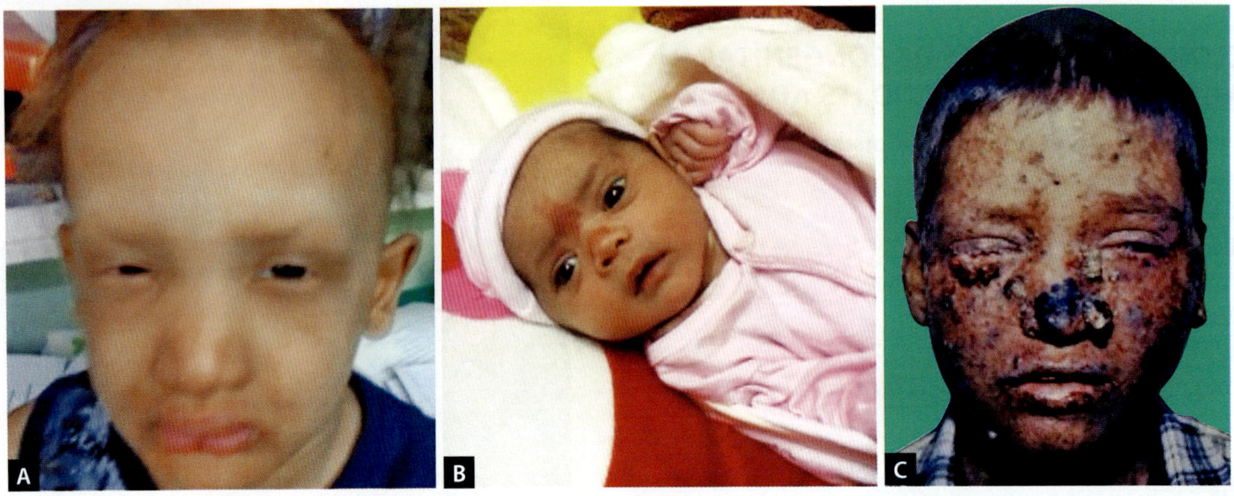

Figs. 3.76A to C: Various types of congenital discoloration of face involving eyes. (A) Albinism; (B) Birthmark; (C) Xeroderma pigmentosa.
Courtesy: (A) Dr A T Dabke; (C) Dr Somen Misra.

The other congenital conditions that produce visible affect are given in **Figures 3.74 to 3.76**. They are: Corneal opacity due to dermoid **(Fig. 3.74)**, proptosis, microphthalmos, coloboma of the lid **(Fig. 3.75)**, abnormal head posture, abnormal pigmentation **(Figs. 3.76A to C)**, albinism, birthmark, and xeroderma pigmentosa.

CONGENITAL ANOMALIES THAT REQUIRE URGENT MANAGEMENT

- Exposure of cornea: Large coloboma upper lid, proptosis
- Bilateral complete cataract
- Advanced unilateral congenital cataract

SUGGESTED READING

1. Banigalla Pati S, Potti S, Marthala H. A rare case of persistent pupillary membrane case based approach and management. Indian J Ophthalmol. 2018;66:1480-3.
2. Basak SK. Essentials of Ophthalmology, 2nd edition. Kolkata: Current Books International; 1999.
3. Bhattacharjee H, Deshmukh S. Soemmering's ring. Indian J Ophthalmol. 2017;65(12):1489.
4. Christy JS, Tagare S. Classical signs of keratoconus. Delhi J Ophthal. 2021;31(1):87-9.
5. Dani Y, Shrivastava AK, Nayak S. Duane's Retraction Syndrome Type III: Rare Case of Strabismus. Proceeding 20th annual CSOS. 2021.
6. Duke Elder S. System of Ophthalmology, Vol. 3, Part 2, 1st edition. London: Henry Kimpton; 1964.

7. Jain AM, Ranjan R, Manayath GJ. A typical superior iris coloboma and retino choroidal coloboma. Indian J Ophthalmol. 2018;66;1474-5.
8. Kumar V, Tewari R, Kumari D. Optic nerve aplasia. Indian J Ophthalmol. 2018;66(1):125-6.
9. Li Y, Shekhar R, Huang D. Corneal pachymetry mapping with high-speed optical coherence tomography. Ophthalmology. 2006;113:792-9.e2.
10. Mann I. Development of Human Eye, 3rd edition. London: British Medical Association; 1964.
11. Mukherjee PK. Clinical Examination in Ophthalmology, 2nd edition. New Delhi: Elsevier; 2016.
12. Mukherjee PK. Ophthalmic Assistant, 1st edition. New Delhi: Jaypee Brothers Medical Publishers; 2013.
13. Mukherjee PK. Pediatric Ophthalmology, 1st edition. New Delhi: New Age International; 2005.
14. Patel P, Singh S. Supernumerary Lacrimal Puncta: A Case Report. Proceeding of 20th annual CSOS. 2021.
15. Qin B, Chen S, Brass R, Li Y, Tang M,Zhang X. Keratoconus Diagnosis with An Optical Coherence Tomography-Based Pachymetric Scoring System. J Cataract Refract Surg. 2013; 39(12):1864-71.
16. Saint-Geniez M, D'Amro PA. Development and pathology of hyaloid, choroidal and retinal vasculature. Int J Dev Biol. 2004;48:1045-58.
17. Saluja G, Bhari A. Brown's Syndrome. Delhi J Ophthalmol. 2020;30:23-7.
18. Sashidhar B. A rare case of persistent pupillary membrane. Indian J Ophthalmol. 2018;66(10):1480-3.
19. Sharma Y, Sudan R, Gaur A. Post traumatic subconjunctival dislocation of lens in Ehler–Danlos syndrome. Indian J Ophthalmol. 2003;51(2):185-6.
20. Szalai E, Berta A, Hassan Z, Modis L, Jr. Reliability and repeatability of swept-source Fourier-domain optical coherence tomography and Scheimpflug imaging in keratoconus.J Cataract Refract Surg. 2012;38:485-94.
21. Uhamwangho OM, Jalali S. Chorio retinal coloboma in paediatric population. Eye. 2014;28:728-33.
22. Usgaonkar U, Chodankar S, Shetty A. Online survey about keratoconus management by optometrists. Indian J Ophthalmol. 2023;71(1):86-90.

CHAPTER 4

Eyes at Birth

Eyes are well developed as sensory organs at birth when compared to their size.

> 60% of afferent input to the central nervous system's higher centers comes through vision.

EYES AT BIRTH

The examination of the eye of a newborn is taken under two circumstances.

1. General; as part of the protocol of the institution where the infant is born.
2. Specific to exclude congenital anomalies that require urgent referral:
   i. Large coloboma on the upper lids.
   ii. White reflex in the pupil.
   iii. Complete cataract.
   iv. Large, hazy cornea.
   v. Proptosis.
   vi. Craniofacial anomalies.
   vii. Critically-ill baby.

> - Premature children not exposed to prolonged oxygenation may be treated as full-term, so far as the eyes are concerned.
> - The eyes attain adult size by 13–14 years. There is no spurt in the increase in the length of the eyeball at puberty.

Each examiner has his/her precedence and protocol of examination for the newborn.

It is better to examine the child in the neonatal nursery with full antisepsis. The room should have a controlled illumination system, i.e., to change ambient light.

At birth, normal eyes are mirror images of each other. Placed at equidistance from the midline, the neonate sleeps almost 18 hours a day, making it difficult to see the structures behind the closed lids without mechanically separating them.

It is a good practice to observe the child's face under diffuse illumination for symmetry and shape of head, birth marks on lids, and proptosis. It is difficult to opine about the presence of ptosis at this stage. The eyebrows are well developed and lighter in color. The orbits are smaller and shallower in proportion to the globe, imparting a sense of bulging in the eyes.

> Though the eyes of newborns are smaller than those of adults, when compared to other organs, they are comparatively larger.

The eyeballs at birth are more spherical than adults, with a diameter ranging between 16.5 and 17.5 mm and a volume of 2.88 mL.

Smaller anteroposterior diameter should make the eye of a newborn pathologically axial hypermetropic by about 20 diopters; this is partially neutralized by index and curvature myopia introduced by the lens of the newborn. The lens of the newborn is almost spherical, introducing index and curvature myopia of about 16–17 diopter, leaving the newborn hypermetropic by 3 diopter, which is gradually neutralized in the next 3 years, leaving the child emmetropic.

The intermarginal fissure of the newborn is 18 mm in length, and the nose bridge is relatively wider; this gives a false impression of esotropia. The fixation is erratic. The lower lid can be pulled down to expose the lower part of the cornea, lower bulbar conjunctiva, and lower fornix. The upper lid is difficult to evert, making inspection of the upper cornea, conjunctiva, and fornix difficult. The levator and orbicularis are fully developed and functional.

The cornea of a newborn is 10 mm in diameter and reaches an adult size of 11.75 mm in 2 years. Corneal diameters <10 mm and >12 mm are abnormal. The cornea is flatter than an adult cornea; the cornea of a newborn is more curved on the periphery, in contrast to an adult cornea.

The sclera is thin and translucent, imparting it a blue tinge. The tinge is due to the underlying choroid; the tinge passes off by 2–3 months postnatal.

The lacrimal gland and the passages are fully developed. About 10% of nasolacrimal ducts may have obstruction due to epithelial debris not cleared at birth. Lacrimal secretions do not materialize before 3–4 weeks postnatal. Hence, there are no tears when the infant cries until 3–4 weeks postnatal. The regurgitation test is negative.

The fornices are fully developed but relatively shallow; the conjunctival tissues are not well developed; the lymphoid tissues are rudimentary; the conjunctiva at birth is sterile; it gets contaminated soon; and all organisms that find access to the conjunctiva are not infective all the time. The pathological organisms, mostly bacteria, are acquired either during birth or soon after birth due to faulty antiseptic and aseptic methods used.

The anterior chamber is fully formed with normally circulating and functioning aqueous. The depth of the anterior chamber is less than that of the adult chamber without impeding aqueous flow. The angle, trabeculum, and Schlemm's canal are formed and functioning. Crypts and ridges on the iris surface are well formed, with a few fine vessels on the periphery without any clinical significance; these vessels disappear in a few months. Persistent pupillary membranes may be found in 10% of eyes; they are symptomless; the color of the iris is variable; heterochromia, when present, may be unilateral or bilateral, sectoral or generalized without any clinical significance.

The normal pupil is slightly eccentric; it is shifted down and medially. This shift is physiological and is considered central. The pupil is circular with a brisk reaction, both direct and indirect. Near-convergence reflexes cannot be tested accurately. The newborn eyes have very high accommodation and convergence.

The lens is almost spherical, imparting a high degree of index and curvature myopia that neutralizes the inherent high axial hypermetropia of the newborn eye. The lens is transparent and may have some remnants of the tunica vasculosa lentis still attached to the posterior surface. It may also have a persistent pupillary membrane that mostly disappears in a few months.

The ciliary body is smaller than in the adult eye, and the choroid is fully developed.

The fundus lacks the pink hue of the adult retina; it is relatively pale; the disc and the peripheral retina are also pale; a few superficial retinal hemorrhages are common without any significance; they disappear in a few days. The retinal vessels are well developed and reach beyond the ora on both the nasal and temporal sides. The macula is not fully developed yet; it stands out against the pale retina. The pale retina makes the underlying choroid more prominent than in adults. The vision is poor; it is estimated to be 1/60. The newborn is able to fix and follow a moving object with a sharp border. The threatening gesture cannot be elicited. The refraction ranges between +3D and +4D. Intraocular pressure is 10 mm Hg.

A brief Comparison between neonatal and adult eye is given in **Table 4.1**.

TABLE 4.1: Comparison between neonatal and adult eye.

Part of eye	***Neonate***	***Adult***
1. Eye brow	Poorly developed and light-colored	Well developed and dark colored
2. Eyeball volume	2.88 mL	7.0 mL
3. Anteroposterior length	16.5–17.5 mm	24.0 mm
4. Refraction (actual)	+2D–+3D	Emmetropic
5. Refraction (estimated)	+21D	Emmetropia
6. Vision	1/60	6/6
7. Orbital rim	Circular	Quadrilateral
8. Interpalpebral aperture	18 mm	30 mm
9. Corneal diameter	10–11 mm	10.5–11 mm
10. *Lens:* i. Shape	Spherical	Ellipsoid
ii. Curvature		
a. Anterior	6 mm	10 mm
b. Posterior	6 mm	6 mm

Contd...

Contd...

Part of eye	*Neonate*	*Adult*
11. *Pupil:* i. Size ii. Reaction	 <2 mm, difficult to dilate Brisk	 2.5–3 mm easily dilate Brisk
12. Anterior chamber	Shallow	Normal depth
13. Angle	Nonoccludable	May be occludable
14. Macula	Not fully developed	Fully developed
15. Disc	Pale	Pink
16. Movement of individual muscles	Bizarre, individual muscles cannot be tested specifically	Regular and smooth individual muscles can be tested specifically

SUGGESTED READING

1. HV Nema. Anatomy of the Eye and its Adnex, 2nd edition. New Delhi: Jaypee Brothers; 1991.
2. Mukherjee PK. Clinical examination in ophthalmology, 2nd edition. New Delhi: Elsevier; 2016.
3. Mukherjee PK. Ophthalmic assistant, 1st edition. New Delhi: Jaypee Brothers; 2013.
4. Mukherjee PK. Pediatric ophthalmology, 1st edition. New Delhi: New Age International; 2005.
5. Salmon JF. Kanski's, Clinical Ophthalmology, 9th edition. New Delhi: Elsevier; 2020.

CHAPTER

5 Retinopathy of Prematurity

Retinopathy of prematurity (ROP) is an acquired, iatrogenic, noninfectious, noninflammatory, subacute, bilateral, potentially blinding, often self-limiting vasculopathy, seen in under weighed, preterm babies, exposed to prolonged concentrated oxygen, without any genetic basis.

To have better understanding of the complex disorder, it is imperative to recapitulate the embryogenesis of retinal vascularization.

Fully developed retina in spite of its high oxygen requirement is avascular up to fourth month (16 weeks) of gestation. There after retinal vessels start sprouting from the hyaloid system of vasculature which till this time is only source of blood supply to intraocular structures. The proximal part of the hyaloid artery represents the future central retinal artery. The central retinal artery divides in to two major arteries, i.e., temporal and nasal; either as a single or two separate branches. Till this time the retinal vessels are solid and get canalized later. The developing vessels are immature vessels, prone to structural change with variation of oxygen concentration. The developing vessels have more endothelial cells compared to other vessels. That makes them vulnerable to proliferation and obliteration. The other noteworthy point is that the basement membrane of the developing vessels are weak, the role of spindle cells in development is not well-elucidated, and they too seem to play some role in genesis of selective neovascularization.

Once the newly formed retinal vessels have sprouted from the hyaloid artery they grow centrifugally on either side of the optic disc; the pace is not equal on the two sides, till the vessels have reached the equator. This happens at 8 months of gestation, by this time the nasal periphery is fully vascularized.

The temporal vessels grow at slower speed, to compensate this retardation they have to continue growing after birth. It takes 4 weeks postnatal, i.e., 40 weeks after conception for these vessels to reach the periphery. Hence, an infant born earlier than 36 weeks lacks vascularization up to extreme temporal periphery. Lesser the gestational age at birth, more are the chances of developing ROP; the dictum in the past was that an infant born before 32 weeks was likely to develop ROP, which is no more considered to be applicable.

Obviously a child born before 32 weeks is underweight also. To save the life of the premature, the infant is put in the incubator with high concentration of ambient oxygen.

It is postulated that concentrated oxygen inhaled by the premature infant leads to vasoconstriction and closure of the arterioles, leading to hypoxia. To overcome this hypoxia the endothelial cells proliferate adjacent to closed capillaries. It takes about 4 weeks to go through the above cycle; by this time the baby is removed from the incubator and the child breaths in the room air. As the oxygen is cutoff; a second wave of changes start acting in the form of neovascularization, some of these newly sprouted vessels are unsupported hence grow in the vitreous to bleed leading to vitreous band formation and ultimately traction retinal detachment with its train of complications.

Following is the natural history of development of ROP.

Premature blood vessels → Exposed to high concentration of O_2 →Vasoconstriction → Occlusion → Hypoxia → Endothelial proliferation → O_2 stopped → Child exposed to normal air → Neovascularization → Vitreous hemorrhage → Traction band → Retinal detachment → Complications of retinal detachment → Blindness

The three factors involved in causing ROP are—prematurity, subnormal weight, and prolonged concentrated oxygen administration. This leads to following riddles.

1. Condition similar to ROP have been reported in full term babies.
2. Premature babies who have not been exposed to high concentration of oxygen too have been reported to have ROP.
3. Role of sudden stoppage of oxygen and irregular flow of oxygen; has not been explored to full extent.

The above questions have lead to explore factors other than prematurity, low birth weight, and hyperoxygenation to be contributory in production of ROP. This leads to examination of role of spindle cells.

The spindle cells are mesenchymal cells that sprout near the developing optic nerve and move toward the periphery. The spindle cell theory is based on the presumption that damaged spindle cells with premature retinal vascularization when exposed to concentrated oxygen release a cytotoxic agent that invades the spindle cells with reduced defense system. This prevents canalization.

Other factor that came under scrutiny was—vascular endothelial growth factor (VEGF.) that is produced in front of the vascular zone and is responsible for development of retina. Stopping of VEGF in natural course or administration of anti VEGF in therapeutic dose has been reported to stop neovascularization.

Deficiency of vitamin E too has been a suspect in production of ROP; the observation has not been substantiated. Though the disorder is sporadic but a genetic predisposition to neovascularization has not been ruled out, additional factors are insulin like growth factor and angioblastic factor.

The highlights of the above observations are:

- The retinal vessels may stop growing at any stage due to ill under stood causes.
- Rarely the temporal retina may be vascularized concurrent with nasal vessels. These retinae will not develop ROP.
- 90% of ROP will have spontaneous regression.
- Spontaneous regression is more common in early stage.
- Shorter the gestation—smaller the baby—more is the risk of ROP.
- Incidence of ROP is inversely proportional to birth weight.
- Administration of oxygen is not sole cause of ROP.
- Short-term administration of oxygen dose not results in ROP.
- Sudden stoppage of oxygen may precipitate worsening of ROP.
- Infant weighing <1,000 g is more likely to develop ROP.

PATHOGENESIS

By eighth month of gestation the developing nasal vessels are almost mature hence not much influenced by extra oxygen but the temporal vessels that have more mesenchymal tissue are still sensitive to extra oxygen. The mature capillaries that have survived the onslaught of hyperoxygenation join to form arteriovenous shunts located at the junction of vascular and avascular area.

In the past the disorder was divided in two phases:

1. *Phase 1:* Also known as hyperoxia—vaso-cessation phase; where there is delayed retinal vascular growth.
2. *Phase 2:* Also known as hypoxia—revascularization phase. This is a stage of release of vaso-stimulating factors after hypoxia caused in phase 1.

Terry 1942 labeled the condition as retrolental fibroplasia, it was soon realized that there were many disorders that also could be called the same. The debate regarding nomenclature continued till an internationally accepted term; ROP was coined in1983–84. This is now universally accepted. This classification was mostly a topographical division to facilitate knowledge of extent, progression/regression of the disorder, and mode of management.

Its components are: Zones, extent, and stage. To this were added terms: plus disease, prethreshold disease, threshold disease, and Rush disease.

ZONES

To demarcate the zones, the retina is divided in three unequal zones; one, two, and three **(Fig. 5.1)**.

The zone one, is the innermost and smallest zone corresponding to posterior pole. It is a circle, with optic

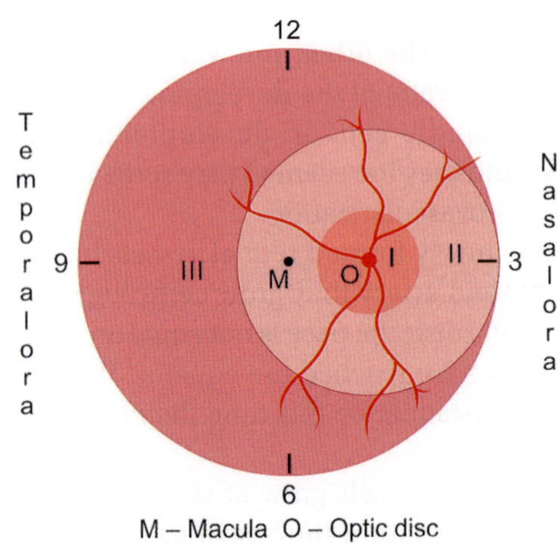

Fig. 5.1: Zones of retinopathy of prematurity.

nerve head as its center, the radius of the circle is two times the distance between the center and the fovea.

The zone two, is larger than zone one, it shares a common center with zone one, its radius is the distance between the center and the nasal ora, its nasal periphery touches the nasal ora at 3 o'clock in the right eye and 9 o'clock in the left eye.

The zone three is the largest zone, it differs from the other two in the sense that it is centered on the macula, with radius equal to distance between macula and nasal ora. It comprises of a concentric space left by the outer border of zone two, it is widest on most temporal ora.

- *Extent:* It is labeled as number of hours on the face of a clock, i.e., 1–12. While noting the extent, it is important to note if the lesions are contiguous or noncontiguous.
- *Staging:* As per norms laid down in Inter National Classification of Retinopathy of Prematurity (ICROP); the disorder has been put in five stages according to severity, i.e., 1–5. In record they are mentioned by numbers. Stage 3 is further divided as mild, moderate, and severe, while stage 4 is divided in to A and B.

The following **Table 5.1** shows stages and their features.

TABLE 5.1: Features and stages of retinopathy of prematurity.

Stages	*Features*
1	Only line of demarcation
2	Ridge formation
3	Extra retinal fibrovascular proliferation
4	A. Subtotal retinal detachment without involving macula B. Subtotal retinal detachment with involving macula
5	Total retinal detachment

Description of Various Stages of Retinopathy of Prematurity (Fig. 5.2)

Stage 1: This consists of a definite pale line between the anterior avascular and posterior vascular retina, it is not raised structure, it is a flat landmark.

Stage 2: The line of demarcation is converted in a definite structure; with height and width. It assumes the curvature of the globe, it has a pink tinge as against paleness of the line of demarcation.

Stage 3: This is stage of development of fibrovascular proliferation projecting above the retina without invading a vascular zone.

Stage 4: This represents an advanced stage of retinopathy, with variable degree of retinal detachment that is mostly tractional in nature, worsened by super added exudation. Initially it may spare the macula; this is labeled as stage 4A. Involvement of macula is called stage 4B.

Stage 5: This is stage of total retinal detachment, the detached retina assuming funnel shape.

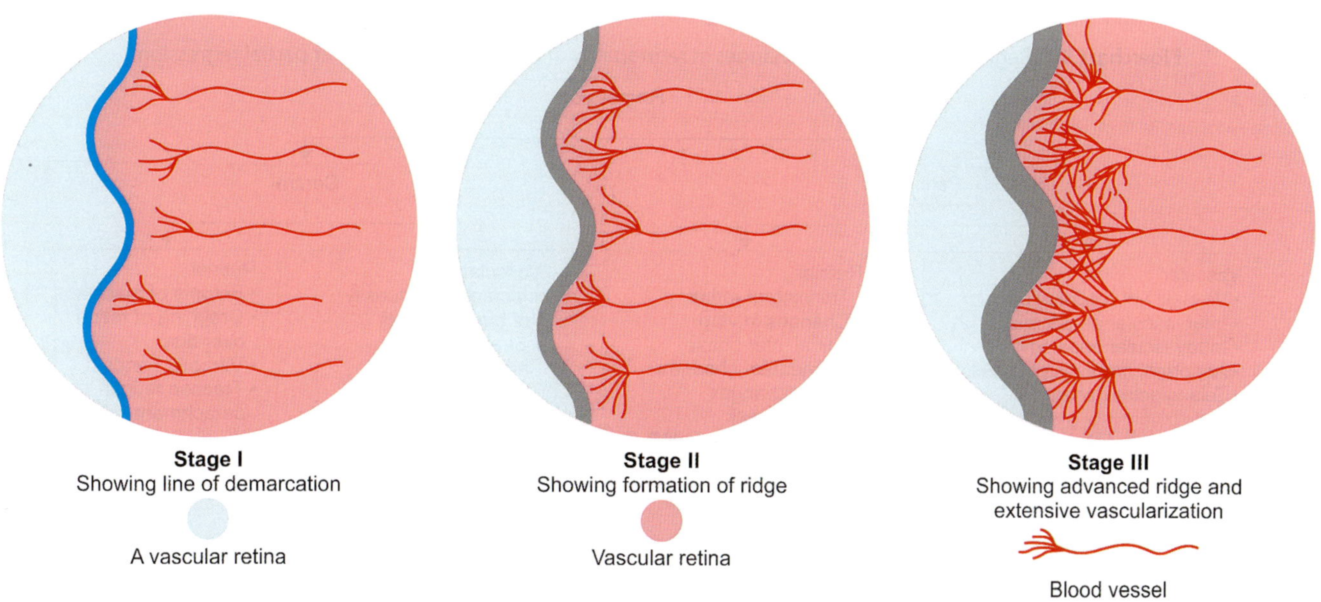

Fig. 5.2: Stages of retinopathy of prematurity.

SPECIFIC TYPES OF RETINOPATHY OF PREMATURITY (TABLE 5.2)

The flowchart depicts regression and residual changes in ROP after partial regression **(Flowchart 5.1)**.

Following are the other changes following complete/partial regression **(Table 5.3)**

No examination for ROP is required at birth even if a child is preterm and underweighed. First examination for ROP. Should be done 4–6 weeks after birth.

Examination of a child suspected to have retinopathy of prematurity

Exception to above are:

- Babies at risk* should have at least one examination in fourth week after birth.
- Babies weighing <1,200 g at birth.
- Babies born with gestational age of 24–30 weeks.

Guidelines for ocular examination of a baby suspected to have ROP

- The examination should be done in neonatal intensive care unit.
- With complete surgical anti sepsis and asepsis.
- By an ophthalmologist well versed in neo natal ophthalmology and retinal land marks of neonatal eye.

TABLE 5.2: Specific types of retinopathy of prematurity.

Condition	***Clinical features***
Prethreshold disease	• Any stage; in zone one with plus disease • Stage 3 in zone two, three contiguous or five noncontiguous. Clock hours involvement with plus disease, it progresses fast hence, requiring frequent examination. If it does not stop at this stage the condition passes in to stage of threshold disease where active treatment is mandatory
Threshold disease detachment	This is the most crucial stage that may pass to subtotal/total retinal if not stopped. It consists of zone 1 and 2, stage 3, extent 5–8 contiguous lesions. Treatment is essential
Plus disease	This is a stage of fast progression, involving both; anterior and posterior segments. There is marked dilatation of veins and arterioles, the iris is swollen due to engorgement of the vessels, this results in rigid constricted pupil that is difficult to dilate, the vitreous may be hazy
Rush disease	Also known as type 2 ROP or aggressive posterior ROP. If untreated it soon passes in stage 5 ROP. It is located most posteriorly with aggressive peripheral vascularization
Regression	80% of cases of ROP will regress, regression can occur at any stage. Clinical features of regression have been divided in two broad groups, i.e., peripheral and central. Each part has again divided in vascular and retina components

Flowchart 5.1: Regression and residual changes in retinopathy of prematurity (ROP) after partial regression.

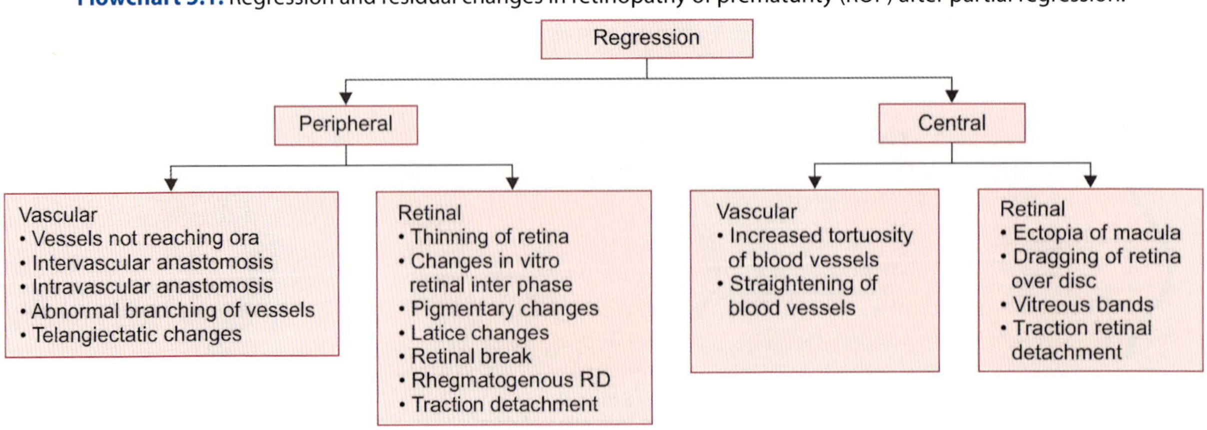

**Babies at risk*

- Premature babies who have been exposed to oxygen for >30 days.
- Premature twins and triplets.
- Babies with respiratory distress.
- Babies with infection.
- Blood transfused babies.
- Babies with intraventricular hemorrhage.

- Preferably by a small pupil indirect ophthalmoscope using: neonatal eye speculum, scleral depression, and plus 28 D lens, under topical anesthesia. As neonatal pupil not only dilates poorly, it requires a combination of cycloplegics of different therapeutic action to get optimal dilatation. The aim should be best dilatation with least side effect. The most popular combination consist of—tropicamide 1% and phenylephrine not >2.5%. Atropine is not recommended in neonates. The frequency of instillation should not exceed more than two times at interval of 15 minutes.
- All findings should be drawn on chart with date for future reference and comparison.
- Inform the parents the exact date of next examination.
- Digital camera like RETCAM can be used for unbiased examination and preservation.

Following pupils dilate poorly (in all ages)—neonatal pupil, congenital microcoria, profuse persistent pupillary membrane, occlusio pupil, seclusive pupil, prolonged use of miotic, neovascularization of iris.

TABLE 5.3: Other changes following complete/partial regression.

Posterior polar	*Others*
Pallor of disc	Myopia
Vitreous haze	Complicated cataract
Vitreous hemorrhage	Secondary glaucoma
Retinal neovascularization	Amblyopia, squint, nystagmus
Retinal hemorrhage	
Rhegmatogenous retinal detachment	

Schedule of Examination (Table 5.4)

- First examination should be between 4 and 6 weeks after birth.
- High risk prethreshold eyes should be subjected to treatment within 3 days of confirmation of findings.
- There after examination depends on clinical findings.

TREATMENT

80% of ROP in zone 3 may regress with some sequel. Treatment of advanced ROP. Involving zone 1 and posterior zone 2 is difficult.

The following **Flowchart 5.2** is one of recommended protocol of management as per zone.

Treatment Available

Treatment of ROP is multifactorial, it should be remembered that all cases do not require treatment. 80% of cases confined to zone 3 have tendency for spontaneous regression. Each child requires a personalized management.

TABLE 5.4: Schedule of examination.

Clinical picture	*Follow-up*
Immature vessels reaching posterior pole	Twice a week
Low risk threshold ROP	Weekly
Minimal prethreshold ROP	Alternate week

Flowchart 5.2: Recommended protocol of management of ROP.

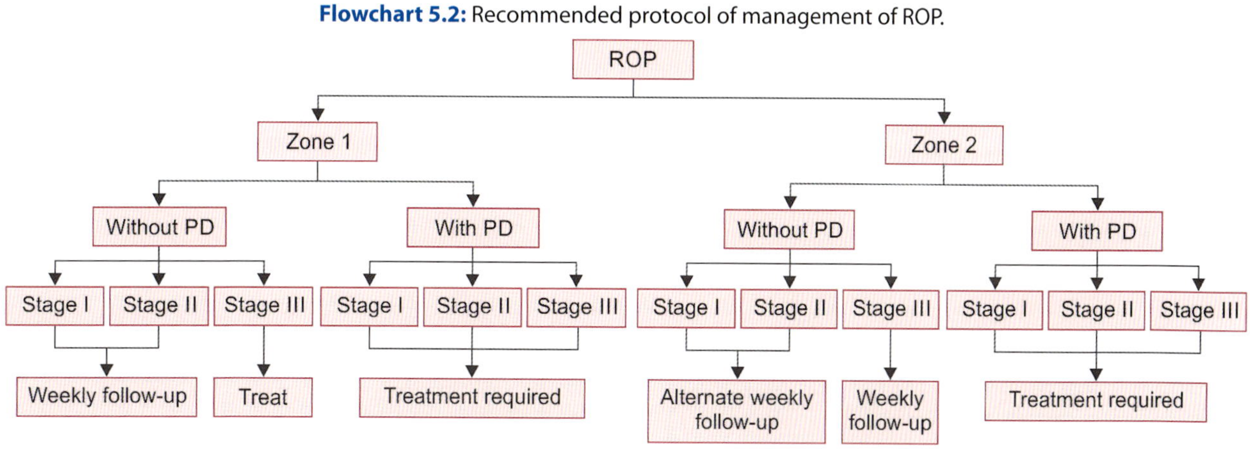

Different institutions follow different protocol. Incidence of ROP is inversely proportionate to birth weight. The rule of thumb is 20% of all premature babies will develop strabismus and refractive error by 3 year.

> There is no known specific treatment, the management is directed to ameliorate the condition, salvage as much vision as possible, and rehabilitate the child.

Following modes are employed, mostly in combination, repeated surgeries, and nonsurgical sessions may be required, they are:

- Cryotherapy
- *Laser photocoagulation:*
    - DIODE 810 nm.
        - Nd Yag 532 nm (both are delivered through indirect ophthalmoscope)
- *Intravitreal anti VEGF:*
    - Bevacizumb, 0.625 mg
        - Ranibizumab, 0.25 mg
- Vitreoretinal surgery
- Management of cataract, glaucoma, squint, and nystagmus
- Rehabilitation

SUGGESTED READING

1. Adams GW, Bates A. Retinopathy of prematurity in Moorfields. In: Jackson TL (Ed). Manual of ophthalmology, 3rd edition. New Delhi: JP Medical publishers; 2020. pp. 635-40.
2. Arvind eye care system. Retinopathy of prematurity, ophthalmological approach. Available from https://aravind.org/diseases/retinopathy-of-prematurity/ [Last accessed February, 2025].
3. Azad R, Trese MT. Textbook of retinopathy of prematurity, 1st edition. Netherlands: Lippincot-Willims and Wilkins; 2011.
4. Cibis GW, Tongue AC, Stass ML. Decision making in pediatric ophthalmology. Mosby: St. Louis Missouri; 1996.
5. Deborah Pavan-Langston. Manual of ocular diagnosis and therapy, 6th edition. Netherlands: Lippincot Williams & Wilkins; 2008.
6. Glen A, Gole MD. International classification of retinopathy of prematurity. Arch Ophth. 2005;123:991-9.
7. Gupta AK, Krishna V. Retinopathy of prematurity in clinical ophthalmology, 9th edition. New Delhi: Elsevier; 2011. pp. 410-8.
8. Hardy RS, Good WV, Dobson V, Palmer EA, Phelps DL, Quintos M, et al. Early treatment for retinopathy of prematurity, clinical trial-presentation by sub group versus analysis within subgroup. Arch Ophth. 2003. pp. 1684-96.
9. Jalali S, Anand R, Kumar H, Dogra MR, Azad R, Gopal L. Programme, planning, and screening strategy in retinopathy of prematurity. Indian J Ophthalmol. 2003;51(1): 89-99.
10. Mukherjee PK. Pediatric ophthalmology, 1st edition. Retinopathy of prematurity. New Delhi: New Age International; 2005.
11. Radhakrishna N, Pai PR. Retinopathy of prematurity. Kerala Jr. Oph xxv 4; 2013.
12. Saxena S. Clinical practice in ophthalmology, 1st edition. New Delhi: J.P. Brothers; 2003.

CHAPTER 6

Leukocoria White Reflex in Pupillary Area (Amaurotic Cat's Eye)

Retinoblastoma, a mostly blinding and occasionally fatal intraocular tumor, is the most common cause of white reflex in the pupillary area in children. Apart from retinoblastoma, there are many causes that render whiteness to the pupil, most of which are occasionally blinding with exceptional fatality.

Till the last century, all white reflexes on the visual axis were called leukocoria, irrespective of their location. This practice continued until they were put into three groups: Prelenticular, lenticular, and retrolenticular. In 1950, it was decided to exclude prelenticular and lenticular lesions from this categorization. Leukocoria was defined as a white reflex in the pupillary area with a clear lens (uniocular or binocular) under 5 years of age. The shortcoming of this classification was that it excluded childhood cataracts from the list, though they are more common than all other causes put together. Cataract is a benign, nonblinding, nonfatal, easily diagnosed, and manageable condition, in contrast to retinoblastoma, a potentially blinding and fatal condition.

As per the previous classification, the list of causes of leukocoria was long.

They can be any of the following alone or in combination:

- *Glioma:*
    - Benign
    - Malignant
- Developmental anomalies
- Inflammatory
- Vascular
- Genetic aberration
- Miscellaneous

The division that followed earlier was glioma and pseudogliomas; the term glioma denoted retinoblastoma on the wrong presumption that retinoblastoma developed from glial tissue. The better term that followed was to divide white reflexes into two classes, i.e., retinoblastoma and nonretinoblastoma. This still failed to separate nonretinoblastomatous conditions from each other, which was needed for specific treatment for each. However, the most acclaimed dictum remains.

> All white reflexes in the pupillary area in children are considered to be retinoblastoma unless proved otherwise.

Thus, leukocoria was divided into two groups:

1. With a clear lens
2. Without a clear lens

This not only took the transparency of the lens into consideration but also laterality, age of first presentation, and heredity.

The list for the first group consists of:

- Persistent hyperplastic primary vitreous (PHPV)
- Coats disease
- Retinopathy of prematurity
- Astrocytic hamartoma
- Familial exudative vitreoretinopathy
- Retinochoroidal coloboma
- Endogenous endophthalmitis
- Incontinentia pigmenti
- Retinal detachment
- Medullated nerve fibers
- Medulloepithelioma
- Pars planitis
- Retinal dysplasia
- Norrie disease

The second group consists of:

- Exudate covering the pupillary area
- Cataract
- Posterior cyclitic membrane

PERSISTENT HYPERPLASTIC PRIMARY VITREOUS

This is the most common nonmalignant cause of white reflex in the pupillary area detected before 1-year, formerly known as persistent fetal vasculature; it is a developmental anomaly of the vitreous. That may be detected even at birth;

the condition is unilateral, and the eye is invariably microphthalmic, which is the clue to the diagnosis, which, on close look, gives a white reflex.

There are two types of PHPV:

1. Anterior
2. Posterior

Anterior Persistent Hyperplastic Primary Vitreous

This is the more common of the two. This is a developmental anomaly of the primary vitreous. Developmentally, vitreous tissue develops in two main stages: Primary and secondary. (See development of vitreous.) During development, the primary vitreous is replaced completely by the secondary vitreous; if the primary vitreous fails to regress, it proliferates, and the condition is called PHPV. This leads to two eventualities: The first is retardation of the growth and development of the eye, and the second is the development of a mass behind the lens that looks white. The remnants of the hyaloid system of arteries may be included in this mesenchymal vitreous. The blood vessels develop at the center of this mass and are visible even under simple oblique illumination at birth. The vessels spread toward the ciliary body and produce notable changes in the ciliary processes. The ciliary processes get attached to the expanding mass, and in a few weeks, the mass starts contracting, pulling the ciliary complex centrally and imparting white color to the pupillary reflex. The contracting mass may stretch the posterior lens capsule as well, which may cause rent in the posterior lens capsule, ending in opacification of the lens and being mistaken for congenital cataracts. The larger the rent, the faster and denser the cataract develops; microscopic rents take more time to develop cataracts.

Clinical Features

The disorder is seen all over the world, in all races, equally in both sexes, without any hereditary predisposition, and in full-term babies with a normal birth weight without exposure to concentrated oxygen for a long time. The affected eye looks smaller than the other and may even be microphthalmic, with a white reflex in the pupil that may be mistaken for a congenital cataract by an untrained resident. The anterior chamber may be shallower than expected and may have a coloboma of the iris and lens or a persistent pupillary membrane. Under mydriasis, a retrolental white mass becomes obvious, to which ciliary processes may be attached; in a few instances, part of the tunica vasculosa lentis may be visible. Generally, the pupil is rigid and difficult to dilate; episodes of hemorrhage are common. Generally, the lens is transparent or may have a small stationary opacity in the posterior part in the case of a small tear in the posterior capsule. In the case of a large rupture, the whole lens becomes opaque and swollen due to the imbibement of fluid that may be present at birth or may take days to weeks to happen; the lens may be swollen enough to cause secondary lens-induced glaucoma. Over time, the swollen lens gets liquefied and ultimately converts into a membranous cataract; this may be mistaken for congenital aphakia. The retina may develop traction detachments. The above is a description of the chronology of PHPV; all the findings may not be concurrent and may not follow the classical course.

Diagnosis

Diagnosis is not difficult in a unilateral small eye in a full-term baby with expected weight without a history of prolonged oxygenation.

The diagnosis is confirmed by indirect ophthalmoscopy with indentation, B-scan ultrasonography, computed tomography (CT), and magnetic resonance imaging (MRI).

Management

The management of PHPV is difficult and time-consuming. There is no test to predict it antenatally; no method to prevent it, no medical treatment, and only available management consists of a series of surgeries that too have unpredictable results.

The aim of the treatment is to salvage as much vision as possible, prevent complications, manage complications present, and take measures to maintain orbital growth. The cataract is managed by a standard microsurgical lensectomy. These cases are not suitable for intraocular lens (IOL). The mass is removed by vitrectomy, and the detachment is repaired by the standard method.

In spite of successful surgeries, visual and cosmetic results are poor.

Posterior Persistent Hyperplastic Primary Vitreous

The term seems to be a misnomer; primary vitreous has hardly any role in its etiopathology; and it is more of a proliferation of the hyaloid vascular system with proliferative bands extending from the disc to the retinal periphery than vitreous proliferation.

The anomaly can be put into two broad classes:

1. Involving the hyaloid vascular system.
2. Papillovitreal bands.

The anomalies of the hyaloid system are: Bergmeister papilla, persistent hyaloid artery, fragmented pieces of hyaloid artery vessel loops, and corkscrew vessels.

Papillovitreal bands: The condition is confined to the posterior pole; the band may rarely reach up to the ora and may develop in any quadrant, the most common being inferior lower. The children with the so-called posterior form PHPV are brought for examination late; the average age of the first visit is seldom <6 years, contrary to the anterior form, which is <1 year. The common features between the two are that both are sporadic and unilateral. The posterior form is not associated with microphthalmia. However, the cornea is generally smaller than normal, and the lens is clear. The child is brought in with either diminished vision, a squint, or both. On examination, the anterior segment was found to be normal with a positive Bruckner test. Retinoscopy reveals hypermetropia that is not correctable, along with a white reflex in the retinoscopy glow. In all cases, the fundus should be examined with an indirect ophthalmoscope, three mirror gonioscopes, B-scan sonography, and CT to help differentiate from retinoblastoma. There is no specific treatment. The vitreous bands are better removed to prevent traction retinal detachment.

RETINOPATHY OF PREMATURITY

For details, *See* Chapter 5.

RETINAL ASTROCYTIC HAMARTOMA

Retinal astrocytic hamartomas are benign retinal tumors of retinal glial cells, generally met with tuberous sclerosis isolated tumors too have been reported. They do not require any specific treatment.

RETINAL DYSPLASIA

The importance of this rare condition lies in the fact that this condition shows rosettes on histopathology, which is a diagnostic feature of retinoblastoma. It is a blinding disease but not fatal, like retinoblastoma. The most accepted theory about its causation is that it is a faulty embryonic differentiation of the inner layer of the optic cup. The eye is generally microphthalmic with a noncataractous white reflex. That is caused either by retinal folds or retinal detachment; the eye generally goes into phthisis. Other associated conditions are uveal coloboma, persistent hyperplastic primary vitreous, recurrent retinal, and vitreous hemorrhages.

NORRIE DISEASE

This is found only in male children. The ocular features are leukocoria, traction retinal detachment, abnormal retinal vasculature, and retinal and vitreous hemorrhages. The associated nonocular defect is neurosensory deafness.

INCONTINENTIA PIGMENTI

This condition is found in both sexes; the males, due to some unexplained causes, die soon after birth; hence all cases reported are in females. The ocular features are: Leukocoria, traction retinal detachment, proliferative retinal pigment epithelium, and occasional uveitis. Systemic involvements include transient skin lesions, dental anomalies, seizures, and mental retardation.

FAMILIAL EXUDATIVE VITREORETINOPATHY

This is a congenital bilateral hereditary disorder. The heredity is variable; it can either be any of the following: Autosomal dominant, recessive, or sex-linked. Many of the family members may be symptomless carriers, making it imperative to examine as many members of the family as possible by indirect ophthalmoscope with scleral indentation and, if possible, by wide-angle fundus fluorescein angiography and RetCam*.

The condition clinically resembles retinal retinopathy of premature, Coats disease, pars planitis, retinal telangiectasias; the conditions require differentiation from each other; and retinoblastoma.

The condition can be divided into vascular and vitreous changes.

The vascular changes are: The changes are thought to be due to abnormal angiogenesis. It is apoptosis (*the process of programmed cell death.*) that hampers the development of retinal vessels that are converted into fibrous bands,

*RetCam is a wide-field digital color imaging system that is not only used to see the fundus but is also used to document the progress of the disease, especially in children.

which later cause traction retinal detachment. The retinal changes consist of subretinal, interretinal hemorrhages, and exudates posterior to the ora serrata, mostly on the temporal side, traction detachment of the retina.

The retinal changes are: The interretinal fluid is converted into hard exudates in the fashion of an arc around the macula; this was formerly called circinate retinopathy, which is not specific and seen in many conditions, hence no more in vogue. The subretinal fluid may cause single or multiple subretinal masses or cause exudative retinal detachment.

The vitreous changes are: Multiple vascular bands all over the vitreous.

Depending on severity and duration, the disorder has been divided into two groups:

1. As per symptoms
2. As per the fundus findings

As per symptoms, the disorder can be mild, moderate, or severe.

Mild cases can be asymptomatic, with complaints of diminished vision, squinting, or both. The children are generally under 5 years of age. On examination, the eyes are noncongested, with a normal anterior chamber, brisk pupil, or relative afferent pupil if there is a marked difference in visual acuity between the two eyes. Bruckner's test may be positive. The lens and vitreous on oblique illumination look transparent. On retinoscopy, there may be grayness in the midst of a pink glow. Striking features are revealed on indirect ophthalmoscopy: The retinal vessels are dilated and tortuous; there may be micro- or macroaneurisms with interretinal or subretinal soft or hard exudates arranged in a wreath-like fashion around the macula.

In moderate cases, most of the lesions at this stage involve both eyes and may not be symmetric, exudative, shallow, or bullous detachments with crystals on the surface and subretinal hemorrhages. Severe cases are generally painful blind eyes. They have total retinal detachment, rubeosis of the iris, nonvascular glaucoma, and complicated cataracts.

As per fundus findings:

Initially, it was categorized as:

- Only exudation
- Exudation with vascular changes
- Angiomatosis was added to the above findings.

The categorization did not include other features; hence, a new classification was put forward.

That divided the disorder into five stages:

1. Stage of telangiectasia only
2. Stage of exudate on or round the macula, along with telangiectasia
3. Stage of partial or total retinal detachment
4. Stages of rubeosis of the anterior uvea, neovascular glaucoma, and complicated cataracts
5. *Stage of pain:* Full blindness

Still more elaborate staging is:

- Avascular periphery
- *Retinal neovascularisation:*
  - Without exudation
  - With exudation
- *Extramacular retinal detachment:*
  - Without exudate
  - With exudate
- *Subtotal macular involvement in retinal detachment:*
  - Without exudate
  - With exudate
- Total retinal detachment

Diagnosis

The anomaly can be diagnosed with certainty even in the early clinical phase with proper evaluation of the retinal periphery by indirect ophthalmoscope of not only the child, generally under 10, but also his family members who may be asymptomatic carriers. Fluorescein angiography of family members helps in clinching the diagnosis. The bands are anchored not only to the peripheral but also to the central retina, dragging the macula. The bands are accompanied by abnormally thick vessels that are the cause of recurrent hemorrhages. The other common feature is the sudden stoppage of peripheral vessels in a rounded manner, leaving an avascular zone beyond the scalloped edge of the vascularized retina with a raised ridge similar to retinopathy of prematurity. Another condition that may be confused with this is persistent hyperplastic primary vitreous. Occasionally, the condition may stop progressing in the early phase, preventing the eye from going blind; however, most unattended eyes pass through the stage of painful blindness.

Management

There is no preventive method as the condition is genetic with positive family history, this makes it essential to examine as many family members as possible to find out asymptomatic carriers and give them genetic counseling.

The treatment is similar to the treatment of retinopathy of prematurity, i.e., cryotherapy, selective laser, lens extraction by standard procedure, and vitrectomy. The prognosis is poor.

COATS DISEASE

The condition was also referred to as Leber's miliary aneurysm and retinal telangiectasia; the first is now considered as forme fruste of Coats disease. There are many conditions that can be put under the second group hence is not considered to be specific. Coats disease is one of the conditions that cause a white reflex in the pupil of a child, hence requiring differentiation from the fatal condition of retinoblastoma and other nonfatal entities that give white reflex; there may be a somatic mutation of other conditions, especially of Norris disease.

Coates disease is an idiopathic, nonhereditary, congenital disorder that is generally not apparent before 5 years of age; it is found in all races, with preponderance among boys (80%). Cases are unilateral in 90% of patients; the children afflicted are full term, with a birth weight of >1,200 g. There is no systemic involvement. The age of the first presentation ranges between 5 and 20. The younger the age of the first presentation severe is the condition and poorer is the prognosis. Spontaneous regression is known. Recurrence years after treatment has been reported.

It is the severest form of retinal telangiectasia, involving not only retinal arteries and veins but chorio capillaries as well. The common vascular changes are tortuosity of vessels, aneurism and neovascularization, recurrent retinal hemorrhages that may culminate in hemophthalmos, the telangiectasia vessels exude lipoprotein-rich fluid that seeps in and under the retina, causing serious detachment and a gray raised mass in the retina that gives a white reflex on retinoscopy and oblique illumination.

The sequence of the condition is:
Abnormal vascular endothelia → Telangiectasia → Aneurism → Defect in blood-retinal barrier → Exudation → Submacular mass → Proliferation of RPE → Increased hemorrhage and exudation → Localized retinal detachment → Subtotal detachment → Total detachment → Blindness.

From time to time, many attempts have been made to put the disorder into classes, groups, and stages for ease of its management. Following is one of the clinical classifications of Coats disease, which is divided into five categories from one to five; the second and third are subdivided into a and b.

1. Retinal vessel telangiectasia and aneurism
2. a. Extra foveal exudate
   b. Foveal exudate
3. a. Partial exudative retinal detachment
   b. Total retinal detachment
4. Secondary glaucoma
5. Blindness

A classification put forward in 1965 is as follows:
- *Stage 1:* Only focal exudates
- *Stage 2:* Massive interretinal exudates
- *Stage 3:* Localized exudative retinal detachment
- *Stage 4:* Total retinal detachment
- *Stage 5:* Neovascularization glaucoma—painful full-blind eye

A more exhaustive classification by Shield et al. is:
- *Stage 1:* Retinal telangiectasia only
- *Stage 2: Telangiectasia and exudates—*
  - Exudation does not involve maculas.
  - Exudation with macular involvement
- *Stage 3: Subtotal retinal detachment—*
  - Macula spared
  - Macula involved
- *Stage 4:* Total retinal detachment with neovascular glaucoma
- *Stage 5:* Blindness

The fundus findings are corroborated with findings from fundus fluorescein angiography, ultrasonography, and CT.

The fundus fluorescing angiograph shows dilated, tortuous vessels with typical light bulb appearance; micro and macro aneurisms; telangiectatic vessels; nonperfusion of capillaries; and nonperfusion of peripheral vessels.

Ultrasonography is the easiest, nonfrightening examination for the child; it is the most helpful method to differentiate retinoblastoma from Coats disease. Coats disease does not show a well-formed tumor mass. A well-marked exudate is a hallmark of Coats disease; there is no intraocular calcification in Coats disease that is common in retinoblastoma. Coats disease may show some cholesterol deposits, which are less refractile than calcium deposits in retinoblastoma.

Computed tomography in Coats disease: Depending on stage, in the early stages, the tumor appears as a solid mass with areas of calcification that have a density similar to bone.

TABLE 6.1: Comparison between Coats disease and retinoblastoma.

	Coates disease	*Retinoblastoma*
Frequency	Rarer than retinoblastoma	Far more common than Coats disease
Age of first presentation	Mostly after 5 years	As early as the first year of life
Limit of first presentation	Rare after 20 years	Rare after 5 years
Family history	Negative	Positive in hereditary form
Sex	More in boys	Equal among boys and girls
Laterality	Mostly unilateral	Unilateral or bilateral
Tissue of origin	Vascular	Retinoblast
Extraocular extension	Nil	Common
White reflex	Late	Early
Retinal detachment	Exudative	Solid
Intraocular calcification	Nil	Present
Spontaneous regression	Possible	Possible
Threat to life	Nil	Potentially life-threatening

Other conditions that require differentiation from Coats disease consist of all the conditions that cause white reflex in the pupillary area: PHPV, parasitic endophthalmitis, Leber's miliary aneurism*, von Hippel-Lindau disease†, ROP, capillary hemangioma of the retina‡, cavernous hemangioma of the retina§, familial exudative vitreoretinopathy, and Choroidal hemangioma.

**Leber's miliary aneurism:* Thought to be a forme fruste of Coats disease. It is the mildest form of Costs disease.

†*Von Hippel-Lindau disease:* Hereditary, benign vascular growth of the retina with involvement of the brain and spinal cord.

‡*Capillary hemangioma of the retina:* Develops near the optic nerve, is unilateral, single-type (central and peripheral), may be associated with von Hippel-Lindau disease, and responds to photocoagulation.

§*Cavernous hemangioma of the retina:* They arise not only from the retina but also from the optic papilla, in small bunches filled with venous blood predisposed to bleeding. On the fundus fluorescein angiograph, they show sluggish flow. Do not require treatment until bleeding occurs.

Magnetic resonance imaging in Coats disease: Depending on the stage of the disease, the findings are similar to those seen in CT but have better resolution and can pick up the earliest changes. It does not show the presence of calcification; it measures the size of the globe that is smaller than its normal counterpart.

Optical coherence tomography (OCT) in coats dieses helps in monitoring macular involvement, showing epiretinal membrane subretinal fluid. It delineates retinal detachment, lipid deposition, and microstructural changes.

Other investigations used to conform to the disorder are indocyanine angiography, structural spectral domain OCT, and OCT angiography.

The conditions that are associated with retinal telangiectasia are:

- Coates disease
- Leber's miliary aneurism
- Von Hippel-Lindau angiomatosis retinae
- Capillary telangiectasia
- Racemose hemangioma of the retina

Difference between Coats disease and retinoblastoma

The most important condition that needs to be differentiated from Coats disease is retinoblastoma.

Table 6.1 highlights the differences.

Management of Coats Disease

Management of Coats disease depends on the duration and stage of the disease, which are divided into two parts:

1. Management of telangiectasia and exudate
2. Management of rubeosis of the iris, neovascular glaucoma, and retinal detachment

The usual protocol is:

Stage	Procedure
Stage 1	Laser photocoagulation
Stage 2	Photo coagulation and cryotherapy
Stage 3	Laser + cryo + retinal detachment surgery

Contd...

Contd...

Stage	*Procedure*
Stage 4	Above + anti-glaucoma management of glaucoma
Intravitreal anti-VEGF* has been tried without uniform result.	

**Anti-VEGF:* Vascular endothelial growth factor is a naturally occurring protein that promotes the growth of new blood vessels. It makes the blood vessels prone to leak. Anti-VEGF medicines act against VEGF by stopping the formation of new vessels and the growth of already present vessels. The most commonly used anti-VEGF drugs in ophthalmology are ranibizumab (Lucentis) and bevacizumab (Avastin). The drugs are monoclonal antibodies that bind VEGF. Out of the two, Lucentis is more effective than Lucentis. The other drugs available are sorafenib, aflibercept, dasatinib, sunitinib, nilotinib, and pazopanib. All are not equally effective; hence, they are not used universally.

OCULAR TOXOCARIASIS

Toxocariasis is a zoonosis* caused by a parasite called *Toxocara canis*, a round worm of dogs of all categories, i.e., domestic, feral, and wild. It is not spread by adult canines but by puppies born to infected mothers. The humans are the accidental hosts, in whom the parasite develops to the third stage without laying eggs. The dogs are the definitive hosts. The puppies born to an infected bitch are responsible for the spread of the disease in children; adults are not immune. An incident in adult human is less than in children. The activated larvae from the mother bitch are passed to puppies in utero via the placenta. By the time the puppies are born, they already harbor the third stage of larvae, which are passed in the puppies' feces, which commonly contaminate the soil and vegetables grown in the contaminated soil. Vegetables and fruits washed in contaminated soil are yet another source of contamination.

The following is the natural history of the disease:
Infected pregnant bitch → Placenta → Puppy growing in utero → Puppy born with third stage → Ova → Passed in feces of puppy → Soil contaminated by ova → Contaminated soil/food consumed by child → Infection → LVM/ocular/systemic → Laraval migrance

The eggs responsible for the disease must be embryonated; the eggs in puppies' stools are not embryonated initially; it takes them about a fortnight to get embryonated. If the nonembryonated eggs are ingested by children or dogs, they remain noninfective and dormant in the soil until consumed. After ingestion, the eggs are converted into larvae. The larvae develop in the lumen of the gut, and from there they find their way to the gut wall, where they are picked up by blood and spread to various parts of the body, i.e., the skin, eyes, liver, lungs, and brain.

Toxocariasis is a chronic multisystemic helminthic disease of children found all over the world, more in developing and underdeveloped countries, mostly due to a lack of awareness, hygiene, and poor medical facilities, both human and veterinary. Children with pet dogs are at higher risk; pica among infants is yet another predisposing factor; and it is equally common among boys and girls. Infection by toxocara is broadly divided into two categories, i.e., systemic and ocular **(Flowchart 6.1)**.

Visceral toxocariasis is the first phase of the disease seen in younger children, with the average age being 2 years. Visceral toxocariasis is caused by antigens liberated by the migrating larvae. The child may be asymptomatic for many months and then develop myriads of symptoms such as anemia, pain in the abdomen, nodules under the skin, hepatosplenomegaly, recurrent respiratory infection, lung infiltrates, wheezing, and frequent seizures. Eosinophilia is common.

Ocular toxocariasis develops in older children with an average age of 7 years, in contrast to 2 years in visceral toxocariasis, more common in boys; unilateral left eye involvement is more frequent. Ocular and visceral toxocariasis do not run simultaneously; there is a gap of 5–6 years between the two. Ocular toxocariasis is rare in adults; ocular involvement may be extensive or localized, and both the uvea and retina may be involved separately or together. The uveal involvement is variable; it could be anterior, intermediate, posterior, or pan uveitis; it may be acute or chronic. The other uveal involvement is granuloma formation, which could be solitary posterior or multiple peripherals.

Chronic anterior uveitis: It is associated with multiple, broad posterior synechiae, posterior cyclitic membrane, and hazy vitreous, exudative retinal detachment. The posterior synechiae may be dense enough to cause a white reflex in the pupillary area. Generally, such uveitis is seen in children between 2 and 9 years of age; in the long run, the lens develops; complicated cataracts and secondary glaucoma are common; and the eye is lost in phthisis/absolute glaucoma. In some cases, the eye may have an acute exacerbation of uveitis mimicking endophthalmitis.

Posterior polar granuloma: It is generally solitary, seen in white eyes in older children. Preretinal gliosis is common;

*Zoonosis is a disease transmitted to humans from animals.

Flowchart 6.1: Various possibilities of toxocariasis.

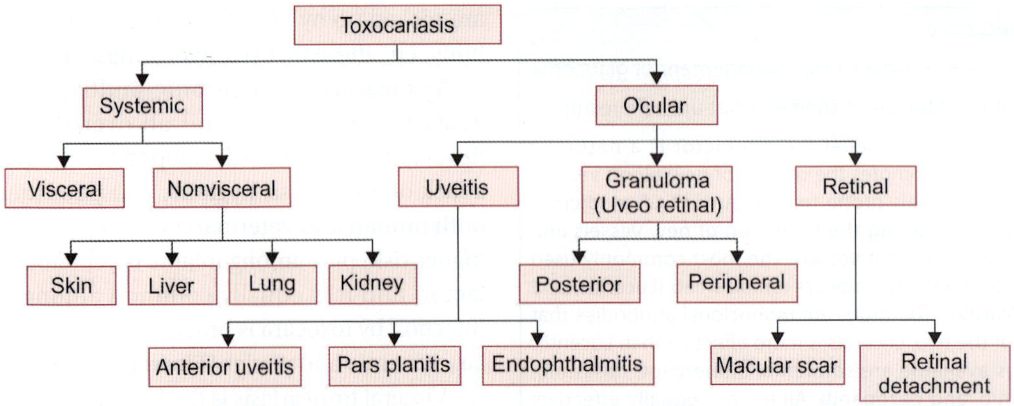

the gliosis is invariably converted into a traction band, causing retinal detachment. The granuloma is hemispheric with convexity toward the vitreous; the granuloma may either be on the macula or in between the macula and the disc. The diameter of the granuloma may be a tiny spot, as large as the disc, or larger. The proximity of the granuloma from the macula influences the visual outcome. Diminished vision is generally the cause that brings the child for consultation; other causes are squint and occasionally a fleeting gray reflex that is confirmed by indirect ophthalmoscopy, examination by +90 D, ultrasonography (USG), and OCT. The condition may be associated with serous retinal detachment and subretinal hemorrhage.

Peripheral granuloma: They are not only seen in older children but also up to the fourth decade in apparently white eyes. The peripheral granulomas too are hemispheric, with varied size and number; vitreous bands are common; the bands may get attached to any structure in the posterior pole, including the macula and the disc; macular adhesion causes dragging of the macula, causing ectopia of the macula; and detachment of the macula. Retrolental gliosis is the cause of the white reflex in the pupil. Peripheral granuloma may often be diagnosed as extensive pars planitis.

Differential Diagnosis

The most important condition that requires to be differentiated is retinoblastoma.

Diagnosis of toxocariasis is facilitated by:

- History of Pica, contact with puppies and kittens
- USG will differentiate it from retinoblastoma.
- *Blood count:* Raised eosinophil count
- Enzyme-linked immunosorbent assay (ELISA)

Table 6.2 depicts a comparison of the clinical features of the common causes of leukocoria.

Management of toxocariasis

The treatment is divided into three parts:

1. Systemic
2. Ocular
3. Prophylaxis

Systemic

- The role of anthelmintics is debatable.
- Treatment of systemic toxocariasis is better left to internist trained in parasitic diseases.
- Commonly used anthelmintics are albendazole, mebendazole, and stromectol, commonly known as ivermectin. Albendazole and mebendazole have been found to be helpful in treating visceral larva migrans.

> Ivermectin was initially developed to combat river blindness (*Wuchereria bancrofti*) and was found to be effective against many intestinal parasites except tapeworm. It is effective against most mites and lice. It does not eradicate flea flukes, flies, and tics; it has no antibacterial or antifungal properties; it is claimed to be effective against some viruses.

Ocular

- Anthelmintics do not cross the blood-retinal barrier hence they have no role in the management of ocular toxocariasis; they even do not have any preventive role either.
- Ocular toxocariasis is treated with cycloplegia and local and periocular steroids.
- Vitrectomy may be required to de-bulk the growth, cut bands, and facilitate renal detachment surgery.

TABLE 6.2: Comparison of the clinical features of causes of leukocoria.

Features	Conditions			
	Retinoblastoma	***Persistent hyperplastic primary vitreous***	***Retinopathy of prematurity***	***Coats disease***
Age of presentation	12 months for bilateral and 18 months for unilateral	At birth	10 weeks postnatal	Infancy or the first decade
Sex	Equal in both sexes	Equal in both sexes	Equal in both sexes	90% males
Laterality	Unilateral 70%, bilateral 30%	Unilateral	Bilateral	Unilateral
Size of the globe	Initially normal, it may become buphthalmic later	Microphthalmic	Normal	Normal
Ciliary processes	Not visible	Visible in most cases	Visible in a few	Not visible
Birth weight	Normal	Normal	<1,500 g	Normal
Prematurity	Nil	Nil	Important factor	Nil
Oxygen supplement	No effect	No effect	Important cause	No effect
Heredity	Significant	No significant	No relation	Noncontributory
Staging and grouping	Significant for management	Not significant	Significant for management	Nonsignificant
X-ray	Intraocular calcification is present in most cases	No calcification	No calcification	No calcification
USG	The tumor is acoustically solid with high internal reflection and calcification	Small size of glow, no calcification	No calcification	No calcification
CT	Depending on stage in early stage, the tumor appears as a solid mass with areas of calcification that have a density similar to bone	Noncontributory	Noncontributory	Shows outline of intraocular changes depending on stage, in the early stage it is normal, later the margin may be mistaken to have retinal detachment, and the edges are well marked. In the late stages, the lesion is hyper dens
MRI	It is the investigation of choice to find out the extension of the tumor that helps in assessing the risk of metastatic	It shows the hyaloid vessel as a tubular structure; total retinal detachment is shown as a funnel; and it delineates the subretinal, retrolental mass, and size of the globe	Noncontributory	Noncontributory
OCT	It can detect the preclinical stage of a posterior pole lesion and has a significant role in intravascular chemotherapy	Not of much use	Use in quantitative and objective assessment	May help in grading the lesion
Metastasis	Common	Nil	Nil	Nil
Extraocular extension	Common	Nil	Nil	Nil
Fatality	May be fatal	Nonfatal	Nonfatal	Nonfatal

Prophylaxis

All house puppies under 6 months should be dewormed as per practice. The role of deworming adult dogs/bitches is debatable.

MEDULLOEPITHELIOMA

Medulloepithelioma of the eye arises from the non-pigmented ciliary epithelium. The two histological classifications are teratoid and nonteratoid; both can be malignant, and 90% of cases are malignant. The non-malignant cases have a tendency to go into malignant form. The condition is unilateral and nonhereditary, seen between 2 and 10 years. The most common presentation is a white reflex in the pupillary area. As the tumor arises from the periphery, the white reflex is not seen in all directions. It may be visible only when the child looks in a particular direction. The condition is often confused with retinoblastoma. The management available in the past was enucleation, which is no more the treatment of choice. Presently, the options are cryotherapy, plaque radiotherapy, and external beam radiotherapy. The role of chemotherapy is not encouraging.

SUGGESTED READING

1. Chandra P, Kumar V. Familial exudative retinopathy. In: Ramamurthy D, Biswas P (Eds). AIOS Ready Reckoner in Ophthalmology, 2nd edition. New Delhi: Jaypee Brothers Medical Publishers; 2017. pp. 476-8.
2. Gillespie SH. Ocular Toxocariasis in Current Ocular Therapy, 5th edition. Philadelphia: W.B. Saunders company; 2000. pp. 97-8.
3. Kaul S, Upaekar M, Mody K, Walinjkar J, Kothari M, Natraj S. Anti vascular endothelial growth factor agent as adjunct in management of Coats disease. IJO. 2010;58: 76-8.
4. Mukherjee PK, Bandyopadhyaya P. Toxocariasis. In: Ocular Microbiology, 1st edition. New Delhi: Jaypee Brothers Medical Publishers; 2010.
5. Mukherjee PK, Bandyopadhyay P. Toxocariasis in Infectious Disease of the Eye, 1st edition. New Delhi: Walters Kluwer; 2010. pp. 294-6.
6. Mukherjee PK. Retinoblastoma in Pediatric Ophthalmology, 1st edition. New Delhi: New Age International; 2005. pp. 471-96.
7. Mukherjee PK. Toxocara infection of uvea. In: Pediatric Ophthalmology, 1st edition. New Delhi: New Age International; 2005. pp. 264-6.
8. Rishi P, Rishi E, Uparar M, Sharma T, Gopal L, Bhende P, et al. Coats disease an Indian perspective. IJO. 2010;58: 119-24.
9. Shield JA, Shield CL, Honavar SG, Demirci H, Carlen J. Classification and management of Coates disease. AJO. 2001;131(5):572-83.
10. Shukla D, Singh G, Sonam M, John PK, Ramaswami K, Perumalswami N. Familial exudative vitreoretinopathy, clinical profile and management. IJO. 2003;51: 323-8.
11. Tasmin W, Augsberger JJ, Shield JA. Familial Exudative retinopathy. Trans Am Oph Soc. 1981;79:211-26.

CHAPTER 7

Retinoblastoma

Retinoblastoma is the most common intraocular malignant tumor in childhood. It is the second most common intraocular malignancy in all ages; it is surpassed by malignant melanoma of the choroid only, which is a malady of late adulthood with an average age of first presentation of 55. The other malignancy of childhood is rhabdomyosarcoma, which, unlike retinoblastoma, is an extraocular disorder arising from striated muscles of the orbit.

In the not-so-distant past, retinoblastoma was considered to be the fastest-growing childhood malignancy that terminated in death unless removed before it became extraocular by enucleation. With the present-day availability of multiple modalities, it is not only treatable but curable, with a 5-year survival rate. In 1896, the death rate stood at 95% that came down to 20% in 1967 in developed countries; in developing countries, it is still pretty high. Modern-day management not only destroys the tumor but also saves the eye many times with salvaged vision, minus recurrence.

No race is immune; it is equally common among boys and girls; clusters of the retinoblastoma gene may be present in some communities; and no endemic zones have been identified. The disorder can be sporadic or hereditary. Statistically, more cases are being reported from developing countries, not due to a spurt in incidence but due to:

- Increased awareness.
- Diminished infant mortality.
- Upward swings in ambient radiation.
- Overall change in the environment.
- Higher rate of survival.
- Treated children reaching reproductive age.
- The treated persons passing the gene on to coming generations.
- Possibility of the presence of an offending gene in a cluster.

Retinoblastoma is considered to be congenital in nature. It may be present at birth but detected later. The visibility of the growth depends on its position and size; a small tumor in the visual axis is visible earlier than one away. Laterality also influences early detection; bilateral cases are detected early. The average age of detection is 18 months in bilateral cases because bilateral cases draw parents' attention early. Most of the bilateral cases seek medical help before the first birthday; the unilateral cases come for consultation a year later. The other cause of early presentation in bilateral cases is their hereditary nature; most probably, the parents have been counseled in the past. Counseled parents are more likely to get their child examined earlier than noncounseled. The average age for seeking medical help is rarely >5 years. The parents may be oblivious to the tumor at an early stage, especially when it is sporadic, and the first consultation may be already too late for the best outcome. Such cases generally come with diminished vision or squinting.

The incidence of retinoblastoma shows a sharp decline after 3 years. The first detection after 7 years is less common. In rare instances, retinoblastoma has been detected in adults; also, the probabilities *are*:

- The person had retinoblastoma in childhood that has undergone spontaneous regression.
- The retinoblastoma cells have remained dormant and suddenly become active.
- Wrong histopathological interpretation of the slide.

> The conditions other than retinoblastoma that show rosette on histopathology are:
> Medulloepithelioma, neuroepithelioma, retinal dysplasia, incontinentia pigmenti, and retinoma.

GENETICS IN RETINOBLASTOMA

A better understanding of genetics has not only led to early diagnosis but also better planning and management. Retinoblastomas are sporadic in 90–95% of cases; the remaining are hereditary. This makes exploring family history mandatory in all cases of retinoblastoma, putting them into two broad groups: Sporadic and hereditary. Thus, a child with suspected retinoblastoma may have a history of retinoblastoma in the family, i.e., parents, grandparents, siblings, or a suggestion of its possibility in the family. Well-counseled parents with a positive family history are more likely to bring their children up earlier than those without.

In cases of positive family history, the following protocol should be followed:

- A child as young as a neonate with a positive family history should be examined with an indirect ophthalmoscope under maximum mydriasis.
- The absence of retinoblastoma at first examination does not rule out the possibility of retinoblastoma.
- Such children should undergo a complete retinal evaluation every 6 months until the age of 3, and thereafter every year up to 7 years.
- These children, when grown up, should be counseled about the possibility of having a child with retinoblastoma.
- Hereditary retinoblastoma has the chance of skipping a generation.
- The reported incidence of retinoblastoma in siblings is as high as 40%.

Flowchart 7.1 Shows genetic variation in hereditary retinoblastoma.

Flowchart 7.1 indicates the following:

- Children with family history have more chances of having children inherit retinoblastoma.
- These children themselves, too, have a chance of children with retinoblastoma.
- Unilateral cases without family history have less chances of passing the gene on to their offspring.
- 40% of offspring born to parents with bilateral involvement are likely to develop retinoblastoma.
- The firstborn with a positive family history is more likely to develop retinoblastoma.
- Children of parents with a positive family history are more likely to have the tumor.
- When retinoblastoma occurs in one of the children of healthy parents, the chances of siblings developing the tumor are less.
- Normal parents with two affected children will have a greater risk of having the disease in more children.
- The reported incidence of retinoblastoma in siblings is as high as 40%.

The retinoblastoma gene is found in the long arm of chromosome 13 in its 14th segment; to be precise, it is labeled as *RB1*, 13q14, and mutation of *RB1* is the cause of the tumor. Gene *RB1* is in fact a tumor suppression gene; its function is to control cell growth and prevent cells from going haywire.

CLASSIFICATION OF RETINOBLASTOMA

Retinoblastoma has neither been put in the category of carcinoma nor sarcoma, yet it shares the malignant properties of both. Some people consider it to be a neural tumor. Children with successfully treated retinoblastoma are at greater risk of developing a second tumor in the form of soft part sarcoma.

Classifying retinoblastoma based on its malignancy potential is a difficult task. Over the last two centuries, many attempts have been made to solve the riddle; till today, it remains an unsolved problem in spite of great strides in the fields of genetics, chemotherapy, and radiation.

Flowchart 7.1: Distribution as per family history.

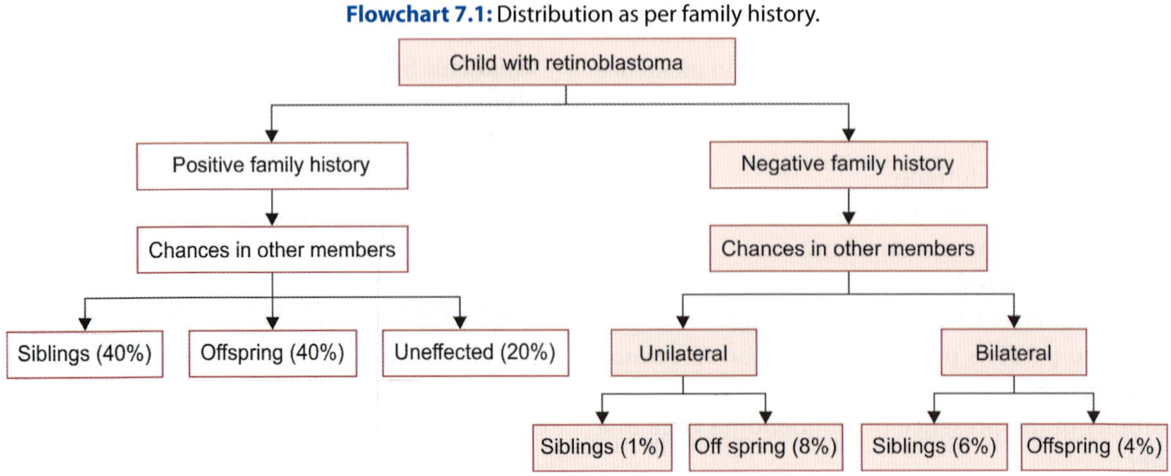

The term glioma was first coined by Virchow; this was before the development of histopathology in general and ocular histopathology in particular. He presumed that the tumor arises from the glial tissue of the retina. It was later realized that the tumors were in fact from specialized cells of the retina called retinoblasts, which were embryonic in nature. Cells before differentiation have occurred in neural and neuroglial cells. The neural cells are rods, cones, bipolar, and ganglion cells, while neuroglial cells are astrocytes and Müller's cells. In 1926, Verhoeff termed the malignancy retinoblastoma, and in science, it is called so.

Some of the classifications are:

- *Agewise:*
  - *Congenital:* It is believed that all retinoblastomas start during the development of the retina; they may not be obvious at birth but become apparent before 3 years of age.
  - Under 5 years (most common)
  - After 5 years (rare)
  - *Adult (doubtful):* The possibilities are: There may be a recurrence after treatment or spontaneous regression. Most of the white reflexes in the pupil after 5 years of being diagnosed as retinoblastoma have turned out to be nonretinoblastoma, with the most common mistaken diagnosis being diktyoma.
  - *Second malignancy:* They are always extraocular, developing years following treatment by external beam radiation or rarely chemotherapy, fatal in 15% of cases, and more common in bilateral cases.

The reported second malignancies are: Osteogenic sarcoma, fibrosarcoma, pineoblastoma, rhabdomyosarcoma, angiosarcoma, and neuroblastoma.

- *Laterality wise:* Unilateral/bilateral
- *Hereditary:* Heritable (germline)/nonheritable (somatic)
- *Cell of origin:*
  - Glioma/nonglioma
  - Retinoblastoma/nonretinoblastoma
- *Location:*
  - Intraocular
  - Extraocular with extension in orbit/central nervous system (CNS)/distant
- *Pathological:*
  - *Gross:* Endophytum/exophytum/diffuse
  - Microscopic

The gross appearance depends on its location in relation to the layers of the retina and its being intraocular or extraocular. It is valid in the early intraocular stage, once the tumor is large enough to obliterate the line of demarcation, it loses its significance. The division has no prognostic value.

Endophytum

Endophytum retinoblastoma is retinoblastoma that arises from primitive photoreceptors and grows toward the vitreous, releasing retinoblastoma cells, called seedlings that are capable of disseminating to all neural and vascular intraocular structures and may start extraocular spread. At this stage, there is no retinal detachment.

Exophytum

Exophytum retinoblastomas arise from cells other than primitive photoreceptors and initially grow into choroid, causing solid or serous detachment, before it breaks through the sclera.

Diffuse Retinoblastoma

This is the least common out of the three types. Commonly seen in boys up to the end of the first decade, these tumors arise on the peripheral retina, hence do not cause a white reflex in the pupillary area and are mistaken for anterior uveitis because they produce pus-like material in the anterior chamber, which is in fact the accumulation of tumor cells (pseudohypopyon) **(Fig. 7.1)**.

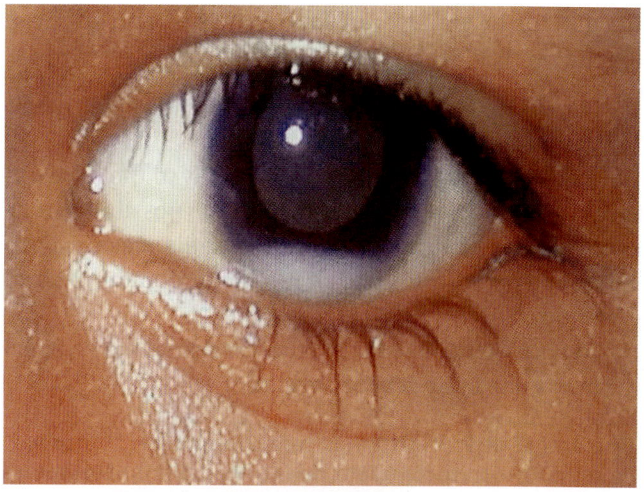

Fig. 7.1: Pseudohypopyon in retinoblastoma
Courtesy: Dr Santosh G Honavar.

Microscopic Grading of Retinoblastoma

The microscopic grading depends on rosette formation and its nature.

The grading is:

- Reese-Ellsworth staging
- Essen staging
- International classification of intraocular retinoblastoma
- Tumor node metastasis (TNM)

Laterality-wise Retinoblastoma

Laterality-wise retinoblastoma may be unilateral and remain so or bilateral at the time of first presentation. Unilateral tumors are generally sporadic; these children are brought for consultation late. Surprisingly, not for retinoblastoma but for diminished vision, squint, or even. With the presumption of cataracts, the average age of the first presentation is 2 years. However, some cases may turn up with a white reflex in the pupillary area; others may not present before the orbit is involved.

Bilateral retinoblastomas are mostly hereditary, with a germinal mutation; one eye may have been involved earlier than the other and have a more advanced disease. Involvement of the other eye is independent of the first and not secondary to it. Children with bilateral involvement seek medical help earlier than unilateral the average age of presentation being 12 months, in contrast to 18–24 months in cases of unilateral, the explanation for the early presentation of bilateral cases is most probably due to parents' awareness about the tumor in the family; either one of the parents or grandparents have suffered and survived the tumor.

Heredity

Heredity plays an important role not only in the development of an affected child but also in the possibility of its occurrence in siblings and offspring. Retinoblastoma can either be sporadic or nonsporadic. The sporadic is more common.

To understand heredity in retinoblastoma, it is essential to know some basic genetics involved:

> The overall genetic pattern in retinoblastoma is autosomal dominant with incomplete penetrance. Retinoblastoma susceptibility gene *RB1* is tumor suppression gene. It is called anti-oncogenic gene.

To develop a tumor, both alleles (copies) should be inactivated. There are three theories of genetics involved.

The various hypotheses are:

- Knudson's two-hit theory
- Matsunaga's host resistance theory
- 13q14 deletion theory

Out of them, the first is more accepted. The main points are:

- To evolve retinoblastoma, two chromosomal mutations are required.
- In the case of heritable retinoblastoma, the first hit is germinal.
- Germinal mutations are inherited and found in all cells.
- The second hit is in the somatic cell.
- Hereditary (germline) retinoblastomas are likely to develop nonocular tumors.
- In unilateral sporadic retinoblastoma, the two hits happen during the development of the retina, hence resulting in a somatic mutation.
- In unilateral, sporadic cases, both hits are somatic.
- There is no risk of the development of a nonocular tumor in unilateral sporadic cases.
- In inheritable retinoblastoma, the tumor is inherited as autosomal dominant.
- Children of survivors have a 50% chance of developing retinoblastoma. Such tumors are mostly bilateral and multiple, each independent of the other.
- 5% of children born to parents who already had a child with retinoblastoma are at a higher risk of developing retinoblastoma.

Matsunaga Theory

This is also known as host resistance theory, which postulates, "At least one mutation is required for manifestation; that depends on host resistance, which is polygenic." The retinoblastoma gene is located in band 14 of the long arm of chromosome 13. 5% of patients with retinoblastoma have karyotype 13q. Patients with 13q14 develop retinoblastoma. Human esterase D is also located in band 13q14, which acts as a marker for the identification of retinoblastoma.

Characteristics of hereditary retinoblastoma:

- The first mutation happens in gametes.
- The first mutation happens in one of the two alleles of the retinoblastoma gene.

- *Mutation happens as:*
    - Inheritance from one of the affected parents
    - Sporadically from one grandparent
- The child has the possibility of a nonocular malignant tumor.
- The second mutation happens in the postzygotic stage.
- The second mutation is the cause of bilateral retinoblastoma.
- 50% of subsequent generations may develop retinoblastoma.
- 66% of hereditary retinoblastomas are bilateral.

Characteristics of nonhereditary (somatic) retinoblastoma:

- The growth is unilateral.
- The growth is unifocal.
- It does not affect offspring.
- Both mutations happen in the same retinal cell after fertilization.

Characteristics of familial retinoblastoma:

- 5–10% of all cases have family backgrounds.
- They are autosomal dominant in nature.
- Abnormality in band 14 of chromosome 13
- 60% bilateral
- There are three to five tumors in each eye.

Genetic Counseling in Retinoblastoma

Genetic counseling should be an integral protocol of the management of retinoblastoma because 40% of siblings and 40% of offspring are likely to develop retinoblastoma if there is a positive family history of tumor in one of the parents. Familial retinoblastoma has a tendency to skip one generation; a child with a unilateral tumor without a family history does not develop retinoblastoma; only 1% of siblings and 8% of offspring have a chance of developing retinoblastoma; the chances of developing retinoblastoma in siblings and offspring rise in bilateral cases without a positive family history.

About the Cell of Origin in Retinoblastoma

For a long time, there have been controversies regarding the cell of origin of retinoblastoma. A group believed them to be glial in origin and called the tumor glioma. The controversy continued until the advent of clinical microscopes and ophthalmoscopes. Verhoeff in 1917 confirmed that the cell of origin was in fact premature photoreceptors that, instead of developing in nonmalignant rods and cones, deviated to a specific form of cells, which he called retinoblasts, the cause of malignancy. In the next few decades, it was realized that all retinal tumors were neither malignant nor did they arise from retinoblast. The percentage of such tumors are far less than their malignant counterpart.

PATHOLOGICAL APPEARANCE OF RETINOBLASTOMA

The appearance is divided into two groups, i.e., clinical and pathological; the latter is further divided into macroscopic and microscopic appearances.

The most obvious clinical feature is the white reflex in the pupillary area, seen even in ambient light and confirmed by retinoscopes and ophthalmoscopes **(Figs. 7.2 to 7.4)**.

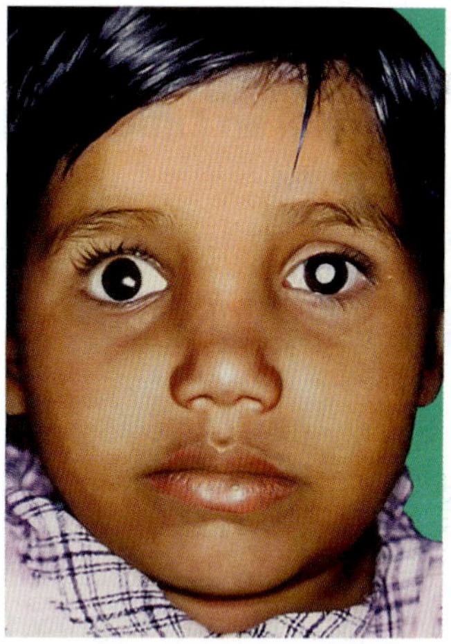

Fig. 7.2: White reflex in pupillary area.
Courtesy: Dr Somen Misra.

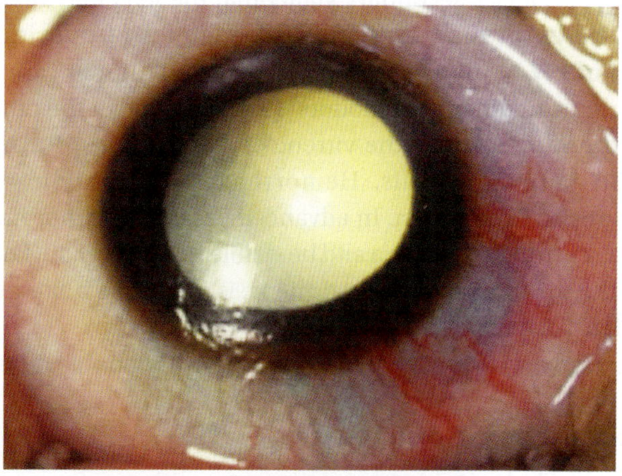

Fig. 7.3: White reflex in pupillary area.
Courtesy: Dr Santosh G Honavar (Retinoblastoma – They Live and See).

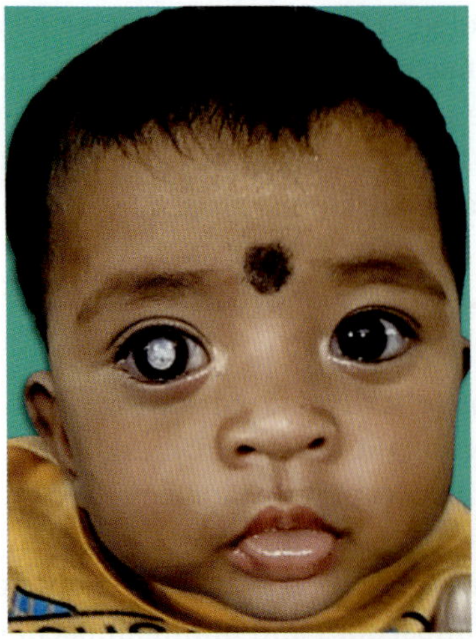

Fig. 7.4: Child with advanced retinoblastoma right eye with small lesion in the left eye.

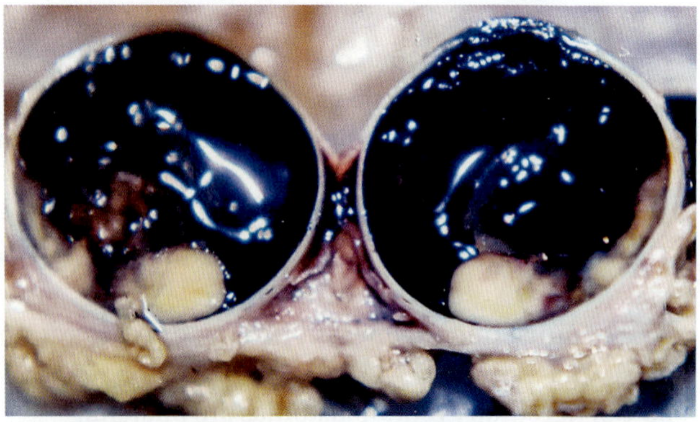

Fig. 7.5: Intraocular retinoblastoma in cut section. *Courtesy:* Dr Somen Misra.

Gross Appearance of an Enucleated Eye with Retinoblastoma

The appearance of the cut section depends on the size and position of the tumor.

The following is the description of a tumor in the vitreous cavity:

The tumor has a pink-white color; it may be solid or fluffy; the surface may be nodular; the retinal vessels are not visible over the surface **(Fig. 7.5)**; in the endophytum variety, initially there may be more than one growth separated from each, the tumors grow to coalesce to form a single larger mass filling the whole vitreous cavity, pushing the iris lens complex or ward.

This causes secondary glaucoma; the lens may retain its clarity or may develop various grades of opacities, ultimately resulting in a complete cataract. In the case of multiple nodules, each nodule is independent of the other and not metastatic; the vitreous is invariably sprinkled with malignant cells. Hemorrhages and patches of necrosis are common. In advanced cases, the tumor may break through the sclera and be visible on its outer surface. In the still-late stage, the optic nerve is seen to be infiltrated **(Figs. 7.6 and 7.7)**.

Figures 7.8 and 7.9 show late stages of retinoblastoma.

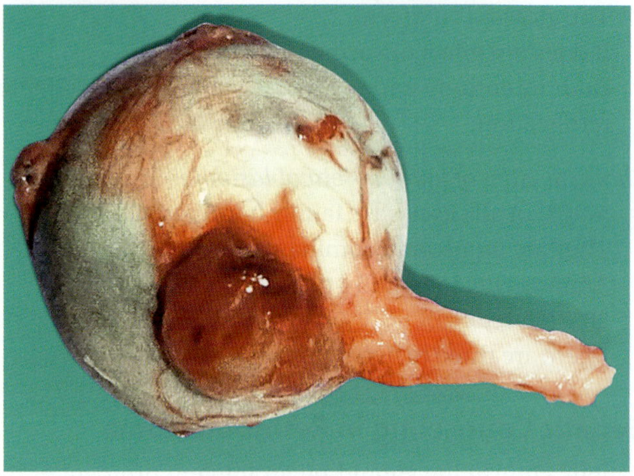

Fig. 7.6: Tumor extruding through sclera without involving optic nerve.
Courtesy: Dr Santosh G Honavar (Retinoblastoma – They Live and See).

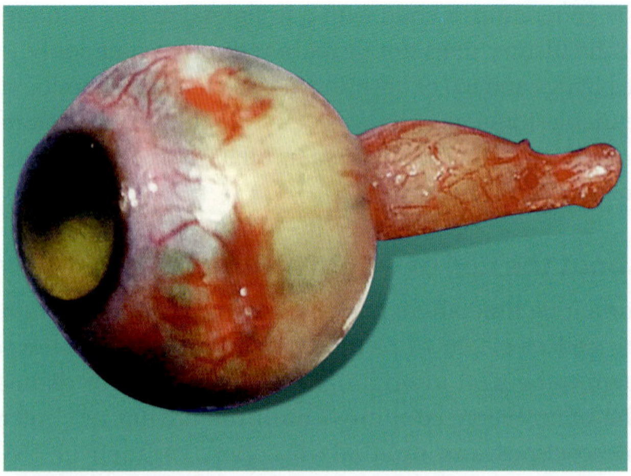

Fig. 7.7: Intraocular retinoblastoma extending in the optic nerve.
Courtesy: Dr Santosh G Honavar (Retinoblastoma – They Live and See).

Microscopic Appearance

Histopathological interpretation of a slide confirms the diagnosis and its stage. Multiple sections taken from various locations should be examined. No microscopic

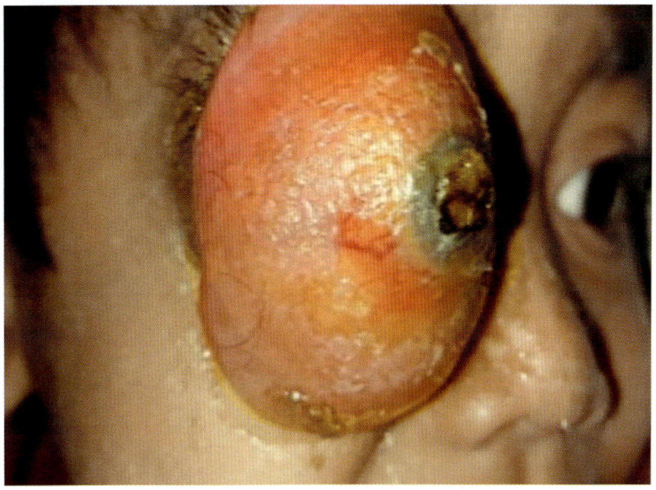

Fig. 7.8: Proptosis in retinoblastoma.

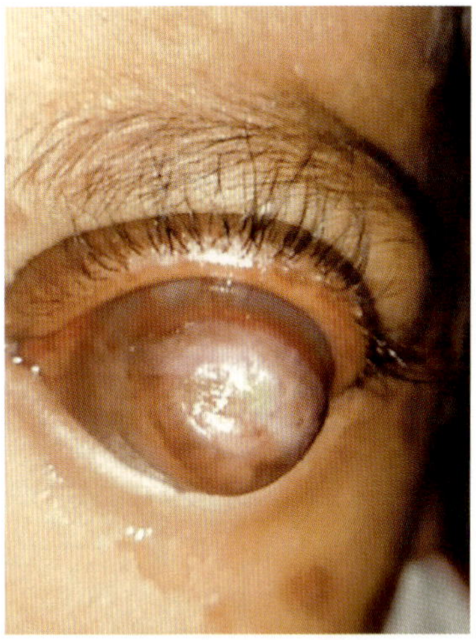

Fig. 7.9: Stage of secondary glaucoma in retinoblastoma.
Courtesy: Dr Kshama Chopda.

examination is considered complete without an examination of the optic nerve. The sections are stained with hematoxylin and eosin; the former stain the nuclei and the later rest of the tissues. No special stain is required other than these. The slides are initially examined under low power, showing an abundance of cells with minimal stroma with plenty of blood vessels. Occasionally, there are patches of necrosis; this happens when growth exceeds the blood supply. In spite of the abundance of necrosis, the inflammatory reaction is minimal. The necrotic area has a tendency to get calcified, which is visible on a plain X-ray and is considered to be diagnostic of retinoblastoma.

The distinct features of retinoblastoma are the rosettes and their variations, i.e., true and pseudorosettes. The true rosettes are well differentiated, while the pseudorosettes are undifferentiated or ill-differentiated structures.

Retinoblastomas arise from specific malignant cells called retinoblasts, which are immature retinal cells of neural origin without oncogenic genes, which are precursors of photoreceptors, i.e., rods and cones, with normal antioncogenic factors. Once the antiretinoblastoma genes are lost, these premature precursors are transformed into retinoblastoma.

The retinoblastoma cell is an oval, semicolumnar cell with a relatively large chromatic nucleus that is decent. The cell has scanty basophils.

The summary of cell differentiation in retinoblastoma is depicted in **Flowchart 7.2**.

Flexner-Wintersteiner Rosette

They are the most common malignant cells seen in retinoblastoma. They are typical of retinoblastoma and not seen in any other malignancy. A typical FW rosette comprises an empty, clear lumen surrounded by a thin membrane. The membrane is the counterpart of the external limiting membrane of the normal retina; the membrane is an essential part of the rosette. The clear lumen contains acid mucopolysaccharide and occasionally a few retinoblasts, but no blood. On the membrane are placed the retinoblasts with hyperchromatic nuclei; the nuclei are shifted away from the lumen. The cells are arranged like petals on a flower, resembling a sunflower. The size of FW rosettes varies from small, with only 5–10 rosettes, to large, with 15–50 retinoblasts round the lumen **(Fig. 7.10)**.

The cells in rosettes resemble the rods and cones. Their presence is evidence of differentiation. The more differentiation, the better the prognosis. There may be a few undifferentiated retinoblasts in a field as well, without forming definite rosettes. It is presumed that less is the age of the patient and more are the rosettes because the number of rosettes is inversely proportional to the duration of the growth. As the retinoblastoma grows, it becomes less differentiated.

Homer-Wright Rosettes

These rosettes resemble FW rosettes in appearance, with the exception that the central lumen, instead of containing clear acid mucopolysaccharide, contains an opaque cobweb of neural frills. They are not exclusive to retinoblastoma; they are seen in medulloepithelioma, medulloblastoma, and neuroblastoma as well **(Fig. 7.11)**.

Flowchart 7.2: Summary of cell differentiation in retinoblastoma.

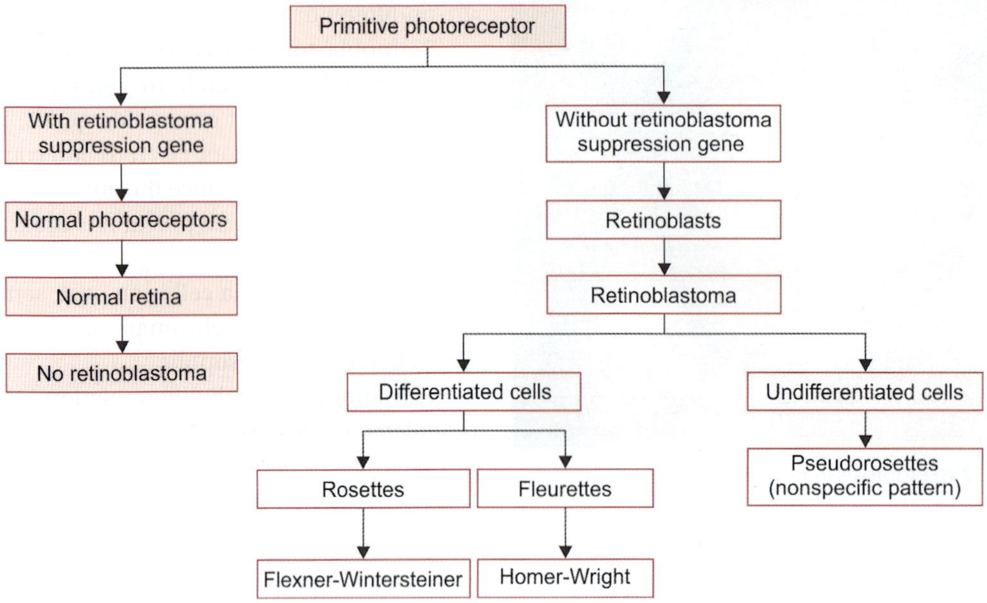

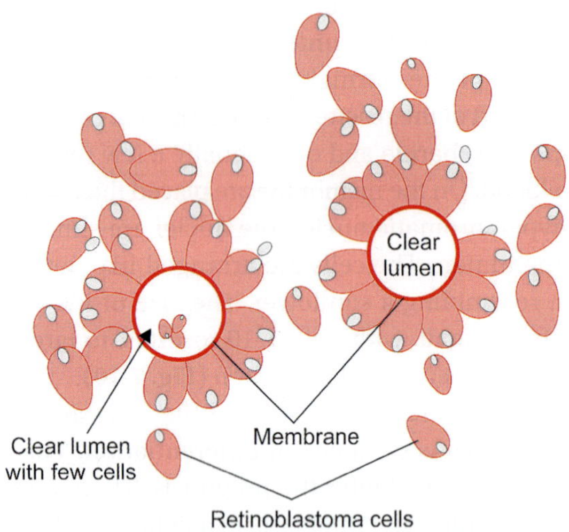

Fig. 7.10: Flexner-Wintersteiner rosette.

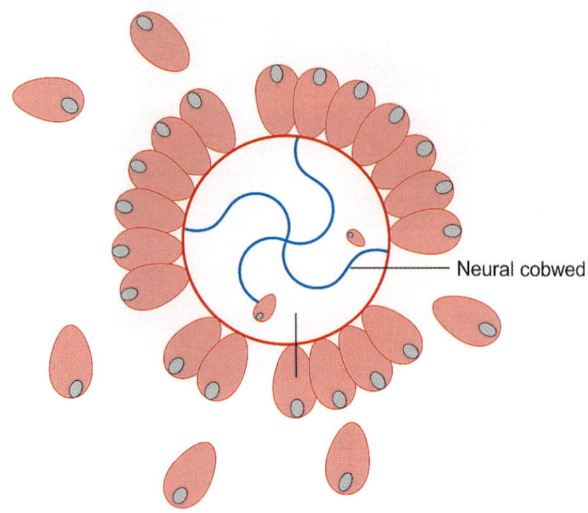

Fig. 7.11: Homer-Wright rosette.

Fleurette

In the two types of cell arrangements discussed above, it has been noted that the retinoblastoma cells are arranged around a lumen in a sunflower pattern called rosettes. In contrast to this, fleurettes are arranged such as miniature bouquets or half-rosettes; they form a bunch of cells with projections that pass through the membrane. The cells forming the fleurettes, which are eosinophilic in nature, represent photoreceptors, as in other cells of retinoblastoma. The presence of fleurettes is an indication of reduced malignancy. Besides retinoblastoma, fleurettes are also seen in benign conditions such as retinoma and retinocytoma **(Fig. 7.12)**.

Pseudorosette

Pseudorosettes are devoid of the specific pattern that is characteristic of rosettes and fleurettes; they are irregularly arranged round blood vessels rather than a clear lumen surrounded by a membrane of rosettes. The pseudo-rosettes may even develop round areas of necrosis. The cells get enhanced nutrition from the blood vessels round which they have grown; this in turn increases the growth of

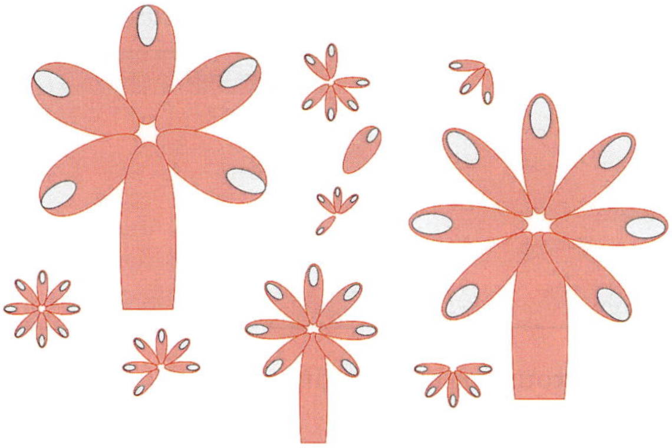

Fig. 7.12: Fleurettes.

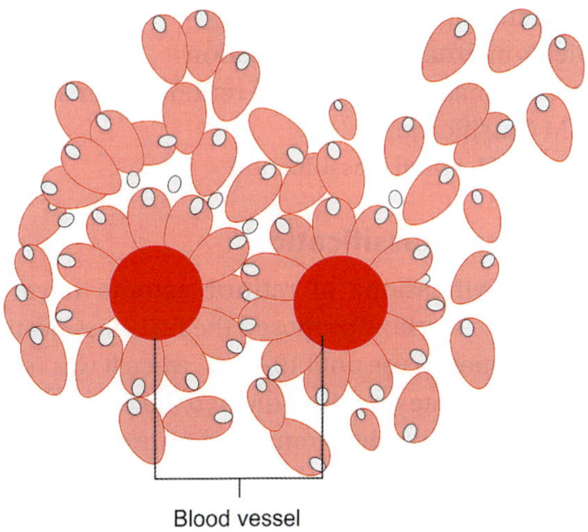

Fig. 7.13: Pseudorosettes.

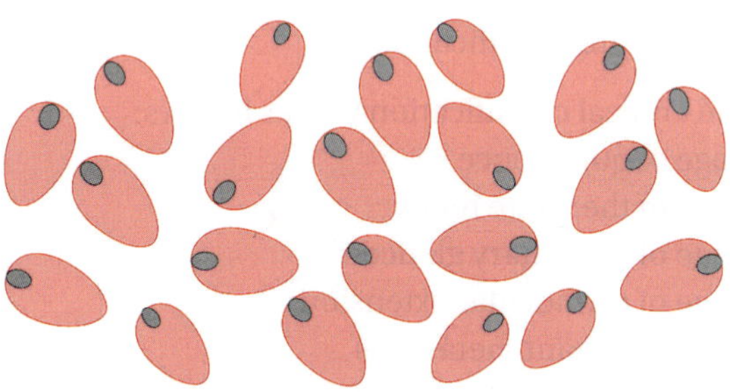

Fig. 7.14: Undifferentiated cells.

the tumor heralding a paradoxical situation of diminished blood supply in a fast-growing tumor that overshoots the blood supply with a state of hypoxia that soon passes into a state of anoxemia and ultimate ischemia by coagulative necrosis and dies with the deposition of calcium that is visible on X-rays, which is strongly suggestive of retinoblastoma. In the advanced stage, the cells fail to form either rosettes or pseudorosettes; they get scattered all over **(Figs. 7.13 and 7.14)**.

PROGNOSIS AND MORTALITY

Prognosis and mortality in retinoblastoma depend on the following factors:

- *Only fleurettes:* Excellent prognosis
- No rosette; poor prognosis
- *Involvement of:*
    - *Choroid:* 25–65% of mortalities
    - *Optic nerve:*
        - No invasion, 8% mortality
        - Invasion up to the lamina: 15% mortality
        - Postlamellar involvement: 44% mortality
        - Beyond the entry of the central retinal artery, 65%

REGRESSION OF RETINOBLASTOMA

Retinoblastomas are known to regress. There are two types of regression, i.e., spontaneous and postradiation.

Spontaneous Regression

Earlier, we have seen that fast-growing retinoblastoma exceeded the blood supply and went into the following states:

Inadequate blood supply – Hypoxia – Ischemia – Death of cells.

Some pathologists attribute this phenomenon to an autoimmune disturbance. The regression leaves a scar similar to postradiation status. Spontaneous regression is also associated with a lowering of intraocular tension that may terminate in phthisis. This makes it mandatory to look into the eyes of parents, grandparents, and siblings for evidence of soft eye or phthisis in all cases of bilateral retinoblastoma in a child with a white reflex in the pupillary area.

Regression following Radiation

This is the end result of successful treatment by radiation, either by external or plaque brachytherapy. Regression following radiation is followed by intensified calcification. There are three patterns of postradiation regression:

1. Avascular with intensified calcification
2. Vessels attenuated without obliteration
3. Combination of the two

Predisposing factors in the regression of retinoblastoma:

- Enhanced calcification
- DNA deposition
- Endothelial proliferation
- Programmed cell death (apoptosis)

Predisposing factors in the severity of retinoblastoma:

- *Cell arrangement:*
  - Pseudorosettes and undifferentiated cells have a poor prognosis.
  - Rosettes have a better prognosis.
  - Fleurettes have the best prognosis.
- *Involvement of the optic nerve:* Once the optic nerve gets infiltrated, the prognosis becomes poor.

Various types of optic nerve involvement include:

- Laminar or prelaminar infiltration
- Retrolaminar infiltration
- Malignant cells are present in the cut end of the optic nerve of the enucleated eye.

Natural history of optic nerve involvement is:
Retina → Optic nerve → Substance of optic nerve → Brain → Subarachnoids space → Leptomeninges → Ventricles → CSF → Spinal cord → Distant metastasis.

Prognosis and Mortality in Retinoblastoma

- Only fleurette — Excellent
- No rosettes — Poor prognosis
- Choroidal involvement — 25–65% mortality
- *Optic nerve involvement:*
  - No invasion — 8% mortality
  - Up to lamina — 15% mortality
  - Postlamina — 44% mortality
  - Beyond entry of central retinal artery — 65% mortality

Five-year survival in various types of optic nerve invasion:

Part involved	*Mortality percentage*
▪ *Optic nerve:*	
• Nil	8–10%
• Up to lamina	15–20%
• Retro laminar	45%
• Distal part of cut end of optic nerve	65%
▪ Choroid	25%
▪ Orbit	90%

SALVAGEABILITY IN RETINOBLASTOMA

To assess the salvageability of retinoblastoma, the cases have been subjected to grouping and staging.

The former is a clinical procedure that indicates the salvageability of the eye; the latter denotes the chances of the child's survivability.

Grouping of retinoblastoma as per risk factors:

Risk	***Group***
Very low	A
Low	B
Moderate	C
High	D
Very high	E

Based on grouping and staging, the following classifications are in vogue:

- Reese-Ellsworth classification
- Essen classification
- International staging
- Shields international classification
- International classification of retinoblastoma
- TNM classification
- St James Hospital classification

Pathological Classification

Various classifications of retinoblastoma have been available since Virchow proposed the first classification in 1864; it remained in use until 1926–27, when it was replaced by a more elaborate one. That divided the tumors into two broad groups: Retinoblastoma and nonretinoblastoma. He established that retinoblastoma developed from a specific malignant cell and coined the term retinoblast. Later, the disorder was given a clinical classification that was followed until a few years ago, when it was replaced by more elaborate classifications.

The old clinical classification was as follows:

- Stage of quiescence
- Stage of the white reflex
- Stage of secondary glaucoma
- Stage of extraocular extension
- Stage of distant metastasis

A modified classification based on its extent in relation is as follows **(Flowchart 7.3)**:

Flowchart 7.3: A commonly used classification of retinoblastoma.

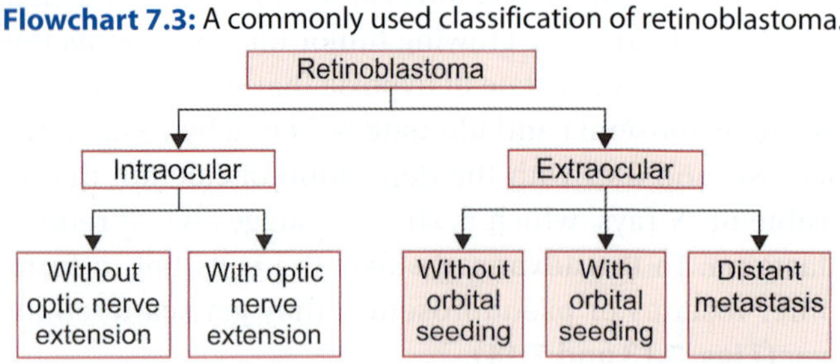

All the classifications mentioned here have failed to fully fill all the parameters that encompass diagnosis, treatment, salvageability of the globe, and overall prognosis.

An ideal classification should have two components:

1. *Salvageability of the eyeball:*
    a. Retaining function
    b. Retaining structure
2. Extent of survival rate

The first comes under grouping, examples of which are: *Reese-Ellsworth* classification and Essen classification. Under second comes the international classification of retinoblastoma. Staging includes clinical evaluation, imaging, and histopathology.

Reese-Ellsworth classification superseded previous classifications; it too has its shortcomings, as it was developed in light of radiation with special attention to external beam radiation without taking into consideration chemotherapy.

Indications for EBR:

- One or more tumor
- One or more tumors involving the optic nerve or macula
- Bilateral
- Diffused vitreous seeding
- Eyes not responding to:
    - Photocoagulation
    - Laser
    - Cryo
    - Transpupillary thermotherapy

Ellsworth divided retinoblastomas into five groups, dividing each group into two stages.

Summary of Ellsworth staging is given in **Table 7.1**.

CALCIFICATION IN RETINOBLASTOMA

- A tumor >10–15 disks in diameter size is likely to develop intralesional calcification.
- Small multicenter growths, though more malignant, do not develop intralesional calcification.
- Regression by radiation is associated with the intensification of intralesional calcification.
- There are three patterns of calcification following external beam radiation, i.e., I, II, and I + II, in the above chart.

The calcified areas are well delineated on tomography; the calcified areas stand out vividly; even small tumors with less calcification not seen on X-rays stand out as bright areas on CT.

Fluorescein angiography is not an essential investigation in retinoblastoma; it is an ancillary investigation in discreet lesions. There is rapid filling of feeder vessels and fast filling of intralesional vessels, followed by fast venous drainage. In the late pictures, the lesions stain brightly due to the leaking of the stain.

The Essen classification is a little more complicated to interpret; hence, it is not used routinely.

Reese-Ellsworth classification has been replaced by a more efficient classification that uses both staging and grouping as parameters.

They are:

- International staging of retinoblastoma
- Shields international classification
- International classification of intraocular retinoblastoma
- TNM classification of retinoblastoma

TABLE 7.1: Ellsworth staging of retinoblastoma.

Group	*Stage*	*Number of tumors*	*Size of tumor*	*Position of tumor*	*Prognosis*
I	A	Single	<4 D	At or behind the equator	Favorable
	B	Multiple	>4 D	Behind the equator	Favorable
II	A	Single	4–10 D	At or behind the equator	Favorable (±)
	B	Multiple	4–10 D	Behind the equator	Favorable (±)
III	A	Any	Variable	Behind the equator	Doubtful
	B	Single	<10 D	Behind the equator	Doubtful
IV	A	Many	>10 D	Anywhere	Unfavorable
	B	Any	Variable	Anterior to ORA	Unfavorable
V	A	Single	Massive	Half of retina	Most unfavorable
	B	Vitreous seeding			Most unfavorable

International Staging of Retinoblastoma

Stage:

1. Tumor completely removed by enucleation
2. Examination of microscopic tissue left after enucleating
3. *Regional extension:*
   a. Frank's orbital extension
   b. Preauricular lymph node (**Figs. 7.15A and B**)
   c. Cervical lymph node.
4. *Metastasis:*
   a. Blood
   b. CNS:
      i. Prechiasmal
      ii. Tumor in the brain
      iii. Extension in leptomeninges

Shields International Classification (Grouping)

Group:

- Retinoblastoma <3 mm at the base and height
- *Retinoblastoma >3 mm at base and height:*
  - <3 mm from foveola and >3 mm × 3 mm in size
  - Subretinal fluid + +
- *Subretinal seeds:*
  - The subretinal seeds are generally <3 mm from the tumor; they can be >3 mm from the tumor.
  - A combination of both is not unusual.
- *Tumor larger than half of the vitreous cavity:*
  - Neovascular glaucoma
  - Hemorrhage in subretinal space, vitreous, and anterior chamber
  - Extension in the optic nerve, choroid, anterior chamber, sclera, and orbit

International Classification of Intraocular Retinoblastoma

International classification of intraocular retinoblastoma divided it into the following groups:

- *Group A:* Multiple tumors <3 mm in the retina without seeding, all tumors 3 mm away from the foveola, and 1.5 mm from the disc.
- *Group B:* All tumors other than in group A, subretinal fluid <3 mm from the tumor without seeding
- *Group C:* Discrete tumors with minimal subretinal and vitreous seeding
- *Group D:* Diffuse tumor with prominent subretinal and vitreous seeding

The following are intraocular retinoblastomas with poor prognosis:

- Growths reaching up to posterior surface of the lens
- Tumors extending into the anterior segment
- Tumors in the anterior vitreous
- Diffuse infiltrative growths
- Vitreous hemorrhage
- Aseptic orbital cellulitis
- Phthisis bulbi.

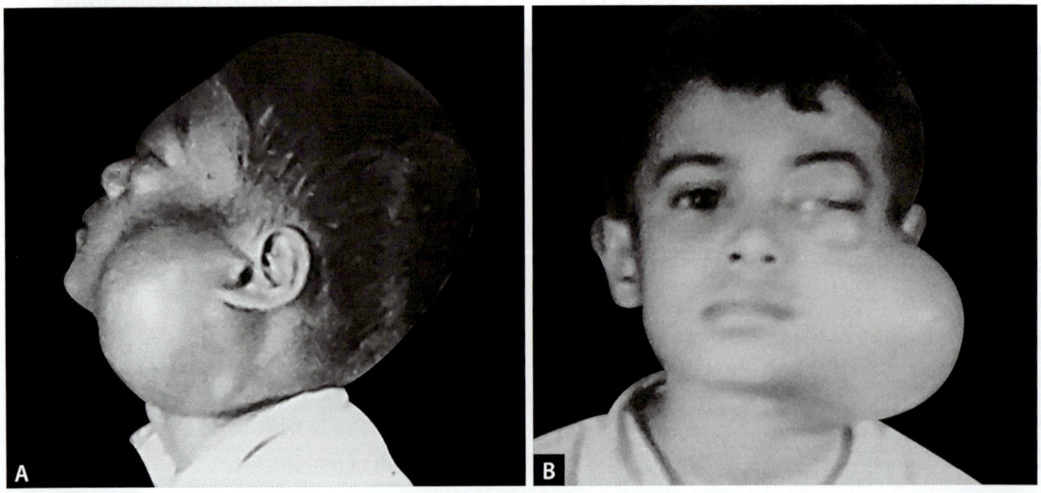

Figs. 7.15A and B: Rare photograph of a child with metastasis of retinoblastoma in the preauricular lymph node.

Tumor Node Metastasis (TNM) Classification

Following is an explanation of the numbers in **Flowchart 7.4** (clinical):

- *T0:* No evidence of the primary tumor
- *T1:* Tumor less than two-thirds of the globe with seeding
- *T2:* Tumor more than two-thirds of the globe with seeding and retinal detachment
- *T3:* Tumor larger than two-thirds of the globe, neovascularization of iris, neovascular glaucoma, tumor invading A C, vitreous hemorrhage, and orbital cellulitis
- *T4:* Involvement of the orbit; CNS involvement; both pre- and postchiasmal
- *N:* Lymph node involvement, both regional and distant
- *M:* Metastasis; intra- or extracentral nervous system; the metastasis can be single or multiple

Following is the explanation of numbers in **Flowchart 7.4** (pathological):

- *PT1:* Intraocular tumor without extension in the choroid or optic nerve
- *PT2:* Tumor with minimal involvement of the optic nerve
- *PT3:* Gross infiltration of the optic nerve and choroid
- *PT4:* Involvement of the optic nerve beyond enucleation
- *PN:* Involvement of regional lymph nodes; preauricular or cervical
- *M:* Metastasis

Classification of Tumor Left after Treatment

The result is expressed as R, where R_0 denotes the absence of a tumor, R_1 means only microscopic evidence, and R_2 denotes clinically obvious residue.

Modified Abramson Grading of Retinoblastoma

- *Intraocular disease:*
  - Involving the retina only
  - Extension: Choroid, up to lamina, sclera, without perforation
- *Orbital disease:*
  - Suspicious orbital lesion/biopsy proved an orbital lesion
  - Preauricular and cervical node involvement
- *Optic nerve disease:*
  - Tumor beyond the lamina, not reaching the cut end of nerve
  - Tumor present in the cut end and beyond
- *Metastatic disease:*
  - Intracranial metastasis with tumor cells in cerebrospinal fluid (CSF)
  - Intracranial growth
  - Hematogenous spreads in bone marrow, bone, and other organs.

Flowchart 7.4: TNM classification.

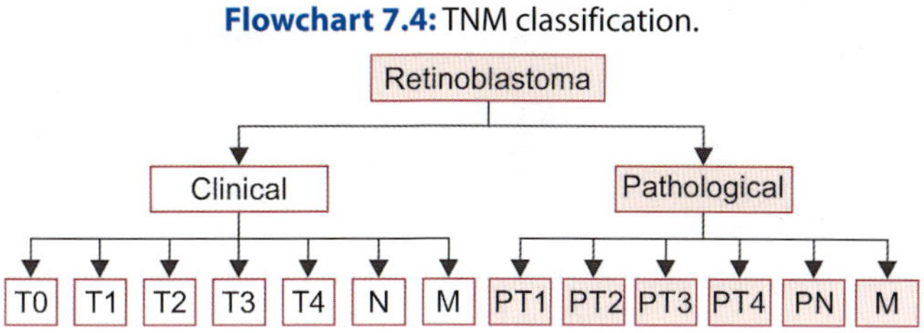

CLINICAL PRESENTATION OF RETINOBLASTOMA

Clinical presentation in retinoblastoma is variable, depending on position, size, and the number of growths. Is it still intraocular, or has it crossed the confines of the globe? Is there evidence of optic nerve infiltration? Is there proptosis? Is it associated with aseptic cellulitis? Is there evidence of metastasis?

Some points worth noting in dealing with a child with retinoblastoma:

- Retinoblastoma is rare.
- Retinoblastoma is not acute.
- Retinoblastoma is rare after 10 years of age.
- Treated retinoblastoma can recur at any age.
- Retinoblastoma can regress spontaneously.
- Retinoblastoma can be hereditary.
- Retinoblastoma can be bilateral and simultaneous.
- With treatment, the child may not only survive but also have vision.
- Hereditary retinoblastoma may develop in siblings and offspring.
- Parents with treated retinoblastoma may bring their normal child for consultation to exclude the possibility of having retinoblastoma.

Symptoms of Retinoblastoma

Symptoms depend on the duration and size of the tumor, the longer the duration, the more pronounced the symptoms and signs.

- *No symptom:* Discovered in a child referred for ophthalmic evaluation for a nonophthalmic cause.
  - The child whose one of the parents has survived retinoblastoma may be brought up to exclude the possibility of the child harboring retinoblastoma.
- *Diminished vision:*
  - *Child with esotropia:* Esotropic children are more likely to harbor retinoblastoma; a growth near the macula is more likely to develop a squint. The closer the growth, the more the macula is affected by the visual loss and the greater the squint, making it mandatory for every child with a squint to have the fundus evaluated with an indirect ophthalmoscope.
  - *Diminished* noncorrectable vision
  - *Leukocoria* parents are more likely to notice a white growth in the pupil in all gazes or a particular gaze.
  - *Pain in the eye:* Pain and redness in the eye are late features of secondary glaucoma.
  - Proptosis may vary between mild to severe and is a late feature.
  - Fungating mass in orbit **(Fig. 7.16)**
- *Other less common features:*
  - Doubtful history of trauma
  - Pseudohypopyon **(Fig. 7.17)**
  - Cellulitis lids **(Fig. 7.18)**
  - Orbital cellulitis **(Fig. 7.19)**.
  - Proptosis **(Fig. 7.20)**
  - Enlarged preauricular and cervical lymph nodes
  - Signs of anterior uveitis
  - Vitreous hemorrhage
  - Phthisis **(Fig. 7.21)**

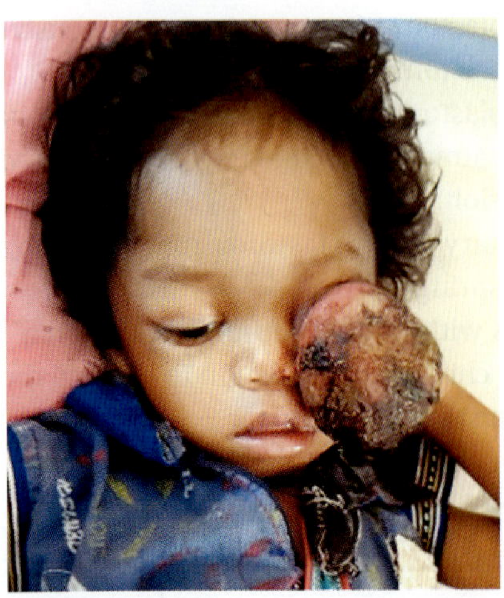

Fig. 7.16: Fungating retinoblastoma in orbit.

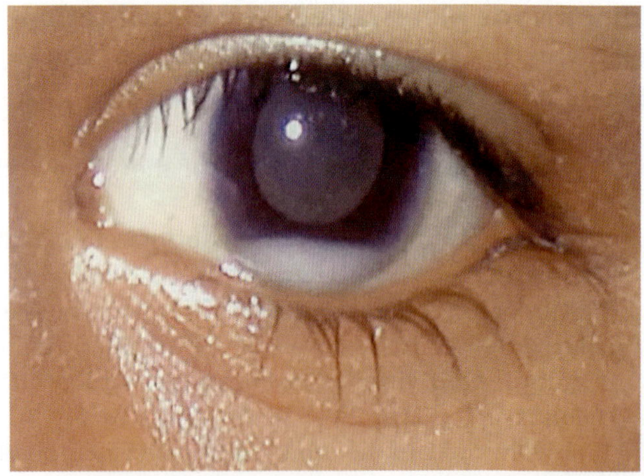

Fig. 7.17: Pseudohypopyon in retinoblastoma.
Courtesy: Dr Santosh G Honavar.

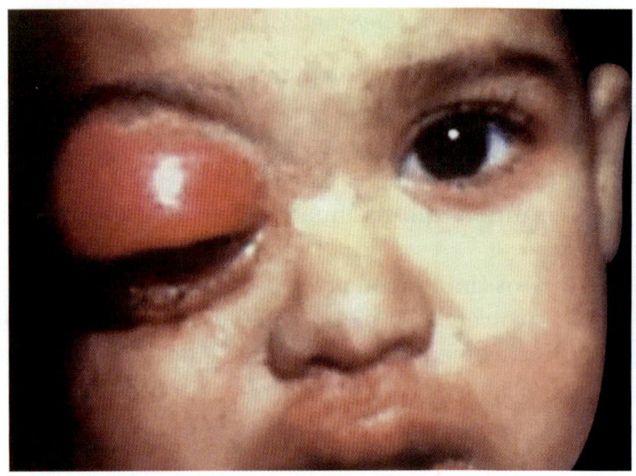

Fig. 7.18: Cellulitis lids in retinoblastoma.
Courtesy: Dr Santosh G Honavar.

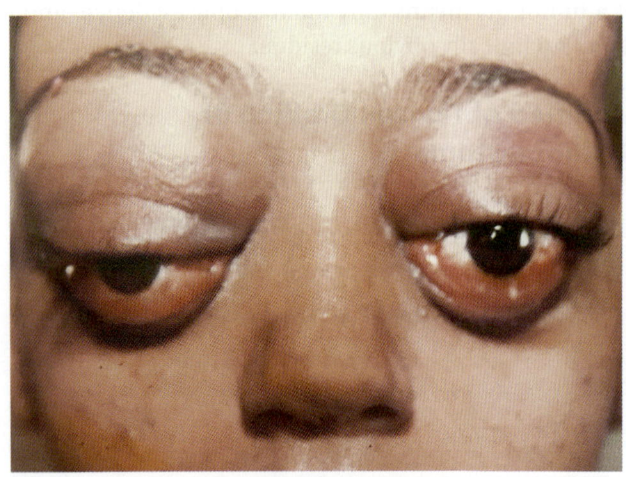

Fig. 7.19: Bilateral orbital cellulitis and proptosis in retinoblastoma.
Courtesy: Dr Somen Misra.

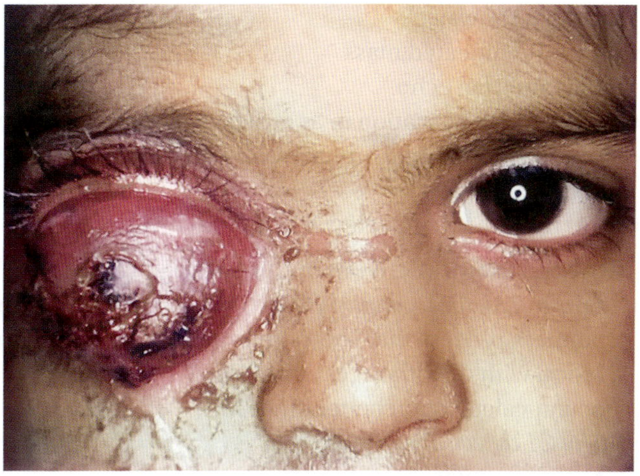

Fig. 7.20: Proptosis in retinoblastoma.
Courtesy: Dr Somen Misra.

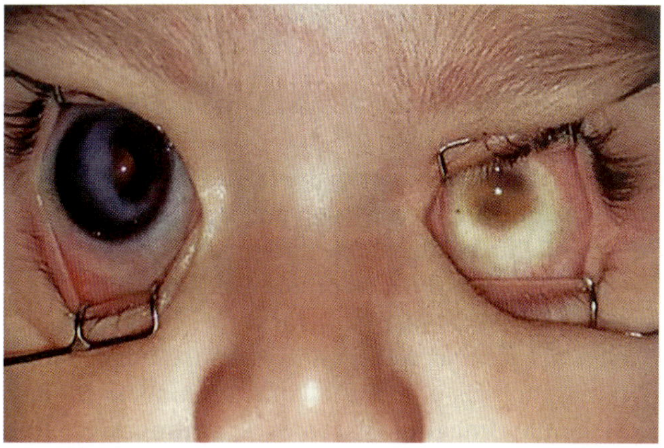

Fig. 7.21: Bilateral retinoblastoma left eye showing phthisis and right eye secondary glaucoma.
Courtesy: Dr Santosh G Honavar.

Diagnosis of Retinoblastoma

Diagnosis of retinoblastoma in its advanced stages is not difficult. The most tricky stage is the stage of white reflex in the pupil, not only for its clinical presentation but also for its social and legal ramifications. There are many conditions that masquerade as retinoblastoma, most of them nonmalignant, some treatable, others not so, and none of them fatal.

The list of nonretinoblastomic leukocoria is as follows (see Leukocoria):

- *Developmental:*
  - Congenital cataract
  - Large uveal coloboma
  - Large, opaque nerve fiber
  - Persistent hyperplastic primary vitreous
  - Congenital retinal fold
- *Trauma:*
  - Traumatic cataracts follow forgotten injuries.
  - Hemophthalmos
- *Inflammatory:*
  - Posterior cyclitic membrane
  - Endophthalmitis
  - Panophthalmitis **(Fig. 7.22)**
  - Toxocariasis and other inflammatory granulomas.
- *Neoplasm:*
  - Retinoma
  - Medulloepithelioma
  - Leukemia
- *Hereditary:*
  - Norrie's disease
  - Congenital retinoschisis
  - Incontinentia pigmenti
- *Unclassified:*
  - Coates disease
  - Retinopathy of prematurity
  - Advanced buphthalmos

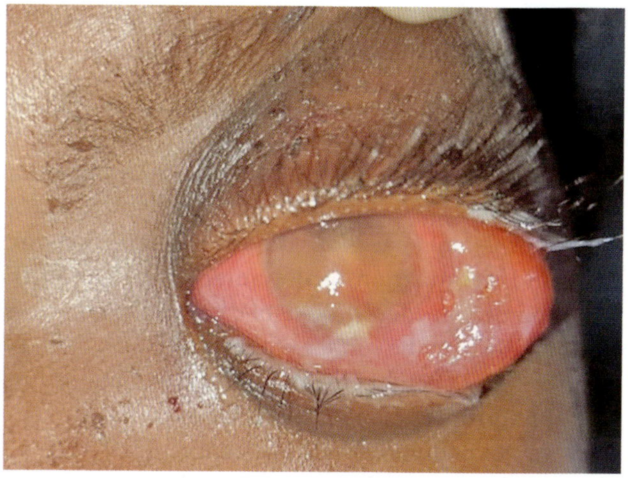

Fig. 7.22: Retinoblastoma was initially thought to be panophthalmitis.

> All eyes with diminished vision in children under 5, all squinting eyes, and all children with a positive family history of retinoblastoma should undergo fundus examination with an indirect ophthalmoscope under maximum mydriasis with scleral indentation if needed under general anesthesia.

Investigations in Retinoblastoma

All investigations should be preceded by noting family history, recording of vision, assessment of error of refraction, and fundus examination; both by direct and indirect ophthalmoscope.

These should be followed by the following investigations:

- *Slit lamp examination:*
  - Clarity of lens to exclude cataracts: Congenital, traumatic, and complicated
  - Retrolental space for vitreous opacities, seeding, and examination of the anterior surface of the tumor if needed with +90 D; generally, no vessels are seen on the surface of the tumor.
  - Anterior chamber for cells both inflammatory and tumor, traces of blood, pseudohypopyon
  - Iris for nodule, neovascularization
  - Angle neovascularization, pseudohypopyon, and malignant nodule
- *Examination under general anesthesia:* Recording of the intraocular pressure (IOP) and detailed examination of fundus
- *X-ray:* orbit (AP) and later, for intraocular calcification, enlargement of the optic foramen. An enlargement means an extension of a tumor in the optic nerve.

> Conditions other than retinoblastoma that cause intraocular calcification (in all ages) are hard, hypermature cataracts, calcification of the choroid, and choroidal osteoma; none of them are seen in children.

- *Ultrasonography (USG)*: Both A and B modes are used; the former is less effective than the latter; both are noninvasive, nonpainful procedures that can be repeated many times; both are devoid of radiation hazards; and both are office procedures **(Fig. 7.23)**.

The B scan shows:

- A well-delineated mass
- High internal echo
- Scattered calcification in as much as 75% of cases
- Diminished normal orbital mass with enhanced tumor mass
- It is not suitable to detect intraneural invasion.

The A scan shows bright internal echoes all over.

- *Computed tomography (CT):* This is a noninvasive, painless process that shows retinoblastoma as a mass lesion with or without calcification. CT picks up intraocular calcification better than USG.
- *The CT detects the following:*
  - Extraocular extension
  - Intracranial extension
  - Trilateral retinoblastoma
  - It does not pick up extensions in optic nerve.
  - 10% of cases do not have calcification large enough to be picked up by CT.
  - A tumor should be at least 2 mm in diameter to be picked up by CT.
- *Magnetic resonance imaging (MRI):* It is indicated to detect intracranial extension and intraorbital invasion. Intraocular tumors look darker than vitreous, and calcified areas look hypointense. The child needs sedation.
- *Optical coherence tomography (OCT):* Ocular coherent tomography is one of the latest entrants in the field of ocular imaging; it too is a noninvasive, nonpainful procedure that can be done without sedation. Children under 5 are not suitable candidates.

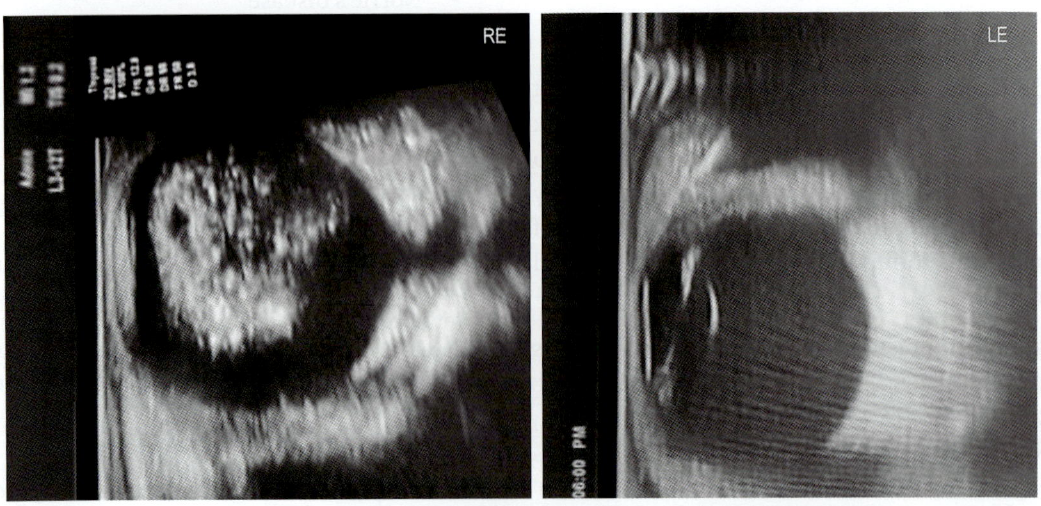

Fig. 7.23: Ultrasonography picture of advanced intraocular retinoblastoma.

The procedure is employed before, during, and after treatment. It is suitable for picking up intraocular calcification, retinal thickening, and disorganization. In retinoblastoma, the posterior layer is thickened, and the neurosensory layer is disorganized. Thickening of the anterior layer is suggestive of astrocytic hamartoma. Vitreous seeds are seen in endophytic retinoblastoma, while exophytic tumors show retinal detachment and subretinal seeding.

- *Funds fluorescein angiography:* This investigation is used sparingly, not because of its less utility but for a practical reason; children do not cooperate.
- *Less frequently used investigations in retinoblastoma are:*
  - RetCam
  - Anterior chamber aspiration for histopathology
  - Lumber puncture for malignant cells
  - Fine needle biopsy of preauricular and cervical nodes
  - Bone marrow aspiration for malignant deposits

VARIANTS OF RETINOBLASTOMA

Trilateral Retinoblastoma (Pineoblastoma)

It is better called pineoblastoma syndrome, which consists of a retinoblastoma along with a specialized malignant tumor of the pineal gland of neuroectodermal origin. The pineoblastoma cells of pineoblastoma differ in appearance from retinoblastoma cells; they are small, trance-lucent blue cells seen in both unilateral or bilateral retinoblastomas with intracranial extension. Some authors consider them to be primary malignant tumors; in bilateral cases, they may be hereditary. The growths can be parasellar or suprasellar in position. They are uniformly fatal; chemotherapy only prolongs life. Quadrilateral retinoblastomas are a more advanced form of pineoblastoma with additional features of suprasellar cisternal involvement.

Cavitary Retinoblastoma

This is seen in regressed retinoblastoma; they show intralesional trance lucent cavity, single or multiple. The cavities are hyperfluorescent on fluorescein angiography and echolucent on USG.

Orbital Retinoblastoma

Orbital involvement by retinoblastoma carries the poorest prognosis, with 70% mortality even with the most intense management, especially in bilateral cases. It generally becomes apparent after 1 month to 2 years of enucleation that all children do not develop orbital retinoblastoma following enucleation yet, making it mandatory to examine the enucleated socket every month following enucleation for the next 2 years.

It has been classified variously:

- Laterality
- In an enucleated socket
- In orbit without enucleation
- As a second malignancy

One of their recent classifications puts them in the following classes:

- Primary orbital retinoblastoma
- Secondary orbital retinoblastoma
- Accidental orbital retinoblastoma
- Overt orbital retinoblastoma
- Microscopic orbital retinoblastoma

Primary orbital retinoblastoma has been defined as an orbital growth diagnosed clinically or radiologically, either as an optic nerve or extrascleral extension (Honavar 2007). The orbital stage of retinoblastoma carries the poorest prognosis in spite of the most aggressive treatment.

The predisposing factors are:

- Perforation of the sclera during enucleation
- Extrascleral extension of growth
- Thickened, nonelastic optic nerve
- Tumor cells in the distal cut end of the optic nerve

The first evidence of orbital retinoblastoma is the gradual shallowing of the socket, followed by a visible, fast-growing mass. The preauricular lymph glands are enlarged, and there may be evidence of distant metastasis. Unattended orbital retinoblastoma ultimately extrudes through the interpalpebral aperture as a fungating mass. Management is dismal, consisting of aggressive chemotherapy and radiation. Orbital exenteration has been given up in favor of chemo and radiational management. Histopathological examination of tissue removed from the orbital mass is essential not only to confirm the diagnosis of retinoblastoma but also to ascertain the nature of other malignancies.

Second Malignancy

The second malignancy is a malignant tumor that develops in a child following successful treatment of retinoblastoma. The second malignancy is neither retinoblastoma nor its extension, or metastasis; it is an independent primary tumor. Children under 1 year, generally treated with radiation, are likely to develop a second malignancy in 35% of cases. Second malignancies in children treated with chemotherapy are less likely to develop second malignancy. The second malignancy develops in the late second decade or early third decade, either in orbit or maybe extraorbital, away from the originally involved eye. 75% are developing in orbit, resting away from the field of radiation. Second malignancies are more common in bilateral cases. The two common malignancies that manifest as secondary malignancies are osteogenic sarcoma and rhabdomyosarcoma, requiring individual management.

> The risk factors in bilateral cases differ from those involved in unilateral cases.

GENETIC RISK FACTORS IN RETINOBLASTOMA

Genetic peculiarities in bilateral cases:

- All bilateral cases should be considered to be hereditary.
- Parents and older siblings may have signs of a healed tumor.
- Asymptomatic parents of bilateral cases should be examined with an indirect ophthalmoscope for evidence of a spontaneously regressed tumor. A regressed lesion looks like a patch of healed chorio-retinitis.
- If the scar really is noninflammatory, the parents are at risk of transmitting the disorder to progeny.
- If no scar is found, then one of the parents may be a carrier, or the child may have a sporadic mutation.
- If there is a positive history of retinoblastoma in the past generation, the parents can pass the mutant gene on to the offspring.

Genetic peculiarities of unilateral retinoblastoma:

- 90% of unilateral retinoblastomas are nonhereditary.
- The person with nonhereditary retinoblastoma does not transmit the gene.
- Even if a remote relative had retinoblastoma in the family of the child with retinoblastoma, the family should be counseled.
- If there is more than one tumor in a sporadic case, counseling should be done.
- Unaffected parents of a child with a unilateral tumor are carriers.

MANAGEMENT OF RETINOBLASTOMA

Managing uniocular retinoblastoma is easier than bilateral. Intraocular tumor carries a 90% success rate; the success rate falls sharply if the tumor breeches the confines of the sclera or invades the optic nerve. The management depends on multiple factors that rarely act singly, more are the predisposing factors, and the poorer are the results.

The following are the factors that influence the outcome:

- *Stage:* Children with uniocular tumors are brought for consultation late; hence, by the time the diagnosis is confirmed, the tumor is pretty advanced, jeopardizing treatment.
- *Laterality:* Uniocular tumors have a better prognosis than bilateral.
- *Age of first presentation:* Generally, younger patients have smaller and fewer growths.
- *Location of tumor:* Peripheral tumors present late; hence, they are in a more advanced stage when examined than central lesions.
- *Extension of the tumor:*
    - Intraocular; tumors confined to the scleral coat are easier to manage than those that have become extrascleral.
    - *Extraocular extension may be in:*
        - Optic nerve
        - Orbit
        - CNS
        - Combination
- *Metastasis:* Tumors with metastasis have a poor prognosis.
- *Stage of retinoblastoma:* (See staging and grouping)

Aims of Treatment

The foremost goal of treatment is to save the life of the child. The second is saving the shape and size of the eye; the next aim is to retain as much vision as possible. The other targets are to prevent metastasis, treat metastasis, manage second neoplasms, provide genetic counseling, and last but not least, provide rehabilitation for the child.

The treatment is divided into two categories:

1. Those require sacrificing the affected eye, i.e., enucleation.
2. Those that spare the eye, i.e., radiation, chemotherapy, and other physical methods such as cryotherapy and laser.

Enucleation

This used to be the standard procedure of management in clinical stages one and two of uniocular growth; the child lived a normal life. This is still a standard protocol in developing countries; in developed countries, it has been mostly replaced by nonsurgical methods. It is generally used in:

- Retinoblastoma without visual potential.
- Tumor, larger than half the globe volume.
- Advanced glaucoma.
- Anterior chamber involvement.

> Choice of enucleation is very individualized, different institutes have different protocols to follow.

Options available to treat and salvage the eye:

- *Physical methods:*
  - *Radiation:* External beam or plaque radiation
  - Transpupillary laser
  - Transscleral cryotherapy is only for small peripheral tumors.
- *Chemotherapy:*
  - *Systemic:*
    - Oral
    - Parental: Selective
      - Intra-arterial
      - Intravenous
  - Regional: Intravitreal, periocular

Management of retinoblastoma is a long-drawn task requiring proper planning based on staging. Till recently, the Reese-Ellsworth classification was the gold standard of treatment; this has been replaced by more advanced strategies.

Commonly used staging protocols are:

- Abramson's staging (1997)
- International classification of retinoblastoma
- International classification of intraocular retinoblastoma
- Tumor node metastasis of retinoblastoma
- International staging system for retinoblastoma
- Modification of Abramson's staging seems to be the latest protocol available.

Tumors sometimes do not follow the usual protocol of staging due to inherent high-risk factors that can be present either in an intra- or extraocular lesion.

- High-risk intraocular factors are:
  - Uveal involvement
  - Optic nerve involvement
  - Scleral infiltrate
- High-risk extraocular factors are:
  - Covert orbital disease
  - Overt orbital disease

The treatment of retinoblastoma is broadly divided into two parts:

1. Intraocular tumor
2. Extraocular tumor

> Extraocular extension is always associated with advanced intraocular tumor.

Management of Intraocular Retinoblastoma

Management depends on:

- Whether the growth is confined to the retina or has invaded other intraocular structures such as the vitreous, uvea, or optic nerve?
- *Location of growth:*
  - Anterior to the equator
  - Involving macula, optic nerve
- *Size:* Small, medium, or large
- *Number:* Single/multiple

The treatment in each group can be:

- *Surgical:* Enucleation and exenteration. Enucleation is preferred in uniocular tumors. In bilateral cases, the eye with a more advanced stage is enucleated, provided there is no overt or covert evidence of extrascleral extension. The other eye is treated with nonsurgical methods.

  Points to remember during enucleation:
  - Gentle handling of the globe to prevent inadvertent dissemination of tumor cells
  - Cut the optic nerve as far as possible from the globe with at least a 5-mm stump.
  - Prevent perforation of the globe
  - Examine the enucleated globe for any growth
  - Exenteration is no more in practice due to its mutilating consequences and inabilities to manage the spread and prevent death.
- Nonsurgical, i.e., chemotherapy, radiation, laser therapy, and cryotherapy

RADIOTHERAPY IN RETINOBLASTOMA

> Retinoblastomas are highly radiosensitive.

The traditional radiotherapy modes are:

- External beam radiotherapy (EBRT)
- Plaque radiotherapy

Out of the two, the former has been used with fairly good results in the past when it was the only nonsurgical method to treat retinoblastoma; in fact, the Reese-Ellsworth classification was based on and developed round this method. EBRT is now a day used sparingly in developed countries but is still widely used in developing countries and is being phased out gradually. In recent years, more effective methods with better results have been used with the aim of directing radiation to the specific tissue, sparing the normal tissue around; that was an inherent drawback of external beam radiation.

The modes available are:

- Intensity-modulated radiotherapy*
- Stereotactic conformal radiotherapy†
- Volumetric modulated arc radiotherapy‡
- Proton beam therapy§

External Beam Radiotherapy

External beam radiotherapy is a multipurpose radiation therapy used for a number of malignant tumors, including retinoblastoma. It uses radiation emitted by cobalt 60, an isotope of cobalt. The radiation is delivered by a machine kept away from the body to deliver radiation from various angles. The method lacks precision for internal radiation. The dose required is 3,500–4,000 cGy** in a divided dose of 200 cGy weekly for 4–5 doses.

Indications of EBRT are:

- Bilateral or unilateral tumor <15 mm but >5 mm
- Multiple tumors
- Tumors with vitreous seeding
- Tumors near the macula
- Tumors near the disc
- Orbital recurrence
- If the tumor is found to have invaded beyond the cut end of the optic nerve
- Where chemotherapy has failed
- Where other physical methods have failed
- If chemotherapy is contraindicated

Complications of External Beam Radiotherapy

Complications are divided into two groups, i.e., early and delayed.

The early problems are:
Ocular surface disorders, cataracts, radiation retinopathy, optic neuropathy, and retardation of orbital growth. The delayed problem is the second malignancy, which is more frequent in bilateral cases.

Brachytherapy

It is also known as plaque therapy or internal radiation therapy. This involves placing a plaque containing a radioactive substance on the surface of the sclera nearest to the tumor.

The two commonly used radioactive substances are: Iodine-125, ruthenium-106, iridium-192, and (rarely) cobalt-60.

Indications of plaque therapy are:

- Eyes that do not respond either to chemotherapy or EBRT
- Recurrences
- Eyes with vitreous seeding

It gives the best result in solitary tumors with a base <16 mm and a thickness <8 mm, 2 mm from the optic nerve, and 2 mm from the macula.

The tumor is located by an indirect ophthalmoscope with scleral indentation. Its thickness is measured by ultrasonography. The method is preferred over *EBRT* because it spares surrounding normal tissues, has minimal effect on the orbit, and prevents cosmetic blemishes.

The plaque containing the isotope is stitched snugly on the sclera nearest to the tumor. The dose of radiation is between 4,000 and 6,000 cGy. The plaque is kept in position

***Intensity-modulated radiotherapy* is a high-precision mode of radiotherapy where computer-controlled liner-accelerated radiation is used to deliver exact radiation to the selected tumor.

†*Stereotactic conformal radiotherapy* is a form of radiotherapy where radiation is directed to the tumor from various angles that the beams meet on the tumor giving it the desired radiation without exposing the normal tissue to excess radiation. It shapes the radiation base to match the shape of the tumor in toto, not in height and width only.

‡*Volumetric modulated arc radiotherapy* requires a radiation-emitting machine that rotates to deliver continuous radiation as per the volume of the tumor.

§*Proton beam therapy* uses positively charged protons in place of X-ray.

**Gy (Gray) is a unit used to calculate the dose of radiation that a patient is exposed to; cGy = 0.01 of a Gy unit. 1 Gy = 100 rads, which is the old unit of radiation.

for 36–72 hours. The dose is calculated by dosimetry*. The radiation received at the apex of the tumor is about 400 cGy.

One of the undesirable effects of plaque therapy is scleral necrosis. The advantages are that the method does not cause bone deformity and does not predispose to a second malignancy.

CHEMOTHERAPY IN RETINOBLASTOMA

Chemotherapy has turned out to be a cornerstone in the management of retinoblastoma in many stages and has replaced surgical options to the minimum; it has gained popularity over *EBRT* and local modes. However, chemotherapy alone is not sufficient to destroy the tumor completely, for which other methods are used to attain an ideal result.

Various methods of delivery are available, including:

- *Systemic:*
  - Oral
  - Intravenous
  - Intra-arterial
- Periocular
- Intravitreal

Commonly used drugs in chemotherapy for retinoblastoma are:

Cyclophosphamide, vincristine, etoposide, carboplatin, doxorubicin, melphalan, and topotecan. Most of the drugs are administered intravenously, in an infusion, or through the central line. Only a few are effective orally; no local drops or ointments are available. The drugs are used single or in combination. A common combination consists of vincristine, carboplatin, and etoposide. The dose is calculated either on the basis of surface area, expressed in per square meter, or by the weight of the patient, in consultation with an oncologist. The drugs are administered on two consecutive days; on the first day, a combination of the above three drugs is given; the next day, only etoposide is administered. Six cycles are required, with a gap of 3 weeks in between. Eyes with serous retinal detachment or vitreous seedlings do not respond to chemotherapy due to the avascularity of the vitreous.

Periocular Chemotherapy

The drug carboplatin is used as a subtenon injection given under the posterior tenon; it is suitable for eyes with vitreous seeds. It enhances the action of systemic chemotherapy.

Intravitreal Injection

Intravitreal injection of a chemotherapeutic agent is not a primary choice; it is used in the recurrence of vitreous seeding following primary treatment. The drug used is melphalan, in doses of 20–30 mg/0.1 mL.

Intra-arterial Injection of a Chemotherapeutic Agent in Retinoblastoma

Systemic chemotherapy is always fraught with complications because it fails to reach the target cells. This happens in plaque therapy also; systemic chemotherapy is akin to *EBRT* in the sense that both lack precision and destroy normal tissues as well. To overcome these shortcomings, a method to deposit concentrated drugs near the target has been developed. The method, in short, is to deposit the calculated amount of drug as near the tumor as possible via the ophthalmic artery. The drug used is melphalan; adding topotecan and carboplatin to melphalan has a synergistic effect with reduced side effects. See clinical pictures in **Figures 7.24 to 7.26**.

Gene Therapy in Retinoblastoma

In the future, gene and stem cell therapy may be used to combat the disease with minimal side effects.

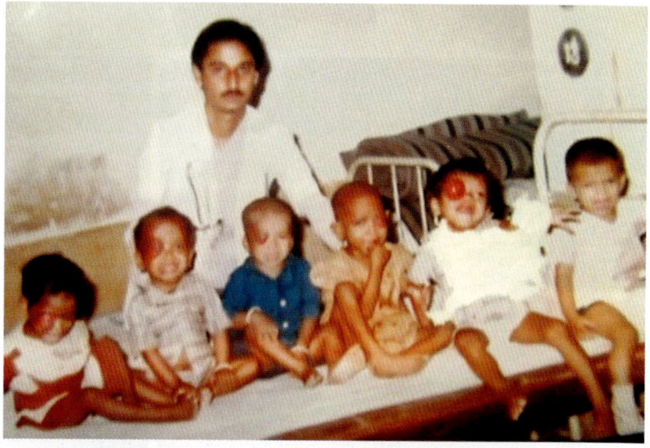

Fig. 7.24: Children with retinoblastoma admitted for chemotherapy.
Courtesy: Dr TC Adwani.

**Dosimetry:* It is the measurement, calculation, and assessment of ionizing radiation.

Orbital retinoblastoma: Points to remember in orbital retinoblastoma **(*Fig. 7.27*)**:

- There are no retinoblasts in orbit, so there is no tumor that can be called a true primary orbital. Generally, the orbital tumor discovered during enucleation is referred to as the primary.
- The most common presentation is proptosis, with or without a fungating mass.
- Orbital retinoblastoma is always an extension of intraocular retinoblastoma.
- The spread of retinoblastoma from the orbit is heterogeneous.
- Orbital retinoblastoma rarely extends backwards
- There are no-formed lymphatics in orbit, hence their spread in the preauricular and cervical glands, which are thought to be hematogenous.
- Orbital retinoblastomas do not get calcified.
- X-rays only show enlargement of the orbit, which has little diagnostic value.
- CT and MRI are better; the latter is preferred over the former.
- Orbital growths not diagnosed before enucleation are labeled as secondary.
- Signs of recurrent orbital retinoblastoma are displacement of the prosthesis and filling of the orbit.

Flowchart 7.5 shows various types of orbital retinoblastoma.

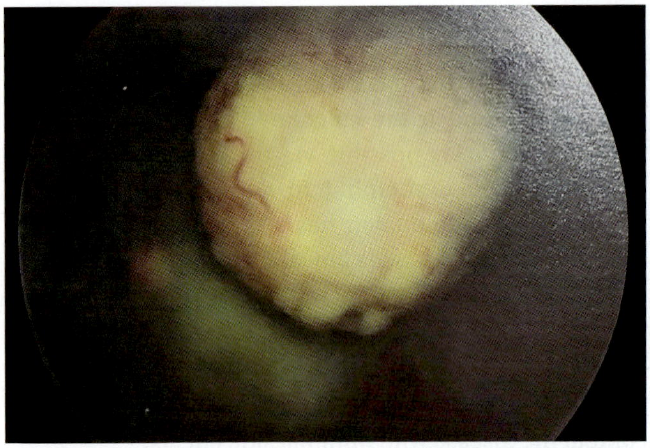

Fig. 7.25: Intraocular retinoblastoma at presentation.

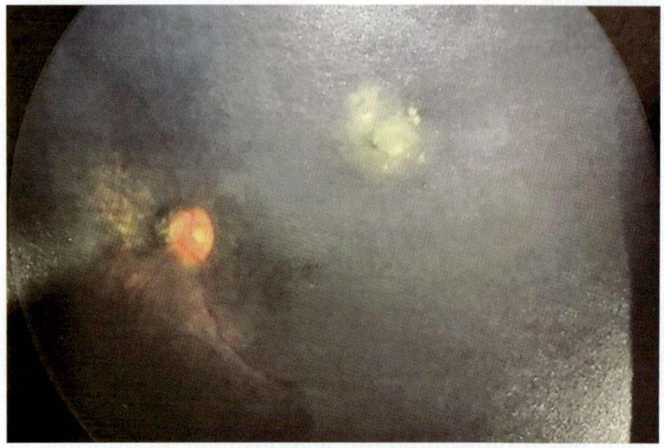

Fig. 7.26: Complete regression after intra-arterial chemotherapy.
Courtesy: Dr Santosh G Honavar, Editor, IJO.

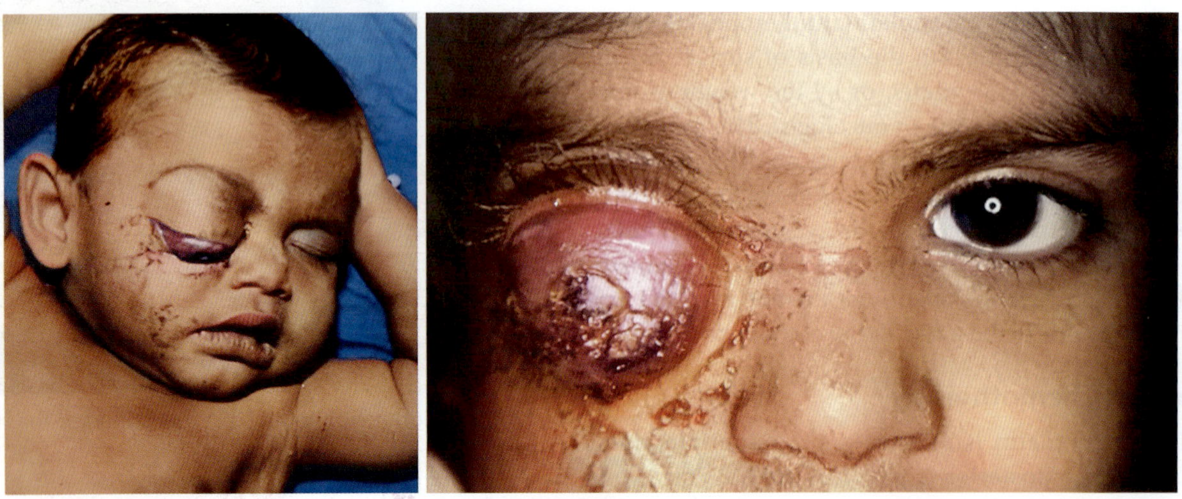

Fig. 7.27: Orbital retinoblastoma.
Courtesy: Dr Somen Misra.

Flowchart 7.5: Orbital retinoblastoma.

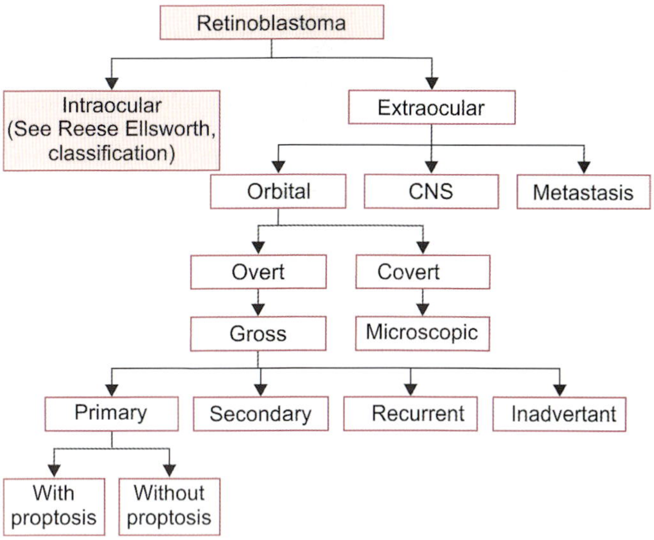

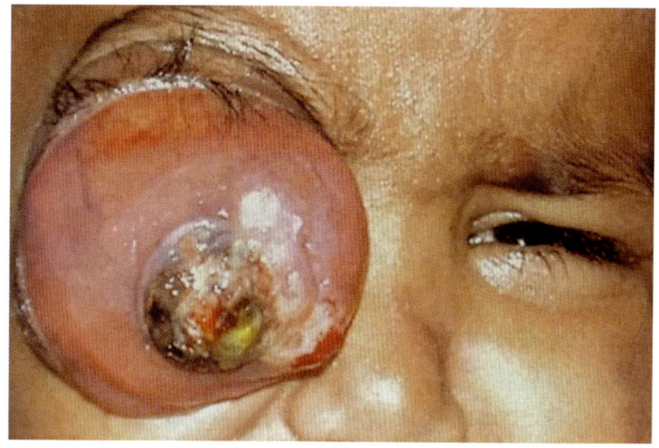

Fig. 7.28: Primary orbital retinoblastoma with proptosis.
Courtesy: Dr Santosh G Honavar (Retinoblastoma – They Live and See) LVPEI.

Primary Orbital Retinoblastoma

The tumor suspected at initial stages before enucleation quantifies to be called primary orbital retinoblastoma. The most common presentation is proptosis with or without a fungating mass, or sterile orbital or lid cellulitis. In rare instances, it can be small enough not to cause proptosis **(Fig. 7.28)**.

Secondary Orbital Retinoblastoma (Fig. 7.29)

This is a previously clinically missed retinoblastoma discovered at the time of enucleation or after enucleation.

Inadvertent Orbital Retinoblastoma

This is not a clinical stage. This is an aftermath of the accidental perforation of the globe during enucleation with the spilling of retinoblastoma cells in the orbit.

Recurrent Orbital Retinoblastoma

Filling of the orbital cavity and displacing the orbital prosthesis following successful exenteration after a few months to years is considered a recurrence of orbital retinoblastoma.

Overt Orbital Retinoblastoma

An unexpected finding of extension in the optic nerve or extra scleral growth is known as overt orbital retinoblastoma.

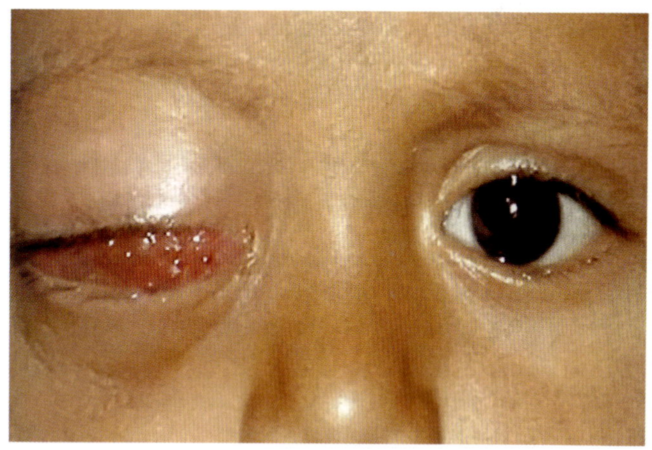

Fig. 7.29: Secondary orbital retinoblastoma with proptosis.
Courtesy: Dr Santosh G Honavar (Retinoblastoma – They Live and See) LVPEI.

Management of Orbital Retinoblastoma

Management of orbital retinoblastoma is less rewarding than treating intraocular retinoblastoma. Once orbit is involved, retaining vision is not possible; even retaining the shape of the eyeball is a far-fetched effort. The aim is to treat the tumor, prevent metastasis, and treat metastasis. Till a few decades ago, the only procedure available was exenteration. This rarely saved the life of the child; even if the child survived, he had a miserable life. This era was followed by the era of EBRT, until chemotherapy was introduced. Chemotherapy is generally supplemented with radiation. The chance of metastasis is 10–15 times more in orbital retinoblastoma than in nonorbital.

The common practice is to start systemic chemotherapy by a regime that employs three drugs: Vincristine, etoposide, and carboplatin. Three to six cycles are generally given, as per standard practice. If treatment is effective, the eye goes into phthisis and is enucleated in due time. If there is no satisfactory result, two more drugs are added.

Management of Metastasis in Retinoblastoma

Metastasis becomes evident within 1 year of a confirmed diagnosis in a treated or partially treated child. Five years of recurrence- and metastasis-free treatment is considered to be a cure. The child may lead a normal life after successful treatment. If the case is hereditary, the patient should be counseled as an adult about the possibility of passing the gene on to the next generation.

The metastatic retinoblastoma does not respond to the usual doses of chemotherapy and radiation; hence, high-dose chemotherapy is required.

FOLLOW-UP PROTOCOL FOR TREATED RETINOBLASTOMA

Different institutions have different follow-up schedules. The following is a protocol based on average practice in developing countries where the dropout rate is very high.

- *First visit:* In the third week
- *Second visit:* After 3 months
- *Subsequent visits:*
  - *First year:* Every 3 months
  - *Second year:* Every 4–6 months
  - *Up to the next 5 years:* Every 6–12 months
  - Thereafter yearly, especially in heritable retinoblastoma and the possibility of second malignancy if the child has received EBRT.
  - The parents should be instructed to report if they feel that the orbit is getting shallow, the prosthesis is getting extruded too often, or the child is developing symptoms of metastasis.

SUGGESTED READING

1. Abraham A, Thirumalairaj K, Gaikwad N, Muthukkaruppan V, Reddy AG, Thangaraj K. Retinoblastoma discordance in families with twins. IJO. 2019;67:436-39.
2. Abramson DH, et al. Neoplasm of the Eye in Cancer Medicine, 4th edition. William and Wilkins; 1997. pp. 1517-38.
3. Albert DM. Historic review of retinoblastoma. Ophthalmology. 1987;94:654-62.
4. Ali MJ, Honavar SG, Reddy VAP. Saudi J Ophthalmol. 2011;25(2)159-67.
5. Arora RS, Eden TOB, Kapoor G. Epidemiology of childhood cancer in India. Indian J Cancer. 2009;46(4):264-73.
6. Ata-ur-Rasheed M, Vemuganiti G, Honavar S, Ahmed N, Hasnain S, Kannabiran C. Mutational analysis of the RB1 gene in Indian patients with retinoblastoma. Ophthalmic Genet. 2002;23:121-8.
7. Biswas J, Das D, Krishnakumar S, Sanmugham MP. Histopathological analysis of 232 eyes with retinoblastoma conducted in an Indian tertiary-care ophthalmic center. J Pediatr Ophthalmol Strabismus. 2003;40:265-7.
8. Camp DA, Dalvin LA, Schwendeman R, Lim LS, Shields CL. Outcome of neonatal retinoblastoma in pre-chemotherapy and chemotherapy eras. IJO;1997;67(12):1997-2004.
9. Chawala B, Singh R. Recent advances and challenges in management of retinoblastoma. IJO. 2017;65:133-9.
10. Das D, Bhattacharjee K, Barthakur SS, Tahilyani PS, Deka P, Bhattachrjee H. New rosette in retinoblastoma. IJO. 2014;62(5):638-41.
11. Ellsworth RM. Orbital retinoblastoma. Trans Am Ophthalmol Soc. 1974;72:79-88.
12. Honavar SG, Gupta R. Retinoblastoma. In: Gupta AK, Krishna V (Eds). Clinical Ophthalmology: Present Perspective, 9th edition. New Delhi: Elsevier; 2011. pp. 526-32.
13. Honavar SG, Maujandavida FP, Reddy VAP. Orbital Retinoblastoma: an update. IJO. 2017;65:435-42.
14. Honavar SG, Singh AD, Shields CL, Demirci H, Smith AF, Shields JA. Post enucleation prophylactic chemotherapy in high-risk retinoblastoma. Arch Ophthalmol. 2002;120: 923-31.
15. Honavar SG, Singh AD. Management of advanced retinoblastoma. Ophthalmol Clin North Am. 2005;18:65-73.
16. Honavar SG.; Intra-arterial chemotherapy for retinoblastoma in low and lower-middle-income countries can we break the barriers? IJO. 2023;71(2):325.
17. Honavar SG. Orbital retinoblastoma in Clinical ophthalmic oncology. 2007;477-83.
18. Kiran VS, Kannabiran C, chakravarthi K, Vemuganti GK, Honavar SG. Mutational screening of the RB1gene in Indian patients with retinoblastoma reveals eight novel and several recurrent mutations. Hum Mutat. 2003;22:339.
19. Kumari N, Jain N, Saboo S, Parthasarathy R, Gupta V, Mahajan A, et al.; Intra-arterial chemotherapy in refractory and advanced intraocular retinoblastoma. IJO. 2023; 71(2):325.
20. Kumar K. Intraocular tumor in AIOS. In: Rammurthy D, Biswas P (Eds). Ready Reckoner in Ophthalmology, 1st edition. New Delhi: J P Brothers; 2017. pp. 369-92.
21. Mruthyunjaya P, Sagoo MS. Retinoblastoma. In: Jackson TL (Ed). Moorfields Manual of Ophthalmology, 3rd edition. New Delhi: Jaypee Brothers Medical Publishers; 2020.

22. Murphree L. Intraocular retinoblastoma – The case for new group classification. Oph Clin Nr Am. 2005;18:41-53.
23. Redler LD, Ellsworth RM. Prognostic importance of choroidal invasion in retinoblastoma. Arch Ophthalmol. 1973;90:294-6.
24. Sanmugam MP. Ocular Oncology. In: Saxena S (Ed). Clinical Practice in Ophthalmology. New Delhi: Jaypee Brothers Medical Publishers (P) Ltd; 2003.
25. Selzer EB, Welch RJ, Jabbour P, Leahy AM, Shields CL. Management of retinoblastoma in older children using intra-arterial chemo-therapy: comparison of outcomes of prechemotherapy and intra venous chemotherapy era. IJO. 2019;67(12):2005-11.
26. Sevel D, Rohm GP, Sealy R. Clinical significance of fleurettes retinoblastoma. BJO. 1974;58-687.
27. Shah PK. Commentary: The challenges of treating retinoblastoma in India. IJO. 2019;67(12):2004-5.
28. Shields CL, Honavar SG, Meadows AT, Shields JA, Demirci H, Naduvilath TJ. Chemoreduction for unilateral retinoblastoma. Arch Ophthalmol. 2002;120:1653-8.
29. Shields CL, Shields JA, Needle M. Combined Chemo reduction and adjuvant treatment for intraocular retinoblastoma. Ophthalmology.1997;104:2101-11.
30. Singh AD, Shields CL, Shields JA. Prognostic factors in retinoblastoma. J Pediatr Ophthalmol Strab. 2000;37:134-41.
31. Sing U. Retinoblastoma. In: AIOS Ready Reckoner in Ophthalmology, 2nd edition. New Delhi: Jaypee Brothers Medical Publishers (P) Ltd; 2017. pp. 521-4.

CHAPTER

8 Disorders of the Lacrimal System

The common adnexal disorders of the eyes in children are: stye, chalazion, blepharitis, and disorders of the lacrimal system. The first three are related to the lid, and the last is related to the lacrimal system.

The function of the lacrimal system is to keep the ocular surface wet and drain the excess wetting agent (tears). The ocular surface consists of the conjunctiva and the cornea. The wetting agent is the tear. To understand the malfunction of the lacrimal system, it is essential to recapitulate the anatomy and physiology of the lacrimal system.

The lacrimal system consists of three parts, i.e.,

1. The secretary system
2. The spreading system
3. The draining part

The last is involved more frequently than the former two put together.

The lacrimal secretary system comprises of:
The main lacrimal gland and accessory lacrimal glands that are not fully developed before 15 years.

LACRIMAL GLAND

There is one lacrimal gland in each orbit, situated at the upper and outer angles of the orbit in a shallow depression called the fossa for the lacrimal gland behind the septum orbital. The gland is a serous gland. The main function of this is to secrete tears. 95% of tears are secreted by the lacrimal gland. The anterior part of the gland is deeply furrowed by the lateral extension of the levator palpebral aponeurosis. This divides the lacrimal gland into two unequal parts: a large orbital and a small palpebral part. The former is neither visible nor palpable under normal conditions. The smaller palpebral part is sometimes visible on everting the lid. The lacrimal gland has about 12 ducts, which start in the orbital part of the gland and pass through the palpebral part to open in the superiotemporal aspect of the upper fornix **(Fig. 8.1)**. Histopathologically, the lacrimal gland has similarities to the other salivary glands. They also share identical pathologies of infection, autoimmunity, and neoplasm.

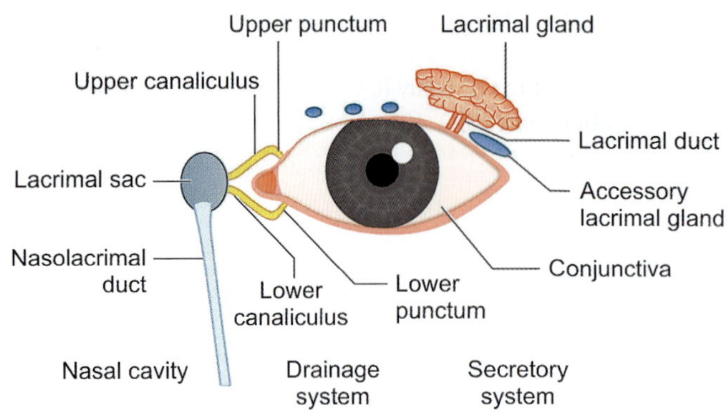

Fig. 8.1: Lacrimal system.

The lacrimal gland gets most of its blood supply from the lacrimal branch of the ophthalmic artery and some amount from infraorbital branch of the maxillary artery. The venous drainage is via the lacrimal vein, which opens into the superior ophthalmic vein. The lymphatic system drains into the preauricular glands. Nerve supply to the lacrimal gland is complicated. It consists of two parts:

1. Sensory supply is via the lacrimal branch of the first division of the fifth nerve.
2. The secretomotor supply is as follows.
   It does not have any motor supplies.

The parasympathetic supply is through the facial nerve, which starts in the superior lacrimal nucleus in the brain stem, from where it descends through the intermediate nerve of the facial nerve → greater superficial petrosal nerve → sphenopalatine nerve → zygomatic branch of the maxillary nerve, which anastomoses with the lacrimal nerve to end in the lacrimal gland. Derangement in this complicated system results in paradoxical tearing, i.e., the crocodile tear, which develops after facial palsy.

Accessory lacrimal glands are relatively small glands that are histologically identical to the main lacrimal gland but not situated in the fossa for the lacrimal gland.

There are two types of them:

1. *Glands of Krause:* They are found in both the lids; in fornices, the upper fornix has about 20 and the lower has only about 8 in number. They open in the upper and lower fornices on the lateral side and secrete tears. They are prone to all the disorders of the lacrimal gland.
2. *Glands of Wolfring:* They are very few, are embedded in the conjunctiva, and are situated in the upper border of the superior tarsus.

SPREADING SYSTEM

The spreading system of tears is as important as the drainage system. The tear is produced in the lacrimal gland and accessory glands and passes into the conjunctival sac at the superolateral fornix. To this are added mucin from the conjunctival goblet cells and lipid from the meibomian glands, forming a three-layered complex that is spread uniformly over the conjunctiva and cornea and then drained out without spilling.

This requires:

- Functioning orbicularis that propels the tear from the superiotemporal aspect across the cornea to the puncta.
- An intact lid margin that prevents the tear from spilling over the lids.
- Puncta in contact with the globe to suck the tears as negative pressure is generated in the sac with every blink.
- An intact lacrimal pump squeezes the sac to expel the teardown, creating a negative pressure that draws tears in via puncta and canaliculi.

Drainage of Tear

The drainage of tears is not a matter of simple gravity. It consists of capillary action, contact of the lid with the conjunctiva, a functioning lacrimal pump, and a healthy ocular surface.

DRAINAGE SYSTEM

The drainage system is divided into two parts, i.e., those involved in direct drainage and those that enhance drainage.

The structures directly related to the drainage of tears are shown in **Figure 8.2**.

- *Puncta:* One in each lid.
- *Canaliculi:* One upper and one lower.

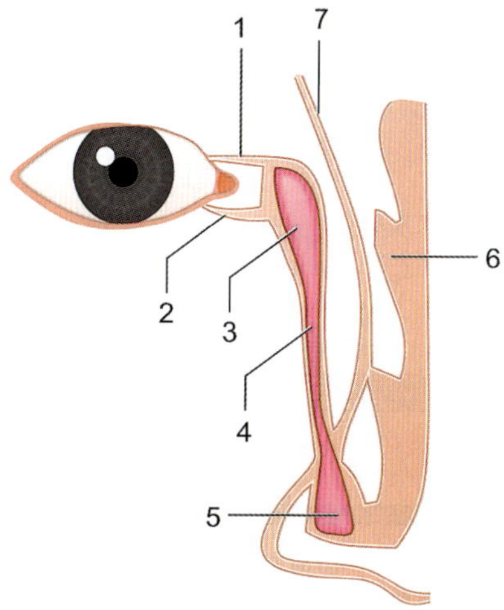

Fig. 8.2: Lacrimal drainage system. (1. Upper puncta and canaliculus; 2. Lower puncta and canaliculus; 3. Fundus of the lacrimal sac; 4. Nasolacrimal duct; 5. Intrameatal end of the nasolacrimal duct; 6. Nasal cavity; 7. Outline of the nose)

- Lacrimal sac.
- Nasolacrimal duct (NLD) in the bony canal.

PUNCTA

There are two puncta, one on each lid. They are pinpoint openings about 1 mm × 1 mm situated about 5–6 mm lateral to the medial canthus in the intermarginal strip. Normally, they lie snug with the globe. Both of them are not visible in normal positions; they become visible only on everting the lids. The lower puncta is better visible than the upper. The lower puncta drain about 80% of the tear.

CANALICULI

There is one canaliculus in each lid. The canaliculi are hollow tubes about 1 mm in diameter. They begin in the puncta. Each canaliculus has two parts, one vertical and the other horizontally slanting. The vertical part is the shorter of the two. The two arms join at an acute angle. The horizontally slanting part is longer than the vertical. It begins at the distal end of the vertical part, then slants toward the sac to open in the sac. The canaliculi may open at two different levels on the lateral wall of the sac with a gap of 1–2 mm in between, or they may join each other before entering the sac and then be opened by a common duct.

LACRIMAL SAC

This is a hollow structure about 15 mm in length and 6 mm wide. The shape is that of an inverted pear.

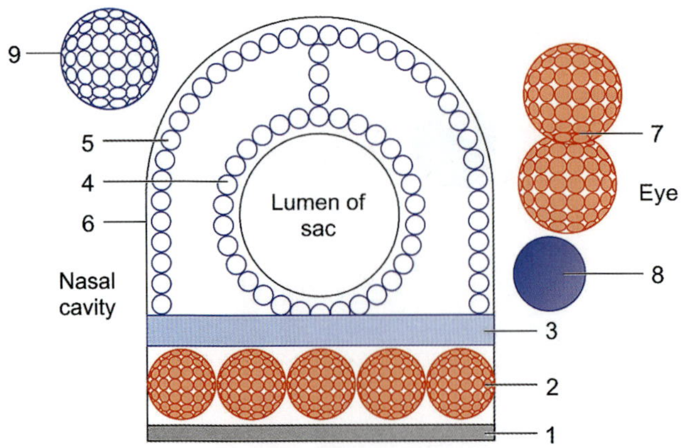

Fig. 8.3: The surgical anatomy of the lacrimal sac and its neighboring structure. (1. Skin over the sac; 2. Orbicularis; 3. Medial palpebral ligament; 4. Lacrimal facia; 5. Periosteum of the lacrimal fossa; 6. Bone of the lacrimal fossa; 7. Orbital part of orbicularis; 8. Angular vein; 9. Ethmoid)

The upper part is round, and the lower part tapers to merge with the NLD. The sac is situated in the lacrimal fossa on the anteromedial aspect of the orbit. The fossa is formed in the frontal process of the maxilla and lacrimal bone, encased in the lacrimal fascia, which is formed by the splitting of the periosteum. The surgical anatomy of the lacrimal sac and its relation to other structures are shown in **Figure 8.3**.

The medial palpebral ligament is placed horizontally over the anterior surface of the lacrimal fascia. Still in front are the fibers of the orbicularis, which lies under the skin. In normal persons the medial palpebral ligament can be palpated as a horizontal cord between the medial canthus and the lateral wall of the nose. This horizontal cord forms the most important surgical landmark in exposing the sac. The rounded part of the sac above the medial palpebral ligament is called the fundus of the sac. The normal sac is neither visible nor palpable. There is no regurgitation of fluid on pressing the normal sac. Regurgitation of fluid is always pathological. The canaliculi open on the lateral side of the sac either separately or by a common duct.

NASOLACRIMAL DUCT

This is a downward extension of the lower end of the lacrimal sac. It is contained in a bony canal. The NLD has two parts: A long intraosseous part that lies snugly in the bony canal and a small intrameatal part that is situated in the mucous membrane of the inferior meatus of the nose.

The direction of the NLD is not straight downward. It is best said to be down, backward, and laterally. Knowledge of the direction is important in passing a lacrimal probe during lacrimal probing. The NLD is not of uniform diameter. There are many areas where the duct is narrower than the rest. These are considered to be valves and eponymed variously. The NLD is relatively narrow in females; hence, they develop NLD obstruction more frequently. The meatus of the NLD is visible through the nose by a nasal endoscope.

BLOOD SUPPLY OF LACRIMAL SAC AND NASOLACRIMAL DUCT

The area round the sac is richly supplied by blood channels. The sac gets its blood supply from ophthalmic, facial, and maxillary arteries. The venous drainage is through the angular vein for the upper part; the lower part is drained by the pterygoid plexus. It is important to locate and isolate the angular vein during dacryocystectomy and external dacryocystorhinostomy (DCR); otherwise, there may be troublesome oozing during surgery.

The function of the lacrimal system is:

- To produce tears.
- Spread it across the ocular surface.
- Drain tear.

TEAR

The tear is produced at a constant rate under the influence of the autonomic nervous system. It requires a delicate balance between the sympathetic and the parasympathetic systems. The amount of normal tear is just sufficient to keep the ocular surface moist. The tear is also drained at a constant rate, which leaves sufficient tear to keep the ocular surface healthy. There is an equilibrium between production and drainage. Production may be increased or decreased under pathological conditions. There is no condition where there is excess drainage.

Normal Tear

The functions of tears are:

- It supplies oxygen to the cornea.
- To keep the cornea and conjunctiva wet and shining with a smooth surface.
- It acts as:
    - An ultra-thin optical layer over the cornea with a thickness of 7–10 mm.
    - Eliminates inborn irregularities of the corneal epithelium.

    - Minimizes the effect of acquired corneal irregularities.
    - The thin tear film over the cornea helps to keep the contact lens in place.
    - The contact lens, the tear film, and the cornea act as an optical complex in the functioning of the contact lens.
- The tear flushes off the ocular surface, excess mucus, minute foreign bodies, mild chemicals, and recently introduced microbes.
- It contains an enzyme lysozyme, which has a bacteriostatic effect.
- It contains the immunoglobulins IgA, IgG, and IgE. Estimates of which have diagnostic significance.
- It acts as a lubricant between the lid and ocular surface.

Tear Film

The tear film is not a single layer of fluid. It has three layers, each with a specific function. They are lipid, aqueous, and mucin layers **(Fig. 8.4)**.

Lipid Layer

The lipid layer is outermost and is secreted by the meibomian glands, the gland of Zeis, and the gland of Moll. The function of the lipid layer is to prevent excess evaporation of the next layer, i.e., the aqueous layer. It also vertically stabilizes the tear film. The lesser-important function is lubrication. It is disturbed in diseases of the lids, specially the posterior blepharitis, which includes various types of meibomianitis.

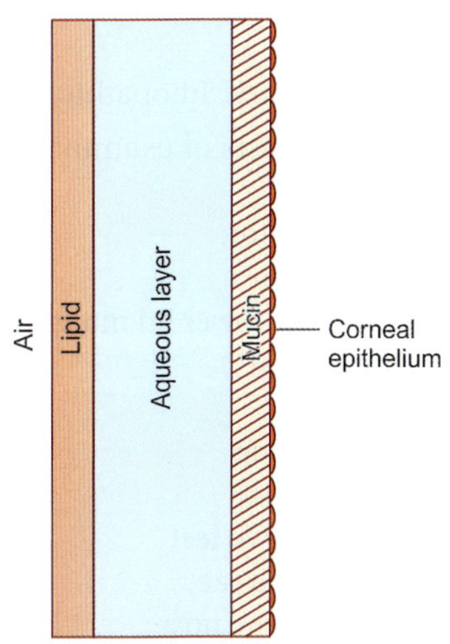

Fig. 8.4: Various layers of tear film.

Aqueous Layer

The aqueous layer is the thickest of all the layers. It is secreted by the main lacrimal gland and accessory lacrimal glands, which are under parasympathetic control.

Mucin Layer

This anchors the aqueous layer to the uneven corneal and conjunctival epithelia. It is mucopolysaccharide in nature and is produced by the conjunctival goblet cells and by the glands of Krause and Wolfring.

The production of tears may be divided into two processes:

1. Basic.
2. Reflex.

1. *The basic* secretion consists mainly of the lipid and mucin layers and is aqueous to a lesser extent. It is a fraction of total tear production.
2. *The reflex* secretion is the major part of the tear film and is under parasympathetic control.

Composition of Normal Tear

The volume of tears present in normal conditions is about 7 µL, which varies with age. It is 3 µm and secreted at a rate of 1–2 µL/min. The pH of the tear is approximately 7.45, which is influenced by diurnal and seasonal factors.

> - The lacrimal gland does not start producing tears before 3–4 weeks after birth.
> - The basic tear is present at birth.

The tear is mostly water mixed with lipids and mucin. It is slightly alkaline and rich in sodium chloride, which imparts a salty taste to the tear. It also contains sugar, urea, and protein. Albumin forms about 60% of total protein, while the rest is shared by globulin and lysozyme. Out of the globulin, the immunoglobulins that are important are IgA, IgG, and IgE. IgA is most abundant. It is produced in the plasma cells of the lacrimal gland. In some external allergic conditions, such as spring catarrh, the IgE concentration is enhanced, and IgM increases in acute infections.

Clinical Features of Disorders of Lacrimal System

- Epiphora
- Lacrimation
- Ocular surface disorders (hyposecretion)
- Infection and inflammation of various parts of the lacrimal system.
- Neoplasm of the lacrimal system

EPIPHORA

Epiphora is one of the two types of watering from the eyes, the other being lacrimation. The two have different etiopathogenesis, yet in present practice, both are taken as interchangeable. Some authors use the term epiphora for chronic watering and lacrimation for acute watering.

> Clinically, epiphora is an overflow of tears in the presence of normal production secondary to faulty drainage; it is a passive, non-neurological process.

Epiphora is brought about by:

- Fault in drainage mechanism, i.e., puncta, canaliculi, or NLD.
- Fault in spreading mechanism, i.e., lid margin.

Fault in drainage: For normal drainage, the lower puncta should be of normal size and in flush with the globe.

The punctal causes that are responsible for epiphora are: Absence of puncta, atrasia of puncta, pinpoint puncta, eversion of puncta, and foreign body in puncta.

The canalicular causes of epiphora:
Similarly, the canaliculi should be patent; the most common cause is traumatic avulsion of the lower canaliculus.

The most common causes of epiphora are:
The most common and important cause of epiphora remains NLD block, which may be congenital or acquired; the most common acquired cause is chronic dacryocystitis. Paradoxically, in epiphora, the sac itself remains unobliterated; the other sac-related causes of epiphora are the absence of the sac following a dacryocystectomy, a failed DCR, or a failed intubation.

> Surprisingly encysted mucocele of the sac and rhinosporidiosis of sac are not accompanied with epiphora.

Epiphora following dacryocystectomy is an unavoidable sequel; it gets reduced over months, most probably reflexively or as a compensatory mechanism.

Spreading mechanism: The tear is propelled from the superiotemporal fornix to the medionasal fornix by the blinking action of the lids. For a proper blink, an intact orbicularis is a prerequisite; an underacting orbicularis is an important cause of epiphora. The second requirement is a lower lid with a sharp inner margin snug with the globe; any derangement in this mechanism will cause epiphora. The causes are coloboma of the lower lid, tylosis, madarosis, and ectropion of the lower lid, severe entropion, and growth of the lower lid.

Symptoms of Epiphora

The only symptom is chronic watering from the eye that may be in one or both eyes; the former is more common than the other. The watering requires constant wiping, leading to uncomfortable excoriation of the outer canthus. Epiphora is more of a social embarrassment than anything else. Every eye with epiphora has a cause behind it, which requires identification and correction. Epiphora is worsened by super-added lacrimation, which is the overproduction of tears.

In epiphora, constant dripping of tears requires constant wiping, which causes social embarrassment. The treatment is directed toward the cause.

Management of Epiphora

Management consists of a detailed history, finding out the cause, and removing the cause.

History: History should include age of onset, laterality, and the association of other features.

Age-wise, it could be:

- *Before 1 month:* Hardly any possibility because tears are not produced before 4 weeks postnatal.
- *After 1 month:*
    - The most common cause is NLD obstruction.
    - Rare congenital atresia of the puncta.
    - Orbicularis is under action due to a birth injury.
- *Second decade:*
    - Untreated or partially treated congenital NLD obstruction.
    - Positive history of chicken pox or measles in childhood.
    - History of bathing in a pond in which buffalos wallow.
    - Craniofacial injury.
- *Beyond the second decade:* Idiopathic.

Finding the cause: It consists of examination of drainage system that include:

- Examination of the lid for:
    - Orbicularis function
    - Examination of the lower lid margin
        - Regurgitation test
        - Taste test
        - Lacrimal syringing
        - Dye clearance test
        - Jones one-and-two test
        - Skin scar over the sac
        - Examination of the nose
        - Imagining

Regurgitation Test

This is a simple, noninvasive office procedure that can be performed even in infants. It consists of applying gentle pressure over the sac; the pressure is directed backward, and the puncta are seen for regurgitation. The following observations are made in **Flowchart 8.1**.

Taste Test

It is a common experience that if a fluid with a distinct taste, such as saline, sour, sweet, or bitter, is instilled in the conjunctiva, the taste of the fluid is felt in the throat after a few minutes. This phenomenon is the basis of the taste test.

To perform the test, one drop of chloroform phenicol ophthalmic drop is instilled in one eye, and the patient is asked to blink a few times to propel the fluid down the NLD. Another drop follows. After 5 minutes, the patient is asked if he has a bitter taste at the back of his throat; a positive answer denotes the patency of ipsilateral NLD.

Flowchart 8.1: Result of regurgitation test.

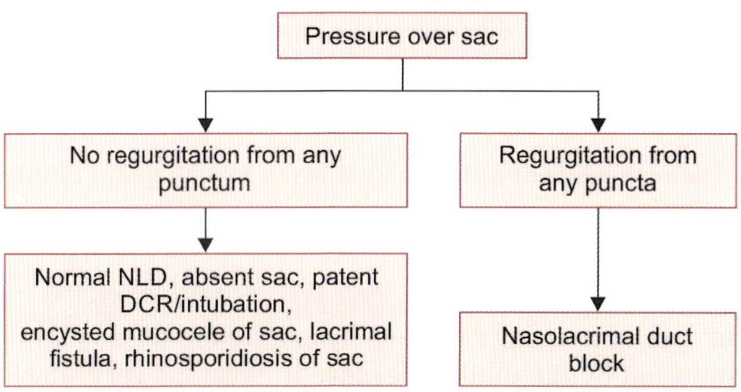

(DCR: dacryocystorhinostomy; NLD: nasolacrimal duct)

A delayed positive result indicates partial obstruction. A negative answer means block. The test is performed in one eye first; the other eye is tested 48 hours later. The test has limited value in small children because they do not express the taste well.

Dye Disappearance Test

This is yet another noninvasive, simple office procedure. To perform the test, one drop of 2% fluorescein sodium is instilled in the eye; the dye should drain out of the conjunctiva in 5 minutes. Nonclearance of the dye is an indication of obstruction to the drainage passage. Examination under a cobalt blue filter gives a better result.

Syringing of the Sac and Nasolacrimal Duct

This is the gold standard among all the tests done to find the patency of the lacrimal drainage system. It is an office procedure done under topical anesthesia in children above ten, following assurance that it will not hurt.

To perform the test, the child is asked to lie down on the examination table under the usual operation light. A drop of local anesthetic agent is put in the conjunctiva to anesthetize the lower puncta. The lower puncta and canaliculus are dilated; take care not to damage them. A lacrimal cannula is passed into the dilated canaliculus; to this is attached a 2 mL syringe loaded with normal saline. The plunger is gently pushed down to force fluid down the sac and NLD. As the saline reaches the child, he reports feeling the taste.

The following **(Table 8.1)** are the interpretations that can be drawn from syringing.

Primary dye test (Jones 1 test): This is a physiological test similar to the dye clearance test. In this test, instead of

TABLE 8.1: Observations and conclusions during the syringing of the sac and nasolacrimal duct.

Observation	***Conclusion***
Saline freely flows in the throat	The following are patent: NLD, DCR, and intubation
Fluid does not reach the throat	NLD and DCR intubations are blocked
Fluid regurgitates through the upper puncta and by the side of the cannula in the lower canaliculus	Both canaliculi and puncta are patent in presence of NLD blocks
No flow of fluid from the upper puncta. Water flows by the side of the cannula	Block in NLD and upper canaliculus
Fluid flows through a hole in the skin	Lacrimal fistula
It is not possible to pass cannula through any puncta	Bicanalicular block

(DCR: dacryocystorhinostomy; NLD: nasolacrimal duct)

observing dye disappearing from the conjunctiva, it is recovered at the nasal end of the NLD.

To perform this test:

1. The nasal mucosa is anesthetized.
2. Two drops of 2% fluorescein are instilled in the conjunctiva.
3. After 1 minute, a cotton-tipped wire probe is introduced under the inferior turbinate, left for a minute, and inspected for the presence of dye. The presence of dye is indicative of patent NLD.
4. If no stain is found on the swab, the next step is to reintroduce it again, and the procedure is repeated every minute for 5-6 times. If no stain is found after six attempts, it is taken that the NLD is blocked.
5. If Jones test one is negative, Jones test two is performed.

Secondary dye test (Jones 2 test): This is not a physiological test. The Jones 2 dye test is performed after a negative Jones 1 test. In this test, the lacrimal drainage system is flushed by syringing. The test is positive if dye is detected on the cotton bud, which suggests functional obstruction of the NLD.

Modified Jones 2 tests consist of instilling the stain as in Jones 2, waiting for a few minutes, and asking the patient to blow the nose on white tissue paper. The presence of dye on the tissue indicates a partial block.

Examination of Orbicularis

In all cases of epiphora, the orbicularis should be examined for under action. Underacting orbicularis causes mild ectropion of the lower lid, causing a loss of snugness of the lid to the globe and precipitating the spilling of teats over the lid margin.

Examination of Lid Margin

The lid should be examined for—tylosis, madarosis, ectropion, and coloboma.

> A small notch in the lower lid can cause intractable, unmanageable epiphora.

Skin Scar, Over the Sac

This is an indication of previous nonendoscopic surgery for NLD obstruction.

> Failed surgeries are the cause of persistent epiphora.

Examination of Nose

The NLDs open under the inferior turbinate. A nasal growth or deformity inside the nose can cause constant epiphora in endemic areas of rhinosporidiosis; it is mandatory to examine for its presence.

Imaging of Sac and Nasolacrimal Duct

Imaging in epiphora has little importance except for computed tomography (CT).

Commonly ordered imagings are:

- X-ray PNS, CT, and MRI.
- Dacryocystography and macro dacryocystography are no longer in vogue.
- Ultrasonography has no place.
- Out of all the above, CT is most useful.

LACRIMATION

Out of two types of watering from the eyes: epiphora and lacrimation, the latter is an active reflex process that involves the lacrimal secretary system with afferent and efferent paths, the former through the fifth nerve and later through the seventh, associated with multiple ocular and a few respiratory disorders. The causes of lacrimation are varied and spread over many ocular tissues, from the lid to the anterior uvea. They are **(Table 8.2)**.

> The management of lacrimation is the management of the primary cause.

HYPOSECRETION

In spite of its being common, hyposecretion of tears is not reported by the patient because it develops very slowly and the patient is not aware that the amount of tear in

TABLE 8.2: Causes of lacrimation.

Part involved	*Causes*
Lid	Foreign body, trichiasis, entropion, ectropion, lagophthalmos, coloboma lids
Conjunctiva	Spring catarrh, acute allergic conjunctivitis, and microbial conjunctivitis
Cornea	FB, abrasion, ulcer, interstitial keratitis, hydrops of the cornea, buphthalmos
Uvea	Anterior uveitis
Limbus	Phlyctenular keratoconjunctivitis
Orbit	Exophthalmos, proptosis
Other causes	Irritating fumes, bright light, and emotion

the eyes is less. What he reports is, in fact, the effect of hyposecretion.

The causes of hyposecretion of tears could be congenital or acquired (in all ages).

1. *The congenital causes are rare.* They are:
   i. Riley-Day syndrome (familial dysautonomia)
   ii. Congenital aplasia of the lacrimal gland
2. *Acquired:*
   i. Surgical removal of the gland
   ii. Senile atrophy of the gland
   iii. Postmumps atrophy
   iv. Systemic diseases
      a. Rheumatoid arthritis
      b. Sjögren's syndrome
      c. Systemic lupus erythematosus
      d. Neoplasm of the lacrimal gland
      e. Leukemia, lymphoma
      f. Stevens-Johnson syndrome
      g. Menopause
   v. *Drugs:*
      a. Parasympatholytics, i.e., atropine and its derivatives
      b. Antihistamines
      c. β-blockers
      d. Oral contraceptives
      e. Many other drugs
   vi. *Local causes:* Vitamin A deficiency; leprosy, pterygium, ectropion, Stevens-Johnson's disease, and chemical burns.

Causes of Deficiency of Various Layers of Tear

See **Table 8.3**.

DRY EYE SYNDROME

Dry eye syndrome was previously known as keratoconjunctivitis sicca. The two overlapped the clinical presentation of each, not encompassing all the features of each group. The condition involves not only tear deficiency but also changes in the epithelium of the conjunctiva and cornea. The changes in the epithelium are inflammatory, brought about by neurogenic causes, the activation of T cells, and the release of cytogenic substances at various levels.

The histopathological changes consist of → destruction of goblet cells in conjunctiva, → enlargement of nongoblet cells in conjunctiva → stratification of epithelium → keratinization.

TABLE 8.3: Various deficiencies of tears and their causes.

Deficiency	***Causes of hyposecretion***
Aqueous	• Lacrimal gland disorder – Congenital – Mumps – Systemic diseases – Systemic medications – Local medication – Surgical removal of lacrimal gland - Radiation - Chemical burns • Diseases of conjunctiva – Scarring of fornices leading to obliteration of lacrimal duct – Trachoma – Leprosy – Stevens–Johnson's disease – Acid alkali burn
Lipid	• Posterior blepharitis • Meibomianitis • Scarring of lid margin – Trachoma – Leprosy - Trauma - Burn
Mucin	• Vitamin A deficiency • Trachoma • Ocular pemphigoid • Stevens–Johnson disease • Local drugs

Histopathological changes lead to:

- Delayed repair of tear break-up
- Dry spots
- Development of filaments on the cornea
- Excess mucus in tears
- Epithelial debris is in tears

Now, it is accepted that the lacrimal gland, conjunctival glands, glands in the lid, and the corneal epithelium act as a single functional unit, and contribute to a healthy tear film. Defects in any way or in combination cause defective tear film.

> The term keratoconjunctivitis sicca is generally used in cases of autoimmune diseases, i.e., rheumatoid arthritis and Sjögren's syndrome.

Sjögren syndrome consist of aqueous deficient dry eye, rheumatoid arthritis, and xerostomia.

The ocular surface disorders have been classified variously. The most frequently used classification is given by Lamp and Holly.

They have divided dry eye syndrome as:

- Aqueous tear deficiency (ATD)
- Mucin deficiency
- Abnormality of lipid
- Disturbed blinking
- Nonwetting of ocular surface due to above four

The latest classification has narrowed the disease into two distinct groups:

1. Aqueous layer deficiency
2. Evaporative surface disorder

Clinical Features

Children under 10 do not suffer from classical dry eye syndrome. That is now a days; referred to as ocular surface disorder, which is a multifactorial disorder considered to be a primary disease. Children suffer more often from vitamin A deficiency, burns, and Stevens–Johnson syndrome, resulting in various degrees of ocular surface disorders.

Dry eye syndrome is a very common ocular disorder the world over (17–25%). It is also the most under-diagnosed or overtreated condition. Its incidence has increased manifold. Primary dry eye is caused due to autoimmune disease or posterior blepharitis. Ocular surface disorder is not a blinding disease. It is equally seen in both sexes. Women of menopausal age have more chances of developing it. In the past, it was thought to be a disease of old age, i.e., in the fifth or sixth decade, but now younger persons are developing the disease. The common factors held responsible for the increase in numbers are prolonged use of computers and pollution. Of course, the role of autoimmune disease in both groups is the same. Many drugs consumed for a long time, including oral contraceptives, are also causes of the disorder.

Symptoms of Dry Eyes

The symptoms are varied. One thing is common: the person is not aware of the fact that he has less tears in the eyes, either due to subnormal production or excess evaporation. One of the paradoxes is that he may complain of an excess of mucus in the eye, which is a compensatory mechanism to counteract hyposecretion.

The common symptoms are:

- Gritty sensation in the eye
- Recurrent redness in the eye
- Persistent redness
- Excessive mucus
- Fluctuating vision

Signs of Dry Eyes

- Surprisingly, in some cases, there may not be any obvious signs unless looked at carefully.
- Variation in level of vision with blinking, after doing near work, or looking at a computer.
- Nonspecific congestion of the conjunctiva that may be mistaken for allergic or chronic infective conjunctivitis.
- *Change in the inferior tear meniscus:* A normal tear meniscus is about 1mm above the lower lid margin. This is best observed on a slit lamp in ambient light, i.e., not putting on the light in the slit lamp; otherwise, it can be seen under a cobalt blue filter following the instillation of fluorescein in the conjunctival sac.
- *Presence of epithelial debris in the tear meniscus:* This is visible in white light from a slit lamp with magnification.
- *Fluorescein dye solution test:* Faint staining of the tear indicates it is less aqueous. Fluorescein may stain the cornea and the conjunctiva.
- Tear film breakup time: normally this is 15–30 seconds. A time of <10 seconds is abnormal.
- *Schirmer's test:* This should be done even before vision is being tested. It measures the tear present in the lower fornix. The wetting of Schirmer paper after 5 minutes indirectly gives the amount of tear present at that particular time. Normal wetting time is 30–35 mm. <10 mm is diagnostic of severe tear deficiency.

Schirmer's Test

There are two types of Schirmer tests: The first measures total tear, i.e., reflex, as well as basal tear. The second is called Schirmer 2, which measures reflex tears.

The Schirmer paper is a strip of Whatman filter paper that is 5.00 mm wide and 35 mm long. The strip is marked with horizontal lines at a distance of 1.00 mm apart **(Figs. 8.5 and 8.6)**.

The paper is bent at right angles at a level of 5.00 mm mark. The test should be done before the lids have been manipulated or light has been thrown in the eye. If the lids have been manipulated, the test is postponed for a few hours. The room light is dimmed and does not need to be switched off. The patient is explained that this is a painless procedure. The patient looks at the distance. The smaller, bent end of the Schirmer paper is gently inserted

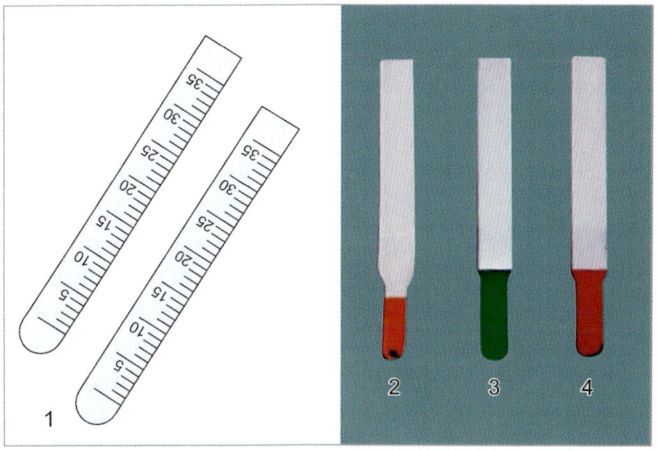

Fig. 8.5: Various types of paper strips used in dry eye: (1) Schirmer's test paper; (2) Fluorescein strip; (3) Lissamine green strip; (4) Rose Bengal strip.

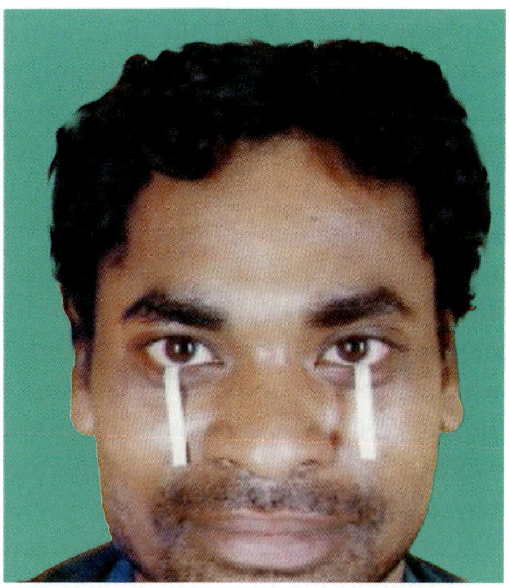

Fig. 8.6: Schirmer's test being performed.

between the lower lid and the globe, away from the cornea, and left there for 5 minutes. The tear starts wetting the paper through capillary action. The strip is removed after 5 minutes, and the wetting is read directly from the scale. In hypersecretion and lacrimation, the whole strip gets drenched in 1–2 minutes.

In normal eyes, the range is 20–35 mm; reading <15.00 mm is suggestive of tear deficiency; reading <10.00 mm is definitely diagnostic.

Rose Bengal

The Rose Bengal test is similar to the fluorescein test. Rose Bengal stains devitalized conjunctiva. The drawback of Rose Bengal is that it causes intense burning. This is avoided by anesthetizing the conjunctiva by paracaine or using the stain Lissamine green, which is not irritable.

Other sophisticated tests are the tear osmolarity test, tear lysozyme assay, tear lactoferrin test, impression cytology, and conjunctival biopsy.

Management of Dry Eye Syndrome

Treatment of dry eye is very illusive when looking at the signs, which are neither sight-threatening nor crippling. However, the symptoms may almost be labeled as annoying and embarrassing. There is no cure for dry eye syndrome. The condition is known to improve without treatment but has never been eliminated.

The main aim of management is to:
1. Replenish tear
2. Preserve tear
3. Reduce the associated inflammatory process

The tear is replenished by a group of drugs. Those are called tear substitutes.

Treatment depends on the severity of the cases.
1. Mild cases may be comfortable with the instillation of artificial tears 3–4 times a day.
2. In moderate cases, the frequency may be raised 6–7 times with lubricant eye ointment at bedtime.
3. In severe cases, the frequency may be as frequent as 1 hourly during waking hours, lubricant ointment at bedtime, and methods to preserve available tears. *This is done by:*
   i. Teaching the person to blink frequently while working on a computer.
   ii. *The humidifier in the AC room:* The humidifier decreases the evaporation of tears; it keeps the eye moist, which stabilizes the tear film, reducing constant irritation, redness, and fluctuation in vision.
   iii. *Punctal occlusion on:*
      - Collagen implant
      - Laser punctoplasty
4. *Ocular inserts:* Hydroxypropyl methyl cellulose inserts release the drug over hours.

ACQUIRED DISORDER OF LACRIMAL SYSTEM

Diseases of the lacrimal system are divided into two parts, i.e., disorders of the secretary system and drainage system.

The first consists of disorders of the lacrimal and accessory glands; the second encompasses disorders of the drainage system; the contribution of the spreading system is relatively small.

The diseases of the lacrimal gland are less common than lacrimal passages.

The clinical presentations of lacrimal gland disorder are:

- Painful swelling of the lacrimal glands.
- Slow, progressive, nonpainful swelling of the lacrimal gland.
- Discharging sinus above the lateral canthus.
- Lacrimation
- Proptosis
- S-shaped curve of the upper lid
- Pseudoptosis
- Ocular surface disorder
- Parotid swelling

The acquired disorders of the lacrimal gland are:

- *Infection:* Dacryoadenitis—acute or chronic
- Autoimmune disorders leading to inflammation of the gland.
- *Neoplasm:* Pseudotumors, benign tumors, and malignant tumors
- Trauma-isolated injuries to the lacrimal gland are rare. It happens following a penetrating injury in the region of the superior orbital rim as part of a gunshot injury, blast injury, or road traffic accident. It may be involved in a craniofacial injury.

Infection of the Lacrimal Gland

The infection of the lacrimal gland is called *dacryoadenitis,* which can be acute or chronic. Any organism can cause dacryoadenitis. The common causes of acute dacryoadenitis are mumps, infectious mononucleosis, herpes zoster, measles, influenza, and gonorrhea. Out of all these, mumps is the most common cause, followed by gonorrhea. Gonorrheal dacryoadenitis is seen in adults; it is metastatic in nature and treated by a systemic antigonococcal antibiotic.

Dacryoadenitis due to the mumps virus is a disease of childhood and teens caused by a single-stranded ribonucleic acid (RNA) virus found only in humans. The disease spreads either by droplets or contaminated fomites. The disease is acquired by inhalation or via conjunctiva. The incubation period is 10–12 days. The disease is associated with other features of mumps, i.e., fever, chill, and painful swelling of both the parotids. The condition can be divided into two broad groups, i.e.,

1. Ocular
2. Systemic

1. *Ocular* involvement can either be extra- or intraocular. The most common ocular involvement is acute dacryoadenitis, which is unilateral and may precede, coexist, or follow parotitis. Involvement of the lacrimal gland causes diffuse, tense swelling on the superior temporal area of the orbit with an S-shaped curve of the pseudoptotic lid and conjunctival congestion. Sometimes, the palpebral part of the gland becomes visible in the superior temporal fornix. Proptosis is rare. Underaction of the later rectus is common.

   The other ocular involvements are superficial and disciform keratitis and episcleritis, most probably as a part of an autoimmune phenomenon. Intraocular lesions are rare when present; they are uveitis and optic neuritis. Infection by mumps gives lifelong immunity. It is fully preventable by prophylactic injection of MMR (Measles, Mumps, and Rubella) at the age of 9 months. Dacryoadenitis due to mumps is a self-limiting disease.
2. *The systemic* involvement of mumps can be parotitis, genitourinary, or central nervous system involvement. The parotitis is ipsilateral to the involvement of the lacrimal gland. Parotid swelling is the first sign of the disease. Parotitis is self-limiting and passes off without any residual effect. There is no specific antiviral drug that is effective against dacryoadenitis or parotitis caused by mumps.
   The most common genitourinary involvements are orchitis and oophoritis, mostly in adolescents. Orchitis is generally unilateral, when bilateral may be the cause of infertility in later life. Central nervous system involvements are variable, seen in 60% of cases in the form of meningitis and encephalitis that resolve fully in a few weeks.

   Treatment consists of hot fomentation, systemic analgesics, and local broad-spectrum antibiotic ophthalmic drops to combat secondary conjunctivitis.

Chronic Dacryoadenitis

Chronic dacryoadenitis is less common than acute dacryoadenitis. It is seen in adults. It may be due to a specific disease such as tuberculosis or syphilis or a nonspecific granuloma like sarcoid. It is unilateral, progresses slowly, and has diffuse swelling in the lacrimal gland.

It is generally painless and presents with mild proptosis with an S-shaped upper lid.

When it is bilateral with diffuse swelling of parotids and submandibular glands, it is called Mikulicz syndrome, which is a symmetrical disease seen in adults. The causes are tuberculosis, leukemia, Hodgkin's disease, and sarcoid. It can cause an ocular surface disorder.

Hydrops of Lacrimal Glands

This is the accumulation of lacrimal secretion inside the gland due to obstruction in all the lacrimal ducts that may be due to infection, spreading from the conjunctiva, scarring of fornices due to thermal or chemical burns, or Stevens–Johnson syndrome. Not seen in children.

Diseases of Lacrimal Passages

Any part of the lacrimal passage from the puncta in the lids to the meatus of the nose may be involved in diseases of the lacrimal passages.

Following is the applied anatomy of the lacrimal passage:
The applied anatomy of the sac is divided into two parts.

1. Involving the upper part
2. Involving the lower part

1. *Involving the upper part:* The upper part consists of the sac, canaliculi, and puncta.
   The sac is the largest part of the drainage system. It is a flattened, club-shaped structure with a lumen; the lumen communicates with canaliculi laterally and the NLD downward; in fact, the NLD itself is a downward extension of the sac. The cavity of the sac normally contains about 20 mm^3 of tear mixed with secretion from the wall of the sac; the contents are just sufficient to keep the cavity patent and distended without being visible or palpable. Pressure over the sac does not result in regurgitation. The sac is snugly encased in a bony lacrimal fossa, with a potential space in between. The lacrimal fossa is lined by periorbita that splits to surround the sac and the NLD as lacrimal fascia. A plexus of fine vessels is visible on the surface of the sac under the fascia. The middle palpebral ligament crosses the sac in the middle of the sac; the sac above the ligament is the fundus of the sac; the remaining is called the body; the junction of the sac and the duct is called the neck.
   The angular vein is an important surgical landmark that runs 8 mm medial to the medial canthus. The other surgical landmark is the medial palpebral ligament, which can be palpated as a horizontal cord under the skin and appears as a white horizontal band when exposed. During surgery, the angular vein should be retracted away from the surgical field to prevent troublesome bleeding.
2. *Involving the lower part:* The lower part of the drainage system is the NLD, which is a downward extension of the sac itself and shares a common development. It has two ill-defined divisions: a longer interosseous part and a small in terminal part. The NLD should be fully developed and canalized at birth; in 10% of newborns, it remains noncanalized, causing so-called congenital dacryocystitis. The direction of the duct has an important bearing on the probing of the NLD. It is downward, lateral, and backward. It has a rich arterial supply and copious venous drainage. The NLD has few constrictions in its course; they are called valves. The most significant of them is the Hasner valve, which is situated at the terminal end of the duct in the nasal mucosa.

The diseases of the lacrimal passage can be congenital or acquired. Out of all congenital anomalies of the lacrimal passage, the obstruction of the NLD is the most common anomaly seen in infants and children. Out of the acquired anomalies, chronic dacryocystitis is the most frequent anomaly. This is followed by laceration of the canaliculi. Malignancies of lacrimal passage are very rare and not seen in children.

Clinical Presentation of an Acquired Disease of Lacrimal Passage

1. *Epiphora:* This is the most common symptoms of lacrimal passage disorder. The causes may be ectropion of the lower lid, eversion of puncta, pin point puncta, and block in the canaliculi, specially the lower canaliculi, chronic dacryocystitis, absence of sac following dacryocystectomy or failed DCR, and NLD block.
2. *Swelling over the sac:*
   i. Painless compressible sac without regurgitation mucocele of sac **(Fig. 8.7)**.
   ii. Painless, compressible swelling with regurgitation.
   iii. *Painless, noncompressible swelling over the sac:* Encysted mucocele **(Fig. 8.8)**.
   iv. Painful swelling over the sac-acute pericystitis **(Fig. 8.9)**.

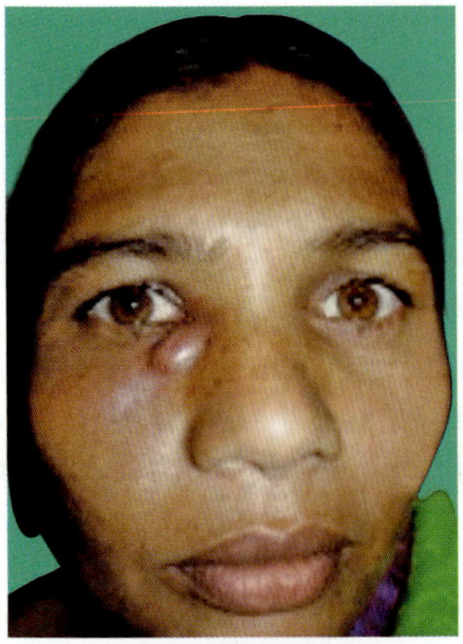

Fig. 8.7: Mucocele of the sac in an adult.
Courtesy: Dr Preeti Gupta.

v. Diffuse, painless swelling extending from the medial canthus to the lower lid rhinosporidiosis of sac (**Fig. 8.10**).
vi. Acute exacerbation of infection over chronic dacryocystitis (**Fig. 8.11**).

3. *Regurgitation:* If the sac is pressed, mucoid, or mucopurulent discharge regurgitates in the conjunctiva (**Fig. 8.12**).
4. *Fistula:* Tears come out of the fistula on the skin surface over the sac (**Fig. 8.13**).
   The causes of fistulas are rupture of the sac after acute pericystitis in adults, congenital fistula, traumatic fistula, and acute pericystitis in newborns (**Fig. 8.14**).
5. *Chronic conjunctivitis:* Conjunctivitis is a common, nonspecific disorder near the medial canthus.

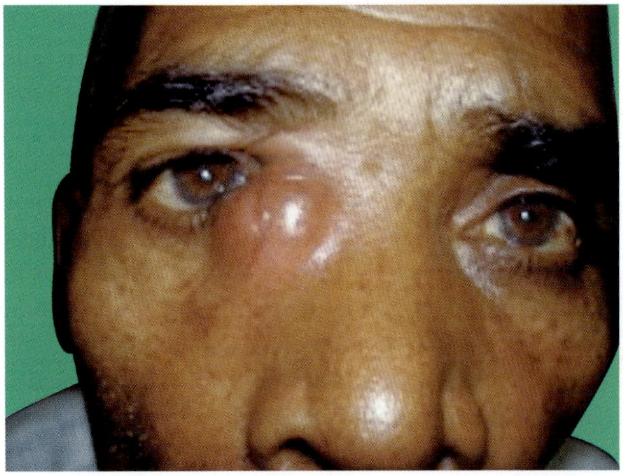

Fig. 8.8: Encysted mucocele of the sac in an adult.
Courtesy: Dr Preeti Gupta.

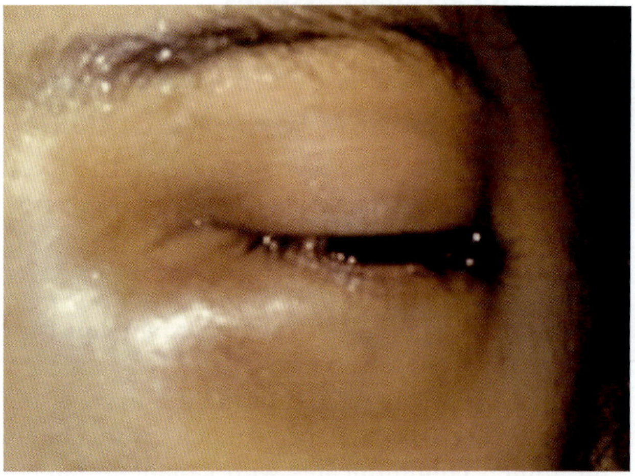

Fig. 8.10: Infected rhinosporidiosis of the sac in adults.
Courtesy: Dr Rakesh Gupta.

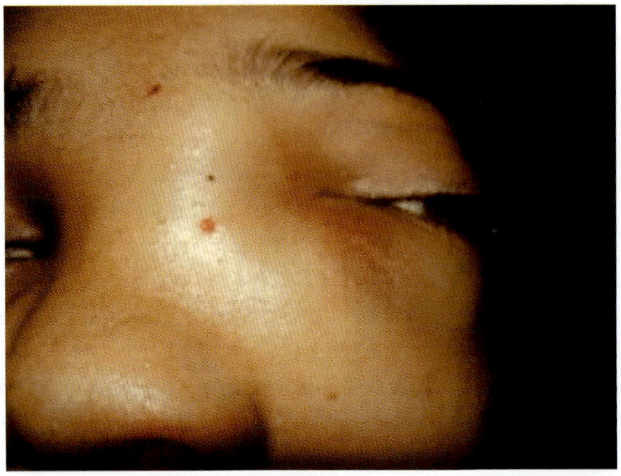

Fig. 8.9: Acute pericystitis of the sac in adults.
Courtesy: Dr Rakesh Gupta.

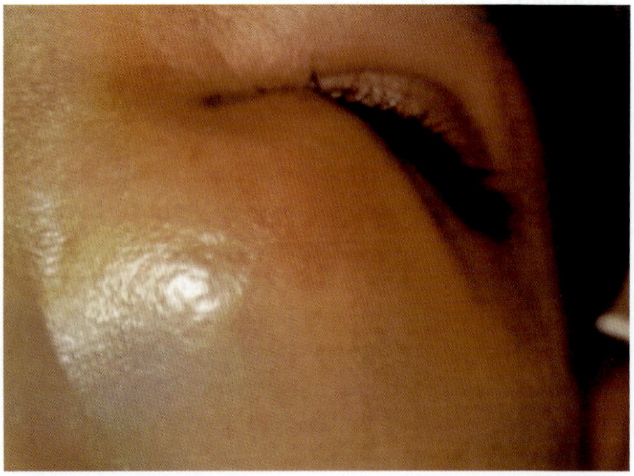

Fig. 8.11: Acute exacerbation of infection over chronic dacryocystitis in adults.
Courtesy: Dr Rakesh Gupta.

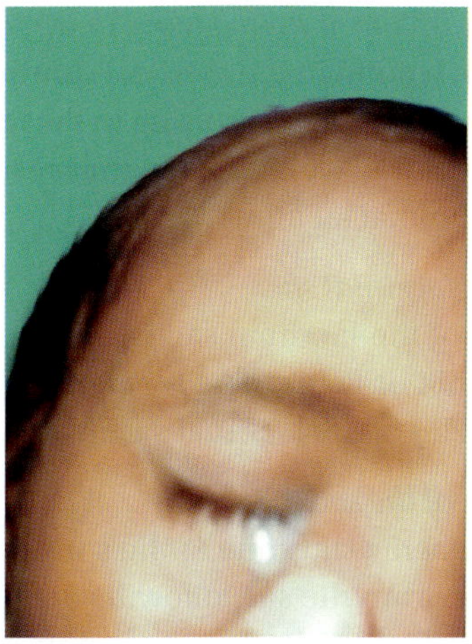

Fig. 8.12: Positive regurgitation in an infant.
Courtesy: Dr Santosh Patel.

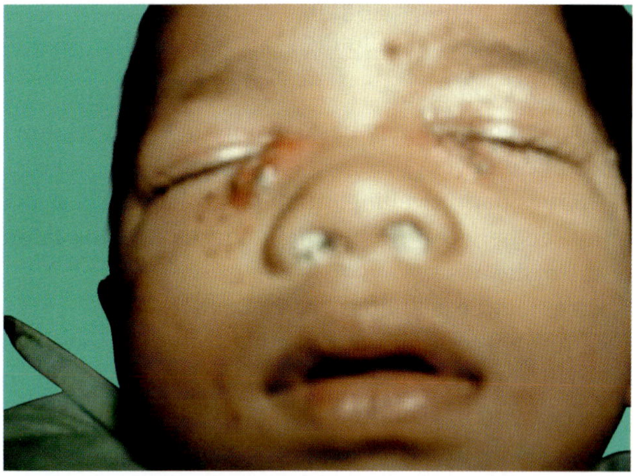

Fig. 8.13: Lacrimal sac fistula in a child.
Courtesy: Dr Preeti Gupta.

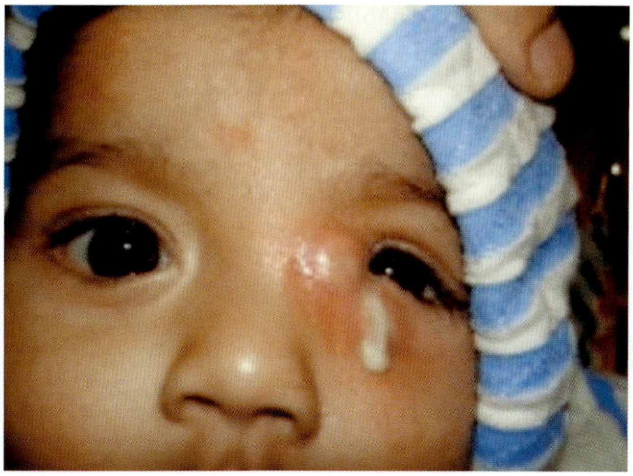

Fig. 8.14: Lacrimal fistula in a child.
Courtesy: Dr Preeti Gupta.

DISORDERS OF VARIOUS PARTS OF THE LACRIMAL PASSAGES

Puncta

- Congenital anomalies may be in the form of an absent puncta or a pinpoint puncta.
- *Eversion of puncta:* The puncta loses contact with the globe. The common causes are Bell's palsy, and ectropion of the lower lid due to any cause.
- A foreign body lodged in the lower puncta.
- A punctal plug may be deliberately put in the puncta to reduce tear drainage in dry eyes.
- The puncta may be obliterated by laser for the same purpose.

Canaliculi

- Congenital anomalies include the absence of canaliculi and the atresia of canaliculi.
- *Injury:* Lacerated wound involving the lid between the medial canthus and puncta.
- Infection of the canaliculi.

Actinomycosis is a rare gram-positive, filamentous, nonacid, fast-anaerobic, and microaerophilic bacteria found in the throat and nose. It is the most common cause of acute canaliculitis. It involves the lower lid more frequently. It is generally unilateral. The diagnosis is confirmed by demonstrating sulfur granules in the regurgitated discharge. The adjacent puncta pouts the condition, which is treated by repeated syringing and local instillation of broad-spectrum antibiotics for a long time.

Transaction of Canaliculi

The common cause of the transaction of the canaliculi is trauma—incised or lacerated wounds of the lids. Trauma of the lower canaliculi is more common and more troublesome than the upper, requiring expert management.

The management of transacted canaliculi requires special microsurgical expertise. If not managed well in the initial stage, it results in persistent epiphora, especially when the lower canaliculus is involved, because 80% of the tears are drained from the lower canaliculi. The canaliculi may get cut either in an incised wound between the punctum and the medial canthus, where the skin, orbicularis, and canaliculus are cut, leaving the posterior lamella intact. In cases of laceration, there is full-thickness disruption of the lid, including the canaliculi.

A lacerated wound is more likely to involve both the upper and lower canaliculi.

The principle of repair of the canaliculi is to anastomose the cut ends without causing stricture.

It consists of:

- Identify the two ends. The distal end is toward the puncta.
- Pass a stent in the canaliculus so the two ends act as a sleeve over the stent.
- Stitch the lid with the usual precautions for lid repair. The two canalicular ends may be stitched by 10-0 sutures or left approximated only without sutures.
- The other alternative is to pass a thin hollow tube from the puncta passing through the ends, which approximate the two ends of canaliculi passing the tube in the sac-down NLD-nose and is made to come out of the external naris.
- If none of the canaliculi can be anastomosed, the next alternative is to anastomose the bulbar conjunctiva to the sac. The procedure is called conjunctivodacryo anastomosis.

Lacrimal Sac

The congenital anomalies of the sac are very few. It may be absent in widespread anomalies of the face, the sac may be small, or it may have a congenital fistula from which tear leaks constantly. In rare instances, it may present as congenital encysted swelling over the sac, often referred to as congenital mucocele of the sac **(Fig. 8.15)**. Gentle pressure over the swelling may force the NLD to block and force the fluid in the cyst to deflate the sac.

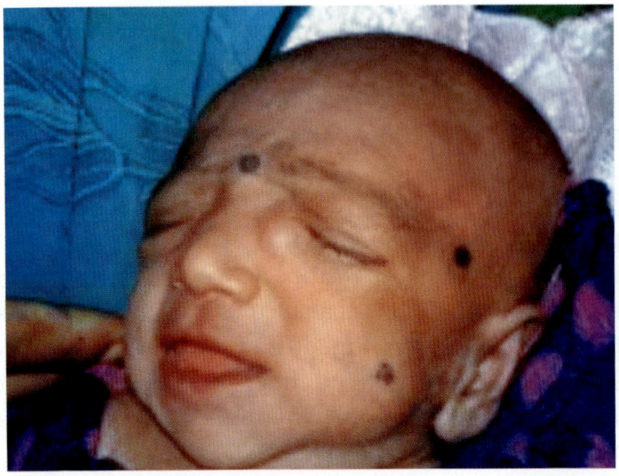

Fig. 8.15: Congenital mucocele of sac.
Courtesy: Dr Preeti Gupta.

The sac may be involved in two ways in trauma:

1. A laceration wound in the medical canthus may cut the anterior wall of the sac, resulting in the leaking of tears. If it is not repaired well, a fistula may result.
2. A severe craniofacial injury.

Infection of the lacrimal sac:

Inflammation of the lacrimal sac is called dacryocystitis. It can be chronic or acute. The former is by far the most common disorder of the lacrimal sac in adults.

Acute infection of the sac:

This is in fact a pericystitis due to the spread of infection to pericystic tissue from the sac following acute exacerbation of chronic dacryocystitis. The common organisms are streptococci, staphylococci, and streptococci pneumoniae. In children, *Haemophilus influenzae* is the most important organism. It requires urgent treatment to prevent lid abscesses and orbital cellulitis.

The clinical features are:

- The patient generally has a history of epiphora due to chronic dacryocystitis.
- There is pain, swelling, redness, and tenderness over the sac between the medial canthus and the lateral wall of the nose.
- There may be cellulitis over the sac area.
- A frank abscess may develop that subsides by systemic broad-spectrum antibiotics, or it may burst on the surface and heal only to recur.
- A nonhealing abscess may be converted into a lacrimal sinus **(Fig. 8.16)** when it does not communicate with the interior of the sac.
    - *Lacrimal fistula:* The infection erodes the wall of the sac and establishes communication between the cavity of the sac and the skin. A granuloma may develop in the fistula **(Fig. 8.17)**.

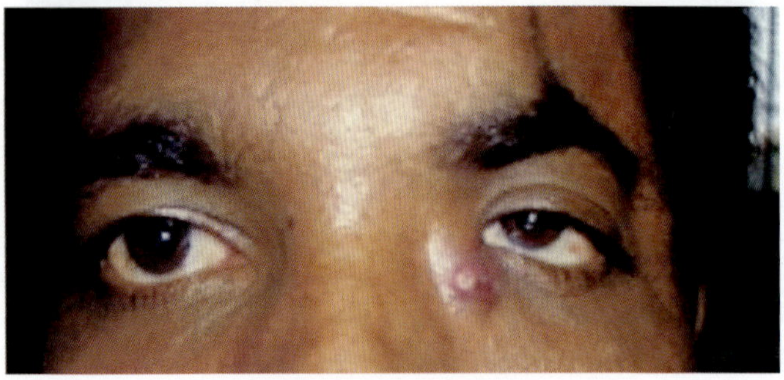

Fig. 8.16: Lacrimal sinus.
Courtesy: Dr Preeti and Rakesh Gupta.

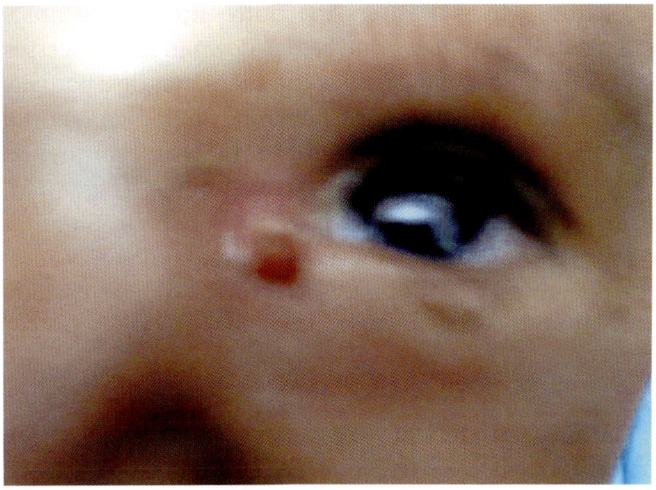

Fig. 8.17: Granuloma protruding through lacrimal fistula.

The presence of a fistula is confirmed by:

i. Fluorescein trickles through the opening when instilled in the conjunctiva.
ii. Fluid comes out of the fistula when lacrimal syringing is performed.
iii. The acute infection subsides with the formation of a fistula; fluid trickles through the opening, reliving epiphora.

The management of acute lacrimal pericystitis is:

1. *Prevention:* This consists of surgical management of chronic dacryocystitis by DCR.
2. *Management of acute pericystitis:*
   i. Broad-spectrum antibiotics by mouth or injection.
   ii. Dry, hot fomentation.
   iii. Drainage of the lacrimal abscess occurs before the sinus develops.
   iv. A fistula will not heal until a DCR has been done.
   v. Excision of the fistulous tract after DCR and closure of the opening in the sac.

Chronic Dacryocystitis

It is the most common cause of epiphora at any age. It is generally unilateral. There are three age groups who suffer from chronic conjunctivitis.

They are:

1. Chronic dacryocystitis in adults.
2. Chronic dacryocystitis in children.
3. Chronic dacryocystitis in infants.

> The basic pathology in all the conditions consists of stasis in the sac, to which chronic infection is added.

The most common cause of stasis is blockage in the NLD, which can be partial or complete. It begins as a partial obstruction, which, when unattended, passes into a complete block. The exact cause of the block is not well understood.

The predisposing factors are:

1. The NLD is genetically narrow. It is unknown to some African tribes. It is also less common among tribes in central India that have a wider nasal bridge.
2. The diameter of the NLD is narrower in females than in males; hence, it is more common in females of all races.
3. Partially treated congenital NLD block.
4. Exanthematous diseases such as smallpox, chicken-pox, and measles occur in childhood.
5. Retrograde chronic infection from the nasopharynx gradually narrows the NLD.
6. Nasal polyp, deviated nasal septum.
7. Craniofacial injury.

> In the absence of stasis, any amount of conjunctivitis does not cause dacryocystitis.

The materials retained following the stasis are:

1. Tear, mucous, lipids, and bacteria.
2. Secretion comes from the epithelium of the sac.

The most common route of microbial invasion is from the conjunctiva. The common organisms are cocci, i.e., streptococci, staphylococci, pneumococci, and *Haemophilus influenzae*, which is a gram-negative bacillus. Mixed inflections are common.

SPECIFIC TYPES OF CHRONIC DACRYOCYSTITIS

Rhinosporidiosis of the Sac

(For Details, See the Following Text)

Rhinosporidiosis of the eye and its adnexa is caused by an organism called *Rhinosporidium seeberi*. The exact order and the family to which the organism belongs have not yet been proved conclusively. In the past, it has been put into different groups, i.e., protozoa, fungi, and algae. At present, it is thought that it belongs to the order Olididiacae. The organism has neither been grown in any medium nor has the disease been produced in animals.

The disease has two forms:

1. That involves the eye and its adnexa.
   i. The common parts of the eye involved are the conjunctiva, lacrimal sac, and sclera.
   ii. No intraocular involved has been reported.
2. Extraocular:
   i. Localized
   ii. Generalized dissemination

The localized lesions can be seen in any part lined by the epithelium, i.e., the urethra, vagina, nose, nasopharynx, trachea, bronchus, and skin. Even bone and skin have been found to be involved.

Conjunctival sporidiosis and dacryo sporidiosis are collectively called oculosporidiosis.

Dacryo Cystosporidiosis

This is a chronic infective disease of the lacrimal sac seen mostly in tropical and subtropical countries. In India, it is found in areas with high rainfall, with high summer temperature, and persistently high humidity. It is a mostly unilateral disease that is more common in children and young adults. Most of the persons with oculosporidiosis have a common habit of taking baths in stagnant community ponds that are shared by water buffaloes, which harbor the organism. Generally, only one or two persons in the family develop the disease, though all the members live in the same environment, including bathing in the same pond.

There are two modes of involvement in the sac:

1. Primary without involvement of the nose.
2. Extension from the nose is via the NLD.

The exact mode of infection and incubation period are not known. The most widely believed theory is that the infective stage of the organism floats in the stagnant pool from where it enters the body through the nose, mouth, and conjunctiva and settles down in blind recesses lined by mucosa. In the case of the sac, it may be a partially closed NLD, either due to partially treated congenital dacryocystitis or dacryocystitis following exanthema. In the case of conjunctiva, it can be fornices **(Fig. 8.18)**, inner canthus, plica semilunaris, and caruncle. Simultaneous involvement of the conjunctiva and sac is rare; the lesion in the conjunctiva may proliferate to cause a chronic granuloma.

The reproduction cycle of the organism is also not very clear.

The initial clinical features are the same as in the catarrhal stage of chronic dacryocystitis, i.e., epiphora and medial bulbar conjunctivitis. Surprisingly, there is no regurgitation. The swelling of the sac is diffuse and may extend under the lower lid. On syringing, the NLD is closed when the infection spreads from the nose but partially open when the infection is via the canaliculi. The skin over the swelling has an orange peel appearance **(Fig. 8.19)**.

The temperature over the swelling has not been raised. Lymph nodes are not enlarged. The patient may have a history of bleeding from the nose. On nasal examination, a granulomatous mass may be visible. If the sac gets infected, as happens many times following syringing, a pericystitis develops that may form an abscess and burst on the surface, and the granuloma may protrude on the skin through the hole **(Fig. 8.20)**.

Management of dacryo sporidiosis is difficult and frustrating; recurrences are common.

There is no known medical treatment. The definitive treatment is the surgical removal of the sac along with the growth totally. This can be done in two ways: external dacryocystectomy and endonasal removal of the sac. Recurrences are common if the growth is partly left.

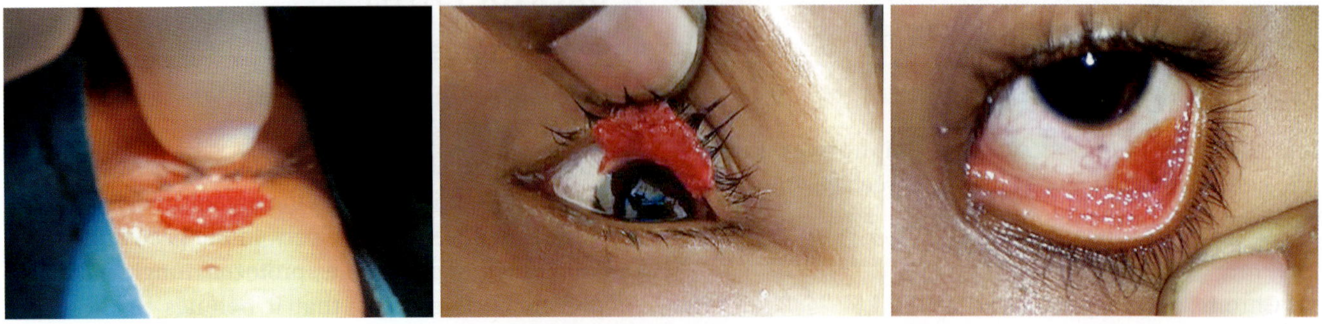

Fig. 8.18: Involvement of conjunctiva in rhinosporidiosis.
Courtesy: Dr Rajesh Awasthi.

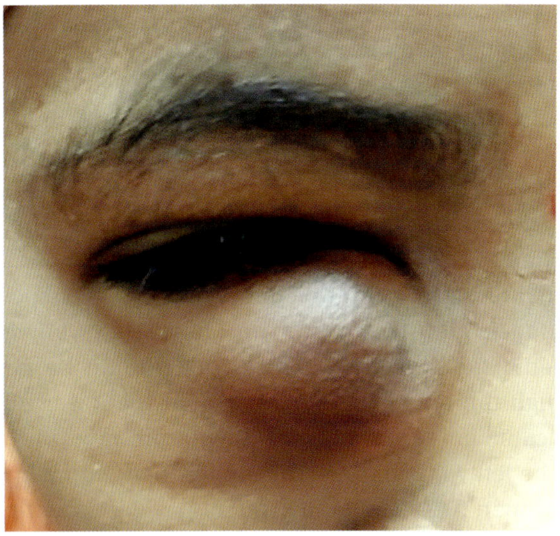

Fig. 8.19: Dacryo cystosporidiosis showing an orange peel appearance.
Courtesy: Dr Somen Misra.

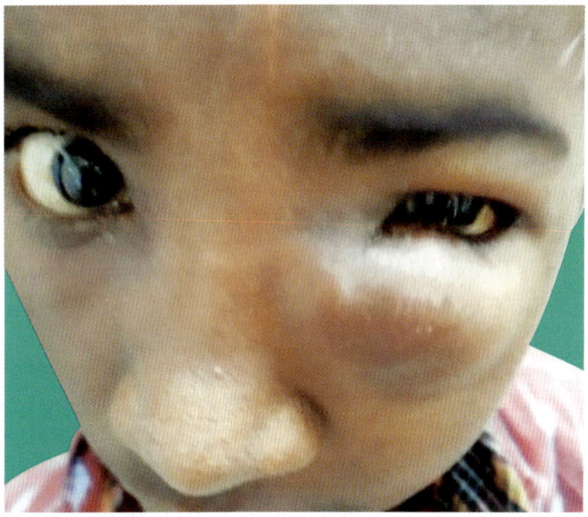

Fig. 8.20: Pericystitis following syringing.

DISORDERS OF NASOLACRIMAL DUCT

The only disorder of the NLD is its congenital obstruction. To understand the mechanism of the obstruction, it is essential to revise knowledge of the development and applied anatomy of the NLD and lacrimal sac.

The lacrimal sac and the NLD develop in a furrow in the frontal process of the maxilla, and the lacrimal bone, beneath the skin, as a solid cord of epithelium. The upper end distends to form the sac, and the lower end gets canalized as the NLD. The canalization starts from both the proximal as well as distal ends. The two ends meet just before birth. The NLD should be fully canalized at birth or within a few days. In some cases, the canalization is not complete, and the two ends do not meet each other but are separated by a membrane or some of the epithelial debris which have not been washed down the NLD at birth.

Failure to canalize the NLD is the cause of congenital NLD obstruction, which is otherwise referred to as congenital dacryocystitis. The obstruction in turn leads to stasis of secretion from the wall of the sac; to this is added mucous from the conjunctiva. As the lacrimal gland does not start secreting tears before 2–3 weeks after birth, initially there is neither collection of tears in the sac nor epiphora. Hence, congenital dacryocystitis does not manifest before 3 weeks after birth.

The congenital dacryocystitis is unilateral in about 75% of cases; bilateral cases due to some ill-understood causes are rare; there may be a positive history among the siblings; even the grandparent may tell that one of the parents of the child had such complaints in infancy. The incidence is more in premature children. It is equally common in boys and girls, in contrast to adult chronic dacryocystitis, which is more common in females. The most common cause of congenital NLD block is an obstruction at the level of the Hasner valve. The other contributing factor is too much epithelial debris in the duct at the time of birth, which generally gets flushed out in a few days.

CONGENITAL NASOLACRIMAL OBSTRUCTION (CONGENITAL DACRYOCYSTITIS)

The symptoms of congenital NLD block are constant watering from the effected eye and mucopurulent discharging.

On examination, there may be slight fullness over the sac, but no mucocele is formed, as is common in adults. Pressure over the sac causes copious regurgitation of mucopurulent material from both the puncta.

> The diagnosis is straight forward in a child born a few weeks ago who develops watering in one eye.

The differential diagnosis includes all causes of watering from the eye of an infant. On the top of the list is ophthalmia neonatorum* which is an emergency. The other causes that constitute a differential diagnosis are: corneal abrasion, keratitis, buphthalmos, orbicularis under action, coloboma of the upper lid, and pin point puncta buphthalmos. Keratitis and corneal abrasions are associated with photophobia.

The dictum is watering from both eyes under 3 weeks is ophthalmia neonatorum. Watering from one eye after 3 weeks is congenital nasolacrimal duct obstruction.

Management

The management of congenital nasolacrimal duct block is as simple as diagnosis; provided it is started before 10–12 weeks of age and carried out as per instruction. Role of mother in carrying out the treatment is most important.

The treatment, which is commonly called massaging of the NLD, is again the wrong term. The procedure involves compressing the sac with external pressure.

The procedure is demonstrated to the mother, who is asked to repeat it in the presence of the doctor. It consists of:

- Clearing the conjunctiva of any discharge by wet swab.
- Applying a gentle press of the small finger of the caregiver over the sac.
- This will cause copious regurgitation from both puncta.
- The regurgitated material is again cleaned.
- A drop of broad-spectrum antibiotic is instilled in the conjunctiva.
- The whole procedure is carried out 5–6 times a day for at least a month.
- After the first 3–4 days of treatment, there will be no regurgitation, but epiphora will persist till the condition has been cured.

This simple procedure, which requires the utmost cooperation of the mother (caregiver), has almost cent percent success.

The success of the procedure depends on compliance, repetition, and continuation.

Those who will not benefit are:

- Improper method
- Infrequency of method
- False sense of cure
- The treatment started after 12 weeks.
- Congenital defect of the bony nasolacrimal canal.

If the condition is not cured in 4–6 weeks, the next alternative is to probe the NLD under anesthesia. The procedure is generally done under short-term dissociative anesthesia administered by an anesthetist well versed in pediatric anesthesia. The probe should be passed through the upper puncta because if the lower puncta and canaliculi are damaged during probing, the child may be left with epiphora for the rest of their life in spite of an open NLD. Generally, single probing is sufficient; if it fails, reprobing is done after 10–15 days. Successes of second and subsequent probing are bleak if the first probing fails. In that case, the child is kept on local antibiotic drops two times a day and evacuating the sac by pressure until the child can undergo either endoscopic DCR or external DCR.

Some ophthalmologists prefer to do probing under topical anesthesia after sedating the child with an oral sedative. The procedure followed is to put one drop of topical anesthetic agent every 5 minutes for three times, wrap the child in a towel snugly to immobilize the child, and proceed with the procedure. This works well in the hands of experienced ophthalmologists. The choice of size of the probe varies per institute. The most common regime is:

- Under 3 years, size 00
- Between 3 and 5 years old (size 0)
- Above 5 years, size 1

Unilateral watering in a child without photophobia in a white eye is most probably a case of congenital nasolacrimal duct block, unless proved otherwise.

The following **Table 8.4** gives a summary of the clinical features of congenital NLD block.

**Ophthalmia neonatorum:* Unlike dacryocystitis, ophthalmia neonatorum develops in the first week and is bilateral. In cases of bacterial infection, the discharge varies from mucopurulent to frank pus laden with causative organisms. The common organisms are bacteria, of many types. The most common organism to cause ophthalmia neonatorum in the past was Gonococcus. The neonate acquired it from the infected birth canal of the mother or due to the absence of asepsis during delivery. The lids are more swollen in bacterial infection than in nonbacterial infection in the ophthalmia neonatorum. The other microbial organism to cause ophthalmia neonatorum is Herpes simplex. $AgNO_3$ drops, which are still used in some centers to prevent ophthalmia; itself can cause chemical conjunctivitis, mimicking ophthalmia neonatorum.

Use of $AgNO_3$ has been replaced by less toxic and more effective betadines. Which is also known as povidone-iodine, which contains 0.5% therapeutically available iodine and other ingredients in water? It is used as a 2.5% aqueous solution only once as a prophylactic measure. In the absence of betadine, any water-soluble broad-spectrum antibiotic eye drop or erythromycin eye ointment can be used.

TABLE 8.4: Summary of congenital nasolacrimal duct block.

Age	*Clinical feature*
At birth	Remains undetected
2–4 months	Epiphora, visible swelling, positive regurgitation test, mucopurulent discharge from the puncta
5 months–1 year	Marked epiphora, mucocele, positive regurgitation test, mucopurulent to purulent discharge
After 1 year	All the above features, to which signs and symptoms of infection can be added, and the patient presents as dacryocystitis or pericystitis

Note: All the cases do not follow the same order at the first presentation. They may have dacryocystitis or pericystitis as an initial complaint. Spontaneous regression is also possible.

The complications of the NLD block are:
The complications of NLD obstruction can be confined to sac and pericystic tissue or involve the cornea and uvea.

Ocular complications can occur at any of the above stages. They are corneal ulcers, hypopyon corneal ulcers, and hypopyon without corneal ulcers. The first two are infective; the most common organism is pneumococci, and the cause of the latter is pneumococcal toxin. The most common organism to be harbored by an infected sac is pneumococci. It is mandatory to examine the sac in all cases of corneal ulcers of all ages.

Congenital Mucocele of Lacrimal Sac (Fig. 8.15)

The congenital mucocele of the lacrimal sac is a far less frequent disorder than the congenital block of the NLD. Most probably, it is the result of simultaneous non-conducting of canaliculi and NLD. The condition is noticed at birth as a bluish swelling between the later wall of the nose and the medial canthus; it is a tense, spherical, noncompressible, and nonreducible swelling that does not increase in size if the infant strains. An increase in size on straining points toward its being a meningocele that is more worrisome than a mucocele of sac and must be attended to early. The congenital mucocele of the lacrimal sac is asymptomatic unless it gets infected; once infected, it behaves like pericystitis and should be treated as such. Occasionally, gentle pressure over the swelling relieves the obstruction, and the swelling deflates, requiring no further treatment.

Chronic Dacryocystitis in Children Above 5 Years

Inflammation of the sac is less frequent than in adults but more common than in infants, equally distributed among boys and girls, as compared to adult dacryocystitis, which is more common among females. Dacryocystitis in adults is a disorder of the third decade, with the incidence reducing with age. Adult dacryocystitis is more likely to be unilateral in contrast to its childhood counterpart, which is invariably bilateral. Dacryocystitis in children manifests more often after the first decade; that does not mean that children under 10 are immune. Dacryocystitis in children can be acute or chronic.

The most common cause of dacryocystitis in children is untreated or partially treated congenital NLD block, resulting in poor evacuation of the sac with stagnation of discharge that gets infected. The most common organism to infect is pneumococci. Invariably, there is a positive history of chickenpox and measles in childhood.

Viruses and fungi are not known to infect sacs in children.

Acute dacryocystitis in children may be simple or associated with pericystitis, which may be converted into cellulitis over the sac between the medial canthus and later wall of the nose; if not treated, getting converted in an abscess that may rupture to result in a sinus, giving relief to the child. If the sinus closes, there are high chances of repetition of the process, with a chance of ending in a lacrimal fistula. Dacryocystitis of all ages do not respond to local instillation of antibiotic drops or application of ointment on the skin; they respond well to systemic, broad-spectrum antibiotics. Pericystic abscesses require surgical draining.

The main pathology of chronic dacryocystitis in adults is similar to dacryocystitis in children, i.e., partially treated congenital nasolacrimal sac obstruction, resulting in stasis of tear and accumulation of secretions from the wall of the sac, to which bacterial infection by organisms of low virulence are superadded. The infection reaches the sac either from the conjunctiva or via the NLD. It may follow chickenpox or measles suffered months or years ago; other less reported causes are midfacial fractures involving the bony nasolacrimal canal. Occasionally, an encysted mucocele that has gone unnoticed may be discovered for the first time. A common cause of chronic dacryocystitis in the second decade in the endemic area is rhinosporidiosis.

Clinical Features

The clinical features of chronic dacryocystitis in the second decade do not differ much from the adult variety, except that the former is more often bilateral. The main symptom is intractable epiphora; sometimes the parents may confess about their knowledge of the presence of symptomless mucocele or mucopurulent discharge on pressure over the sac, and sometimes an adolescent may present with full-blown pericystitis.

Investigations

Not many investigations are required.

Commonly ordered investigations are:

1. *Lacrimal syringing:* This is a simple outdoor procedure that can be performed in children as young as five following proper counseling under topical anesthesia or under ketamine (a dissociative anesthetic agent). It only indicates the presence of the block and its extent, i.e., complete or partial, but not the level of the block.
2. *Imaging:*
   i. *X-ray skull:* Not indicated.
   ii. *X-ray paranasal sinuses (PNS):* Useful in detecting fractures of the bony nasolacrimal canal.
   iii. *Dacryocystography:* Simple or macro dacryocystography (no more in vogue).
   iv. *Computed tomography (CT):* This procedure has replaced all other imaging methods. It is better than a magnetic resonance imaging (MRI). It can be used to enhance the results of dacryocystography.

Management of Chronic Dacryocystitis in Children

Treatment of chronic dacryocystitis does not differ from that of adults.

> Pus in the sac is always a threat to the cornea and uvea.

The acute phase, whenever present, should be treated with a suitable antibiotic. This always does not prevent recurrence. To prevent recurrence, broad-spectrum antibiotic drops are prescribed to be instilled in the ipsilateral conjunctiva once a day for the next 3 months, unless definitive treatment in the form of surgery has been done. The definitive surgery in chronic dacryocystitis is a DCR, either external transcutaneous or internal endoscopic. Simple dacryocystectomy is not a good option; it is better avoided. Another alternative is intubation of the NLD either through the fundus of the sac or by the standard method used to do DCT, i.e., incising the anterior wall and passing a short stent in the NLD. The other method is to pass a thin silicon stent through the canaliculus.

RHINOSPORIDIOSIS OF THE SAC IN CHILDREN (DACRYO SPORIDIOSIS)

(See in previous text as well)

Rhinosporidiosis of all ages is confined to a population indigenous to the particular endemic area that is besieged by this infection, unless the person has acquired the disease in the endemic area and migrated to a nonendemic area. The endemic areas are spread over some countries that share common features, such as high humidity due to high annual rainfall, lots of water bodies, and the staple diet being rice. They share a common water body to bathe with water buffaloes, which are considered to be reservoirs of the infective stage of the organism. People use the same water for cooking, drinking, washing, and ablution. These countries are tropical and subtropical topographically. The two countries from which the most cases have been reported are India and Sri Lanka. In India, the distribution is patchy; the maximum number of cases have been reported from Chhattisgarh and Kerala. The other states to report are Odisha, Jharkhand, and West Bengal.

The infection is caused by an organism, *Rhinosporidium Seeberi* (*Rhinosporidium Kinealy*), that has not been classified properly; initially, it was thought to be a protozoa, then a fungus, and algae, unless in 1973 it was put in the order of olipidicae. Some microbiologists relate them to mycobacteria, others to cyanobacterium even .The disease rhinosporidiosis has not been produced in humans as well as animals. It has not been cultured either; the organism is found in water and soil. It has two stages in the life cycle, i.e., trophocytes and sporangia **(Figs. 8.21 and 8.22)**.

The sporangia are believed to be the infective stage. The infection is chronic; no acute episode has been reported. The exact mode of infection, incubation period, and mode of spread are not clear; there is no report of spontaneous cure, and recurrence following incomplete treatment is the rule. The common presumption is that humans acquire the disease after repeated baths in stagnant water laden with the infective stage of *Rhinosporidium*. The organism can find its way into the body through any epithelium-lined surface exposed to the atmosphere, ocular or extraocular. The ocular structures involved besides the lacrimal sac are the conjunctiva and sclera; scleral involvement is <5% of conjunctival involvement. Most of the time, scleral involvement is associated with conjunctival involvement; however, isolated scleral lesions have also been reported. The combined involvement of the conjunctiva and sac is commonly seen between 5 and 15 years old. Orbital involvements have not been reported, in spite of reports of involvement of paranasal sinuses. Surprisingly, involvement of the skin, the largest epithelial surface, is also infrequent; bone involvement is perplexing. Systemic involvement is generally in adults; they most probably acquired the disease in childhood. The incidence is slightly higher in boys.

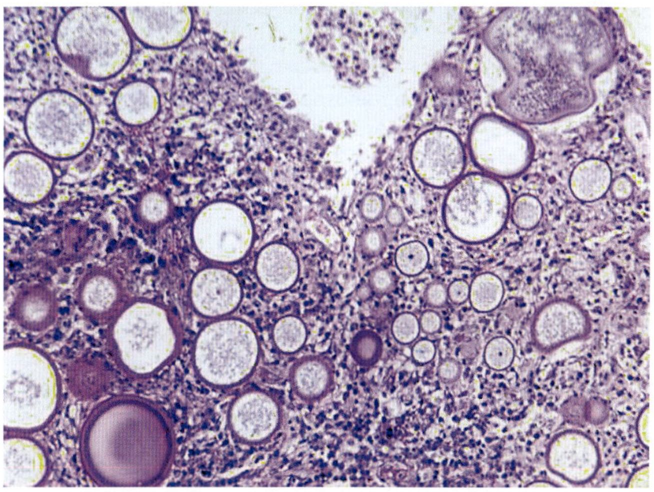

Fig. 8.21: Histopathological section through typical granuloma of *Rhinosporidium*.
Courtesy: Professor V Sudershan.

The other organs inflicted are:

- *Respiratory:* Nasopharynx, trachea, lungs, and paranasal sinuses.
- Parotid duct.
- *Genitourinary:* Urethra, vagina.

Mode of Presentation

The disease presents in one of the following modes:

1. Ocular
2. Systemic:
   i. Respiratory
   ii. Extra respiratory

Ocular involvement **(Fig. 8.23)**, *confined to the adnexa, can be:*

1. Isolated conjunctival.
2. Isolated involvement of sac.
3. Combination of the above two.
4. Scleral.

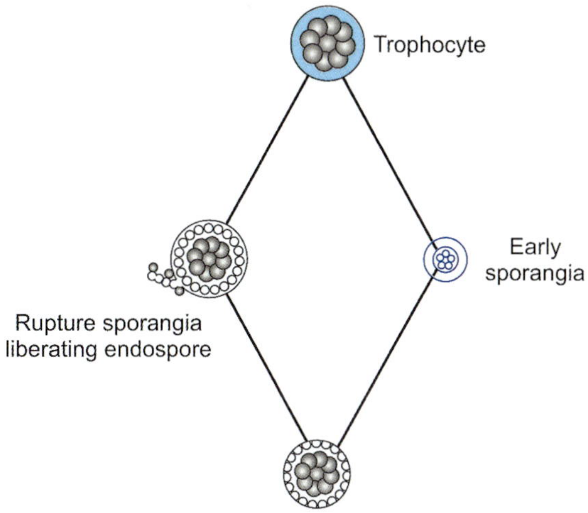

Fig. 8.22: Simplified natural history of *Rhinosporidium*.

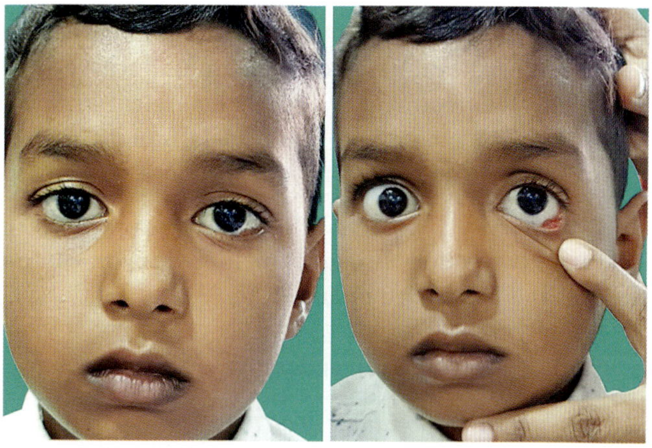

Fig. 8.23: Rhinosporidiosis of the tarsal conjunctiva lower lid visible on eversion of lower lid.
Courtesy: Dr LN Madaria.

- Isolated involvement of conjunctiva is called conjunctivo–sporidiosis.
- Isolated involvement of the sac is called dacryo sporidiosis.

Clinical Presentation of Dacryo Sporidiosis

1. Initially, the child may be symptomless except that he occasionally has bleeding from the nose and, on examination, is found to have sac involvement, or vice versa.
2. Diffuse, nontender, compressible swelling over the sac region, without epiphora or regurgitation.
3. A patent NLD in dacryo-cysto-rhinosporidiosis explains the phenomenon.
4. Diffuse swelling under the lower lid **(Fig. 8.20)**.
5. Orange peel appearance of skin over the swelling **(Fig. 8.19)**.
6. Epiphora will ensue if the growth extends in NLD, either from above or below.
7. On syringing, the swelling gets inflated without regurgitation.
8. The inflated sac can be flattened by gentle pressure.
9. Occasionally, the sac can get infected following syringing or probing.
10. A large conjunctival growth may extend in the nose via the sac or in the orbit **(Fig. 8.24)** and may be confused with neoplasm.
11. The growth may protrude through a fistulous tract **(Fig. 8.25)**.
12. In bilateral cases, involvement on both sides is independent of each other.

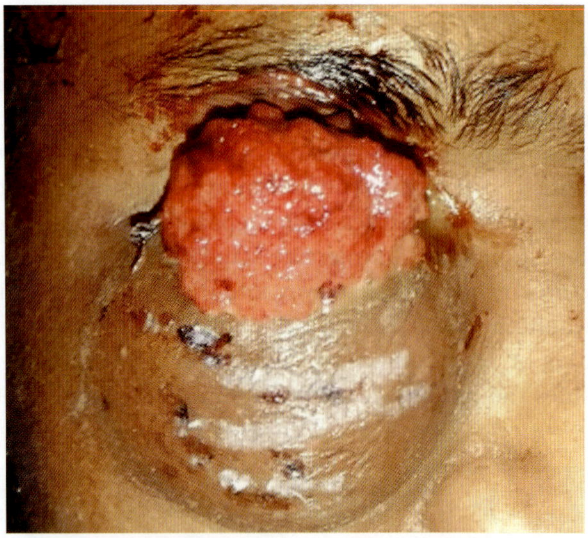

Fig. 8.24: Unusually large rhinosporidium of granuloma of lower conjunctiva extending in nose and orbit.
Courtesy: Professor ML Garg.

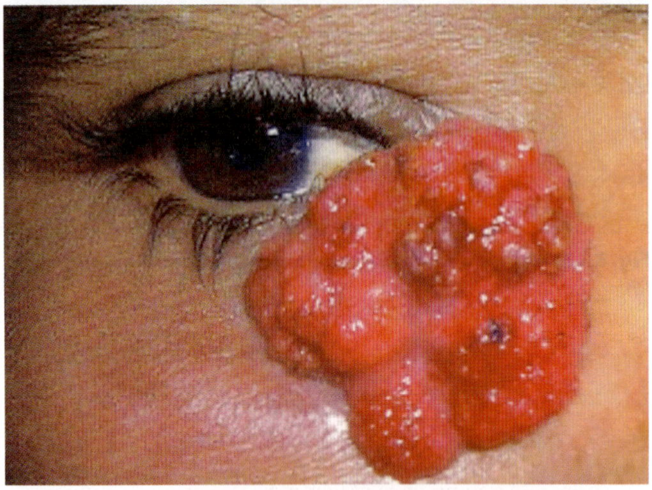

Fig. 8.25: Rhinosporidiosis granuloma extruding through the wall of sac.

Management of Rhinosporidium of Sac

There is no medical treatment for the disorder. Many drugs have been used from time to time with uniform results. The definitive treatment is complete surgical removal of the growth; incomplete removal is fraught with a chance of recurrence, which may be more difficult to manage.

There are two routes through which the growth can be reached and removed; they are:

1. Trance cutaneous
2. *Nasal:* The second is an endoscopic surgery.

The riddle of rhinosporidiosis of all types consists of:

- The disease inflicts only a few families utilizing the same environment and depending on the same source of water.
- Only a few people in the same family get the infection; sometimes only one or two children out of many may be infected.
- Adults generally do not contract a disease unless they have had it since childhood.
- A successful removal prevents a recurrence.
- Involvements of unrelated systems, i.e., respiratory and genitourinary, have not been reported with involvement of the sac.

Incidence can be minimized by:

1. Consuming only potable water.
2. Segregating the water supply for human and animal consumption.

SUGGESTED READING

1. Ahaluwalia KB. Culture of the organism that cause rhinosporidium. J Laryngol Otol. 1999;113(6):523-8.
2. Ali MJ. Chronic dacryocystitis in AIOS. In: Rammurthy, Biswas P (Eds). Ready reckoner ophthalmology, 2nd edition. New Delhi: JP Brothers; 2017. pp. 641-2.
3. Ali MJ. Pediatric dacryocystorhinostomy. IJO. 2017;65(10):1008-09.
4. Awasthi RK. Rhinosporidiosis: A case study in Chhattisgarh – Personal communication.
5. Bharathi M, Ramakrishnan R, Maneksha V, Rao R. Comparative bacteriology of acute and chronic dacryocystitis. Eye. 2008;22:953-60.
6. Billore OP. Rhinosporidiosis 1st edition. New Delhi: AITBS Publishers and distributors; 1996.
7. Bothra N, Rath S, Mittal R, Tripathy D. External D.C.R. for isolated rhinosporidiosis. A suitable alternative to dacryo cystectomy. IJO. 2019;67(5):665-8.
8. Das C, Das S, Chatterjee P, Bandhopadhyay SN. Series of atypical Rhinosporidiosis: our experience in Western part of West Bengal. Indian J Otolaryngol Head Neck Surg. 2019;71:1863-70.
9. Grover A, Kaur S. Principal of Oculo plastic surgery. In: Grover A (Ed). Oculoplastic surgery practical guideline: CME Series no 5 AIOS. New Delhi: JP Brothers; 2001.
10. Grover A. Management of nasolacrimal duct block in children how is it changing. IJO. 2017;65:910-1.
11. Gupta RK, Singh BP, Singh BR. Rhinosporidiosis in Central India: a cross-sectional study from a tertiary care hospital in Chhattisgarh. Trop Parasitol. 2020;10:120-3.
12. Kamal S, Ali MJ. Primary acquired nasolacrimal duct obstruction and secondary nasolacrimal duct obstruction. Principle and practice of lacrimal surgery. India: Springer; 2015.
13. Karthikeyan P, Vijayasundaram S, Pulimoottil D. A retrospective epidemiological study of Rhinosporidiosis in a rural tertiary care Centre in Pondicherry. J Clin Diagn Res. 2016;10:4-8.
14. Karunaratne WA. Rhinosporidiosis in man. London: The Athlone Press; 1964.
15. Kims U. Congenital nasolacrimal duct block in–A.I.O.S. Ready reckoner ophthalmology, 2nd edition. New Delhi: JP Brothers; 2017. pp. 631-40.
16. Kim U. Congenital nasolacrimal duct block in AIOS. Ready reckoner ophthalmology 2nd edition, New Delhi: JP Brothers; 2017. 637-41.
17. Kuriakose ET. Rhinosporidiosis of the eye. BJO. 1963; 47:346.
18. Likhari K. Acute dacryocystitis in AIOS. In: Rammurthy, Biswas P (Eds). Ready reckoner ophthalmology, 2nd edition. New Delhi: JP Brothers; 2017. pp. 643-7.
19. Mishra D, Bhushan P, Sinha BP, Bhaskar G, Rao R. External dacryocystecto rhinostomy conventional surgery versus Pawar implant, A comparative study. IJO. 2019.
20. Mishra LK, Gupta S, Pradhan SK, Baishakh MR. Lacrimal sac rhinosporidiosis. Plastic aesthetic research. 2015;2: 353-6.
21. Misra S, Misra N, Nagarkar NM, Meshta R. Clinical presentation, Ophthalmological spectrum (Rhinosporidiosis) in Rhinosporidiosis. Singapore: Springer nature; 2022. pp. 47-58.
22. Mukherjee PK, Bandyopadhyay, Preeti. Infectious diseases of lacrimal sac infectious diseases of eye, 1st edition. New Delhi: Wolter Kluwer; 2010. pp. 43-5.
23. Mukherjee PK, Bandyopahyay, Preeti. Rhinosporidiosis in Ocular microbiology, 1st edition. JP Brothers: New Delhi; 2010. pp. 115-9.
24. Mukherjee PK, Jain PC, Mishra RK. Exanthemata, a cause of chronic dacryocystitis in children. IJO. 1969;17:27-30.
25. Mukherjee PK, Jain PC. Intubation of nasolacrimal duct with polythene tube. IJO. 1967;20(1):16-9.
26. Mukherjee PK, Shukla IM, Deshpande A, Deshpande M, Praveena Kher. IJO. 1983;30:513-4.
27. Mukherjee PK. In: Frauenfelder ET, Roy FH (Eds). Rhinosporidiosis in current ocular therapy, 5th edition. Philadelphia: W.B. Saunders company; 2000. pp. 66-7.
28. Mukherjee PK. Inflammation of lacrimal sac in Paediatric ophthalmology, 1st edition. New Delhi: New age international; 2005. pp. 92-3.
29. Mukherjee PK. Rhinosporidiosis sac in paediatric ophthalmology, 1st edition. New Delhi: New age international; 2005.
30. Pandey N. Rhinosporidiosis in Eyes in systemic disorders. In: Nema HV, Venkatesh P, Sharma YR, Nema N.
31. Saha J, Basu AJ, Sen I, Sinha R, Bhandari AK, Mondal S. Atypical presentations of Rhinosporidiosis: a clinical dilemma? Indian J Otolaryngol Head Neck Surg. 2011; 63:243-6.
32. Singh M, Sharma M. Manpreet K, Grewal AM, Yadav D, Handa S, et al. Nasal endoscopic features and outcome of nasal endoscope guided binocular for congenital nasolacrimal duct block. IJO. 2019;67(7):1137-42.
33. Sinha A, Phukan JP, Bandyopadhyay G, Sengupta S, Bose K, Mondal RK, et al. Clinicopathological study of rhinosporidiosis with special reference to cytodiagnosis. J Cytol. 2012;29:246-9.
34. Tiwari R, Karthik K, Dhama K, Shabbir MZ, Khurana SK. Rhinosporidiosis: a riddled disease of man and animals. Adv Anim Vet Sci. 2015;3:54-63.

CHAPTER 9

Disorders of Lid in Children

The main functions of the lids are—protective, cosmetic, and spreading tear film over the ocular surface without spilling. The protective function is supplemented by the eyebrows. In newborns, the eyebrows are scanty. Normal eyebrows are separated from each other by a gap that ranges between 1–2.5 cm **(Fig. 9.1)**.

Altered distance between two eyebrows has no clinical significance except in a rare congenital anomaly called Cornelia de Lange syndrome. That consists of a monobrow with excess hair, peculiar facial appearance, pre- and postnatal growth retardation, mental retardation, and multiple upper limb deformities **(Figs. 9.2A and B)**.

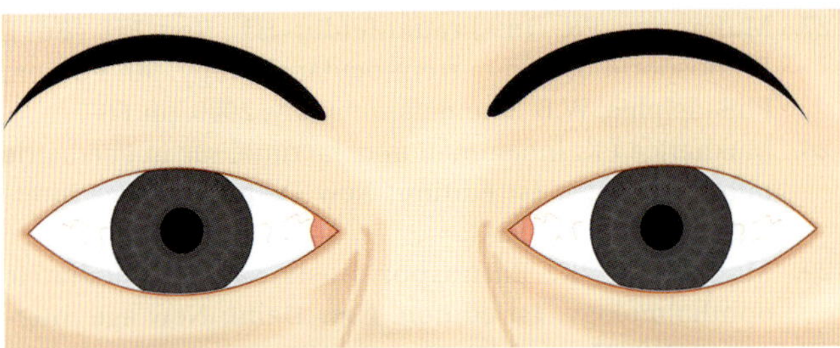

Fig. 9.1: Normal eyebrow.

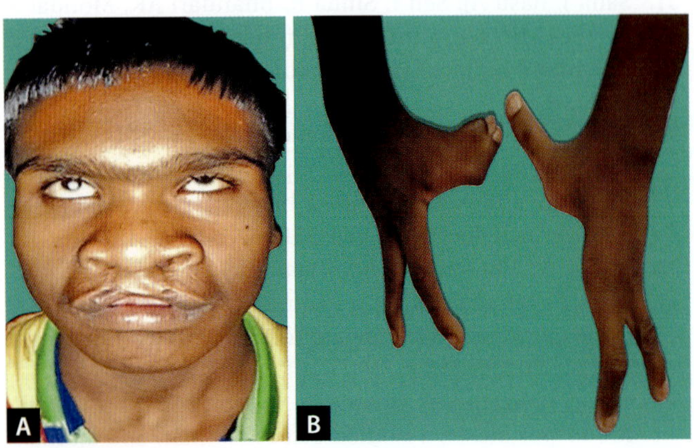

Figs. 9.2A and B: A case of incomplete Cornelia de Lange syndrome.
Courtesy: Professor ML Garg.

In normal children, the two eyebrows are symmetric with a broader medial end. The brows are arched upwards and tapper laterally to dip down slightly above the outer canthus over the later orbital rim. Rarely are the brows fused in the midline over the nose bridge; the condition is called synophrys.

In synophrys, there is excess hair in the fused eyebrows; the junction of the two eyebrows has concavity upwards, while the portions on either side have convexity upwards on either side **(Figs. 9.3A and B)**.

The normal eyebrows form smooth symmetrical arches over the eyeball, as shown in **Figure 9.4**; the eye brows are raised in ptosis **(Figs. 9.5 to 9.7)**. **Figure 9.6** shows unilateral ptosis with unilaterally raised eyebrows. **Figure 9.7** shows bilateral severe ptosis with bilaterally raised eyebrows. The eyebrows are flattened in lagophthalmos, as shown in **Figures 9.8 and 9.9**.

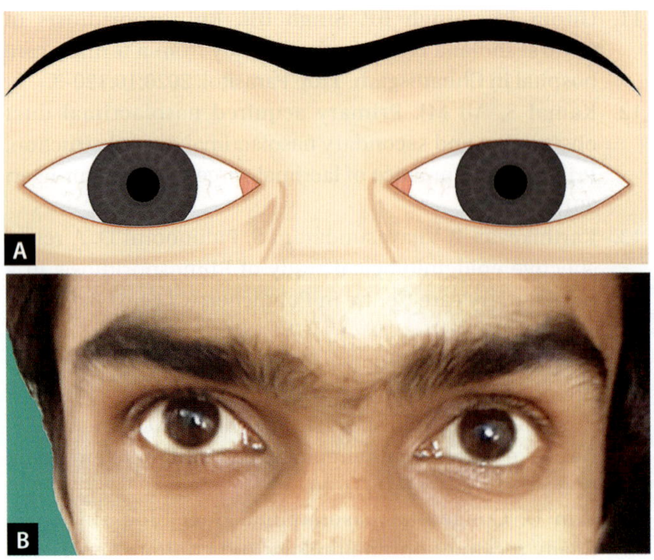

Figs. 9.3A and B: Synophrys.

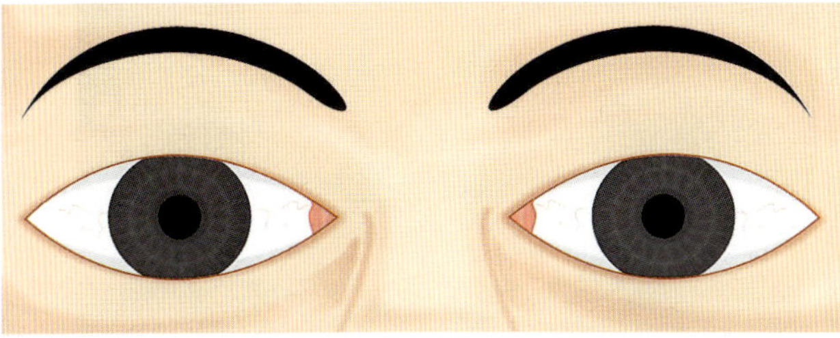

Fig. 9.4: Normal eyebrow.

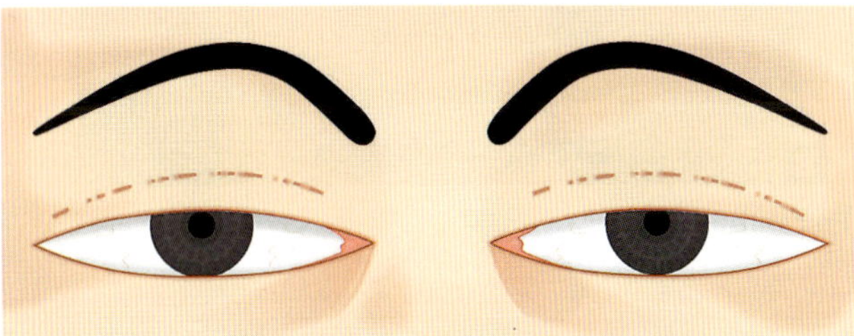

Fig. 9.5: Bilateral ptosis. Both eyebrows raised.

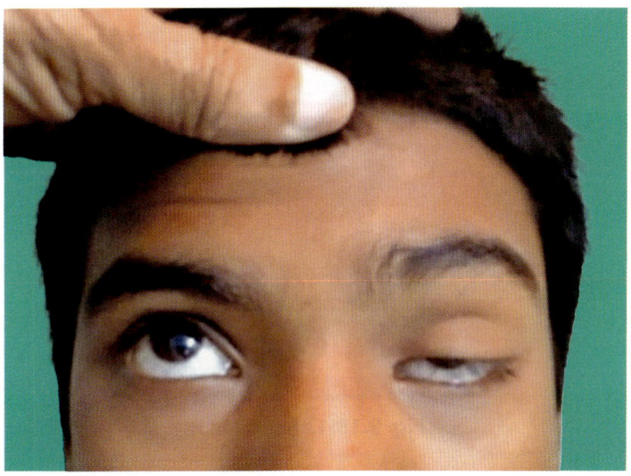

Fig. 9.6: Congenital left ptosis eyebrow raised.

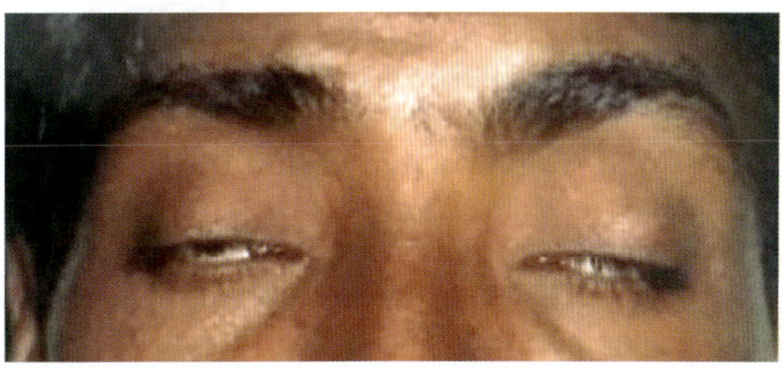

Fig. 9.7: Bilateral sever ptosis both eyebrows raised.

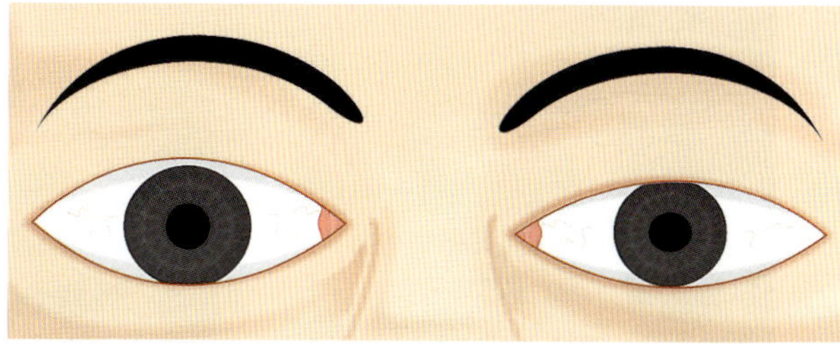

Fig. 9.8: Right lagophthalmos, right eyebrow flattened and IPA widened.

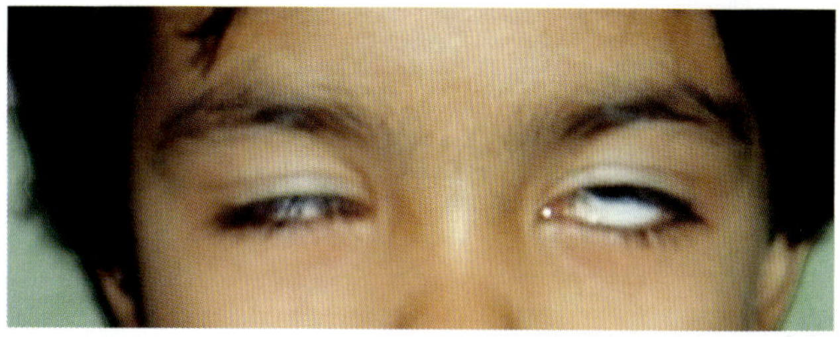

Fig. 9.9: Bilateral lagophthalmos in a child.

TABLE 9.1: Disorders of the lid.

Congenital	*Acquired*
Ptosis	Infection
Epicanthus	Inflammation
Telecanthus	Injury
Blepharophimosis	Myogenic
Coloboma	Abnormal movements
Ankyloblepharon	Lagophthalmos
Distichiasis	Pseudoptosis
Epiblepharon	
Euryblepharon	
Phacomatosis	

Disorders of the lid in children are fairly common. The most common acquired lid disorder among children is stye, followed by chalazion and blepharitis. The most frequent congenital anomaly is ptosis. Malignancies of the lids are rare in children. Phacomas that are benign are more common than malignant tumors in children.

The disorders of the lid can broadly be divided into two groups, i.e., congenital and acquired, as given in **Table 9.1**.

Congenital anomalies of the lids depend on the involvement of the tissues and the location of the pathology in the lid margin, muscles, nerves, and blood vessels.

The skin of the lid involved produces:

- *Structural:*
  - Epicanthus **(Figs. 9.10A and B)**
  - Epiblepharon (rare)
  - Blepharochalasis (**Fig. 9.11**; Not seen in children).

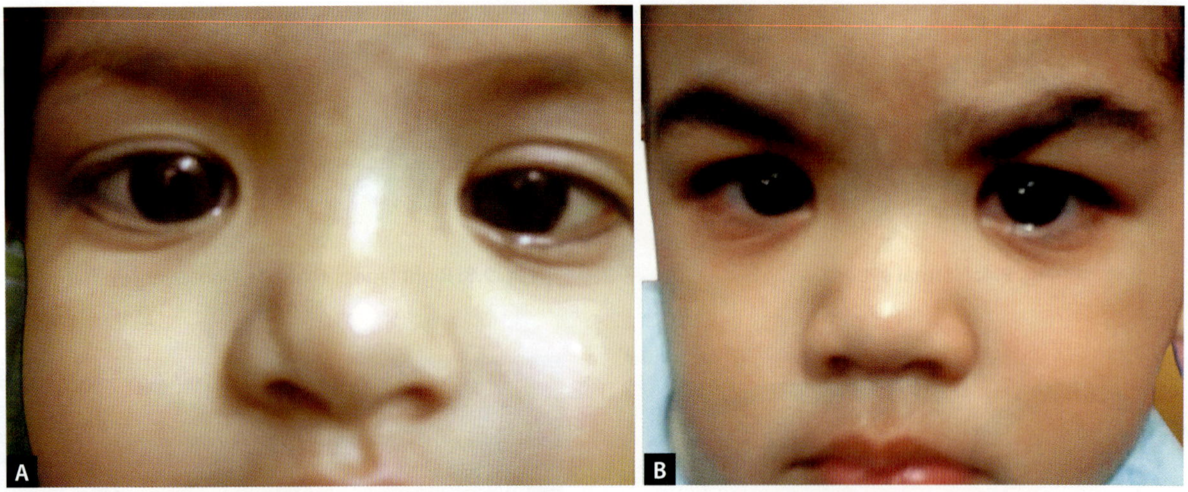

Figs. 9.10A and B: Epicanthus.

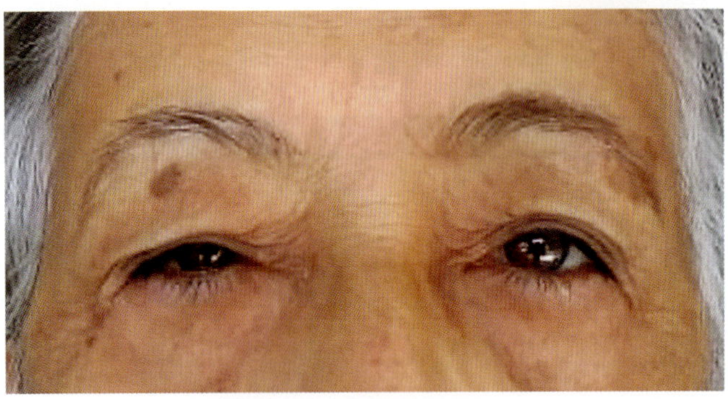

Fig. 9.11: Blepharochalasis.

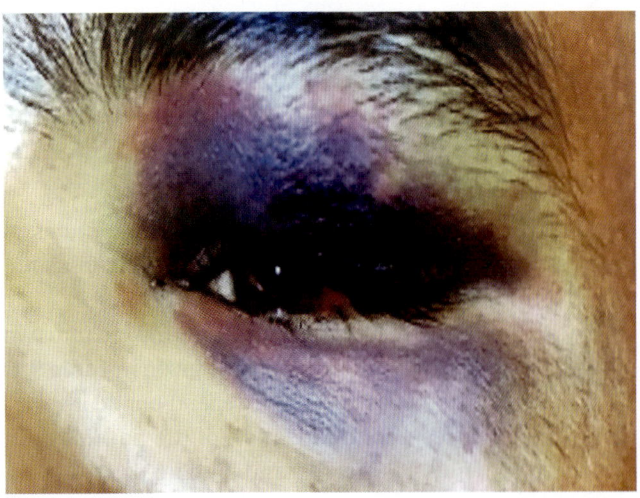

Fig. 9.12: Ecchymosis of the lids.

- *Color:*
  - Ecchymosis **(Fig. 9.12)**
  - Cafe-au-lait (**Fig. 9.13**; port-wine stain)

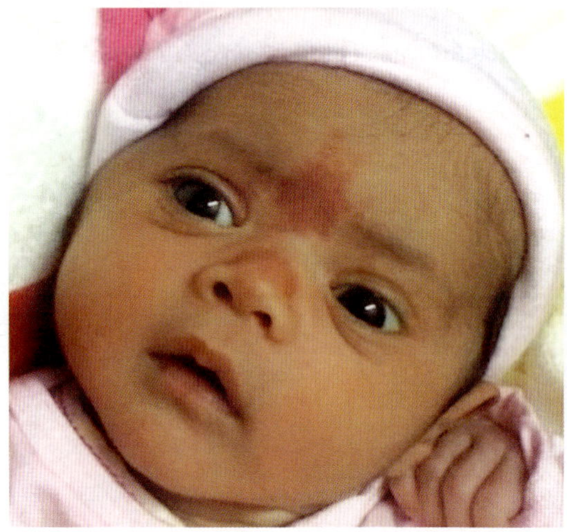

Fig. 9.13: Cafe-au-lait.

  - *Hypopigmentation:*
    - Albinism **(Fig. 9.14)**
    - Vitiligo **(Fig. 9.15)** (not seen in children)
    - Leprosy (not seen in children)
    - *Poliosis:* Poliosis is the whitening of the skin, eyebrows, and lashes. Rarely, it can be congenital.
  - *Hyperpigmentation:*
    - Hyperpigmentation **(Fig. 9.16)** can be congenital, may involve conjunctiva, and lasts for life.
    - Other causes are genetic, atopic, allergic contact dermatitis, and spring catarrh **(Fig. 9.17)**.
- *Infection:* Herpes zoster, herpes simplex, chickenpox, measles, molluscum, and boils
- Allergy **(Fig. 9.18)**.

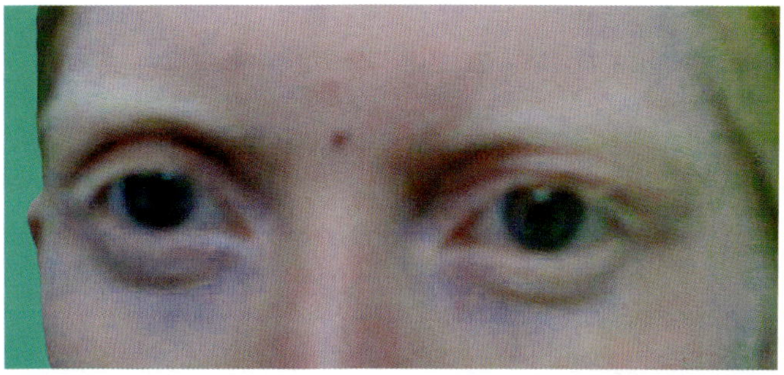

Fig. 9.14: Total albinism.

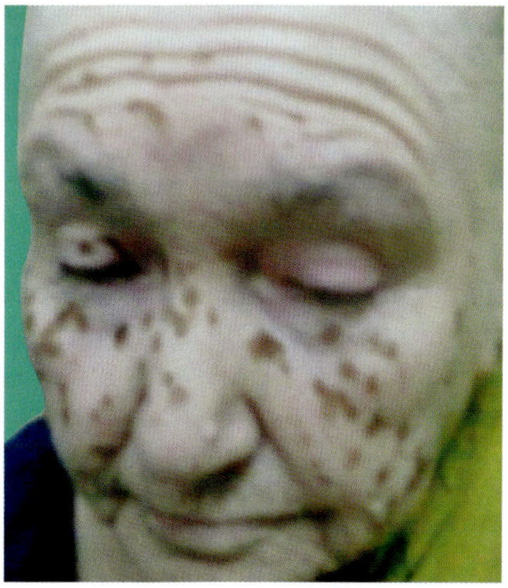

Fig. 9.15: Acquired vitiligo in adult.

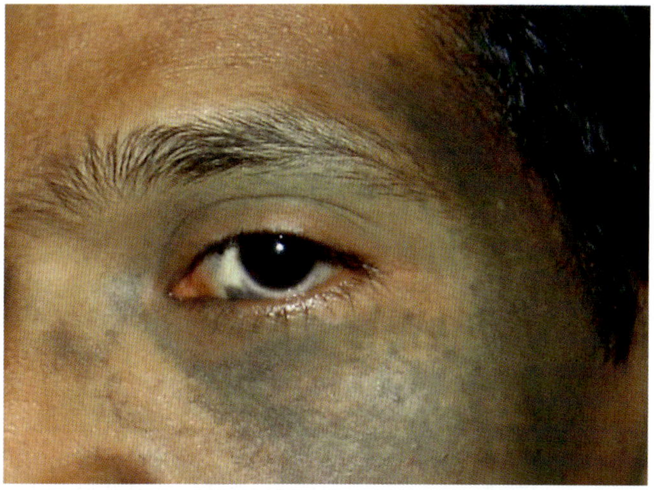

Fig. 9.16: Hyperpigmentation of the skin with conjunctival involvement.

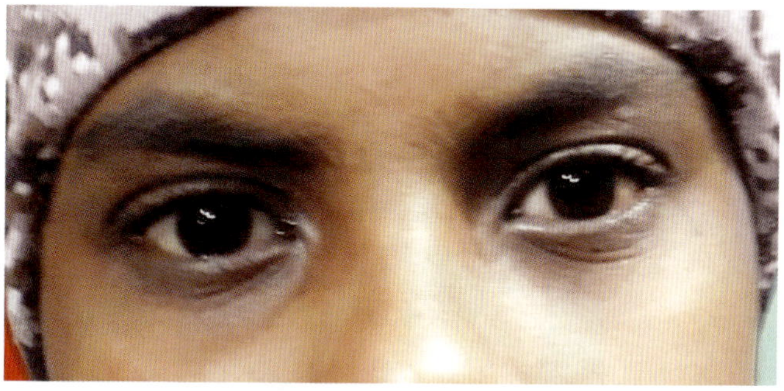

Fig. 9.17: Hyperpigmentation of lids in spring catarrh.

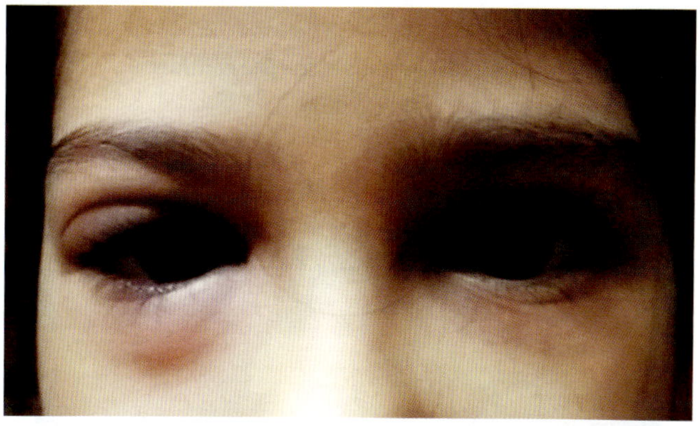

Fig. 9.18: Hyperpigmentation of lids due to unknown allergy. *Courtesy:* Dr Prakash Lunkad.

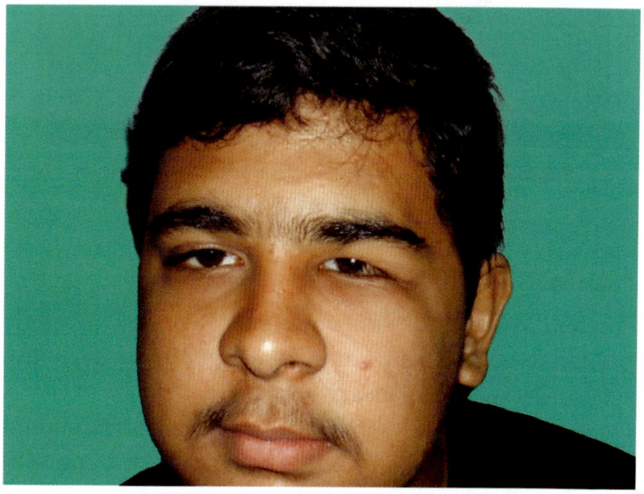

Fig. 9.19: An operated case of congenital neurofibroma.

- *New growth:*
  - *Benign—Phacomatosis:*
    - Hamartomas **(Fig. 9.19)**
    - Choristoma **(Figs. 9.20 to 9.22)**
  - *Malignant:*
    - *Primary:* Rhabdomyosarcoma
    - *Secondary:* Neuroblastoma

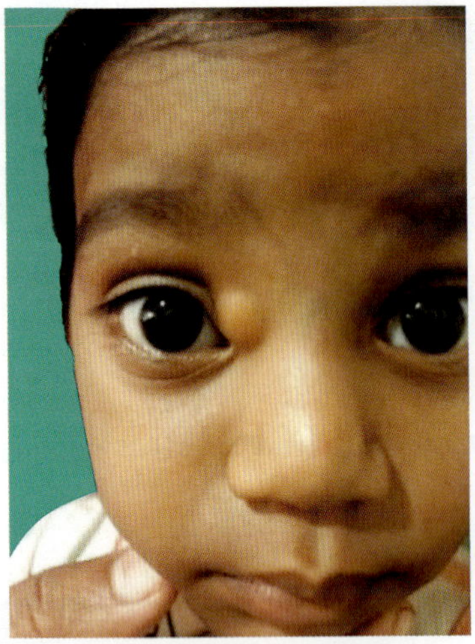

Fig. 9.20: Dermoids at medial canthus.
Courtesy: Dr Santosh Patel.

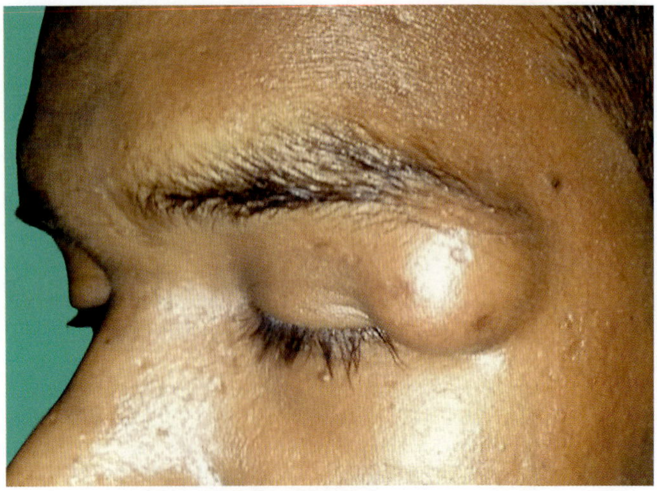

Fig. 9.22: Dermoid at outer canthus.

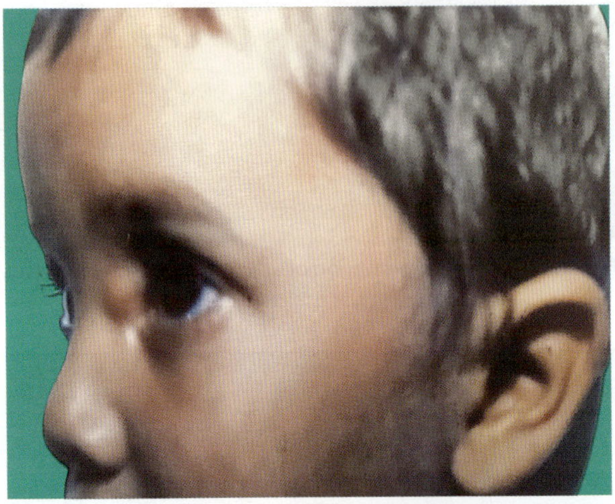

Fig. 9.21: Dermoids at medial canthus (lateral view).
Courtesy: Dr Somen Misra.

DISORDERS OF LID MARGIN

Congenital anomalies are common; they may be subtle enough to go unnoticed or grow enough to be seen and felt. Congenital anomalies may be:

- *Ankyloblepharon:* Ankyloblepharon is an infrequent sporadic congenital anomaly of the lid margin; it is adhesion between the upper and lower lids, partially or completely by tag of skin (for details, refer **Figure 9.38**).
- *Coloboma:* The coloboma of the eye is congenital partial or total absence of tissue forming the lids. They are topographically classified depending on the amount of tissue involved, as shown in **Figures 9.23 and 9.24**. For details, see below.

> The total absence of lids is called ablepharon, which is very rare. The absence of an interpalpebral aperture with the presence of eyelashes is called cryptophthalmos, where the skin of the lids is continuous over the eyeball.

- *Abnormal lashes:*
  - Distichiasis*
  - Trichiasis (rare)
  - Entropion (rare)
- *Infection:*
  - *Nonspecific:* Stye, cellulitis, abscess, and gangrene
  - *Specific:* Herpes simplex, herpes zoster, chickenpox, and molluscum
- *Disorders of muscle:* The two common disorders of the muscles of the lids are ptosis and lagophthalmos. The former is a disorder of the levator supplied by the third nerve, and the latter is a disorder of the orbicularis supplied by the seventh nerve. The ptosis can be congenital or acquired. Congenital lagophthalmos is rare; when present, it is generally bilateral and partial **(Fig. 9.26)**.

Distichiasis* is a congenital anomaly of the lashes, which arise from the meibomian gland opening and are directed backward, as shown in **Figure 9.25, while normal lashes arise from the skin epidermis, contain sebaceous glands, and are directed forward with convexity toward the globe.

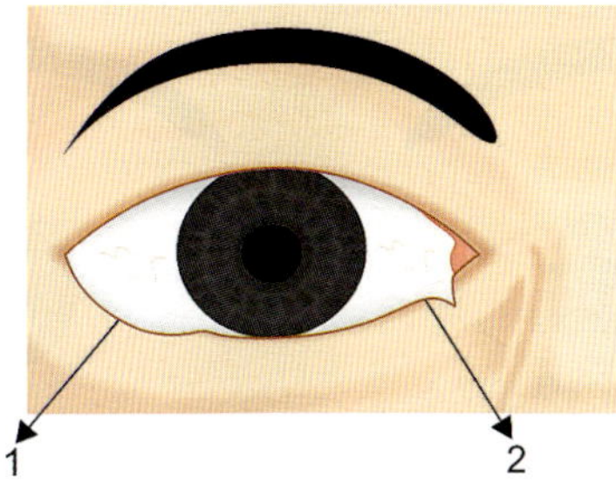

Fig. 9.23: *Coloboma of lids:* (1) Shallow coloboma lower lid; (2) Notch coloboma lower lid.

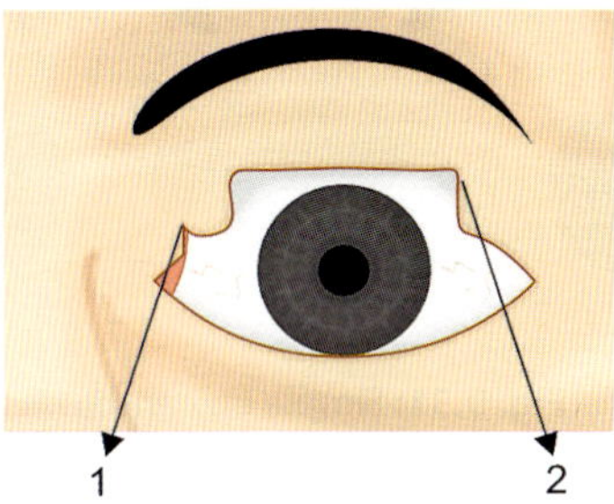

Fig. 9.24: *Coloboma of lids:* (1) Notch coloboma upper lid; (2) Large full-thickness coloboma upper lid.

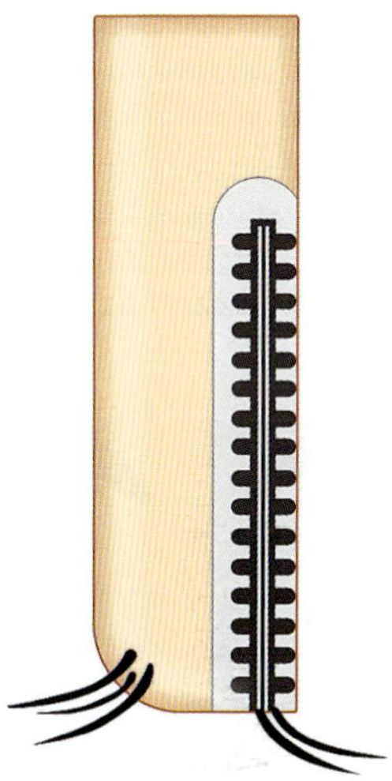

Fig. 9.25: Distichiasis.

Ptosis: Congenital ptosis can be due to the involvement of levator palpebral superior Muller's muscle or nerve supply to the levator. The levator anomaly may involve aponeurosis, muscle, or rarely both.

Lid retraction:

1. *Congenital:* Down syndrome and Duane's syndrome **(Fig. 9.27)**
2. *Acquired:* Thyroid eye disease (not seen in children)

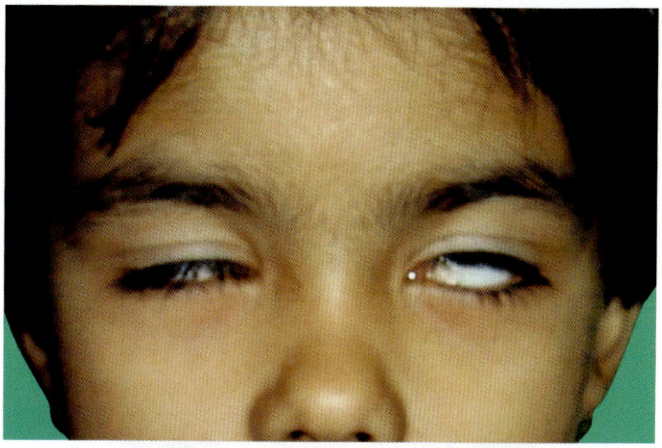

Fig. 9.26: Bilateral and partial congenital lagophthalmos.

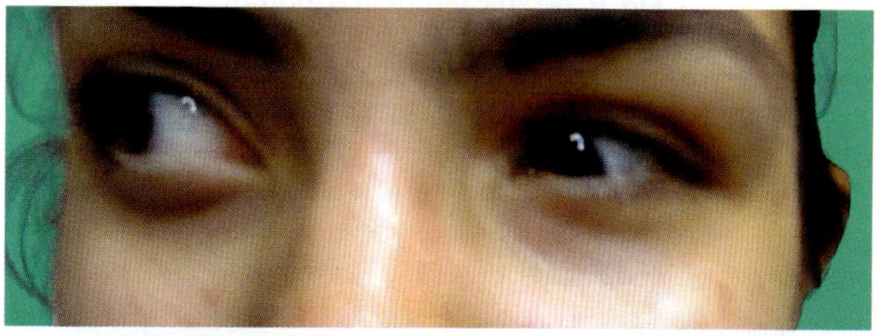

Fig. 9.27: Duane's syndrome right IPA widens on looking right.

Other congenital anomalies of the lid consist of:

- Ptosis
- Epicanthus
- Telecanthus
- Blepharophimosis
- Microblepharon
- *Ptosis*
- *Epicanthus:* It is a common congenital anomaly of the face. Though it is congenital in nature, its presence is felt only after the 1st year. The child is brought for consultation as a case of squint. It is a self-resolving phenomenon without any clinical significance except pseudoesotropia that disappears with the disappearance of epicanthus **(Figs. 9.28 and 9.29)**. In some races, it does not disappear with age, and patients may demand its surgical correction more for cosmetic reasons than any other. Epicanthus is nothing but a fold of skin without any other tissue on the medial side of the medial canthus.

Generally, it is an isolated congenital anomaly; however, it is an essential feature of blepharophimosis syndrome and a feature of Down's syndrome. It is generally bilateral and symmetric. It is equally common among boys and girls.

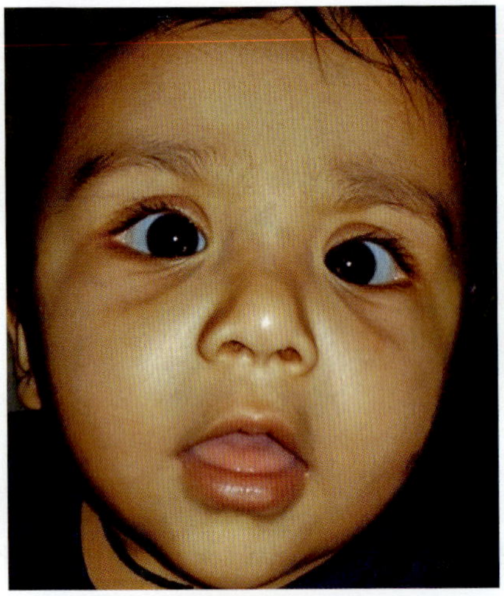

Fig. 9.28: Epicanthus at 6 months.

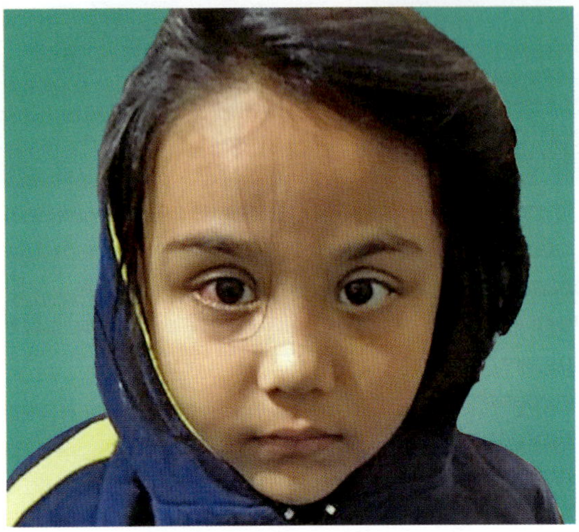

Fig. 9.29: At 3 years.

Epicanthus has been divided into five categories as per its position and extent.

They are:

1. Simple epicanthus **(Fig. 9.31)**
2. *Epicanthus inversus:* The skin fold starts from the crease of the lower lid **(Fig. 9.32)**.
3. *Epicanthus superciliaris:* The skin fold starts just below the eyebrow **(Fig. 9.33)**.
4. *Epicanthus tarsalis:* The skin fold starts just above the tarsal plate.
5. Epiblepharon is considered to be an extended form of epicanthus tarsalis.

The above conditions are shown in **Figures 9.30 to 9.33**.

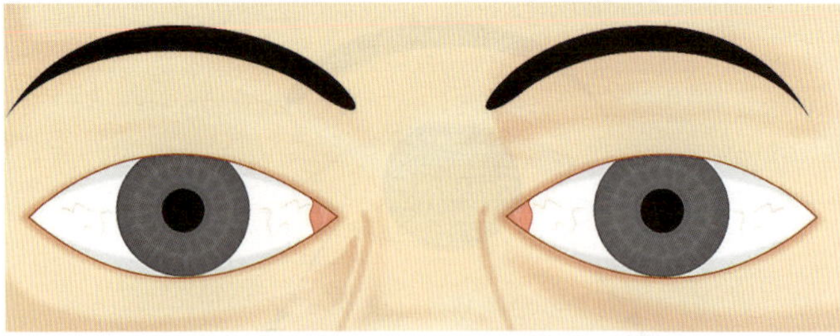

Fig. 9.30: Normal eye.

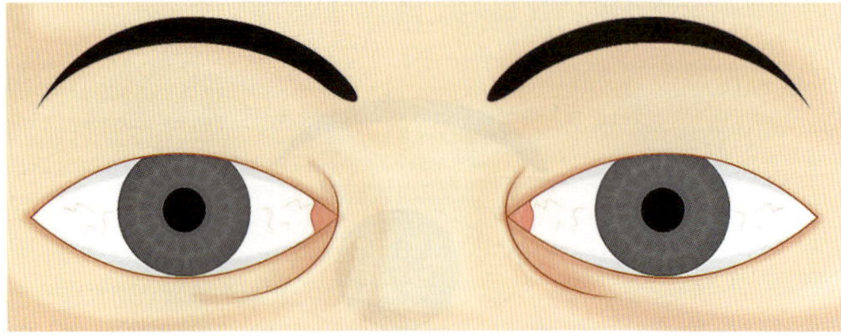

Fig. 9.31: Simple epicanthus.

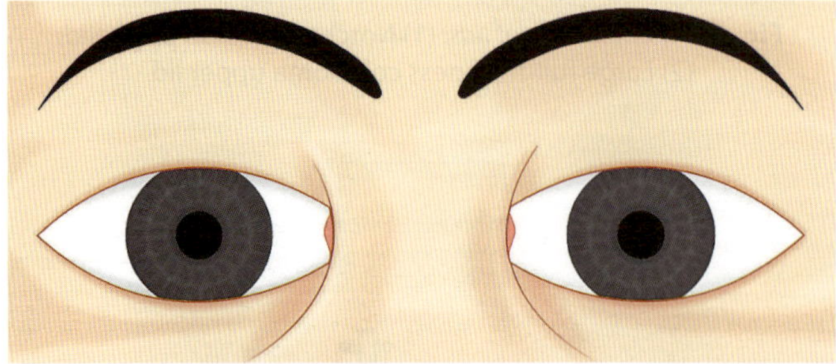

Fig. 9.32: Epicanthus inversus.

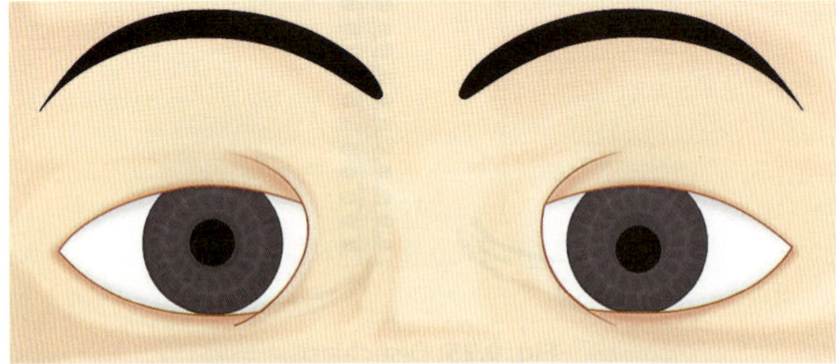

Fig. 9.33: Epicanthus superciliaris.

Figures 9.31 to 9.33 show various types of epicanthus.

1. *Simple epicanthus:* Epicanthus is generally sporadic and not transmitted to future generations; rarely can it have an autosomal dominant trait. The child is brought for consultation, fearing that the child has squinted **(*see* Fig. 9.28)**. The epicanthic fold can be obliterated by compressing it against the nose bridge by examiners thumb and index finger, abolishing pseudoesotropia.

Most of the simple epicanthic folds do not require any treatment. Treatment is required if it does not resolve by 3 years. The only treatment available is surgical, that should be delayed until facial maturity has taken place. It takes about 10–12 years for facial bones to stop molding. There are many surgical procedures. They are basically variants of Z-plasty or VY-plasty.

2. *Epicanthus inversus:* This is less common than simple epicanthus; it consists of a skin fold arising from the medial lower eyelid, going up to the upper lid. It may be associated with blepharophimosis, ptosis, and epicanthus inversus syndrome. It is not to be confused with telecanthus. It is an autosomal dominant disorder of the midface. The only treatment is surgical correction for cosmetic reasons **(Fig. 9.34)**.
3. *Epicanthus superciliaris* is the rarest of the above epicanthic folds; it consists of a vertical skin fold extending from the lower surface of the eyebrow and extending up to the infraorbital rim covering the caruncle **(*see* Fig. 9.33)**.
4. *Blepharophimosis* is an overall reduction of the interpalpebral fissure, both in length and width, giving an appearance of a small slit-like interpalpebral fissure **(Fig. 9.35)**. Isolated blepharophimosis is rare. More common is a combination of extraocular features, which is better called blepharophimosis syndrome.

The condition is bilateral and symmetric. The child is brought in for evaluation for a weird look. The child keeps the chin up and the brows raised. This is to compensate for severe ptosis that is an integral part of the syndrome. The ptosis is congenital, bilateral, severe, and symmetric, associated with epicanthus inverses and telecanthus; the child has a pseudoesotropia. The extraocular muscle, Muller's muscles, and orbicularis are normal.

A combination of ptosis, telecanthus, epicanthus inversus, and blepharospasm is called the Komoto's tetrad.

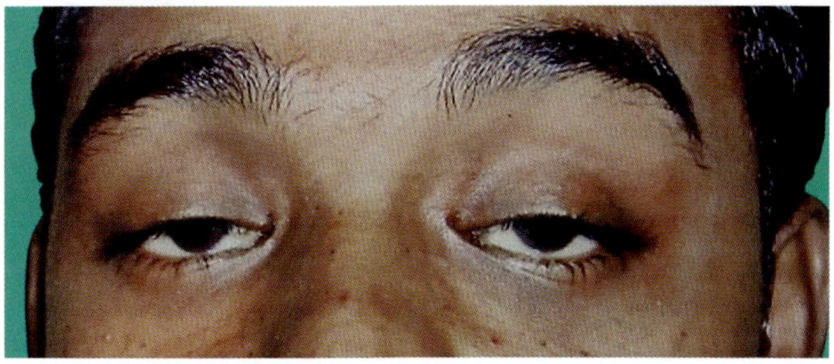

Fig. 9.34: Photo showing epicanthus inversus, ptosis, with raised eyebrow.

The treatment consists of a series of surgical procedures.

5. *Telecanthus:* Telecanthus is not a true anomaly of the lid, it is congenital lengthening of medial palpebral ligament. That shifts the medial canthus laterally, the usual intracanthal distance is half the interpupillary distance **(Figs. 9.36 and 9.37)**. In telecanthus, this is increased. In many ways, it resembles hypertelorism which is a congenital anomaly of orbit with lateral displacement of orbit.

Telecanthus is bilateral. Association of telecanthus and epicanthus is common. Telecanthus is symptomless without any clinical significance, accept cosmetic blemish, it is common in Waardenburg syndrome (white forelock, hypertelorism, heterochromia, and deafness). No treatment is required for telecanthus.

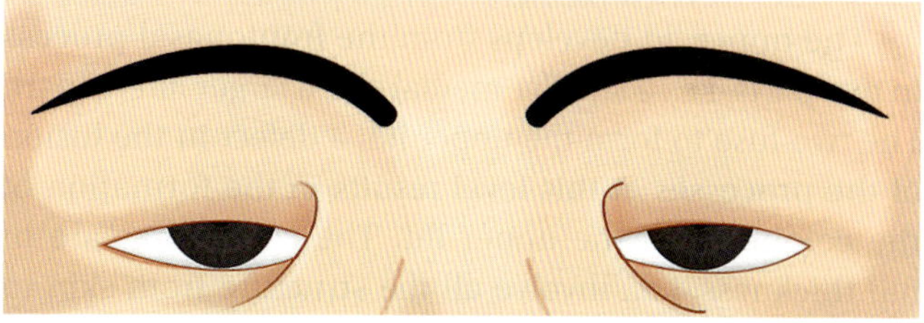

Fig. 9.35: Blepharophimosis epicanthus inversus and telecanthus.

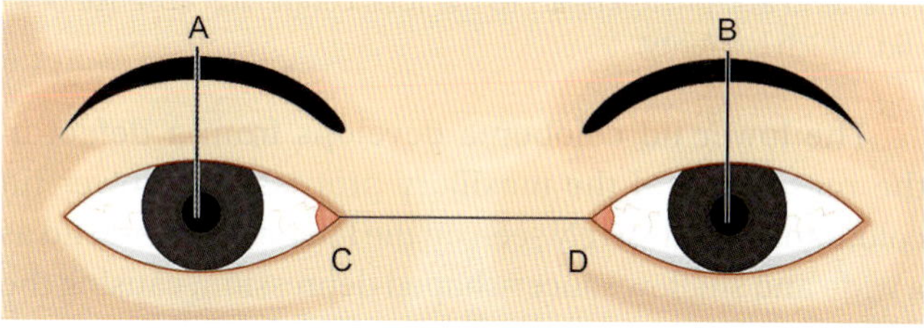

Normal intracanthal distance
A-B = Interpupillary distance
C-D = Intercanthal distance
Normal intercanthal distance = ½ interpupillary distance = AB = 2CD

Fig. 9.36: Normal intercanthal distance.

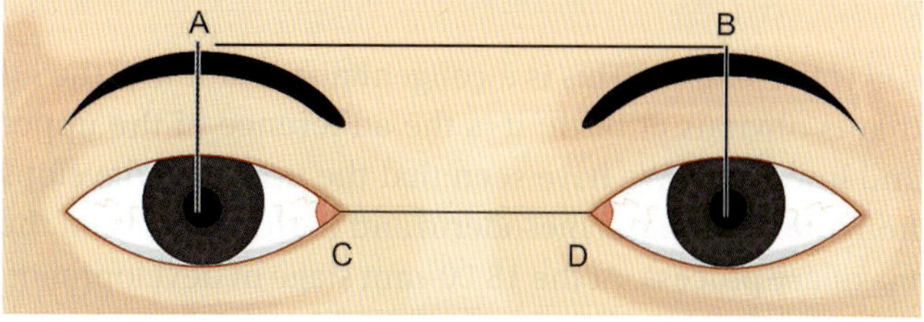

Telecanthus
Intercanthal distance CD is more than interpupillary distance AB

Fig. 9.37: Telecanthus.

The coloboma of the lids in children can be acquired or congenital. The former is mostly traumatic or surgical. The loss of tissue may be a small portion of the lid or a total avulsion of the lid.

Avulsion of the lids is a true emergency.

To understand the congenital coloboma of the lid, it is essential to recapitulate events that lead to the formation of the lids. The lid has dual origins, i.e., ectoderm and mesoderm. The skin and conjunctival epithelium develop from the ectoderm, while the rest of the lid develops from the mesoderm.

Most of the congenital anomalies of the lids happen during the 2nd month of pregnancy, either in isolation or in association with other clefting syndromes. The development of the lids, in short, is as follows:

The upper lid develops from the frontonasal process in two parts, i.e., a smaller medial and a larger lateral part. The two fuse to form the upper lid; a defect in the fusion of the processes at this level results in the formation of the coloboma of the upper lid. The colobomas are of full thickness, i.e., involve all the structure from skin to conjunctiva in various sizes; they are of three types (as shown in **Figure 9.23**).

The term ablepharon refers to the total congenital absence of a lid, which is a rarity.

The lower lid coloboma develops from a defect in the mesoderm of the maxillary process. The lower lid coloboma is exclusively seen on the lateral half of the lid as a wide and shallow saucer-shaped depression, causing the tear to dribble in spite of intact lacrimal drainage.

Microblepharon is a congenital short lid that causes lagophthalmos. The child sleeps with the eyes slightly open, exposing the lower cornea.

Large colobomas present at birth are true emergencies because they make the cornea vulnerable to exposure.

Ankyloblepharon: This is a congenital condition of the lid that is obvious at birth; it is the adherence of the upper and lower lids. We have seen that the upper lid develops from the frontonasal mesoderm and the lower lid from the maxillary process. At the 18.00-mm stage of development, the mesodermal mass for the lid folds is covered by the ectoderm that forms the skin of the lid.

The interpalpebral fissure is not fully formed till late; it is covered by a fused upper and lower lid between the 3rd and 6th months; thereafter, the two lids separate, beginning from the middle. At birth, the lids are fully developed with normal movement and a fully formed interpalpebral aperture. If separation is not complete, some strands of skin remain attached, bridging the interpalpebral aperture, resulting in ankyloblepharon.

As the condition is visible at birth, the term adnatum is suffixed. The frills contain only skin with a few fine blood vessels; the frills are very small, between one and half a dozen **(Figs. 9.38A and B)**.

They are best snipped soon after birth to free the lids.

Distichiasis is a rare anomaly of lashes of both the lids; it is more common in the upper lid. In a normal lid, the lashes arise in front of the opening of the meibomian orifices in two–three rows. In cases of distichiasis, the meibomian openings are replaced by lashes, leaving a clear intermarginal surface in-between the normal and abnormal rows. The lashes grow backwards in contrast to normal lashes that grow forward away from the cornea.

The number of abnormal lashes may vary from single to many. The lashes rub on the cornea and conjunctiva, causing lacrimation. The condition must be differentiated from trichiasis that is an acquired and far more common condition.

Management of distichiasis consists of epilation or laser destruction of the lash follicle; this is effective only when a few lashes are involved and otherwise a plastic repair is required.

Epiblepharon: This is a congenital condition of an extra horizontal fold of skin in any of the lids parallel to the

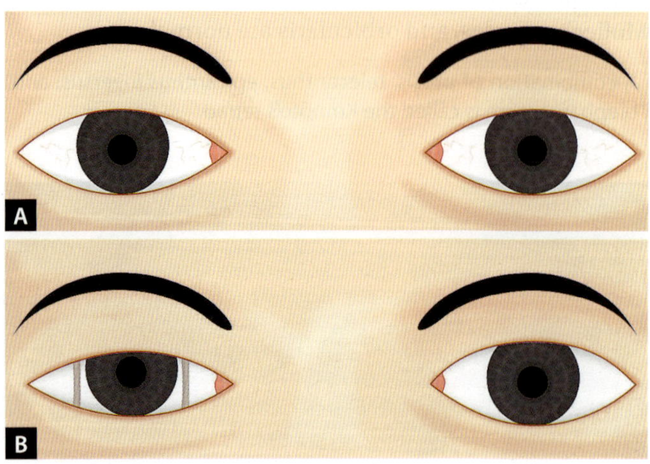

Figs. 9.38A and B: (A) Normal eye; (B) Ankyloblepharon right eye.

lid margins. It is occasionally associated with congenital entropion of the lower lid.

Euryblepharon: In this condition, the interpalpebral fissure is congenitally enlarged; the enlargement is uniform, giving it a staring look. The outer canthus is displaced laterally; the condition should be differentiated from more serious conditions like proptosis, thyroid ocular disease, and lagophthalmos. Occasionally, the coloboma of the lower lid mimics euryblepharon.

Phacomatoses: The word is used to represent a group of benign new growths of mixed origin, i.e., ectoderm/mesoderm. They are congenital in origin and may not be obvious at birth. Few of them have discoloration of the skin, i.e., port-wine spots, Café-au-lait spots, and ash-leaf spots, i.e., Sturge–Weber syndrome, neurofibromatosis, respectively. All phacomata are hamartomas.

Hamartomas are benign congenital new growths of normal tissue that are designated to be present at the site under consideration. They are slow-growing and may be localized or scattered. Lesions at other locations may be a direct extension of the first growth or independent of it. The cells of hamartomas grow to maturity without reproducing; hence, they are self-limited. The examples are Sturge–Weber syndrome and neurofibromatosis.

Choristomas: Like hamartomas, choristomas, too, are benign congenital growths that develop in embryonal cells in parts where they should not belong, for example, the dermoids.

The following is a list of phacomata seen in children:

Condition	Eponyms
• Neurofibromatosis	Von Recklinghausen disease
• Encephalotrigeminal angiomatosis	Sturge–Weber's syndrome
• Angiomatosis retinae	Von Hippel–Lindau disease (not seen on lids)
• Tuberous sclerosis	Bourneville disease (do not involve lids)
• Ataxia telangiectasia	Louis–Bar syndrome

Neurofibroma: Neurofibroma is a hamartoma of the peripheral nerve sheath. It is present at birth as a café-au-lait spot anywhere on the body. The fully developed neurofibroma does not manifest before the 2nd year and thereafter grows for a few years to reach its maximum dimension and stops growing without extending into other tissues. It does not metastasize unless it turns malignant, which is rare. Neurofibroma is not known to disappear spontaneously. The condition is autosomal dominant; it may be sporadic sometimes **(Figs. 9.39A to D)**.

Genetically, they are put into two distinct clinical types, i.e., NF-1 and NF-2.

Type 1 is eponymized by Von Recklinghausen syndrome.

It is due to a mutation on chromosome 17. It has ocular, cutaneous, and central nervous system involvement.

The ocular lesions are:

Lid: Cafe-au-lait spot, plexiform growth causing pseudoptosis with a typical *S-shaped* curve of the lid margin

Conjunctiva: Plexiform growth

Iris–Lisch nodule: Lisch nodules are seen on the anterior surface of the iris, rarely more than two or three in number. The nodules are melanocytic hamartomas; they may increase in number to four or five, do not increase in size, do not interfere with vision or cause glaucoma unless present at an angle, and do not require any treatment.

Lens: 40% of cases have posterior subcapsular opacity; the relation between the opacity and neurofibroma is not clear.

Retina: Retinal nodule (rare)

Optic nerve: Glioma of the nerve or chiasma.

Orbit-pulsating exophthalmos due to faulty development of the sphenoid

Cutaneous lesions (café-au-lait patch), single to multiple in number, plexiform neurofibroma

Type 2 neurofibroma: Type 2 neurofibroma is due to a mutation in chromosome 22; it has less ocular features than central nervous system (CNS); hence, it is also referred to as central neurofibromatosis. In contrast to type 1, it does not involve the optic nerve. The cranial nerve involved is the eighth, in the form of a glioma. Eighth nerve involvement is bilateral. It may be seen in first-degree relatives. Type 2 neurofibromatosis is often associated with meningioma and schwannoma.

Posterior subcapsular opacity is the only ocular manifestation.

Criteria for the diagnosis of neurofibromatosis type 1:

- Cafe-au-lait spot
- Neurofibroma anywhere in the body, including the lids

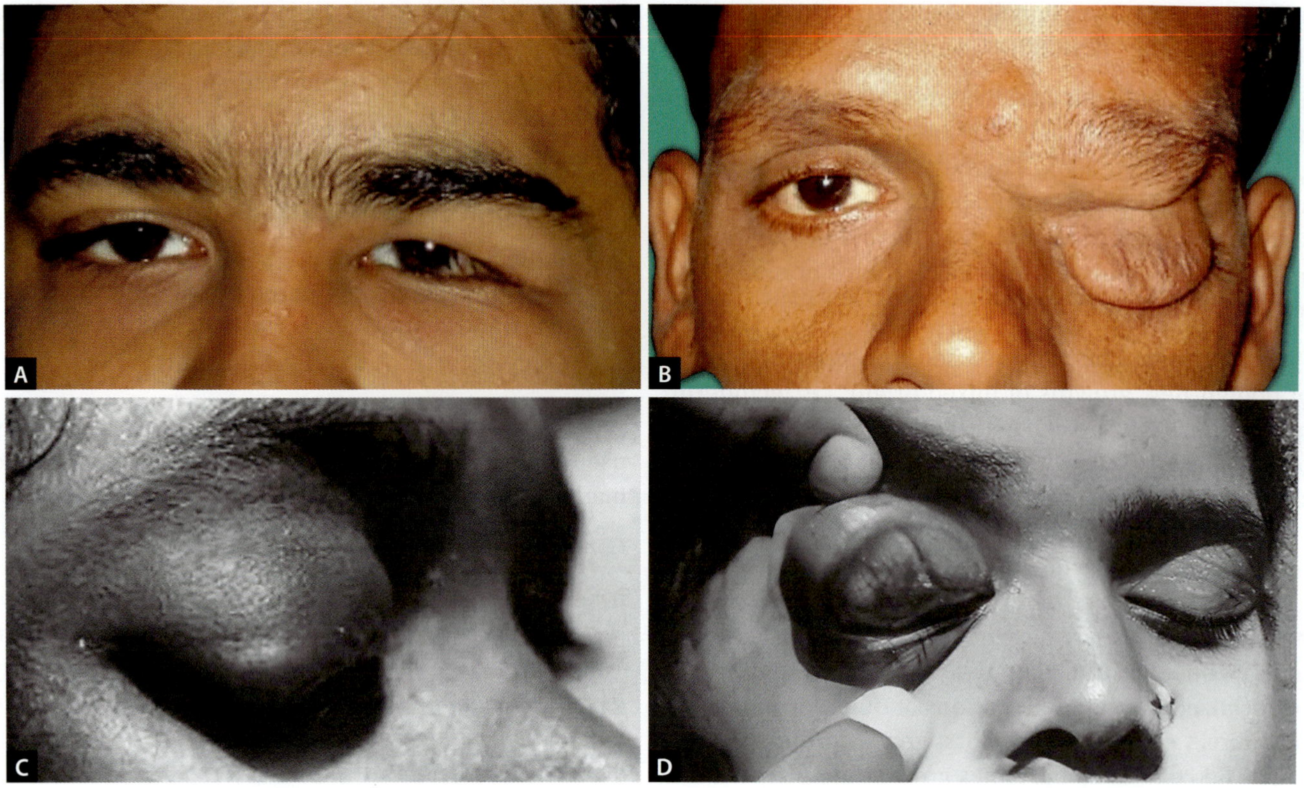

Figs. 9.39A to D: Neurofibroma of the lids. All the above cases had congenital origins.

- At least one plexiform neurofibroma anywhere in the body
- Optic nerve glioma
- At least two nodules in the iris
- Pulsating exophthalmoses due to sphenoidal dysplasia
- Evidence of NF-1 in at least one first-degree relative
- Other features are schwannoma, glaucoma, retinal hamartoma, thickened cranial nerves, and a tendency to malignant change.
- Neurofibromatosis is an autosomal dominant trend in 50% of cases.
- May have an orthopedic problem.

Criteria for the diagnosis of neurofibromatosis type 2:

- Unilateral neurofibroma
- Evidence of neurofibroma in first-degree relatives
- Posterior subcapsular opacity in the lens
- Unilateral acoustic neuroma
- Multiple meningiomas

Note: All features sited above need not be present in all cases. A combination of more than two features is highly suggestive of both types.

The following features are confirmatory:

- Six or more café-au-lait spots >5 mm in children and 15 mm in adults
- Axillary and inguinal freckles
- Two or more neurofibromas
- One plexiform lesion
- Types 1 and 2 are not known to coexist.

Investigation required:

- X-ray orbit for enlargement of the optic canal in the glioma of the optic nerve
- *CT:* Orbit and skull
- Gadolinium enhanced the MRI orbit and skull.
- Histopathological confirmation from a skin biopsy

Sturge-Weber syndrome: Sturge-Weber syndrome is a congenital disorder that is evident at birth and involves the eyes, skin, and central nervous system. All systems need not be affected at the same time. It can be monosystemic or polysystemic. Incomplete features are not exceptions.

Though the syndrome is grouped under hamartoma phacomatosis (mother spot), it differs from all of them by not being hereditary. The cases are sporadic without family history, which is prominent in neurofibromatosis.

As per the presentation, the syndrome is put into flowing groups:

- Involving the eye, skin, and CNS (encephalocranio-cutaneous)
- Involving eye and skin, sparing CNS (oculocutaneous)
- Involving the CNS and a skin-sparing eye (encephalo-cutaneous)

Eyes are always involved when skin is affected; isolated ocular involvement has not been reported.

The cause of the syndrome is not well understood. It seems to be a mix-up of cells from the cephalic neural crest and mesodermal mesenchymal. This is explained on the basis of the following factors:

- The syndrome is basically an abnormality of the vasculature of the meninges, skin, and choroid.
- Vasculatures of intraocular structures other than choroids are not affected.
- It is the endothelium of the vasculature that is at fault.
- The endothelia of medium and fine vessels are involved, which are derived from mesoderm.
- From the cephalic neural crest, develop facial skin, pia mater, choroid, and smooth muscle of the vessels. All these tissues are involved in Sturge-Weber syndrome.
- When the developing cephalic neural crest and mesodermal mesenchymal interact, clinical features develop.

The syndrome is seen among children of all races in both sexes equally; the condition is generally unilateral and present at birth and may be monosystemic or polysystemic; hence, the clinical features could be cutaneous or ocular.

Cutaneous: The cutaneous changes are common; they could be port-wine stain **(Fig. 9.40)** or nevus flammeus on the forehead, scalp, lids, and conjunctiva. The stain is the cause of a typical birthmark due to an excess of capillaries under the superficial skin. 95% of birthmarks are present at birth as dull red patches with irregular borders. The size varies in dimension, so in number, the patches do not increase in size or number with age. They only change hue.

The stain may be small or extensive enough to cover the forehead, scalp lid, conjunctiva, and episcleral. The color is due to an excess of capillaries under the superficial layer of skin. The cutaneous features are present in 95% of cases at birth as dull red patches with irregular borders; the size varies in dimension, as do the numbers. The patches do not increase in size or number. They only change the

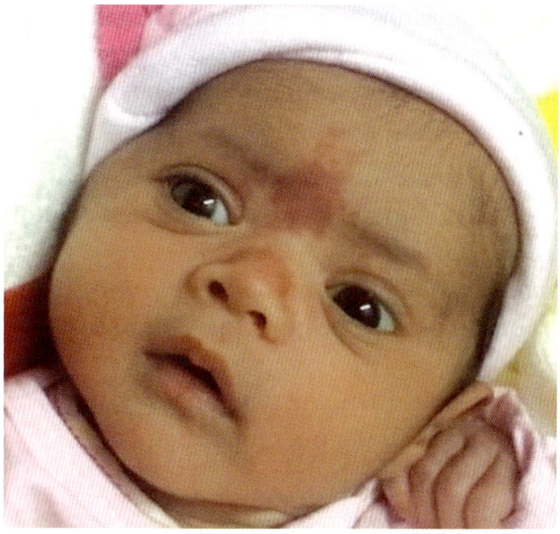

Fig. 9.40: Port-wine stain syndrome.

hue; the color changes to a darker shade with age; they last a lifelong presence on the distribution of the trigeminal nerve. 90% of cases are unilateral; bilateral cases, when present, are more serious.

Ocular involvement: Ocular involvements are many; out of them, glaucoma and choroidal hemangiomas are vision-threatening.

- *Lid:* Port-wine stain may involve both lids, generally unilaterally. Bilateral cases are more vision-threatening and are associated with other congenital anomalies of the eye. The cutaneous involvement in Sturge-Weber syndrome does not cause ptosis, which is common with neurofibromatosis.
- *Conjunctiva:* Dilatation of conjunctival and episcleral vessels
- Episcleral vascular growth
- Increases episcleral pressure
- *Iris:* Heterochromia in 10% of cases
- *Glaucoma:* The most important ocular involvement of the syndrome in congenital glaucoma which is resistant to medical treatment, surgical results are also not encouraging. Half the children with Sturge-Weber syndrome develop glaucoma, which is ipsilateral to port-wine stain; children without skin involvement generally do not develop glaucoma. Incidence of glaucoma is more likely if both lids have cutaneous involvement. It is imperative to subject the child to a complete ophthalmic examination as soon as the child is suspected to have Sturge-Weber syndrome for glaucoma. Glaucoma may be present at birth and mistaken for primary congenital glaucoma. Glaucoma

generally develops by 2 years of age; a raised intraocular pressure (IOP) is detected.

Before 2 years of age is more damaging than developing later.

The glaucomatous change consists of:

- Watering this may be mistaken as congenital naso-lacrimal duct block.
- *Photophobia:* This is due to a rupture in Descemet's membrane. May be mistaken as—trauma or keratitis.
- *Cornea:*
  - Larger than 12 mm in diameter
  - Rupture in Descemet's membrane
  - Clouding
- *Globe:* Buphthalmos
- *Angle:* It is better to measure angle by gonioscope under general anesthesia.
- Tension is generally very high. Tension >23 mm is a red flag. Tension is better recorded under general anesthesia.
- *Other ocular changes:*
  - *Choroidal hemangioma:* Choroidal hemangiomas are unilateral, ipsilateral to cutaneous changes with typical tomato catch-up appearances, and may be extensive enough to involve half of the retina. Posterior pole is often involved.
  - Retinal vessels develop arteriovenous anastomosis or may simply be tortuous.
  - Other changes due to raised intraocular tension are: myopic shift, anisometropia, amblyopia, field, and fundus changes.

The central nervous system changes:

- The neural changes are due to angiomatous malformation of the leptomeninges, ipsilateral to cutaneous and ocular changes.
- The malformations are seen on the occipital and posterior parts of the parietal globe of the brain.
- The cortex under the vascular malformation develops progressive calcification. The calcification may even spread to the temporal and frontal lobes. The expanding angiomatous growth causes convulsions that may be localized or generalized.
- Convulsions are seen as frequently as in 80–90% of children with Sturge–Weber syndrome. It starts in the first few months and becomes worse. About half of children with Sturge–Weber syndrome have some mental retardation.
- Other neurological changes are hemiplegia and homonymous hemianopia.

> A newborn with an unexplained convulsion and port-wine stain should be considered to be suffering from and investigated for Sturge–Weber syndrome.

Investigation:

- All children not responding to usual treatment for convulsions should be suspected of having Sturge–Weber syndrome and examined for port-wine stains and ocular changes.
- A plain X-ray of the skull often shows intracranial calcification.
- The CT skull shows a double-lined pattern of intracranial calcification, which is parallel to the convolution of the brain.
- MRI is not as effective a diagnostic tool as CT.

Management:

- Cutaneous manifestations do not require any specific treatment other than counseling.
- CNS involvement is best treated by a neurologist.
- The glaucoma is difficult to treat; medical treatment is not very effective; surgical treatment alone is equally futile; a combination of surgery and medicine is the only choice left.
- All efforts should be made to salvage as much vision as possible by managing errors of refraction and amblyopia.

Less common phacomas of childhood are ***(Table 9.2)****:*

- Angiomatosis retinae
- Tuberous sclerosis
- Ataxia telangiectasia (Louis–Bar)
- Wyburn–Mason syndrome

All the above conditions are congenital, become obvious in the first decade, and may be diagnosed on routine fundus examinations. They differ from neurofibroma and Sturge–Weber syndrome by not having cutaneous involvement. They have not only ocular and CNS involvement but also a visceral component. The ocular manifestations appear earlier than the systemic ones. All are slow-progressing but may be fatal.

INFECTION AND INFLAMMATION OF THE LIDS

Infections and inflammation of the lids may involve:

- Only skin
- Lid margin
- Subcutaneous tissue
- More than one of the above

TABLE 9.2: Clinical presentation of other less common conditions.

Syndrome	*Von Hippel–Lindau*	*Bourneville*	*Wyburn–Mason*
Other names	Angiomatosis retinae	Tuberous sclerosis	Ataxia telangiectasia
Nature	Hamartoma	Hamartoma	Hamartoma
Laterality	Bilateral	Bilateral	Unilateral
Heredity	Plus	Plus	Plus
Onset	First decade	First decade	Congenital
Progression	Progressive	Progressive	Progressive
Ocular involvement	Retinal hemangioma, arteriovenous shunt, macular star, and disk swelling	Hamartoma of the retina, drusen of the disk, and mulberry astrocytoma	Racemose hemangioma of the retina, episcleral, and CNS hemangioma
Cutaneous involvement	Rare. When present, there are vascular ecchymotic nevi	Angiofibroma, ash-leaf spot, and fibroma tongue	Pulsatile vascular nevus
Systemic involvement	• CNS—cerebellar hemangioma • Visceral—various types of malignancies	Intracranial calcification, hamartoma of the kidney and heart, convulsions, and mental retardation	Racemose hemangioma in mid-brain

(CNS: central nervous system)

Infection of the skin of the lid: Infection of the skin of the lid can be localized to the lid, i.e., boil, abscess, and cellulitis. It may be part of an infection of the face, i.e., herpes zoster ophthalmicus, herpes simplex, molluscum, measles, or chickenpox.

The infection can be:

- *Bacterial:* Both cocci and bacilli, the former being more frequent
- Viral
- Fungal

Bacterial infections are far more common than viral and fungal infections put together. Fungus infections of the lids are rare.

Bacterial Infection

The bacterial infection of the skin of the lid may involve the skin away from the lid margin or may involve the lid margin only. It is more often acute and caused by pus-forming organisms. Bacilli rarely involve the skin of the lid; chronic cutaneous involvements are caused by tuberculosis, syphilis, and leprosy.

The bacterial infection of the lid can be—boil->cellulitis-> abscess.

Boils

Boils of the lids are common in children. They generally involve the upper lid. They may be accompanied by folliculitis of the face. They are more common during the summer and early rains, developing as small, tender nodules under the skin and soon developing pus. The boil may be single or multiple, may be in one lid or both lids; it may be seen on both sides simultaneously. The most common organism is staphylococcus. Other frequent organisms that cause infections of the skin of the lid are *Streptococci* and *Haemophilus*. *Haemophilus* is more severe than the other two. A boil may subside without treatment, may be followed by another, or there may be a crop of boils. If the boil does not subside, it causes cellulitis of the lid. The laxity of the skin of the lid and the abundance of blood vessels make it an ideal place for inflammatory fluid to accumulate, making it more visible and symptomatic.

Cellulitis

The cellulitis of lid in children starts as diffuse painful swelling, warm to touch, may be tender, tense, and hyperemic, causing pseudoptosis to obliterate IPA (**Figs. 9.41 and 9.42**). The lids can be separated easily, the globe is not involved, there is no proptosis, movements are normal.

Abscess

Abscess generally follows cellulitis, where the exudate is converted to frank pus, gravitating to the most dependent part. At this stage, there is no scope for pus to get absorbed. If inflammation is not managed, the abscess bursts on the surface of the lid, giving prompt relief from pain, and the swelling subsides. The treatment of an abscess is to drain the swelling at the thinnest and most dependent part with a stab incision when fluctuation develops. It is better to give medical treatment a try before making an incision. The usual management consists of dry hot fomentation and broad-spectrum anti-staphylococcal and

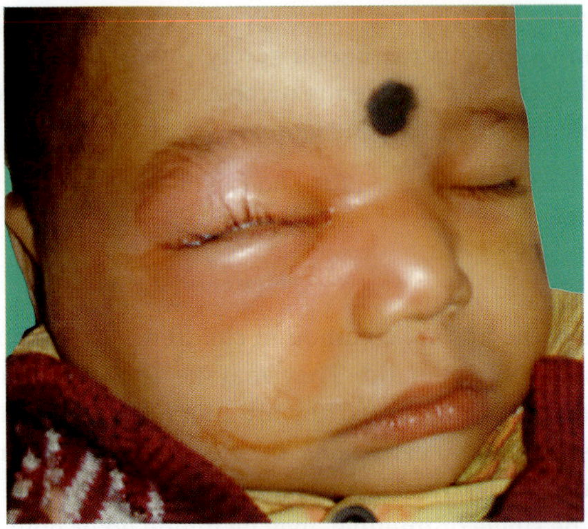

Fig. 9.41: Cellulitis lid in an infant a boy.

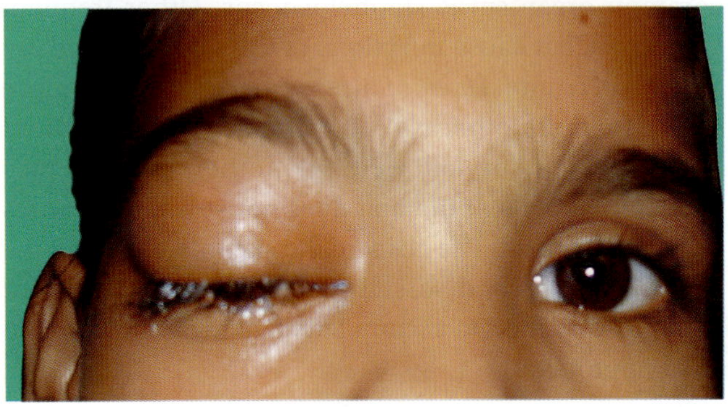

Fig. 9.42: Cellulitis lid in a boy.

anti-Haemophilus antibiotics as per the weight of the child under 12 years. Local antibiotics have no role. Mild oral analgesics are sufficient to control pain.

Viral Infection of the Lids

The common viruses that infect the skin of the lids in children are:

- Herpes simplex
- Herpes zoster ophthalmicus
- Molluscum contagiosum
- Varicella
- Measles
- Vaccinia
- Lymphogranuloma venereum

Herpes Simplex

The overall incidence of herpes simplex infection is increasing. It is natural that more and more number of cases of herpes simplex in children are being reported. It may involve the skin, mucocutaneous junction, and mucous membrane, all of which are mild and hence often missed. They are self-limiting. However, systemic involvement, when present, is more severe and may be fatal. Generally, a newborn is protected by the antibodies present in the mother for the first 6 months. Hence, it is uncommon to get a herpes simplex infection in neonates. Intrauterine infection of lids with the herpes simplex virus is rare. Acquired infection from the maternal birth canal is more common. In the absence of maternal antibodies, neonatal lid lesions are caused by the type II herpes simplex virus. Neonatal infection may involve the eye and adnexa in the following ways:

- Infection of the skin of the lids
- Infection of the conjunctiva
- Infection of the cornea

The lids of children after 6 months are more frequently infected, either as a primary or recurrent infection of the lid. The primary lesions develop between 6 months and late teens. In teens, the incidence increases with age due to precocity. Lid infections in children are caused by contact with an infected person.

The primary lid lesions are generally unilateral, more common in the lower lid; bilateral cases are not exceptions. The lesions are in clusters on the skin or the lid margin. Lid margin involvement is associated with catarrhal conjunctivitis and keratitis.

In children, the primary involvement of the cornea is mild and self-limiting. It may be superficially punctuate or microdendritic in nature. Children with atopia are prone to developing eruptions that look like eruption of chickenpox. Normally, the eruptions are self-limited and disappear without scaring, unlike herpes zoster. Herpes simplex does not cause post-herpetic neuralgia in spite of *H. simplex* and *H. zoster* belonging to the same group and having a common natural history of lying dormant in the trigeminal ganglion following primary infection and traveling down during reactivation. The activated viruses are responsible for recurrence, mainly in the cornea. 60% of children become seropositive by 6 years; this rises to 90% in adults, out of which only 1% are likely to develop keratitis in later life that may take months to years to manifest. The corneal lesions, when present, are milder and more self-limiting than in adults, without requiring any specific treatment. The lid lesions also do not require any treatment; they are self-healing. There is no vaccine against *H. simplex* either.

Herpes Zoster in Children

The infection is caused by a pox virus called varicella zoster that causes chickenpox in children and herpes zoster in adults. Chickenpox is more common in children than in adults. The incidence is reversed in adults. More adults suffer from herpes zoster than chickenpox. The incidence of chickenpox is negligible after 30 years of age. The incidence of herpes zoster in adults increases with age. Neonates do not suffer either from chickenpox or herpes zoster. This is in contrast to herpes simplex, which is common in neonates.

Zoster virus is a DNA virus structurally similar to chickenpox virus; both of them are neurotropic; the zoster and simplex have similar morphology with differences in antigen. The chickenpox and herpes zoster give life-long immunity in immune-competent persons. It is claimed that if a child is immunized against chickenpox, they will not develop herpes zoster later; a specific vaccine is under trial for adults over sixty against zoster. No vaccine is available against herpes simplex. Chickenpox has a predominant cutaneous manifestation; herpes zoster ophthalmicus has pronounced ocular involvement with localized skin involvement that is confined to single dermatomes that do not cross the midline. Central nervous system involvement in cases of zoster infection is less frequent; herpes zoster infection can be pre-eruptive, eruptive, or post-eruptive. The last is called postherpetic neuralgia; it is less severe in children and shorter-lived than in adults. A varicella infection is neither painful nor followed by post-varicella neuralgia. Herpes zoster infection may leave an area of hypoesthesia or anesthesia in the area supplied by the involved dermatome, which is not met with in varicella. The inclusion and elementary bodies are similar in the two. In rare condition, both chickenpox and zoster may coexist, incubation period in two is same.

Herpes zoster infection of the eyes and its adnexa is clinically known as herpes zoster ophthalmicus. It is localized to the distribution of the fifth cranial nerve **(Figs. 9.43A and B)**. Out of the three branches of trigeminal, the first is most commonly involved, the second branch is less commonly involved, and the involvement of the second division, which is rarer, does not include the eyes and its adnexa.

The third branch is rarely involved in immune-deficient persons; all the branches may be involved simultaneously in immune-compromised. Only a twig of the trigeminal may be involved in a mild infection or in a child with some immunity **(Fig. 9.44)**.

> Ophthalmic involvement accounts for 20% of all cases of zoster infection.

The most remarkable feature of zoster infection is that it does not cross the midline and is confined to a single dermatome. The latency of the disease is perplexing. The most accepted theory is that the child has suffered a subclinical attack of chickenpox in the past, which has not provided with sufficient immunity, and the virus has traveled to the Gasserian ganglion, where it has remained dormant. With the lowering of immunity, the virus is activated sufficiently to cause herpes zoster.

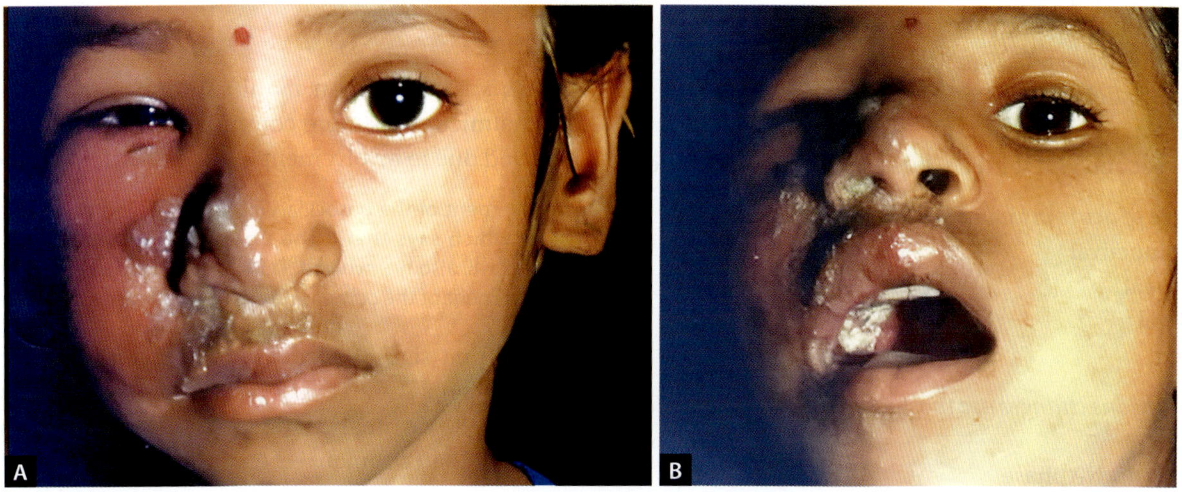

Figs. 9.43A and B: Involvement of the second division of the fifth cranial nerve without involving the eyes.
Courtesy: Dr Madan K Deshpande.

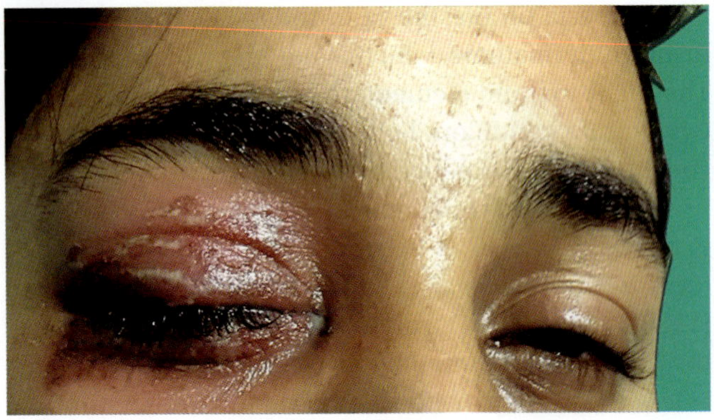

Fig. 9.44: Herpes zoster involvement of a twig of the first division of the fifth cranial nerve in an adolescent.

Besides the trigeminal ganglion (Gasserian ganglion), the other ganglia, i.e., the ciliary and otic, may also be affected, causing mydriasis and cycloplegia in the first instance and Ramsay–Hunt syndrome in the second. Other cranial nerves that do not have extra medullary ganglions may rarely be involved, most probably not due to viral invasion but as an autoimmune response independent of latency. This happens once the initial infection is on its way to subsidence. Involvement of the cervical sympathetic is rare; there are scant reports of the Argyll Robertson pupil in herpes zoster; still rare is contralateral hemiparesis, that is thought to be autoimmune.

Mode of presentation:

The incidence of herpes zoster in children is far less than in adults, in spite of both sharing the same etiopathology and clinical features.

The clinical presentation is divided into the following three stages:

- Stage of acute infection and its complications
- Stage of delayed effect
- Stage of residue

The second and third are less spectacular in children.

The stage of acute infection is further divided into:

- Conjunctival
- Corneal
- Scleral
- Uveal

The cutaneous changes are most marked and diagnostic. They are:

- Pre-eruptive phase
- Eruptive phase
- Post-eruptive phase

In the pre-eruptive phase, the child complains of ipsilateral hemicrania, malaise, and fever. The onset is acute, and the skin over the dermatome where the eruption will develop is edematous and hyperemic. At this stage, the skin sensation is retained. Hypoesthesia, followed by anesthesia, develops in the post-eruptive phase. The pre-eruption stage may be taken as the prodromal stage of the eruption that lasts for 4–5 days. Afterwards, actual eruptions start developing as papules and pass through stages of vesicles and pustules. Fully developed vesicles have stark similarities to the vesicles of chickenpox, which take 10–15 days to dry up and crusts to fall off. Fallen crusts leave shallow, hypopigmented craters. The pits heal within a few days to weeks, lesions at the lid margin leave notches, and a notch at the lower lid causes permanent epiphora.

By this time, cutaneous sensations get dulled and pass on to the state of cutaneous anesthesia, the cutaneous sensation rarely returning to the pre-eruption state. In adults, it may be a lifelong feature.

Stage of eruption: This spreads over a large hemifacial skin, extending from the tip of the nose to the mid cranium. The conjunctiva is congested, and the cornea may also be involved in a moderate way. Nonspecific conjunctivitis is universal; it may develop some vesicles that may be mistaken as phlycten. Secondary infection of conjunctiva is frequent.

One of less common feature is ptosis to begin with; it is pseudoptosis that generally passes off with the subsidence of edema. In a few instances, the levator gets entangled in inflammation and loses its action; the other cause is neuritis, to cause ptosis.

Keratitis

Keratitis is a common manifestation of herpes zoster ophthalmicus; it is more common if the tip of the nose is involved due to involvement of the nasociliary branch.

> Involvement of the nasociliary branch is called the Hutchinson sign, which says that if the tip of the nose is involved, the cornea will also be involved. This is not always true; there can be involvement of the cornea without involving the tip of the nose.

The first sign of corneal involvement is diminished corneal sensation, even before actual lesions have developed. Corneal involvement is more commonly epithelial than stromal.

The epithelial changes are: Punctate lesions, microdendrites, and filamentary keratitis. The punctuate lesions start on the periphery and stain with fluorescein and Rose Bengal; the later gives a better stain. The dendrites and microdendrites are mostly transient, occasionally invading stroma, resulting in deep keratitis, nummular, or disciform. The deeper corneal lesions are suspected to be autoimmune in nature. They do not respond to local or systemic antiviral drugs but to steroids. If a secondary infection sets in, the lesion is converted into a frank bacterial ulcer, leaving a permanent central scar and impeding vision. The absence of corneal sensation predisposes to bacterial invasion.

Episcleritis

About one-third of cases will develop episcleritis, which is generally overshadowed by more prominent lid and conjunctival signs. They are often mistaken for zoster vesicles. Scleritis is a more serious matter that may become sclerokeratitis or sclerouveitis. Intraocular lesions can otherwise develop without scleral involvement. Intraocular involvement is more common and severe if all the branches of the first division of the trigeminal are affected. The intraocular lesions invariably cause anterior uveitis.

Retinal lesions are rare; when present, they are—perivasculitis, retinitis, hemorrhages, and exudates. Optic neuritis is still rare.

Uveitis is nongranulomatous; it may develop along with keratitis or scleritis. Circumciliary congestion is overshadowed by conjunctivitis. Unexplained pain should arouse suspicion of uveitis. Slit lamp examination reveals flare, cells, and KPs. Hypopyon is rare; the aqueous fluid may be tinged with blood. One of the not well-understood phenomenon of iridocyclitis is ischemic necrosis of the iris, causing partial or full-thickness loss of the iris, resulting in pseudopolycoria and a distorted pupil. The other cause of irregular pupils is associated with iridocyclitis. Cyclitis causes a lowering of IOP, leading to a soft eye that may terminate in phthisis. In contrast to this, peripheral anterior synechiae and trabeculitis are responsible for the rise in pressure, ending in secondary glaucoma.

Neurological involvement:

- All cranial nerves, from the second to the seventh, can get involved in herpes zoster.
- The nerves that are likely to be involved can be put into two groups, i.e.:
  1. Those with extramedullary ganglion: Third, fifth, and seventh
  2. Those without extramedullary ganglion: Second, fourth, and sixth
- Cervical sympathetics are rarely involved.

The nerves with extramedullary ganglion are directly invaded by the virus during the initial subacute attack, only to lay dormant till the immunity is good. As immunity declines, the infection manifests as herpes zoster ophthalmicus in the case of the fifth nerve and Ramsay-Hunt syndrome* in the case of the seventh nerve. Involvement of the ciliary ganglion is less frequent; when involved, it manifests as cycloplegia; still, rarely, there may be an Argyll-Robertson pupil.

Other cranial nerves are most probably involved in autoimmune reactions.

The dissimilarity lies in the fact that herpes zoster ophthalmicus spares orbicularis, which is a predominant feature in Ramsay-Hunt syndrome.

Clinical presentation of Ramsay-Hunt syndrome: The syndrome is milder, has a short clinical span, is self-limited, and does not require antiviral treatment.

Typical presentation consists of rashes similar to those of zoster ophthalmicus present on the pinna, external auditory canal, and tympanic membrane. Pain in the ear is a constant feature, as is unilateral loss of hearing that may be permanent. As far as the eyes are concerned, it is limited to mild-to-moderate ipsilateral orbicularis palsy, leading to lagophthalmos with its usual features of lacrimation, conjunctivitis, and exposure keratitis, with the cornea retaining its sensation.

Postherpetic neuralgia: Postherpetic neuralgia is the most frustrating part of herpetic infection. It is a pain that develops on the dermatome, which had an eruption during

---

**Ramsay-Hunt syndrome:* This is rarely seen in children. Though caused by the herpes zoster virus, it is not related to herpes zoster ophthalmicus, yet they have some similarities:

- Both are caused by the herpes zoster virus.
- Latency
- Involvement of the extramedullary ganglion
- Unilateral
- Involvement of a single dermatome
- Loss of cutaneous sensation in the postherpetic period

the attack. Almost all patients are likely to develop this malady. The older the patient, the more severe the pain is. It is milder or absent in children, and lesions away from the head are less painful. The pain is felt a few days after the vesicles have dried. Stabbing in nature may be continuous or episodic; it is akin to trigeminal neuralgia lasting for a few months to years. One of the paradoxes of pain is the absence of cutaneous sensation, resulting in anesthesia dolorosa. The treatment is frustrating and ineffective and may be very severe. The usual treatment consists of analgesics at the least dose that gives maximum relief. The other medications include tricyclic antidepressants, gabapentin, and pregabalin. Electrodes may be placed around the area of pain to create artificial neurons that send "nonpain" signals to the brain; local infiltration in the effective area has been given up in favor of electrodes.

Sequel to an acute attack: The sequels are many; some of them are unwelcome lasting for the rest of the life, as seen in the areas that have withstood the onslaught of the infection. They are:

- *Lid:* Hypo- or hyperpigmented scar, trichiasis, madarosis, entropion, ptosis that may be restrictive or neurological, and coloboma of the lid margin.
- *Conjunctiva:* Recurrent secondary bacterial conjunctivitis, ocular surface defect, mucus-secreting conjunctivitis, and scar
- *Sclera:* Recurrent scleritis
- *Intraocular pressure:* Secondary glaucoma
- *Cornea:* Corneal changes are many and may be the cause of visual loss. They can be broadly categorized into the following groups without clear-cut demarcation between two adjacent groups: concurrent with eruption, posteruptive, and late **(Table 9.3)**.

TABLE 9.3: Chronology of corneal involvement in herpes zoster.

Category	*Time of onset*	*Clinical presentation*
Concurrent	2–3 days	Peripheral keratitis, punctate keratitis
	4–6 days	Multiple dendritic ulcers
	6–7 days	Stromal edema, fold in the Descemet's membrane, kp$^{\pm}$ hypopyon$^{\pm}$, hyphema$^{\pm}$, secondary glaucoma
	10–15 days	Stromal infiltration, nummular opacity, and disciform keratitis
Posteruption	4 weeks	Peripheral gutter perforation$^{\pm}$
	4–8 weeks	Vascularization and thinning of the cornea
	8–12 weeks	Scleritis, elevated mucus plaque over the epithelium
	12 weeks	Corneal haze, punctate erosion, oval deep opacity
	12–16 weeks	Disk-shaped stromal haze without epithelial defect; may have immune ring round the opacity
	After 16 weeks	Exposure keratitis
Late	1–2 years	Seen following extensive cornel involvement, deep vascularization
	>2 years	Permanent endothelial following direct invasion by virus, patchy epithelial separation from Bowman's membrane

Mucus Plaque

About 15% of eyes infected by herpes zoster ophthalmicus suffer from this malady. Mucus plaque develops after 1-3 months, and the eye has become quite. This is associated with a loss of corneal sensation. Another associated corneal change is disciform keratitis; the development of mucus plaque may be delayed by as much as 4-5 months. The plaque consists of accumulated mucus over the epithelium, either as a single plaque or as scattered plaques. The plaque can be removed with ease. The plaque is otherwise self-limiting and is shed automatically, leaving a stromal haze that passes without any treatment.

Differential diagnosis: A fully developed case of herpes zoster ophthalmicus is rarely missed due to its characteristic distribution: not crossing vesicles, not crossing the midline, and developing on a particular dermatome. In the initial stage, it can be mistaken for chickenpox, allergic dermatitis stye, cellulites lid, or insect bite.

Management: The management of herpes zoster ophthalmicus in children basically does not differ from that of adults, except for the fact that postherpetic neuralgia is milder and less common in children and anesthesia dolorosa is rare. Some of the deep scars may become permanent as tell-tale sign of a childhood infection.

Management is divided into two parts:

1. Local
2. Systemic

The local lesions requiring treatment are—skin, conjunctiva, lid margin, sclera, cornea, and glaucoma.

Skin:

- During the first 48 hours, a cold compress gives temporary relief to burning sensations and pain.
- *Eruption phase:* It is better to avoid lotions, sprays, and ointments containing home remedies like turmeric, lime, or formulas containing antibiotics, starch, and calamine. They form thick scabs that result in deep and larger scars without any relief from pain. The best way is to put the child under a mosquito net or put a thin cloth covering the face; this lowers the chances of secondary infection. The most important treatment at this stage is to apply a 5% ointment of acyclovir three to four times a day.

Conjunctiva: Conjunctivitis is a constant feature; it may even start before the eruptions have started developing or with the eruption. It can be nonspecific or secondary to bacterial invasion. The conjunctivitis is self-limiting; however, some clinicians use acyclovir ocular ointment routinely at this stage. Broad-spectrum antibiotic drops are used empirically.

Lid margin: Occasionally, a vesicle develops too close to the lid margin, causing a notch; a notch in the upper lid is of no consequence; a notch in the lower lid causes troublesome epiphora for the rest of life; this malady has no treatment.

Keratitis: Keratitis is common if the tip of the nose is involved, subepithelial, and scattered; occasionally, there are micro-dendrons that may turn into frank ulcers with loss of epithelium. The cornea is hypoesthetic or is completely devoid of sensation, which is a bad sign of a predisposing secondary bacterial infection.

Above features make the management of keratitis in herpes zoster ophthalmicus a difficult task. The subepithelial lesions do not respond either to antivirals or antibiotics but to steroids or nonsteroidal anti-inflammatory drugs. Adding cycloplegic to steroids helps in preventing and treating uveitis, giving much-needed relief from pain.

Sclera: This is often masked by conjunctival and ciliary congestion and is treated by steroids.

Anterior uvea: Anterior uveitis is treated with frequent steroid drops and atropine. Atropine in children should be used with usual precaution.

Secondary glaucoma: Secondary glaucoma is rare in children and, when present, is treated by β-blockers and local carbonic anhydrase inhibitors.

Systemic manifestation: Postherpetic neuralgia tops the list of systemic manifestations. It is milder, self-limiting, and short-lived in children and can be managed by oral analgesics. Other systemic complications are restricted to the nervous system; they are transient multiple cranial nerve palsy and contralateral hemiparesis, both of which are pretty frightening to parents who should be counseled about their benign character.

Chemotherapy in herpes zoster ophthalmicus: There is no antibiotic that is effective against the herpes virus. There are a limited number of antiviral drugs effective against herpes zoster; they are virostatic, needing large frequent and prolonged administration. The drug most commonly used is acyclovir. In children, it should be used as per the weight of the child and not empirically. The other drug used is valaciclovir, which is a pro-drug of acyclovir. More drugs are under trial for zoster treatment, like famciclovir, that helps in reducing the effects of stromal keratitis and uveitis. Systemic antiviral drugs should be used in consultation with a pediatrician.

Varicella (Chickenpox)

Chickenpox is a common viral disease in childhood. It mainly inflicts skin and rarely mucous membrane; systemic infection is rare; when present, it may prove to be fatal. It is caused by the human herpes virus; it is a double-stranded DNA virus.

Most common age group to be infected is between 5 and 15 year in both sexes all over the world. There may be epidemics of the disease. The same virus that, after a latency period as long as years, causes herpes zoster in adults. In contrast to zoster, chickenpox is not confined to a single dermatome; it rarely involves the face and neck, and ocular involvement is minimal.

The disease starts with malaise, fever, and headaches, followed by eruptions that go through the *following stages*: macules—papules—vesicles—pustules—scab formation. It takes a few days for the scabs to fall, leaving them without scars or hypopigmentation. The infection imparts permanent immunity to the child. Ocular involvements are fewer and milder than herpes zoster ophthalmicus. *They are*—rashes on the skin and conjunctiva; superficial keratitis. Unlike herpes zoster and simplex, corneal sensations are not diminished. Conjunctivitis is the first to appear. The conjunctiva may actually develop papules that may be mistaken as phlycten. Conjunctivitis is nonspecific and self-limited, as is keratitis; lesions on the lid margin may end up as notch coloboma. Another cause of epiphora is post-chickenpox chronic dacryocystitis, which may take months to years to manifest.

Management: In underdeveloped countries, chickenpox is taken lightly as a natural feature for which no medical help is sought; the child only gets some folk medicines that sometimes prove to be deleterious. Two shots of the anti-chickenpox vaccine impart lifelong immunity.

No antibiotic or antiviral is effective against chickenpox, either. Conjunctivitis is treated with usual antibiotics; keratitis is managed with antibiotics and cycloplegia; and steroids have no role in treating chickenpox.

Molluscum Contagiosum

This is a chronic infection of the skin and mucous membrane caused by a virus of the pox group; it is a DNA virus, and humans are its only reservoir. Though the term contagious is suffixed to it, the disease is the least contagious out of all pox viruses; it is nonfatal with limited skin involvement in immune-competent persons. The disease is acquired following intimate body contact, sexually or otherwise; there may be a spread of lesions from one part of the body to other by way of autoinoculation. It has no systemic involvement either. Its incubation period is about 1 month from the day of inoculation. The point of entry is a scratch on the skin or mucous membrane anywhere on the body; the face is a frequent site. In the eye, the lower lid is the most common site to be infected. The exact cause of this selective involvement is not well explained **(Figs. 9.45A and B)**.

A typical lesion is a vesicle that grows slowly without pain, itching, redness, or tenderness. It starts as a pinhead vesicle and gradually assumes a dome-shaped, tense swelling with umbilication at the vertex. The color varies from creamy white to brown. The number varies from single to multiple; in an immune-competent child, it may be as many as ten to twenty, involving both the lids.

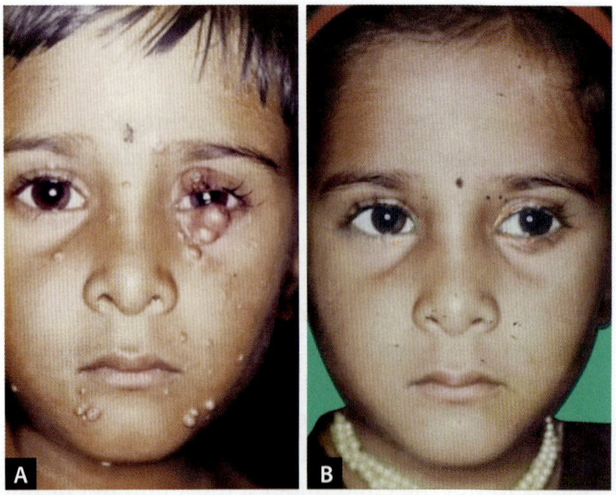

Figs. 9.45A and B: Molluscum of face and lids before and after treatment.
Courtesy: Dr Somen Misra.

In immune-compromised patients, the whole face may be covered with numerous vesicles of different sizes. Unlike herpes zoster, the lesions do cross the midline and are not confined to a particular dermatome. In spite of its long duration, there is no lymphadenopathy. Squeezing a vesicle exudes a cheesy white material. A lesion on the lid margin causes chronic conjunctivitis and keratitis without involving the uvea that is common in herpes zoster ophthalmicus.

Skin lesions heal over months without scarring, pigmentary changes, or loss of sensation; that is another permanent feature of zoster infection.

Diagnosis: Diagnosis is easy due to the peculiar morphology, number, absence of pain, tenderness, and not being confined to one dermatome, crossing the midline.

Differential diagnosis consists of—herpes zoster, vaccinia, and chickenpox milia* in immune-competent children. In immune-compromised cases, it can be mistaken for pyogenic granuloma, warts, and even basal cell carcinoma.

There is no vaccine against the disease, and no antibiotic has been effective against it. No antiviral drug is required for immune-competent children. Immune-compromised children require intravenous Cidofovir; acyclovir is not effective against the virus. Intravenous anti-HIV is mandatory, along with anti-molluscum treatment, when the child has AIDS.

*Milia are infrequent transient cysts consisting of subepidermal keratin of a white milky color in various numbers seen mostly on the face and may be on the lids. It is self-limiting, not requiring any specific treatment.

If there are a few vesicles, the management consists of puncturing the vesicles, expressing the content, and cauterizing the wall of the vesicle with carbolic.

Chronic Bacterial Infection of Skin the Lid

Common chronic infections that involve lids are—tuberculosis, leprosy, and syphilis.

The last two are not seen in children.

Tuberculosis: The incidence of tuberculosis of the lids is higher in developing countries because of the higher incidence of pulmonary tuberculosis in these countries in general and in children in particular. Tuberculosis of the lids are considered to be extrapulmonary; however, some cases can be secondary to pulmonary tuberculosis as well. Tuberculosis of the lids can be localized to the skin or may be an extension of tuberculosis from the lid. The involvement of the lower lid due to its proximity to the ala of the nose is more frequent. The lid can be involved in the following ways:

- Primary (rare)
- Extension from nose
- Hematogenous
- Autoinoculation
- Spread from tarsal plate

Various types of cutaneous tuberculosis of the skin of the lids are:

- Lupus vulgaris
- Scrofuloderma
- Tuberculoma

Lupus vulgaris: Out of all tubercular lesions of the skin, lupus vulgaris is the most common form seen in children. It generally starts in childhood and heals or spills over into adulthood. Untreated cases may last 4–5 years and heal, leading to deformities. It is taken lightly by parents because of slow progress, a self-limited course, and the absence of pain. The lesion starts in the skin as an abrasion, which, if contaminated by tubercular bacilli, gets converted into lupus. The other mode is the extension of the lower lid from the nose. The lesion starts as a pea-sized translucent nodule, which, when pressed against a glass slide, leaves a translucent mark. There may be more than one nodule at a given time that may join to form a larger nodule that ultimately ulcerates with granulation on the floor with a well-marked boundary. The ulcer may be limited to one lid, or all lids may be involved. The ulcer does not remain confined to the skin and may deepen to invade deeper layers up to the conjunctiva. The lesion may extend from canthus to canthus and cause a coloboma, exposing the globe.

Tuberculoma is the least common tubercular involvement of a child's lid and is caused due to a metastasis from a distant primary lesion; it could remain nodular or may ulcerate. The diagnosis should be confirmed by histopathology. The disorder may be confused with—large chalazion, neurofibromatosis, nonspecific ulcer, or even ring worm.

Antitubercular treatment should only be initiated following histopathological confirmation. Treatment should include at least three antitubercular drugs.

DISORDERS OF LID MARGIN

Disorders of the lid can be seen at all ages. They could be congenital or acquired. The common congenital conditions are—ptosis, epicanthus, ankyloblepharon, coloboma, entropion, and distichiasis **(Fig. 9.46)**. The acquired conditions can be infectious or noninfectious. The infectious disorders can be acute stye and infected chalazion. The chronic disorders consist of various types of blepharitis. Beside infection and inflammation, the lid margins can be involved in trauma and new growths. The lid margins in children are not known to develop malignancy.

The lid margin shares the epithelium of both the skin and conjunctiva. The intermarginal strip is in fact a transient zone between the two; this makes them prone to get infections of from both. The situation is worsened by the presence of lashes in front and the tarsal opening a little behind. The lashes grow in three to four rows along the rounded border; the glands of Zeis and Moll also open in this region; and the meibomian ducts open away from the lashes near the sharp edge of the lid **(Fig. 9.47)**. All these factors make the lid margin an ideal location for microbes to grow and thrive.

The infection of the lid margin is divided into two groups:

1. Infection round the base of the lashes
2. Infection of the glands of Zeis and Moll
3. A combination of the two is not uncommon.

Infection round the base of lashes are: Stye and blepharitis

> Chalazion is not an infectious condition of the base of the lashes; they are chronic granulomas of the meibomian glands.

Stye

Styes are the most common painful conditions of the lid margin in children. 20% of children suffer from styes

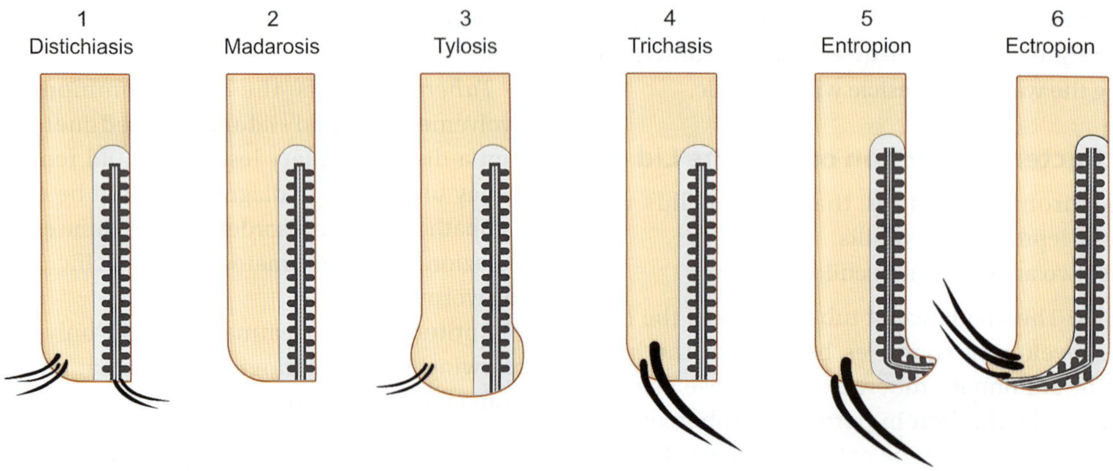

Fig. 9.46: Various pathological conditions of the lid margin seen in all ages. Conditions shown in diagrams 4, 5, and 6 are not seen in children.

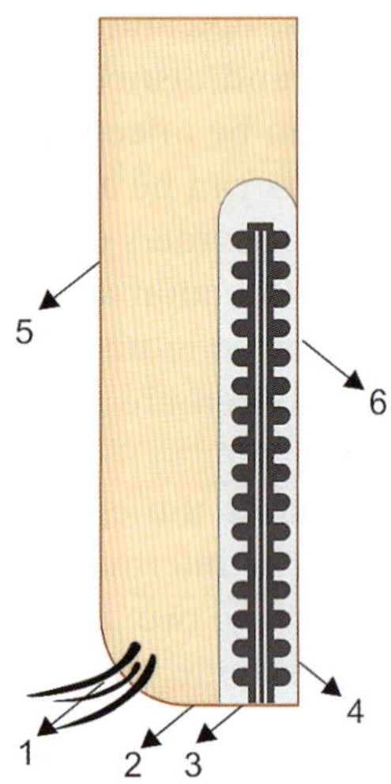

Fig. 9.47: Various parts of normal lid. (1: Lashes; 2: Intermarginal strip; 3: Meibomian opening; 4: Meibomian gland; 5: Skin; 6: Conjunctiva)

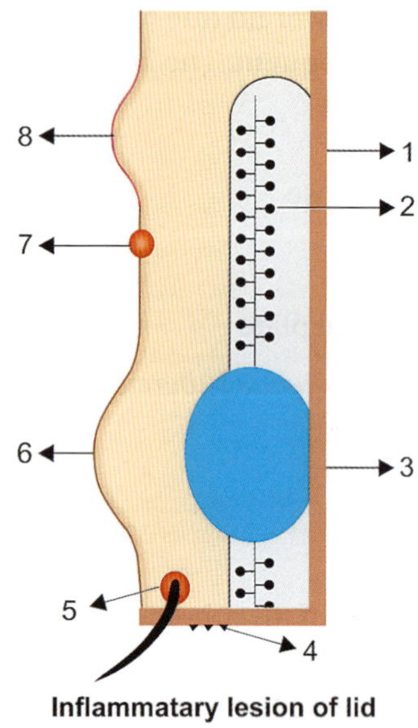

Fig. 9.48: Various types of acute and chronic inflammatory conditions of the lid margin. (1: Tarsal conjunctiva; 2: Tarsal gland; 3: Calazion; 4: Blapharitis; 5: Stye; 6: Bulge in the skin over calazion; 7: Boil; 8: Lid abses)

sometimes or other under 15 years; they are most frequent between 5 and 15, equally common in boys and girls all over the world. Styes after 15 become less common. Styes being infectious do not have a definite genetic background; however, positive family history is common among parents or siblings **(Fig. 9.48)**.

Pathologically, a stye is an acute recurrent staphylococcal infection of the glands of Zeis and Moll without involving meibomian glands or ducts; allergy has no part to play.

Best way to locate the position of a stye in the lid is to move the index finger of the examiner along the lid margin. As soon as the fingertip crosses the stye, the child whines. The number of styes may vary from single to many at the same time; a single stye may resolve spontaneously or may enlarge to cause cellulites; multiple styes do not resolve; they are more painful and cause more cellulites; six to seven recurrences are common; it is not uncommon to get all the lids involved; styes are more common in the upper lids due to the presence of more lashes and their glands. Styes in the canthi are more painful than in the middle of the lid. Styes of the outer canthus are more frequent than inner canthus; the styes of the outer canthus are most painful. Styes are more common following measles. It is not unusual for stye and chalazion in the same lid. Styes of various grades and locations are shown in **Figures 9.49A to I**.

Acute conjunctivitis is very common with stye, so is preauricular lymphadenopathy. Predisposing factors in the production of styes are—positive family history, uncorrected errors of refraction, muscle imbalance, malnutrition, an unhygienic environment, and a recent attack of measles.

Management

Repeated attacks of stye in various combinations make management frustrating; moreover, a single stye may occasionally not reoccur even without treatment.

The most practiced regimen of treatment consists of:

- Dry hot fomentation three to four times a day till the stye subsides.
- Mild oral analgesic

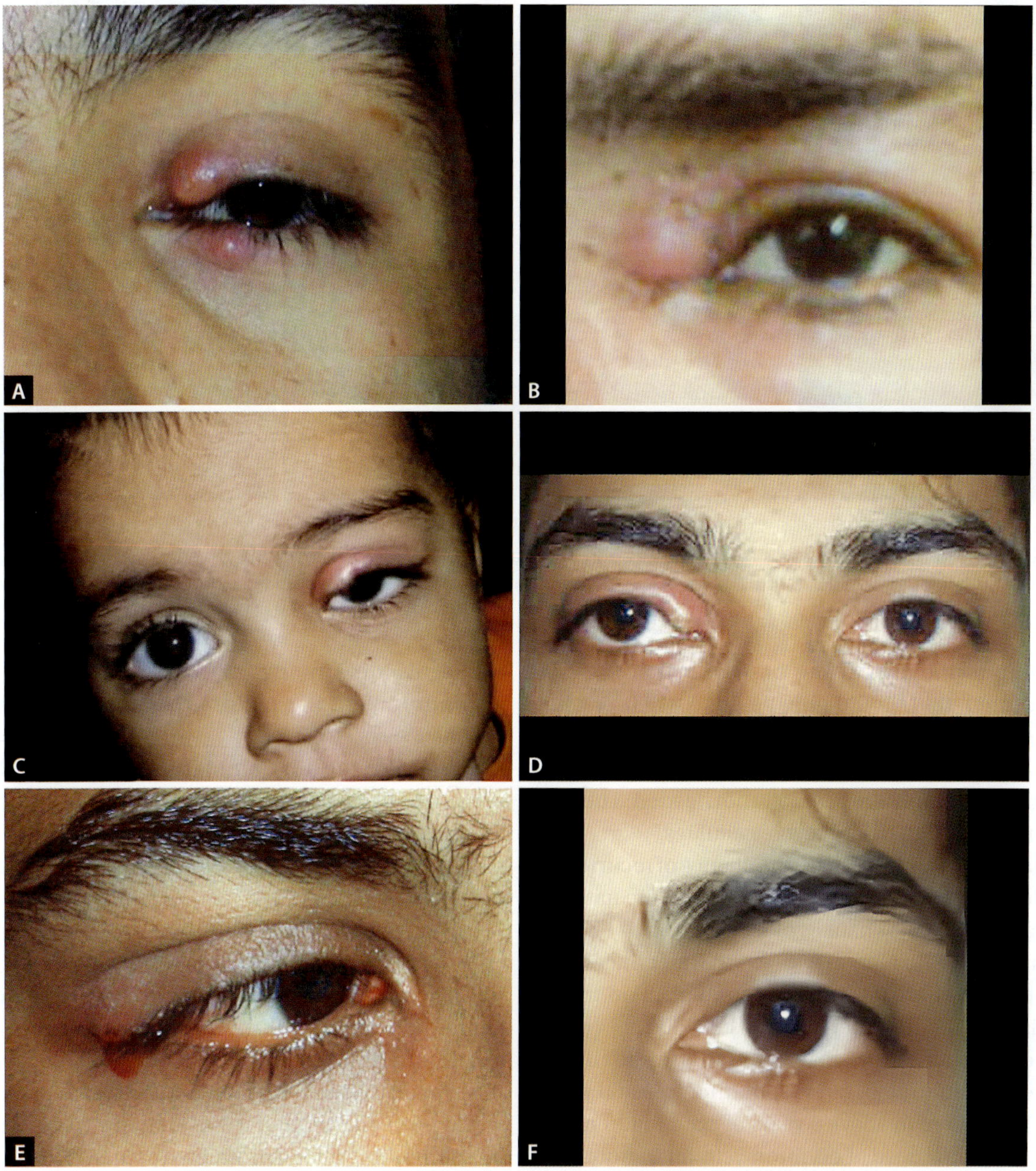

Figs. 9.49A to F

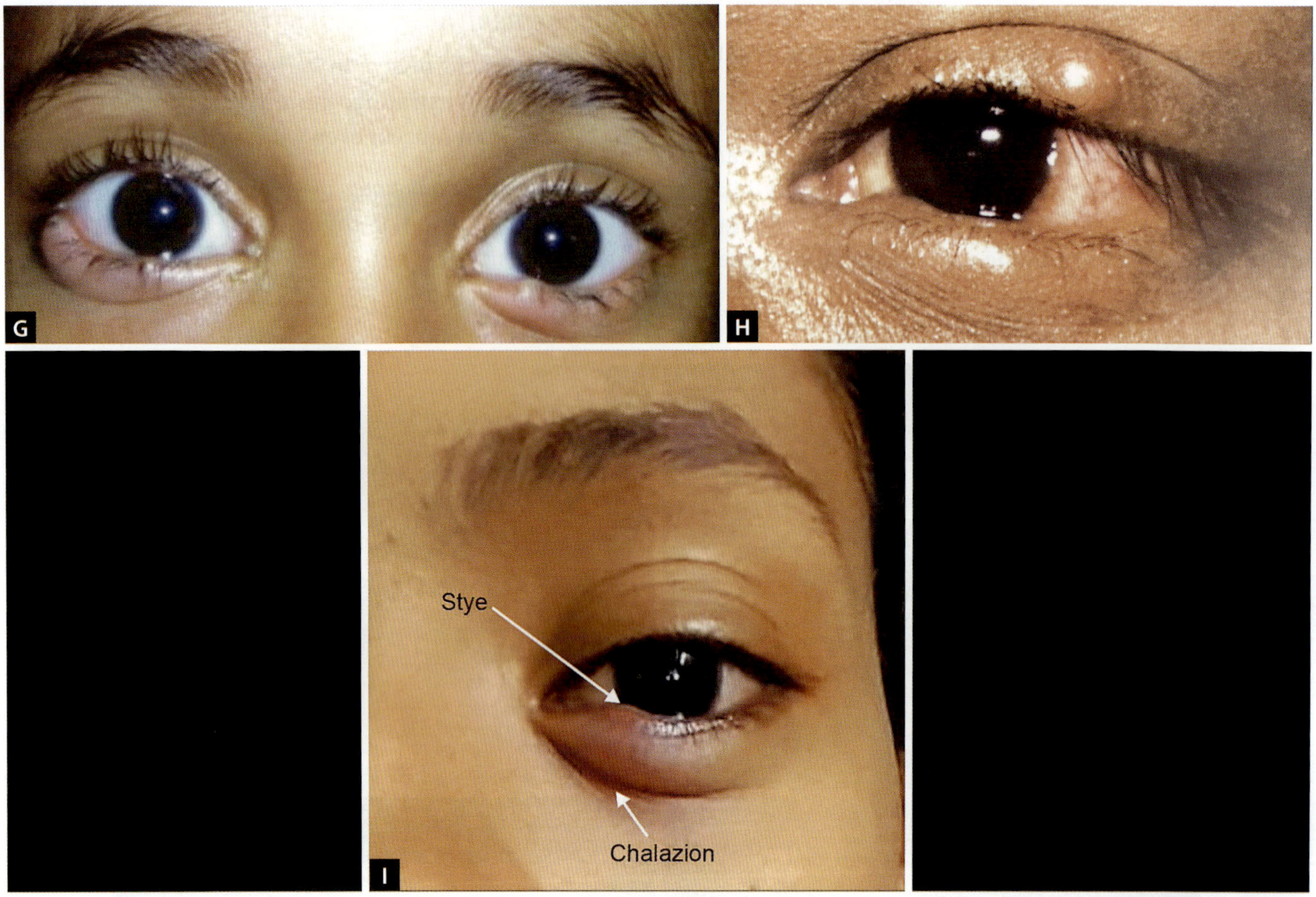

Figs. 9.49G to I

Fig. 9.49A to I: (A to D) Unilateral styes at various location and stages; (E) Stye at outer canthus bleeding; (F) Healed stye lower lid; (G) Bilateral simultaneous styes; (H) Multiple styes in the lower lid and a chalazion in the upper lid; (I) Persistent chalazion and recurrent stye in the same lid.

- Epilating of the lash at the base of which the stye has erupted, this should only be done when pus has formed at the base of the offending lash.
- Local broad-spectrum antibiotics drop frequently.
- Systemic antibiotics are generally not needed. They are indicated only if there are severe cellulites.
- Regular face washing reduces the chance of recurrence, and deworming and immunization under the national program reduce the chances of recurrence.
- Cleaning of the lid margin with warm water once a day and rubbing of broad-spectrum antibiotics on the lid margin for 3 months after stye has subsided.
- Oral doxycycline at a dose of 50–100 mg daily for 2 weeks in children is not responding to usual treatment in children in above 8 years of age. Children may be put on a low dose of erythromycin for 2 months in consultation with pediatrician
- Regular deworming
- Immunizing the children against measles reduces chances of stye.

Logically, any inflammation of the lid should be considered blepharitis; however, in clinical practice, only inflammation of the lid margin is called so, encompassing structures between the rounded anterior edge and sharp posterior border.

Blepharitis

It is a common, chronic, mild, and nonpainful condition of the lid margin. All the lid margins can be involved single/simultaneously or in different combinations. It is equally common among boys and girls in all races the world over, and though it is a long drawn disorder, it can be self-limiting after a protracted course.

Anatomically, it is divided into two types, i.e.:

1. Involving structures between lashes and the opening of meibomian glands
2. Involving structures from the meibomian opening to the posterior lid margin

The second classification is based on appearance:

- Nonulcerative
- Ulcerative

Recent classification divides blepharitis in following types **(Table 9.4)**.

Another classification:

- Anterior that encompasses 1, 2, 3, and 5 of the above classification.
- Posterior includes 4 and 5 of the above classifications.

Children mostly suffer from anterior blepharitis. In children, blepharitis is better discussed in traditional divisions into squamous and ulcerative blepharitis.

Squamous Blepharitis

This is the milder of the two and is taken as a synonym for seborrheic blepharitis. It is so in conspicuous that parents take it as physiological. It is more common after 10 years in both sexes and is generally associated with seborrhea of the eyebrows, nasolabial folds, and scalp **(Fig. 9.50)**.

It is presumed to be a malfunction of the Zeis gland. The scales are situated at the base of the lashes and can be brushed off with ease without any ulcers or bleeding points. It causes chronic conjunctivitis and punctuate keratitis. Recurrent styes are a common occurrence.

TABLE 9.4: Recent classification of blepharitis.

Type	*Clinical features*
1. *Staphylococcus*	Most common form, more in females, acute inflammation of short duration present with dry scales and crusts
2. Seborrheic	Few glands are effected, oily scales++
3. Combined 1 + 2	More oily scales, increased meibomian secretion
4. Meibomianitis	Inflammation superimposed on seborrheic blepharitis, enhanced meibomian secretion
5. Primary meibomianitis	Associated with chronic skin disorder like rosacea
(The above classification is more useful in adults than children)	

Ulcerative Blepharitis

Ulcerative blepharitis is more visible and symptomatic than the nonulcerative variety. It is more difficult to manage. It has more complications. It too involves all the lids, with the upper lid being involved more frequently. It can be unilateral or bilateral; when unilateral, the other eye too gets involved later **(Figs. 9.51 and 9.52)**.

Once the disorder sets in, it lingers for many years and passes off automatically, with or without complications. The course is shortened by treatment. Recurrences are common. It may start as early as 3 years of age, but is more common in older children and adolescence. The exact cause is not well established. The most frequently blamed factors are staphylococcal allergy and its toxin.

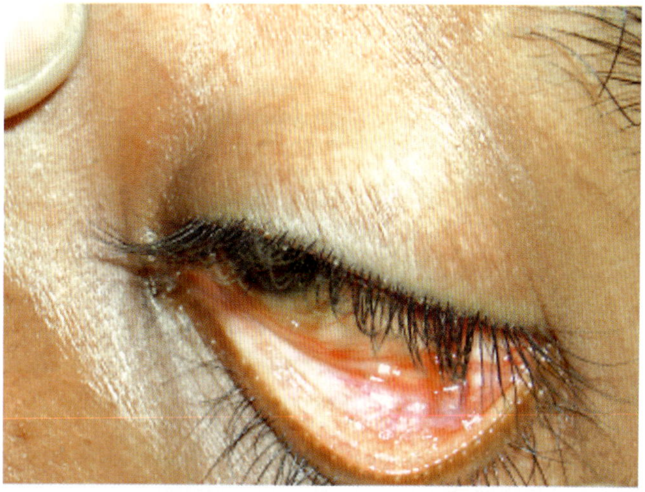

Fig. 9.50: Squamous blepharitis.

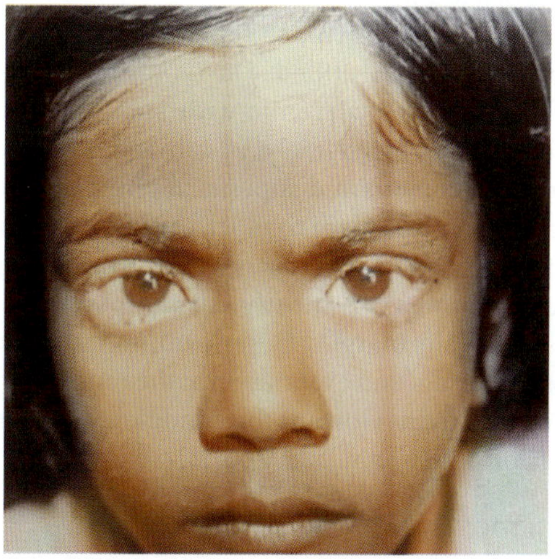

Fig. 9.51: Bilateral ulcerative blepharitis.
Courtesy: Dr Somen Misra.

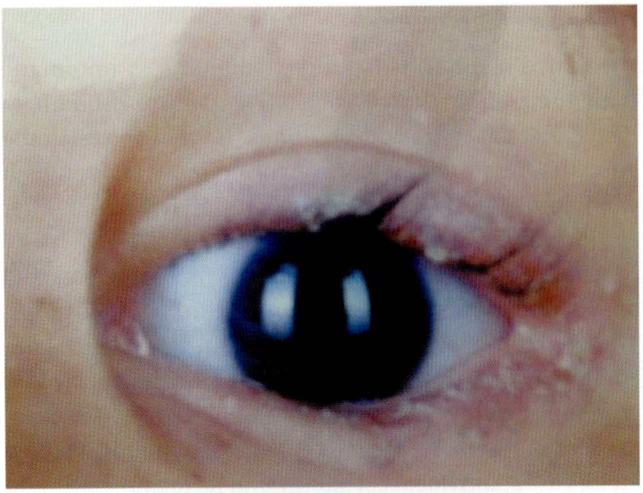

Fig. 9.52: Unilateral ulcerative blepharitis.

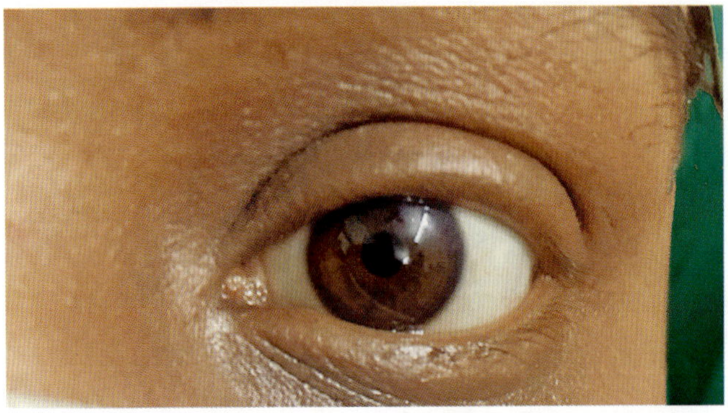

Fig. 9.53: Madarosis following ulcerative blepharitis.

The clinical findings consist of—yellow crusts at the bases of lashes; hyperemia of the lid margin; on the long run, there may be madarosis **(Fig. 9.53)**; tylosis; and trichiasis of a few lashes.

The crusts are difficult to remove unless moistened in warm water or scrubbed. On removal of crusts, the underlying skin is hyperemic with small hemorrhagic points that do not bleed freely. It is always associated with chronic conjunctivitis and superficial punctuate keratitis. Older children often learn to pluck the lashes and rub the lid margin to get rid of the scales worsening the condition.

The symptoms are mostly cosmetic due to visible crusts on the lid margin. Other symptoms are chronic redness, watering, and excoriation at the outer canthi. The presence of keratitis worsens the condition. The condition is nonvision-threatening.

Management

Management of all blepharitis are difficult, prolonged, and without immediate relief. This is applicable to all ages; there is no single regime to suits every case. Each individual requires a different protocol. Thus, treatment of squamous differs from ulcerative.

- *Treatment* of squamous blepharitis is basically management of seborrhea; it consists of control of dandruff of the scalp and eyebrows, cleaning of the hands and face, and application of broad-spectrum antibiotic ointment on the lid margin at least for a month.
- *Treatment* of ulcerative is more elaborate; it consists of:
  - *Removal of crusts:* The lid margin is moistened with warm water for a few minutes, and the crusts are scraped mechanically at least twice a day.
  - Application of broad-spectrum antibiotics to the lid margin. Erythromycin and bacitracin are claimed to be better than other antibiotics.
  - Children who do not respond are put on oral antibiotics for 7–10 days in consultation with pediatrician. The common antibiotics used as ointments or oral tablets are erythromycin and doxycycline. Children under 8 years old are not administered doxycycline.
  - Children should be made aware of the cleanliness of their hands and faces.
  - All children should undergo refraction under cycloplegia and be dealt with accordingly.
  - Parents should be counseled about the nonblinding nature of the disease and its prolonged treatment.
  - Steroids are required only locally in recalcitrant cases.

Parasitic Blepharitis

Two types of parasites, i.e., lice and mites, cause blepharitis. Lice infestation is more common than mite infestation. The terms pediculosis and phthiriasis are often used as interchangeable terms. Three types of lice—*Pediculosis corporis, P. capitis*, and *P. pubes*—cause blepharitis. The last, i.e., *P. pubes* (crab lice), is the most common cause.

The child gets an infection of *P. capitis* from playmates; the other two are acquired from parents or other caregivers.

The exact duration from infestation to manifestation is not known. The symptoms depend on the lice population on the lids and the duration of their presence. The lice cling to the base of the lash and the skin in between, the number varying between a few to many of different ages. When numerous and fully mature, the parasites are visible on daylight without magnification on the lashes and the lid margin **(Fig. 9.54)**.

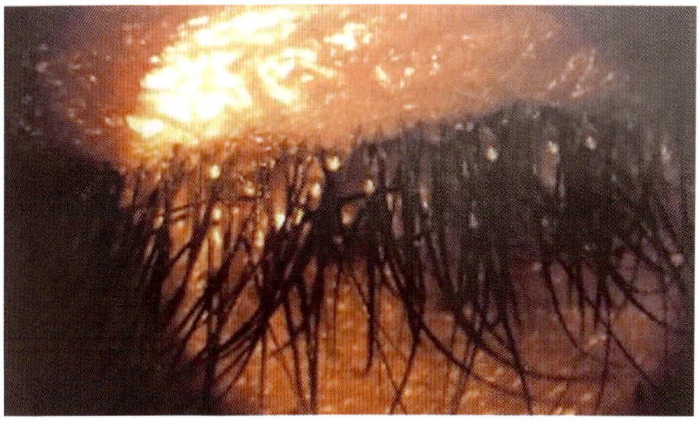

Fig. 9.54: Lice on the lid margin.
Courtesy: Dr SC Batalia.

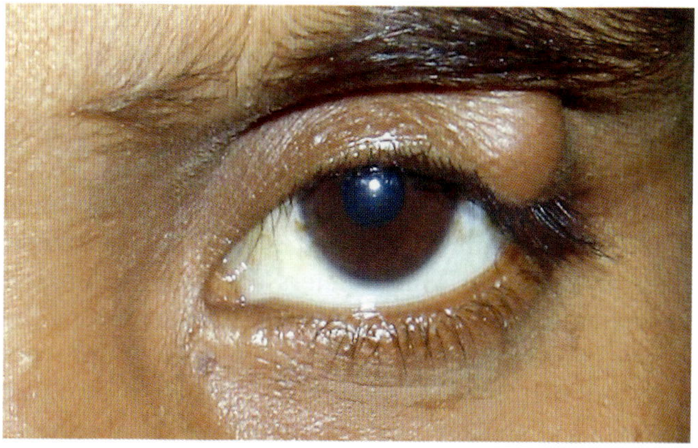

Fig. 9.55: Noninfected chalazion.

The symptoms are—visible parasites on the lashes and the lid margin; itching; redness of the lid margin; and chronic blepharoconjunctivitis.

Management:
- Treatment should be directed to all possible contacts.
- In cooperative children, the lice can be picked up with epilation forceps.
- Application of diluted pediculicide on the lid margin three times a day for about a week. The commonly used pediculicides are benzene hexachloride (1%) and permethrin (1%). Fluorescein sodium (20%) applied two times gives a good result.
- *Ivermectin:* The role of this multipurpose drug in pediculosis is not well established; the recommended dose is 200 μg/kg of weight in two doses at a 7-day interval. It should not be given to children under 15 kg.

Chalazion

The chalazia are not true disorders of the lid margin; they are disorders of the tarsal glands that open on the lid margin. In contrast to styes, they are not acute staphylococcal infections either; they are granulomatous changes in meibomian glands. The chalazia are slow-growing, painless, firm, nontender, spherical subcutaneous preconjunctival nodules fixed to the conjunctiva that give a blue tinge when the lid is everted, and the skin can be moved on the nodule **(Fig. 9.55)**.

All the above features are changed if the chalazion gets infected; the most common organism to infect is staphylococcus, which makes it painful and tender.

The chalazia are universal, equally common in boys and girls; all lids are liable to be effected, they are more frequent, numerous, and large in the upper lids due to the more and larger meibomian glands in the upper lids; the number of chalazion may vary from single to many **(Fig. 9.56)**.

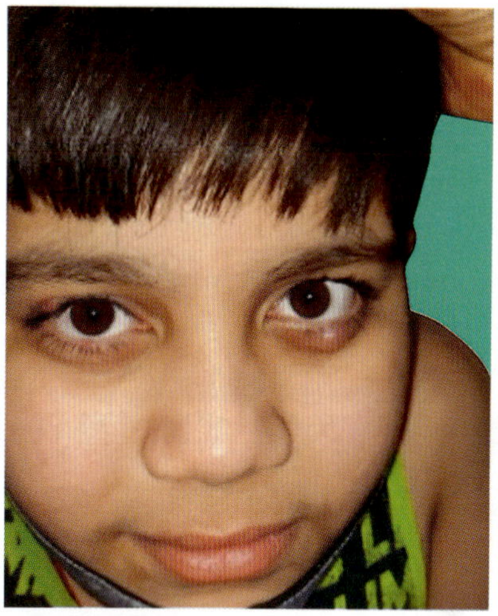

Fig. 9.56: Chalazion of all the lids of various stages.

Recurrences are common, but there may be chalazion that resolves spontaneously not to recur; chalazia does not develop in the same location a second time.

Chalazia are not genetic; however, positive family history is common among parents and siblings. The common age group that develops chalazion is 5–20; chalazion have been seen in children <5 years as well. Persons above 20 are not immune to them; 50% of people over 50 years of age with chalazion are likely to be diabetic.

> Persons in the same age group with repeated chalazia carry the risk of developing malignancy of the tarsal gland. Chalazion in children has no chance of malignancy of the tarsal gland.

An infected chalazion is called hordeolum internum or suppurative chalazion; these are more tender and painful than stye; an infected chalazion situated near the lid margin may masquerade as a large stye **(Fig. 9.57)**.

Chalazion has a different look on skin and conjunctival surfaces. The appearance differs from location to location and number **(Figs. 9.58 to 9.60)**.

On the skin surface, it is a smooth, spherical nodule not fixed to the skin but adherent to the tarsal plate. Their size varies from two millimeters to a centimeter, and there are no cellulites round a chalazion. On everting the lid, the conjunctiva over the chalazion is flat, translucent with a bluish tinge, and there is no tissue protruding unless the chalazion bursts on the conjunctival surface. The protruded mass is sessile, joined to the underlying chalazion; it is compressed between the globe and lid, which makes it flat. Burst chalazion of the lower lid has a different look; though it remains sessile, it is not flat but rounded. In contrast to a burst chalazion of the upper lid, which is flat with an irregular margin mimicking capillary hemangioma or rhinosporidiosis **(Figs. 9.61 and 9.62)**.

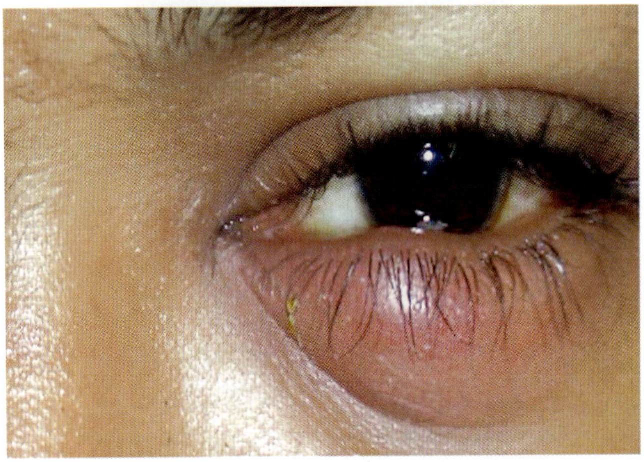

Fig. 9.57: Infected chalazion.

Pathology of Chalazion

Chronic, low-virulent organisms creep into the meibomian duct from the lid margin, inducing low-grade inflammation with swelling of the epithelium of the duct, narrowing, and then obstructing the duct. This leads to a stasis of secretion above the block. The meibomian secretion, being rich in lipids, acts as a foreign body, irritating the gland. The irritant stimulates the formation of foreign body granuloma, similar to tubercular granuloma without cassation. There is no capsule round the granuloma.

Probable changes in a fully formed chalazion are:
- Chalazion grows slowly.
- Becomes stationary
- Regresses slowly, or the material in the nodule liquefies to convert the chalazion in a tarsal cyst **(Figs. 9.63 and 9.64)**.
- Bursts on the conjunctival surface
- Protrusion of the granuloma through the tarsal opening (rare)
- Ruptures through the skin (rare)
- A nonresolving chalazion may get infected and converted into hordeolum internum, which is very painful and requires systemic antibiotics and analgesics.

The first two are common in children; the others take months to years to happen.

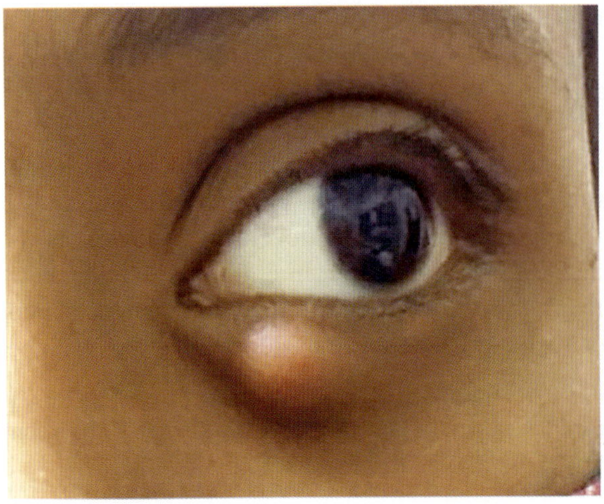

Fig. 9.58: Chalazion as seen from skin surface.
Courtesy: Dr Gunjan Saluja Bhatia.

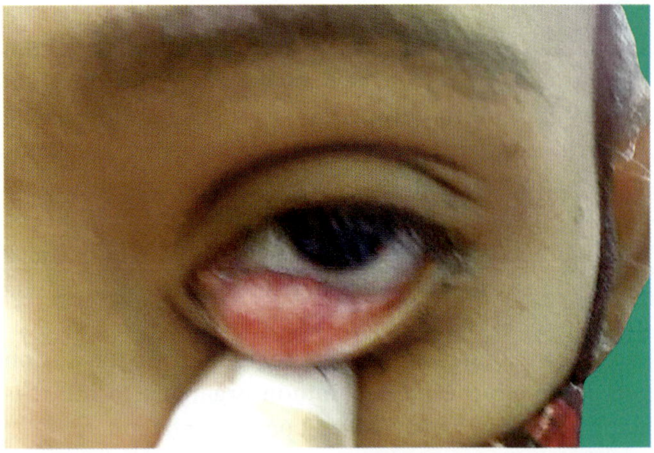

Fig. 9.59: Large chalazion of lower lid as seen from conjunctival surface.
Courtesy: Dr Gunjan Saluja Bhatia.

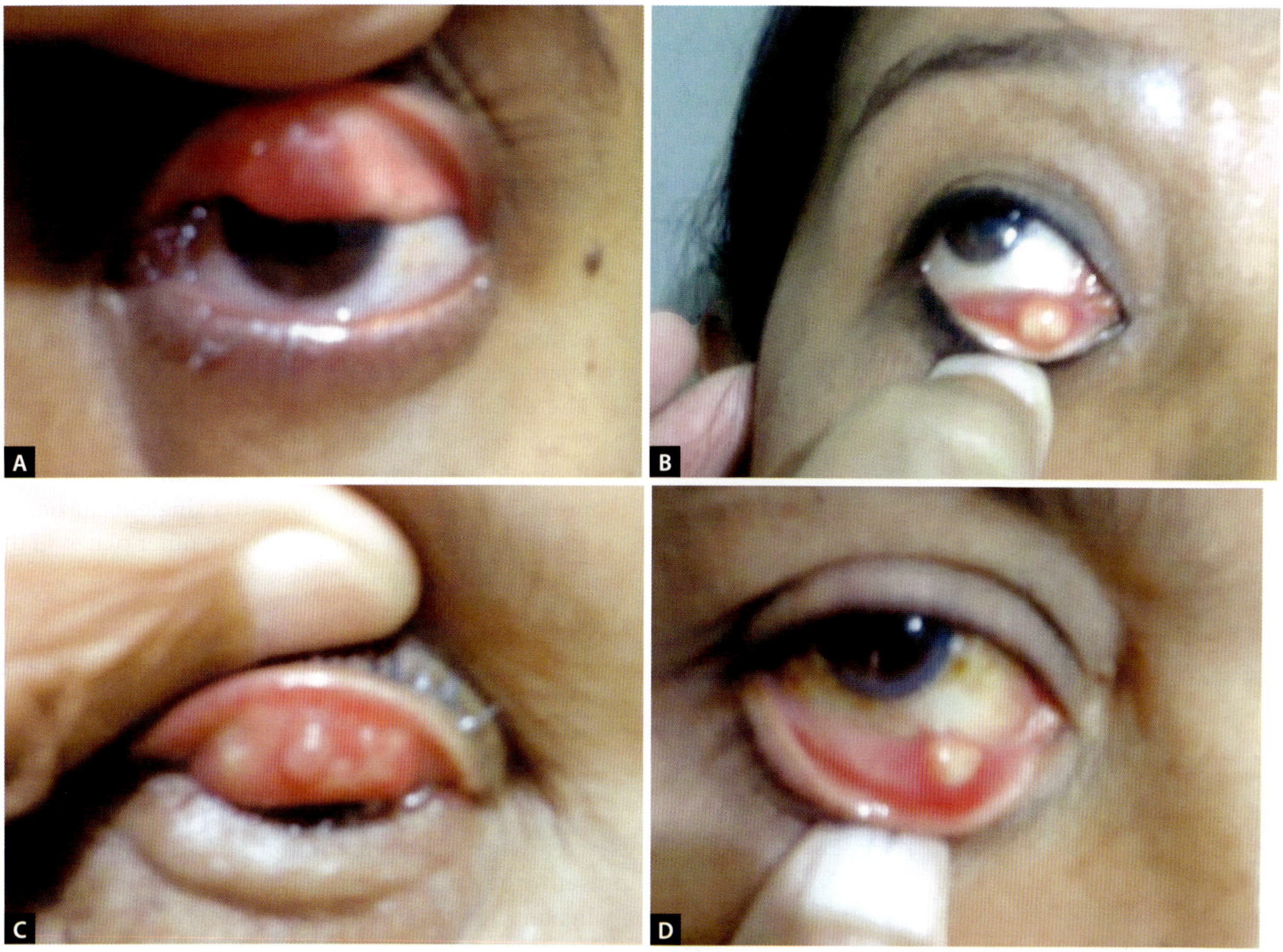

Figs. 9.60A to D: Photograph showing various types of chalazia seen from the conjunctival surface.

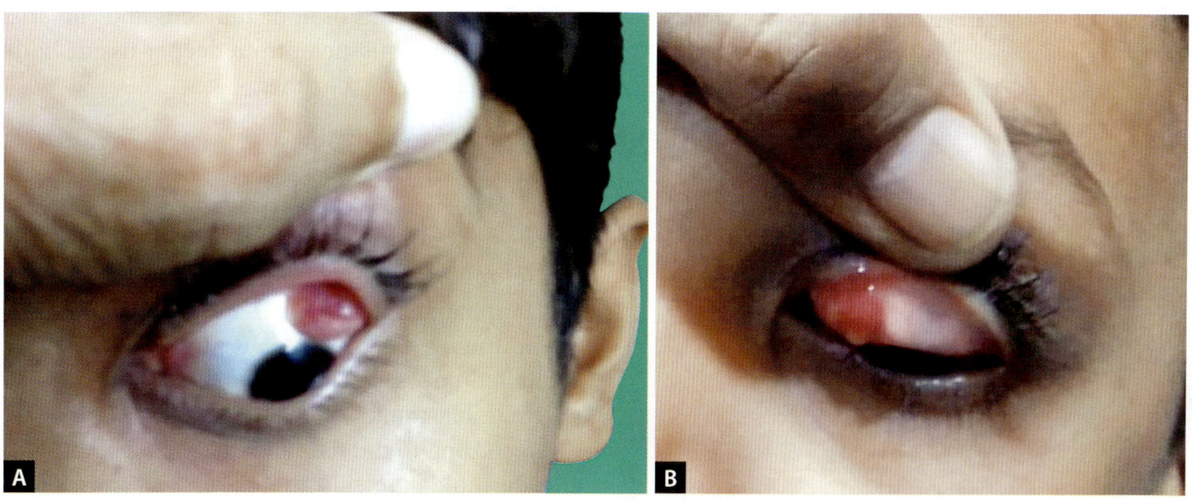

Figs. 9.61A and B: Burst chalazion upper lid.

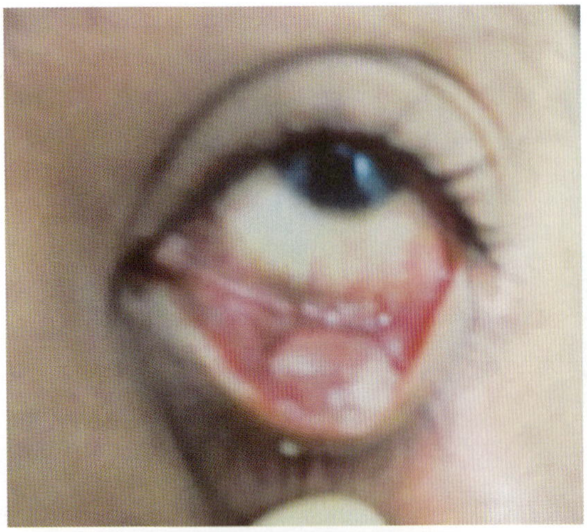

Fig. 9.62: Burst chalazion lower lid.

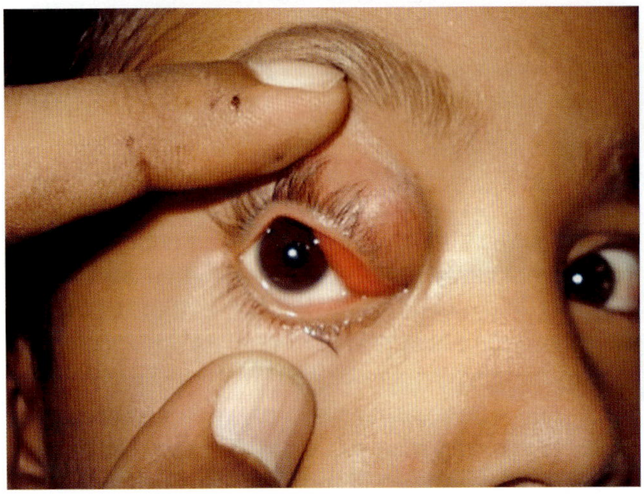

Figs. 9.63: Large tarsal cyst developing in chalazion.

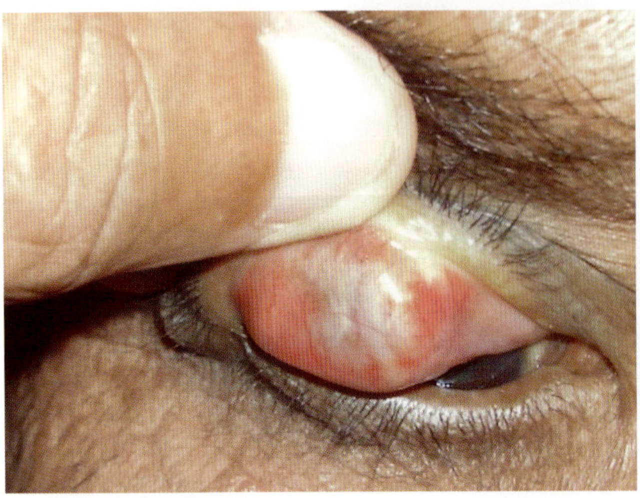

Figs. 9.64: Tarsal cyst seen from conjunctival surface.

Management of Chalazion

- There is no medical treatment for chalazia, and antibiotics have no role in the management of chalazia unless they are infected.
- Small stationary chalazia do not need any treatment.
- Chalazia larger than 3 mm require treatment by way of dry hot fomentation for 5 minutes morning and evening for 5–7 days; this is claimed to liquefy the granuloma that facilitates its absorption.
- Chalazia larger than 4–5 mm requires definitive treatment.
- The definitive treatment is incision, curettage, and carbolization of the interior of the curettage wall.
- It should be impressed up on the caregivers that the procedure was directed toward a single chalazion; it will in no way prevent chalazion at other places in the same lid in the future.

Other procedures available are:

- Intralesional injection of triamcinolone acetonide every fortnight for three times.
- High-frequency laser.

TUMORS OF LID IN CHILDREN

New growths of lids in children are infrequent; when present, they are mostly congenital and benign; rare malignant growths are either extensions from neighboring structures, i.e., orbits, or still rarely secondary. Some of the growths that look like they were acquired are in fact congenital with late presentation. Topographically, they are either cutaneous or noncutaneous and can arise from either superficial tissue or from deeper tissue, both being capable of invading the other.

The common growths are:

- Nevi
- Strawberry nevi (capillary hemangioma)
- Nevus flammeus (port-wine stain)
- Neurofibromatosis
- Lymphangiomas
- Dermoid
- Rhabdomyosarcoma
- Neuroblastoma

According to the tissue involved, nevi, neurofibroma, and dermoids are skin tumors arising from the dermis or epidermis. Hemangiomas, lymphangiomas, and nevus flammeus are vascular; dermoids are choristomas. Neurofibromas and hemangiomas are hamartomas.

Nevi are common, benign congenital tumors of infancy and childhood that may be obvious at birth or become apparent later. They may be flush with skin or slightly raised and pigmented; the color has a tendency to darken at puberty. They do not change much in size and do not develop malignancies. The lid margin is the most common site for their development; it may involve both lids simultaneously. Generally, no treatment is required unless it is too large; in such a situation, surgical excision is the treatment of choice.

Capillary Hemangiomas (Strawberry Nevi)

Capillary hemangiomas are benign, mostly transient, unilateral congenital tumors seen in children; they are nonheritable tumors, situated in the preseptal area; growths are noncapsulated rarely; they do not invade orbit like its counterparts, the cavernous hemangiomas, which have a preponderance for orbit and are capsulated; cavernous hemangiomas are seen in adults only, without skin involvement.

Capillary hemangiomas are pretty common at birth as a red cutaneous blotch that turns brighter and may increase in size when the child strains. The other mode makes the tumor visible only by 3 months. The growths vary in shape and size, ranging from a small strawberry stain to a tumor a few inches in diameter. The tumor has a fixed cycle of growth and regression. The mass increases in size for the first 6 months, then stabilizes up to 2 years and regresses gradually; the regression is completed by 7 years. Though the tumor does not generally grow backwards, it may grow in both lids, giving them a bluish tinge similar to the ecchymosis of lids. Involvement of the upper lid produces pseudoptosis with a typical S-shaped curve. The pseudoptotic lid induces amblyopia in two ways, i.e., by covering the pupil and causing irregular astigmatism due to the irregular pressure exerted by the thick and heavy lid. The tumor is composed of blood vessels, blood-filled channels, and their proliferating endothelia. The condition rarely invades orbit. In such a situation, proptosis develops.

Small, self-limiting lesions do not require any treatment. Nonregressing tumors are best treated by β-blockers; that is the first line of treatment. β-blockers are administered orally or as topical drops. The latter is less effective; the most common β-blocker used orally is propranolol. The role of β-blockers is not well understood. In most of the children, β-blockers reduce the chances of an increase in growth, for which the most accepted theory is that β-blockers and adrenergic receptors, like propranolol, cause narrowing of the vessels, thus reducing blood supply. The locally used β-blocker is timolol maleate 0.5%, rubbed over the growth three times a day. It takes about a fortnight to show the effect. Oral β-blockers in children should be used with caution in consultation with a pediatrician.

Nevus Flammeus (Port-wine Stain)

These are congenital benign vascular tumors spread over the distribution of the trigeminal nerve, as a flat, dark pink discoloration that does neither blench on pressure nor disappear over time.

Two percent of children develop Sturge–Weber syndrome that includes glaucoma in one-third of cases. It must be differentiated from capillary hemangioma.

Neurofibromatosis

See **Figures 9.39A to D**.

Lymphangiomas

These are rarer congenital nonmalignant growth not always confined to lid, they may develop in conjunctiva as well. Histopathologically they are endothelium lined vascular channels. They manifest generally by 4–5 years of age as bluish noncompressible growth that does not show spontaneous regression. They are liable to bleed on minor trauma resulting in subconjunctival hemorrhage, ecchymosis, pseudoptosis, and proptosis. They are difficult to remove surgically. CO_2 laser is better option.

Dermoids

Dermoids are congenital, slow-progressing choristomas. They are not true growths of lids; the common site for a dermoid to develop is junction of orbital bones **(Figs. 9.65A to D)**; the most common location is superior-lateral orbital rim, followed by the superior nasal orbital rim. The growth presents as a round, subcutaneous, firm, nontender mass attached to the periosteum. The growth may show a spurt in size in puberty, but they do not develop malignant changes. The dermoids are innocuous; they cause only cosmetic blemishes, for which surgical removal is the best option. Steroids have no role; β-blockers have been tried without uniform results.

Rhabdomyosarcoma

Rhabdomyosarcomas are more often found in orbit rather than in lids. They arise from striated muscles;

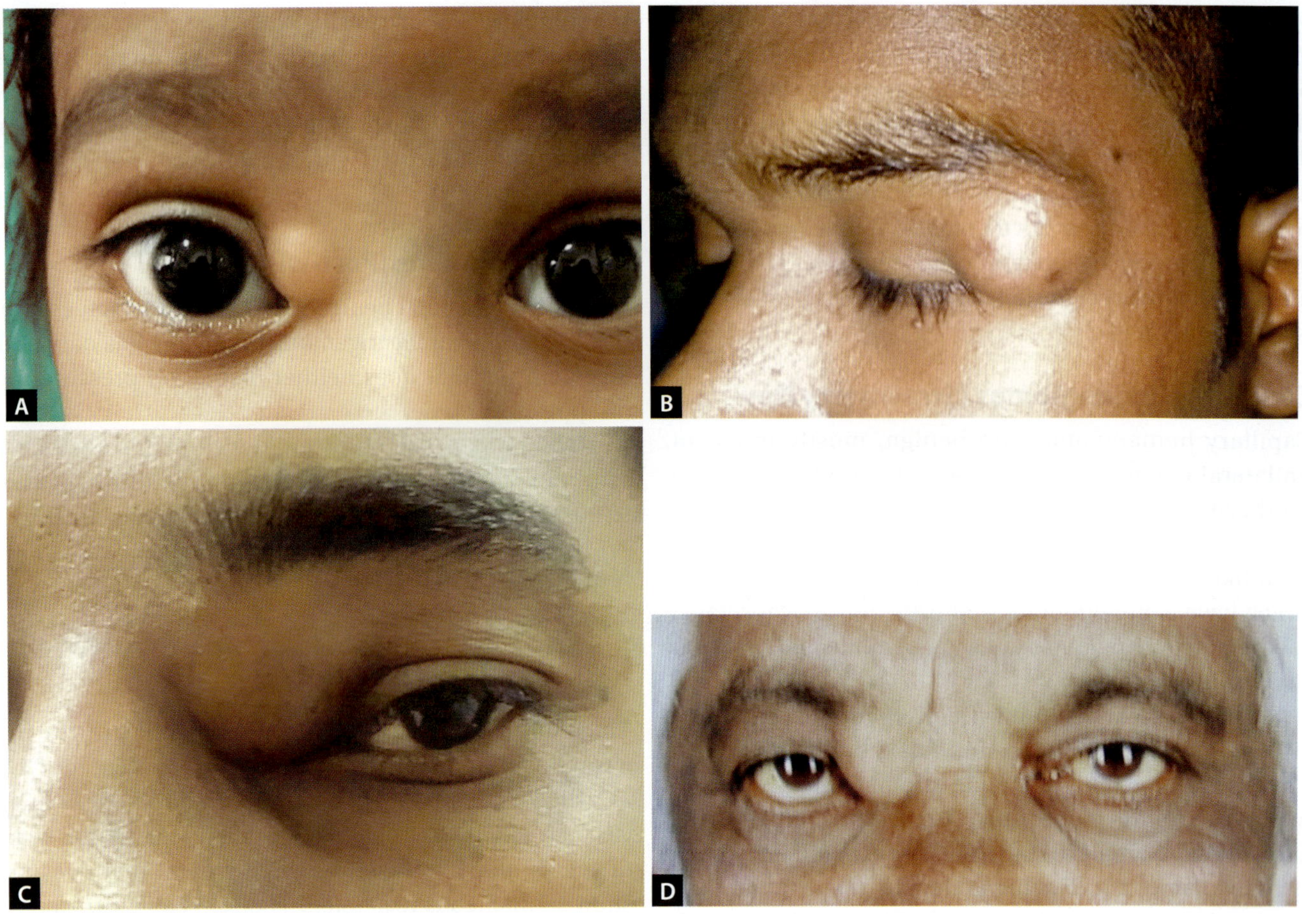

Figs. 9.65A to D: (A) Dermoid in a child; (B to D) Dermoid in adults, first noticed in childhood.

hence, lids are not exempted. They are rare in the first year of life. They are highly malignant but amenable to chemotherapy, and they are radiosensitive.

Neuroblastoma

Neuroblastomas are metastatic tumors of the lid; they are fatal tumors arising from the sympathetic chain. Fast growing lid tumors with ecchymosis should be suspected to be neuroblastoma, unless proved otherwise.

Neurofibromas

Neurofibromas are congenital hamartomas that are generally diagnosed in the second year or later; isolated involvement of the lid is less frequent. Neurofibroma can be localized, diffuse, or plexiform. The first is more common; plexiform neurofibromas are the largest and most extensive. The lid is mostly plexiform in nature, which makes it cosmetically unacceptable. Pathologically, the neurofibroma have been put into two types, i.e., Type 1 (NF-1) and Type 2 (NF-2). The shape and size vary from a small nodule to a mass large enough to cover the pupil, resulting in amblyopia. There is no treatment except for partial surgical removal.

XERODERMA PIGMENTOSA

This is an autosomal recessive malignant condition with a precancerous phase of childhood and young persons of both sexes. Persons inflicted do not survive beyond the third decade. It has been reported as early as 1 year; generally, siblings are also inflicted **(Fig. 9.66)**.

The disorder equally involves tissues of both ectodermal and mesodermal origin; all parts of the body exposed to natural ultraviolet rays are genetically predisposed. Prolonged exposure to artificial ultraviolet lights, too, has been occasionally blamed. The disease mostly involves the skin and central nervous system, along with the eyes and their adnexa. The cause of the disorder is the failure of the nucleotide to salvage DNA damaged

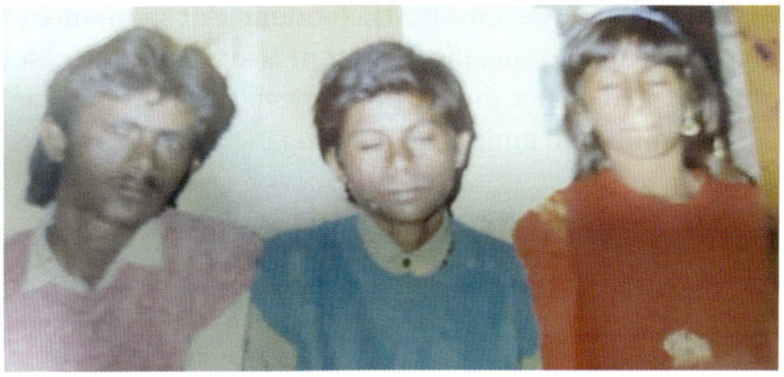

Fig. 9.66: Sibling with xeroderma pigmentosa.
Courtesy: Dr SC Batalia.

by ultraviolet rays. The disorder has three overlapping components **(Figs. 9.67A and B)**.

1. Cutaneous
2. Ocular
3. Central nervous system

The cutaneous changes being the most widely spread and earliest to develop, first to draw attention, the first being intolerance to sunlight. This is followed by diffuse red patches on the exposed boy parts, maculae, bullae, telangiectasia, and nodules. The skin is atrophic. The nodules may be mistaken as melanomas. The child is likely to develop other malignancies like epithelioma, epidermoid carcinoma, basal cell carcinoma, and true melanoma. The new growths are multicentric; on long run, they may metastasize to other parts of the body to cause death. Benign growths are not uncommon.

80% of children with the disease have ocular involvement; all the parts of the eye exposed to sun rays, i.e., the lids, conjunctiva, and cornea, are affected in various combinations. The skin of the lid is first to be involved; the lid involvements are—atrophy of the skin, freckles, telangiectasia, and malignant and nonmalignant tumors.

The conjunctival changes are seen on the exposed part; they include chronic hyperemia, ocular surface disorder, xerosis, bilateral pterygium, and neoplastic and non-neoplastic growths. Occasionally, there is ulceration that may end in symblepharon.

Corneal changes are initially seen on the exposed part, hence more marked in the lower part. The corneal involvement leads to lacrimation, photophobia, and blepharospasm. The exposed parts of the cornea get vascularized.

Management is difficult; there is no specific treatment. All that is available is palliative, directed toward minimizing troublesome symptoms; they include frequent use of lubricants to keep corneas moist and soft-colored contact lenses to provide much-needed respite from glare and photophobia. The patients are provided with large, anti-ultraviolet-colored glasses large enough to cover the lids and sides of the eyes. When outdoors, the children should wear full-sleeved shirts, trousers, socks, gloves, and wide-rimmed hats. Anti-UV lotions and creams are recommended to cut the effects of UV rays.

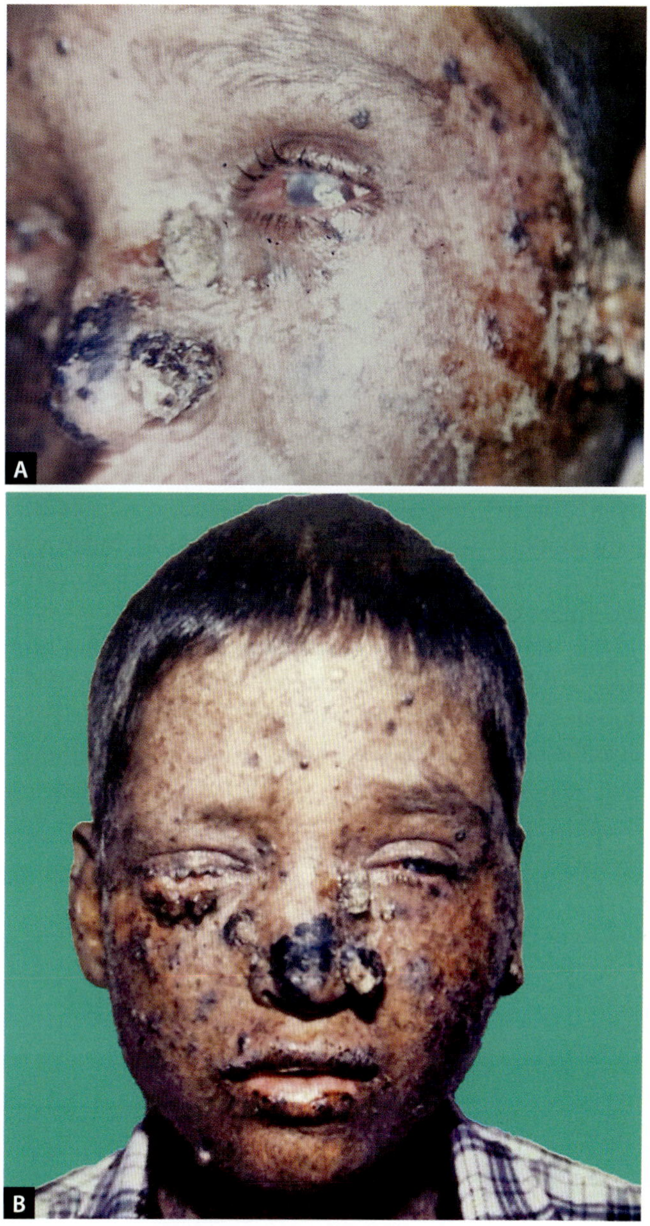

Figs. 9.67A and B: Extensive xeroderma pigmentosa in adults noticed since childhood.
Courtesy: Dr Somen Misra.

Commonly used drugs are zinc oxide, titanium dioxide, and chemicals containing para-aminobenzoic acid.

Xanthogranuloma Juvenile

This is a rare benign cutaneous and ocular manifestation; it is mostly self-limiting. Tumor of infancy and childhood. They are either present at birth or become obvious after 5 years.

The ocular lesions may be extra- or intraocular and may be accompanied with cutaneous or systemic lesion. The lesion have tendency to spontaneous regression.

The extraocular lesions are solitary tumor of the lid or extraocular muscle. Orbital lesions are less common.

The intraocular lesions are confined to the anterior uvea. The iris may show an asymptomatic nodule that may suddenly bleed without any attributable cause. The hyphema generally resolves; otherwise, it may cause secondary glaucoma.

The skin lesions vary in size from pinhead to 3–4 mm; they are firm and dome-shaped, and the color of the nodule varies from yellow to orange. They are scattered all over the body, including the lids.

As most of the lesions have a tendency for spontaneous regression and no specific treatment is available, the cases are managed as per the part of the eye involved by usual local steroids and antiglaucoma drugs.

SUGGESTED READING

1. Agrawal NK, Bhattacharya V. Xeroderma pigmentosa. In: Kanski JJ, Thomas DJ (Eds). Eyes in Systemic Disorders, 1st edition. New Delhi: Wily India; 2015.
2. Freedman J. Xeroderma pigmentosa. In: Fraunfelder FT, Roy FH (Eds). Current Ocular Therapy, 5th edition. Philadelphia: W.B. Sunders & Co.; 2000.
3. Heidary G, Kazlas M. Pediatric Ophthalmology, Juvenile Xanthogranuloma. In: Deborah PL (Ed). Manual of Ocular Diagnosis and Therapy, 6th edition. Philadelphia: Lippincott Williams & Wilkins; 2008. p. 306.
4. Jethani J. Paediatric eye in various systemic syndromes xeroderma pigmentosa. In: Ramamurthy D, Biswas P (Eds). AIOS Ready Reckoner in Ophthalmology, 2nd edition. New Delhi: Jaypee Brothers Medical Publisher; 2017.
5. McCulley JP, Dougerty J, Deneau DG. Classification of chronic blepharitis. Ophthalmology. 1982;89:1173-80.

CHAPTER 10

Mobility Disorders of Lid in Children

The mobility disorders of the lid can be:

- That narrows the interpalpebral aperture (IPA)—ptosis and blepharospasm
- Those that widen IPA—lagophthalmos and lid retraction
- Associated with synkinetic movements of the lid (jaw winking)
- *Others:* Lid apraxia, myoclonus, and twitching

PTOSIS

Ptosis is a common disorder of the upper lid in all ages where the upper lid margin is placed at a lower position in relation to the limbus **(Figs. 10.1 to 10.6)**.

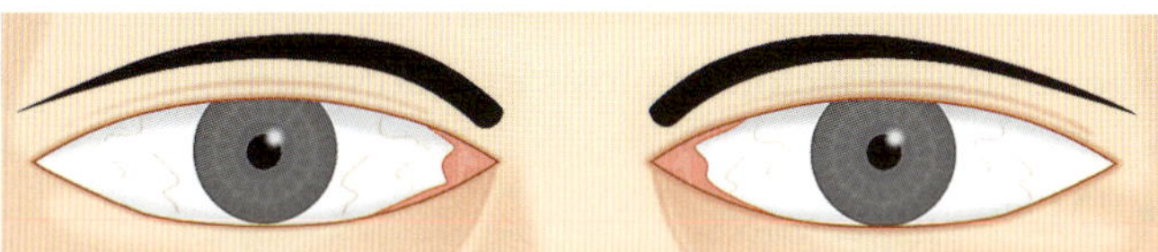

Fig. 10.1: Eyes without ptosis.

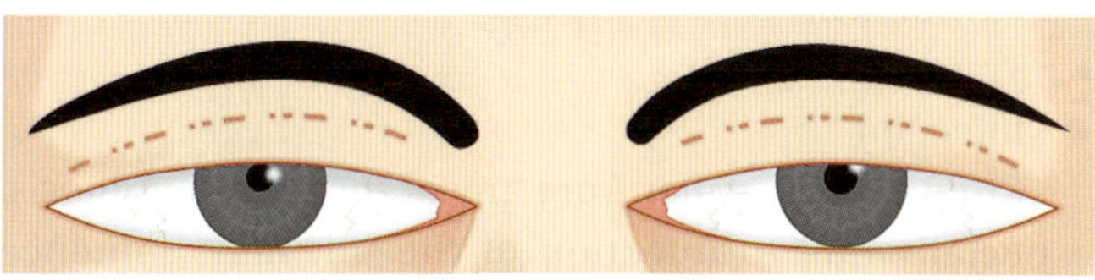

Fig. 10.2: Ptotic eyes.

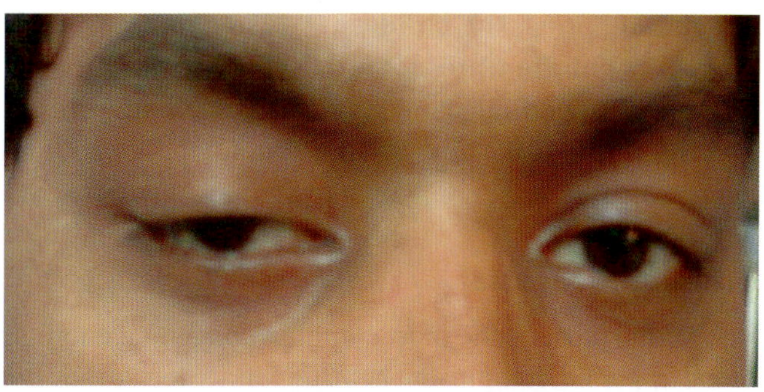

Fig. 10.3: Unilateral severe ptosis.

The nonptotic lid covers 2.00 mm of the upper lid, and the lower lid just touches the lower pole of the limbus **(Fig. 10.7)**. This leaves a clear space in front of the cornea,

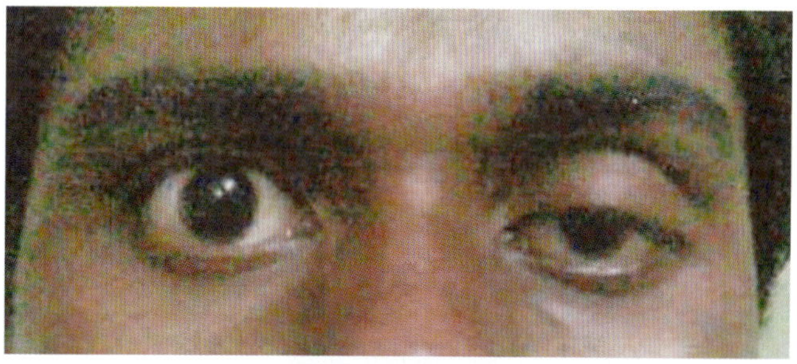

Fig. 10.4: Unilateral moderate ptosis.

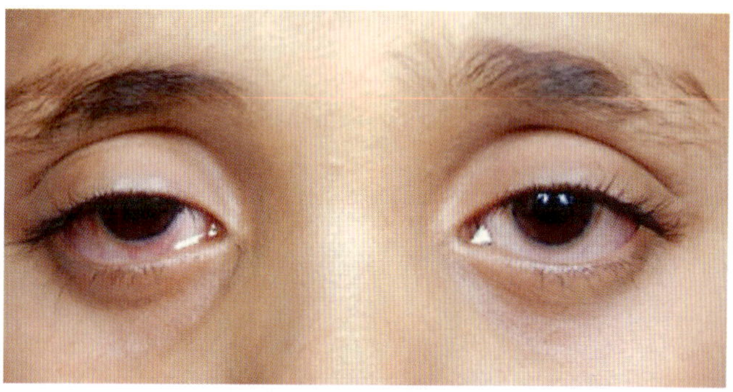

Fig. 10.5: Bilateral moderate ptosis.

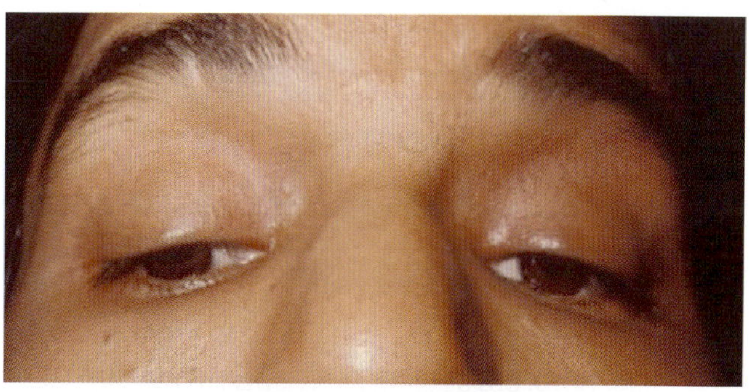

Fig. 10.6: Bilateral severe congenital ptosis.

in the interpalpebral fissure. If the upper lid covers >2.00 mm of the upper limbus in the primary position, it is considered to be ptotic **(Fig. 10.8)**. In contrast to this, if the lower lid margin covers even 1.00 mm of the lower limbus, it is abnormal, and the condition is called reverse ptosis or upside-down ptosis **(Figs. 10.9 and 10.10)**. Reverse ptosis is far less common than upper lid ptosis. The most common cause is Horner's syndrome.

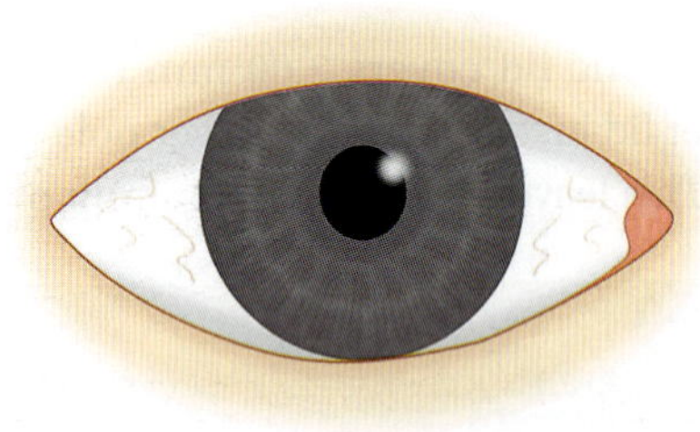

Fig. 10.7: Normal upper lid covering 2.00 mm of cornea. The lower lid touching lower pole of cornea.

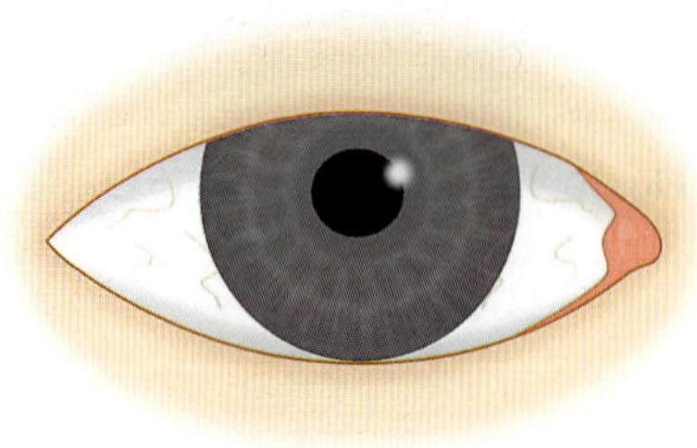

Fig. 10.8: Ptotic lid covering more than 2.00 mm of cornea.

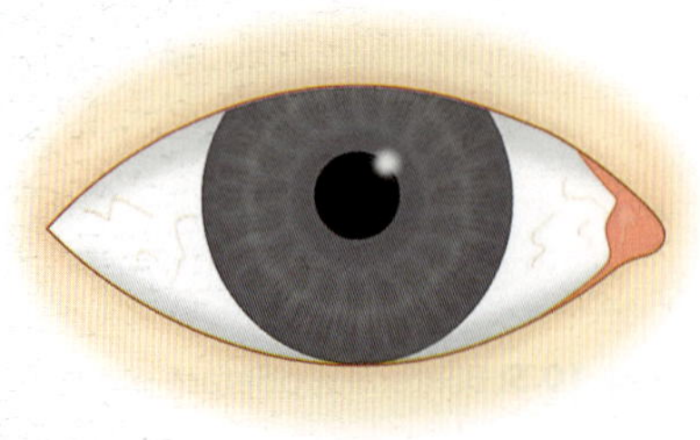

Fig. 10.9: Normal position of upper lid.

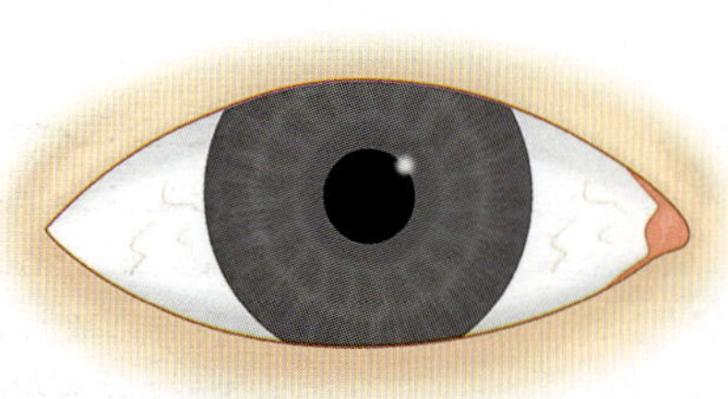

Fig. 10.10: Upside down ptosis lower lid covering 1.00 mm of lower pole of cornea.

The clear space in front of the cornea is called the interpalpebral fissure, which is wide in the middle and gradually narrows on either end. The IPA of a newborn is 8.00 mm wide and 18.00 mm long. The adult IPA is 9.00 mm wide and 30.00 mm long.

Ptosis is found in all ages, from neonates to ripe old age. It can be congenital or acquired **(Flowchart 10.1)**.

> Congenital ptosis is more common in children. All ptoses in adults are acquired, barring the ptosis that has not been attended to at a young age.

A ptosis is said to be true when the fault lies in any of the retractors (elevators) of the upper lid. The retractors of the upper lid are the LPS and Müller's muscles. The LPS is a striated muscle supplied by the third cranial nerve; it is responsible for 85–90% of elevation. The remaining elevation is due to the action of Müller's muscle, a non-striated muscle supplied by the sympathetic nerve. The Müller's muscle neither has a definite insertion nor an origin. It lies under the LPS and can be reached either from the conjunctival fornix or transcutaneously for surgical purposes. The latter gives a better and more predictable result. Each group mentioned in **Flowchart 10.1** has a distinct feature, etiological factor, and management.

The etiological factors of ptosis in children are:

- Congenital
- Myogenic
- Aponeurotic
- Neurogenic
- Mechanical
- Traumatic
- Infection

Children may suffer from any of them. Pseudoptosis, especially due to infection of the lid, may influence the clinical features of congenital ptosis. Mechanical ptosis, a common form of ptosis, is more frequent than congenital ptosis in children. Most of the pseudo-ptoses in children are acquired **(Fig. 10.11)**. Except for some congenital hamartomas such as neurofibromatosis **(Figs. 10.12 and 10.13)**, hemangiomatosis, and lymphangiomatosis.

Congenital Ptosis

Congenital ptosis is the most common congenital anomaly of the upper lid. It is present at birth. Milder forms may not be noticed by parents, especially when they are bilateral

Flowchart 10.1: Broad classification of ptosis in all ages.

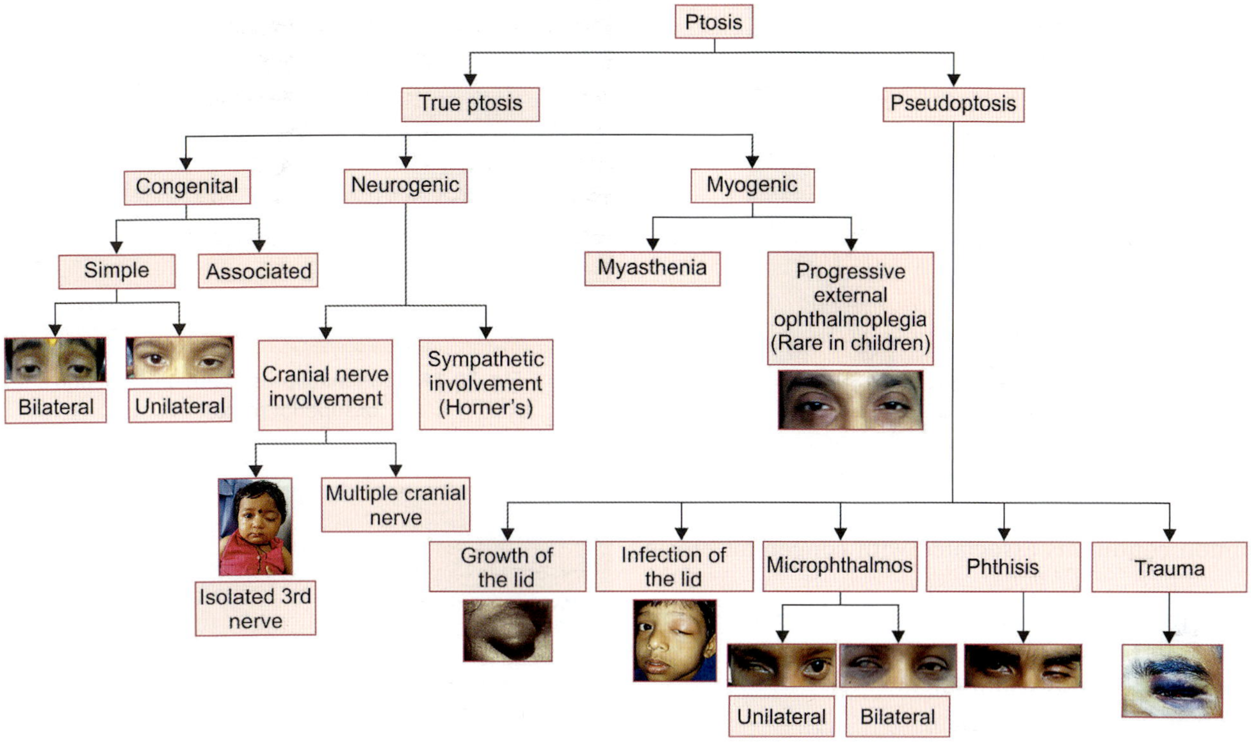

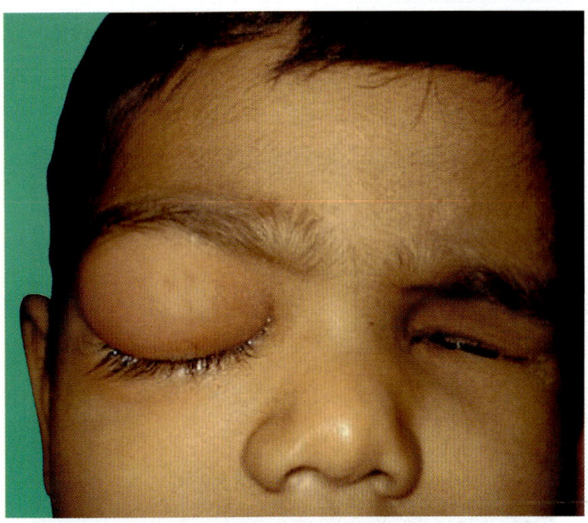

Fig. 10.11: Pseudoptosis due to cellulitis upper lid.

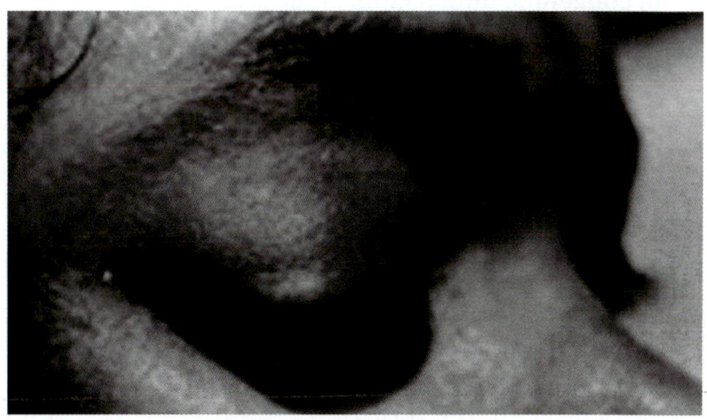

Fig. 10.12: Neurofibroma of upper lid in a child since birth.

and symmetric. Unilateral congenital ptoses draw attention more frequently. Congenital ptosis is responsible for 75% of all ptoses seen in children, widely distributed the world over without any racial preponderance. It is equally seen among boys and girls. There may be a positive family history in parents/grandparents. It is not uncommon to find ptosis among many of the siblings. The exact cause of the condition is not well understood. The most common hypothesis is that it is a congenital myopathy with fibro-fatty infiltration of the levator muscle with intact aponeurosis.

Congenital ptoses are stationary. They may be the only malformation or may be associated with other congenital anomalies. The former is called simple congenital ptosis.

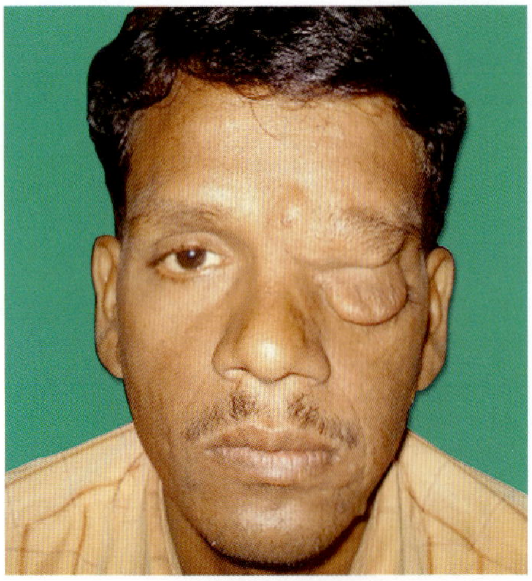

Fig. 10.13: Neurofibroma in an adult present since birth.

Common conditions associated with congenital ptosis are:

- Concurrent ipsilateral superior rectus under action **(Figs. 10.14 and 10.15)**
- Blepharophimosis syndrome
- Marcus Gunn's jaw is winking.

The congenital ptosis may be associated with the following abnormal movements as well:

- Lifting of upper lid in attempted abduction
- Paradoxical retraction of upper lids of the affected side in congenital underaction of the sixth nerve.
- Pseudo-Graefe sign*.
- Lid retraction on occlusion of contralateral eye

Symptoms of Congenital Ptosis

The only complaint for which the child is brought for consultation is a cosmetic blemish of a narrow palpebral fissure. Uniocular blemish attracts attention earlier than bilateral unless the latter is gross.

Otherwise, the infant may be brought with alternate opening or closing of the lid while sucking. This happens on one side only (Markus Gunn syndrome). The child may be brought in with bilateral chinky eyes. A toddler or preschool child may be brought with raised eyebrows and a head tilted back with ptosis **(Fig. 10.16)**.

Rarely a child may be brought for correction of diminished vision and found to have moderate ptosis.

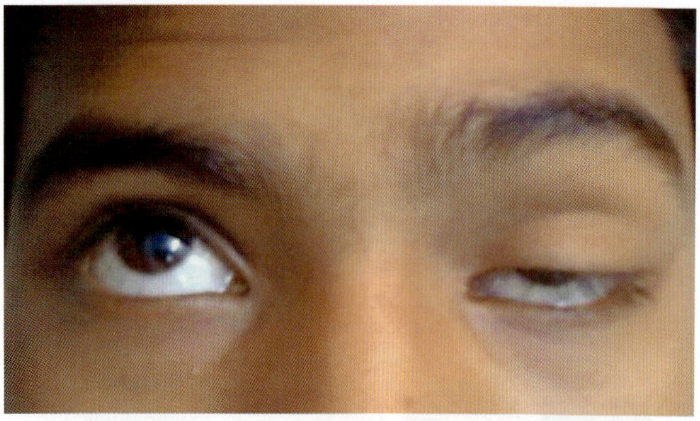

Fig. 10.14: Congenital ptosis with under action of superior rectus.

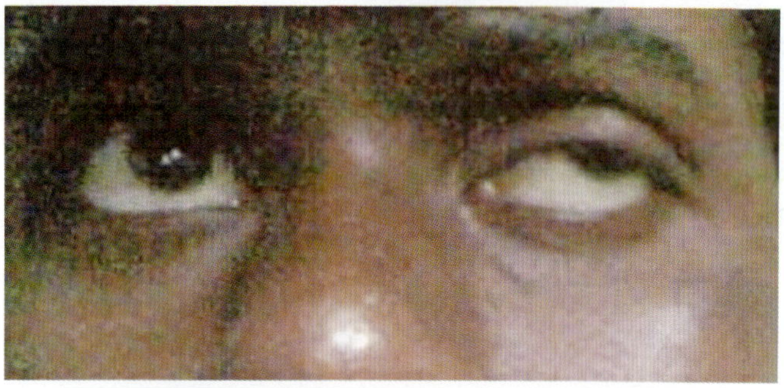

Fig. 10.15: Congenital ptosis with good superior rectus action.

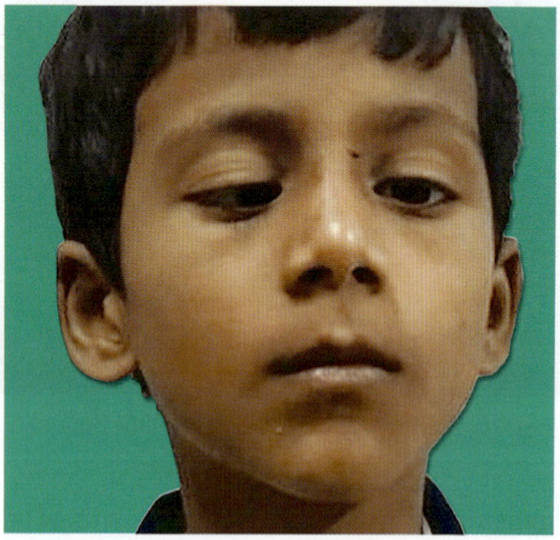

Fig. 10.16: Child with moderate bilateral ptosis, raised eyebrow, and head tilted back.

*A *pseudo-Graefe* sign should be differentiated from Graefe's sign seen in thyroid eye disease. Graefe's sign consists of a lagging of the upper eyelid in the downward gaze. A pseudo-Graefe's sign shows a similar lag but is due to aberrant regeneration of fibers of the oculomotor nerve (III) into the elevator of the upper lid.

Evaluation of Ptosis in Children

Evaluation begins with a detailed history. It should enquire:

- *History:*
  - Whether present at birth (congenital) or developed later (acquired), this is necessary because the amount of surgical correction in congenital ptosis cases differs from the acquired. It is better to undercorrect acquired ptosis than congenital ptosis.

  The dictum is

> - Operating a congenital ptosis as acquired will lead to under correction.
> - Operating an acquired ptosis as congenital will lead to over correction.

  - Most of the pseudoptosis is acquired, except for benign conditions involving the globe. The hamartomas of the lid that are congenital may be associated with pseudoptosis.

> - *Lid:* Cellulites, hematoma
> - *Globe:* Microphthalmos, micro cornea, enophthalmos, phthisis, perforation of globe, anophthalmos, enucleated socket, and eviscerated socket
> - *Orbit:* Fracture floor orbit
> - Hypertropia

Causes of pseudoptosis are:

- *Family history:* Positive family history goes in favor of congenital ptosis.
- *History of trauma:*
  - *Birth trauma:* Ptosis following birth trauma may present as congenital ptosis.
  - *Trauma latter:*
    - May cause injury to the aponeurosis.
    - Traumatic hematoma presents as pseudoptosis.
    - Chemical and thermal injuries can cause pseudoptosis.
- *History of variation:* Goes in favor of myasthenia
- *History suggestive of neurological deficit:* Rarely congenital

  A careful history is followed by a complete examination of both eyes, with special reference to the examination of the lids, which includes:

- Visual acuity without lifting the lid
- Visual acuity after lifting the lid
- Improvement of vision following lifting of the lid denotes severe ptosis covering the pupil
- Refraction under cycloplegia
- Exclusion of amblyopia
- Fundus examination
- Examination of extraocular muscles, especially the superior rectus
- Bell's phenomenon*.
- *Examination of the pupil:* A constricted pupil with mild ptosis should arouse suspicion of congenital Horner's syndrome†.

The permanent features consist of:

- *Ptosis:*
  - Not more than 2.00 mm due to the involvement of Müller's muscle
  - Well-maintained lid crease
  - There is no lid lag on up gaze.
  - The action of levator palpebral superior (LPS) and superior rectus is normal.
- *Upside-down ptosis of the lower lid:* This is due to poor sympathetic supply to the retractor muscles of the lower lid.
- *Enophthalmos:* This is more of a pseudoenophthalmos than true, the contributory factors of which are ptosis of the upper lid and upside-down ptosis concurrently.
- Narrowing of IPA.
- *Miosis:* The pupil of the affected side is small but not pinpoints which is best observed in dim light.

**Bell's phenomenon* is a physiological phenomenon present in all persons. This is an up-and-out movement of the eyeball in an attempt to close the lids. In cases of superior rectus under action, Bell's phenomenon is either lost or reduced. The absence of Bell's phenomenon in the case of ptosis is an absolute contraindication for any type of ptosis surgery.

†*Horner's syndrome* is also called sympathetic ptosis due to the involvement of the sympathetic chain anywhere from the hypothalamus to the globe. The incidence of Horner's syndrome is less in children than in adults. It can be congenital or acquired. Some authors believe that there is no congenital syndrome. The conditions labeled as congenital are in fact acquired due to trauma to the brachial plexus associated with Klumpke's paralysis‡. Besides birth trauma, accidental injury to the neck, enlarged lymph nodes in the neck, cavernous sinus diseases, and orbital inflammation may contribute to sympathetic ptosis in children. The features of Horner's syndrome can be broadly divided into permanent and transient features.

‡*Klumpke's paralysis:* It is a form of paralysis involving muscles of the forearm and hand, resulting from brachial plexus injury.

The pupil does not dilate with 4% cocaine but dilates with hydroxyamphetamine.

- *Anhidrosis:* Ipsilateral
    - *Heterochromia:* Ipsilateral. The affected side is lighter, and this is considered to be characteristic of congenital Horner's syndrome in children.

The transient signs are:

- Reduced intraocular pressure (IOP)
- Increased accommodation with no change in convergence and pupillary light reflex
- Dilatation of conjunctival vessels and facial vessels

This should be followed by an examination of ptosis proper:

- *Face:* Raised eyebrows:
    - Persistent—congenital ptosis
    - Transient—pseudoptosis
- *Head posture:* Head tilted back. This phenomenon helps to:
    - Increase upper field.
    - The child utilizes the chink of the pupil left clear by the ptotic lid for better vision. (Pinhole effect).
- Blepharophimosis syndrome
- Jaw winking syndrome*.

Evaluation of Lid Function

- Examination of LPS
- Examination of IPA in front of the pupil
- Height of upper lid crease
- Examination for lid lag

> Lid lag is confirmatory sign of congenital ptosis.

- Excursion of the upper lid is the difference in the level of the upper lid margin in down and up gaze. This is called MLD, i.e., margin limbus distance **(Fig. 10.18)**.

> Levator function is assessed to plan type of surgery. Height of IPA indicates severity of ptosis.

The normal excursion is 12.00 mm. The lid excursion is graded as:

- Good (8–12 mm)
- Moderate (5–7 mm)

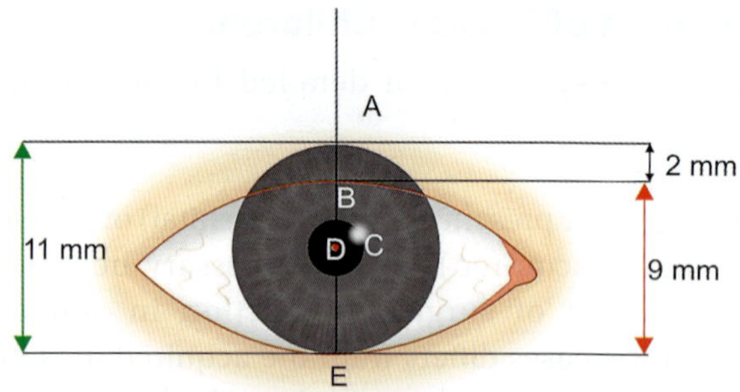

Normal position of lid in relation to the cornea.

AE = 11.00 mm, diameter of cornea
AB = 2.00 mm, distance of normal upper lid from limbus
BE = 9.00 mm, width of interpalpebral aperture
C = Pupil
D = Central corneal light reflex
BD = Distance between upper lid and cornea light reflex

Fig. 10.17: Normal dimension of IPA in relation to cornea and pupil.

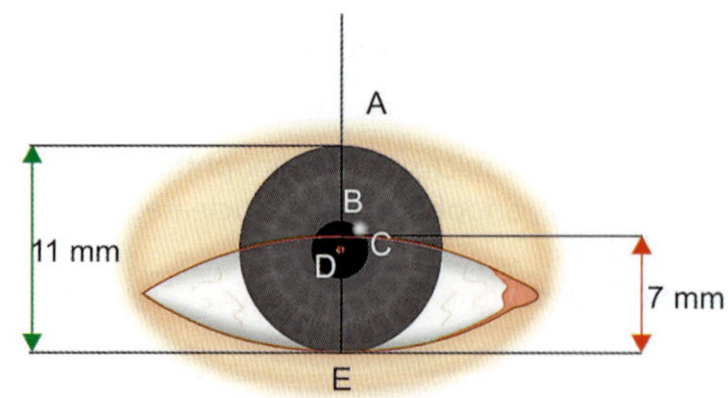

Measurement of ptosis—Margin limbus distance (MLD)

AE = 11.00 mm, diameter of cornea
D = Central corneal light reflex
AC = Distance of drooping lid from upper limbus
CE = 7.00 mm, width of palpebral aperture
AC-AB = 2.00 mm, is ptosis

Fig. 10.18: MLD in a ptotic eye.

- Poor (<4.00 mm)
- Absent

The other measurements are MRD-1 and MRD-2 **(Fig. 10.19)**.

MRD is an acronym for margin reflex distance, where R is the position of the central corneal reflex. It is the distance between the corneal reflex and the center of the lid margin. M is said to be positive if some clear cornea

Jaw winking syndrome (Marcus Gunn syndrome):* It is a congenital phenomenon seen in unilateral ptosis, where the ptotic lid elevates with the movement of the jaw. It is a congenital misdirection of motor supply to the external pterygoid and levator. This results in the widening of the IPA during chewing or moving the jaw from side to side **(Fig. 10.17). Though it is common in congenital ptosis, it can be seen in children even without ptosis. It automatically resolves by the age of 10–12.

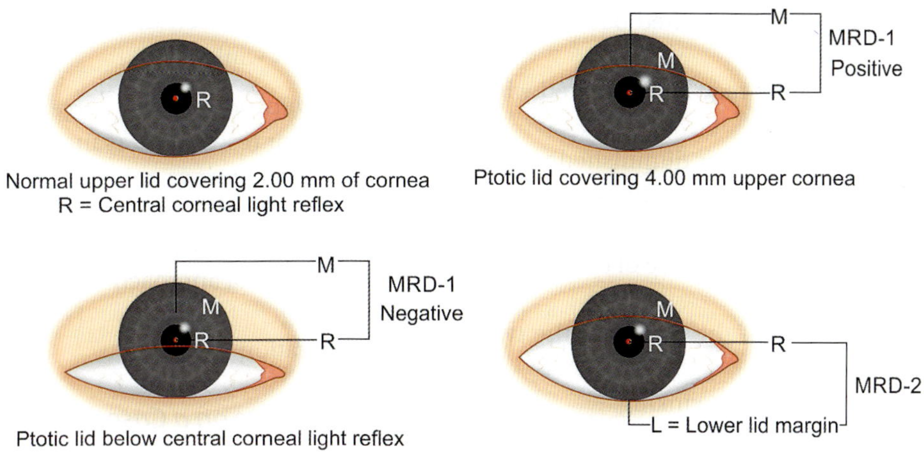

Fig. 10.19: Measurement of MRD 1 and 2.
Note: This is done primary position.

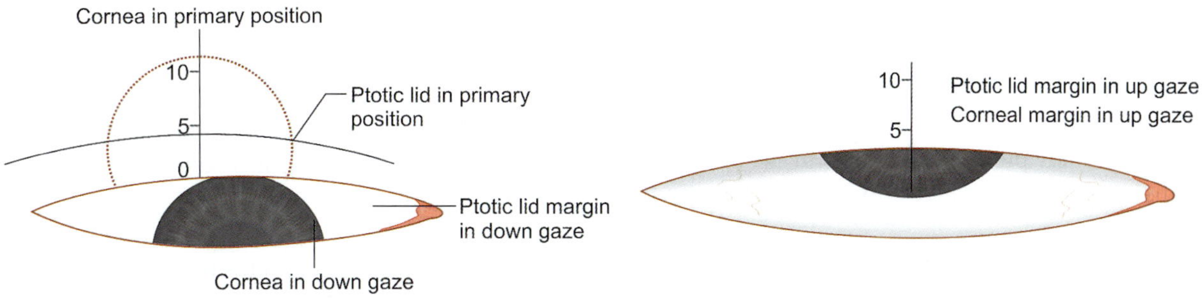

Fig. 10.20: Position of the ptotic lid in up and down gazes.

is visible between R and M. If M comes down below R, it is noted as negative **(Fig. 10.20)**. The other grading is based on the amount of ptosis, i.e., mild (2.00 mm or less), moderate (3.00 mm), and severe (>4.00 mm).

Various types of measurement in ptosis are given in **Box 10.1**.

Phenylephrine Test

Slight elevation of the ptotic lid following the instillation of phenylephrine indicates normal action of Müller's muscle. A positive phenylephrine test predicts a favorable result following the Fasanella-Servat operation. The test is not very accurate.

Characteristics of congenital ptosis:

- It may be missed at birth as the neonate sleeps almost 16–18 hours a day.
- It may be missed if it is bilateral, moderate, and symmetric.
- It is unilateral more often (75%).
- When bilateral, it is generally asymmetric.
- The total absence of levator function in the absence of birth trauma is a strong indicator of congenital third nerve palsy.

BOX 10.1: Various types of measurement in ptosis.

Measuring margin-reflex distance

MRD I:

- Bring the eyes of the patient and the observer to the level
- Ask the patient to fix a distant object
- Bring fixation light in between the patient and the observer
- Note the position of the corneal reflex
- Measure the distance between the corneal light reflex and the center of the upper lid. This measurement is called positive
- If the corneal light reflex is obstructed by the drooping lid, note the position of the drooped lid and elevate it until the corneal light reflex becomes visible and this distance is measured as negative

MRD II: It is the distance between the corneal light reflex and the lower lid at the primary position

MRD III: It is the distance between the corneal light reflex and the upper lid in up gaze

- A child with ptosis keeps his head tilted back and his brows raised.
- In a few cases, bilateral ptosis may be associated with blepharophimosis syndrome.
- Ptosis per se is not responsible for diminished vision unless the lid covers the pupil fully. In such cases, assisted lifting of the ptotic lid reveals good vision.
- Associated astigmatism is a major cause of diminished vision in ptosis.
- Astigmatism and occlusion of the pupil are the two main causes of amblyopia.
- Ptosis may be associated with jaw winking.
- More levator resection is needed to correct congenital ptosis than in acquired ptosis.
- Ptosis surgery is the definitive treatment to correct congenital ptosis.
- It is better to wait 4–5 years to plan surgery because it is difficult to reach reliable measurements under 4 years. The exception is total congenital ptosis, which requires a sling operation.
- The congenitally ptotic lid is higher in the lower gaze because the fibrotic changes do not relax fully in the down gaze.
- Lid lag is a sure sign of congenital ptosis.
- The minimum resection required is as follows:
  - Initial minimum 11.00 mm resection gives 1.00 mm of elevation of the lid.
  - Thereafter each resection of 3.00 mm gives 1.00 mm of elevation.
- Squint if present should be corrected before ptosis surgery, especially the vertical squint.
- Combination of the amount of ptosis and levator function decides the type of surgery to be performed.
- The points discussed above may not be in the same order as depicted above in all cases.

A commonly used mnemonic for the preoperative evolution of ptosis is:

DESTINY:

- *D:* Droop-amount of ptosis
- *E:* Extrusion
- *S:* Superior rectus
- *T:* Tearing
- *I:* Iliff test for LPS function*
- *N:* Nerve-corneal sensation
- *Y:* Yawn-Jaw winking

A broad classification of ptosis surgery:

- Tarso levator resection (Fasanella-Servat operation)
- Müller's resection
- *Levator shorting:*
  - External approach
  - Conjunctival approach
  - Tucking
- Sling operation

When to Operate on a Case of Congenital Ptosis?

A case of congenital ptosis should be operated on when accurate measurements can be taken; this is not possible before 1 year of age. The best time to operate is after 4 years unless there is bilateral complete ptosis, which requires a sling operation.

Points to remember in congenital ptosis:

- Lid lag is a sure sign of congenital ptosis.
- A well-formed supratarsal crease denotes aponeurotic ptosis.
- The absence of the Bells phenomenon indicates that the ipsilateral superior rectus is under action.
- In neurogenic ptosis, levator action is inversely proponent to nerve impulse.
- The combination of the amount of ptosis and levator function decides the type of surgery to be performed.

Note: The type of surgery is highly personal. Various institutes have their own protocols.

Table 10.1 is a rough guide to the type of surgery in squint.

Table 10.2 summarizes the indications and outlines of procedures of various surgeries.

TABLE 10.1: Types of surgery in squint.

Levator action	*Grade*	*Surgery*
Normal	Mild	Fasanella-Servat
Good	Moderate	Levator resection
Poor/absent	Severe	Sling operation

**Iliff test* is performed to find levator function. To perform the test; the upper lid of the infant is everted, as the child looks down the lid should revert back on its own if the levator action is sufficient.

TABLE 10.2: Indications and outlines of procedures of various surgeries.

Surgery	***Outline of procedure***	***Indications***
Fasanella-Servat	Transconjunctival excision of Müller's muscle with excision of the upper part of the tarsus, some length of LPS, and some conjunctiva	• Mild congenital ptosis, Horner's syndrome, and residual ptosis following initial surgery • Any ptosis with moderate levator function
Levator resection: • Eversbusch	Easier to master, gives a good lid crease, performed from the skin surface, a large amount of levator can be resected, followed by the attachment of the cut end of the LPS to the tarsus	Any ptosis with moderate levator function
• Blaskovics	Difficult to master but as effective as Eversbusch. In both procedures, a large amount of levator aponeurosis is resected and attached to the upper end of the tarsus	Any ptosis with moderate levator function
Frontalis sling operation	The action of the frontalis is not affected in any ptosis this faculty is utilized to correct severe ptosis transcutaneously by a sling, that lifts the tarsus up. Various materials are used to form the sling that may be natural or artificial. It is better to perform bilateral surgery to maintain symmetry, even in unilateral cases	Myopathic ptosis, Markus Gunn syndrome, and very poor levator function. In Marcus Gunn syndrome, both sides are operated on simultaneously

Some points to remember regarding congenital ptosis:
- Lid lag is a sure sign of congenital ptosis.
- A well-formed supratarsal crease denotes aponeurotic ptosis.
- The absence of Bell's phenomenon indicates that the ipsilateral superior rectus is under action.
- In neurogenic ptosis, levator action is inversely proportionate to nerve impulse.

Surgery for Congenital Ptosis

Selection of cases for ptosis surgery in children:

- *Counseling of the caregiver/parents:*
  - *Regarding correction:* Under correction/overcorrection
  - Operation of contralateral apparently normal lid in the case of sling operation in unilateral severe ptosis
  - Regarding the use of general anesthesia
- *History*:
  - Find out if the ptosis is congenital or acquired.
  - If acquired, find out if it is true or pseudoptosis, all pseudoptoses do not require surgery.
  - Many pseudoptoses require multiple surgeries.
  - In cases of acquired ptosis, no surgery is contemplated unless ptosis has been stationary for at least 6 months. This is more relevant in neurogenic and traumatic ptosis.
- *Examinations that require special attention:*
  - Best corrected vision to exclude amblyopia.
  - Exclude blepharophimosis, syndrome, and Jaw-winking syndrome.
  - Test for Bell's phenomenon—absence of Bell's phenomenon is a contraindication for all ptosis surgeries.
  - *Corneal sensation:* The absence of corneal sensation is contraindicated for ptosis surgery.
  - Ocular surface disorders should get appropriate attention.
  - Exclude vertical diplopia by the cover test.
  - *Test action of extraocular muscles:* Underacting extraocular muscles cause diplopia if the pupil is not covered, which is masked by the downcoming lid in ptosis. Following lid surgery, the pupil is uncovered. This may precipitate uncomfortable diplopia.

Complications of congenital ptosis surgery:

1. Undercorrection
2. Overcorrection
3. Abnormal lid fold
4. Ectropion
5. Entropion
6. Prolapse of conjunctiva
7. Exposure keratitis

Blepharophimosis Syndrome

This congenital anomaly of the lids is less common than simple congenital ptosis. It is:

- Autosomal dominant/sporadic in nature
- Strong family history
- Bilateral

- More often symmetric
- Severe ptosis
- Poor levator function
- Epicanthus inversus
- Telecanthus
- Blepharophimosis (small IPA, both in length and height)
- Pseudosquint
- 5% of children with congenital ptosis have blepharophimosis, to some degree or other
- There is no associated systemic disorder.
- Flat nose bridge
- Congenital ectropion of the lower lid
- Hypoplasia of bony orbital margin
- The Komoto tetrad consists of ptosis, blepharophimosis, telecanthus, and epicanthus inversus.

Diagnosis

Diagnosis is not difficult due to specific appearance as shown in **Figure 10.21**.

Treatment of Blepharophimosis

Treatment is divided into:

- *Treating telecanthus:* This is best done by a faciomaxillary surgeon.
- Correction of epicanthus
- Correction of the squint
- Correction of ptosis

Neurogenic Ptosis

Neurogenic ptosis in children can be present at birth due either to congenital third nerve palsy or congenital Horner's syndrome, both of which are uncommon. The former is more frequent out of the two. The third nerve palsy is most of the time complete, involving the pupil. A unilateral miotic pupil with mild ipsilateral ptosis is a hallmark of sympathetic involvement, causing Horner's syndrome. Congenital ptosis due to third nerve involvement is less common than acquired. In children, ptosis may be the first sign of third nerve involvement (**Figs. 10.22A and B**). Mydriasis with ptosis is more confirmatory. The lesions may be supranuclear, nuclear, fascicular, basilar, or peripheral. The supranuclear lesion results in mild ptosis, miosis, and gaze palsy. Nuclear congenital third nerve palsy is still rare; when present, it manifests as bilateral superior rectus weakness due to the proximity of the two nuclei. Lesions of the fascicle cause Benedikt* and Weber syndromes†. Trunk lesions are seen in the lesions of the cavernous sinus.

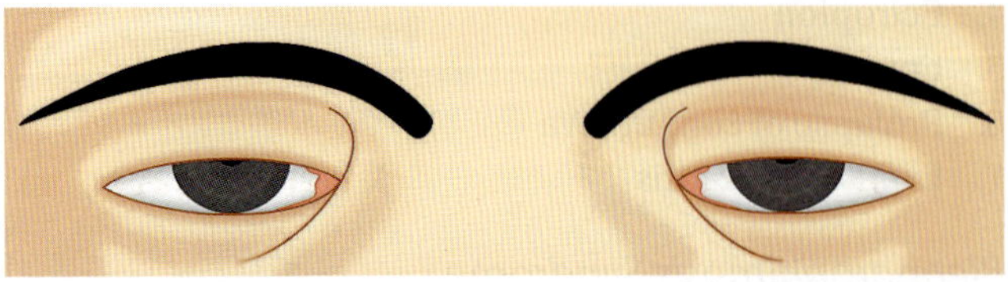

Fig. 10.21: Typical appearance of blepharophimosis.

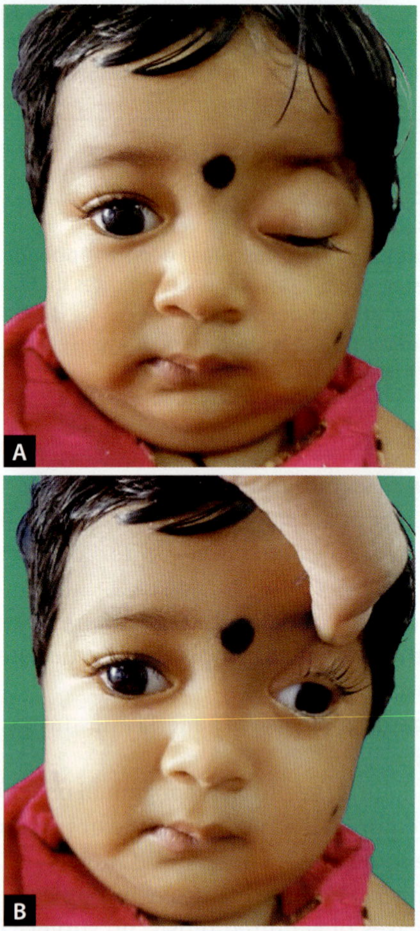

Figs. 10.22A and B: Total ptosis in a child with acquired third nerve palsy.
Courtesy: Dr Anand Deshpande.

**Benedikt syndrome* is caused due to lesion at the midbrain that results in ipsilateral oculomotor nerve palsy, contralateral hemiparesis, contralateral cerebellar ataxia, and tremor. It is generally seen in adults.

†*Weber syndrome* consists of ipsilateral third nerve palsy with contralateral hemiparesis due to a vascular lesion in the midbrain. It is generally seen in adults.

Acquired neurological conditions that may cause ptosis are:

- Birth trauma
- Infection (most common)
- Inflammation
- Intracranial neoplasm

All of them should be differentiated from pseudoptosis, which outnumbers them all put together.

APONEUROTIC PTOSIS IN CHILDREN

Aponeurotic ptosis is less common in children. When it is present, it is mostly traumatic. Congenital aponeurotic ptosis is exceptional. When present, it is due to a failure of attachment of the distal part to the tarsal plate. This results in ptosis of varying degrees and underaction of the levator. Birth trauma may be mistaken for a congenital cause. In the case of aponeurotic ptosis, there is either thinning or stretching of the aponeurosis of LPS; a combination of both may be present; and rarely, there is actual disinsertion of the levator from the tarsus. Frank laceration of the levator muscle or its aponeurosis requires different management from senile aponeurotic ptosis. The lacerated muscle or its aponeurosis should be repaired by primary suture without tampering with the orbital septum. Damage to the septum is invariably associated with retraction of the globe and lid lag, both worsening ptosis.

Myogenic Ptosis

The two myogenic ptosis found in children are myasthenic ptosis and chronic progressive external ophthalmoplegia. The former is more common than the latter.

Myasthenic Ptosis (Dysmyogenic Ptosis)

Myasthenia gravis is an autoimmune disease due to a fault at the myoneural junction secondary to reduced acetylcholine at the postsynaptic receptors of striated muscles. It spares smooth muscles, including the iris and ciliary muscles.

Myasthenia gravis can be divided into two broad categories:

1. Ocular
2. Systemic

Generally, ocular symptoms proceed systemically. 80% of ocular myasthenic patients develop systemic symptoms over the next 2 years. A chance of systemic involvement after 2–3 years is uncommon. Ocular and systemic involvement can be concurrent. In adults, myasthenia can develop at any age. Children are not immune to myasthenia. Children born to a myasthenic mother may develop neonatal myasthenia. Myasthenia is sporadic. However, it may be seen in many members of the same family. Myasthenia is more common in females than males at a ratio of 2:1. Age-wise, myasthenia can be childhood myasthenia or adult myasthenia.

Myasthenia in children differs from those seen in adults. It may be transient neonatal or persistent neonatal. The former develops in children born to mothers who have myasthenia. The latter is seen in children without a myasthenic mother. Juvenile myasthenia develops after 10 years of age, the natural history of which does not differ from adult myasthenia.

Myasthenia may progress relentlessly or may be intermittent. Occasionally, it is self-limited and passes off without any treatment or sequel.

Characteristics of myasthenic ptosis:

- Ptosis may be the only sign of ocular involvement.
- It may be associated with diplopia.
- Both may run concurrently or one may follow the other.
- *The ptosis is mostly:*
  - Mild to moderate, never complete
  - Ptosis becomes more pronounced following physical exercise. It is the least on awakening and increases by evening.
  - Degree of ptosis is variable.
  - Variability may be demonstrated by following a simple, noninvasive test as an office procedure.

Variability Tests for Myasthenia

Variability tests for myasthenia are described in **Table 10.3**.

Other tests to confirm ocular myasthenia:

Other tests to confirm ocular myasthenias are therapeutic, like Pyridostigmine test and Tensilon.

Therapeutic trial to confirm myasthenia:

- *Oral prostigmin or pyridostigmine.* They are available as oral tablets. A test is performed as an outdoor procedure. The action of pyridostigmine starts within 10–30 minutes and includes the undoing of ptosis and the abolition of diplopia. If this happens, the child is prescribed oral pyridostigmine in consultation with a pediatrician.
- *Tensilon (edrophonium) test. To perform the test:*
  - Caregivers/parents are counseled about the efficacy of the drug and its side effects.
  - An informed consent is taken.

TABLE 10.3: The list of variability tests for myasthenia.

Test	*Procedure*
Lid twitch test	The excursions of the lid are noted, and the child is asked to look down for 15–20 seconds. Then it is asked to fix a distant target quickly. If the lids overshoot the previous leaf and then fall down, it is considered to be positive
Lid fatigue ability test	The extent of ptosis is noted by usual methods, the child is asked to look up for a few minutes, worsening of ptosis is considered positive
"Peek" sign	This is effective in asymmetric ptosis, where one lid droops more than the other; if the more ptotic lid is lifted mechanically, the less drooping lid develops more ptosis
Cold test	Keep an ice cube over the ptotic lid for 2 minutes. On removal of the ice cube, the lid is found to be markedly elevated; it remains elevated for 15–20 seconds only to fall to its original level
Testing the action of the orbicular	A combination of ptosis and underaction of the orbicular is suggestive of myasthenia. Though there is poor action of the orbicularis, it is never complete. As in seventh nerve palsy, when the child is asked to close the lid forcefully, the examiner tries to separate the lid with the index finger and thumb of only one hand. A normal orbicular will not permit the lid to be separated. A myasthenia lid will open up with ease

- *It is mandatory to have the following measures available for emergency:*
  - *Intravenous atropine:* 0.5–1.0 mg
  - Arrangement for resuscitation
  - Cardiac monitor
  - It is preferred to have a pediatric anesthetic to perform the test.
  - Tensilon is available as a 10 mg clear solution for intravenous injection.
  - Load a syringe with 10 mg of Tensilon, inject 2 mg in the intravenous line, and observe ptosis.
  - If no effect is observed, the remaining 8 mg is injected slowly, and the amount of ptosis is compared with the preinjection level.
  - Stop the test if there is an adverse reaction to the test dose.

The following types of responses are noted in the Tensilon test:

- No improvement
- *An improvement:* Most common and diagnostic
- Worsening, i.e., small tropia becoming large tropia
- *Reversal:* The squint shifts to the other eye.

The last two responses are not seen in true myasthenia.

1. *Diplopia in myasthenia:* Diplopia may be the first symptom that the child complains of in myasthenia. The cause of diplopia is paralysis of extraocular muscles, which may follow or precede the involvement of the levator. Like ptosis, diplopia too is variable. Vertical diplopia, though less common, is more troublesome than horizontal diplopia. Diplopia becomes more marked after exertion. Hence, the child complains of diplopia more often in the evening. Diplopia may be absent in the morning. The test described above may also be tried to test the variability of extraocular muscle involvement.
2. *Squint in myasthenia:* Children may present with squints of various types and degrees. There is no rule of thumb to predict the order of extraocular muscle involvement. The child may have phoria; exophoria is the most common latent deviation. The tropia may be mistaken for a more serious neurological defect such as central gaze palsy or internuclear ophthalmoplegia. The medial rectus is the most commonly isolated and involved muscle. Multiple extraocular muscle involvement is common, i.e., muscles of the face, mastication, and laryngeal muscles. There may be nystagmoid movement. Involvement of the thymus is common.

Differential Diagnosis of Myasthenia in Children

All children with variable ptosis, diplopia and mild lagophthalmos with normal pupil should be suspected to be myasthenia unless proved otherwise.

The conditions that come into differential diagnosis are:

- Simple, chronic, progressive external ophthalmoplegia
- Complicated chronic progressive ophthalmoplegia, i.e., involving the heart and laryngeal muscles
- Internuclear ophthalmoplegia
- Dysthyroid myopathy
- Myotonic dystrophy

Outline of Treatment for Myasthenia in Children

Myasthenia in children generally progresses but can be kept under control with medical treatment with ancillary optical support. Surgery is rarely required. In many cases, myasthenia in children is self-limiting. Still, it should be treated to avoid cosmetic embarrassment and the chances of diplopia-related accidents.

The medical treatment consists of:

- *Anticholinesterase (pyridostigmine and neostigmine):* The effect of pyridostigmine starts in 10–20 minutes following oral administration. The effect lasts for 4 hours. Hence, the drug has to be repeated every 4 hours. Neostigmine is less effective than pyridostigmine. It takes 2–3 days for neostigmine to be effective. The side effects of the anticholinesterase drugs can be reduced by the simultaneous administration of parasympatholytic drugs (such as atropine).
- Steroid tablets (prednisolone)
- Immunosuppressive drugs (azathioprine) (It takes weeks to months before it becomes effective; till that time, anticholinesterase drugs in reduced doses may be used.)
- Other drugs used are:
  - Cyclosporine
  - Cyclophosphamide
  - Tacrolimus

All the drugs should be administered under the supervision of a pediatrician.

Optical

The child learns to close one eye to avoid diplopia. The optical treatment consists of the prescription of ptosis crutches, provided the child tolerates them. Frequent variations of diplopia make the use of prisms impractical. Surgery should not be tried till ptosis/squint has been stable without medication. Thymectomy has been claimed to give good results in refractory cases, but only in properly selected cases.

Chronic Progressive External Ophthalmoplegia

This is considered to be a disorder of adults **(Figs. 10.23A and B)**, which in fact starts by the end of the first decade. It has been observed even in children <10 years of age. It can be sporadic and nonfamilial. It is associated with mutations in mitochondrial DNA. As the name suggests, it is a chronic, relentless paralysis of extraocular muscles, including the levator. It spares the orbicularis, Müller's muscle, and intrinsic muscles of the eye. It is bilateral, symmetric, and starts with mild ptosis.

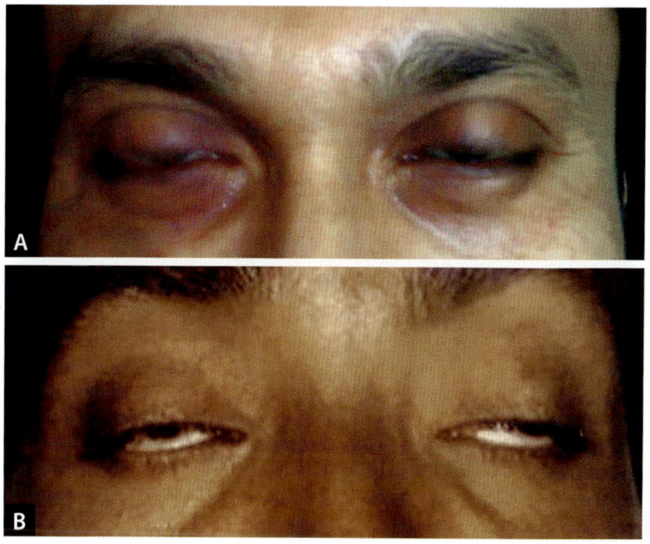

Figs. 10.23A and B: Chronic progressive external ophthalmoplegia in adults, the condition started in the second decade.

Childhood-progressive external ophthalmoplegia has the following components:

- Ophthalmic
- Cardiac

Ophthalmic: The ophthalmic component consists of progressive external ophthalmoplegia and peripheral retinal degeneration. It should be differentiated from myasthenia, thyroid ocular disease, and bulbar palsy. It starts as a mild ptosis, developing so slowly that for years, ptosis may go unnoticed. However, old photographs may betray the presence of ptosis. Extraocular muscles get involved years after the onset of ptosis. The squint is bilateral and symmetric; hence, the patient does not complain of diplopia. Gradually, all the muscles lose function, and the eye gets fixed, most commonly in the primary position. The patient keeps the head tilted back to offset the effect of ptosis and uses the chink of the IPA to improve vision. Ultimately, the pupil gets occluded by a down-coming immobile lid. As there is no movement of the globe, the patient moves the head from side to side to improve the temporal field. As long as only extraocular muscles are involved, the condition is designated as ocular myopathy. With the involvement of striated muscles other than extraocular muscles, the condition is called ophthalmoplegia plus. The pupil, accommodation, and vision remain intact. There is no error of refraction that can be attributed to the condition. The condition may involve only the eyes or may be associated with systemic diseases in later life. There is no treatment for the condition. Ptosis surgery is contraindicated. Ptosis crutches may be of help, provided the patient accepts them.

Cardiac: Cardiac changes in progressive external ophthalmoplegia are often missed in children that can prove to be fatal in later life. The cardiac involvement is multifactorial and may be AV block, QT prolongation, ventricular tachycardia, and syncope. This makes it mandatory to get a cardiac evaluation done by a cardiologist.

Pseudoptosis

Drooping of the upper lid with a normally acting levator and Müller's muscle is called pseudoptosis. It is invariably unilateral. When it is bilateral, it is mostly due to anomalies in the globe, congenital or acquired. The conditions are microcornea, microphthalmos, and phthisis which are shown in **Table 10.4**.

Table 10.4 gives various causes of pseudoptosis.

Alternate classification of ptosis and pseudoptosis (unilateral and bilateral):

- *Congenital:*
  - Simple ptosis (only the levator is involved)
  - *Complicated congenital:*
    - With the superior rectus under action
    - With synkinetic movement
    - Blepharophimosis syndrome
    - Retraction syndromes
- *Acquired:*
  - *Edema of the lid:*
    - Infection—lid abscess
    - *Inflammatory:*
      - Chalazion
      - Tarsal cyst
    - *Allergic:*
      - Edema
      - Drug-induced edema
      - Severe spring catarrh
  - *New growth:*
    - Neurofibromatosis
    - Hemangioma
    - Lymphangioma
    - Sturge–Weber syndrome
  - *Neurogenic:*
    - *Third nerve palsy:*
      - Nuclear
      - Trunk
    - External ophthalmoplegia
    - Horner's syndrome
  - *Myogenic:*
    - Myasthenia gravis
    - Myopathies
    - Chronic progressive external ophthalmoplegia
  - *Aponeurotic:*
    - Trauma to LPS aponeurosis
    - Disinsertion of LPS aponeurosis
  - *Trauma:*
    - Black eye
    - Laceration of LPS
    - Fracture orbit
  - *Miscellaneous:*
    - Anemia
    - Hypoproteinemia

TABLE 10.4: Causes of pseudoptosis.

Causes in Lid	***Globe***	***Orbit***	***Miscellaneous***
Edema of lid: • Allergic • *Inflammatory:* – Multiple chalazia – Tarsal cyst – Lid abscess • Nephrotic syndrome • *New growths:* – Hemangioma – Neurofibroma – Sturge–Weber syndrome – Inflammatory growths	• *Congenital anomalies:* – Microphthalmos – Microcornea – Anophthalmos • *Postinflammatory:* – Phthisis/enophthalmos – Atrophic bulbi • Eviscerated socket • Enucleated socket	Fracture floor of orbit	• Duane's retraction syndrome • Ipsilateral hypotropia • Contralateral hypertropia • Contralateral lagophthalmos

Management of Congenital Ptosis

> There is no medical treatment for congenital ptosis; those improving with medical treatment are in fact acquired and most probably pseudoptoses.

The management of congenital ptosis is divided into parts.

- Surgical
- Ptosis crutches

1. *Surgical*

2. *Ptosis crutches:* These are mechanical devices fitted behind the upper part of a spectacle frame in the form of a horizontal bar long enough and wide enough to create a horizontal crease in the upper lid to lift the lid at a desired level above the pupil. The greatest drawback of the crutches is that they prevent a normal blink; the eyes remain open, giving a weird look **(Figs. 10.24A and B)**.

Other mobility disorders of the lid in children:

- Lagophthalmos
- Lid retraction
- Blepharospasm
- Blepharoclonus
- Lid tick
- Apraxia

Lagophthalmos in Children

Blinking is a physiological protection mechanism to protect the eye from external substances, i.e., solid, liquid, gas, or microbia. The other function of the blink is to spread the tear over the ocular surface. Blinking can be defined as the synchronous opening and closing of the lids. The neonates blink less frequently. The two striated muscles that take part in blinking are the levator and orbicularis. Out of the two parts of the orbicularis, the palpebral part is more involved in blinking. The upper lid has a major role in blinking. Müller's muscle has no part to play in blinking.

There is a delicate balance between the action of the levator and the orbicularis. The former is involved in retraction (opening of the upper lid), and the orbicularis is involved in closing both lids. In a situation where the power of the levator surpasses that of the orbicularis, lagophthalmos sets in. It can be subtle enough to be missed, like micro lagophthalmos, which is a congenital, subtle lagophthalmos where all the layers of the lid are deficient or so advanced that the lids just fail to come down. The eyeball rolls up due to Bell's phenomenon. Bell's phenomenon is retained in lagophthalmos in contrast to ptosis, where Bell's phenomenon is either absent or weak.

Lagophthalmos is seen at all ages **(Fig. 10.25)**. It can be congenital (rare) or acquired. It can be unilateral or bilateral, with the former being more common than the latter. The causes of lagophthalmos can be broadly divided into two groups, i.e., neurological and mechanical. In the former, there is an underaction of orbicularis. In the second, the orbicularis function is retained, losing its ability to approximate the lids due to mechanical factors such as proptosis, thyroid ocular disease, scars, and large coloboma.

All lagophthalmos present at birth need not be congenital. The commonest cause of lagophthalmos in neonates is birth trauma. The congenital causes are mostly genetic

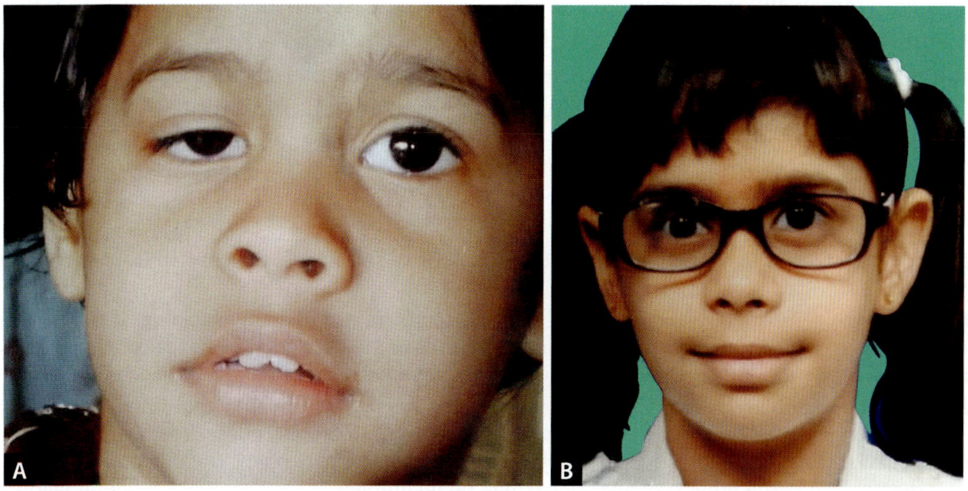

Figs. 10.24A and B: Right moderate congenital ptosis corrected by crutch fitted in spectacle.

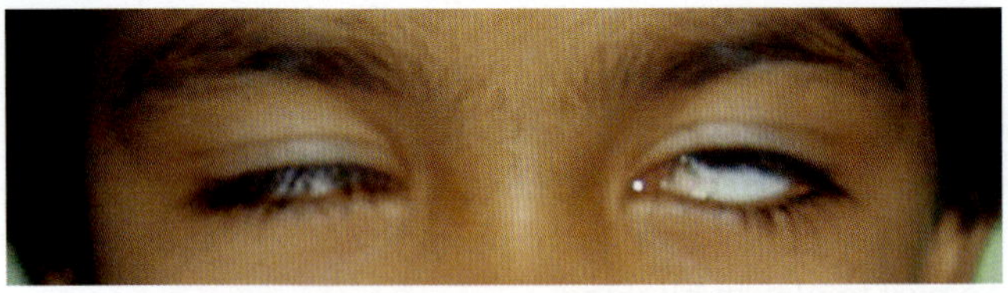

Fig. 10.25: Bilateral lagophthalmos in a child.

and associated with the congenital action of other cranial structures.

The cranial nerve involved in causing lagophthalmos is the seventh cranial nerve. The lesion can be anywhere from the fascicle of the seventh nerve to the orbit. The nerve may be involved in isolation or with other cranial nerves. Combined lesions of the sixth and seventh nerves are common. It can also be associated with the underaction of the fifth and twelfth nerves can be accompanied by lesions of other neural tracks. Supranuclear and nuclear lesions of the seventh nerve do not involve the orbicularis. Pontine lesions involving the seventh nerve cause ipsilateral sixth nerve palsy, absent or diminished conjugate movement on the same side, and contralateral hemi paresis. This is called Foville syndrome. Millard Gubler syndrome consists of the above features minus conjugate gaze palsy. The above two syndromes in children are mostly due to pontine glioma. Fracture base of the skull and basal meningitis are two causes of seventh nerve palsy due to the involvement of roots of the seventh nerve that involve the eighth nerve as well, resulting in diminished hearing, loss of taste in the anterior two-thirds of the tongue, and poor tear production. However, sometimes, orbicularis may be spared. Lesions at the cerebello-pontine angle (rare in children) cause ipsilateral facial weakness and hyperacusis. Geniculate ganglion lesions cause Ramsay Hunt syndrome, consisting of lagophthalmos with hyperacusis due to Herpes Zoster infection (rare in children).

Causes of Lagophthalmos in Children

The causes of unilateral lagophthalmos in children can be:

- *Trauma*:
  - Birth trauma—forceps delivery
  - *Surgical:*
    - Overcorrection of ptosis
    - Too much recession of the inferior rectus
    - Plastic repair of the upper lid
    - Surgery on mastoid
  - *Accidental:*
- *Infection:*
  - Herpes Zoster
  - Acute otitis media
  - Chronic otitis media
  - Meningitis
  - Other viral infections—herpes simplex, Epstein Barr virus, cytomegalovirus, mumps, and rubella
  - Lyme disease in endemic areas*
  - Leprosy—not seen in children
- Autoimmune diseases—Bell's palsy
- *Mechanical:*
  - Large coloboma of the upper lid
  - Proptosis preventing closure of lids
  - Scar on the skin of the lid

Causes of Bilateral Lagophthalmos in Children

- *Trauma:*
  - Birth injury
  - Accidental
  - Surgical
  - Closed head injury (brain stem injury)
- *Congenital:*
  - Microblepharon and euryblepharon
  - Moebius syndrome†
  - Nocturnal lagophthalmos‡

**Lyme disease* is caused by the microorganism Borrelia Burgdorferi, a type of spirochete, transmitted from some animals to men in an endemic area.

†*Moebius syndrome* is a rare congenital bilateral facial palsy. The child at birth has difficulty suckling. It is permanent in nature. The patient cannot smile or frown, has poor blinking, and cannot move the eyes in the horizontal plane, causing bilateral convergent squints. The sixth and seventh cranial nerves are not well developed; however, other cranial nerves may also be affected.

‡*Nocturnal lagophthalmos* is the inability to keep the lids closed during sleep. It is a benign condition. The child may not be aware of it, but the caregivers may notice. As the condition has very few symptoms, the parents may not seek advice. Rarely, there may be watering and redness due to an ocular surface defect that heals during the day when the eyes are open. The most common cause seems to be the vertical shortening of the upper lid. The other probable cause may be incomplete improvement of bilateral lagophthalmos following treatment.

- Melkersson-Rosenthal syndrome*
- Guillain-Barré syndrome†
- Goldenhar syndrome‡
- *Others:*
  - Brain stem glioma
  - Myasthenia
  - Thyroid eye disease
  - Cicatricial lower lid ectropion
  - Patient on live support system
- *Infection:* Leprosy (Most common cause of bilateral lagophthalmos above 20 years. It is not seen in children.)

Bell's Palsy

This is the most common type of unilateral lower motor neuron lagophthalmos in children. Involvement of the other eye is rare when present; it does not occur simultaneously. In two eyes, there may be a gap of months to years between the two episodes. Bell's palsy under 5 years and above 60 is a rarity. It is equally seen in both sexes. There is no genetic predilection. It is sporadic.

The attack is acute and may be preceded by pain in the ear. The most common presentation is as follows: The child gets up from sleep with unilateral watering and an inability to close the affected eye. Pain in the ear may be present. Parents are invariably associated with exposure to the cold. In 2–3 days, the condition assumes a full-blown picture of classical Bell's palsy, which involves both the upper and lower half of the ipsilateral face. The features can be put into three groups: Static, dynamic, and visceral signs.

The static signs are those signs that pertain to the face. They are:

- Flattening of the frontal furrow
- Flattening of the eyebrow
- Wide IPA
- Difficulty in closing the lids
- Mild ectropion of the ipsilateral lower lid
- Drooping of the angle of the mouth
- Shifting of the contralateral angle of the mouth to the other side
- Flattening of the nasolabial and infraorbital creases
- Drooling of saliva
- No loss of sensation
- Normal movement of the other muscles than orbicularis
- Conjunctival congestion
- Exposure keratitis

The dynamic signs are:

- Inability to close the lids
- Intact Bell's phenomenon
- Inability to whistle
- Inability to frown
- Inability to blow the cheek

The visceral signs consist of:

- Diminished tear and saliva production
- In spite of the hypoproduction of tears, there is watering in the affected eye—both epiphora and lacrimation. The former is due to improper drainage of tears; the latter is secondary to exposure to keratitis and exposure conjunctivitis.
- In the long run, the conjunctiva can get keratinized and may develop xerotic spots.

Etiology

The exact cause of Bell's palsy in children is obscure. The commonly proposed causes are viral infection, post-vaccination status, and autoimmune disorders. The lesion lies in the peripheral facial nerve as it courses through the facial canal. The pathology causes edema in the nerve substance. This causes throttling of the nerve in a narrow, rigid bony canal. The condition is self-limiting. It passes off gradually, leaving no trace in most of the cases in 2–3 months. However, in a small percentage of cases,

---

**Melkersson-Rosenthal* syndrome is a neuromusculocutaneous congenital disorder in children. In adults, it may be acquired. The classical features are:

- Recurrent bilateral peripheral facial palsy
- Puffiness of the face
- Swelling of the upper lid
- Fissured tongue (Lingua plicata)

†*Guillain-Barré syndrome:* The exact cause is not known. It manifests days after a systemic bacterial infection or vaccination. It is a neurological cause due to an autoimmune disorder that involves peripheral nerves. Ocular features consist of bilateral facial palsies.

‡*Goldenhar syndrome:* Goldenhar syndrome is a rare congenital condition characterized by abnormal development of the eye, ear, and spine. It is also known as oculo-auriculo-vertebral syndrome.

full recovery is not attained. Such cases should undergo a detailed neurological workup. Bell's palsy in children in their late teens should be watched for nonimprovement and investigated for myasthenia, otitis media, pontine glioma, and posterior fossa neuroma. Rarely, direct trauma to the lateral orbital rim and mastoid may present as unilateral orbicularis palsy and be mistaken for Bell's palsy.

Management of Bell's Palsy in Children

There is no specific treatment for Bell's palsy because:

- The exact cause of the disorder is not known.
- There is no effective antimicrobial drug to cure it.
- Anti-inflammatory drugs have not proven to be effective.
- The role of steroids is questionable.
- The disorder has a self-limiting course.

The methods employed to manage Bell's palsy are only ameliorative. Their purpose is to relieve symptoms and prevent complications. The complications are:

- Exposure keratitis, which may get converted into frank corneal ulcer with its usual complications
- Exposure conjunctivitis
- Dryness of the conjunctiva
- Keratinization of the ocular surface
- Unpleasant watering

The methods used are:

- Assurance about its benignness
- Prevent local infection by frequent broad-spectrum antibiotic drops by day and ointment of the same antibiotic at night.
- Lubricant in gel form
- Lids may be sutured by a simple stitch or temporary tarsorrhaphy may be done.
- Corneal ulcers, when present, should be treated by the usual, accepted methods.
- Considered physiotherapy to improve the function of the orbicularis by:
  - Monophasic electrical stimulation
  - Physiotherapy by a specially trained physiotherapist

Both of the above have not been found to give uniform good results.

Lid Retraction

The normal upper lid covers the superior 2.00 mm of cornea, and the lower lid just touches the periphery of the lower pole of the cornea. Thus, no part of the sclera above or below is visible when the child looks straight ahead. The upper lid follows the globe as it looks down. Failure of the upper lid to follow the globe in downward movement is called lid lag. Similarly, if a normal child looks straight, the upper lid keeps the upper 2.00 mm covered. Any exposure of the strip of sclera above or below is designated as lid retraction **(Figs. 10.26 to 10.28)**.

The lid retraction is mostly acquired. Rarely can it be present at birth, passing within a few weeks of birth. In spite of the lid retraction, the child retains the action of the orbicularis in such a situation. This is considered physiological. Such widening of the IPA is more common in preterm babies. A newborn may widen the IPA if the ambient light is suddenly switched off. Lid retraction can be true or false. The true lid retraction is caused by overaction of the retractors of the upper lid. The lid retraction can be unilateral or bilateral. Bilateral retractions need not be symmetric **(Fig. 10.28)**.

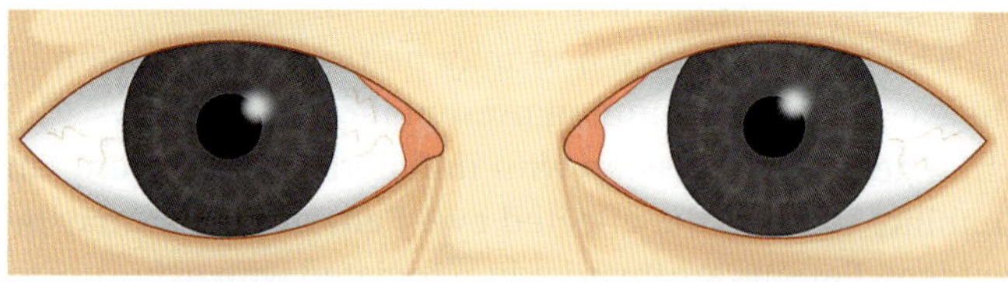

Fig. 10.26: Normal eye—upper lid covering 2.00 mm of upper cornea and touching lower limbus.

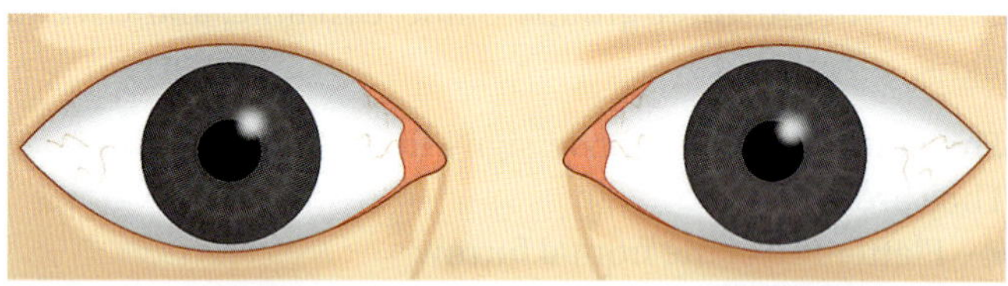

Fig. 10.27: Bilateral lid retraction showing 2.00 mm bare sclera above and 1.00 mm bare sclera below.

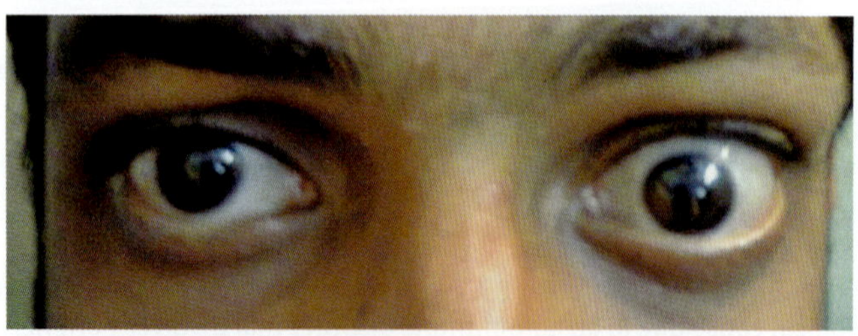

Fig. 10.28: Bilateral asymmetric lid retraction in thyroid eye disease.

The causes of lid retraction at all ages are:

- Myogenic
- Neurogenic
- Mechanical
- Pathological

Proptosis gives the appearance of pseudo-lid retraction; such retraction does not always show the baring of the sclera that is present in true lid retraction. The eyeball is extruded out of the socket, depending on the cause. Contralateral ptosis may give an appearance of lid retraction during the initial days of neurogenic ptosis when an attempt to lift the ptotic lid results in ipsilateral lid retraction. Similarly, in the initial days of weakness of the orbicularis, it may be mistaken for lid retraction.

Neurological causes of lid retraction are:

- Closed head injury
- Dorsal mid-brain lesion (Parinaud syndrome–Collier sign)
- Markus Gunn syndrome
- *Hydrocephalus:* Sunset sign
- Bulbar poliomyelitis
- Encephalitis
- Aberrant regeneration of the third nerve (not seen in children).
- Cyclic third nerve palsy (not seen in children).

Therapeutic causes of lid retraction:

- *Local:*
  - Phenylephrine
  - Apraclonidine
- *Systemic:*
  - Prostigmin (diagnostic and therapeutic)
  - Tensilon (diagnostic)
  - Thyroid extract to the mother suffering from hyperthyroidism at the time of delivery

Myogenic causes are:

- Congenital lid retraction
- Grave ophthalmoplegia (rare in children)
- Congenital hyperthyroidism
- *Post-traumatic:*
  - Surgical overcorrection of ptosis
  - Excess of superior and inferior rectus recession
  - Surgical coloboma of the upper lid following entropion correction
  - Accidental avulsion of the lid

Mechanical causes are:

- Proptosis
- Exophthalmos
- Postinflammatory scar
- *Post-trauma:*
  - Thermal burn
  - Acid/alkali burn
  - Radiation

Pathological Causes of Lid Retraction

Barring mechanical lid retraction in proptosis, all causes are nonocular. The nonocular causes can be myogenic or neurogenic. Examples of myogenic lid retraction are thyroid eye diseases caused by sympathetic stimulation of Müller's muscle, the exact cause of which is not known. The lid retraction may be enhanced by the instillation of sympathomimetic drugs and reduced by the instillation of sympatholytic drugs. Lid retraction in thyroid eye disease is generally bilateral and symmetric. The features of sympathetic lid retraction are just the reverse of sympathetic underaction, as seen in Horner's syndrome, i.e., mild ptosis, upside-down ptosis, enophthalmos, and miosis.

The features of sympathetic lid retraction are:

- Widening of IPA
- Deepening of the supratarsal crease
- Dilated pupil
- Mild exophthalmos
- Visible sclera above and below the cornea

The neurological causes of lid retraction are: Midbrain signs, when put together, are designated as Collier signs that consist of bilateral lid retraction, convergence deficiency, conjugated up gaze, retraction nystagmus, and dissociated light reflex.

Clinical Presentation

Patients with mild, bilaterally symmetrical lid retraction may not be aware of the conditions and may even deny their presence when pointed. Newborns who are especially premature may be brought on with periodic lid retraction. The sunset sign is a prominent sign in hydrocephalus; otherwise, a child with lid retraction may have a staring appearance. Exposure to the globe may lead to watering, foreign body sensations, and redness. All older children with lid retraction should be investigated for thyroid disease and retrobulbar mass.

Management

There is no specific treatment for lid retraction except for the management of systemic conditions. Surgical treatment consists of the weakening of the levator and Müller's muscles. Local lubricant drops and gels frequently help the child.

Apraxia Lid

It is a rare neurological nonparalytic disorder of the upper lid seen mostly in adults. When present in children, it may be confused with a psychosomatic disorder. The cause is the suppression of the levator that opens the lid with the activation of the orbicularis. The patient is unable to initiate the opening of the lid. The lids are to be separated manually. The patient throws the head back, and the brows are arched as in complete ptosis. However, the lids may sometimes open suddenly on command. In between the episodes of underaction of the levator, the structure and function of the lid are normal without ptosis or blepharospasm. It is confirmed by electrophysiological tests.

Myoclonus

Myoclonus of the lid or lid myoclonia is the most common form of seizure, with repeated jerks of the lids with the eyeball rolling up.

Lid Twitch

- Stress
- Fatigue
- Eye strain
- Dry eyes
- Allergy

Blepharospasm

Blepharospasm is the involuntary, bilateral, forceful closure of both the lids simultaneously. It is divided into two broad classes. The first more frequent is called primary or peripheral blepharospasm, without any neurological importance. The reflex is initiated following irritation of peripheral sensory twigs of the fifth nerve, it is generally associated with photophobia. It is commonly seen in children. The most common cause of reflex blepharospasm in children is phlyctenular keratoconjunctivitis. The other causes are corneal foreign bodies, corneal abrasion, corneal ulcer, interstitial keratitis, buphthalmos, hydrops of the cornea, ultraviolet keratitis as seen in welding, arc burn, snow blindness, and anterior uveitis. The reflex blepharospasm can be abolished by local instillation of anesthetic agents; the exact path of the phenomenon is not well established. Secondary, or central, blepharospasm is not seen in children. It is called essential blepharospasm.

Blepharoclonus

Blepharoclonus is a rhythmic closure of the eyelid of uncertain origin, that could be central, peripheral, or psychological. It is not to be confused with tic, which is mostly functional and seen in children; the condition is self-limited.

SUGGESTED READING

1. Allen C, Rubin P. Blepharophimosis-Ptosis-Epicanthis Inversus Syndrome (BPES): Clinical Manifestation and Treatment. Int Ophthalmol Clin. 2008;48(2):15-23.
2. Baldwin H, Manners R. Congenital Blepharoptosis. Ophthal Plast Reconstr Surg. 2002;18(4):301-7.
3. Beard C. Müller's superior tarsal muscle: anatomy, physiology, and clinical significance. Ann Plast Surg. 1985; 14:324-33.
4. Beard C. "Congenital Ptosis" in Ptosis. St. Louis, MO: CV Mosby Company; 1976. pp. 91-115.
5. Berke R. The surgical correction of congenital ptosis. Trans Pa Acad Ophthalmol Otolaryngol. 1961;14:57-61.
6. Berke RN. Results of resection of the levator muscle through a skin incision in congenital ptosis. AMA Arch Ophthalmol. 1959;61(2):177-201.
7. Cherian V, Foroozan R. Benign unilateral apraxia of eyelid opening. Ophthalmology. 2010;117(6):1265-8.
8. Daily RA. Epicanthus in Current Ocular Therapy, 5th Edition, Editors Fraund-Felder FJ, Roy F. Hampton-WB Saunders, Philadelphia; 2000.
9. Glatt HJ, Putterman AM, Fett DR. Comparison of 2.5% and 10% phenylephrine in the elevation of upper eyelids with ptosis. Ophthalmic Surg. 1990;21:114-22.
10. Grover AK, Bageja S, Chandrakar N. (2021). Ten Tips for the Beginner to Examine a Patient of Ptosis. [online] Available from https://www.eophtha.com/posts/ten-tips-for-the-beginner-to-examine-a-patient-of-ptosis [Last accessed February, 2025].
11. Harley RD. Abnormalities of Lid Function in Pediatric Ophthalmology, Vol. II, 2nd edition. Philadelphia: WB Saunders; 1983. pp. 807-14.
12. Jebasingh YK, Menon KB, Jawahar M, Gobinathan S, Balasubramanian S, Shanbhogue KR. Apraxia of lid opening. Ann Indian Acad Neurol. 2006;9:163-5.

13. Kearsey C, Fernando P, D'Costa D, Ferdinand P. The use of the ice pack test in myasthenia gravis. JRSM Short Rep. 2010;1(1):14.
14. Kim JY, Park KD, Richman DP. Treatment of myasthenia gravis is based on its immunopathogenesis. J Clin Neurol. 2011;7(4):173-83.
15. Lee MJ, Oh JY, Choung HK, Kim NJ, Sung MS, Khwarg SI. Frontalis Sling Operation using a silicone rod compared with preserved fascia lata for congenital ptosis. Ophthalmology. 2009;116(1):123-9.
16. Mirzai H, Baser E. Congenital Horners' syndrome and the usefulness of the apraclonidine test in its diagnosis. Indian J Ophthalmol. 2006;54:197-9.
17. Mukherjee PK, Dongre RC. A case of acquired facial diplegia, macular oedema, and lingua plicata ("Melkersson-Rosenthal syndrome"). Indian J Ophthalmol. 1973;21: 36-9.
18. Mukherjee PK. Clinical Examination in Ophthalmology, 2nd edition, Gurgaon (India): Elsevier; 2016.
19. Mukherjee PK. Essentials of Neuroophthalmology, 1st edition. New Delhi: Jaypee Brothers; 2010.
20. Mukherjee PK. Ophthalmic Assistant, 1st edition. New Delhi: Jaypee Brothers; 2013.
21. Nair AG, Patil-Chhablani P, Venkatramani DV, Gandhi RA. Ocular myasthenia gravis: a review. Indian J Ophthalmol. 2014;62(10):985-91.
22. Satyakaran. Lid Retraction in Step-by-Step Neurophthalmology: Clinical Examination and Diagnosis, 1st edition. New Delhi: Jaypee Brothers; 2006. pp. 183-8.
23. Singhal BS, Bhatia NS, Umesh T, Menon S. Myasthenia gravis: a study from India. Neurol India. 2008;56(3):352-5.
24. Verity DH, Priscilla Mathewson. Ptosis in the Moorfields Manual of Ophthalmology; Third Edition, Ed. Timothy L. Jackson, JP Medical Publisher, New Delhi (2020).

CHAPTER 11

Disorders of Orbit in Children

Before discussing disorders of the orbits, it is better to recapitulate applied anatomy and the development of orbits.

APPLIED ANATOMY OF THE ORBIT

Orbits are two spaces, one on each side of the nose. The bones of the face and skull surround it from all sides except the front. Each orbit has an appearance of a truncated pyramid with a circular base anteriorly and an apex toward the cranium. The base is more circular in children than in adults. It is worth noting that the widest part of the orbit is not the actual rim but a few millimeters behind it*; this corresponds to the maximum diameter of the globe. The medial walls of the two orbits are parallel to each other; the distance between the two walls in adults is 25.00 mm. An increased distance between the two walls is called teleorbitism. The lateral walls are inclined to each other and, if projected backward, meet at imaginary points in the cranium, forming an angle of 90° with each other. The term exorbitism is occasionally used to denote the protrusion of the eyeball due to a lack of orbital space.

The relation of the orbital walls is: The roof is under the anterior cranial fossa and the frontal sinus, the floor lies above the maxillary sinus; the medial wall is formed by the walls of the sphenoidal, ethmoidal sinus and middle cranial fossa. Outside the lateral wall are the temporalis and middle cranial fossa.

The following diagrams show the bones that form the walls of the orbit and the various fissures and foramina of the orbit **(Fig. 11.1)**.

Imaginary outline of orbits:

1. Frontal
2. Sphenoid
3. Zygomatic
4. Maxillary
5. Ethmoid

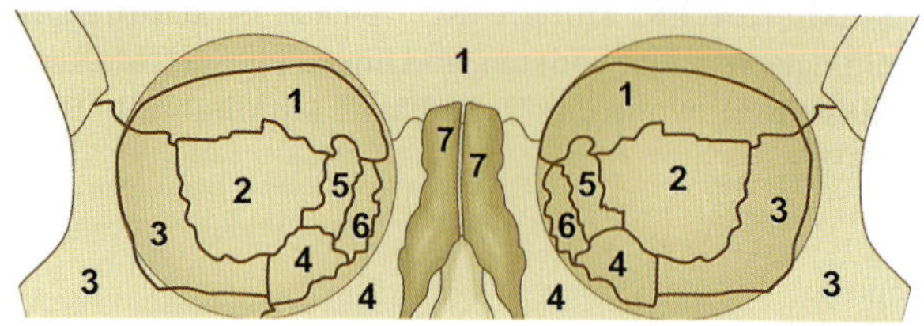

Fig. 11.1: Various bones forming orbit as seen from the front.

6. Lacrimal
7. Nasal (not a part of the orbit, palatine is not shown)

Clockwise, the rim is divided into four segments: (1) Superior, (2) medial, (3) inferior, and (4) lateral. The first is formed solely by the frontal bone; the others are formed by two bones each. The medial rim is formed by the lacrimal and maxillary bone; the inferior rim is formed by the maxilla along with the zygomatic bone; the lateral rim is formed by the zygomatic and the frontal.

Weak spots on the rim of the orbit: The sutures on the orbital rim are relatively weak spots and are likely to break under pressure, direct or indirect. These are: Frontomaxillary, zygomaticomaxillary, and frontozygomatic sutures; the last is the most frequent suture to be affected. Similarly, the weakest bone in the orbit is the ethmoid, but the most common site to suffer a blow-out fracture is the posterior medial part of the floor.

WALLS, FISSURES, AND FORAMEN OF ORBIT

Each orbit is formed by the following bones of various sizes and thickness:

- Frontal
- Sphenoid
- Lacrimal

**The rim of the orbit:* All the bones that constitute the walls of the orbit do not participate in forming the rim topographically; the rim is divided into four parts without any specific line of demarcation.

- Ethmoid
- Maxilla
- Zygomatic
- Palatine

The orbit lies above the maxillary sinus and below the anterior cranial fossa; the medial wall is formed by the lacrimal, palatine, ethmoid, and sphenoid bones. The frontal sinuses are situated in the frontal bone above. The orbits are surrounded by air sinuses from all sides except the lateral. The orbital surface of the paranasal sinuses (PNSs) is as thin as paper; virulent microorganisms can traverse the paper-thin bones of the paranasal (paraorbital) sinuses, especially the ethmoid sinuses.

Some of the PNSs are present at birth. The others develop later and grow slowly. Early to develop are the maxillary and ethmoidal sinuses. At birth, they are filled with fluid, which is later replaced by air over the years; by the seventh year, the fluid is fully replaced by air, and the sinuses reach adult size. The frontal sinuses are last to develop and remain smaller than adult size up to adolescence. The maxillary sinus is the largest and the sphenoidal smallest. The orbit communicates with the brain through the superior and inferior orbital fissures and the orbital apex. The blood vessels and nerves travel through these portals from the brain to the orbit.

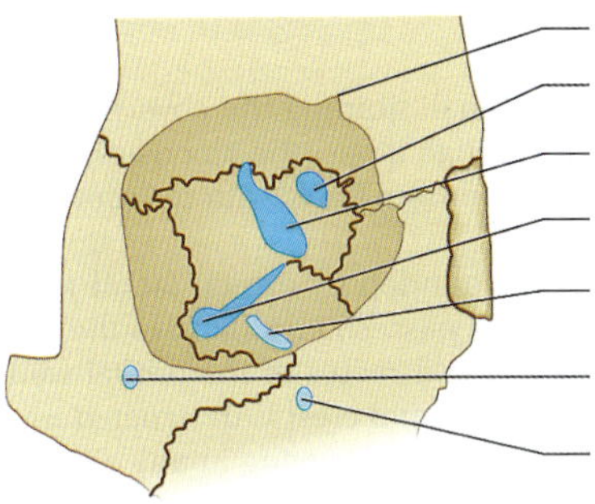

Fig. 11.2: Sutures, fissures, and foramens of the orbit.

Figure 11.2 shows various sutures, fissures, and foramens of the orbit.

Superior Orbital Fissure

This is a space that looks like an inverted comma between the roof and the lateral wall of the orbit. It is bounded by the greater and lesser wings of the sphenoid, and the annulus of Zinn sits astride the fissure, i.e., a part above an inside and the other outside the circle. The fissure communicates with the middle cranial fossa. Through it pass lacrimal, frontal, trochlear nerves and ophthalmic veins **(Fig. 11.3)**.

Inferior Orbital Fissure

This is an elongated gap below the superior orbital fissure, extending laterally. It is formed superiorly by the greater wing of the sphenoid; the inferior border is formed by the maxilla, palatine, and zygomatic bones. Through it pass the maxillary division, trigeminal nerve, zygomatic nerve, and inferior ophthalmic vein **(Fig. 11.3)**.

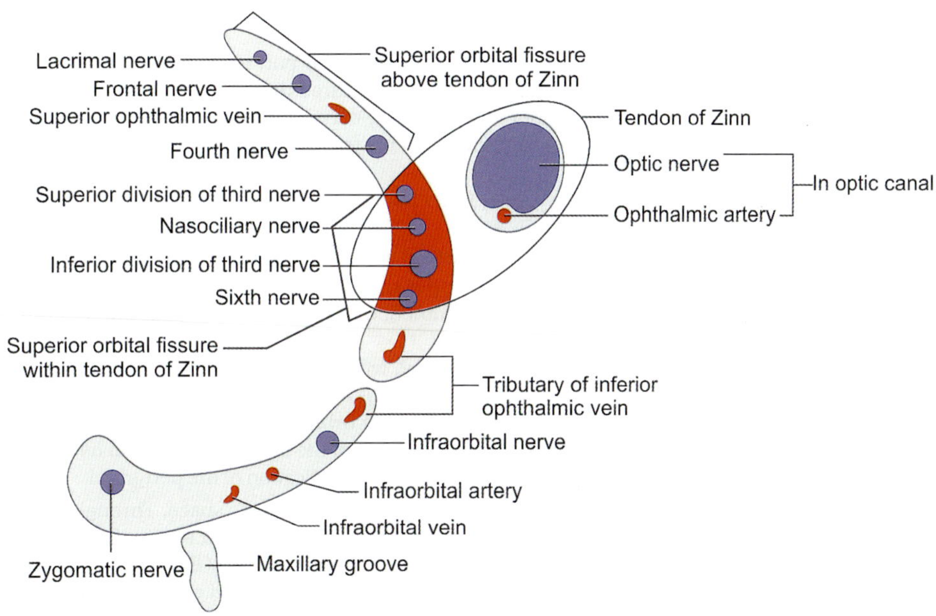

Fig. 11.3: Orbital fissures with their content.

Orbital Apex

The orbital apex is where the bones of the orbit meet, it is the posterior most part of the orbit, and it is a junction of orbit and cranium. Through it pass the nerves and vessels from the cranium to the orbit. The extraocular muscles except the inferior oblique take their origin from this area. As this is a small area through which important vessels and nerves pass, any disorder at this level causes multiple cranial nerve palsies, singly or in combination. The optic foramen is nasal to the orbital apex, through which the optic nerve passes from the orbit to the brain. The superior orbital fissure is lateral to the apex **(Fig. 11.4)**.

The contents of orbits are: The eyeball is the most important and largest single content of the orbit; it is covered by Tenon's capsule* and attached with the extraocular muscles, blood vessels, and nerves. The optic nerve traverses between the optic foramen and the back of the globe. The orbital fat surrounds the globe all round, and the ciliary ganglion† lies in the orbital fat. The walls are lined by periorbita. The orbital septum‡ divides the orbit into two unequal parts, i.e., a small preseptal and a large retroseptal.

Surgical Spaces of the Orbit

The orbit is divided into five surgical spaces: Three potential and two apparent. The former are the periorbital, subtenon, and subarachnoid spaces. The remaining are intra- and extraconal spaces. The spaces have great clinical importance; they help in restraining infection, inflammation, and neoplasms until their boundaries are breached. The involvement of each space has specific significance **(Figs. 11.6 and 11.7)**.

Periorbital Space

This is the most peripheral surgical space of the orbit; it is a potential space between the bony wall and its

---

**Tenon's capsules:* Tenon's capsule is a thin fascia that extends from the limbus to the back of the eyeball, joining the covering of the optic nerve. At the limbus, it merges with subconjunctival and episcleral tissue to form a strong bond. Through it pass the blood vessels and nerves. It merges with the fascia of extraocular muscle, the sclera lies within the capsule; and the capsule moves freely with the movement of the eye.

The space between the capsule and the sclera is called Tenon's space§, the Tenon's capsule is surrounded by orbital fat all-round, and the Tenon capsule is converted into a tube-like, ill-defined structure in which the extraocular muscle passes like a hand in the glove. The capsule sends extensions beyond muscles and called ligaments. The lateral extension from the lateral rectus to the orbital wall is called the lateral ligament, which acts as a check ligament. The extension from the medial rectus to the lacrimal crest is designated as the medial check ligament. The function of the check ligaments is to give stability to the globe, preventing it from sagging in any direction, and they also prevent excessive movement of the globe.

The extension from the sheath of the medial rectus is fused to the extension of the aponeurosis of the levator palpebral superior. Similarly, an extension from the inferior rectus is attached to the poorly developed lower palpebral ligament. The expansion from the superior oblique is attached to the trochlea. The expansions from the lateral and medial recti are joined by extensions from two obliques to form a hammock-like sling called the Lockwood ligament.

†*Ciliary ganglion:* Ciliary ganglion is an important ganglion situated at the posterior part of the orbit, in front of the apex between the optic nerve and the lateral rectus. The ophthalmic artery is lateral to it. It has three roots, i.e., parasympathetic from the third nerve, sympathetic from the cervical sympathetic, and sensory root from the nasociliary nerve **(Fig. 11. 5)**.

The parasympathetic root, also known as the motor root, supplies the constrictor pupillae and ciliary body. Paralysis of this causes mydriasis and cycloplegia.

The sympathetic roots supply dilators, pupillae, and blood vessels. Its paralysis causes miosis. It reaches the ciliary ganglion through the long ciliary nerve.

‡*Orbital septum:* This is a strong elastic tissue that spreads across the orbital rims with a window called the interpalpebral fissure. It starts from the periorbita, in the upper part, it ends 10–15 mm above the upper tarsus plate and merges with the aponeurosis of the levator. In the inferior part, it gets attached to the inferior capsulopalpebral ligament of the lower lids. It ends about 6 mm away from the lower tarsal plate.

It divides the orbit into two spaces. The anterior space is called preseptal, while the other is called retroseptal. The former is shallower than the latter and contains orbicularis muscle covered by the skin of the lids. It is devoid of fat but capable of accumulating a large amount of inflammatory fluid and blood. The retroseptal space houses the rest of the orbital contents, with the largest bulk being orbital fat. The space is also capable of accumulating fluid, air, and deposits. The importance of the orbital septum is in its ability to prevent the spread of infection and inflammation from one space to the other. It is presumed to be a modification of the periorbita.

§*Tenon's space:* The potential space between Tenon's capsule and the sclera is called Tenon's space. Through which pass the tendons of the extraocular muscle before they are attached to the sclera. It is traversed by ciliary vessels and nerves, from the cranium to the eyeball, the venae vorticosae travel back through this space. The space normally does not contain any fluid but may accumulate inflammatory fluid in it. The accumulation of fluid in the posterior part pushes the eyeball forward. The space is used to give anterior and posterior sub-Tenon's injections of antibiotics, steroids, and anesthetic agents.

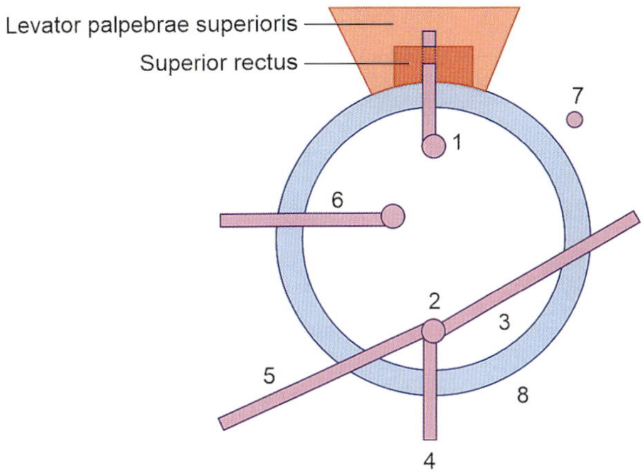

The upper division of the third nerve supplies the superior rectus and levator palpebrae superioris[a].

- Lower division of the third nerve
- Branch of the lower division of the third nerve supplying the medial rectus
- Branch of the lower division of the third nerve supplying the inferior rectus
- Branch of the lower division of the third nerve supplying the inferior oblique
- The sixth nerve supplying the lateral rectus
- Fourth nerve
- Imaginary line showing the orbital apex

Fig. 11.4: Distribution of the cranial nerve at the orbital apex.ww
Note: [a]The levator palpebrae superioris gets its motor nerve supply from the upper division of the third nerve after it has passed through the superior rectus **(Fig. 11.4)**.

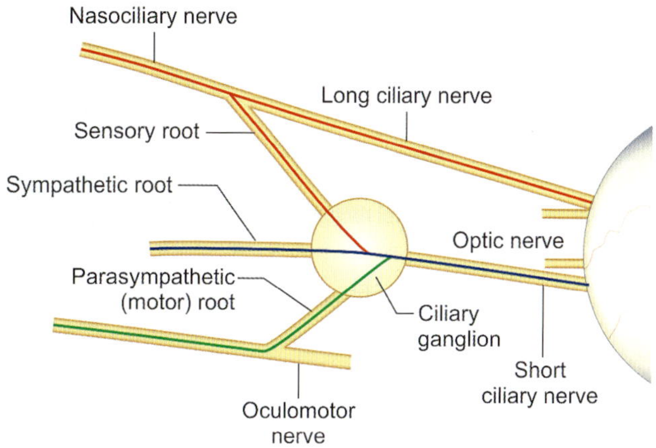

Fig. 11.5: Connections of ciliary ganglion.

periosteal covering*. The accumulation of blood and pus and the presence of a tumor elevate it from its attachment, making a bulge toward the orbital cavities. This pushes the eyeball away from the swelling. The tumors can either be benign or malignant. They are tumors arising from the bones of the orbit, leukemia deposits, dermoids, meningiomas, and mucoceles arising from various PNSs. The other common fluid to accumulate is blood. The diagnosis is confirmed by computed tomography (CT) and magnetic resonance imaging (MRI).

The following structure passes through the ring: The optic nerve, the oculomotor nerve, the abducens nerve, and the nasociliary nerve. The trochlear nerve travels outside the ring and is hence not anesthetized following retrobulbar injection of an anesthetic agent **(Fig. 11.8)**.

Peripheral Space

This is an apparent space between the periosteum and the muscle cone and is bounded anteriorly by the septum orbital, tarsal plates, tarsal ligament, and aponeurosis of the levator. The frontal, lacrimal, and ethmoidal nerves pass through this space. The most important structures to pass through these spaces are the superior and inferior ophthalmic veins. The superior ophthalmic vein, due to its constant position, is used in orbital venography.

---

*The periosteum covering the bones of the orbit is commonly referred to as the periorbita; it is continuous with the periosteum of the face and forehead; it is loosely attached to the bony wall of the orbit with a potential space in between; it accepts round the edges of the superior and inferior orbital fussers, the optic foramen. At the edges of the optic foramen, it mingles with the covering of the optic nerve, anteriorly and continues as the dural covering of the optic nerve; leaving a subdural space all round the nerve. Posteriorly, it enters the cranium through the optic foramina to merge with the intracranial durra. At the anterior inferior rim of the orbit, it splits to form the lacrimal fascia. At the superomedial border of the rim, it is modified to form the trochlea; the other modifications of the periorbita are the orbital septum, common tendon of Zinn[†], suspensory ligament of Lockwood[‡], medial and lateral ligaments of the orbit.

[†]*Common tendon of Zinn:* This is a fibrous circular structure formed by condensation of periorbita at the apex of the orbit. It straddles across the superior orbital fissure. From the ring arise the four recti. The superior oblique originates outside the ring. The inferior oblique takes its origin from the inferior orbital rim.

[‡]*Suspensory ligament of Lockwood:* This is a blending of the sheaths of the inferior oblique and inferior rectus muscles, resulting in a thickened fascial structure. That forms a hammock under the globe, extending from the medial canthal ligament to the lateral orbital tubercle. It is formed by the fusion of the capsulopalpebral fascial sheaths in front of the inferior oblique muscle. The function of the ligament is to prevent the globe from sagging down in the absence of the floor of the orbit.

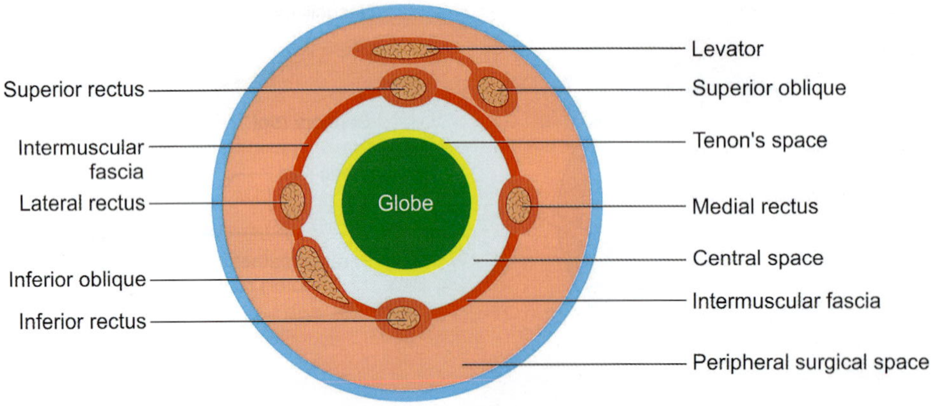

Fig. 11.6: Various surgical spaces in the coronal plane.

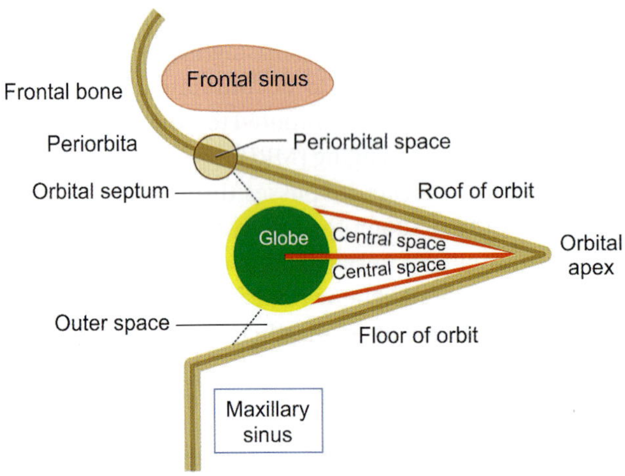

Fig. 11.7: Various surgical spaces in the sagittal plane.

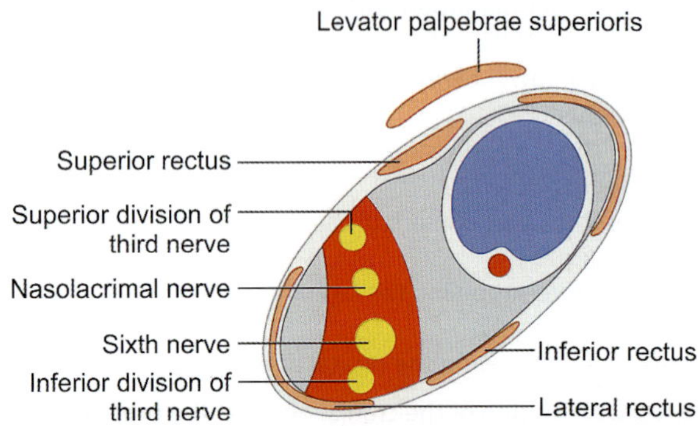

Fig. 11.8: Relation of origins of extraocular muscles, optic canal, the second part of the superior orbital fissure, and nerve in it in the circle of Zinn. The obliques do not originate from the circle of Zinn.

The *orbital venography** is used to differentiate between intraconal and extraconal lesions. The space contains superior and inferior oblique muscles, which, in contrast to the four recti, do not participate in forming the muscle cone of the orbit. The lacrimal gland lies on the superotemporal periphery of the space, the space continues with the posterior part of the central cone. Any growth or fluid accumulating in the space pushes the eyeball away from the mass; it may push the eyeball forward as well. It is best seen on CT and MRI. It is best explored by transnasal endoscopy.

Central Space

This is a visible conical space surrounded by four recti and their intramuscular attachments. The apex of the cone is toward the apex of the orbit, and the base is formed by the posterior surface of the globe. The space bound by the extraocular muscles and their septa is called the intraconal space, and the space outside the cone is called the

**Orbital venography* is an imaging technique to differentiate between intraconal and extraconal lesions by injecting a radiopaque die in the frontal vein, followed by a series of X-rays. Simple orbital venography is no more in vogue and has been replaced by MRI venography and CT venography. The principle behind the technique lies in the fact that the superior ophthalmic vein is one of the veins with a constant position sufficient to be considered a surgical landmark. When injected with a radio opaque dye, it forms a parallelogram in the axial view of imaging. Changes in the shape of the parallelogram are utilized to differentiate intra- and extraconal growths. In an intraconal lesion, the angle of the parallelogram is more obtuse and said to be open. The second and third parts of the ophthalmic vein are raised in an extraconal lesion; when the angle of the parallelogram is 90°, it is called a closed or collapsed parallelogram. Orbital varices, cavernous hemangioma, neurofibroma, and malignant growths may show abnormal branching from the ophthalmic veins.

extraconal space. As the attachments of the muscles are deficient at the posterior part of the cone, the boundaries between the two spaces are lost at this region. The optic nerve traverses from the apex of the orbit to the back of the globe, and the following structures also pass through: The space-long and short posterior ciliary nerves and veins; the ciliary ganglion with its roots and ciliary nerves; the two divisions of the third nerve; the nasociliary and ophthalmic arteries; the space inside the cone and outside the cone is filled with orbital fat. The growth arising from any of the structures inside the cone will result in axial proptosis. The most common growth in children is glioma of the optic nerve, followed by capillary hemangioma. Meningioma is rare in children; in adults, meningioma outnumbers the glioma of childhood.

> It was previously thought that there is no formed lymphatic in orbit. It is now thought to be otherwise, and there is evidence of presence of lymphatics in orbit.

For Development of Orbits and Orbit at Birth (*See* Chapters 2 and 4).

CONGENITAL ANOMALIES OF THE ORBIT

From the above, it is clear that congenital anomalies of orbits are common; some so mild that they are considered to be within normal limits, and neither the parents nor the child complain about them.

They can be put under the following groups:

- Craniofacial malformation
- *New growths:*
  - Hamartoma—hemangioma, neurofibroma, and lymphangiomas
  - Choristomas—dermoid, epidermoid, and teratoma
- *Herniation of brain and its covering in orbit:*
  - Meningocele
  - Meningoencephalocele
- *Developmental defect of eyeball:*
  - Microphthalmos
  - Anophthalmos
- *Position of orbit in relation to midline*:
  - Hypertelorism
  - Hypotelorism
- Miscellaneous

Craniofacial Malformation

Craniofacial malformations have been classified in various ways.

They can be:

- Those associated with proptosis, i.e., oxycephaly, Crouzon syndrome, and Apert syndrome
- Those without proptosis

Both can be with ocular involvement and without ocular involvement.

The common conditions with ocular involvement are:

- *Craniofacial dysostosis:*
  - Crouzon syndrome
  - Apert syndrome
- *Branchial arch syndromes (mandibulofacial dysostosis):*
  - Treacher-Collin syndrome
  - Franceschetti syndrome
  - Goldenhar syndrome
  - Hallermann-Streiff syndrome
  - Pierre-Robin syndrome
- Median cleft face syndrome.

The congenital anomalies of the skull influence congenital anomalies of the orbit by way of premature fusion of the cranial suture, which may be at the base or the apex. The sutures are coronal, sagittal, lambdoid, and frontal **(Fig. 11.9)**.

> The premature fusions of cranial sutures are called craniostenosis/craniosynostosis, for clinical purpose they are considered to be interchangeable.

Closure of:

- Sagittal sutures result in scaphocephaly, which results in a narrow, long, keel-shaped skull. This is the most common form of craniostenosis.
- Coronal suture results in brachycephaly, which results in skull with short, broad, flat forehead.

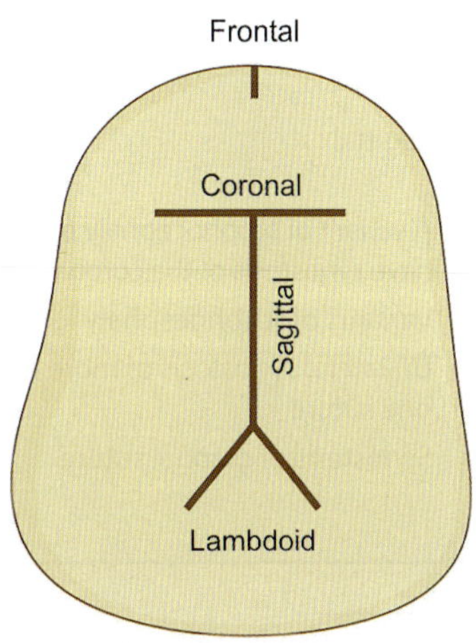

Fig. 11.9: Diagram showing various cranial sutures seen from above.

Flat head syndrome (plagiocephaly) can be congenital or acquired; neither of them causes ocular or brain damage or retarded growth. The back of the skull is flat; the flattening is more on one side, generally with anomalies of the ipsilateral orbit, which is pushed upward, and the maxilla. The ears are pushed anteriorly. The acquired form is seen in infants who habitually sleep on the occiput.

Fusion of the frontal suture hardly causes any orbital deformity.

Other deformities of ophthalmic interest are dolichocephaly, trigonocephaly, microcephaly, and hydrocephalus.

> The premature closures of cranial sutures are based on Virchow's law, which says that.
> "During craniosynostosis, skull growth is restricted to a plane perpendicular to the affected, prematurely fused suture and is enhanced in a plane parallel to it."

The other points worth noting in craniostenosis are:

- The growth of the cranium depends on the growth of the brain.
- The shape of the orbit is influenced by the shape of the skull.
- The brain grows most rapidly during the first 6 months after birth.
- The growth of the brain is complete by the second year.
- The fontanelles get closed after 18 months.
- The closure of the fontanelle is caused by the growth of bones from the periphery.
- Sutures do not fuse fully till puberty.

Table 11.1 shows a summary of craniostenosis of ophthalmic interest.

Hydrocephalus

Hydrocephalus is a condition of too much cerebrospinal fluid (CSF) in the ventricles, either due to obstruction in the circulation of normally produced CSF or excess production of CSF, as in choroidal plexus papilloma (rare). Hydrocephalus can either be congenital or acquired. The congenital causes are aqueductal stenosis, **Dandy Walker syndrome*, encephalocele, and meningoencephalocele. Common acquired causes are mostly infections, i.e., tubercular meningitis or other bacterial meningitis, and intraventricular and extraventricular tumors.

It creates a situation that is the opposite of craniosynostosis. In hydrocephalus, the cranial sutures open up,

TABLE 11.1: Craniostenosis of ophthalmic interest.

Type	*Sutures closed*	*Shape of the skull*	*Ocular changes*
Oxycephaly	All coronary sutures show maximum synostosis	Vertically elongated	Shallow orbit, bilateral proptosis, dislocation of the globe ±, squint, both concomitant or restrictive, nystagmus, diminished vision, papilledema, and optic atrophy
Hypertelorism	None	No change in the skull, and the intraorbital distance is wider than normal	No specific finding except pseudo divergent squint, diminished vision ±
Microcephaly	All	Smaller than normal compared to face receding of for head, high vertex flat occiput	Microphthalmia, microcornea, coloboma of the uvea, and cataract
Scaphocephaly	Sagittal	Anteroposteriorly elongated and narrow transversely	No specific change
Brachycephaly	A variant of scaphocephaly may have synostosis of the coronal suture	Same as above	No specific change
Dolichocephaly	Variants of scaphocephaly	Same as above	No specific change
Plagiocephaly	Unilateral synostosis of more than one suture	Unilateral slant of the skull	Congenital cataract
Trigonocephaly	Synostosis of coronal suture	Poorly developed for head, excessively developed posterior half of skull	Hypotelorism and optic atrophy

**Dandy-Walker syndrome:* Dandy Walker syndrome is caused by congenital anomalies of the cerebellum. The cerebellum fails to develop normally and may remain small or partially developed. Resulting in retardation of growth, flaccid muscle/spasticity of muscles, ataxia, and enlargement of the head due to the associated hydrocephalus.

causing expansion and thinning of the skull bones. The clinical picture of hydrocephalus depends on the age of onset and the cause.

Hydrocephalus can be one of the following: Communication and noncommunication. The first has an obstruction outside the ventricle, and the second is inside.

The clinical picture also depends on the extent of the closure of the fontanelle. If the fontanelles are open, the child will have an enlarged head without much rise in intracranial pressure. Once the fontanelle has closed, the skull stops expanding with the building up of intracranial pressure. The child develops symptoms of raised intracranial pressure in the form of headache and vomiting, with changes on the cranial walls visible on an X-ray. Untreated, the child develops bilateral papilledema and its aftermath; still, late ataxia is added to the above symptoms. Children with unattended hydrocephalus are likely to develop squints, abnormal pupillary reactions, and ultimately blindness.

The possible sites of obstruction can be any of the following:

- Aqueduct of Sylvius
- Foramen of Magendie
- Foramen magnum

With impeded CSF, the intraventricular pressure rises to press the brain between the ventricle and cranial wall, resulting in the expansion of the cranium. The skull above the eyebrows expands mostly, the forehead looks prominent, and the skin over the skull is stretched and glossy. The fontanelles are stretched and bulging, the eyeballs are pushed down, the lower lids are pulled up, and the eyeball seems to hide behind the lower lid, giving a sunset appearance to the cornea. The face looks triangular under the expanding head. The head may be too large for the child to hold it upright.

Management

There is no medical treatment. The only surgical method available is creating a shunt between the ventricle and abdomen; the prognosis is bad.

The Clinical Features of Orbital Disorders (at All Ages)

There are some orbital disorders that begin in childhood and spill over to adulthood, i.e., capillary hemangiomas, lymphangiomas, neurofibroma, dermoids, teratoma, optic nerve glioma, and neurilemmoma (Schwannoma).

> Cavernous hemangioma and neurilemmoma are tumors of adulthood; thyroid eye disease also does not inflict children under 10.

The orbital disorder may be congenital or acquired. The acquired conditions outnumber the congenital conditions. The disorders may be unilateral or bilateral; some of the unilateral cases ultimately become bilateral. When bilateral, they need not be of the same duration; they need to be symmetric and of the same duration.

The common causes of unilateral acquired disorders are: Orbital cellulitis pseudotumor (rare in children), orbital abscess, hematoma, emphysema, retained foreign bodies, parasitic cyst, secondaries, congenital cystic eyeball, dermoids, neuroblastoma, and nephroblastoma.

The acquired disorders can be acute, chronic, or recurrent (pseudotumors), the cause of acute involvement is generally infective or traumatic. The fast-developing symptoms are seen in neuroblastoma, rhabdomyosarcoma, leukemia, lymphangiomas, and pseudotumor.

Dermoids and optic nerve gliomas are slow-progressive.

The abnormal contents that influence the orbital disorders are: Foreign bodies, parasitic, cysts, blood, air, pus, and new growth.

The *new growth* may be primary (rhabdomyosarcoma), an extension from surrounding structures, or an extension from the globe (retinoblastoma). **Flowchart 11.1** shows various possibilities for the growth of orbit.

CLINICAL FEATURES OF ORBITAL DISORDERS

Topographically, they can be divided into two broad groups depending on their position in relation to the orbital rim and the shape of the globe.

- *Protrusion*:
  - Proptosis
  - Exophthalmos
- *Retraction*:
  - Cryptophthalmos
  - Anophthalmos (anopia)
  - Microphthalmos
  - Microphthalmos with cysts
  - Nanophthalmos
  - Enophthalmos (an abnormal retro displacement of the globe)
  - Phthisis bulbi
  - Buphthalmos

Flowchart 11.1: New growths of orbit.

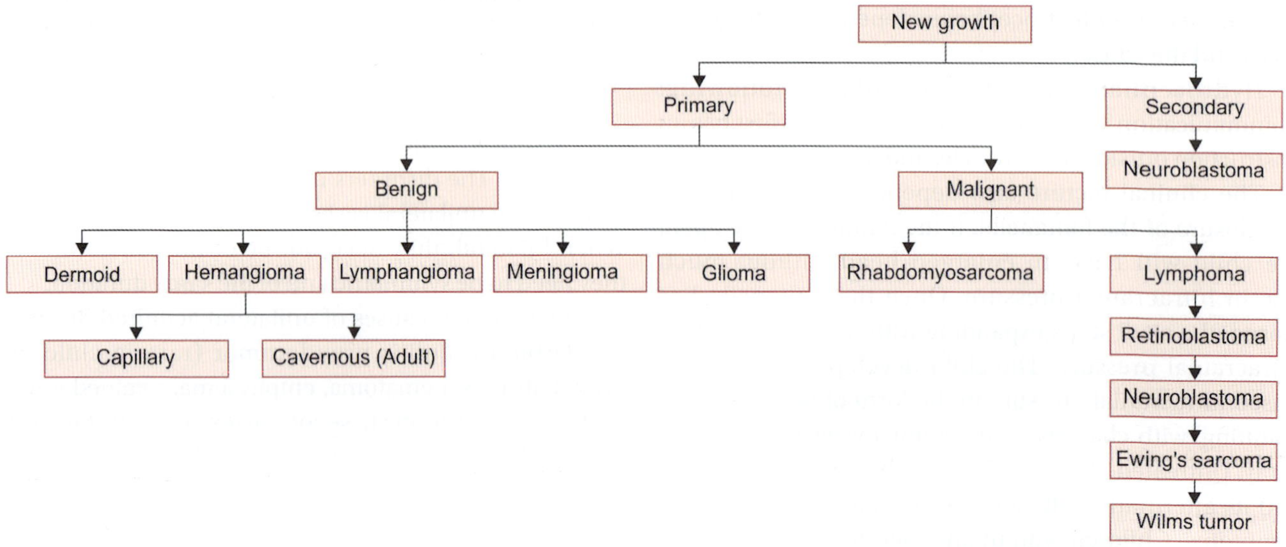

- Staphyloma (corneal and ciliary)
- Pseudo proptosis (disorder lies in the other eye)
- Hypoglobus*
- *Miscellaneous*:
  - Silent sinus syndrome†
  - Orbital compartment syndrome‡

It is divided into two types:

1. Hemorrhagic
2. Nonhemorrhagic

The nonhemorrhagic causes are:

- Orbital cellulitis
- Emphysema (less likely)
- Carotid cavernous fistula **(Fig. 11.10)**
- *Malignancies:*
  - Primary—rhabdomyosarcoma
  - Secondary—neuroblastoma

The hemorrhagic causes are:

- *Orbital:*
  - *Trauma:*
    - Accidental—fracture of orbit

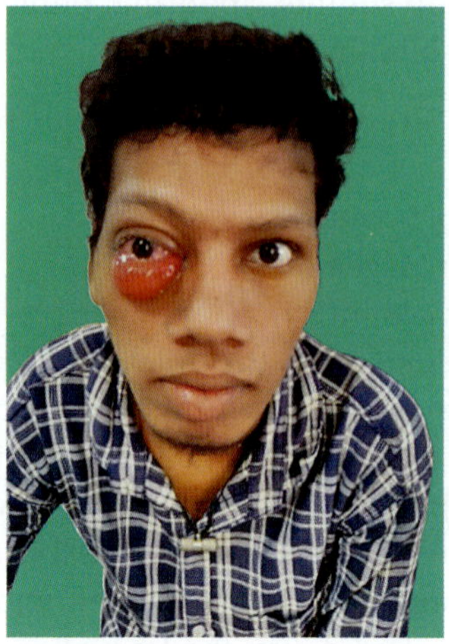

Fig. 11.10: Carotid cavernous fistula.
Courtesy: Dr Somen Misra.

    - Surgical—retrobulbar and sub-Tenon's injection of anesthetic agents and drugs
- *Vascular anomalies:*
  - Carotid cavernous fistula
  - Orbital varices

**Hypoglobus* means the lower position of the globe; it may or may not be associated with enophthalmos. The most common cause is fracture of the floor of the orbit and silent sinus syndrome.

†*Silent sinus syndrome:* Silent sinus syndrome represents an ever-increasing retraction of the globe with an inferiorly displaced globe; it is unilateral and rare and may be seen in infancy; the most common cause being congenital ipsilateral hypoplasia of the maxilla, resulting in unilateral ptosis, hypoglobus, and asymmetry between two eyes.

‡*Orbital compartment syndrome:* This consists of diminished vision, restricted movement of the eyeball, proptosis, relative afferent pupillary defect (RAPD), and ptosis due to an acute rise of the intraorbital pressure sufficient to cause obstruction of the central retinal artery that causes hypoxia of the retinal circulation and diminished vision. The causes of the condition are: Retrobulbar hemorrhage, surgical emphysema, acute edema of the retroocular structure due to trauma, infection, or inflammation such as orbital cellulitis, orbital abscess, and pseudotumors. The condition is an ophthalmic emergency. This is an acute and progressive form of ophthalmic emergency brought about by a sudden and sustained increase in intraorbital pressure.

- *Systemic diseases*:
  - *Blood disorders*:
    - Anemia
    - Leukemia
    - Hemophilia
    - Purpura
  - *Systemic infection:* Malaria
  - *Noninfectious conditions (in adults only)*:
    - Advanced atherosclerosis
    - Hypertension
    - Aneurism of ophthalmic artery
- *Hamartomas*:
  - Hemangioma
  - Lymphangioma

Mechanism of Production or Orbital Compartment Syndrome

The causes must be large and extensible enough to raise intraorbital pressure beyond the physiological limit. The orbit is a small space with rigid walls all-round except in front; that constitutes the base of the orbital pyramid; this is formed by the septum orbital, reinforced by the orbicularis. The septum itself is not a continuous structure; it has a horizontal aperture called an interpalpebral aperture. This is the space that shows the earliest signs of the syndrome in the form of proptosis and chemosis of conjunctiva with restricted or absent movement of the globe. As the intraorbital pressure rises, the following things can happen:

- Proptosis
- Swelling of the lids
- Congestion of lids
- Chemosis of conjunctiva
- Restricted movement of the globe
- *Vascular changes*:
  - Ischemia of the optic nerve
  - Ischemia of the retinochoroidal complex
  - Central retinal vein obstruction
  - Central retinal artery obstruction
- Diminished vision, the causes of which are:
  - Exposure keratitis
  - Edema of the cornea
  - Raised intraocular tension—the causes of which are raised episcleral pressure and compromised uveoscleral flow.
  - Optic neuropathy
  - There are various types of ischemic vasculopathy.
  - Error of refraction

Clinical Features

The most common cause of the syndrome is the collection of blood/exudate in the retrobulbar space; hence, the clinical features depend upon the amount of fluid in the retrobulbar space and its position. Hemorrhage in the cones causes more and early proptosis. A small hemorrhage may take a benign course of mild proptosis, a loss of a few lines on Snellen's chart.

Small hemorrhage may resolve gradually or rarely and form a blood cyst without any visual loss. Large hemorrhages cause early and sometimes permanent loss of vision.

Symptoms

- Pain in the eye, tenderness on the orbital rim, and frontal headache
- Fast-growing proptosis
- Hemorrhagic conjunctiva protruding through the interpalpebral fissure
- Diminished vision

Signs are:

- *Lid:*
  - Tense, swollen, and red without tenderness
  - Pseudoptosis/lid retraction
  - Mechanical lagophthalmos
  - Ecchymosis
  - Surgical emphysema
- *Proptosis:* Generally axial
- Absent movement of the globe
- Exposure keratitis
- Hazy cornea
- Raised intraocular pressure
- Diminished or absent vision
- Afferent relative pupil
- Disc changes

Diagnosis

It depends on history, systemic examination, ocular examination, and imaging.

Imaging in ocular compartment syndrome consists of ultrasonography (USG), CT, and MRI.

X-rays may be used as a screening method to detect fractures of orbital walls and intraorbital foreign bodies.

Management

Management depends on the amount of blood in the orbit. Small clots do not require any recurrence treatment except counseling and observation. Proptosis in blood dyscrasias is best managed by a hematologist. Medical treatments in the form of systemic and local antibiotics are not effective except in infective conditions. However, systemic carbonic anhydrase tables and local antiglaucoma drugs may reduce intraocular tension. In acute and rapidly increasing proptosis, antiglaucoma treatment should be initiated as soon as possible. Lateral canthotomy and cantholysis are most effective. Blind insertion of wide bore needles and cannulas are better avoided.

White Orbital Syndrome

This happens in a fracture of the orbital floor without fracture of the adjacent rim and without external signs of injury. This causes raised intraorbital pressure that may lead to orbital compartment syndrome.

"White-eyed" Blow Out Fracture

This is seen commonly in children under 18 years, mostly in boys following small single or multiple fractures following blunt injury to the lid; the globe may also be traumatized, and thin and poorly calcified bone of the orbit in children is the most probable cause of its occurrence in children. It presents with vertical diplopia and enophthalmos, herniation and entrapment of orbital soft tissues, and restrictive strabismus without external signs of injury. The diagnosis is confirmed by CT. One of the important complications is oculocardiac reflex that, if not attended, may prove to be fatal. The condition is overlooked in cases of more serious craniofacial injuries.

Clinical Presentation of Orbital Disorder (in All Ages)

It consists of six Ps, in combination or isolation. Multiple features are more common than solitary.

> *The six Ps of orbital disorders are:* Pain, proptosis, progress, palpability, pulsation, and paraorbital features.

> *To this, the following should be added:* Restriction of movement, ptosis (rare), lagophthalmos, lid retraction, and pupillary changes diminished vision, conjunctival congestion, conjunctival chemosis, fundus changes, rise of intraocular tension, rise of intraorbital pressure, positive findings on imaging, and systemic diseases.

Pain

Pain is a relative sensation; children have a greater threshold of pain. Slow, progressive lesions are generally devoid of pain. Some of the conditions that are associated with pain are acute in onset and progressive. They are:

- Acute orbital cellulitis
- Orbital abscess
- Periorbital abscess
- Orbital and periorbital hematoma
- Exposure keratitis
- Cavernous sinus thrombosis
- Trauma

Conjunctival Congestion

Conjunctival congestion can either be active or passive. The former is due to infection and the second to proptosis, caused by impeded venous returns secondary to growth in the orbit or raised episcleral tension.

Conjunctival Chemosis

This is generally seen in thyroid eye disease, which by itself is uncommon in children. When present, the patient is generally in late teens.

Diminished Vision

A child with orbital disorder may or may not have diminished vision. In cases of preseptal cellulitis, the child is unable to see not due to disease but mechanical hindrance in the visual axis caused by pseudoptosis; in such cases, vision should be recorded by lifting the edematous lid. Generally, a child with a preseptal lesion has good vision.

The other causes of diminished vision in orbital disorders are:

- Error of refraction
- Amblyopia
- Squint
- Corneal changes
- Optic nerve involvement

Errors of refraction in orbital disorders are caused by:

- Change in corneal curvature due to pressure of the lids and growth
- Change in the curvature of the globe
- Mass pushing, the posterior pole forward

Amblyopia: If the visual axis remains obstructed by an overhanging edematous lid, the child may develop amblyopia within weeks to months. Even with a clear visual axis, the child may develop amblyopia due to an associated error of refraction, muscle imbalance, and optic nerve involvement.

Squint: Squint is common in orbital disorders. It can be concomitant/restrictive/paralytic; the causes of concomitant squint are associated errors of refraction, amblyopia, and opacities in the media, and optic nerve changes.

The causes of paralytic squints are isolated trunk lesions of individual cranial nerves and combined lesions of more than one cranial nerve. Restrictive squint is common in thyroid eye disease due to pushing of the globe by the increasing mass, infiltration of the muscle, and error of refraction.

Corneal changes: Corneal changes in orbital disorder are brought about mostly due to exposure, which can vary from ocular surface disorder to abrasion, superficial keratitis, foreign bodies, to frank or fulminating corneal ulcer. Less common changes are due to compromised corneal sensation.

Optic nerve involvements: They consist of optic atrophy, both primary and secondary. It may be caused due to pressure on the optic nerve substance or stretching of the nerve. Orbital disorders are rarely to cause classical papilledema, when present papilledema is unilateral and caused by pressure on the central retinal vein.

Lid changes in orbital disorders:

- *Edema:* The most common orbital disease is edema of the lid, which is more common and severe in the upper lid. However, the lower lids are not always spared. The most common cause of lid edema is acute preseptal cellulitis.
- *Ptosis:* Both types of ptosis, i.e., pseudo- and true ptosis, are met with disorders of the orbit. The former is more common than the latter. The most common cause is preseptal cellulitis. The other mechanical causes are neurofibromatosis and capillary hemangioma. The cause of true ptosis is neurogenic due to the involvement of the third nerve in isolation or combination with the fourth and sixth nerves in orbital apex syndrome, superior orbital fissure syndrome, or cavernous sinus thrombosis.
- *Lagophthalmos:* True paralysis of the seventh nerve rarely occurs in orbital disorders. The common cause of the inability to close the lids is mechanical protrusion of the globe due to proptosis, which may be acute or slowly progressive. Trauma to the zygomatic arch may be the other cause.
- *Lid retraction:* The most common cause of lid retraction in orbital disorders is thyroid eye disease, depending on the severity and duration of thyrotoxicosis. It may begin as mild unilateral retraction to severe bilateral retraction of both the lids. Such changes are rare before 20 years.

Proptosis versus Exophthalmos

In the past, the two terms were discussed separately. Proptosis was defined as active propulsion of the eyeball mostly forward in any direction by a mass in the orbit, and exophthalmos was considered to be passive protrusion of the globe in any direction and used exclusively in thyroid eye diseases. Presently, the two terms are used as synonyms and interchangeable. However, it is better to use the term exophthalmos for thyroid eye disease because the two conditions do not share the same clinical features, except for prominent eyeballs.

Proptosis

Proptosis is an important clinical feature of orbital disorders. It is not only a sign but also a symptom. It could be mild and innocuous or blinding and life-threatening.

It could be congenital or acquired, unilateral or bilateral when bilateral need not be symmetric. A proptosis is said to be uniocular if there is a difference of >2.00 mm between the exophthalmometry measurements of two eyes with one eye normal. Proptosis is measured by a set of instruments called exophthalmometer that measure the distance between the lateral orbital margin at the level of the outer canthus and the vortex of the cornea when the child looks straight ahead. It can be measured in both sitting and supine positions. This is an outdoor procedure. The normal exophthalmometry measurement is 12–21 mm in adults. A child's eye, due to its relatively larger size in comparison to an orbit, seems to be proptosed.

All prominent eyes are not proptosis.

The most common cause of unilateral proptosis in children is orbital cellulitis **(Figs. 11.11 and 11.12)**.

The other common causes are:

- Rhabdomyosarcoma
- Optic nerve glioma **(Fig. 11.13)**
- Capillary hemangioma
- Lymphangiomas
- Dermoid
- Varix
- Secondary neuroblastoma
- *Retinoblastoma extension from* **(Fig. 11.14)**:
    - Globe
    - Orbital

The most common cause of bilateral proptosis is leukemia, but other causes are metastasis from:

- Neuroblastoma
- Burkett's tumor
- Ewing's sarcoma
- Nephroblastoma
- Histiocytosis
- Leukemic deposit **(Fig. 11.15)**

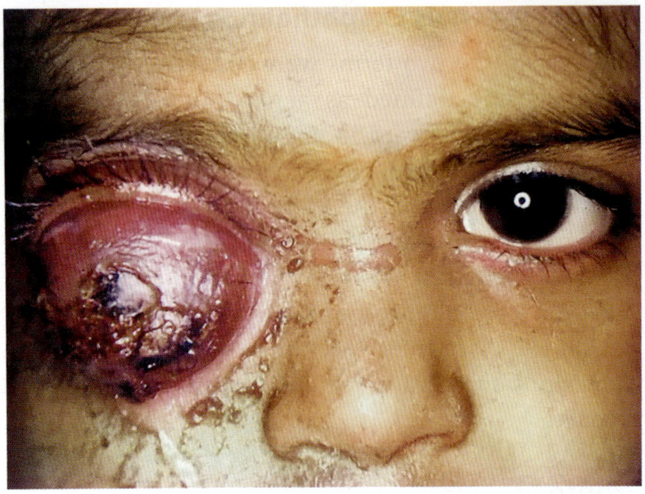

Fig. 11.11: Unilateral proptosis in advanced orbital cellulitis.
Courtesy: Dr Somen Misra.

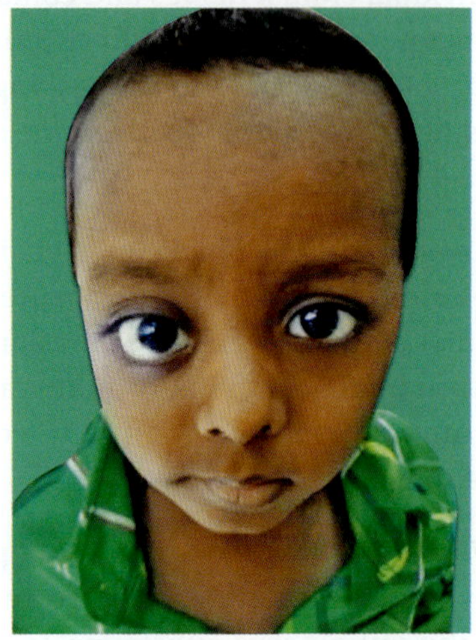

Fig. 11.13: Right-sided moderate proptosis due to small optic nerve glioma.

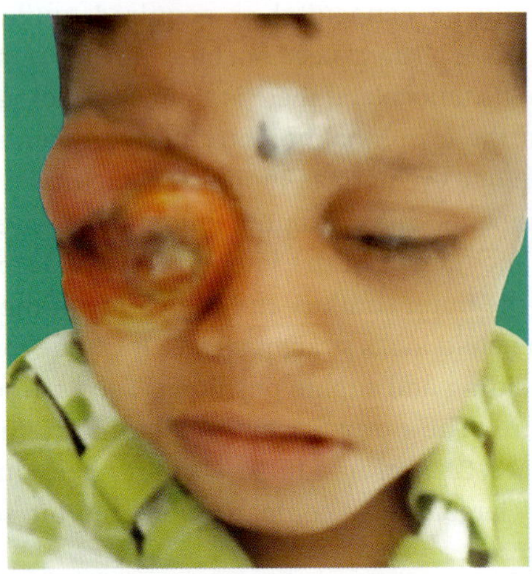

Fig. 11.12: Unilateral proptosis due to unknown growth orbit.
Courtesy: Dr Somen Misra.

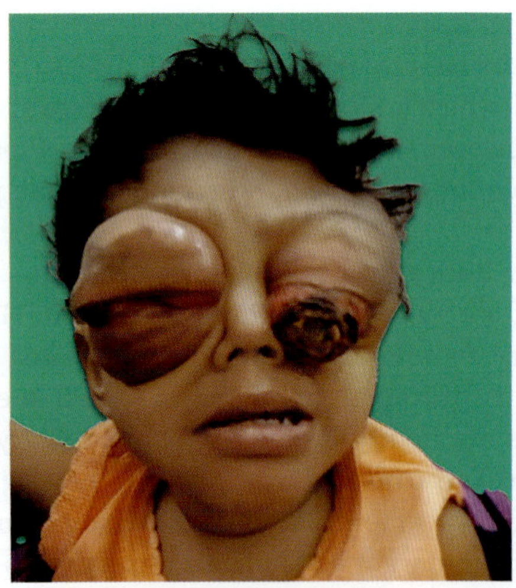

Fig. 11.14: Bilateral proptosis due to orbital retinoblastoma.
Courtesy: Dr Somen Misra.

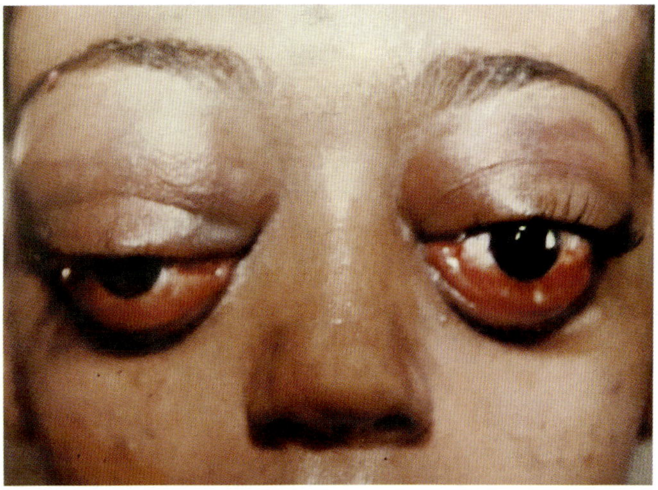

Fig. 11.15: Bilateral proptosis in leukemic deposit. *Courtesy:* Dr Somen Misra.

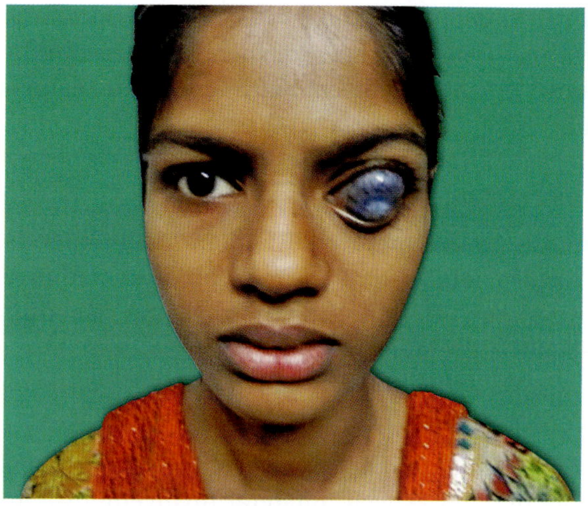

Fig. 11.16: Pseudoproptosis.

Pseudoproptosis

A unilateral prominent eye within normal exophthalmometry may look like a case of proptosis if the fault lies in the other eye.

The condition is called pseudoproptosis.

The causes are contralateral:

- Ptosis
- Anophthalmos
- Enophthalmos
- Microphthalmos
- Phthisis bulbi
- Ipsilateral causes are buphthalmos and large ciliary staphyloma **(Fig. 11.16)**.

Mechanism of Production of Proptosis

There is an inherent balance between the volume of the bony orbit and its contents, and as long as the balance is maintained, there is no proptosis. The proptosis will result if:

- The volume of the orbit is too small to accommodate the normal contents, as seen in congenitally small orbits.
- Its contents are too voluminous in comparison to normal intraorbital space. It may be congenital or acquired.

The congenital causes of proptosis are:

- Meningocele
- Meningoencephalocele
- Dermoids
- Epidermoids
- Teratoma
- Microphthalmos with cystic eyeball (rare)
- Optic nerve glioma (average age of detection is 7–8 years)
- Orbital hemangioma (manifest in the early second decade)
- Orbital varix (manifest in the early second decade)
- Fibrous dysplasia

The acquired causes of proptosis are:

- Infection
  Inflammation
- Trauma
- Retained foreign body
- Cavernous sinus thrombosis
- *Malignancies:* Primary/secondary

The infections responsible for proptosis in children are:

- Orbital cellulitis
- Orbital abscess
- Orbital periostitis
- Panophthalmitis
- Cavernous sinus thrombosis

Inflammations responsible for proptosis in children are:

- Orbital pseudotumor (rare)
- Foreign body granuloma

Trauma

Both penetration as well as blunt injuries directly or indirectly to the orbital structures/periorbital structure can cause proptosis due to retrobulbar hemorrhage, hematoma, emphysema (transient, rare in children), retained intraocular foreign body, and carotid cavernous fistula.

Retained Intraorbital Foreign Body

Proptosis by an intraorbital foreign body depends on its size, location, sterility, duration, association with hemorrhage, hematoma, emphysema, secondary infection, and granuloma formation.

Cavernous Sinus Thrombosis

Cavernous sinus thrombosis is not only vision threatening. It may be fatal as well. Bilateral involvement is more common; however, it is not unusual for it to start in one eye and remain confined to the same eye for some time.

Malignancies

The moist common primary malignancy of orbital contents in children is rhabdomyosarcoma; other less common are: Reactive lymphoid proliferation, histiocytosis, and Burkitt's lymphoma. The secondary malignancies consist of metastatic deposit and extension from neighboring structures that are rare in children; more common is extension from the globe in the case of advanced retinoblastoma.

The following is the list of common orbital secondaries in children:

- Neuroblastoma
- Nephroblastoma
- Ewing's tumor
- Orbital retinoblastoma
- Wilms tumor
- Leukemia

Details of the Infections Responsible for Proptosis in Children

Orbital Cellulitis

Orbital cellulitis is an acute infection of intraorbital structures by microorganisms. The most common group of microorganisms are: Bacteria, both cocci and bacillus, the former is more common than the latter. Recently, there has been a spurt in acute, fulminating orbital cellulitis due to infection by mucormycosis in patients suffering from COVID-19 or post-COVID periods **(Figs. 11.17 and 11.18)**.

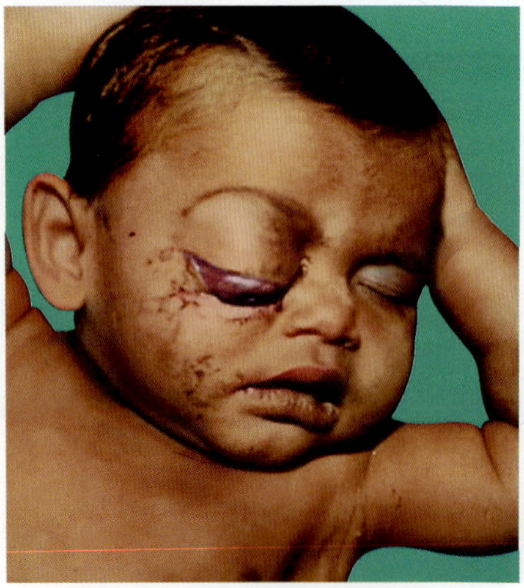

Fig. 11.17: Orbital cellulitis in an infant.
Courtesy: Dr Somen Misra.

The common organisms responsible for orbital cellulitis are pneumococci, *Staphylococcus aureus*, *Streptococcus pyogenes*, and *Haemophilus influenzae*. The last is the most common pathogen in children and is often ampicillin-resistant. 80% of the cellulitis caused by *H. influenza* is seen in children. In older children, sinus infections are more common causes of orbital cellulitis. Ethmoidal sinusitis tops the list of sinus infections to cause cellulitis in children. The frontal sinus is rarely responsible under 10 years. In children under 5 years, acute dacryocystitis caused by pneumococci is the most common periorbital disease to cause orbital cellulitis. The other causes of infection are generalized bacteremia and retained intraorbital foreign bodies. Organic foreign bodies are more prone to cause orbital cellulitis than nonorganic ones. Any virulent infection in a malnourished or immune-compromised child can precipitate orbital cellulitis.

> Classical orbital cellulitis is an ophthalmic emergency that may not only be vision threatening but fatal as well.

The next group consists of fungi that cause cellulitis in children. The common fungi are mucor and aspergillus. The fungal infection carries a high risk of fatality, especially in immunocompromised children. The most devastating fungal infection is by mucor mycosis in persons suffering from COVID, which has not been reported in children. The viruses are not known to infect intraorbital contents.

The orbital septum in adults acts as a barrier between preseptal and orbital contents; hence, the chances of

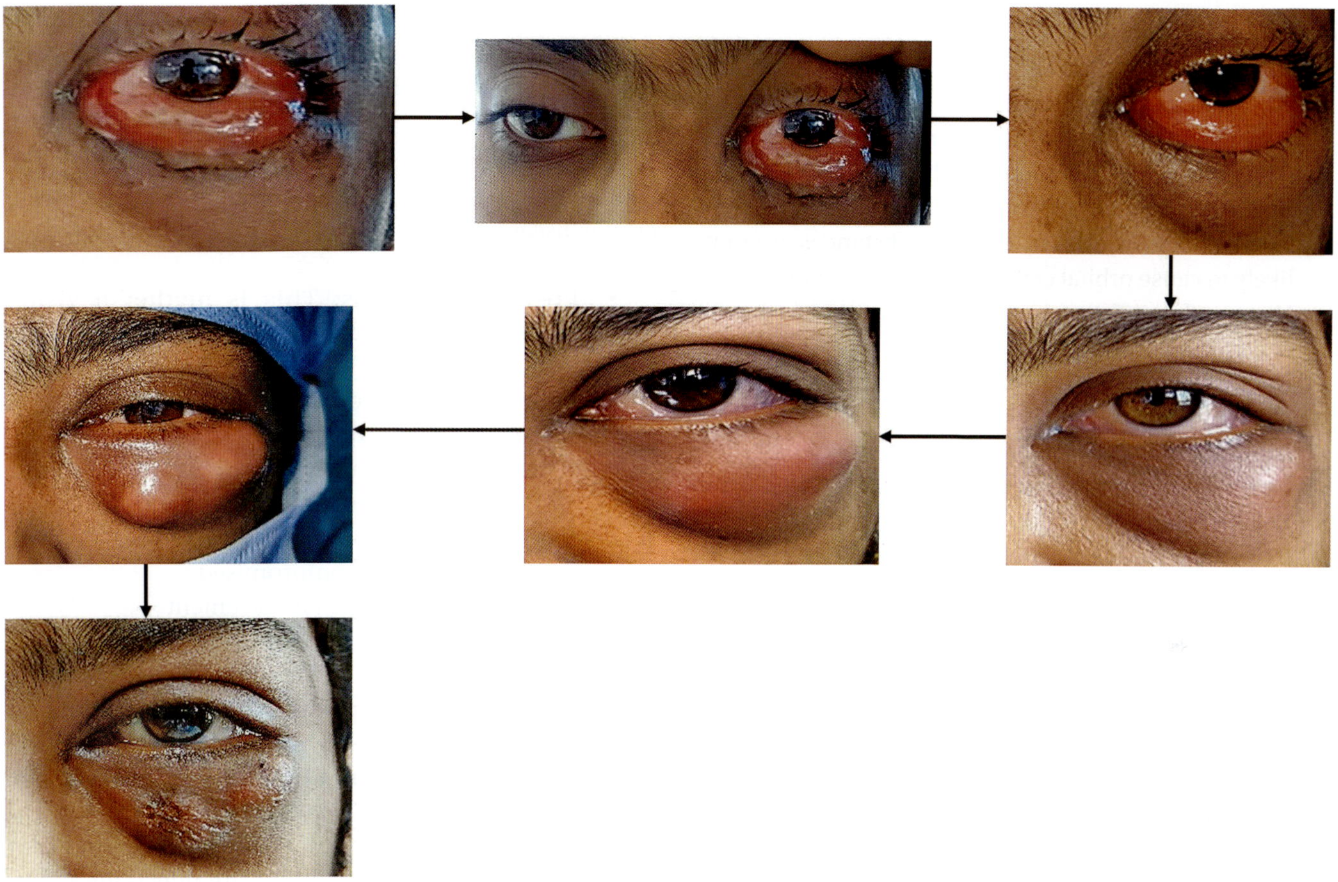

Fig. 11.18: A series of photographs of a case of orbital cellulitis that developed an abscess in the lower lid. *Courtesy:* Dr Bhanu Priya, Professor Ankur K Shrivastava, and Dr Somen Misra.

infection spreading from preseptal to retroseptal space in adults is less. In contrast to this, the orbital septum in children is poorly developed; hence, preseptal infection may find its way into the retroseptal space, easily causing orbital cellulitis in children. A blood culture is mandatory in children suffering from orbital cellulitis, especially if they are suspected to be immune compromised or malnourished with fever. Orbital cellulitis in children can be seen between infancy and adolescence. The younger the patient, the more severe the infection.

Orbital cellulitis is acute in onset with fever, malaise, orbital and periorbital pain, and headache. Generally unilateral, starting with fast-developing proptosis and lid swelling that may masquerade as preseptal infection. A bluish-red hue of the swollen lid is a strong feature of infection by *H. influenzae.*

Fast collection of pus in a closed compartmental orbit causes severe pain and headaches; it pushes the eyeball forward, resulting in fast-growing proptosis. The proptosed globe may endanger the cornea to exposure to keratitis that may soon develop ulceration with its train of usual complications such as frank ulcer, hypopyon endophthalmitis, or even panophthalmitis.

The loss of mobility in a case of orbital cellulitis is due to:

- Accompanied inflammation of extraocular muscle
- Neuritis of nerves in the orbit
- Expanding fluid in a tight orbital compartment
- The condition is worsened with retained organic foreign bodies.

The conjunctiva is chemosed and may bulge through the lid aperture.

The pupil is dilated due to the involvement of the optic and third nerves. The vision falls fast.

Deterioration of vision with a dilated pupil points toward involvement of the optic nerve, central retinal artery, and venous obstruction.

Diagnosis

The diagnosis of orbital cellulitis is relatively easy if the following points are kept in mind:

- The child is malnourished, immune compromised, suffers from type 1 diabetes, and has a history suggestive of penetrating injury with or without a retained foreign body. Injuries by organic substances are more likely to cause orbital cellulitis than nonorganic.
- History of rapidly growing unilateral proptosis in an ill child
- Immobile eye with fixed pupil or relative afferent pupil defect
- Normal or slightly swollen lids
- Chemosis of conjunctiva
- Positive changes on imaging

Investigation

- *Total blood count:* Results of the total blood count are nonspecific except for high leukocytosis in a child with fever; this points toward an acute infection.
- Smear and culture of conjunctival discharge are invariably negative unless there is a discharging sinus in the fronix.
- Smears and culture from the tract leading to the retained foreign body are more specific.
- *Imaging of the orbit and PNSs:*
  - *X-ray:* X-ray PNSs that used to be the only available imaging process a few decades in the past have taken a back seat. It is still relevant for the presence of an intraorbital foreign body, compound fracture of PNSs, fracture of other orbital walls, fluid level in PNSs, and air in orbit. Air in the orbit may be from the fractured PNSs or an offending gas-forming organism.
  - USG has limited utility in orbital cellulitis as an imaging tool; however, it is an alternative imaging system that is quick and can be done without anesthesia and without risk of radiation. It is mostly used to differentiate between periorbital and orbital cellulitis.
  - *CT scan:* It has proved to be the most useful imaging procedure in orbital cellulitis. It delineates not only the orbital contents but also the fluid level in the PNSs, air in the orbit, and the presence of subperiosteal pus.
  - *MRI:* It gives information regarding not only orbital contents but also information regarding involvement of cavernous sinuses. The T2W fat-suppressed sequence is especially useful for the detection of orbital infections.

Differential Diagnosis

Differential diagnosis consists of the following groups of orbital diseases:

- *Infections:*
  - Preseptal cellulitis: This is neither a vision threatening nor a fatal disorder. The hallmarks of the disorder are:
    - Swelling of the lid, mostly upper
    - Conjunctiva is not chemosed under a swollen, drooping lid.
    - The cornea is bright.
    - Movements are normal.
    - The vision is not compromised.
    - No anterior segment involvement
  - Cavernous sinus **(Fig. 11.22)**
  - *Panophthalmitis:* The disease starts from intraocular structures and spreads to peribulbar structures, commonly following the perforation of a corneal ulcer and trauma, both surgical and accidental.
- *New growths:* The common new growths that may masquerade as orbital cellulitis are infections superadded to:
  - Rhabdomyosarcoma
  - Leukemia
  - Secondaries
  - Orbital retinoblastoma

Management of Orbital Cellulitis

- Orbital cellulitis is an ophthalmic emergency at all ages, more so in children. It is better to hospitalize the child. A team comprising ophthalmologists, pediatricians, and ear, nose, and throat (ENT) consultants should supervise the treatment.
- The management is mostly medical, with the usual ancillary support.
- Medical treatment consists of age-matched systemic antibiotics and permissible analgesics.
- *Antibiotics:* The Most appropriate will be to administer antibiotics as per smear and culture from a discharging sinus. A smear report is available within a few hours. It indicates if the organisms are cocci or bacilli, and its staining property, the smear also reveals if the infection is mono- or multiorganism.

- The culture takes a day to many days to give a definite result; hence, the safest strategy is to start empirically with either a single or a combination of antibiotics that will cover both gram-positive and -negative organisms.
- The antibiotics are initially given intravenously, generally twice a day as per the weight of the child, at least for the first 3 days in the hospital, and then the child is put on oral antibiotics.
- Steroids, with usual precautions, are started after an initial improvement that takes about a week. The role of steroids is to hasten the resolution of associated myositis and neuritis. This helps improve vision, regain muscle function, and prevent fibrosis.
- The result of recovery is hampered due to the development of orbital and periosteal abscess formation. This requires surgical drainage after the pocket of pus has been precisely located by CT and MRI. Blind drainage should be avoided as it may encourage dissemination.

A Complication of Orbital Cellulitis

Complications can be:

- *Local:*
  - Subperiosteal abscess*
  - Orbital abscess[†]
  - Periorbital cellulitis
  - *Sinus formation:* Sinus formation per se is rare without intraorbital retained.
  - Unattended foreign bodies
- *Systemic:*
  - Meningitis
  - Cavernous sinus thrombosis[‡]
  - Central retinal vessel obstruction

A blind procedure without proper localization is fraught with the danger of the dissemination of infection.

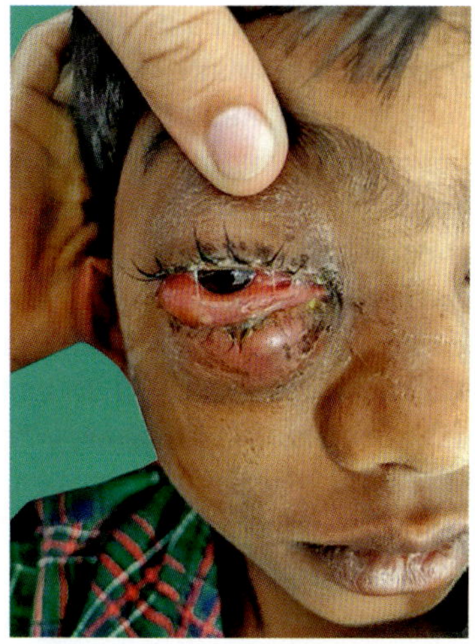

Fig. 11.19: Orbital abscess pointing through lower.

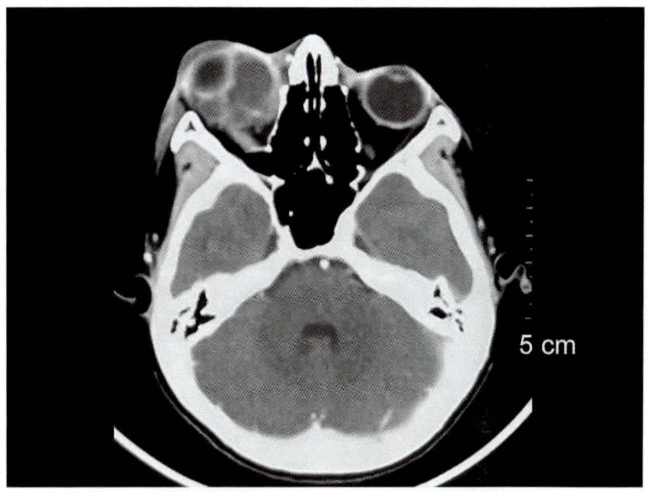

Fig. 11.20: CT showing lid peribulbar orbital abscess.

It acts as a reservoir of venous blood from the areas drained by it. The veins forming and draining the cavernous sinus do not have valves that make them vulnerable to infection. The sphenoidal sinus forms the inferior relation.

**Subperiosteal abscess:* This is rarer than orbital cellulitis; primary subperiosteal abscess is still frequent. It is commonly due to the spread of infection from orbital cellulitis.

†*Orbital abscess:* This happens if the orbital cellulitis is not eliminated completely; a residual pus may develop a pseudo-coat, converting it into a pocket of pus. If the abscess is intraconal, it will cause a mild to moderate tense axial proptosis, and an extraconal abscess will cause eccentric proptosis as per its position. The best management is to drain the abscess following accurate localization by CT/MRI **(Figs. 11.19 to 11.21)**.

‡*Cavernous sinus thrombosis:* Applied anatomy of the cavernous sinus.

Cavernous sinuses are a pair of large venous channels situated on either side of the sphenoid, longitudinally extending from the superior orbital fissure to the tip of the petrous bone. It is formed by splitting the dura with multiple loculi that give it a spongy look on the section. It acts as a reservoir of venous blood from most of the cranium, face, nose, throat, ear, and mouth; the vessels that join the sinus anteriorly are the superior and inferior ophthalmic veins, the central retinal vein, and the sphenopalatine vein. The sinus drains posteriorly through the superior petrosal vein and inferior petrosal vein into the lateral sinus and ultimately into the jugular vein **(Fig. 11.22)**.

The pituitary gland in the sella lies under the chiasma. The Gasserian ganglion is situated at the posterior aspect outside the sinus. The two sides of the sinus communicate with each other through the transverse sinus. The walls are uneven, making it an ideal site to develop thrombus. Each internal carotid, accompanied by a sympathetic nerve, lies in the substance of the sinus on each side of the sphenoid. The sixth nerve too lies in the substance, infero-lateral to the internal carotid **(Figs. 11.23 and 11.24)**.

The rest of the oculomotor nerves are embedded in the lateral wall of the sinus. The third nerve is on top, followed by the fourth below, and the two branches of the fifth nerve are inferior to the fourth. The fourth nerve changes its course in the anterior part of the sinus to become superior to the third nerve. This portion of the fourth nerve above the third nerve has a small course.

Cavernous sinus thrombosis is in fact a form of thrombophlebitis, consisting of thrombus formation on the walls and loculi of the sinus to which acute infection has been added; the reverse is also possible. The sinus gets infected from the areas draining by various veins, as shown in the drawing above.

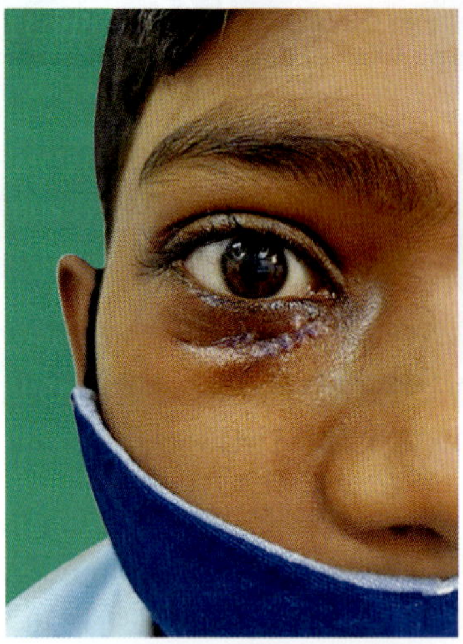

Fig. 11.21: Same case after draining through anterior orbitotomy. *Courtesy:* Dr Somen Misra.

In the preantibiotic era, cavernous sinus thrombosis used to be fatal in all cases, irrespective of age. Children were more prone than adults, and even today, the prognosis is immune-suppressed and malnourished, and children on antimetabolites carry a poor prognosis. A small boil or furuncle in the danger zone could cause the dreaded disease. The danger zone prone to cause cavernous sinus thrombosis lies in the nose, PNSs, skin, and lids **(Fig. 11.25)**.

The infection starts acutely with fever, malaise, headache, and vomiting. The condition, commonly referred to as cavernous sinus thrombosis, follows an acute bacterial infection. The cases that survive the initial onslaught pass into a stage of chronic granuloma, generally in the anterior cavernous sinus, that may spread to the superior orbital fissure, causing Tolosa Hunt and orbital apex syndromes, which are not fatal. A third type of disorder is septic thrombosis following a head injury or surgical intervention.

The signs consist of lid-swelling, redness and chemosis of the conjunctiva, fast-growing painful proptosis, loss of ocular movement, and diminished vision. The cause of diminished vision depends on the involvement of the cornea and optic nerve. The optic nerve may show minimum to severe papillitis and papilledema. Swelling of the disc is more common in otic involvement; papilledema is more common in bilateral proptosis. Swelling and tenderness over the mastoid indicate emissary vein involvement; the other importance of a tender mastoid is that it heralds contralateral involvement. The first sign of bilateral involvement is a sixth nerve palsy in the apparently normal another eye. 50% of cases are bilateral.

The condition is potentially vision- and life-threatening, hence an ophthalmic emergency. The diagnosis of cavernous sinus thrombosis is easy in an ill child with high pyrexia, headache, proptosis, and an immobile globe.

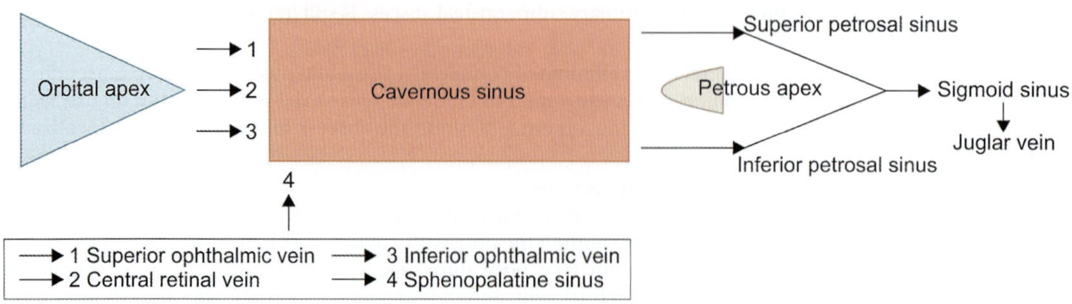

Fig. 11.22: The afferent and efferent veins of the cavernous sinus.

The most important condition to be differentiated from cavernous sinus thrombosis in children is orbital cellulitis, which is unilateral. Orbital cellulitis itself can be a cause of cavernous sinus thrombosis. The two conditions are best differentiated by CT and MRI. X-rays are hardly of any significance except in cases of head injuries.

Management

The condition should be treated as a medical emergency. The child should be admitted to the pediatric intensive care unit and administered a broad-spectrum antibiotic intravenously with ancillary support. The cornea should be protected from exposure to keratitis. The condition carries a uniformly poor prognosis.

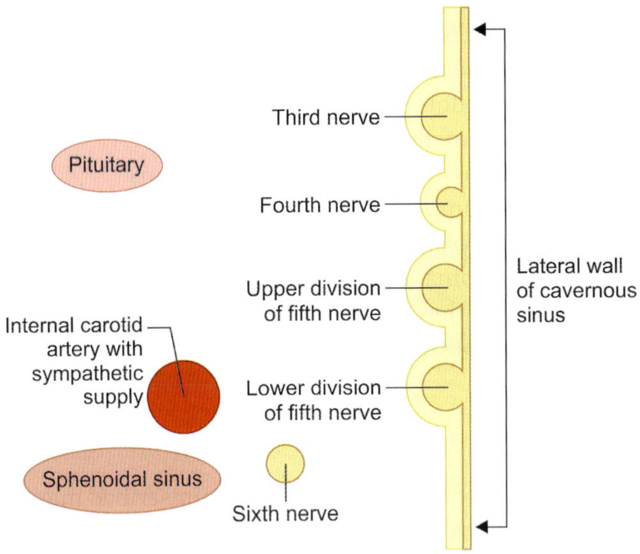

Fig. 11.23: Relation of internal carotid and oculomotor nerves in cavernous sinus.

Malignant Tumors of the Orbit in Children

Malignant tumors can either be primary, metastatic, or an extension from neighboring and intraocular structures. The most common primary malignant orbital tumor in children is rhabdomyosarcoma.

Rhabdomyosarcoma

The average age of presentation is 8 years; it has been reported in newborns as well, seen equally in all races, and slightly more frequent in boys. There is no known genetic predilection.

The lesion is unilateral. It presents as a case of fast-growing proptosis with ptosis. The expanding mass can initially be reached by insinuating a finger between the globe and the orbital wall. This becomes difficult as the mass involves the whole of the orbital space. The proptosis is generally forward and lateral.

Rhabdomyosarcoma can be classified in two ways:

1. Histopathology
2. Clinical

Histopathology of Rhabdomyosarcoma

The tumor arises from pluripotential mesenchymal tissue present in the orbit and not from the striated extraocular muscle. It is also known to arise in the vicinity of lids.

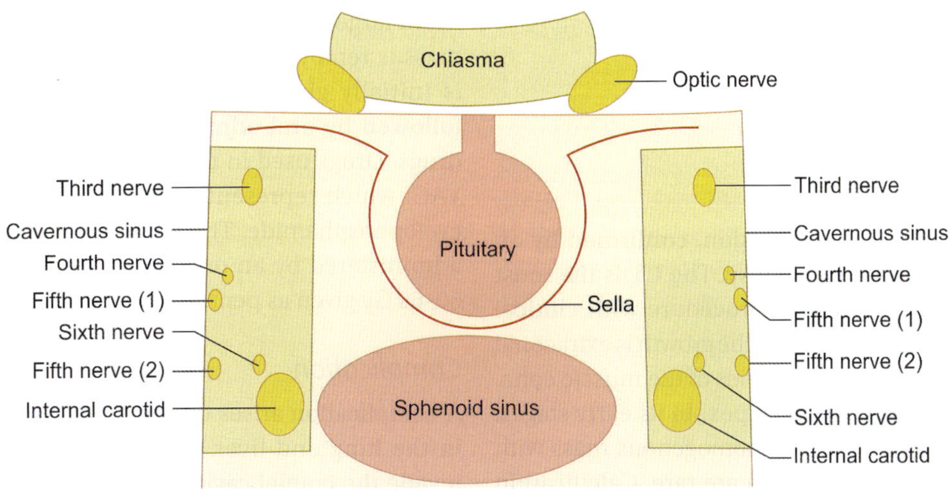

Fig. 11.24: Section showing relation to chiasm, pituitary sphenoid sinus, and wall of cavernous sinus.

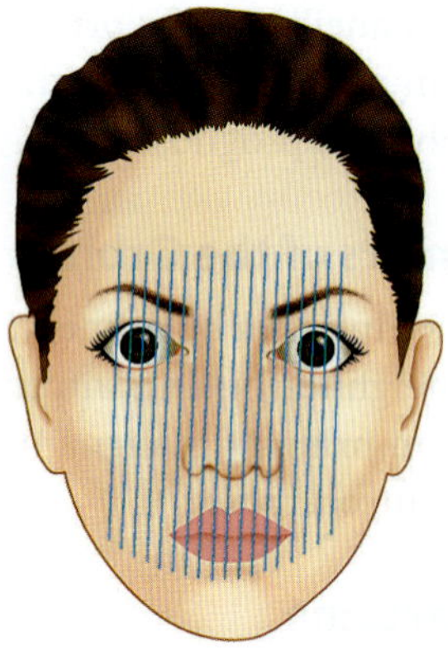

Fig. 11.25: Danger zone to cause cavernous sinus thrombosis.

Histologically, the tumor is divided into 5 forms: Embryonic, alveolar, botryoid embryonal, spindle cell embryonal, and anaplastic. Though all the types have been reported among children, the embryonal form is most common among children. The alveolar type is mostly seen in the lower part of the orbit and is most malignant, with a bad prognosis; botryoid is less common. The regional lymph nodes are involved more commonly in alveolar types.

The most common route of distant metastasis is hematogenous; the most common organ involved in rhabdomyosarcoma is the lung. Other organs to be affected are the brain and bones.

Clinical

Clinically, it has been divided on the basis of resectability into four grades.

The grades are:

- Localized disease
- Regional disease
- Gross residual disease after resection
- Distant metastasis

Diagnosis

The diagnosis is clinical by exclusion, confirmed by an ancillary test of imaging and biopsy. The CT is the most common confirmatory imaging procedure with clinical and prognostic importance. On CT, the growth is extraconal unless it has breached the boundaries of the muscle cone, which is more common near the apex. In its early stages, it is a well-circumscribed, ovoid, homogenous mass with an irregular surface. Calcifications are rare. Calcification is seen only when the orbital bones have been invaded. MRI is helpful in detecting extraocular invasion and extraorbital extension. The feature of MRI is homogeneous on T1WI but hyperintense on T2WI. B-scan USG gives low to medium reflectivity in a well-defined mass. The X-ray orbit is noncontributing; however, the X-ray chest is useful to exclude metastasis in the lungs.

> A child with fast-growing unilateral painless proptosis with ptosis and fairly good ocular movement and a normal blood count is most probably a case of rhabdomyosarcoma.

Differential Diagnosis

Rhabdomyosarcoma should be differentiated from the following conditions:

- Leukemic deposit
- Metastatic neuroblastoma
- Orbital pseudotumor (rare in children)
- Capillary hemangioma
- Cavernous hemangioma (rare in children)
- Lymphangioma
- Early stages of an orbital abscess
- Retinoblastoma and Burkitt's lymphoma are not true metastases; they are extensions from the eyeball and maxilla, respectively.

Treatment

- Surgery
  - Complete removal of a well-circumscribed mass
  - Debulking
- Radiation
- Chemotherapy
- Combination

Radiation and chemotherapy are given if the tumor is too large to be debulked; once the size is reduced, the mass is removed mostly by excision. The chemotherapy is initially given intravenously weekly for 5–6 doses, followed by oral administration of the combination of drugs. Drugs used in rhabdomyosarcoma are acronymed VAC, which represents vincristine, actinomycin D, and cyclophosphamide. The radiation and chemotherapy are administered by an oncologist. The dose of radiation is 50–60 Gy given as per the practice of the institutions.

Complication

A complication arises due to the fast spread of the tumor in the lung and liver. A posteriorly placed tumor may invade the cranial cavity. An apparent complete removal of the tumor surgically is not always a guarantee against recurrence; hence, the practice is to give a combination of chemotherapy and radiation following the surgical removal of the tumor.

Neuroblastoma

Neuroblastoma is a malignancy of childhood; the average age of presentation is 7 years. It has been reported even under 1 year of age. It is most probably a congenital tumor arising from neural crest cells involving the paraspinal sympathetic ganglion and adrenal glands. Rarely does it originate in the orbital sympathetic element. It is the proliferation of immature sympathetic ganglion cells. The tumor arising from orbital sympathetic elements is a primary orbital tumor, while those arising from adrenal and paravertebral sympathetic chains cause secondaries in orbit. The child with secondary neuroblastoma may present to the ophthalmologist initially with fast-growing bilateral proptosis and ecchymosis and be found to have primary in the abdomen or chest. Secondaries in the orbit are far more common than primary neuroblastoma of the orbit; they do not invade the globe.

The typical presentation is a child with bilateral ecchymosis, which is invariably connected to either an imaginary injury or a real trivial injury. On examination, the child has proptosis, generally axial. Initially, other ocular examinations do not reveal any contributory features. The pupils do not show white reflexes. The ocular changes, when present, are due to proptosis. On palpation of the abdomen, a mass may be felt, which is confirmed by CT. The X-ray chest may show a widening of the mediastinum. The growth not only involves the orbital cavity but also invades the orbital walls. The zygomatic bone is the most common orbital bone to be involved. The growth can also involve the cheek. The liver is involved in hematogenous spread.

Diagnosis is by exclusion. However, a child with bilateral ecchymosis, proptosis, and a lump in the abdomen most probably has a metastatic neuroblastoma that is confirmed by X-rays of the chest, which show paravertebral lymph nodes, USG shows mass in the abdomen; CT and MRI give more definitive information. A positive fine needle aspiration shows rosette formation, which is confirmatory.

> Other malignancies that show rosette formation on histopathology are: Retinoblastoma and medulloepithelioma. There are some rare benign retinal tumors that also form rosettes; they are retinoma, retinal dysplasia, and incontinentia pigmenti. The retinoma produces more fleurettes than rosettes.

As per metastatic behavior, there are two types of metastatic neuroblastoma:

1. Hutching type
2. Pepper type

The former has a predilection for the orbit, and the latter spreads to the liver.

Differential Diagnosis

There is no condition except metastatic neuroblastoma that presents with bilateral ecchymosis and proptosis in a child under 10 years old. However, orbital retinoblastoma may present with bilateral orbital mass; such cases are preceded by leukocoria. Fortunately, cases of bilateral orbital retinoblastomas have become rare.

The other orbital malignancy is rhabdomyosarcoma, which is unilateral and not accompanied by ecchymosis.

Thus:

- Fast-growing bilateral proptosis with ecchymosis is a case of metastatic neuroblastoma.
- Moderately growing bilateral proptosis with a history of leukocoria is a case of orbital retinoblastoma.
- Fast-growing unilateral growth without ecchymosis or leukocoria is a case of rhabdomyosarcoma.
- A slow-growing unilateral axial proptosis is most probably a case of glioma of the optic nerve.

Other conditions that merit inclusion in the list of differential diagnoses are:

- *Malignancy:* Burkitt's lymphoma, metastatic Wilms tumor, metastatic Ewing's sarcoma, and leukemia
- *Benign growth:* Capillary hemangioma and optic nerve glioma
- *Infection:* Orbital cellulitis, panophthalmitis, and cavernous sinus thrombosis
- *Trauma:* Black eye and retrobulbar hemorrhage

Treatment

Treatment of neuroblastoma consists of surgery, chemotherapy, and radiation. Surgery alone is not very effective. A better option is to give a full course of chemotherapy either as a primary treatment or to reduce the size of the growth before surgery and postsurgical palliation. Commonly used drugs are vincristine, cyclophosphamide, danyelza, dinutuximab, naxitamab, and unituxin. Similarly, radiation can be given to debulk the growth before surgery alone or with chemotherapy.

Ewing's Sarcoma

This is a metastatic tumor of the orbit of doubtful origin. Previously, it was thought to develop from primitive neuroectodermal cells. Now, they are supposed to arise from neural crest mesenchymal stem cells. They commonly arise from muscles. They may arise due to the rearrangement of chromosomes.

The most common site of primary tumor is a long bone; it does not develop in bones of the cranium, and hence the orbital involvement is always metastatic. It is one of the malignancies that develop following radiation therapy for retinoblastoma.

It is commonly seen in the second decade but may be present in children under 10.

The orbital manifestations are proptosis and swelling of soft orbital tissue that contribute to the development of proptosis and pains in and around the orbit. It may be associated with fever, which is a misleading finding, and the case may be wrongly thought to be an infective process. The diagnosis is confirmed by CT, MRI, and a fine needle biopsy.

The vision is not always compromised. The overall prognosis is bad. The treatment is mostly chemotherapy.

Differential diagnosis consists of both primary and metastatic growths of the orbit; they are orbital retinoblastoma, neuroblastoma, and lymphoma of bone rhabdomyosarcoma.

Other treatments consist of radiation, autologous bone marrow transplants, and stem cell therapy.

Burkitt's Lymphoma

Burkitt lymphoma is a non-Hodgkin's lymphoma of rapid progress thought to be of virus origin; the virus commonly causing the disorder is the Epstein-Barr virus. It is seen in all ages, with predilection in children between 7 and 10 years. Immunosuppression is supposed to be a contributing factor, and boys and girls are equally affected. It has been reported in many countries, mostly in central Africa.

It is sporadic and starts in the maxilla, from which it creeps into the orbit, causing proptosis pain, swelling of the lids, and ballooning of the conjunctiva without ecchymosis. Its clinical presentation is similar to that of metastatic neuroblastoma, which is always associated with ecchymosis. Burkitt tumor is rarely bilateral.

It shows predilection for orbit sparing the eyeball. The change in the eyeball is secondary to proptosis and not malignancy.

In late stages, it may invade the central nervous system and prove fatal. It is radiosensitive and responds to chemotherapy. Recurrences are common and life threatening.

Histiocytosis

Histiocytosis is a relatively uncommon tumor, mostly seen in children with ocular and systemic involvement.

Histiocytosis is a systemic disease of the special cells of the WBC, also known as Langerhans cell cytosis. That is commonly seen in children with ocular and extraocular findings alone or in combination. The disease starts in infancy and early childhood. The common orbital features are eosinophilic granulomas of the orbital wall. It causes bilateral asymmetric.

Proptosis is generally associated with diabetes insipidus. It is treated by chemotherapy **(Fig. 11.26)**.

In the past, they have been confused as Hand-Schuler-Christian disease and eosinophilic granuloma. Presently, it is referred to as Langerhans cell cytosis. Langerhans cells are derived from bone marrow; they are present in many tissues in the body besides the orbit. It is claimed that it is not a malignancy but an autoimmune disease that responds to steroids. It causes bilateral proptosis, may involve bones of the orbit, and diabetes insipidus is a common accompaniment due to the involvement of the posterior pituitary. The malady may involve intraocular structures; treatment consists of systemic steroids, anticancer drugs, and radiation.

Hodgkin's Lymphoma

This malignant disorder is seen generally above 5 years of age; the incidence increases with age and is maximum in the late years of the first decade; it is more frequent in boys. It is amenable to chemotherapy and radiation.

Optic Nerve Gliomas

Optic nerve gliomas are encountered between birth and age 20. They have not been reported in the third decade; hence, they are called juvenile pilocytic astrocytoma on the basis of histopathology. As they have a propensity to involve the visual tract, they are also called optic pathway gliomas. In fact, they are low-grade, slow-progressing brain tumors that are hamartomas in origin. They rarely turn malignant; the malignant variety is called glioblastoma. 25% of optic nerve gliomas are associated with neurofibromatosis type 1. Optic nerve gliomas without associated neurofibromatosis do not follow any genetic pattern **(Fig. 11.27)**.

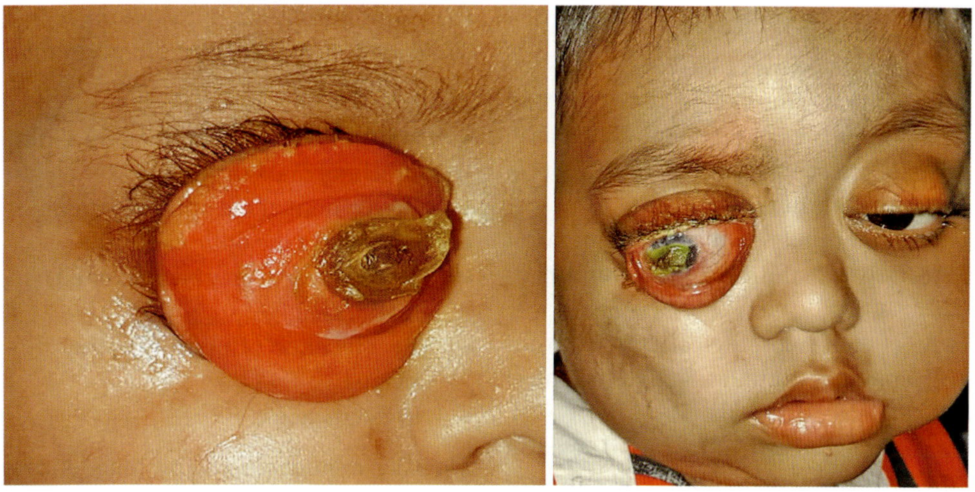

Fig. 11.26: Child with histiocytosis.

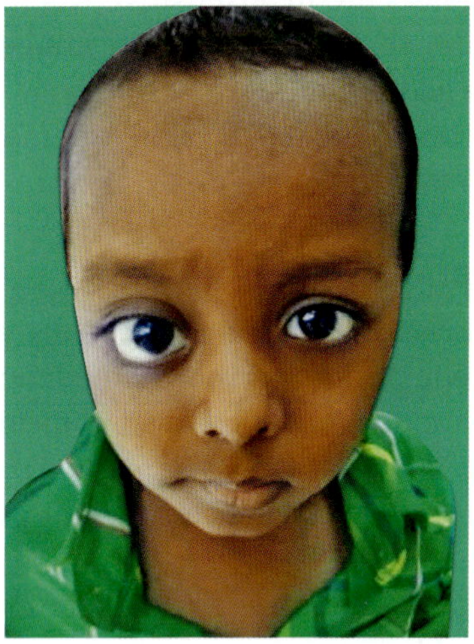

Fig. 11.27: Right-sided optic nerve glioma producing unilateral, slow-growing proptosis.

The association of neurofibroma type 1 with optic nerve glioma is so common that a child with a café-au-lait spot with unilateral slow-growing proptosis is a candidate for optic nerve glioma unless proved otherwise.

Only one-fourth of gliomas involve the orbital part of the optic nerve; the rest develop in the intracranial part and chiasma.

The intracranial type may extend into ventricles to find its way to the hypothalamus. Such tumors produce raised intracranial tension and papilledema, they are not only vision threatening but fatal unless treated. Fortunately, they are slow progressing; hence, they do not cause early death.

Clinical Presentation

The most common age of presentation is under 5 years. The parents complain that one eye of the child is larger and more prominent. On examination, the child has mild to moderate unilateral axial proptosis. The child may have diminished vision ranging from loss of one line to 6/60, depending on the extent of involvement of the optic nerve. The ipsilateral eye generally has a variable degree of squint with normal movements. There is no ptosis or lagophthalmos. The eyes are externally normal. Initially, the pupillary reaction is normal; in later years, the child may have an afferent pupillary defect. The onset of an abnormal pupillary reaction denotes the beginning of optic atrophy that may be primary or postpapillae edematous. The onset of papilledema means the presence of visual tract involvement with infiltration in the ventricle or even the hypothalamus.

The age of chiasmal involvement is more than that of nerve involvement, i.e., the second decade, and may be associated with symptoms of central nervous involvement. The presence of café-au-lait spots on the skin and Lisch nodules on the iris are suggestive of the presence of neurofibroma type 1.

The growth of the orbital part has a typical spindle shape. Anteriorly, it rarely reaches the optic nerve head and may extend back into the intracanalicular part of the nerve. Extension of growth in the intracanalicular part causes enlargement of the optic foramen and canal.

As the growth is intraconal, it produces axial proptosis. The growth is not palpable; the proptosis is nonreducible and does not increase with the Valsalva maneuver.

Diagnosis

Diagnosis depends on the following points:

- The clinical presentation of unilateral slow-growing, mild-to-moderate proptosis in an apparently healthy child under 10 years of age with Café-au-Lait Sport is strongly suggestive of optic nerve glioma.
- Diminished vision and optic nerve changes manifest after months to years of the first presentation of proptosis.
- The above findings with neurological deficits point toward the involvement of the chiasma that may have corresponding field defects.
- Signs and symptoms of raised intracranial tension are seen in the involvement of the ventricle and hypothalamus.
- Blood count and biochemical tests are noncontributory.
- Real diagnostic tools are imaging devices: X-ray, USG, CT, and MRI.

X-ray

- Rhese view reveals the presence of retrobulbar growth.
- A more specific change is seen in the X-ray of the optic foramen; both foramina should be pictured for comparison.

The features of which are:

- An optic foramen >7.5 mm is suggestive of optic nerve glioma extension in the foramen. The normal diameter of the optic foramen is 6.5 mm.
- A difference of >1.5 mm between the two is suggestive of a tumor on the side with a larger foramen.
- The enlargement is uniform.
- The lip of the enlarged foramen is sclerosed with a shining look.
- The canal is not enlarged because the growth rarely invades the canal. In contrast to this, enlargement is common in retinoblastoma, which has a tendency to become intracranial via the optic canal.
- Involvement of the sella is seen in the involvement of the chiasma*. In such a situation, the sella loses its circular appearance, i.e., is replaced by a J-shaped deformity.

Ultrasonography of optic glioma: B-scan reveals the presence of fusiform retrobulbar homogenous mass.

Computed tomography

- Computed tomography shows diffuse retrobulbar, intraconal mass that involves the optic nerve.
- Enlargement of the optic foramen
- Widening of the optic canal
- The optic nerve may be thickened, lengthened, kinked, and buckled.
- The presence of neurofibroma type 1 may become obvious.
- No calcification

Magnetic resonance imaging: Magnetic resonance imaging is better than the other imaging methods described above; it shows intracranial extension better than seen in CT. The tumors are hyposensitive when T1-weighted and hyperintense on T2, and the images are better enhanced by gadolinium. MRI also reveals intracranial extension. A combination of CT and MRI may be required sometimes.

Management

- *No treatment:* If the proptosis is slow-growing with mild to moderate loss of vision without nervous system involvement, it is best observed clinically. Repeated MRIs over the years is the best method of observation, along with fundus and field examinations.
- *Treatment is required*:
    - If the eye has vision but is not aesthetically acceptable.
    - A blind proptosed eye with pain due to exposure may be operated on through an orbitotomy or craniotomy. The aim should be to spare the nerve and remove as much as possible of the growth piece meal. Endoscopy that is removable gives a better result.
    - Radiation is used if there is evidence of intracranial extension. Radiation is fraught with chances of radiation-induced central nervous system disorder; the possibility of a second malignancy cannot be ruled out.

**Chiasmal glioma:* It is generally independent of orbital tumors, though both share the same histopathology. The chiasmal glioma may extend into the third ventricle or even the hypothalamus and optic tract. The involvement of the chiasma does not produce a typical bitemporal field defect, which is a sure sign of pituitary adenoma. In contrast to bilateral hemianopia, field changes in chiasma glioma are irregular; they are more akin to field changes seen in optic neuritis. Involvement of the third ventricle and hypothalamus produces a syndrome consisting of obesity, diabetes, precocious puberty, dwarfism, and panhypopituitarism. Chiasmal glioma is best treated by chemotherapy.

- Chemotherapy has a better result than radiation. The commonly used drugs are actinomycin D and vincristine. The newer drugs presently available are: MEK inhibitors and bevacizumab.
- Chemotherapy may be supplemented with radiation.
- The overall result of the treatment is uncertain.

Leukemic Deposits in Children

Lymphoblastic leukemia is more common to involve the orbit than other types; it not only involves the orbit but is also known to involve intraocular structure. The deposits are bilateral, mostly involving the posterior segment in the form of retinopathy. Myeloid leukemia is a major cause of leukemic retinopathy, which is not seen in children. The child with a leukemic deposit in the orbit has thrombocytopenia and anemia, bleeding from the gums, and epistaxis. The condition is treated with chemotherapy and radiation **(Fig. 11.28)**.

Orbital Varices

They are relatively rare congenital malformations of the veins of the orbit that may spill over the conjunctiva. In this condition, there is dilatation of congenitally deformed venous channels in the orbit. It could be primary or secondary. The primary is congenital in nature, causing uniocular, intermittent, nonpulsatile proptosis. The proptosis is present at birth but generally noticed in early infancy when the child strains or lowers the head. It may be associated with dilated vessels in the conjunctiva, lid, or scalp. One of the prevailing theories is that the varices are, in fact, variations of capillary hemangioma or lymphangioma. The varices keep on increasing slowly until puberty, then stop growing. The X-ray picture shows an enlarged orbit, round phleboliths, and prominent vascular markings in the frontal bone. USG shows dilatation in the superior ophthalmic vein. CT and MRI are better options **(Fig. 11.29)**.

Meningioma of the Optic Nerve

Meningeal involvement by a new growth is relatively rare in children compared to glioma. It is far more common in adults that too, in the mid-fifties, and in females.

Meningiomas are benign tumors covering the optic nerve. They can be broadly divided into two groups, i.e., intracranial and intraorbital. The tumors arise from arachnoid cap cells and meningothelial cells. The intracranial growths are seen in adults and may have a widespread distribution with different clinical presentations, i.e., parasagittal meningioma, sphenoidal ridge meningioma, and cavernous sinus meningioma.

The intraorbital meningiomas are seen in children. The child is brought on with a loss of vision and a mild proptosis of slow progress. Early loss of vision with a pupillary defect prompts parents to bring the child for consultation.

> A child with mild proptosis preceded by loss of vision and pupillary abnormalities is most probably suffering from meningioma of the optic nerve.

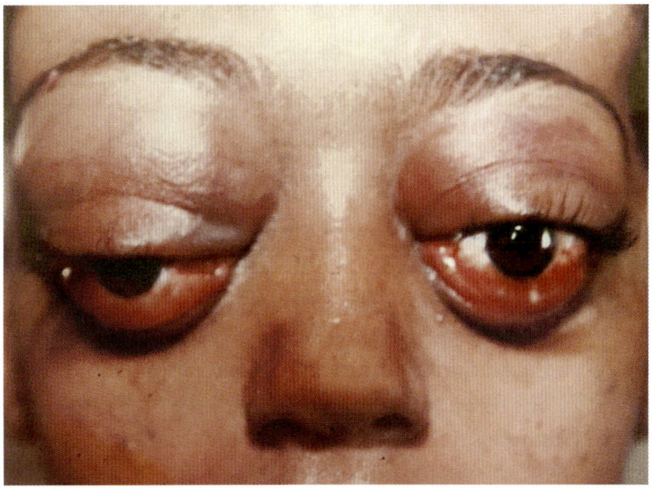

Fig. 11.28: Bilateral proptosis due to leukemic deposit. *Courtesy:* Dr Somen Misra.

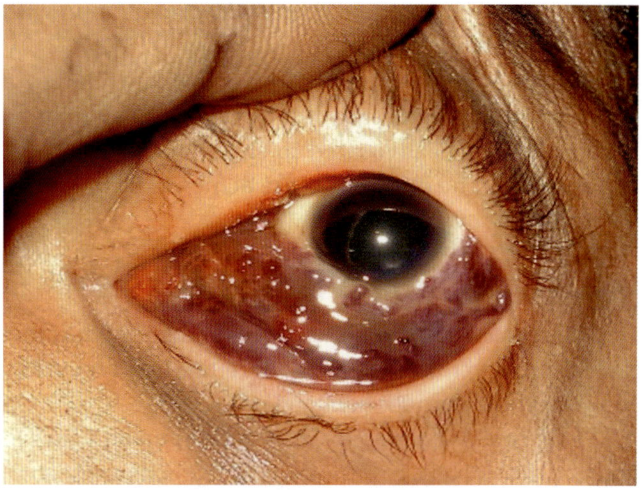

Fig. 11.29: Orbital varices with conjunctival involvement. *Courtesy:* Professor ML Garg.

On examination, the child has variable, noncorrectable visual defects, squint, and afferent pupillary defects. On fundus examination, there is a variable degree of pallor of the disc with optociliary vessels.

The presence of diminished vision, pale disc, and optociliary vessels form a triad not seen in other conditions. Rarely, there may be associated disc edema, which points toward intracranial growth. A long-standing meningioma has the tendency to break out of the optic nerve sheath and invade the orbital contents. Once the meningioma becomes extradural, it turns invasive, requiring early intervention.

Diagnosis

- The main differential diagnosis consists of optic nerve gliomas.
- The triad of diminished vision, pale disc with optociliary vessels, should raise the suspension of intraorbital optic nerve meningioma.
- An early loss of vision with mild proptosis points toward meningioma of the optic nerve.
- The diagnosis is confirmed by imaging that shows tubular enlargement of the optic nerve with a tram track change in the sheath and calcification.

Treatment

The meningiomas are not sensitive to chemotherapy but respond to hormonal therapy because about 70% of meningioma cells contain both estrogen and progesterone receptors. This explains the increase in size of tumors in pregnancy and breast feeding; this forms the basis of antiestrogen/progesterone therapy in consultation with an endocrinologist.

Hormone therapy is not recommended for children.

The meningiomas are not very radiosensitive as well. Radiation is advocated to stabilize the growth of meningioma. The best results are achieved by definitive surgery.

Hemangioma of the Orbit

Hemangiomas are yet another group of hamartomas that have a predilection for orbit. There are two types, i.e., capillary and cavernous hemangiomas.

The former is commonly seen in children and later in adults. Occasionally, cavernous hemangiomas are seen in the second decade. Both types are congenital. Capillary hemangiomas may be detected at birth or soon after. The two verities have distinct clinical features and separate modes of management.

Capillary Hemangioma

They are the most common hamartomatous orbital growths in infants and may be present at birth or detected later. The growth may involve the orbit, lids, skin of the face, and other parts of the body. A combination of orbit and lid is frequent. So much so that some of the orbital tumors may be thought to be arising in the lids. This happens due to the purple-blue discoloration of the skin of the lid. Histopathologically, the capillary hemangiomas are blood-filled endothelial channels without a true capsule. The growth is commonly diffuse and rarely localized, and it may be confused with cavernous hemangioma. The growth is more commonly present in the superonasal aspect of the anterior orbit and may be continuous with lid growth. The growth on the lid is referred to as a strawberry spot. The tumor has three stages of involution, i.e., a stage of rapid growth, a stage of stability, and a stage of regression. The first is seen in the first year of life; the second lasts for the next 2–3 years; and the last takes about 4–5 years to be over. The deeper lesions are not visible; they cause proptosis as per their location, and the growths disappear with age due to the inherent property of involution.

Topographically, the growths are put into three broad groups:

1. Present in the anterior orbit as a purple subcutaneous mass that becomes pink on straining
2. A visible strawberry lesion on the superonasal anterior orbit
3. A nonvisible mass deep in orbit with mild to moderate proptosis

Diagnosis

- The diagnosis of a strawberry lesion is straightforward
- Difficulty arises with occult lesions, which are best diagnosed by various imaging methods:
  - *X-ray:* It is not very specific; it may show uniform enlargement of the orbit without a bony defect.
  - *USG:* B-scan USG is better than X-rays in delineating the mass, which has an irregular shape that blends with the surrounding intraocular tissue.
  - *CT:* It reveals the presence of irregular mass as in an X-ray. The appearance is sharper than an X-ray.

A contrast study may show feeding vessels and vascular architecture.

- *MRI:* This is better than the above imagings when done by fat suppression; a T1-weighted image with gadolinium and fat suppression is a better option; on a T2-weighted protocol, the tumors look hyperintense against a hypointense surrounding.

Differential diagnosis: The conditions that are often mistaken as capillary hemangiomas are:

- Cavernous hemangiomas, which are seen in adults and are well capsulated
- Port wine stain (nevus flammeus) in Sturge–Weber syndrome
- Early stage of rhabdomyosarcoma

Management

Management is divided into two parts:

1. Management of the growth
2. Management of errors in refraction and amblyopia

Management of the growth: In managing the growth, it should be kept in mind that the growth is benign and self-limiting due to its inherent involution, stabilization, and regression. The whole process may take as long as 5–6 years. The parents should be counseled about its benignity and self-limitation. If the growth is large or grows relentlessly, which is rare, it is treated with a steroid, either intralesional or oral. It takes weeks to months to disappear following interlesional injection; the benefit of steroid therapy should be weighed against the side effects of steroids in infants and children. Other nonsteroidal therapies available are beta blockers. The most common beta blocker used is propanol as an oral tablet or syrup in consultation with a pediatrician. Timolol, yet another beta blocker commonly used in the management of glaucoma, may be used as drops in the eye or gel (0.5%) rubbed over the growth two to three times a day. It takes months to be effective. The exact action of beta blockers in the management of capillary hemangioma is not well understood. The common theories are: Inhibition of angiogenesis, and vasoconstriction.

The other modalities available are:

- Cryo application
- Radiotherapy
- Yttrium-Aluminum-Garnet (YAG) laser photocoagulation
- Surgical

Management of errors in refraction and amblyopia: Large capillary hemangiomas, mostly of the lids, are generally associated with errors of refraction, amblyopia, and squints of various grades and types, all of which require management with suitable methods.

Cavernous Hemangiomas

Cavernous hemangiomas are also hamartomas, mostly found in the third decade and upward. They are solitary, well-defined, and capsulated, in contrast to capillary hemangiomas, which are noncapsulated and ill defined. Though congenital anomalies are rarely seen in children, when they are present, they are unilateral. An adult in the third decade with slow-growing unilateral, painless proptosis with restricted movement and diminished vision should undergo imaging. On B-scan USG, a well-demarcated intraconal lesion is characteristic. CT and MRI are more specific; they show moderately well-circumscribed intraconal swelling.

Management

There is no specific treatment; steroids are effective, as are beta blockers. Slow-growing proptosis with mild to moderate nonprogressive visual loss should be observed; otherwise, eyes with symptoms should undergo complete removal by the appropriate method.

Lymphangioma

They are hamartomas seen in children; they are vascular and not lymphatic, as the term may suggest, and develop from vascular mesenchyme independent of arterial or venous connection. However, they may have a lymphatic element incorporated. The incidence of lymphangioma of the orbit is lower than that of hemangiomas. They are seen not only in the orbit but also in the conjunctiva and other parts of the head and neck. They may present as cystic growths of the palate, cheek, or upper respiratory tract.

There are two modes of presentation. The first is chronic, and the other is acute.

The first presents as slow-developing uniocular proptosis. The progress may continue for years without hampering vision.

The second mode is acute in onset, superimposed on a preexisting lesion, manifesting as painful proptosis due to rupture of the vessel-like channels. The channels may dilate and form cysts with lymph-like fluid or dark blood. The acute episode of proptosis is secondary to the rupture of blood cysts. The blood in the cysts has a dark color; hence, the cysts are called chocolate cysts. Arterialization of the vessels is another common change.

The growths are infiltration without metastasis; if the growth invades the orbital apex or the blood spreads backward, various types of paralytic squints develop. Pressure on the optic nerve may cause diminished vision.

Rupture of cyst is self-limited. There are no treatments except palliatives. The cutaneous lesions are best dealt with by dermatologists.

Differential Diagnosis

- Black eye
- Hematoma orbit
- Orbital emphysema
- Hemangioma
- Rhabdomyosarcoma
- Neuroblastoma
- Orbital cellulitis
- Pseudotumor orbit

ORBITAL PSEUDOTUMOR (IDIOPATHIC ORBITAL INFLAMMATION)

Orbital pseudotumors comprise a group of chronic inflammatory disorders that clinically behave as neoplasms but are not being so. Typical features of malignancy are not seen on histopathology. The exact cause of the disorder is not known; they are considered to be a form of localized lymphocytic infiltration of autoimmune origin.

It may be seen at any age. In children, it is mostly seen in the second decade; incidence increases with age; and the maximum cases are met in the fifth and sixth decade. When present in children, 50% are bilateral.

The usual presentation is subacute, painful unilateral proptosis with restricted movements, diplopia, and chemosis of the conjunctiva, depending on position, size, and duration of the growth. The mass may or may not be palpable. The condition is known to subside without going into a chronic stage or may become smoldering or intermittent. Prolonged course, not responding to treatment, passes into the stage of an immobile globe, diminished vision, and ptosis.

The lesion is an infiltrative mass in the orbital fat. Besides orbital fat, it may involve any or all orbital tissues. The position of the diffuse mass varies from the anterior orbit to a deeper level near the apex of the orbit. The mass may grow back in the anterior cavernous sinus.

Depending upon the position of the mass, the condition is classified as—anterior cavernous sinus syndrome, superior orbital fissure syndrome*, and orbital apex syndrome†. Occasionally, the mass may be extensive enough to fill the entire orbital cavity. The most common presentation is mild to moderate proptosis, the direction of which depends on the position of the growth. It may present as a case of isolated myositis. The optic nerve, in spite of its passage through the mass, is not infiltrated but may be compressed. Rarely, the lacrimal gland, too, may be involved.

The pseudo-orbital tumor begins with acute onset and follows any of the following clinical courses:

- Subside without sequelae over weeks to months.
- Become intermittent.
- Subsides and recurrences.
- Gradually die down over years, leaving a frozen orbit due to fibrosis of extraocular muscle.

A pseudotumor of the orbit may be idiopathic or associated with scleritis, myositis, chronic dacryoadenitis, rheumatoid arthritis, Crohn's disease, systemic lupus erythematosus, nonspecific granuloma, vasculitis, reactive lymphoid hyperplasia, and anterior cavernous sinusitis.

Differential Diagnosis

A definitive diagnosis is by exclusion, confirmed by histopathology of a piece removed either surgically or by fine needle aspiration. The investigation commonly ordered consists of USG, CT, and MRI. That shows thickening of the uveoscleral complex, flattening of the posterior scleral curve, abolishment of the posterior

**Superior orbital fissure syndrome:* This is also known as Tolosa-Hunt syndrome or anterior cavernous sinus disease. The syndrome is a localized chronic inflammation of bones, forming superior orbital fissures and structures passing through them. The structures commonly involved are cranial nerves passing through the fissure, resulting in the paralysis of multiple cranial nerves. The condition should be differentiated from: Carotid cavernous fistula, chronic cavernous sinus thrombosis, Wegener granuloma, pituitary apoplexy, sarcoidosis, and mucormycosis.

†*Orbital apex syndrome:* This is a more extensive form of superior orbital fissure syndrome involving the optic foramen in general and the optic nerve in particular. The superior orbital fissure syndrome generally does not involve the optic nerve, which is the hallmark of orbital apex syndrome. The changes may be mild to moderate papilledema with its sequelae.

V-shaped feature, thickening of extraocular muscles, thickening of the optic nerve, and widening of the superior orbital fissure.

The condition is rarely seen in children under 15 years of age.

The condition must be differentiated from:

- Specific conditions of sarcoidosis and tuberculosis
- Thyroid eye disease
- Wegner granuloma
- Rhabdomyosarcoma
- Secondaries in orbit
- Parasitic cyst of the orbit

Treatment

- There is no specific treatment.
- Surgery is not indicated unless the globe is threatened.
- The surgical procedure followed is debulking of the mass by endonasal endoscopic procedure.
- The management is palliative, comprising of:
    - Systemic steroids
    - Antimetabolites
    - Low-dose radiation

Systemic steroid therapy is the cornerstone of management. Systemic steroids are effective most of the time, especially in acute and subacute phases. The initial dose varies between 60 and 80 mg of prednisone per day over a week. If there is a favorable result, the drug is gradually tapered over several weeks to prevent relapse. It may be administered as a single dose daily in consultation with a pediatrician.

A cytotoxic agent could be considered only if systemic steroids prove to be ineffective. The cytotoxic agents do not show immediate results; they take days to weeks to be effective; hence, the practice is to combine them with gradually tapering steroids. The commonly used drugs are chlorambucil, cyclophosphamide, methotrexate, cyclosporine, and azathioprine, in consultation with a pediatric oncologist.

Low-dose radiation may be required, along with steroids and cytotoxic drugs. Antibiotics per se do not have any role in the management of pseudotumors.

Mucormycosis of the Orbit

Mucormycosis of the orbit is generally seen in old, debilitated, immunocompromised patients with diabetic coma, renal failure, and those who have undergone a transplant. It is commonly seen in persons with ADIS. There is a sudden rise in cases of mucormycosis in persons of all ages suffering from COVID-19 or post-COVID syndrome **(Figs. 11.30 and 11.31)**.

As the children do not suffer from corona or corona-related conditions, the mucormycosis in them is not corona-related but other conditions listed above. The disorder is hyperacute, blinding, and life-threatening. The disease is caused by a fungus called *Rhizopus*. It starts in the nasopharynx, spreading to the orbit, causing black crusty lesions in the nasopharynx, orbit, and conjunctiva. The cranial nerves, from the third to the sixth, are commonly involved. The diagnosis is straightforward in an immunosuppressed, debilitated person by the presence of typical black growth in the conjunctiva and orbit. The diagnosis is confirmed by an examination of the biopsy, which shows typical nonseptate branching hyphae.

The treatment is frustrating. This is an ophthalmic emergency that should be managed by a team of ENT

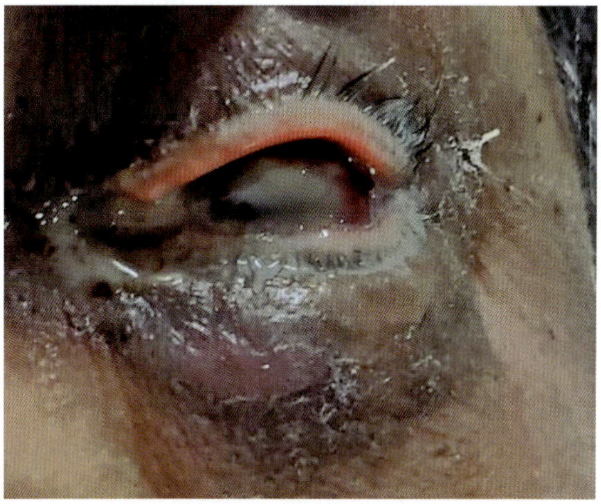

Fig. 11.30: Mucormycosis orbit in a patient suffering from COVID-19.
Courtesy: Professor Vijaya Sahu.

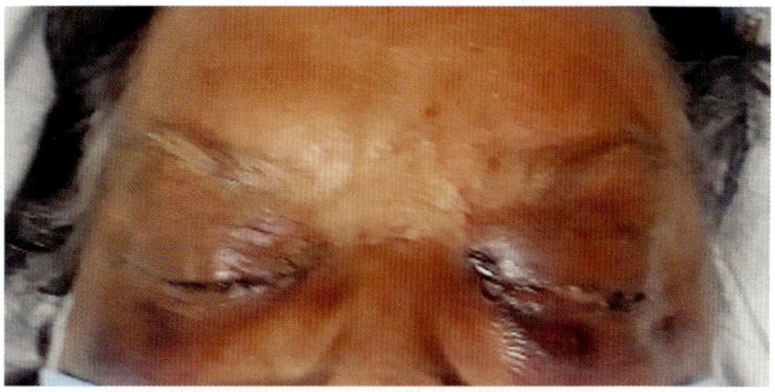

Fig. 11.31: Mucormycosis orbit in a patient suffering from COVID-19.
Courtesy: Dr Somen Misra.

specialists, mycologists, and internists. The treatment consists of the correction of systemic disease and intravenous antifungal drugs, such as high doses of amphotericin B. Early debridement may be able to contain the infection. However, exenteration may occasionally be the last hope to save a life.

The age-wise distribution of childhood proptosis is mentioned in **Table 11.2**.

Clinical Features of Proptosis (in All Ages)

The orbit has been called Pandora's Box because it contains a multitude of tissues surrounded by many structures, the disorder of which influences the structures in the orbit. Orbits may, however, be inflicted by primary infection, inflammation, and neoplasm; thus, it is natural that orbital disorders will have many clinical features. Proptosis, being the most prominent disorder, shares many clinical features of not only the orbit but also surrounding structures. The most common among them are:

- *Pain:* Pain is a relative term; its severity differs from person to person. Children have a greater threshold for pain. They may not complain until it is unbearable; a nonverbal child may not be able to express pain or cry. Pain in proptosis depends on the extent and progress of proptosis. A slow-growing proptosis, as seen in the glioma of the optic nerve, may not cause pain until the cornea is exposed; a fast-growing proptosis such as acute orbital cellulitis and cavernous sinus thrombosis may be very painful and reported early.
- *Diminished vision:* Diminished vision also varies with the extent of proptosis. It may precede or follow the development of proptosis; it may vary from a loss of a few lines to a total absence of vision. The causes of diminished vision are:
    - Error of refraction: An *error of refraction* is caused. Due to the compression of the eyeball at various locations, it generally produces astigmatism that is irregular; a shift of the retina forward causes relative hypermetropia.
    - Fundus changes: *Fundus changes* range between mild edema of the disc to frank papilledema and optic atrophy of various grades and vascular changes.
    - Squint: *Squint* in proptosis is generally restrictive due to the involvement of extraocular muscles and their nerve supply. Errors in refraction contribute to concomitant squints. Paralytic and restrictive squints may cause diplopia.
    - Amblyopia: *Amblyopia* is common in children due to error or refraction, muscle imbalance, and fundus changes. Amblyopia may develop even in loss of vision by two to three lines.
    - Changes in the cornea: *Changes in the cornea* cause diminished, painful vision due to exposure.
- True ptosis, per se, is not part of proptosis; it happens only if the upper division of the third nerve is involved. Pseudoptosis develops with edema of the lids.
- Lagophthalmos in proptosis is mechanical; it is caused when a bulging eyeball prevents the lid from coming down.
- Corneal changes are late and seen following exposure. They range from superficial abrasions to sloughing corneal ulcers; corneal involvement may occur in loss of corneal sensation.
- Pupillary changes consist of a relative afferent pupillary defect due to optic nerve involvement.
- The rise of intraocular pressure happens due to pressure from extraocular causes and the rise of episcleral pressure.
- The rise of the intraorbital pressure takes place due to an extraocular expending orbital lesion. Unlike intraorbital pressure, there is no clinical method to measure intraorbital pressure.
- Fundus changes depend on the involvement of the optic nerve. It may be optic atrophy or papilledema and their consequences. The other changes are central retinal artery obstruction and central retinal vein stasis.
- Positive changes in imaging.

TABLE 11.2: Age distribution in unilateral and bilateral proptosis.

Age	*Unilateral*	*Bilateral*
Under 10 years	Congenital cystic eye ball	Craniosynostosis
	Rhabdomyosarcoma, retinoblastoma, neuroblastoma, capillary hemangioma, lymphangiomas, neurofibroma, dermoid, optic nerve glioma, meningocele, and leukemia	Leukemia, Hodgkin's lymphoma, cavernous sinus and thrombosis, neuroblastoma
Above 10 years	They behave like disorders of early adulthood	They behave like disorders of early adulthood

Clinical Examination of Proptosis

Like all disorders, evaluation of proptosis should be preceded by history of the disease as follows:

- *History:*
  - *Age of onset:* Proptosis can be present at birth as congenital anomalies of the cranium and face; there are various types of craniostenosis, meningocele and meningoencephalocele, and microphthalmos with congenital cysts. Besides these deformities, there may be some congenital new growths such as dermoid, epidermoid, teratoma, and hamartomas. Some of the malignant growths seen in infancy are rhabdomyosarcoma and Burkitt lymphoma. Common secondaries that cause proptosis in infancy and childhood are neuroblastoma, Ewing's tumor, Wilms tumor, and leukemia. Orbital retinoblastoma also manifests in childhood and causes fast-growing proptosis. The other new growths that cause proptosis are orbital varix and fibrous dysplasia. The acquired conditions are mostly infectious; they are orbital cellulitis, orbital abscess, cavernous sinus thrombosis, panophthalmitis, and retrobulbar hemorrhage. Intraorbital foreign bodies and intraorbital granulomas are less common in childhood. Orbital pseudotumors are seen in the late first decade and second decade.
  - *Mode:* Sudden onset is seen in acute orbital cellulitis, panophthalmitis, cavernous sinus thrombosis, and trauma with retrobulbar hemorrhage. Primary and secondary tumors have moderate to fast progress.
  - Congenital anomalies have slow to very slow progress.
  - Recurrences in retinoblastoma, rhabdomyosarcoma, neuroblastoma, and leukemia are frequent following initial successful treatment.
  - Pain is frequent in acute infective lesions such as orbital cellulitis, orbital abscess, cavernous sinus thrombosis, or fast-expanding masses. Orbital abscesses are the most painful. Pain, lacrimation, and photophobia are caused due to exposure keratitis. Unexplained pain always points toward raised intraocular pressure.
  - Diplopia means paralytic or restrictive strabismus.
  - *Diminished vision:* Loss of vision in proptosis is an indication of optic nerve involvement, either as optic nerve glioma or pressure-induced optic atrophy/papilledema.
- *Clinical examination:*
  - *Evaluation of vision:* A recording of vision should precede all examinations, not only for diagnosis but also to record the progress of the condition. The legal aspect of visual acuity should not be overlooked.

> In a nonverbal child, a bright cornea, normal anterior chamber, brisk direct and indirect pupillary reaction, clear media, absence of error of refraction, and normal fundus denote good vision, except in cases of cortical blindness.

  Slow deterioration of vision is seen in craniostenosis, optic nerve glioma, and capillary hemangioma. In optic nerve glioma, loss of vision precedes proptosis, and corneal involvement is generally associated with a painful loss of vision. Fundus changes that include optic neuropathy, hemorrhage in the retina and vitreous, and the development of a curvature error of refraction are some other causes of subnormal vision.

  - *Pupillary reaction:* A relative afferent pupillary defect denotes ipsilateral optic nerve involvement. As in optic nerve glioma, cavernous sinus thrombosis, Tolosa Hunt syndrome, and orbital apex syndrome. A dilated pupil indicates internal ophthalmoplegia and absent vision.
  - *Inspection:* A fully established proptosis can be diagnosed by simple inspection, but that is not sufficient to pinpoint the cause of proptosis, on which depends its management. The first condition that requires differentiation is pseudoproptosis. The cause of pseudoproptosis may lie in the same eye or the contralateral. The ipsilateral causes could be in the lids or the eyeballs. The ipsilateral causes in the lid could be edema, hematoma or lid retraction, and lagophthalmos. The conditions on the globe that mimic proptosis are pathological myopia, ciliary staphyloma, and unilateral advanced buphthalmos. The contralateral causes that may be mistaken for proptosis in the normal eyes are mild ptosis, microphthalmos, phthisis, and enophthalmos.
  - *Laterality:* The next step is to ascertain if the proptosis is unilateral or bilateral; if bilateral, it is equal and symmetrical on both sides.

    The causes of unilateral proptosis in children are:
    - Orbital cellulitis
    - Orbital and periorbital abscess
    - Early stage of cavernous sinus thrombosis
    - Rhabdomyosarcoma

- Optic nerve gliomas
- Capillary hemangioma
- Lymphangioma
- Dermoids
- Orbital injury
- Congenital anomalies (rare)

The causes of bilateral proptosis in children are:

- Craniofacial dysostosis
- Systemic condition
- The systemic conditions are leukemia, bilateral retinoblastoma, cavernous sinus thrombosis, neuroblastoma, and secondary deposits.

- *Direction of proptosis:* The direction of proptosis gives a clue to the position and cause of proptosis in relation to the globe. The eyeball may be displaced axially or eccentrically. The latter can be unidirectional or a combination.

  The causes of axial proptosis lie in the muscle cone. The most common cause is glioma of the optic nerve. The other causes are pus in the muscle cone, parasitic cysts in the muscle cone, and foreign bodies in the muscle cone.

  The causes of eccentric proptosis lie outside the muscle cone. They are generally from the walls of the orbit, lacrimal gland, or sinuses. A growth from the medial wash pushes the eyeball laterally and forward; similarly, a growth from the lateral wall pushes the eyeball in the opposite direction; a growth from the lacrimal gland will push the eyeball forward; and inferomedially, the growth of the maxilla causes forward and upward displacement.
- *Position of the lid:* Normally, the upper lid covers the superior cornea by 1.00 mm, the lower lid touches the lower pole of the cornea, and no strip of sclera is visible between the cornea and lid. A visible strip of cornea is strongly suggestive of proptosis unless proved otherwise. The other cause of bare sclera without proptosis is lid retraction.
- *Visible pulsation:* Normally, the proptosed globe does not show any pulsation; an eye with pulsation is suggestive of a retrobulbar vascular mass in the muscle cone, which is variably associated with axial proptosis.
- *Palpation:* Palpation in proptosis is divided into two parts, i.e., palpation of the orbital margin and palpation of orbital mass.
  i. The orbital margin is smooth without any projection or defect except the superior orbital notch, and rarely, in the trochlea, a palpebral protuberance or deficit is pathognomonic.
  ii. Anteriorly placed masses are easily palpable. To palpate a mass, the index finger of the examiner is insinuated between the mass and the orbital wall. If the finger cannot be insinuated, the growth must be arising from the wall or PNSs. The most common lesions in children are meningocele, encephalocele, and dermoid. The other lesions seen in adults are growths of the lacrimal gland and mucocele or PNSs.
- *Compressibility of the proptosis:* The child is asked to look straight and close the lids; the examiner applies gentle pressure over the closed lids sufficient to push the globe backward. If the child winces the globe the tendered, in such cases the procedure should be abandoned. Otherwise, a compressible mass means a cystic or vascular growth; solid tumors are noncompressible.
- *Cough impulse:* Cough impulses are seen in meningo and meningoencephalocele.
- *Valsalva maneuver:* The procedure is absent in all cases of proptosis except in large capillary hemangioma and varices of the orbit.
- *Forced duction test:* The test is generally done to differentiate between neurological squint and restrictive squint; it is clinically important for thyroid eye disease.
- *Imaging: The various imagings ordered are:*
  - *X-ray:*
    - Skull: AP, lateral, and special positions. Especially to see the optic foramen and superior foramen orbital fissures. For evidence of fractures and retained foreign bodies.
    - PNSs
    - X-ray, chest for secondaries, and widening of the mediastinum
  - USG
  - CT
  - MRI

The above imaging may be sufficient when used alone or may require various combinations.

- *Therapeutic trial:* Sometimes, the administration of steroids reduces proptosis, mostly in pseudotumors of the orbit.

DISORDERS OF ORBIT DUE TO RETRACTION OF GLOBE

The conditions are:

- Anophthalmos
- Enophthalmos

- Microphthalmos
- Nanophthalmos
- Phthisis
- Associated with retraction syndromes

The conditions can be congenital or acquired.

The congenital conditions are anophthalmos, microphthalmos, microphthalmos with cysts, and nanophthalmos.

The acquired conditions are put into a group of conditions that are collectively called enophthalmos. The causes, or enophthalmos, are: Phthisis bulbi, punctured wound of the globe, retraction syndromes, and fracture of the floor of the orbit.

Table 11.3 shows the outline of congenital anomalies of the globe.

Anophthalmos

The term anophthalmos should logically be used to denote the congenital absence of all the structure of the eyeball and its attachments. This happens due to the nondevelopment of cerebral neuroelements from which the eyeball and its immediate attachments develop, leading to the complete absence of neural and mesodermal tissues in the orbit with a normal or near-normal orbit. Such a situation is extremely rare, and the possibility of total absence of the eyeball has been questioned because, on exploring such cases, traces of ocular tissue have been frequently found. Hence, the term was replaced by a better term, clinical anophthalmos, which means the presence of vestigial ocular tissues in the socket.

Anophthalmos has been divided into two groups:

1. Related to the development of the forebrain and the malformation of the anterior part of the neural tube
2. The degeneration of the optic vesicle after its formation may be due to intrauterine infection or trauma. The condition has an array of genetic possibilities in the form of genetic mutations. The mutation is brought on by prenatal and environmental exposure to X-rays, chemicals, drugs, toxins, viruses, and radiation.

TABLE 11.3: Congenital anomalies of the globe.

Basic fault in	*Result*
Formation of an optic vesicle	Anophthalmos
Invagenation of the optic cup	Coloboma with a cystic eyeball
Closure of fetal fissure	Coloboma of uvea
Separation of lids	Cryptophthalmos

Anophthalmos may be:

- *Inherited:* Recessive, dominant, or sex-linked; trisomy 13, 14, 15
- Sporadic
- Associated with craniofacial malformation syndrome
- Associated with congenital multiorgan syndromes

Anophthalmos can be unilateral or bilateral; when unilateral, the other eye may be normal; however, it is more often microphthalmic.

The absence of an eyeball has far-reaching consequences for the development of the orbit and anterior visual path. The presence of an eyeball of normal size is a prerequisite for the development of an orbit. An anophthalmia, or severe microphthalmia, is a hindrance to the development of the orbit. Which in turn affects the development of the face as well.

With anophthalmia, the orbit remains small in all dimensions; it is shallow and conical, and the depth is generally <12.00 mm at its deepest part. The orbital rim is small, and the optic foramen and canal are poorly developed. The small orbit is associated with small lids. The lids are small in height as well as length; both the retractor and constrictors of the lids are malformed, and this leads to a small, slit-like interpalpebral aperture. The lids retain some movement. The lacrimal system may be normal or partially absent. Small orbits and changes in the musculature of the lids result in the shallowing of the fornices.

The differentiation between true anophthalmos and extreme degrees of microphthalmos is academic. CT and MRI show underdeveloped or absent chiasma. This is more common in bilateral cases. In the past, amniocentesis and CT were done in the second trimester as tools of prenatal diagnosis. Presently, amniocentesis has been abandoned.

Management

No visual improvement is possible. The aim is to maintain the symmetry of the face and keep the socket deep enough to fit a cosmetic shell by conformers of gradually increasing size that will enhance the development of the orbit. Attempts are made to rectify other congenital defects. The parents should be informed that the artificial eye has been put in for cosmetic reasons and not for visual purposes. The child should be raised as a visually handicapped child, as per the national guideline.

Microphthalmos

Microphthalmos is the most common congenital anomaly of the globe. Clinically, an eye smaller than two-thirds of the age-matched normal eye is microphthalmic. Another dimension that is taken into consideration is axial length. An eye with an axial length <16 mm is also considered to be microphthalmic. It can be inherited or sporadic. It can be transmitted both as recessive or dominant.

Microphthalmia has been classified into various types.

The commonly used classification is as follows:

- Pure microphthalmos (nanophthalmos)
- Complicated microphthalmos are associated with cataracts, glaucoma, retinal detachment, iridocorneal anomalies, corectopia, ectopia lentis, myopia, congenital retinal detachment, and persistent hyperplastic primary vitreous.
- Colobomatous microphthalmos without cystic eyeball
- Colobomatous microphthalmos with cystic eyeball

Clinical Feature of Microphthalmos

Microphthalmos can be unilateral or bilateral; when unilateral, the other eye may be normal or with minimal changes **(Fig. 11.32)**.

Unilateral microphthalmos Bilateral microphthalmos Bilateral microphthalmos with pseudoptosis

The microphthalmic eyes may not have vision, or vision may be very poor; that is just the ability to perceive light. The interpalpebral aperture is narrow; there is pseudoptosis with retained lid crease; the eyeball lies deep and set with movement; it may have nystagmus. The orbit is generally smaller than normal.

Management

Management of microphthalmos is as difficult as in anophthalmos; however, artificial scleral shells may be successful in minimal microphthalmia. Children with severe loss of vision should be trained as visually challenged.

Nanophthalmos

This rare congenital anomaly of the globe is also called pure microphthalmos because the eyes do not have any developmental lacuna except for failing to keep pace with normal growth. This retardation of normal growth may start even before the child is born. Some authors prefer to call it simple microphthalmos.

This is a bilateral disease seen in full-term infants and diagnosed either as complaints of small eyes or any of the manifestations of poor distant as well as near vision with squint and amblyopia.

The cause of diminished vision is axial shorting of the globe, which is compounded by a flat cornea.

The globe is reduced in size in all meridians. The posterior segment is disproportionately short. A nanophthalmic eye is said to be a normal eye with reduced dimension all-round with hypermetropia, which may be as much as 15D to 20D. The size of the lens is age-matched, but larger in comparison to the volume of the eye. Phakic child with aphakic correction is the term often used to describe a nanophthalmic child, as the child requires distant glasses as high as +6D to 8D.

All the ocular structures are of a smaller size except the lens. The cornea is smaller than its expected size, and the anterior chamber is shallow. The lens is larger when matched with the other structures prone to develop cataracts in the third decade. The sclera is thicker than normal. The thickened sclera throttles the venae vorticosae.

The eyes have poor vision due to high axial and curvature hypermetropia. The shallow anterior chamber and small pupil are predisposed to various types of glaucoma. In spite of being a small hypermetropic eye,

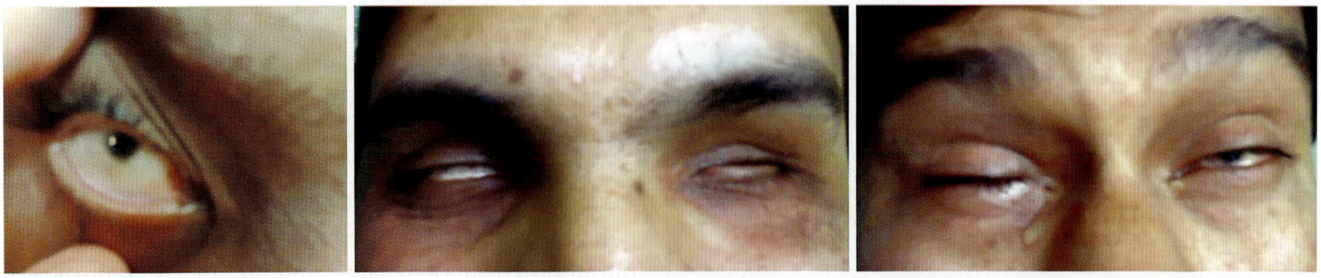

Unilateral microphthalmos — Bilateral microphthalmos — Bilateral microphthalmos with pseudoptosis

Fig. 11.32: Various types of simple microphthalmos.

the nanophthalmic eyes are predisposed to retinal detachment.

The nanophthalmic eyes are prone to develop uveal effusion syndrome* following a penetrating wound that may be surgical or accidental. Hence, all cares to avoid uveal effusion should be taken during any intraocular surgery and managed if it occurs.

The first step in the management of a nanophthalmic child is to correct refractive error and manage amblyopia by standard methods.

The child may require near addition to distance correction.

Abnormal Sclera

The two abnormalities of the sclera that predispose to uveal effusion syndrome are thickened sclera and throttling of venae vorticosae. The normal thickness of the sclera is 0.5 mm at the limbus and 1 mm round the disc. It is thinnest at the attachment of extraocular muscles that is 0.4 mm. In the case of nanophthalmos, it is raised to 2–3 mm behind the scleral spurs, the thickness is best measured by ultrasonic biomicroscopy and anterior segment optical coherence tomography (OCT). The investigations that may pinpoint the cause of nanophthalmos are USG, CT, and MRI.

Management

Management of uveal effusion syndrome in nanophthalmos is difficult and frustrating. The best solution is to anticipate its possibilities in all nanophthalmic eyes prior to intraocular surgery and to keep the intraocular pressure low during surgery with systemic and local antiglaucoma drugs. The commonly used systemic drugs are carbonic and hydrase inhibitors orally and mannitol intravenous during and after surgery. Local antiglaucoma drugs that reduce the production of aqueous and increase uveoscleral outflow are used; constriction of the pupil should be avoided. A peripheral iridectomy is supposed to reduce the chances of glaucoma. Once the condition has been diagnosed, treatment consists of dilatation of the pupil by atropine and frequent use of local steroids. Various surgical methods have been used to alleviate the raised tension, which may be as high as 80.00 mm Hg with unexplained pain. The surgical procedures used are guided paracentesis, anterior vitrectomy, sclerotomy, and extensive vitrectomy with drainage of subchoroidal fluid. Occasionally, the condition has been reported to be self-limiting.

Microphthalmos with Cysts

A congenitally small eye with cystic protrusion through a coloboma, mostly in the lower part, is called a microphthalmos with cyst. The anomaly starts at the optic vesicle stage, with the arrest of the growth of the eyeball along with the protrusion of the retina through the gape. Large posterior colobomas are more likely to cause protrusion than the anterior. The pathology is disorganization of the developing neuroectoderm, changes in the intraocular vasculature, and glial proliferation. The size and position of the cyst vary with the size and position of the coloboma. The cyst may be a small protrusion or large enough to occupy the whole of the orbit, pushing the small eyeball backwards. A microphthalmos with a cyst does not cause true proptosis because the eye never protrudes. The most common presentation is a small bulge in the lower lid.

The whole lid may be stretched over the cyst, and due to stretching, the lid looks translucent and bluish. It is sporadic in nature and mostly unilateral.

Enophthalmos

Enophthalmos is a common orbital disorder, which, in its milder form, may not be noticed on a cursory look. It may be unilateral or bilateral. Unilateral enophthalmos may be mistaken for contralateral exophthalmos or ipsilateral ptosis. It may be familial, which is generally of no clinical significance.

Enophthalmos has been defined in various ways. The most commonly used definition is "abnormal retro displacement of the globe in the orbit due to increased volume of the orbit, decreased intraorbital mass, or anomalous action of the orbital part of the orbicularis and other extraocular muscles."

**Uveal effusion syndrome:* The uveal effusion syndrome is a combination of symptoms that may develop in any eye after any penetrating injury, accidental or surgical. The common factors contributing to the disorders are thickened sclera in small eyes and deranged uveal venous drainage; the uveoscleral drainage is also compromised. Though penetrating injuries are common causes of the syndrome, it has been reported following a blunt injury with an intact globe. The other causes are chronic uveitis, leaking wounds, and hypotony due to any cause. It is inevitable in nanophthalmos following intraocular surgery. Occasionally, no cause can be attributed to the malady. It may affect one or both eyes and progress unless treated well.

The basic mechanism or production of enophthalmos is the disparity between the volume of the orbit and the volume of the intraorbital contents. It can happen if the orbital volume is larger than normal with a normal volume of intraorbital contents, and vice versa. It can be congenital or acquired; the former is also called primary, for which no definite cause or causes can be determined. It constitutes <1% of cases of enophthalmos. Most of the causes of enophthalmos are acquired; they can be put into the following groups:

- *Increased orbital volume:*
    - Congenital (rare)
    - *Expansion of orbital volume:*
        - Fracture of the orbital floor
        - Silent sinus syndrome
        - Surgical removal, floor, or orbit
        - Maxillary hypoplasia
        - Absence of a sphenoidal wing (neurofibromatosis)
- *Reduced volume of orbital contents:*
    - Microphthalmos and its variations
    - Orbital varices
    - Postradiation status
    - Phthisis bulbi
    - Constantly leaking wound
    - Overfiltering bleb
- *Traction to extraocular muscles:*
    - *Postsurgical:*
        - Excessive resection of recti muscles
        - Postinflammatory fibrosis of extraocular muscles
        - Metastatic (breast cancer—not seen in children)
        - Retraction syndromes
        - Orbital fat atrophy
- *Others:*
    - Horner's syndrome
    - Marfan syndrome
    - Age-related loss of fat
    - Familial deep-set eyes

Clinical Features

Clinical features depend upon the extent of enophthalmos and laterality.

Parents may not notice mild enophthalmos in bilateral cases unless it is realized that the child has diminished vision or a squint. An eye is designated as having pseudo-enophthalmos when the nonenophthalmos eye is thought to be larger.

Signs

Signs also vary from eye to eye; the child may have fairly good vision or there may be total loss of vision. The interpalpebral aperture is narrower than normal; there is pseudoptosis; the anterior curvature of the upper lid is flattened with a retained lid crease; the size of the globe may vary from pin point to <8.00 mm; and, in post-traumatic cases, there may be signs of a blow-out fracture or an orbital floor.

Differential Diagnosis

A differential diagnosis consists of clinical anophthalmos and an eviscerated socket.

Treatment

- All cases of enophthalmos, especially when mild and bilateral, do not require treatment.
- Blow-out fractures are semi-urgent surgical procedures.
- Postinflammatory (phthisis) should be put on topical steroids, and if needed, atropine may be added.
- A prosthesis may be required for cosmetic purposes; the other function of a prosthesis is to stimulate the growth of the orbit.

Hypoglobus

The term hypoglobus is a nonspecific term to denote the position of the glove lower than normal due to a fracture of the floor and the entrapment of inferior extraocular muscle in the fracture. Logically, an eye pushed up should be called a hyperglobus.

ORBIT FOLLOWING VARIOUS SURGERIES

Enucleated Socket

Enucleation of the eye consists of the removal of the globe with its contents without opening the globe and leaving all peribulbar and intraorbital structures. The opposing extraocular muscles may be stitched to each other, i.e., medial rectus to lateral rectus and superior to inferior. The obliques are left free. Various types of implants are available to which the muscles can be stitched. The conjunctiva is stitched over the stump of the muscles horizontally, and a conformer is put over the conjunctiva to keep the fornices deep. The enucleated stump lacks movement. The muscles, if left unstitched, cause shallowing of the orbit, making it difficult to put an artificial eye **(Fig. 11.33)**.

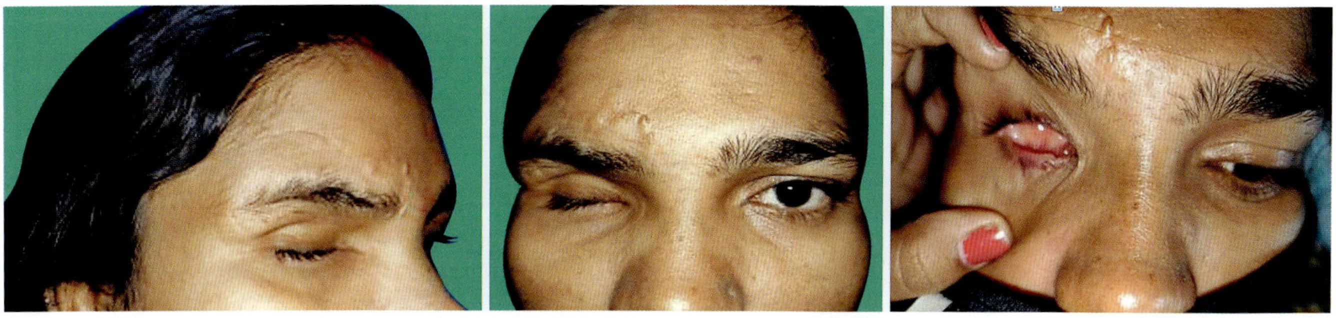

Fig. 11.33: Enucleated socket in an adult.
Courtesy: Shalvika Gupta and Professor Ankur K Shrivastava.

The enucleated sockets result in pseudoptosis, enophthalmos, and flattening of the lid curvature with a retained lid crease **(Fig. 11.34)**. The conjunctiva retains its usual pink color, but the depth of the fornices is variable. A deep fornix is a prerequisite for the good fitting of an artificial eye **(Figs. 11.35 and 11.36)**.

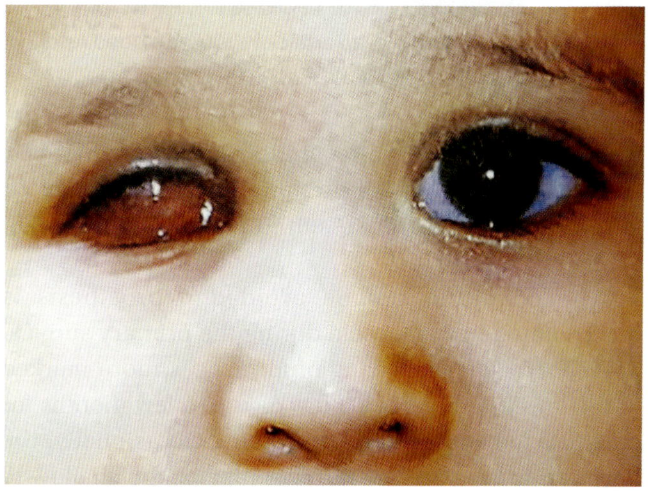

Fig. 11.34: Enucleated socket after removal of the globe.
Courtesy: Dr Santosh G Honavar (Retinoblastoma—They Live and See, LVPEI).

The artificial eye following enucleation without an integrated prosthesis lacks normal movement.

Eviscerated Socket

Evisceration of the globe is an operation where the cornea and intraocular contents of the globe are scooped out, leaving the scleral shell, extraocular muscles, blood vessels, and nerves. The scleral wound is stitched. A prosthesis put in the empty scleral shells gives a better appearance and full movement; the conjunctiva is stitched over the sclera. Evisceration is contraindicated in intraocular malignancy; the most common indication is panophthalmitis, followed by endophthalmitis not responding to usual treatment and a disorganized globe following a penetrating injury. The surgery leaves a good fornix with a sufficient fit and an artificial eye with movement.

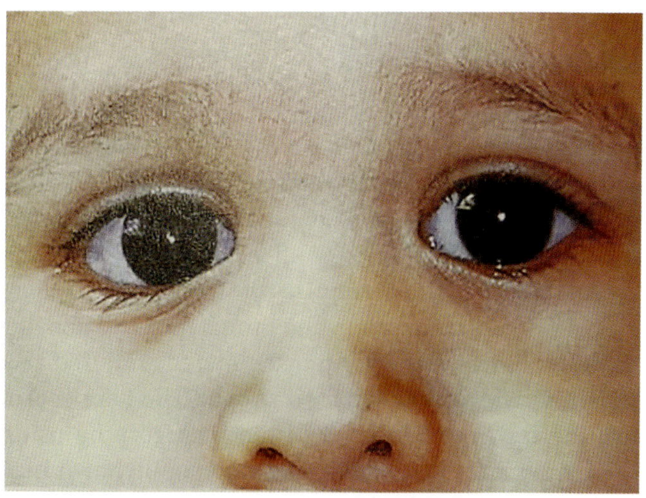

Fig. 11.35: The same socket showing good fitting of artificial eye.
Courtesy: Dr Santosh G Honavar (Retinoblastoma—They Live and See, LVPEI).

Anophthalmic/Enophthalmic Socket (Contracted Socket, Postenucleation Socket Syndrome)

Anophthalmic sockets are also referred to as contracted sockets or postenucleation socket syndrome. It is the most unwanted but avoidable situation for enophthalmos, with reduced orbital content resulting in diminished orbital volume with a decrease in the depth of fornices, mostly lower fornices. It is associated with the tilting of the superior fornix posteriorly, creating a relatively deep

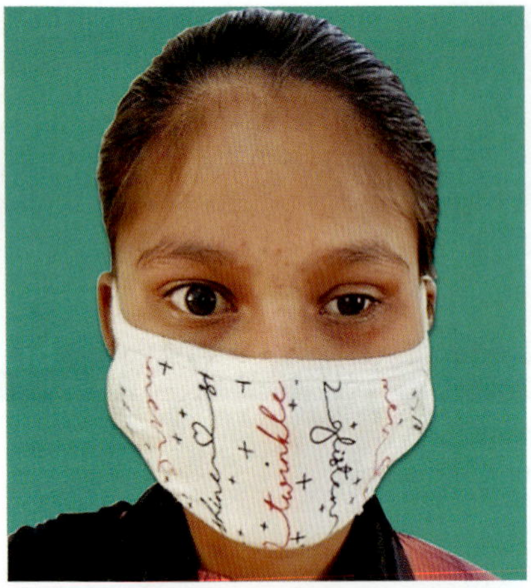

Fig. 11.36: Girl fitted with an artificial eye with a good result.
Courtesy: Professor SL Adile.

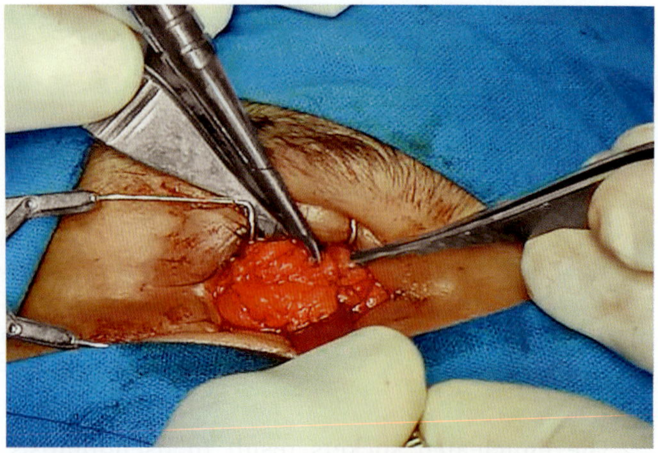

Fig. 11.37: Dermis fat graft during surgery.
Courtesy: Shalvika Gupta and Professor Ankur K Shrivastava.

superior sulcus. The other findings are pseudoptosis, elongation, and laxity of the lower lid, and shallow or absent lower fornix that result in an inability to retain ocular prostheses.

The condition can be avoided if prosthesis is incorporated in the muscle during the primary surgical procedure. The shallowing of fornices is more marked in the lower part; it takes a few days to a few months for a contracted socket to develop fully. Occasionally, the lower lid is everted. The fornices may be too shallow to retain a prosthesis; the prosthesis may be thrown out in an attempt to close the lids. The treatment is oculoplastic reformation of the fornices, and dermal fat grafts have shown encouraging results **(Figs. 11.37 and 11.38)**.

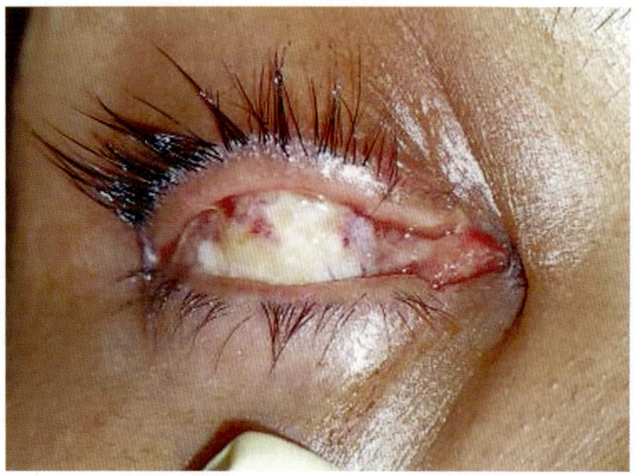

Fig. 11.38: End result after a month.
Courtesy: Shalvika Gupta and Professor Ankur K Shrivastava.

Exenterated Socket

This is the most undesirable and ghastly effect of an ophthalmic surgery; it is indicated in primary malignancy, secondary deposits, extension from the globe, and PNSs in the orbit, not responding to usual anticancer methods. It comprises the removal of all structures in the orbit except the bones. That comprises the lid, lacrimal system, eyeball with its connection, and orbital fat. Occasionally, the anterior leaf of the lids may be spared and used as a skin graft with an intact blood supply. The bare socket may be repaired following primary surgery by using the temporalis muscle with its blood supply, or it may undergo a skin graft after a few days to weeks. One of the indications that requires exenteration is post-COVID mucormycosis **(Fig. 11.39)**.

ORBITAL TRAUMA

The most common effect of trauma on the orbit is the fracture of various walls and rims, either in isolation or in combination. They are seen from childhood to ripe old age. Most of them occur in the second to fifth decade, more frequently in males of all races. The common causes are sports injuries, brawls, road traffic accidents, and blast injuries. They can be unilateral or bilateral; they may be isolated orbitals or associated with a craniofacial injury. They may be trivial enough to go unnoticed or ghastly **Flowchart 11.2** depicts various types of fractures in the orbit.

Summary of the tripod fracture of the orbit:

- On X-ray and CT, the fractures are seen to run through the:
  - Zygomaticomaxillary suture

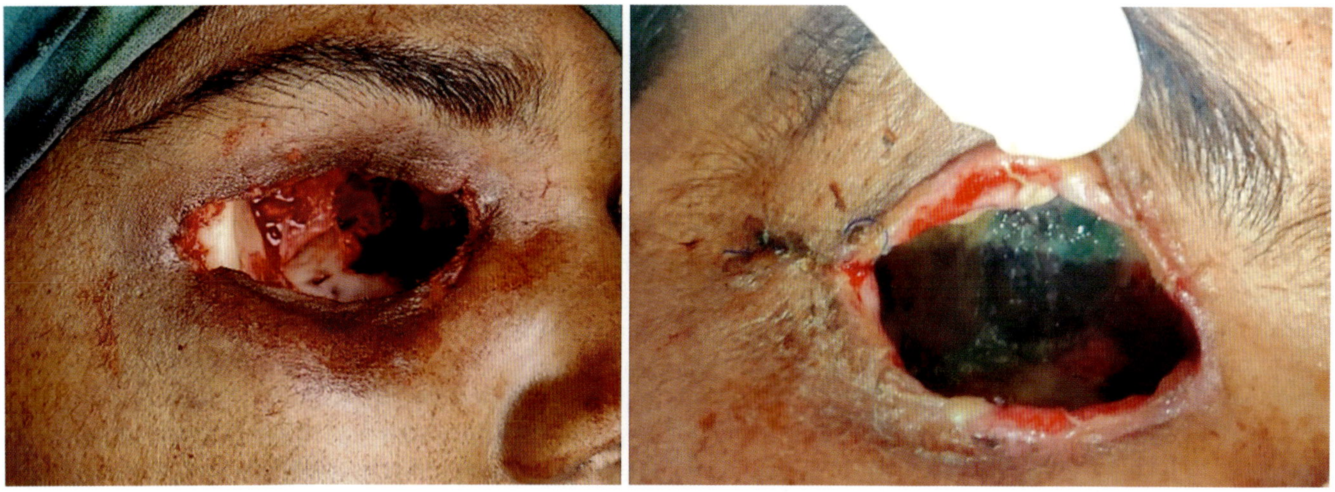

Fig. 11.39: Recently exenterated socket in post-COVID mucor infection in adult.
Courtesy: Dr Somen Misra and Professor Vijaya Sahu.

Flowchart 11.2: Types of orbital fractures.

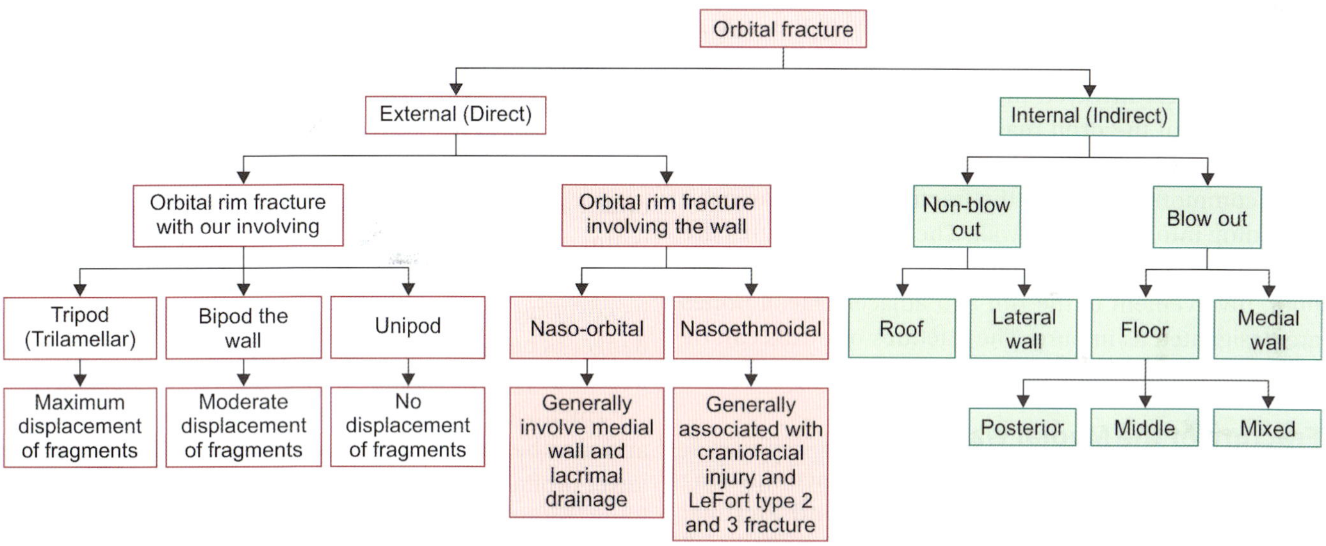

- Zygomaticofrontal suture
- Zygomaticotemporal suture

- Flattening of malar eminence
- Palpable step at the suture line
- Diplopia (frequent)
- Ptosis (less common)
- Displacement of lateral canthus *downwords*
- Trismus
- Positive forced duction test

Note:

- Surgery is indicated in cases with clinically detectable displacement, trismus, or cosmetic blemish.
- Craniofacial and ocular involvements get priority over orbital injuries.

It is imperative to revise the osteology of the orbit before discussing the intricacies of orbital fracture and its management. The orbit consists of the roof, lateral wall, floor, and medial wall in a clockwise fashion in the left eye; the sequence is reversed in the right eye. The pyramidal orbit has an apex and a base; the apex communicates with the brain and transmits important structures from the brain to the eyeball. The orbit has two fissures, i.e., a superior orbital, an inferior orbital, and an inferior orbital groove. The superior orbital fissures transmit the third, fourth, two divisions of the fifth nerve, and the sixth nerve beside the sympathetic nerve and vessels. No structure enters the orbit via inferior orbital fissures, which act as the exit of the maxillary division of the fifth nerve. The walls are bony, but the base of the pyramid lacks bones. The base is attached to and surrounded by the rim of the orbit. The rim is formed by the thickened anterior end of the orbital walls; it is the strongest part of the orbit. It is an oval aperture; it is almost circular in newborns but becomes quadrilateral in adults. Incidentally, it is not the widest part of the orbit; the widest part of the orbit lies 0.5 mm to 1.00 mm behind the edge of the rim. It corresponds to the equator of the globe, and the equator of the globe happens to be the widest part of the eyeball. The base is formed by the orbicularis, levator, tarsal plate, ligaments of the lid, ligaments of the eyeball, and orbital septum, with a horizontal opening called the interpalpebral aperture.

The most common traumatic disorder of the bony orbit is fracture. The fracture can be limited to the walls of the orbit, with or without involving the rim. It is common for PNSs to get involved in a fracture of the orbit; any of the walls of the orbit may be involved in fracture, in isolation or combination with the adjoining wall, and the most common example is the fracture floor of the orbit extending into the medial wall. The orbital fractures are called pure when they involve only the walls, roof, and floor. Involvement of the rim and adjacent facial bones are designated as impure. The fractures or orbits can be simple, comminuted, or compound.

Fracture of the Medial Wall

The medial wall is the longest of all the walls, encompassing the ethmoidal and sphenoidal sinuses and lacrimal passage. It is most vulnerable to blow-out force. The wall formed by the PNSs is paper thin that is liable to cave in or out in cases of raised intraorbital pressure. Behind the paper-thin walls lie the ethmoidal and sphenoidal air cells. The dehiscence of these bones leads to the escape of air from them into the orbit, causing emphysema of the orbit, resulting in bulging of the lids and conjunctiva. The emphysematous skin and chemosed conjunctiva produce crepitation on pressure, which is a diagnostic feature of orbital emphysema. The escape of air through the fractured bone is associated with the escape of fluid from the sinuses. The infected fluid may cause orbital cellulitis, a common complication of a fracture of the medial wall. The third event is entrapment of the medial rectus in the fracture, causing esotropia, diplopia, a positive forced duction test, and a positive Valsalva maneuver. An isolated medial wall fracture is rare. It is generally associated with fractures of the floor, more often associated with blows to the nose than not. A fracture of the bony nasolacrimal canal may be an associated feature.

Fracture Floor

The fracture floor of the orbit is the most common fracture, met with blunt injury to the orbital rim. The floor has deficiencies such as inferior orbital fissures and inferior orbital grooves that lie between the lateral wall and the posterior end of the floor. The floor fracture is called direct when the inferior orbital rim is involved and indirect when the inferior rim is intact. Indirect fractures are also called blow-out fractures or pure orbital fractures. The various types of floor fractures include LeFort type 2, type 3, tripod fracture, and white eye blow-out fracture. The orbital plate of the maxilla, which forms a large part of the floor, is involved in the LeFort fracture.

Table 11.4 shows various types of LeFort fractures.

They may follow either a blunt or penetrating injury.

The walls of the orbit converge posteriorly to form the apex of the orbit, and through the apex passes the bony optic canal. The anterior circular termination of the canal is the optic foramen. The posterior part of the canal is intracranial. The optic canal transmits the optic nerve with its covering and ophthalmic artery; the optic nerve is in danger of being throttled by bony spicules and hematoma in case of a fracture of the bony canal.

The fracture of the floor of the orbit is mostly indirect and may be isolated or associated with a fracture of the lower orbital rim. The most common mode of trauma is a blunt, rounded, hard, or semisoft object with a diameter more than the diameter of the orbital margin. They are common sports injuries; the offending projectiles are cricket, tennis, hockey, and golf balls. There are two theories to explain the mechanism or blow-out fracture.

They are:
- Hydraulic theory
- Buckling theory

TABLE 11.4: Various types of Le Fort fractures.

Type	*Bone involved*	*Orbital involvement*
1	Maxilla	Nil
2	Nasal, lacrimal, and maxilla	Medial orbita wall
3	Multiple craniofacial bones	Lateral wall, floor medial wall

The hydraulic theory is based on the presumption that when intraorbital pressure rises above a tolerable level, the floor and medial walls give way. The rise of intraorbital pressure is brought about by a round object with a diameter more than the diameter of the rim. In contrast to this, the buckling theory is based on the presumption that the stronger orbital rim absorbs the force of the blow up to a certain level. When the pressure exceeds the tolerable level, the force is passed to the paper-thin bones that give way. The fracture is not only transmitted to the floor but may involve the medial wall as well. The fracture of the floor and medial wall is a common occurrence; both may be associated with soft tissue injury, retrobulbar hemorrhage, surgical emphysema, and entrapment of extraocular muscles, i.e., medial rectus in the case of medial wall fracture and inferior rectus and inferior oblique in the case of floor fracture. Entrapment of all three muscles is a rarity. The fracture of the floor may be a linear fracture only without caving down the floor in the maxillary sinus. Such an event is generally associated with prolapse of the orbital floor in the maxillary sinus; this causes hypoglobus, enophthalmos, vertical diplopia, and a positive force duction test. The diplopia may be transient or permanent. The latter is due to entrapment of the inferior rectus and oblique, while transient diplopia is due to swelling of soft tissue. The permanent diplopia is relieved only by surgical intervention.

The enophthalmos are often masked by temporary exophthalmos. The causes of temporary exophthalmos are surgical emphysema, retrobulbar hemorrhage, and swelling of soft tissue.

Clinical Feature

Clinical features depend upon the severity of the impact and the time lapse between injury and consultation.

The clinical features are:

- Edema of the lids, ecchymosis of the lids, surgical emphysema, chemosis of the conjunctiva, and subconjunctival hemorrhage
- Transient, moderate exophthalmos
- Late development of enophthalmos <2.00 mm. Enophthalmos may be stationary or may keep regressing over 6 months and then stabilize. Progressive enophthalmos is due to traumatic degeneration and fibrosis of orbital soft tissue.
- Hypoesthesia in the distribution of the inferior orbital nerve
- *Diplopia:* (1) Up gaze; (2) Down gaze; (3) Double diplopia: The combination of diplopia in up and down gazes is called double diplopia and must be differentiated from double elevator palsy*.
- Positive forced duction test
- Diminished vision due to associated changes in the globe.

Clinical Feature

Symptom

- Vertical diplopia
- Vertical tropia
- Abnormal head posture
- Ptosis
- Diminished elevation of affected eye

Signs

All the above symptoms are associated with absent Bells phenomena and positive forced duction tests.

Differential Diagnosis

- Brown syndrome
- Congenital fibrosis
- Paralysis of the upper division of the third nerve
- Vertical retraction syndromes
- Progressive external ophthalmoplegia

Diagnosis of Fracture Floor of Orbit

All cases of blunt injury by a rounded, hard object with proptosis, surgical emphysema, crepitus over the lids, restricted gaze, hypoesthesia in the lower lid, and cheek

---

Double elevator palsy (mono-ocular elevation deficiency):* Double-elevator palsy is a rare palsy, mostly congenital. It presents as diminished movement of the eye in the upper gaze due to the combined weakness of the ipsilateral inferior oblique and superior rectus muscles in one eye. On rare occasions, it may be associated even with adduction or abduction are affected, where elevation in the horizontal axis is also faulty. It is due to the underaction of the two elevators of the eye, i.e., the superior rectus and inferior oblique, above the horizontal plane **(Fig. 11.40).

In a still-rare case, a tight and fibrosed inferior rectus may present with similar pictures. Primary supranuclear palsy with secondary inferior rectus inhibition too may simulate DEP. However, some authors doubt the involvement of both elevators and think they are predominantly under the action of the superior rectus.

The condition can be congenital or acquired. The congenital conditions are sporadic. Rarely, this may follow trauma, mid-brain tumors, acoustic neuroma, and a cerebrovascular accident. Out of all traumas, this is the only cause in children.

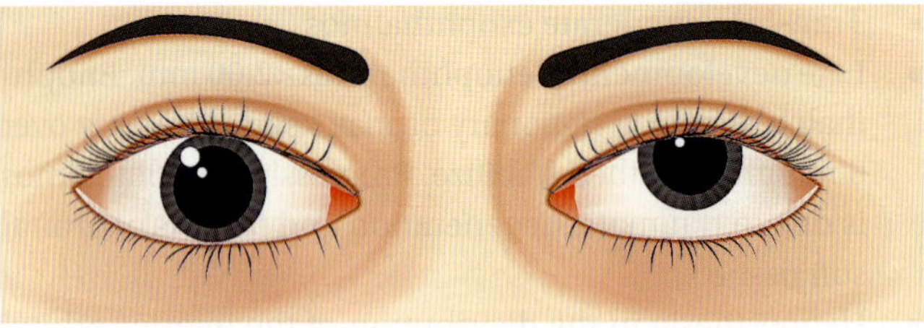

Fig. 11.40: Mono-ocular elevation deficiency.

should be suspected to have a fracture of the floor of the orbit. This is true if the child reports within the first week following the injury. After 10 days, proptosis is gradually replaced by enophthalmos, and double diplopia becomes more pronounced.

The fracture was confirmed by X-rays and CT in the coronal and axial planes, taken as 2.00 mm slices. This will not only delineate the fracture but also show prolapse of orbital contents in the maxillary sinus; this feature is called droplet signs. A trap door fracture of the floor with an entrapped inferior rectus also becomes evidence.

X-rays and PNS (Waters View) were the only imaging options available before CT, USG, and MRI came into vogue. MRI is less effective than CT.

Indications for surgical intervention:

- Significant entrapment
- Persistent enophthalmos >2.00 mm
- Persistent hypoglobus
- Fracture involving 50% of the floor and medial wall
- LeFort fractured two and three
- Persistent pain
- Diplopia is >20% of the primary position.

Ocular injuries get priority over orbital fractures.

Orbital Rim Fracture

The rim of the orbit is more likely to giveaway under direct hit by a blunt object, the diameter of which is greater than the diameter of the rim. This is also known as an external orbital fracture. Such fractures are invariably associated with fractures of the orbital walls, nose, and ethmoid. Any or many parts of the rim may be involved simultaneously. Single fractures are more common than multiple fractures. The common sites to be involved in lateral wall fracture are through the zygomaticofrontal suture and the zygomaticomaxillary suture, which are the weak parts of the rim. A fracture in this region is called a tripod fracture due to the involvement of three projections of the

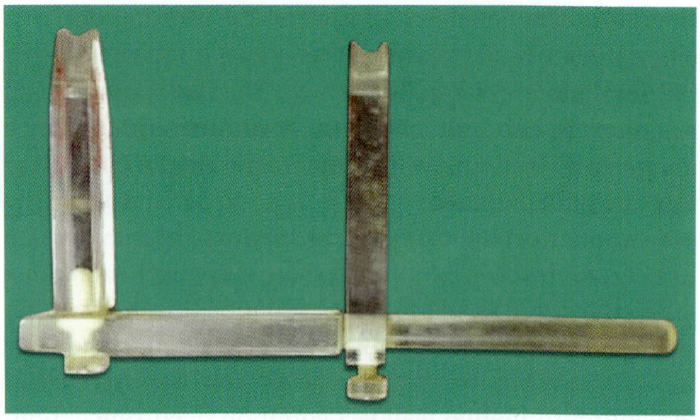

Fig. 11.41: Exophthalmos meter.

zygomatic bone. Linear fractures do not cause disjunction. Forceful blows are associated with the displacement of the zygomatic process.

The displacement is a combination of medial, inferior, and posterior rotations.

The naso-orbital fractures are associated with fractures of the lacrimal bone and bony nasolacrimal canal, disrupting the lacrimal drainage system. The involvement of the medial canthal ligament results in telecanthus and downward sagging of the medial canthus.

LeFort two and three fractures are associated with nasoethmoidal fractures.

Clinical Presentation

- Clinical presentation depends on the location of the fracture; it consists of a history of craniofacial trauma and trauma to the rim by a blunt object with a diameter more than the diameter of the rim.
- *Tripod fracture results in:*
  - Flattening of malar prominences
  - On palpation of the rim, a stepped depression is felt.
  - Trismus
  - Displacement of the outer canthus
  - Ptosis
  - Crepitation on pressing the lids
  - Passive edema of the lids
  - Chemosis of conjunctive
  - Restricted movement of the eye
  - The other tests are diplopia charting, force duction testing, and exophthalmometry.

Figure 11.41 shows one of the commonly used exophthalmos meters.

- *Imaging*:
  - X-rays of the PNS, Caldwell, and Waters orbits show the presence of fractures, displacement of fragments, and rotation of the zygoma.
  - *CT:* This is the imaging of choice; coronal views with 2.00 mm slices are most commonly used. CT, besides conforming to X-ray findings, will also reveal subtle fractures of the floor and medial wall. Three-dimensional reconstructions are preferred over plain CT.
  - *MRI:* It will show cranial injury besides orbital fracture when performed with contrast, especially optic nerve swelling and edema of its covering.
  - *USG:* In the absence of a CT facility, USG may be performed, but its results are not as precise as CT.

Management

Generally, a fracture of the rim without displacement is not an ophthalmic emergency; however, it is a potential threat to vision. The management is surgical and consists of undoing displacement with stabilization of the fragments, generally done by craniofacial surgeons.

Orbital Roof Fracture

Isolated fractures of the roof are rare in children. The fracture happens due to direct trauma over the brow. Orbital roof fractures are mostly seen in extensive skull injuries or localized fractures of the frontal bone. Orbital roof fractures present with ecchymosis of the upper lid and subconjunctival hemorrhage; the posterior border of the subconjunctival hemorrhage is not visible because subconjunctival blood trickles downward. Both ecchymosis of the lid and subconjunctival hemorrhage may take about 24–48 hours following injury to develop because that is the time for the blood to gravitate down from the scalp to the lid and conjunctiva. The ecchymosis may spread over the contralateral orbit in a few days.

The presence of crepitus in the lids and conjunctiva denotes the involvement of the frontal sinus. CSF rhinorrhea may develop immediately or days later. The globe may be displaced downward and forward. The superior oblique muscle may be traumatized, resulting in vertical diplopia.

A posterior extension of trauma may involve the optic bony canal, either as a fracture or a hematoma in the lumen, resulting in *traumatic optic neuropathy**.

The mechanism involved is the transmission of force from the site of injury to the optic nerve. The site of injury is always away from the optic nerve and blunt. The kinetics of indirect traumatic optic neuropathy are not well understood.

The presumptions are:

- Contusion of the optic nerve
- Hemorrhage in the optic canal
- Tearing of the dura covering the optic nerve due to a pull on the optic nerve. The dura of the optic nerve is actually a continuation of the periorbita.
- Edema of the optic nerve
- In rare instances, the optic nerve may be avulsed from the globe, causing a sudden loss of vision.

The direct form of traumatic optic neuropathy is due to an actual injury to the optic nerve in the orbit or the canal following a penetrating injury behind the globe. Isolated lesions are less common. It is generally associated with an anterior cranial or craniofacial injury. The presenting symptoms are often missed due to a more severe craniofacial injury.

Symptoms

The symptoms of traumatic optic neuropathy vary in two types.

1. The typical natural history of indirect traumatic optic neuropathy is that its presence is felt after a few days to weeks following a trivial injury to the outer side of the superior orbital rim. The symptom that brings the child for consultation is diminished vision, ranging between loss of a few lines on the Snellen chart to the absence of light perception without any other external finding except RAPD. RAPD is the single most common clinical finding that leads to the presence of indirect traumatic optic neuropathy.

**Traumatic optic neuropathy:* This is caused by acute, sudden injury to the optic nerve, which may be direct or indirect. The indirect injury is generally away from the optic nerve, i.e., the orbital rim or forehead. These trivial injuries are more common to cause traumatic optic neuropathy than severe and direct injuries. It is more common in males, with one-fourth being children. The original injury is seldom grave, a small but forceful injury on the outer side of the superior orbital rim is the commonest injury to result in traumatic optic neuropathy. Road traffic and sports injuries are often responsible for indirect traumatic optic neuropathy.

2. The direct type is often missed due to the overwhelming signs and symptoms of cranial and craniofacial injuries. The child, recovering from the effects of an acute injury, realizes a loss of vision in one eye. Involvement of both eyes is not uncommon in crush injuries to the head. The clinical presentations are the same as in indirect traumatic optic neuropathy.

Signs

The triad of loss of vision, RAPD, and ophthalmoscopic findings are the cornerstones of the disorder.

The ophthalmoscopic finding depends on time laps, the type of first examination, and the extent of the injury. A classical ophthalmoscopic finding is a pale disc with normal central retinal vessels. The color change of the optic nerve head varies from pallor to chalk white disc.

Treatment

Treatment of traumatic optic neuropathy is controversial. Medical treatment should be initiated within 48 hours of the injury. The regime is a bolus injection of intravenous methylprednisolone at a dose of 30 mg/kg at a rate of 5.4 mg/kg/h for 24 or 48 hours, followed by protocol as followed in the institute in consultation with a pediatrician.

Surgical management consists of deroofing of the optic canal within 48 hours of injury, which is rarely possible. The result of surgical intervention is not always very encouraging.

Lateral Wall Fractures

Lateral orbital wall fractures are the least common due to their thickness. It is generally seen in severe maxillofacial injuries and crush injuries of the cranium and has a minimum intraorbital manifestation.

Orbital Apex Fracture

The orbital apex is not a well-defined structure. It is an area where all the walls of the orbit converge. Its clinical importance lies in the fact that all the vessels and nerves of the eyeball traverse through this narrow space. All the extraovular muscles except the inferior oblique take their origin in its vicinity. Its posterior proximity to the cavernous sinus makes it vulnerable to intracranial lesions.

The fractures involving orbital apexes are part of a larger condition of craniofacial injury. The fractures involving the orbital apexes are broadly divided into two groups, i.e., those with intact optic nerves and those with involvement of optic nerves, which can be with or without displacement of fragments.

The fracture passing through the orbital apex invariably involves extraocular muscles and/or their nerve supply. The most important feature of a fracture involving the orbital apex is the development of a carotid-cavernous fistula*. Fractures involving orbital apexes are generally managed by neurosurgeons and craniofacial surgeons.

Direct Fistula

The most common cause of direct fistula is intercavernous injury to the carotid. The less common cause is a spontaneous leak from the internal carotid, which is rarely seen in children. The still-rare cause is a congenital anomaly.

The post-traumatic high-flow fistula is an acute cranial event that may become obvious within a few hours to a few days following injury. It is invariably unilateral, rarely bilateral, and carries a poor prognosis for all ages. All the vascular tissue, intra- or extraocular, is involved. The venous channels are dilated while the arterial channels are attenuated. There may be arterialization of the veins in the long term. Venous stasis is seen as:

- Chemosis, hyperemia, and passive congestion of the conjunctiva with prominent episcleral veins.
- Pulsatile axial proptosis with bruit. The pulsations are synchronized with the heartbeat and can be stopped by applying ipsilateral pressure over the carotid in the neck. If the media are clear, the pulsation can be seen on ophthalmoscopy.
- Signs of anterior segment ischemia manifest as edema of the corneal epithelium, circumciliary congestion, flare, cells in AC, and a semi-dilated, sluggish pupil.

Carotid-cavernous fistula (see* ***Fig. 11.10**):* A carotid-cavernous fistula is not a primary orbital lesion. The orbit and its contents suffer secondary to the malady. The lesion is retro-orbital, associated mostly with a fracture at the base of the skull. The internal carotid artery traverses the cavernous sinus without communicating with the venous blood surrounding it. In cases of trauma, there is a rent in the wall of the internal carotid or its branches, i.e., the meningeal and dural branches. Rarely, the external carotid is indirectly involved. As per the size of the hole in the internal carotid and the amount of blood spurting from it, the condition is clinically divided into two types:

1. High flow (direct fistula)
2. Low flow (indirect fistula)

In the long run, there is neovascularization of the iris, followed by patches of iris atrophy.

- Raised intraocular tension. The rise in intraocular pressure is multifactorial.
  They are:
  - Raised episcleral pressure
  - Iris neovascularization
  - Anterior segment ischemia
  - Secondary narrow angle
- Diminished vision is caused due to corneal edema, anterior segment ischemia, and cataracts. About one-fifth of cases develop secondary cataracts, raised intraocular tension, and venous stasis retinopathy.
- Extraocular muscle palsies cause ophthalmoplegia, the causes of which may be neurogenic or myogenic. The former is part of anterior cavernous sinus involvement, or superior ophthalmic fissure syndrome. The most common cranial nerve to be involved is the sixth, followed by the third and fourth. The myogenic causes are supposed to be hypoxia, leading to passive edema of the muscle.

Management

The treatment of carotid cavernous fistulas is outside the domain of ophthalmology. It is best managed by neurosurgeons. Some of the small leaks get obliterated without any intervention over weeks or months. The other options are ligation of the carotid and embolization of the artery.

Indirect Fistula

They are less frequent than direct. They are seen in adults, mostly in menopausal women with hypertension. They are low-flow, generally unilateral, with a less dramatic presentation than their direct counterparts. Though it is put under the term carotid cavernous fistula, it does not involve the cavernous sinus directly. The arterial blood flows through the dural and meningeal branches of the external/internal carotids in the case of an indirect fistula.

The precise causes of the low-flow fistula are not well established. Common predisposing factors are: Congenital anomalies, mild head injuries in the past, and hypertension.

The clinical features are milder.

- The first to occur is a unilateral dilated episcleral vessel.
- Subtle or mild proptosis.
- Dull ipsilateral pain.
- Diminished vision.
- Raised IOP.
- Ophthalmoplegia.

Most of the patients recover without much treatment, i.e., management of hypertension.

Table 11.5 shows a summary of various imagings ordered in the fracture of the orbit.

They are X-ray, CT, MRI, USG, and color Doppler imaging.

Orbital tomography: Orbital tomography is a technique that identifies the level of interest in orbit, blurring out structure above and below the level of interest. That gives a clear picture of the lesion. There is a long list of conditions under which this method is employed. Some of the indications are given here: Small fractures and

TABLE 11.5: X-ray and CT ordered in orbital fractures.

X-ray	
X-ray view	***Part imagined***
Waters view	• Orbital floor and roof • Zygomatic bone and temporal arch
Lateral view	• Various walls, rims, and craniums • Intraorbital, intraocular, and intracranial foreign bodies • Relative position of a foreign body
Rhese view	• Optic canal • Size of the optic foramen • Spicule in a fracture of the optic canal
Caldwell view	• Paranasal sinuses • Superior orbital fissure • Sphenoid ridge • Intraorbital and intraparanasal foreign body
X-ray skull	• Fracture fontal bone • Intracranial foreign body
Computed tomography (CT)	
View	***Part imagined***
Axial	• Most useful for anatomical changes, contrast between orbital fat, muscles, and bone • Intraocular and intraorbital foreign bodies • Intraocular calcification
Coronal 2 mm slice (cuts)	• Roof and floor of the orbit • Muscles • Muscle compartment • Optic nerve and paraoptic tissue
3D construction	The whole of the skull and orbit

their extent. It is done in coronal, sagittal, and transverse sections of the skull from the vortex down to the base of the skull; 1.00–2.00 mm cuts are required for optic nerve injury, intraocular foreign body, orbital foreign body, blowout fracture, muscle incarceration, hematoma, rupture of the globe, optic canal, dislocation of the lens vitreous hemorrhage, retinal and choroidal detachment, fractured sinuses, and some other indications.

Magnetic resonance imaging: This is a noninvasive process of imaging that does not use either X-ray or ionizing radiation. It gives high-resolution images not only of the intraorbital structures but also of the intracranial visual paths in all planes. It is contraindicated in suspected intraorbital, intracranial ferromagnetic foreign. It can be used without or with fat suppression. It is not a good procedure to delineate intraocular/orbital calcification. Bone changes are better visualized in CT. MRI and CT are complementary to each other. MRI is better at detecting intracranial lesions.

Color Doppler imaging: Color Doppler imaging (CDI) has no role in the diagnosis of an orbital fracture. It is best utilized to study the hemodynamics of cases of intraorbital vascular disorders following orbital injury. It is commonly used in congenital vascular anomalies of the orbit, central artery, and vein, occlusion of the cranial arteries, and carotid artery disease, most of which do not manifest in children.

Ultrasonography: Ultrasonography is less useful than CT and MRI in the diagnosis of fractures of the orbit.

INTRAORBITAL FOREIGN BODIES

Intraorbital foreign bodies are common following blast injury, penetrating injury with a broken piece of the offending object, gunshot injury, and a pellet from an air gun. They are seen at all ages, but more common after 10 years onward. Both sexes are involved in war injuries; otherwise, they are more common in males in their prime.

The symptoms are variable depending on the factors discussed above. An inert, sterile small particle may present with a point of entry and remain asymptomatic; it may be large enough to cause proptosis that may be stationary or may be processed to cause an urgent situation requiring surgical intervention, i.e., surgical compartment/compressive syndrome.

Clinical Features

Clinical features depend on the time lapse between the accident and the examination. It may be short or may be as long as months before a large protruding intraorbital foreign body is too obvious to diagnose; the child is generally brought for consultation within hours. A deep, small, inert intraorbital foreign body may present with recurrent redness, mild proptosis, or even a discharging sinus.

Diagnosis

Diagnosis requires:

- Complete history of symptoms and description of the accident. The child may not be expressive enough. An eyewitness may be more helpful.
- *Physical examination:*
  - *Ocular:*
    - RAPD when the globe is intact
    - Ruptured globe
  - Adnexal
  - Face
  - ENT
  - Neurological
- *Imaging:*
  - Radiology
  - USG
  - CT
  - MRI

Radiology

X-rays remain the most useful, convenient, and cheap screening method to locate a radiopaque intraorbital foreign body. It has the advantage of examination of PNSs and intracranial structure as well.

The first picture should be a lateral exposure that will denote the presence of a radiopaque foreign body, its position, size, and shape. It will also show the number of foreign bodies and the distance of foreign body/bodies from the orbital and cranial fractures **(Figs. 11.42 and 11.43)**.

Ultrasonography

It is a handy, inexpensive method of imaging. It gives a two-dimensional image and is more effective in locating anterior orbital foreign bodies. It is more sensitive than an X-ray in many ways; it does not indicate the composition of a foreign body. Besides orbital foreign bodies, it can detect

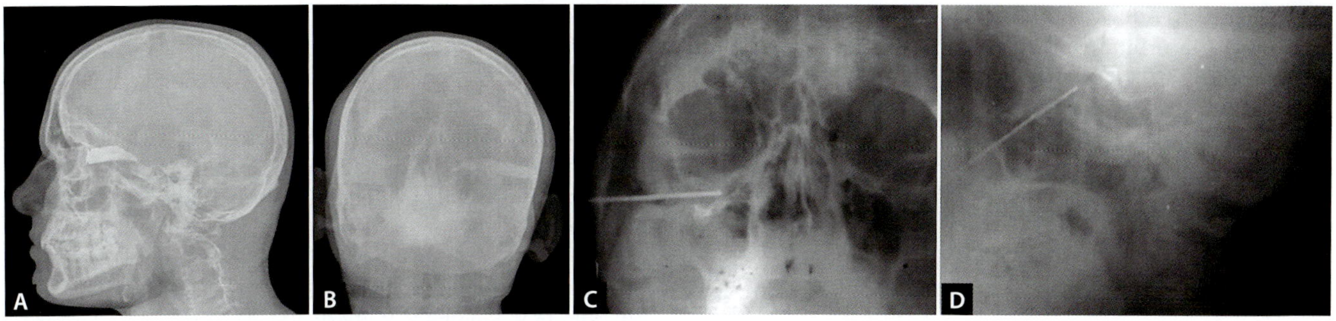

Figs. 11.42A to D: Two views of a metal foreign body lodged in orbits.

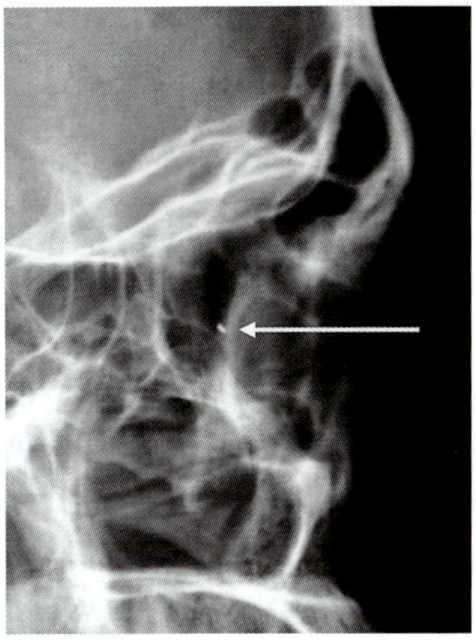

Fig. 11.43: Small foreign body in the orbit just behind the globe.

associated intraocular features like retinal detachment and vitreous hemorrhage.

Computed Tomography

This is the most sensitive imaging method to see and locate an intraorbital foreign body as small as 0.06 mm. It is used in three planes depending upon the part of the orbit, tissue or interest, and location of the foreign body. The intensity depends on the nature of the foreign body.

- *Glass and plastic:* Low intensity
- *Graphite and stone:* High intensity
- *Metal:* Hyperintensity

Computed tomography also delineates bony fractures, orbital abscesses, intraocular lesions, and cranial and intrasinus extensions of the orbital foreign body.

The planes used are axial, coronal, and sagittal. The axial plane is best for optic nerve lesions and foreign bodies in the vicinity of the optic nerve and between the globe and the optic canal. The coronal plane is used for extraocular muscles, intraconal foreign bodies embedded in the floor, and fractures of the floor.

A combination of axial and coronal planes is used to construct a three-dimensional view that is most useful to localize intraorbital foreign bodies.

Management

The management of the intraorbital foreign body depends on the time lapse between presentation and occurrence; it is influenced by its speed, size, number, position, composition, and radio density. All intraorbital foreign bodies do not require intervention. An inert, small, sterile, foreign body not involving optic nerves or muscles may be left without intervention. Organic foreign bodies are most likely to be infected. In contrast, high-speed inorganic foreign bodies are generally sterile. The removal of intraorbital foreign bodies requires a team of ophthalmic surgeons and neurosurgeons. All cases should receive antitetanus prophylaxis and an appropriate broad-spectrum antibiotic. Orbital foreign bodies with globe involvement should be preceded by the management of ocular morbidity.

SUGGESTED READING

1. Asif JA, Pohchi A, Alam MK, Athahar Y, Ahmad R. An Intraorbital Foreign Body. IJO. 2014;52:1098-100.
2. Babar TF, Hussain M, and Zaman M. Clinicopathologic study of 70 enucleations. J Pak Med Assoc. 2009;59(9):612-14.
3. Bajaj MS, Pushker N, Chaturvedi A, Betharia SM, Kashyap S, Balasubramanya R. Orbital space-occupying lesions in Indian children. J pediatr Opthalmol Strabismus. 2007;44:106-11.
4. Bakhshi S, Gupta S, Gogia V, Ravindranath Y. Compliance in retinoblastoma. Indian J pediatr. 2010;77;535-40.
5. Bavishi AK, Patel CK, Nagarimuni CH. Double elevator palsy. IJO. 1997;27(4):135-7.

6. Bhate M, Adewara B, and Bothra N. Strabismus in pediatric orbital wall fractures. Indian J Ophthalmol. 2023;71(3):973-6.
7. Edmund M, Mury AT, Durrani MO. Disorders of the Anophthalmic Eye in the Oxford Hand Book of Oph, 4th edition. Oxford: Oxford University Press; 2018. pp. 696-7.
8. Fredick DR. Special Subjects of Paediatric Interest, In General Ophthalmology, 15th edition. Connecticut: Appleton & Lange; 1999. pp. 330-2.
9. Goriyar A, Pandey N, Patel S, Verma A, Sahu R. A rare case of congenital teratoma. Proceeding of the 20th annual CSOS; 2021.
10. Hardy TG, Rose GE. Orbital Trauma in Moor Fields Manual of Ophthalmology, 3rd. New Delhi: Jaypee Brothers Medical Publishers; 2020. pp. 126-31.
11. Krishna G. Contracted sockets (etiology and types). Indian J Ophthalmol. 1980;28:117-20.
12. Mamalis N. In: Roy F. Globe, In current ocular therapy, 5th edition. Philadelphia: WB Sanders; 2000. pp. 455-6.
13. Mukherjee B, Goel S, Subramaniam N. An unusual intraorbital foreign body and its management. IJO. 2011;59: 59-60.
14. Mukherjee PK. Disorder of Orbit in Pediatric Ophthalmology, New Delhi: New Age International; 2005. pp. 673-719.
15. Naik MN, Tourani KL, Chandra Sekhar G, Honavar SG. Interpretation of computed tomography imaging of the eye and orbit. A systematic approach. Indian J Ophthalmol. 2002;50(4):339-53.
16. Salmon JF. Orbital trauma in Kanskis Clinical Oph, 9th edition. New Delhi: Elsevier; 2020. pp. 894-5.
17. Sheild C, Sheild JA. In: Fraunfelder FT, Roy HT (Eds). Orbital Rhabdomyosacoma in Current Ocular Therapy, 5th edition. Philadelphia: WB Saunders Company; 2000.
18. Shukla Y. In: Shukla B, Natrajan S. (Eds). Paediatric Ocular Trauma in Management of Ocular Trauma, 1st edition. New Delhi: CBS Publishers; 2005. pp. 288-94.
19. Sihota R, Sujatha Y, Betharia SM. The fat pad in dermis fat grafts. Ophthalmology. 1994;101(2):231-4.
20. Sihota R, Tandon R. Injury of the Orbit in Parsons' Diseases of the Eye, 23rd edition. New Delhi: Elsevier; 2020. pp. 44-45.
21. Singh AK. An unusual intraorbital foreign body. Delhi Jr. Oph. December 2016.
22. Singh V, Kaur A, Agrawal S. An unusual intraorbital foreign body. IJO. 2004;42:64-5.
23. Suryawanshi M, Desai W, Suryawanshi R. Orbitocranial wooden foreign body, Jr. Clinical Oph Res. 2014;2:105-8.
24. Vanikieti K, Preechawat P, Poonyathalang A. Pediatric primary optic nerve sheath meningioma. 2015;8:159-63.
25. Vathsalya V, Alam MS, Subramanian N, Subramanian KK, Biswas J, Mukherjee B. Clinical spectrum and clinicopathological correlation of pediatric orbital tumors: 20 years of experience from a tertiary eye care center. IJO. 2024;72(2):249-57.

CHAPTER

12 Disorders of Conjunctiva in Children

CONJUNCTIVA

The conjunctiva is the mucous membrane of the eye. It lines the inner surface of the lid and the outer surface of the globe, leaving the cornea clear. The conjunctiva at the lid margin blends with the skin of the lid and conjunctival epithelium continue with the corneal epithelium. The junction where the conjunctiva meets the cornea is called the limbus. The conjunctiva is joined indirectly to the nasopharynx via the lacrimal sac and nasolacrimal ducts. Thus, infections of the nasopharynx and skin have an easy access to the conjunctiva.

> The conjunctiva is so well endowed with lymphoid tissue that the complex is a veritable bisected lymph node lined by epithelium.

Histologically, conjunctive tissue has two layers, i.e., epithelium and stroma.

1. The epithelium is superficial to the stroma. Underneath the stroma lies the sclera. The stroma is connected loosely to the sclera by an ill-defined fibrous coat called episcleral tissue. The epithelium is multilayered. The number and character of epithelial cells vary in number and character at different locations of the conjunctiva. The number of cells varies between 2 and 5, and the type ranges from squamous to columnar.

   Table 12.1 shows various layers and cells at various parts of the conjunctival epithelium.

   The melanocytes are present in the basal layer. The basal cells have a thin basement membrane that separates the epithelium from the stroma. The normal epithelium is nonkeratinized; it gets keratinized when exposed to the atmosphere. The epithelium also contains goblet cells, the gland of Manz, and the crypts of Henle. These are not true glands; they are unicellular bodies, and the goblet cells are scattered all over the conjunctiva. The glands of Manz are seen at the limbus; the crypts of Henle are seen mostly in the tarsal conjunctiva; they may be found in the fornix and bulbar conjunctiva as well. These glands secrete mucin in the tear film.

TABLE 12.1: Layers of conjunctiva and types of cells present in them.

Part of the conjunctiva	*Number of layers of epithelium*	*Types of cells*
Intermarginal conjunctiva	5	Stratified squamous
Tarsal conjunctiva	2	• Superficial-columnar • Deep-flat
Fornix	3	• Superficial-columnar • Middle-polygonal • Deep-cuboidal
Bulbar conjunctiva	3	Same as above
Limbus	5–6	Stratified squamous

2. The stroma forms the main bulk of the conjunctiva. It is divided into two parts without any definite line of demarcation in between. The two layers are: (a) Adenoid layers and (b) fibrous layers.
   a. The adenoid layer contains lymphatic cells in the form of fine meshwork in which the lymphocytes are embedded; the adenoid layer is most developed in the fornices. The adenoid layer is not present at birth; it takes 2–3 months for it to develop fully. This is the cause of the absence of follicular reactions in newborns, even with severe infections.
   b. The fibrous layers contain elastic tissue and collagen in a fine meshwork, in which lie the conjunctival vessels and nerves. It is loosely attached to the Tenon's capsule below in the form of ill-defined episcleral tissue. It is very thin in the tarsal conjunctiva **(Fig. 12.1)**.

Other Glands of the Conjunctiva

These groups of glands are larger than the above-mentioned mucin and aqueous-producing glands. They are collectively called accessory lacrimal glands.

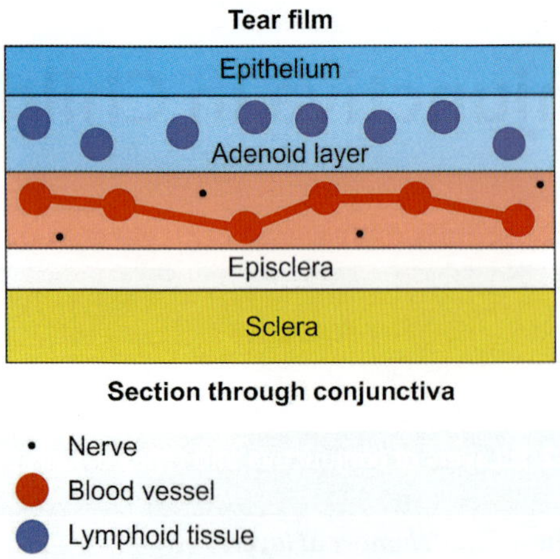

Fig. 12.1: Various layers of conjunctiva.

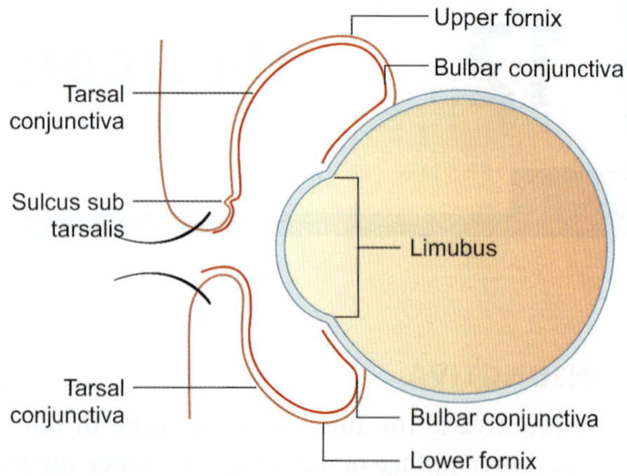

Fig. 12.2: Various parts of the conjunctiva.

They produce a sufficient amount of aqueous to keep the tear film intact when the main lacrimal gland has been extirpated. They share the inflammatory and pathological changes common to the lacrimal gland. Development-wise, they are similar to the development of the main lacrimal gland. The main lacrimal gland starts developing at 8 weeks, and the accessory lacrimal gland develops at 12 weeks as an invagination of epithelioid columns deep in the orbit from the fornices.

The glands are:
Glands of Krause and glands of Wolfring. The glands of Krause are about 40–45 in number and situated in the fornices, with more in the upper fornix.

The glands of Wolfring are fewer than the Krause glands, situated along the upper border of the superior tarsus and the lower edge of the inferior tarsus.

Topographical Parts of the Conjunctiva

Anatomically, the conjunctiva is broadly divided into three parts, i.e., the palpebral conjunction, the bulbar conjunctiva, and the fornix. The palpebral conjunctiva can again be divided into intermarginal, tarsal, and orbital parts; the bulbar part is divided into the scleral part, limbus, plica, and caruncle **(Fig. 12.2)**.

The palpebral conjunctiva extends from the anterior lid margin to the fornix in both lids. Before it transforms into a fornix, it passes through parts, i.e., the tarsal and orbital parts.

The Marginal Conjunctiva

It extends from the base of the eyelashes anteriorly to the sulcus subtarsalis. It is a transient zone between the skin of the lid and the conjunctiva; hence, it shares disorders of both structures. It is firmly attached to the lid margin and cannot be peeled from the lid margin. The conjunctiva on the lid margin is perforated by the opening of the meibomian glands throughout the length. The two puncta open at the medial and lid margins. The sulcus subtarsalis is a shallow groove about 2.00 mm from the sharp edge of the posterior lid margin, running along the lid horizontally. It is better developed in the upper lid. The sulcus subtarsalis is a common location for small foreign bodies to be lodged. The foreign bodies rarely get lodged in the lower groove.

> A patient with small foreign bodies rarely feels their presence in the lid; he always thinks that the foreign body is in the cornea.

Tarsal Conjunctiva

The tarsal conjunctiva in the upper lid extends from the sulcus subtarsalis to the upper orbital border of the tarsal plate. It covers the inner surface of the lid. It is firmly attached to the tarsal plate. The attachment is so strong that the conjunctiva cannot be peeled off the tarsal plate, and no fluid can accumulate under it. It is a common site for both papillae and follicles to develop. The normal tarsal conjunctiva is transparent. The blood vessels and tarsal glands are visible through the tarsal conjunctiva; the diseased conjunctiva obscures the tarsal plates. The common conditions that obscure the tarsal glands are multiple follicles, papillae, edema, hyperemia, membrane scarring, and scaring. The tarsal conjunctiva starts from the poorly developed sulcus to the proximal part of the lower fornix.

Orbital Conjunctiva

This part of the palpebral conjunctiva extends from the upper edge of the tarsal conjunctiva to the beginning of the fornices as a narrow strip. It is loose enough to be picked up. The unstriated muscle of Muller lies just beneath this part of the conjunctiva in the upper lid.

Bulbar Conjunctiva

The bulbar conjunctiva is the largest part of the conjunctiva, extending from the limbus to the fornices above and below; it forms medial and lateral canthi on either side. Most of the bulbar conjunctiva is covered by the lid, leaving a small, spindle-shaped area visible. At the limbus, it is formally attached to the Tenon's capsule up to the insertion of the ocular muscle. The conjunctiva epithelium traverses the limbus to become continuous with the corneal epithelium, which makes the cornea vulnerable to conjunctival infection. The bulbar conjunctiva covers the sclera for about 15.00 mm from the limbus. Its attachment to the sclera becomes weak toward the periphery; it can be picked up from the sclera with ease, away from the limbus. The laxness of the bulbar conjunctiva away from the limbus is a suitable site to give a subconjunctival injection. This laxity is also the cause of the accumulation of a large amount of fluid, producing chemosis of the conjunctiva. The bulbar conjunctiva is profusely supplied with blood vessels, which are visible to the naked eye. An increase in the number and dilatation of these vessels makes the transparent conjunctiva, which is white with few blood vessels hyperemic. Which is commonly referred to as pink eye. The bulbar conjunctiva is not only transparent but also moist and glistening. Normal bulbar conjunctiva does not stain with any of the stains. It is nonkeratinized, becoming keratinized only when exposed for a long time. On exposure, it gets desiccated and dry, losing its usual luster.

The common causes are: Proptosis, lagophthalmos, exophthalmos, ectropion, and large coloboma. The most common cause of loss of luster in children, especially in developing countries, is xerosis due to vitamin A deficiency in the form of a Bitot spot.

Limbus

The limbus is an ill-defined zone that encircles the corneal periphery. It is the junction of the cornea on one side and the conjunctiva, Tenon's capsule, and sclera on the other side. It is richly supplied with blood vessels and is the only source of blood to the peripheral cornea. Hypoxia of the limbal vessel has a deleterious effect on the cornea. Which is frequent in acid and alkali burns. The limbus is a rich source of stem cells for the corneal epithelium.

The limbus has great surgical value, especially in glaucoma surgery. The annulus of the limbus does not have a uniform width all round. It is widest superiorly and narrow on either side.

The surgical limbus is divided into two surgical zones by three lines.

The lines are: Posterior, middle, and anterior.

The limbal lines:

- The limbal lines are concentric with each other and the corneal periphery.
- The posterior limbal line lies over the scleral spur, 2.00 mm away from the anterior on the limbal line. It is demonstrable on scleral scatter mode of biomicroscopy.
- The anterior represents the termination of Tenon's capsule and the conjunctiva. It overlies the end of Bowman's membrane.
- The middle lines lie in between the above two. It represents the end of Descemet's membrane and overlies Schwalbe's line. On slit lamp examination, it looks blue. Beneath the limbus lies the trabecular meshwork.

Caruncle

The caruncle is a triangular nodule in the medial canthus between the medial ends of the two lids; it lies medial to the plica semilunaris. As per development, it is a part of the lower lid that gets separated from the lower lid during the development of the lower canaliculus. On histologically, it is a transient zone between the skin and conjunctiva. It functions as a mucocutaneous junction. Hence, it shares the disorders of both the skin and mucus membrane in the form of growth. It is covered by stratified squamous epithelium, and few hairs develop on it. The conjunctival elements present in the caruncle are goblet cells, Krause's grands, and sweat glands.

Pica Semilunaris

It represents the vestigial third lid of the lower animals. It is a curved fold of conjunctiva with concavity toward the cornea. The border is rounded. The plica has a shallow, blind recess underneath. That disappears if the eye is rotated laterally. Histologically, it is similar to the conjunctiva and shares all the disorders of the conjunctiva. It is not known to have any definite function **(Fig. 12.3)**.

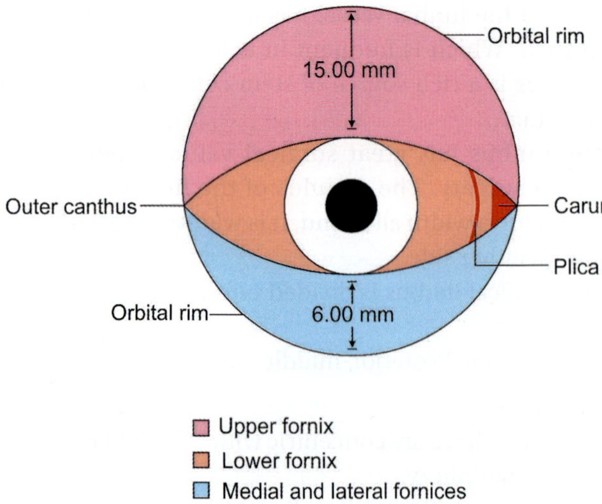

Fig. 12.3: Various parts of the conjunctiva.

Fornix

The fornix is a circular space all round the globe, formed by conjunctiva due to mergers of the orbital part of the tarsal conjunctiva and the peripheral part of the bulbar conjunctival. The caruncle and plica invade the space on the medial side at the level of the medial canthus. It is divided into four unequal parts without any definite line of demarcation; they are the superior, inferior, medial, and lateral fornixes. The superior fornix is the largest and deepest. Its depth is maximum at 12 o'clock, reaching almost the orbital margin, which is roughly 15.00 mm from the superior limbus. The depth gradually tapers on each side. On the outer side of the superior fornix are attached fibers of the levator palpebral superior. All the fornices except the superior can be examined by pulling the lower lid. The inferior fornix and lateral fornix become visible if the patient turns the globe to the side opposite the fornix being examined, i.e., if the lateral fornix is to be examined, the child is asked to look medially and vice versa. The superior fornix is examined by the technique of double eversion. The superior fornix, being the deepest, is a common site for foreign bodies to be lodged. It is a common site for lost contact lenses to rest. The inferior fornix is smaller than the superior. The inferior border reaches the inferior orbital rim. The maximum depth is 6–8 mm at the 6 o'clock position. It can be examined with ease by just pulling the lower lid down and asking the child to look straight up. This is the place where eye drops should be instilled. It may also harbor foreign bodies, which can simply be picked up after pulling the lower lid down.

The lateral fornix is a small, ill-defined space in the horizontal plane; it is about 14 mm from the limbus. The medial fornix is also an ill-defined area fully occupied by the caruncle and plica.

Blood Supply to the Conjunctiva

The conjunctiva has an abundant arteriolar supply. The larger vessels may be visible in normal conjunctiva; they become dilated following the slightest insult. The rich blood supply of the conjunctiva is responsible for the quick healing of conjunctival wounds. The blood supply of the conjunctiva follows the embryonal development of the lid and its blood supply. The conjunctiva is supplied by the peripheral and marginal arcades of the lids and the anterior ciliary artery. The tarsal conjunctiva is supplied by twigs from the peripheral and marginal arcades of the lids. The bulbar conjunctiva is supplied by anterior conjunctival arteries arising from the anterior ciliary artery. The other source of blood supply is from the posterior conjunctival arteries that arise from the arcades of the lids. The anterior and posterior conjunctival branches anastomose with each other.

Venous Drainage

The venous drainage of the conjunctiva is intimately related to the venous drainage of the lids. They are far more in number than the corresponding arteries. They drain into the superior and inferior ophthalmic veins.

Lymphatic Drainage

The conjunctiva is very rich in formed lymphatic channels; the lymphatics from the lateral half drain in the preauricular and remaining in the submandibular lymph glands.

Nerve Supply

The conjunctiva is less sensitive to all stimuli compared to the cornea. The conjunctiva gets its nerve supply from the first division of the fifth nerve.

Development of Conjunctiva

In short, the development of the conjunctiva is dependent on the development of the lids, just as the development of the cornea is; it is not possible for the cornea to develop independently.

The conjunctiva has two sources of development, i.e., ectoderm and mesoderm. The epithelium develops from the surface ectoderm, and the rest from the mesoderm.

The congenital anomalies of the conjunctiva are rare. The common anomalies are choristomas, congenital pigmentation, epitarsus, lymphadenoma, telangectasia, and pigmentation.

Conjunctival Choristomas

Choristomas are common congenital anomalies of the conjunctiva. Choristomas are a group of congenital disorders. They comprise tissues that are normal in nature but present at places where they are not supposed to be; they have been called normal tissues at abnormal locations. This is in contrast to hamartomas, which are normal tissues at a normal location; both types are present in the conjunctiva. Examples of choristomas are dermoid and dermolipomas, while an example of hamartomas is congenital telangiectasia. Most of them have systemic involvement. Examples of hamartomas are Rendu-Osler disease and Sturge-Weber syndrome. The choristomas and hamartomas may be present at birth or may become visible in childhood and adolescence. The choristomas have been observed with microphthalmos, optic nerve anomalies, macular hypoplasia, and Goldenhar syndrome.

Dermoids

Dermoids are choristomas that are of two types, i.e., cystic and solid; the former are found either in the orbit or at the orbital rim and not in conjunctiva. The conjunctival dermoids, due to their frequent location at corneoscleral junctions, are commonly referred to as limbal dermoids. The most common site for a conjunctival dermoid to develop is the inferior temporal quadrant of the limbus, but it may be seen in other quadrants as well **(Fig. 12.4)**. Rarely do they develop on the cornea without involving the conjunctiva. Lid colobomas are common with large dermoids.

The size of the dermoid may be very small or large enough to cover almost the whole of the cornea and protrude through the interpalpebral fissure. They are dome-shaped circular growths that generally do not grow in size, unlike cystic orbital or periorbital dermoids that show a spurt in size during puberty. The dermoid never develops malignancy. The limbal dermoids straddle the limbus. The surface of the dermoid is rough. The conjunctiva cannot be moved over the growth; the growth itself is fixed to the underlying sclera and cornea. Rarely do they grow inside the iris or ciliary body; they are also known to develop on the caruncle. The color of the dermoid is dirty white; sometimes, there may be pigmentation on the vortex of the dermoid. It is common to find a few hairs growing out of the dermoid.

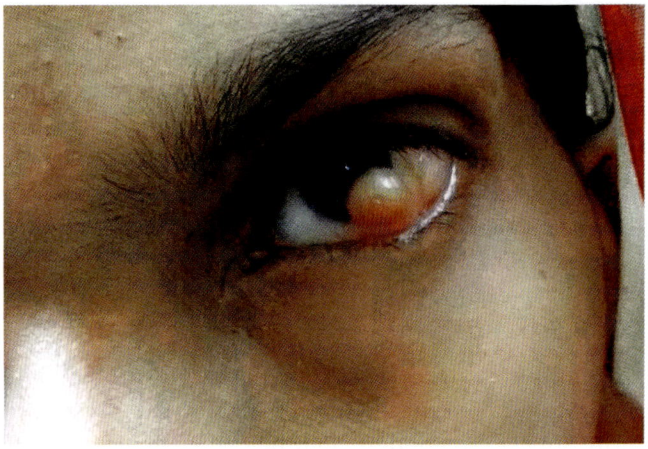

Fig. 12.4: Dermoid of the conjunctiva.

On histopathology, the dermoid comprises both ecto- and mesodermal elements. The ectodermal tissues are hair, sebaceous glands, nerve fibers, and smooth muscle. The mesodermal structures are blood vessels and cartilages.

The symptoms of the dermoids are:

- *Cosmetic:* A white growth against a black background is bound to draw the attention of the onlooker and make the child aware of it.
- *Diminished vision:*
  - If the dermoid is large enough to cover the visual axis, it causes considerable visual loss.
  - Even small dermoids cause irregular astigmatism.
  - The dermoids may be associated with developmental errors of tissue and the second bronchial arch; the chief among them is Goldenhar syndrome.*

**Goldenhar syndromes:* The syndrome consists of a limbal dermoid, a preauricular appendage, and an aural fistula. The other possible ocular involvements are coloboma of the upper lid, microphthalmos, and coloboma of the uvea. The systemic anomalies are hypoplasia of both the jaws and macrostomia. The condition is unilateral.

Treatment of dermoid: Small dermoids do not require any treatment. Large dermoids are better shaved off the cornea and sclera. The disadvantage of the procedure is that it leaves a circular corneal opacity which requires separate management; removal does not effectively cure astigmatism. Other difficulties with limbal dermoid are that contact lenses cannot be fitted, and refractive surgery is contraindicated.

Dermolipomas

Dermolipomas are less frequent choristomas than dermoids. They are mostly unilateral and present at birth. Small dermolipomas may be missed at birth only to become obvious later. They become more prominent and visible if the eye is moved opposite the dermolipoma, i.e., temporal growth becomes more obvious when the child looks medially, and a superotemporal dermoid becomes more visible as the child looks down **(Fig. 12.5)**.

The common sites are the superotemporal and later canthus, never reaching the limbus. They may be stationary or increase in size with age. It is common for superotemporal dermoid to extend back in the orbit between the superior and medial recti; being soft in consistency, they do not produce proptosis. The growths are smooth, soft, and yellowish in color; the conjunctiva vessels are prominently visible over the growth; and the conjunctiva can be moved over the growth. The growth is irreducible and does not change in size during the Valsalva maneuver. They contain a large amount of adipose tissue.

They are better left undisturbed; incomplete removal is always followed by recurrence. They should only be removed when facilities for orbital and neurosurgical procedures are available. Incomplete removal may damage the levator, superior and medial rectus, and lacrimal gland.

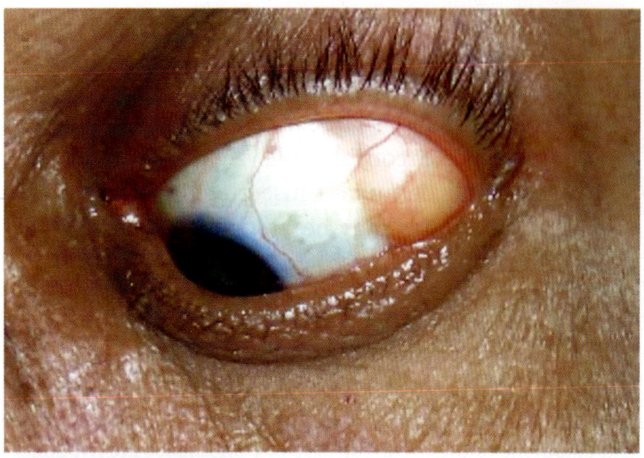

Fig. 12.5: Dermolipoma present since childhood.

Conjunctival Lymphadenoma

These are rare hereditary anomalies with solid conjunctival edema and solid edema of the limbs.

Epitarsus

In this rare anomaly of the tarsal conjunctiva, there is an added fold of conjunctiva over the normal tarsal conjunctiva with a blind recess in between. The pouch may harbor foreign bodies or inflammatory cells. Microbes may find access to the blind pouch, causing recurrent conjunctivitis. The condition does not require any specific treatment except for the evacuation of the inflammatory material from time to time.

Microbiology of Normal Conjunctiva

Conjunctiva is never devoid of microflora except for the first few hours of birth. Sterility is lost if:

- Maternal passage is infected.
- Attending persons are infected.
- The water used to give baby baths or the swab used to clean the lids are contaminated.
- Instillation of nonstandard anti-infective drops. (Folk medicine)

All the organisms present in the conjunctiva are not always pathogens. Some of them may remain nonpathogens, but some of them can get converted into disease-causing organisms. The organisms that do not cause disease are called commensal saprophytes. Saprophytes can be divided into two broad groups. The first group consists of *Staphylococcus aureus*, *Staphylococcus epidermidis*, diphtheroids, and *Propionibacterium*. The second group consists of those microbes that can be isolated from time to time only; the conjunctiva in between two positive results is found to be devoid of microorganisms. The growth of the organism in the culture varies according to the presence of the organism. Such organisms are called transient microbes; the organism can be bacterial or fungal. The common transient fugal floras are *Candida albicans*, *Penicillium*, *Aspergillus*, *Fusarium*, and *Blastomyces*.

The common bacteria that can be isolated from an asymptomatic conjunctiva are *Staphylococci* (except *S. aureus*), *S. epidermidis*, *Hemophilus*, *Escherichia coli*, *Klebsiella Branhamella*, and *Pseudomonas*.

The frequent commensals are *Scaphirhynchus albus*/*Citrus*, diphtheroid, Morax-Axenfeld, and *Corynebacterium xerosis*.

> Fungal infections of the conjunctiva are rare. The viruses are always pathogenic.

Most of the microbes that cause conjunctival disease are exogenous; only a few organisms can spread by an endogenous route. Such organisms are *Gonococci*, *Meningococci*, *Staphylococci*, *Streptococci*, and *Dysentery bacilli*.

The conjunctival microbial diseases are:

- Infective conjunctivitis
- Infection superimposed on allergic conjunctivitis
- Infection developing in local or systemic immune suppression
- Granuloma
- Ulcer (rarest among all above)

The functions of the conjunctivas are:

- To cover the sclera in the anterior half
- Supply blood to the periphery of the cornea.
- Supply mucus to the tear film.
- Fornices act as reservoirs of tears.
- Conjunctiva acts as a barrier to small foreign bodies from getting embedded in the sclera.
- The conjunctiva supplies stem cells to the cornea.
- The conjunctival epithelium is continuous with the corneal epithelium; hence, it is a predisposing factor in corneal ulcers.

Physical Signs Associated with Disorders of the Conjunctiva in Children

The eye may have one or many signs at a given time; it may be unilateral or bilateral, with both eyes developing the same at the same time or with a gap in between different times. The unilateral case may remain unilateral, or the other eye may be involved later. The signs may be symmetric or asymmetric.

An example of the first is the presence of localized subconjunctival hemorrhage, Bitot's spot, or pinguecula. Examples of the second are conjunctival congestion and discharge, with petechial hemorrhages.

The common signs of conjunctival disorders in children are:

- Change in colors of the conjunctiva
- Change in transparency of conjunctiva
- Edema (chemosis) of conjunctiva
- Discharge
- Hemorrhage in the conjunctiva or subconjunctival tissue
- Follicles
- Papillae
- Membranes
- Xerosis
- Scaring
- Degeneration
- Ulcer
- Granuloma
- Cysts
- Neoplasm (rare)
- Keratinization
- Adhesions
- Lymphadenopathy

The Color Changes in Conjunctiva

The color changes in conjunctiva can be due to the following conditions:

- Hyperemia of conjunctiva
- Hemorrhage
- Pallor of conjunctiva
- Pigmentation of conjunctiva

The normal conjunctiva is transparent enough to make the sclera visible through it. The visible sclera imparts white color to the eye in the interpalpebral aperture. The meibomian glands in the tarsal conjunctivas are visible as bluish lines in normal conjunctiva.

The conjunctiva is richly endowed with blood vessels, both arteries and veins. This vascularization is more in the fornices, mostly by fine capillaries. When the larger blood vessels dilate, they also cause dilatation of the capillaries. Dilatation of blood vessels is called conjunctival hyperemia or conjunctival congestion.

Conjunctival congestion can be brought about by active dilatation of arterioles or passive dilatation of veinules. The former is more common.

The congestion can be:

- Conjunctival
- Ciliary
- Mixed

Mixed conjunctival and ciliary congestion is not uncommon. It is not difficult to identify an isolated type of congestion, but difficulty arises when both types of congestion are present at the same time, which is generally referred to as red eyes by laypersons.

Conjunctival congestion, which is also known as conjunctival injection, can be unilateral or bilateral. The latter is more frequent than the former. In cases of unilateral congestion, the other eye soon develops congestion and follows the course taken by the first. Conjunctival congestion can be generalized or localized. In generalized congestion, all the parts of the conjunctiva, i.e., the bulbar, palpebral, and fornices, are involved. The congestion is most visible on the bulbar conjunctiva. The generalized congestion begins in the fornix and spreads in the bulbar and tarsal conjunctival areas **(Figs. 12.6A and B)**.

In bulbar conjunctiva, it is more marked on the periphery, fading toward the cornea. Conjunctival congestion can be acute or chronic. The color of acute hyperemia is bright red in color and invariably associated with discharge. The vessels involved in conjunctival congestions are posterior conjunctival arteries and their corresponding veins, which are tortuous, branch profusely, and may anastomose with each other. The flow of blood is from the fornix to the limbus in the case of bulbar conjunctiva. The flow can be obliterated by pressing over the conjunctiva in the periphery or instilling drops of a local vasoconstrictor. The effect of the vasoconstrictor passes in a few minutes, and the conjunctiva returns to the hyperemic stage. Severe conjunctival congestion may be associated with chemosis of the conjunctiva, subconjunctival petechial hemorrhage membrane, and pseudomembranes. The most common cause of conjunctival hyperemia is conjunctivitis that can be infective or allergic. Besides these two, there is a type of benign, nonallergic, noninfective conjunctiva that is called simple hyperemia.

Simple Hyperemia

This is less common in children; it is a mild congestion with little or no tearing, without discharge or itching, generally bilateral or universal. It presents as mild congestion on awaking this type of congestion passes in a few minutes. The other causes of simple hyperemia are: Lack of sleep, cold or hot wind, fumes, dust, uncorrected errors of refraction, especially hypermetropia, small degree of astigmatism, the wrong spectacle, and muscle imbalance. Reflex hyperemia is common and frequent in the common cold as is emotion and mechanical irritation of the conjunctiva by inturned lash. Entropion, conjunctival foreign bodies in the conjunctiva. Most of the time, no cause can be pinpointed. Such cases are mostly familial. The condition does not require any active treatment; simple astringents and lubricants may be sufficient. Local use of vasoconstrictors is of no use. The first step to ameliorate the condition is to correct errors of refraction and muscle imbalance.

Localized Conjunctiva Hyperemia

The localized conjunctival hyperemia is more specific and requires treatment. The common causes of localized conjunctiva congestion in children are shown in **Figure 12.7** and enlisted as follows:

- Local trauma
- Phlycten

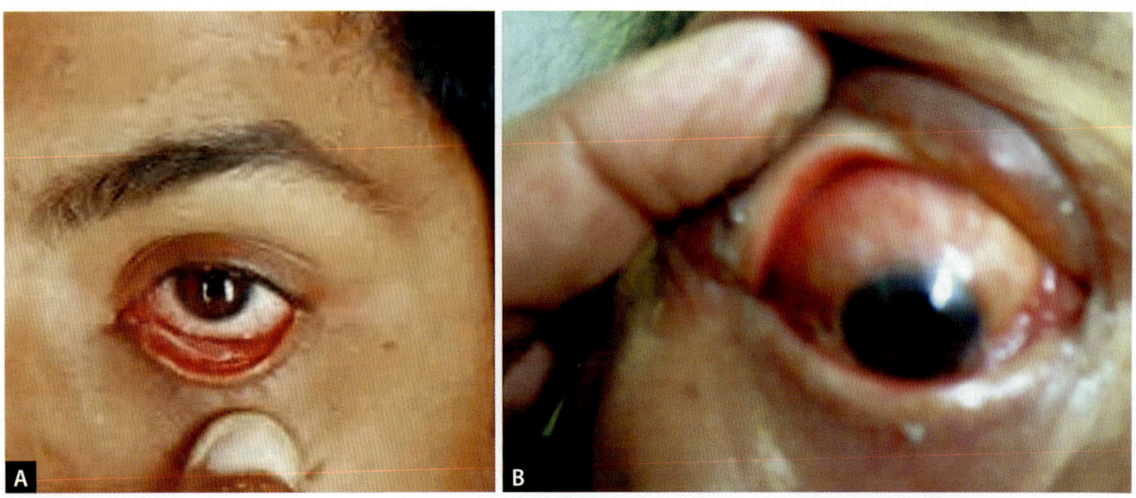

Figs. 12.6A and B: Two types of conjunctival congestion. (A) Conjunctival congestion of lower fornix and tarsal conjunctiva; (B) Bulbar conjunctival congestion.

- Limbal spring catarrh
- Circumciliary congestion
- Superior limbic conjunctivitis
- Episcleritis (in older children)
- Angular conjunctivitis
- Conjunctivitis lacrimal
- *Granuloma:*
    - Infective granuloma
    - Foreign body granuloma
- *New growth:*
    - Hemangioma
    - Papilloma

Passive Conjunctival Congestion

Passive conjunctival congestion is less common in all ages and still less frequent in children. Passive congestion is caused by impeded venous flow, mostly due to mechanical obstruction or increased blood viscosity. The conjunctival capillaries are less effected than veinules and veins. Passive congestion lacks the bright red colors of active congestion, which is brought about due to active dilatation of capillaries. The conjunctival passive congestion has a dark colored bluish hue. The causes can be ophthalmic or systemic.

The ophthalmic causes are in the globe or in the orbit. The systemic conditions are brought about by diminished venous returns between venous drainage and the heart.

The most common intraocular cause is obstruction of the anterior ciliary veins, as in generalized high intraocular pressure in absolute glaucoma or intraocular malignancy. Raised intraocular pressure itself blanches the conjunctiva, against which the veins stand out prominently as caput medusae **(Fig. 12.8)**.

The orbital causes consist of:

- Intraorbital inflammation
- Intraorbital neoplasm
- Thyroid eye diseases
- Carotid cavernous fistula
- Orbital thrombophlebitis
- Cavernous sinus thrombosis

The systemic causes are:

- Right-sided heart failure
- Pressure on the neck vein
- Mediastinal growth
- Polycythemia
- Multiple myeloma

Treatment is directed toward the causes.

Ciliary Congestion (Circumcorneal Congestion)

Ciliary congestion is, in fact, not a part of conjunctival disease. It is secondary to inflammation of the cornea, uvea, or an acute or sustained rise in intraocular tension **(Figs. 12.9A and B)**.

However, it is common to confuse circumciliary (corneal) as conjunctiva congestion and vice versa.

Both types of congestion may coexist. The circumciliary congestion is due to acute dilatation of anterior ciliary and radial episcleral vessels, denoting inflammation of anterior uvea.

> Posterior uveal inflammations do not cause circumciliary congestion. The presence of circumciliary congestion points toward impending pan uveitis.

The condition, as the name suggests, develops around the cornea and not over the ciliary body. It is lighter than conjunctival congestion, which is of a dull pink hue (violaceous).

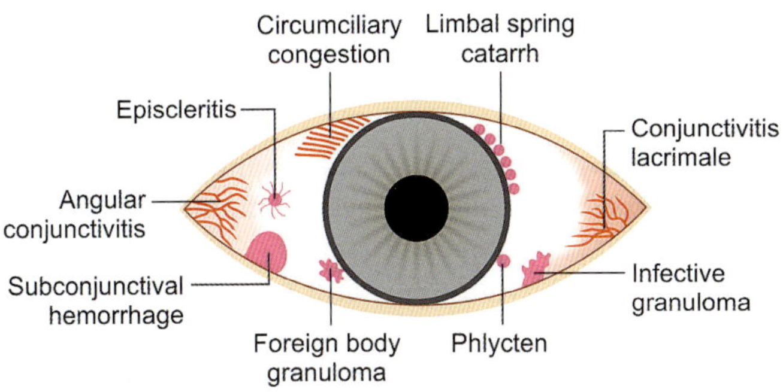

Fig. 12.7: Various types of localized conjunctival congestion in children.

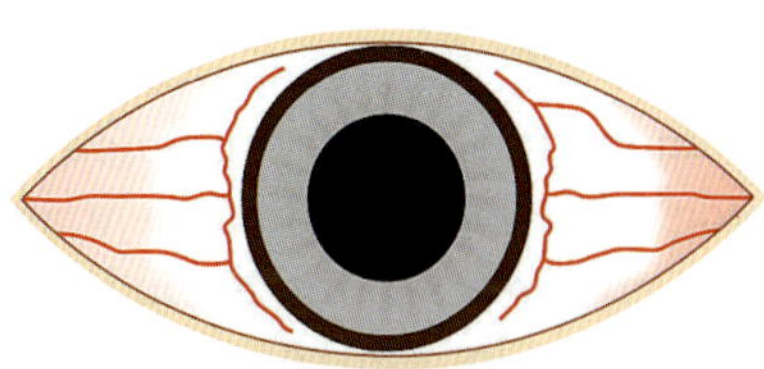

Fig. 12.8: Episcleral congestion causing caput medusae.

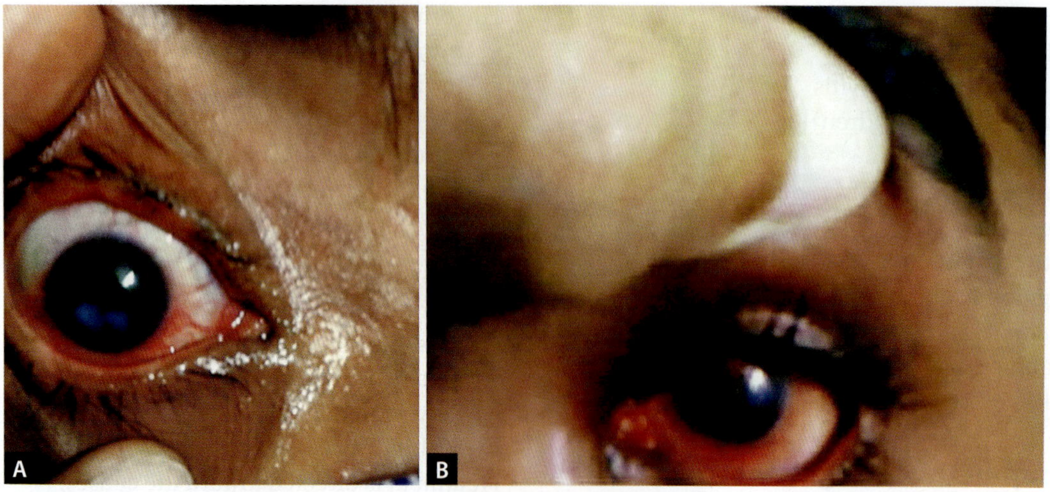

Figs. 12.9A and B: Two types of circumciliary congestion. (A) Circumciliary congestion in corneal ulcer; (B) Circumciliary congestion without corneal ulcer.

It is better referred to as a circumcorneal flush. The vessels are finer than conjunctival, straight, and rarely anastomosing; the flow of blood is from center to periphery; the vessels do not obliterate with gentle pressure; and they do not blanch with local vasoconstrictors. It is invariably associated with ciliary tenderness and signs of uveal irritation, i.e., KP, flare, and photophobia.

The causes are:

- Anterior uveitis; more marked in acute iritis
- Corneal infection and inflammation are deep enough to involve the endothelium.
- Acute congestive glaucoma

Comparison between conjunctival, ciliary, and episcleral congestion is shown in **Table 12.2**.

Pigmentation of Conjunctiva

Pigmentation of the conjunctiva may be congenital or acquired. The congenital form may be localized to the conjunctiva or be associated with pigmentation of the lids spreading over the cheeks **(Fig. 12.10)**.

The most common pigment that imparts colors to the conjunctiva is bilirubin, giving yellow color to the transparent conjunctiva. It is very common in newborns; that is physiological, requiring no treatment, and the yellow discoloration is most marked on the bulbar conjunctiva. For the conjunctiva to look discolored, the pigment may be in the conjunctiva or in the sclera. It can be seen in all ages; it is bilateral and is referred to as jaundice in common parlance.

The other systemic conditions that cause discoloration of conjunctivas are malaria, antimalaria drugs, and yellow fever. The discoloration in malaria is due to hemosiderin. Discoloration in conjunctiva can be seen in Addison's disease as well.

The other causes are melanocytic lesions of the conjunctiva, congenital, or acquired. Some metals also cause discoloration of the conjunctiva, i.e., silver causes argyrosis; discoloration by iron is called siderosis.

Loss of Transparency of the Conjunctiva

Conjunctiva loses its transparency in chemosis of conjunctiva, conjunctival congestion, subconjunctival hemorrhage, xerosis, keratinization, and scar formation. The loss of transparency of the conjunctiva due to scar formation is most marked in the trachoma and pterygium. In trachoma, the scar is in the form of a star-shaped white area, obscuring the view of the tarsal glands. The scarring in trachoma is not seen in children, so is obscuration by pterygium.

The following list of pathological processes causes loss of transparency in conjunctiva and corresponding disorders.

- *Conjunctival congestion:* Acute conjunctivitis
- *Chemosis:* Acute allergy, severe conjunctivitis, endophthalmitis, and panophthalmitis
- *Membrane:* Membranous and pseudomembranous conjunctivitis
- *Hemorrhage:* Subconjunctival and interconjunctival due to severe infection, local trauma, and craniofacial injury

TABLE 12.2: Comparison between various types of conjunctival congestion.

Features	*Conjunctival*	*Ciliary*	*Episcleral*
Vessels involved	Posterior conjunctival	Anterior ciliary arteries	Anterior ciliary veins
Distribution	From fornix to limbus	Limbus to fornix	Periphery to cornea
Flow of blood	Centripetal	Centrifugal	Centrifugal
Branching of vessels	Profuse	Limited or nil	Nil
Effect of weak vasoconstrictor	Instant blanching	No or late	No blanching
Color	Bright red	Violaceous	Bright
Tortuosity of vessels	Tortuous	Straight	Tortuous
Mobility of conjunctiva	Vessels move with conjunctiva	Do not move with conjunctiva	Do not move with conjunctiva
Subconjunctival hemorrhage	May be present	Absent	Absent
Chemosis of conjunctiva	May be present	May be present	Absent
Cause of congestion	Diseases of conjunctiva	Disease of the iris ciliary body and an acute rise in intraocular pressure	Absolute glaucoma, obstruction of venous flow from the head and neck

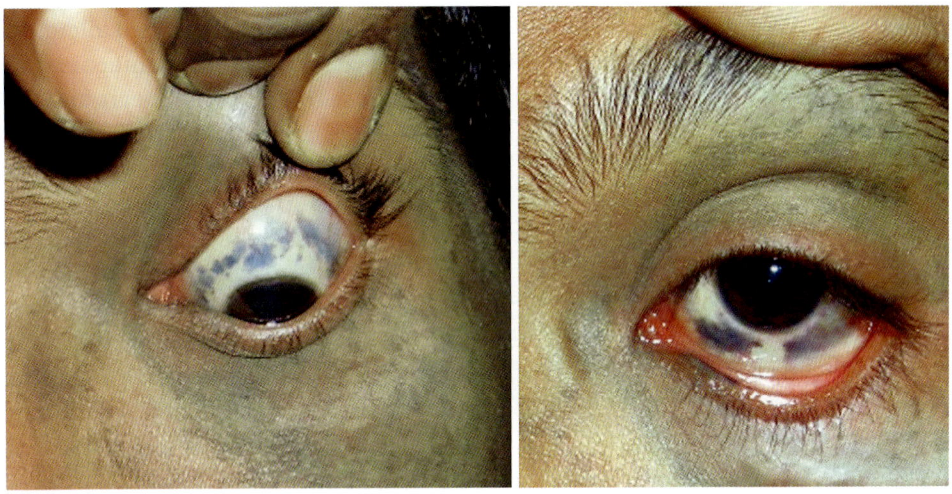

Fig. 12.10: Congenital melanosis.

- *Scaring:* Trachoma, trauma, conjunctival growth, and pterygium
- *Subconjunctival deposit:* Steroid and scleral implant
- *Dryness:* Xerosis, Bitot's spot, and keratinization

Conjunctival Chemosis

Physiologically, there is no fluid either under or in the substance of normal conjunctiva. The stasis of fluid in the conjunctiva is called the chemosis of the conjunctiva. It causes soft, transient, translucent bulging of the conjunctiva and the accumulation of fluid underneath. There is either increased permeability of arterial blood supply or impeded venous drainage. Deranged lymphatic drainage also causes chemosis, which is called solid in contrast to soft edema of vascular origin. An example of lymphedema is congenital lymphedema of the conjunctiva.

The conjunctival chemosis can be mild, moderate, or severe, depending upon the accumulation of fluid in and under the conjunctiva. In mild chemosis, the conjunctiva has a glossy appearance; in moderate chemosis, the conjunctiva is lifted from the sclera with a water-laden translucent appearance. In severe chemosis, the conjunctiva is enormously swollen and may be edematous enough to protrude in or out of the interpalpebral aperture. It is generally congested with copious watering. Chemosis due to systemic conditions is generally bilateral and chronic.

The chemosis can be unilateral and remain so, or it may be bilateral. The chemosis is least marked in the tarsal conjunctiva and more marked in the bulbar conjunctiva and fornices. Its presence in fornix is not well visible due to the large space available. In the bulbar conjunctiva, the chemosis stops at the limbus, but the accumulation of fluid continues; hence, the conjunctiva assumes the appearance of a doughnut round the limbus. It is not uncommon for the chemosed conjunctiva to spill over the cornea sufficient enough to obscure the corneal details; this happens most in acute exogenous allergic conjunctivitis, ophthalmia neonatorum, and panophthalmitis. If the chemosed conjunctiva remains exposed for sufficient time, it may get dry and keratinized as is seen in thyroid exophthalmos.

The causes of chemosis can be:

- *Ocular:*
  - *Conjunctival:*
    - Allergy
    - Infection
- *Orbital:* Intraocular and peribulbar inflammation such as orbital cellulitis, cellulitis lid, and acute dacryocystitis. Fracture of the paranasal sinuses causes emphysematous edema of the conjunctiva, where the conjunctiva is raised with crepitus.
- *Systemic:* Thyroid eye disease, hypersensitivities to drugs and food, and angioneurotic edema.

Treatment

- Edema caused by exogenous allergens subsides within a few minutes. Instillation of a weak steroid gives prompt relief.
- Mild chemosis due to no apparent cause may be treated with local vasoconstrictors and lubricants.
- Chemosis secondary to infection requires treatment of the primary cause by antimicrobials.
- Systemic conditions require treatment of the primary cause by an internist.
- Surgical emphysema due to fractured paranasal sinuses does not require any treatment except reassurance.

Conjunctival Discharge

Discharge is a very common manifestation of conjunctival disorders. It is caused by infection and inflammation. Conjunctival discharge consists of tears, mucus, inflammatory cells, and microorganisms, rarely blood and foreign bodies. Discharge in adults contains more tears than mucus, which is more common in children. Discharge in newborns up to 2–3 months is devoid of tears; it is mainly mucus, inflammatory cells, and microorganisms. As seen in the ophthalmia of newborns, the most common example of copious discharge is gonococcal ophthalmia neonatorum. According to composition and consistency, the discharge is divided into the following types:

- *Watery:* This is mostly a tear with little or no mucus seen in viral, chemical, and allergic conjunctivitis and soon gets converted into mucoid discharge.
- *Mucoid:* This consists of tears and mucus, seen in mild bacterial conjunctivitis but more prominent in allergic conjunctivitis, i.e., vernal or atopic keratoconjunctivitis, or ocular surface disorder.
- *Ropy:* This is characteristic of spring catarrh, where the child may say that when he tries to wipe the discharge, it comes out in the form of a white string. A less common and missed disorder is mucus fishing syndrome.*
- *Mucopurulent discharge:* The discharge is thick with mucus, and inflammatory cells may cause the lids to stick during sleep. It is seen in bacterial and chlamydial conjunctivitis.
- *Purulent discharge:* This is seen in hyperacute conjunctivitis, mostly gonococcal **(Fig. 12.11)**.
- *Blood-tinged discharge:* The usual conjunctival discharge is either colorless or white. It may get blood tinged in the case of membrane-forming conjunctivitis or conjunctivitis associated with petechial hemorrhage.

**Mucus fishing syndrome:* It is an ill-understood, disgusting symptom; needing removal of excess mucus from the conjunctiva. This is mostly seen in ocular surface aqueous deficiency disorder and spring catarrh, or perennial allergic conjunctivitis. This starts following trauma to the bulbar conjunctiva, which results in the production of reflex tearing and mucus. The cycle of trauma-mucus production-removal-trauma goes on, and the patient develops an involuntary reflex of mucus removal. The patient denies the habit. The traumatized conjunctiva stains with rose Bengal, mostly on the nasal side of the conjunctiva. The treatments consist of counseling the patient about the condition and avoiding the habit of removing the mucus. The underlying cause of ocular surface disorder and allergic status should be treated adequately.

Subconjunctival Hemorrhage

Subconjunctival hemorrhage is in fact inter conjunctival hemorrhage in the stroma of the conjunctiva and seeps to the sclera.

It is a common and frightening condition due to bright blood standing out prominently against white sclera. A large subconjunctival bleeding is referred to as a subconjunctival hematoma, which, when large, may break through the epithelium and cause bleeding from the conjunctiva. Most of the subconjunctival hemorrhages are sudden **(Figs. 12.12 and 12.13)**.

The subconjunctival hemorrhage may develop anywhere in the conjunctiva. The hemorrhage in the interpalpebral fissure is most visible and makes the patient seek medical help; even a small speck of hemorrhage draws patients' or onlookers' attention.

The hemorrhages in the hidden part of the conjunctiva, i.e., the upper tarsal and upper fornix, may go unnoticed. The conjunctival hemorrhage can be unilateral or bilateral.

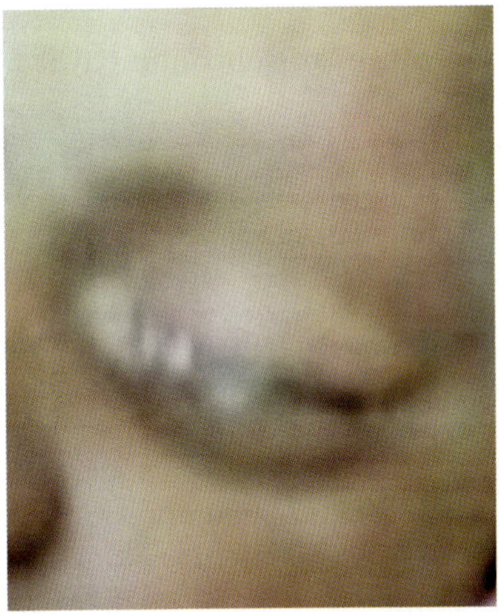

Fig. 12.11: Purulent discharge.

The size of the subconjunctival hemorrhage varies from a few millimeters to large enough to cover the whole of the conjunctiva where the outer border of the hemorrhage is not visible.

Subconjunctival hemorrhage per se is painless except in cases of direct trauma to the conjunctiva. Subconjunctival hemorrhage may occur at any age. In newborns, it is caused due to birth trauma and improper instrumentation. The subconjunctival hemorrhage may be the sole sign and symptom, or it may be associated with periocular and systemic disorders.

The subconjunctival hemorrhage is generally noninfective, but some microbial conjunctivitis are associated with petechial hemorrhages, i.e., pneumococcal and viral conjunctivitis. Trauma is the most common cause of subconjunctival hemorrhage. The trauma may be so trivial as not to be remembered by the patients or may be associated with a severe craniofacial injury. Thus, subconjunctival hemorrhage can be traumatic or nontraumatic.

The traumatic causes may be conjunctival, orbital, scalp, or cranial, which could be frontal or basal.

The nontraumatic causes are:

- *Microbial conjunctivitis:* Bacterial/viral
- *Rupture of conjunctival vessels:*
  - Secondary to the sudden rise of intrathoracic pressure—whooping cough
  - Bleeding from telangectasia, papilloma, and conjunctivo sporidiosis

Direct Trauma to the Conjunctiva

Direct trauma to the conjunctiva is mostly accidental. The trauma may be in the form of a small foreign body that may or may not be embedded or a large, lacerated wound. The amount of subconjunctival hemorrhage is not always proportionate to the extent of the wound.

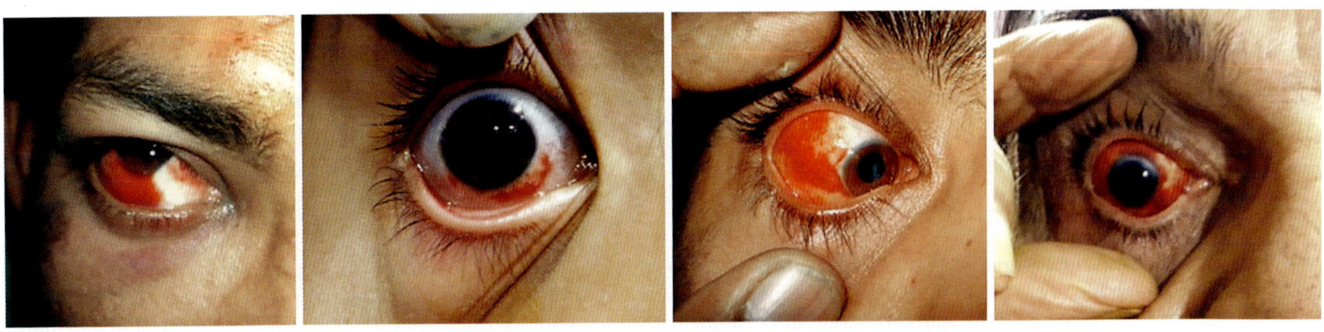

Fig. 12.12: Various types of subconjunctival hemorrhage without ecchymosis of the lid.

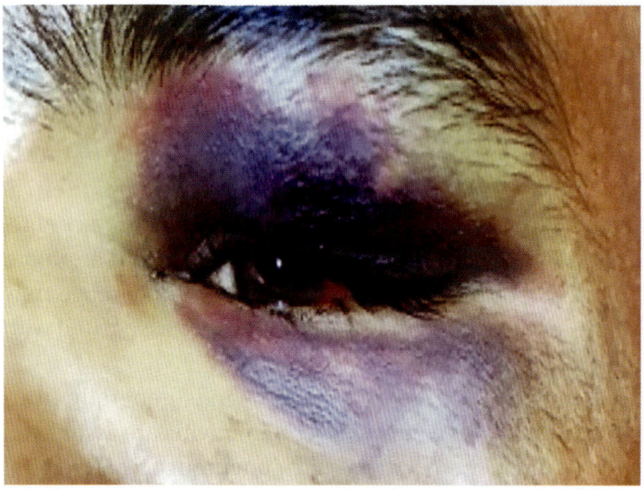

Fig. 12.13: Extensive subconjunctival hemorrhage with ecchymosis of lids following a road traffic accident.

All surgical wounds do not cause subconjunctival hemorrhage. Large surgical incisions surprisingly do not cause subconjunctival hemorrhage.

Orbital Trauma

The most common cause of subconjunctival hemorrhage is the fracture of the orbital wall, the apex of the orbit, and paranasal sinuses. The subconjunctival hemorrhage in the case of a fracture involving the orbit becomes evident a few hours after the actual trauma. It takes time for the blood to trickle down to the conjunctiva from the site of the actual fracture; the farther it is from the conjunctiva, the longer it takes to become visible. The blood either trickles along the orbital wall or the recti. The blood travels from the periphery toward the cornea; hence, the peripheral edge is not visible. Conversely, any subconjunctival hemorrhage where the periphery is not visible with a history of injury should be suspected due to the fracture orbit and investigated. Fractures of the paranasal sinuses are often associated with conjunctival emphysema.

Head Injury

All head injuries do not result in subconjunctival hemorrhage. The two types of head injuries that are commonly associated with subconjunctival hemorrhage are scalp injuries involving the frontal bone and the base of the skull.

The scalp injury causes moderate to severe subconjunctival hemorrhage that trickles down from above in the lid and conjunctiva. Hence, ecchymosis of the upper lid is so common in scalp injuries **(Fig. 12.13)**. Some of the blood trickles down the conjunctiva in a few hours. The upper periphery of the subconjunctival hemorrhage is not visible.

Subconjunctival hemorrhage following a fracture of the base of the skull also develops a few hours after the accident due to the same cause and does not have a visible peripheral border. It is generally associated with epistaxis and bleeding from the ears.

Remote Injuries

Multiple fractures of long bones the pelvis, and crush injuries of the chest and abdomen cause streaks of subconjunctival hemorrhage, mostly in the forearms. Such injuries are generally associated with Purtscher retinopathy.*

Nontraumatic causes of subconjunctival hemorrhage are:

- Infections
- Rupture of conjunctival vessels
- Rupture of conjunctival telangectasia
- Systemic condition

Infections: Some of the microbial conjunctivitis, bacterial or viral, causes subconjunctival hemorrhage, mostly in the form of petechiae that may join to form a large confluent hemorrhage. The organisms causing subconjunctival hemorrhages are seen in pneumococcal conjunctivitis, membranous and pseudomembranous conjunctivitis, hemophilus conjunctivitis, and Koch-Week conjunctivitis. The common viruses responsible for subconjunctival hemorrhage are adenoviruses 70, coxsackievirus, and adenoviruses.

Rupture of conjunctival vessels: The most common cause of subconjunctival hemorrhage in nonimmunized children is whooping cough. It used to be so common before immunization against whooping cough became

**Pustscher retinopathy* is not a primary conjunctival disorder. It is also known as traumatic retinopathy, a rare microvasculopathy caused by the obstruction of fine blood vessels in the retina and subconjunctiva in the fornices. The features are many white retinal spots round the optic nerve spreading to the fovea; the spots are less frequent at the paravascular areas, where they are replaced by superficial hemorrhage. The condition is generally seen following severe injuries to large bones and the thorax.

compulsory that every parent who brought a child with subconjunctival hemorrhage was asked if the child was suspected to be suffering from whooping cough, the answer to which was not always very correct; hence, all nontraumatic, noninfectious subconjunctival hemorrhages were suspected to be due to whooping cough, and the child was referred to an expert in childhood infectious diseases unless proved otherwise. The cause of subconjunctival hemorrhage in such a situation is not the organism but the sudden rise of venous pressure in the conjunctiva. It does not require any treatment except reassurance. The child should be referred to a pediatrician.

Rupture of conjunctival telangectasia: This is rare.

Systemic condition: Systemic conditions that cause subconjunctival hemorrhage are thrombocytopenic purpura, leukemia, and aplastic anemia.

Treatment

- Traumatic subconjunctival laceration unless large does not required any treatment except reassurance and usual antibiotic drops. It must be explained to the patient that it will take 7–10 days for the hemorrhage to clear.
- If the outer border of the subconjunctival hemorrhage is not visible, the patient should be subjected to a neuroophthalmic workup. Computed tomography (CT) and magnetic resonance imaging (MRI) may be required.

Follicles

The conjunctiva is rich in lymphoid tissue, and any injury to the conjunctiva is a microbial or chemical cause of the proliferation of lymphoid tissue under the epithelium. The proliferating lymphoid tissue causes the formation of small nodules that project on the surface. They range between 0.5 and 2.00 mm in diameter, are pale in color, and no blood vessels pass over the follicles but are seen round the base of the follicles. Each follicle consists of an active germinal core with hyperplasia of lymphoid tissue **(Fig. 12.14)**.

There are no lymphoid tissues in the conjunctiva at birth; it takes 2–3 months to develop them. Hence, there is no follicular reaction in the conjunctiva of newborns up to 3 months. The follicles are seen in fornices and palpebral conjunctiva. They do not develop on the bulbar conjunctiva but may develop at the limbus in the trachoma. The presence of follicles in the conjunctiva is not always diagnostic, especially in the lower fornix and lower tarsal conjunctiva. Their presence in the upper tarsal conjunctiva is suggestive of chronic viral and chlamydia infections. A combination of follicles and conjunctivitis is loosely referred to as a nonspecific term for follicular conjunctivitis. This is mostly seen in children and is self-limiting. Follicles can be acute or chronic. Chronic folliculosis lasting >4 weeks is called chronic follicular conjunctivitis.

The following is the list of common causes of follicles in all ages:

- *Viruses:*
  - *Adenovirus:*
    - Pharyngoconjunctival fever virus
    - Epidemic keratoconjunctivitis fever
  - *Enterovirus:* Acute hemorrhagic conjunctivitis
  - *Herpes:*
    - Zoster
    - Simplex primary/secondary
  - Newcastle disease
  - Influenza virus
  - Molluscum
- *Chlamydia:*
  - Inclusion conjunctivitis
  - Trachoma

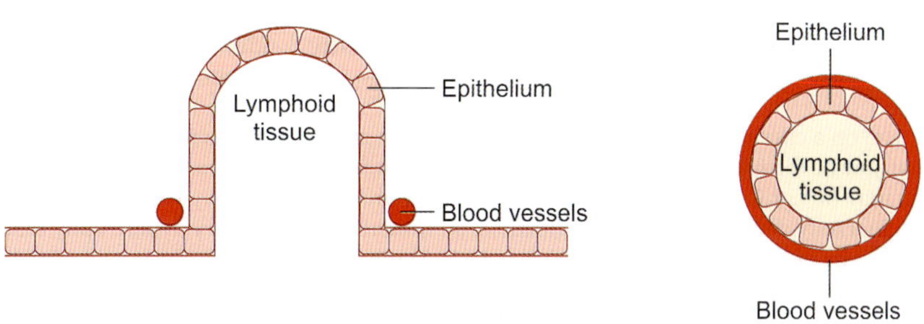

Fig. 12.14: Histology of a typical follicle.

- Parinaud's oculoglandular syndrome*
- *Bacterial:*
    - Streptococci
    - Moraxella
    - Treponema
- *Toxic:*
    - Atropine
    - Miotics
    - Adrenergic drugs
    - Sulpha
    - Aminoglycosides
    - Idoxuridine

The number, size, and position vary with the type of conjunctivitis, its duration, severity, and causative factor. The usual size of follicles and their numbers are variable. The number varies between a few and dozens.

The follicle must be differentiated from the papillae. The follicles themselves do not require any specific treatment except in chlamydia conjunctivitis.

Papillae

Papillae are caused by a vascular reaction to an offending factor that is generally allergic in nature and may be bacterial, drug-induced, or mechanical. Papillae are also seen in chronic blepharitis and floppy eye syndrome.†

The development of papillae differs from the formation of follicles, which are lymphoid proliferations without any blood vessels in the substance.

In the case of papillae, the inflamed conjunctiva gets anchored to the tarsal plate or limbus by fine fibrous septa, followed by the proliferation of fine vessels that lift the stroma and epithelium. The blood vessels reach the basement membrane of the epithelium. The tuft of blood vessels is surrounded by a swollen stroma and epithelium. The epithelium is hyperplastic; it is common to find inflammatory cells in the papillae. On the outer surface, the papilla has a velvety appearance; the top is flat with a hexagonal configuration. The papillae are larger than the follicles; the size ranges between 1.00 mm and 5.00 mm across **(Fig. 12.15)**.

The common allergic causes to give rise to papillae are:

- Perennial and seasonal conjunctivitis
- Spring catarrh
- Atopic keratoconjunctivitis
- Superior limbic keratoconjunctivitis‡

**Parinaud's oculoglandular syndrome:* This is an uncommon, often missed, and wrongly treated unilateral condition that involves the conjunctiva as well as the lymph nodes that drain it. The conjunctival lesion is a chronic granuloma that is surrounded by follicles all-round with a tendency to ulcerate; the common causes are tuberculosis, syphilis, lymphogranuloma venereum, and cat scratch fever.

The treatment is of the organism causing the granuloma. (The condition is not to be confused with neurological Parinaud's syndrome, which is a supranuclear disorder.) Parinaud's oculoglandular syndrome is rare in children.

†*Floppy lid syndrome:* This is basically a disorder of the upper lid where the conjunctiva gets involved secondarily. The exact cause of the disorder is not clear. The patient with the syndrome is generally obese, of both sexes. The upper lid is lax; the tarsal plate has a rubbery softness that makes eversion of the upper lid easier than the normal lid. The problem, which is chronic, starts when the upper lid gets everted without any effort during sleep. The prolonged eversion exposes the tarsal conjunctiva, which becomes hyperemic with papillae formation. The condition becomes worse if the bed sheet or pillow rubs over the everted lid. It is not associated with any local or systemic disorder. The symptoms are a foreign body sensation, watering, and redness of the exposed conjunctiva. Most of the time, the lid gets automatically corrected or may be repositioned back without effort. The condition is not seen in children.

There is no specific treatment; lubricant eye ointment may be instilled before going to sleep. Antibiotic drops are given to prevent secondary infection, though taping of the upper lid is generally advised; it is cumbersome and not effective. The best result is achieved by shortening the upper lid horizontally.

‡*Superior limbic keratoconjunctivitis:* This is a chronic, recurrent allergic disorder with irregular remissions and exacerbations. The condition may last for a few months to many years, even without treatment, or resolve spontaneously, leaving no sequelae. The exact cause is not known; it is more common in elderly women with thyroid dysfunction who may have ocular surface disorder as well; it has been reported in persons in the second decade as well. One eye may be involved more than the other. Seasonal variation does not seem to influence. No allergen, external or systemic, has been corelated to the condition. The condition has symptoms disproportionate to the signs.

The symptoms consist of foreign body sensations, watering, mucus discharge, photophobia, and even blepharospasm. There may be mild ptosis with good levator action.

The signs are so minimal that, on a casual look, the eye may look normal. On careful examination, the upper bulbar conjunctiva at 12 o'clock has a sectorial congestion that may be mistaken for localized circum corneal congestion because the congestion is more marked at the limbus and fades toward the fornix, may be confused with episcleritis or a transparent foreign body with conjunctivitis. Absence of tenderness excludes scleral involvement. In a fully developed disorder; the tarsal conjunctiva has papillary hypertrophy that gives a velvety appearance and may be mistaken for a tarsal type of partially treated spring catarrh. The bulbar conjunctiva is thickened, and the limbus has hypertrophied papillae. The corneal changes are localized to the upper cornea which consist of superficial vascularization, erosion, and filamentary keratitis.

There is no specific treatment. Soft contact lenses give maximum comfort. Other helpful therapy is the use of lubricant drops by day and ointment at night. Steroids do not seem to have any role. The patient may volunteer to say that she has used a steroid without relief.

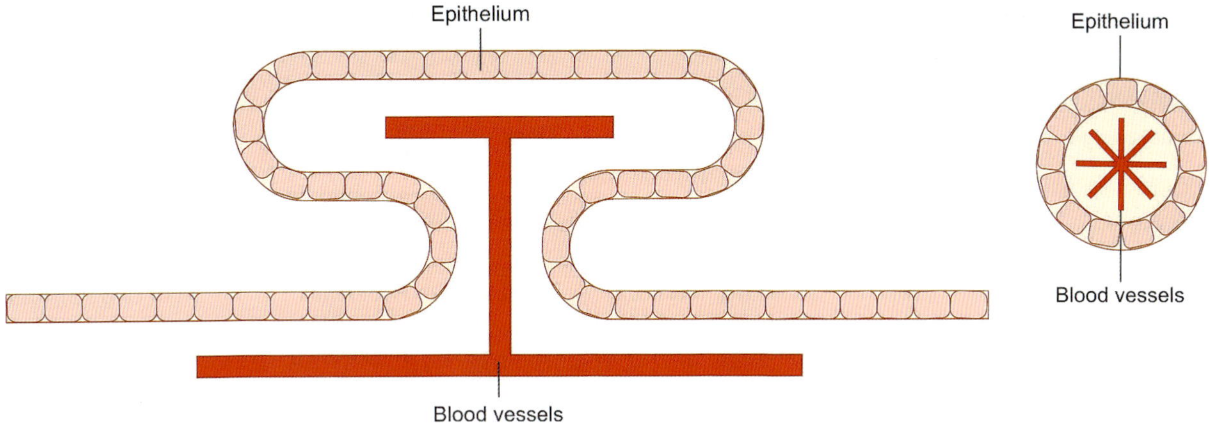

Fig. 12.15: Histology of typical papilla.

Giant Papillary Conjunctivitis

Papillae on the upper tarsus and limbus are more common in spring catarrh, while papillae in the lower tarsus are more frequent in atopic and allergic conjunctivitis. When the papillae, due to prolonged inflammation, lose the septa separating them, they become large and called giant papillae. The size of the papillae in such cases may be as large as 2.00 mm across. The most common cause is mechanical, as seen in soft contact lenses, exposed nylon sutures, and ocular prosthesis. It can also be seen in spring catarrh, atopic conjunctivitis, and floppy lids. The treatment depends on the offending cause. A change of contact lens gives immediate relief. The nylon sutures are best removed and the shape of the prosthesis changed; steroids do not seem to play much role; lubricant, vasoconstrictor, and antihistamine drops give better results.

Table 12.3 shows the comparison between various types of allergic conjunctivitis (All ages).

Membrane Formation in Conjunctiva

Conjunctival inflammation severe enough to damage conjunctival vessels and the surface of the epithelium is associated with the leak of fibrin and exudative material to which inflammatory cells and necrotic material are added that is converted as coagulum and deposited under the already edematous and damaged epithelium; this white glossy substance is called the conjunctival membrane. The membrane is generally in patches on the tarsal conjunctival and fornices. In severe cases, it may develop all over the conjunctiva. If the membrane can be wiped off the surface with ease without bleeding, it is called a pseudomembrane. If the membrane is deeply anchored to the conjunctival epithelium, it cannot be removed with ease. An attempt to peel it is associated with hemorrhage, and the condition is called a true membrane. The condition is called membranous conjunctivitis. Diphtheria used to be the most common cause before universal immunization became compulsory.

> In a nonimmunized child, all membranes should be treated as diphtheria unless proven otherwise. All cases proved to be diphtheritic and should be treated by a person trained in infectious diseases.

It is not always possible to differentiate the two; it is presumed that a true membrane is nothing but a severe form of pseudomembrane. The following box summarizes the main difference between the two:

> 1. Membranous conjunctivitis involves the growth of true membranes into the conjunctival epithelial surface, resulting in significant bleeding upon peeling the membranes.
> 2. Pseudomembranous conjunctivitis membranes are more superficial, with no growth into the conjunctival epithelium, and can be removed with minimal bleeding.

The causes of membrane formations are:

- *Bacterial:*
  - *Corynebacterium diphtheriae*
  - Beta-haemolytic streptococci
  - *Gonococci*
  - Pneumococci
  - *Staphylococci aureus*
- *Viral-epidemic keratoconjunctivitis*
- Allergic–Spring catarrh (rare)
- *Others:*
  - Stevens–Johnson syndrome
  - Ocular pemphigoid

TABLE 12.3: Various types of allergic conjunctivitis and their differences.

Sr. no.	Clinical condition	Age	Sex	Onset	Season	Allergen	Symptoms	Treatment
1.	Acute allergic	All	Both	Hyper acute	All	Many	Itching, FB sensation, watering, and chemosis of conjunctiva	Weak steroid drops three times a day for 24 hours
2.	Seasonal allergic	All	Both	Subacute, chronic course	Particular season	Variable	Hyperemia conjunctiva and mild itching	Mast cells stabilizer, weak solution of steroid, and oral long-acting anti histamine
3.	Perennial allergic	All	Both	Chronic	Through out of year	Variable	Itching and excoriation of angle	Mast cell stabilizer
4.	Spring catarrh	3–5 years	More in boys	Variable	Summer	Many	Intense itching and watering	Strong steroid for a few days, followed by weak solution of steroid for months, and mast cell stabilizer for months
5.	Giant papillary hypertrophy	Any, more common in adults	Both	Chronic	Any	Contact lens, contact lens preservative, and nylon suture	Pseudoptosis, minimal itching, FB sensation, and persistent redness	Change contact lens and contact lens preservative; remove offending foreign body, contact lens hygiene
6.	Atopic conjunctivitis	Any, more common between second and fifth decade	Both	Chronic	Not specific	Not specific	Similar to recurrent spring catarrh	Mast cell stabilizer

- Ligneous conjunctivitis
- Alkali burn
- Graft versus host disease

The end results of true conjunctival membranes are: Xerophthalmia, ocular surface disorder, symblepharon, trichiasis, and entropion.

Scaring of the Conjunctiva

Scaring of the conjunctiva may involve all the layers of the conjunctiva; it may anchor the conjunctiva to the underlying structure. The causes can be traumatic or inflammatory. The traumatic causes are improper suturing of the conjunctiva and an unattended lacerated wound. The trauma can be surgical or accidental; the other cause of scar formation is a chemical burn.

The most common inflammatory cause is trachoma, where the scar anchors the conjunctiva to the tarsal plate and deforms the lid due to contracture. The tarsal scar in trachoma stands out as white subconjunctival stars, best seen in the upper tarsal conjunctiva (trachomatous scarring is not seen in children).

Spring catarrh, too, is rarely known to cause scarring of the conjunctiva.

Other causes that cause mild to severe conjunctival scarring are Sjogren syndrome*, ocular pemphigus, epidermolysis bullosa, toxic epidermal necrolysis,

**Sjogren syndrome:* This is a systemic autoimmune disease that compromises a triad of symptoms: kerato conjunctivitis sicca (dryness), dryness of the mouth, and arthritis. The disorder is not seen in children.

other bullous conditions, graft versus host disease,* and Steven–Johnson syndrome.[†]

Xerosis

Xerosis refers to the dryness of the conjunctiva; this may involve the cornea as well. Involvement of the cornea along with the conjunctiva is called xerophthalmia. Which, when severe, results in keratomalacia or the melting of the cornea. This is very common in malnourished children and should be differentiated from dry eye (ocular surface disorder), which by itself is a separate entity. Xerosis has been classified differently in the following groups:

- Epithelial xerosis
- Parenchymatous xerosis
- Idiopathic

Epithelial Xerosis

This is caused by vitamin A deficiency without the presence of any other diseases in the eye that may contribute to the dryness of the conjunctiva. The fault lies in the goblet cells that are destroyed. Associate squamous metaplasia is the cause of the keratinization of the conjunctiva. The columnar cells are converted into stratified squamous epitheliums, and the loss of goblet cells that are already present; worsens the condition.

Conjunctiva is thrown in vertical folds on either side of the limbus. The folds become more evident if the child looks laterally. The conjunctiva shows abundant growth of nonpathogenic *Corynebacterium xerosis.*

It may be associated with or without Bitot's spot.[‡] Xerosis does not depend on the presence of the main lacrimal gland. It does not happen even in the absence of the lacrimal gland. Conversely, xerosis is present in the presence of a normal lacrimal gland. It is very common for a child to have diminished night blindness with xerosis of the conjunctiva; however, xerosis may precede night blindness.

WHO classification of xerophthalmia:

- *X1A:* Conjunctival xerosis
- *X1B:* Bitot spots
- *X2:* Corneal xerosis
- *X3A:* Corneal ulceration/keratomalacia, involving less than one-third of the cornea
- *X3B:* Corneal ulceration/keratomalacia, involving more than one-third of the cornea
- *XS:* Corneal scars due to xerophthalmia
- *XF:* Xerophthalmic fundus

Parenchymatous Xerosis

Parenchymatous xerosis is seen in the diseased eye. The common causes are chemical burn, trachoma, diphtheria, ocular pemphigus, Stevens–Johnson syndrome, exophthalmos, inability to close the eye due to anchoring of the tarsal conjunctiva to the bulbar conjunctiva, proptosis, lagophthalmos, ectropion, and coloboma of the lids.

The following is the WHO recommendation for the treatment of xerophthalmia:

The principle of management is:

- Treat early symptoms to avoid the development of severe complications.

**Graft versus host disease:* This follows bone marrow transplantation, where the transplanted cells destroy the host cells. It is a serious systemic disorder. In the eye, conjunctival involvement is seen in the acute phase, i.e., within 100 days of transplant, which may range between hyperemia and sloughing of epithelium, papillae, and membrane formation, which ultimately leads to cicatrization of the conjunctiva with its sequelae and ocular surface disorder. It may be associated with blood in the tear.

[†]*Steven–Johnson syndrome:* This is an acute vasculitis of the conjunctiva and other mucosa of the body. This is brought about by acute allergic reactions brought about by the consumption of many drugs; the main among them are sulphonamides, penicillin, and other antibiotics and antianalgesics such as phenylbutazone. The conjunctiva is involved in half the cases that may develop membranous conjunctivitis with mucopurulent conjunctivitis; in severe cases, the cornea may be involved. The corneal involvement is more marked if the eye develops extensive symblepharon in a long run; it causes trichiasis, xerophthalmia, entropion, and symblepharon. It can inflict at any age.

[‡]*Bitot's spot:* This is a white spot (whiter than the sclera). Raised triangular spot on the conjunctiva in the interalpebral aperture. It is not seen under the lids. The base of the spot is toward the cornea, 2–3 mm away from the limbus. Most of the time, it is bilateral. The surface of the spot is slightly elevated than the surrounding conjunctiva. It moves with the conjunctiva; no blood vessels grow over it. Its surface is foamy; the foamy material can be partially wiped off only to recur; the spot does not stain with the usual staining material but stains with Kajal (kohl) or Surma. It is mostly seen on the lateral side, is generally associated with vitamin A deficiency, and resolves with the administration of vitamin A, within 2–5 days without any trace. Rarely it can be seen without vitamin A deficiency in older children. That is generally unilateral and not associated with night blindness and does not improve with the administration of vitamin A.

- Vision can be saved, provided the ulceration is limited to less than a third of the cornea and the pupil is spared.
- Even if the deficiency has already led to keratomalacia and irreversible loss of sight in one eye, it is imperative to administer treatment in order to save the other eye and the life of the patient.

Retinol (Vitamin A) Oral

Table 12.4 gives oral doses of retinol in children and pregnant mothers.

Prevention

Systematically administer retinol peroral to children suffering from measles (one dose on days 1 and 2).

In areas where vitamin A deficiency is endemic, routine supplementation of *retinol* orally is as per **Table 12.5**. The oral vitamin A is available either as drops or capsules. Each capsule contains 200,000 IU. In the case of children, the capsule is punched, and the drug is directly put in the mouth. This is applicable until the child learns to swallow the capsule.

To avoid overdose, find out if the child has already received a preventive dose of vitamin A under the national program of prevention of vitamin A deficiency. The program is carried out under the National Rural Health Mission (NRHM) by Accredited Social Health Activists (ASHA) health workers in Anganwadi, or primary health centers. The information can be seen on the health card issued to each child/expectant mother. If the child has already received the usual dose, the child/expectant mother is not administered an additional dose. Vitamin A, being non-water-soluble, remains in the body and can cause toxicity that includes raised intracranial pressure that results in the bulging of fontanelles in infants, headaches, nausea, vomiting, and, in severe cases, impaired consciousness and convulsions. These adverse effects are transient; they require medical surveillance and symptomatic treatment if needed.

Vitamin A deficiency is rare in breastfed infants under 6 months.

TABLE 12.4: Doses of retinol in different ages.

Age	*Dose*
Children <6 months	50,000 IU (2 drops) once daily on D1, D2, and D8
Children 6 months to <1 year	100,000 IU (4 drops) once daily on D1, D2, and D8
Children ≥1 year and adults	200,000 IU (one capsule) once daily on D1, D2, and D8

Note: The letters D1–D8 show the days of administration of retinol.

TABLE 12.5: Doses of vitamin A in different ages.

Age	*Dose*
Children <6 months	50,000 IU (2 drops) single dose
Children 6 months to <1 year	100,000 IU (4 drops) every 4–6 months
Children 1 to <5 years	200,000 IU (one capsule) every 4–6 months
Women after delivery	200,000 IU (one capsule), single dose

In pregnant women, treatment varies according to the stage of illness.

- *Diminished vision in reduced light or Bitot's spots*: 10,000 IU once daily or 25,000 IU once weekly for at least 4 weeks. Do not exceed the indicated doses (risk of fetal malformations).
- If the cornea is affected, the risk of blindness outweighs the teratogenic risk. Administer 200,000 IU once daily on day 1, day 2, and day 8.

Corneal lesions are a medical emergency. In addition to the immediate administration of retinol, treat or prevent secondary bacterial infections with 1% tetracycline eye ointment, one application twice daily (do not apply eye drops containing corticosteroids), and protect the eye with an eye pad after each application.

Degeneration of the Conjunctiva

The conditions that are discussed under the degeneration of conjunctiva are nearer to dystrophy than degeneration. They are bilateral and almost symmetric; the persons have a family history without trauma, infection, or inflammation.

The conditions are:

- Concretion
- Pinguecula
- Pterygium

Concretion

They are also known as lithiasis, which is a misnomer. They are not depositions of calcium either. They develop over months, mostly in upper tarsal conjunctiva, roughly 1 mm in diameter, arranged irregularly in clusters, and are white in color but not calcified. They are, in fact, accumulations of inspissated mucus and epithelial cells deposited in the crypts of Henle. The exact cause is not known, but there may be a positive family history. They are seen from the second decade onward; the incidence increases with age, and they are more common in males. Most of the time, the patient is not aware of their presence, which is discovered on everting the lids. Rarely do the concretions rub against the cornea, causing a gritty sensation. They can be removed easily, only to recur. They are better left untouched. However, in the case of nonhealing corneal ulcers, they must be removed.

Pinguecula

This is supposed to be a degeneration of conjunctiva with frequent positive family history, never more than one in each eye, mostly on the lateral side, slow progressing, nonvision-threatening, almost symptomless. The only symptom is cosmetic, in the form of a yellowish-white nodule a little away from the limbus in the interpalpebral fissure. It is not met with before the third decade; the incidence rises with age; hence, it is supposed to be an aging process. New nodules do not develop after 40 years of age. One of the contributing causes is exposure to sunrays. The exact mechanism of production for pinguecula is not known. It is presumed that exposure to ultraviolet rays leads to the formation of a substance called elastin in the fibroblast of the conjunctiva. There is hyalinization of the superficial layers of the stroma. If the *pinguecula itself, or conjunctiva, rounds, it gets infected. The pinguecula stands out white amidst the red conjunctiva. Due to some unexplained reason, pterygium is known to develop on preexisting pingueculae. Noninflamed pinguecula is best left undisturbed. In cases of infection of the conjunctiva, conjunctivitis should be treated with the usual antibiotic drops.* If the patient insists on getting rid of it due to cosmetic reasons, it should be removed and the gap covered by the surrounding conjunctiva.

Pterygium

Pterygium is a subconjunctival fibrovascular proliferation of tissue that spreads over the cornea at the limbus. It is more common in tropical counties between 35° north and 35° south latitudes and is unevenly distributed. It is more common in dry, sandy, hot weather in places that get plenty of sunshine, leading to longer exposure to ultraviolet rays. It is more common in males; there may be a positive family history; some communities have more frequency than others. It was rare before 30 years, and new pterygia do not develop after 60 years. The eyes with pinguecula are more prone to develop pterygium. It is more common on the nasal side of the interpalpebral fissure; less commonly, it may develop on the temporal side. In such cases, the eye may have two pterygia, one on each side of the limbus. Isolated temporal pterygium is far less common. More than one pterygium on the same side is not met with.

The exact etiology of pterygium is not known.

The predisposing factors are: Family history, male, age above the third decade, climate, and exposure to ultraviolet rays. Some of the other presumptions are: Caused by the human papilloma virus and mutations in the tumor suppression gene.

Histology of a pterygium shows hyperplasia of proliferating subconjunctival tissue and vascularization—hyalinization of the subepithelial tissue and increased fibroblast.

Clinically, pterygia have been divided into two groups, i.e., more common true pterygium and less common pseudopterygia. A true pterygium should be differentiated from a pseudopterygium.

Pseudopterygium: Pseudopterygium is a sequelae to severe inflammation of the conjunctiva developing anywhere on the limbus. It may be considered a pseudo-symblepharon, where the adhesion is between the tarsal conjunctiva and cornea. It is generally unilateral and nonprogressive. The shape of the pterygium is more like a rhombus with a narrow arm on the cornea. It is seen at any age and does not produce much astigmatism; it develops when severely inflamed and chemosed conjunctiva overhangs the cornea and gets adherent to the corneal epithelium. As the inflammation subsides, most of the conjunctiva regresses, leaving only a tag of conjunctiva. The attached tag is called pseudopterygium. There is a clear space between the undersurface of such a band and the sclera; the gap is large enough for a probe to be passed between the pseudopterygium and the sclera. A simple excision of the pseudopterygium is sufficient to remove the growth with no recurrence, which is common in true pterygium.

The true pterygium has been divided into three parts without any definite line of demarcation between the two adjacent parts. They are the head, neck, and body. The head is the rounded apex of the triangular pterygium.

The whole of the pterygium fans out toward the periphery from the head. It seems to drag the superficial vessels with it into the progressive pterygium. In atrophic pterygium, the head becomes parchment-like, translucent, and white, losing many of the vessels. The head is the advancing end of the pterygium. It buries into the Bowman's membrane and superficial stroma. The neck is an ill-defined part that lies over the limbus between the head and the remaining part, which is referred to as the body. The body is the largest and most bulky part of the pterygium. It spreads from the limbus to the canthus. Its outer edges may spread beyond the interpalpebral aperture.

A white area 1.00 mm ahead of the head is called the cap of the pterygium. It is more marked in progressive pterygium. The deposition of iron in front of the head is called the Stocker's line, while infiltration in front of the head is called Fuchs spots.

As per progression, the pterygium can be:

- Roundlet pterygium
- Progressive (active)
- Nonprogressive (stationary)
- Regressed (atrophic)
- Recurrent

Roundlet pterygium: The roundlet pterygium is the earliest clinical feature of a pterygium. Which is often misdiagnosed as phlycten in younger persons. It is a rounded, raised, white nodule at the limbus without much hyperemia. It may, in the long term, get converted into a true pterygium that may pass into the next state of progressive pterygium.

Progressive (Active): Progressive pterygium **(Fig. 12.16)** is hyperemic with prominent vessels, thick and flashy; with infiltration ahead of the apex, the head encroaches toward the pupil in a few months or years.

In less common instances, it may deviate upward, bypassing the pupil.

Nonprogressive (Stationary): The nonprogressive pterygium is less fleshy and less hyperemic, with infiltration in front; the condition does not grow further **(Fig. 12.17)**.

Regressed (Atrophic): The regressed pterygium has a translucent appearance with a small body; the head is white like parchment **(Fig. 12.18)**.

Recurrent: The pterygium that develops following incomplete removal is called recurrent pterygium. It is more aggressive and more visible than the original

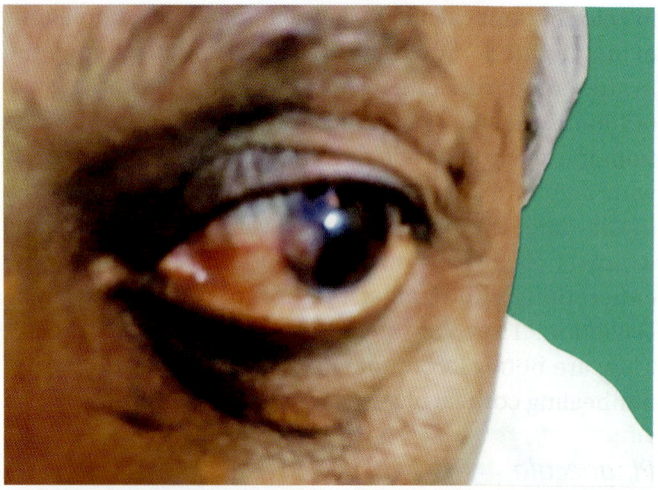

Fig. 12.16: Active pterygium.

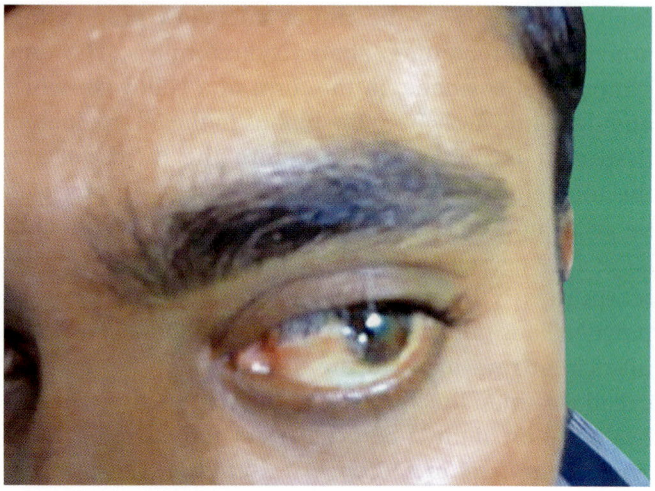

Fig. 12.17: Stationary pterygium.

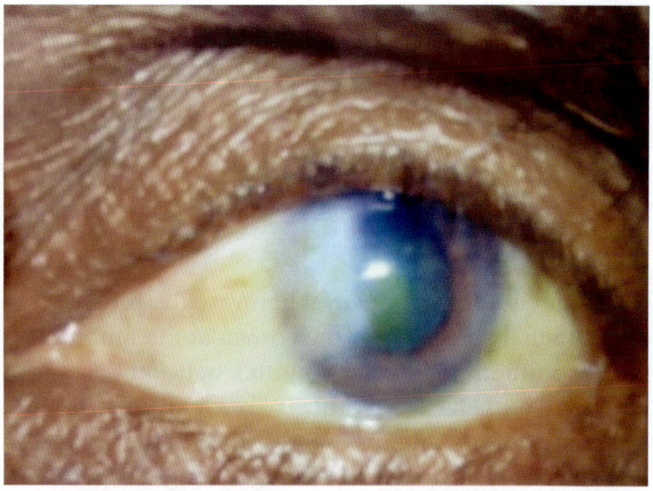

Fig. 12.18: Atrophic pterygium.

progressive pterygium. Various strategies that are in vogue to prevent recurrence are: Operating under magnification; maintaining planes of tissue frequent and prolonged use of local steroid, azithromycin-mitomycin combination; subconjunctival and intraoperative metomycin C steroid; and 5 fluorouracil subconjunctival, anti-VEGF, autologous serum, and local argon laser. Systemic doxycycline and menocycline have also been tried. The rationale for the use of doxycycline is based on the presumption that, besides being an antibiotic, it has anti-inflammatory and anticollagenase properties and acts on meibomian lipid and vascular stabilizing properties. Other procedures employed are conjunctival autografts that may be free or rotatory, amniotic membrane grafts, lamellar corneal grafts, and radiation by strontium 90. Fibrin glue can be used in place of sutures. One of the strategies followed is acronymed PERFECT, where P stands for pterygium, E for extended removal, F for followed-up, E for extended, and CT for conjunctival transplant.

Sequelae

There is hardly any complication in pterygium except irregular corneal astigmatism that is not corrected by surgical removal. Removal of pterygium by any method leaves a corneal opacity under the head. The other complications are infection and cystic degeneration. A phlycten-like translucent cyst may develop at the head; calcium deposit on the pterygium is a rare occurrence. There is no relation between pterygium and malignancy. Any malignancy encroaching on the pterygium has no direct relation to the existing pterygium.

Symptoms

- Cosmetic blemishes are the foremost cause that makes a person consult an ophthalmologist to get rid of the stigma.
- Recurrent localized redness between the limbus and medial canthus
- There may be mild epiphora due to an ocular surface defect and abnormal tear breakup time.
- *Diminished vision:*
  - Due to astigmatism induced by pterygium, it may be regular or irregular; astigmatism with the rule is more common; and astigmatism may be simple, compound, or even mixed.
  - Occlusion of the pupil by the pterygium
- Diplopia

Pterygium per se does not cause diplopia because pterygium is lax enough to have unrestricted movement of the globe. Diplopia in the pterygium may be considered to be iatrogenic following injury to the medial rectus during excessive dissection of the subconjunctival fibrous tissue.

Signs

The signs of pterygium are variable depending on the stage of pterygium, its duration of superimposed infection, and recurrence **(Figs. 12.15 to 12.17)**.

Differential Diagnosis

A true pterygium should be differentiated from a pseudopterygium.

In the initial stages of development, the hyperemia of the pterygium may be mistaken as angular or lacrimal conjunctivitis. There is a difference between pterygium and pseudopterygium, as shown in **Table 12.6**.

Conjunctival Ulcers

Ulcers of the conjunctiva are rare; they may happen in cases of mild chemical injury when infected. It can occur in severe bacterial infections such as pneumococcal conjunctivitis; the removal of a membrane can also cause the formation of conjunctival ulcers, breakdown of phlycten (self-limited), or chronic granuloma.

Conjunctival Granuloma

Granulomas of the conjunctiva are more common than ulcers; they are chronic, generally painless, and may be flat, sessile, or pedunculated. They may arise anywhere on the conjunctiva.

The common causes are:

- *Traumatic:* Retained foreign body
- *Inflammatory:* Burst chalazion **(Fig. 12.19)**
- *Infective:* The infections causing granuloma are chronic; the common causes are leprosy, tuberculosis, syphilis, conjunctivo sporidiosis, conjunctivitis nodosa, actinomyces, and lymphogranuloma venereum. These conditions are not seen in children except for rhinosporidiosis **(Fig. 12.20)**. The most common infective granuloma in children is conjunctivo sporidiosis.

TABLE 12.6: Difference between pterygium and pseudopterygium.

Feature	*Pterygium*	*Pseudopterygium*
Age	Between the third and sixth decade	Any
Sex	More males	Both
Family history	May be present	Noncontributory
Pathology	Fibrous vascular and proliferative	Postinflammatory
Ultraviolet rays	May be the cause	No relation
Position	In the interpalpebral aperture	Anywhere on the limbus
Progression	May progress	Stationary
Shape of the apex	Rounded	Rhomboid
Presence of cap	+/–	Absent
Probe test	Probe cannot be passed under the pterygium	Can be passed in most cases
Prevention	Nil	Can be prevented if acute infection is managed well
Treatment	Surgical and laser	Surgical
Recurrence following surgery	Frequent	Nil

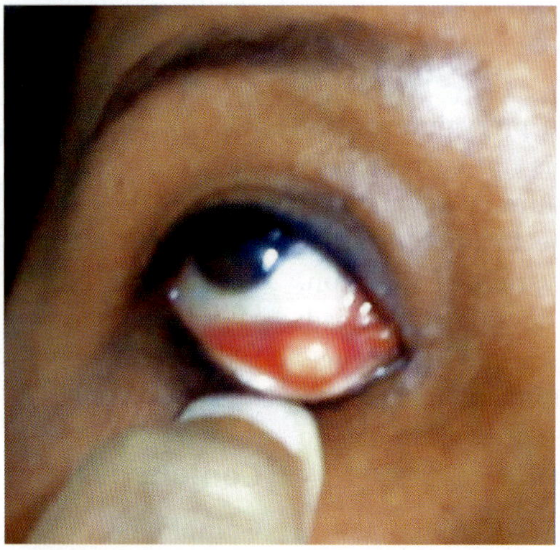

Fig. 12.19: Burst chalazion lower lid.

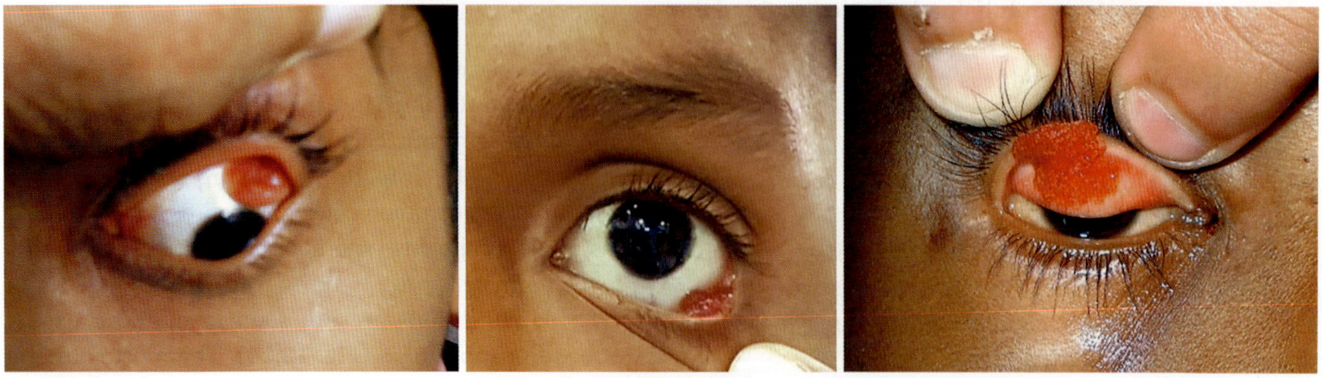

Fig. 12.20: Various types of conjunctival sporidiosis.
Courtesy: Professor LC Madaria.

Pyogenic Granuloma

This is not a true granuloma; it is a vascular growth.

Cystic Lesions of the Conjunctiva

The cysts of the conjunctiva can be congenital or acquired.

The most common congenital cyst is the cystic epibulbar dermoid.

The acquired can be traumatized, retained, or parasitic. The traumatic cysts are: Filtering blebs, leaking corneoscleral wounds covered by conjunctiva, and implantation cysts.

Parasitic cyst: The most common parasitic cyst is cysticercus, which is more common in the left eye near the medial canthus **(Fig. 12.21)**.

Keratinization of Conjunctiva

In this condition, the normal wet, shiny conjunctiva is replaced by a dull, dry conjunctiva.

The common causes are xerophthalmia, exposure of conjunctiva in the large coloboma of the lid, ectropion, and proptosis.

Adhesion between two surfaces of the conjunctiva: The most common example is symblepharon **(Fig. 12.22)**, where the tarsal conjunctiva gets adhered to the bulbar conjunctiva and rarely to the cornea. This happens more commonly on the lower lid. The adhesion may be small and narrow, or the whole of the lid may get adhered to the bulbar conjunctiva. When both lids are adhered to the globe, the condition is called total symblepharon. The common causes are membranous conjunctivitis, alkali burn, Stevens-Johnson syndrome, and ocular pemphigus. The symblepharon causing shallowing of the fornices is referred to as posterior symblepharon; the most common cause is advanced trachoma, which is not seen in children.

Lymphadenopathy with Conjunctival Diseases

Conjunctiva is very rich in lymphatic supply. Enlargement of preauricular and submandibular lymph nodes are seen in some infective conjunctivitis and neoplasm of the conjunctiva. Enlargement of preauricular glands is more common than submandibular glands.

All conjunctiva infections are not associated with lymphadenopathy. Only a few causes enlargement of preauricular glands, lymphadenopathy can be seen in acute as well as chronic infections of conjunctiva. The common infections are staphylococca, diphtheroids, vaccinia, adenovirus, inclusion conjunctivitis, and gonococcal conjunctivitis in adults.

Chronic conjunctivitis diseases that cause enlargement of lymph nodes are tuberculosis, syphilis, leprosy, and lymphogranuloma venereum.

The common nonconjunctival causes of enlargement of lymph nodes are stye, infected chalazion, cellulitis lid, and orbital retinoblastoma. The two syndromes related

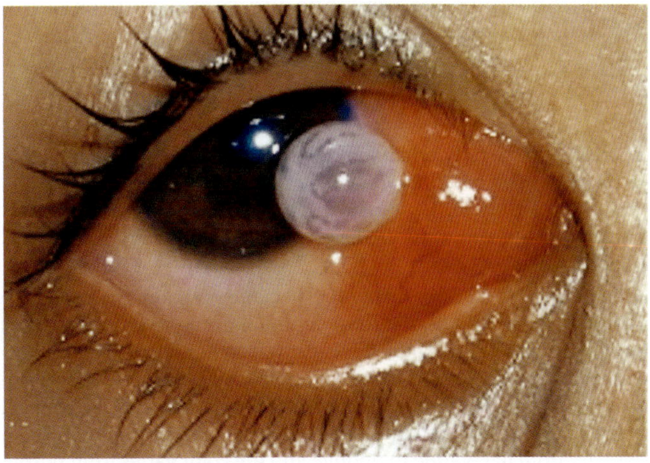

Fig. 12.21: Cysticercus cyst of conjunctiva.

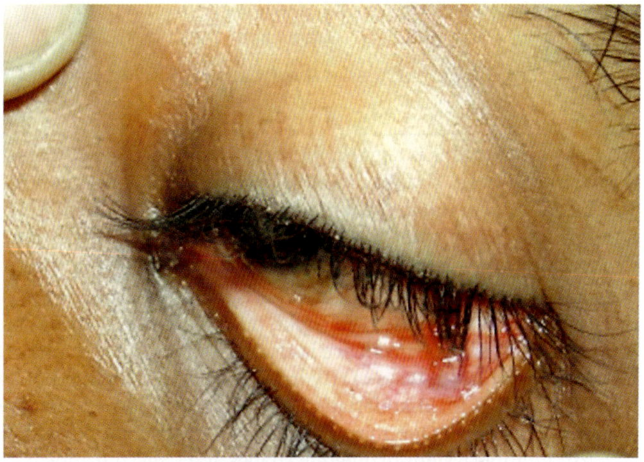

Fig. 12.22: Symblepharon.

to lymphadenopathy are Parinaud's oculoglandular fever and Beal's syndrome.*

No active treatment is required. Astringent drops and lubricants offer relief.

Nodules at or Around the Limbus

The common nodules at the limbus are **(Fig. 12.23)**:

- Limbal phlycten
- Limbal spring catarrh
- *Filtering bleb:* Surgical or accidental
- Iris prolapse
- Limbal dermoid
- Foreign body granuloma
- Intercalary staphyloma
- Amyloidosis (not seen in children)
- Cystic degeneration of the pterygium head (not seen in children)
- Squamous cell carcinoma (not seen in children)
- *Intraepithelial epithelioma:* Bowens disease (not seen in children)

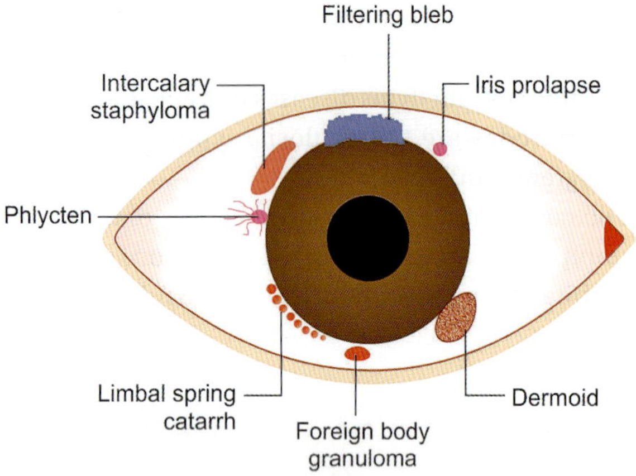

Fig. 12.23: Nodules at the limbus in children.

Neoplasm of Conjunctiva

The structures of the conjunctiva are of a varied nature, i.e., ectodermal as well as mesodermal. It is rich in various types of cells, blood vessels, lymphatic, and nerve tissues; hence, it is prone to developing hosts of neoplasms of different origins. The growth can be congenital or acquired. Examples of congenital growths are epidermoids, dermolipoma, and neurofibroma. The newly acquired growths are seen in adults. They can be benign, potentially malignant, or frankly malignant. Extensions from the lids are common; secondaries exclusively in conjunctiva are extremely rare.

The following is a list of new growths of conjunctiva (in all ages):

- *Benign tumors:* Choristoma and hamartomas, papilloma, pyogenic granuloma, hemangioma, and lymphangioma
- *Precancerous tumor:* Intraepithelial epithelioma
- *Malignant tumors:* Malignant melanoma, squamous cell carcinoma, basal cell carcinoma, conjunctival lymphoma, and Kaposi sarcoma†

Note: All malignant tumors of the conjunctiva are seen in adults.

Symptoms of Conjunctival Disorders in Children

Any of the following, alone or in combination, may be present. The degrees of involvement in the two eyes are not always similar.

- *Redness:*
  - *Unilateral or bilateral:* In the case of unilateral, the other eye develops the same features soon, especially in infections and allergic conditions.
  - Localized/generalized

**Beal's syndrome:* This is acute conjunctivitis; the causative organism responsible is not fully understood. The most common theory is that it is a virus disease. The condition has an acute onset that may become bilateral. The condition is mostly seen after the second decade. The lids are edematous; the conjunctiva is congested, including the plica and caruncle. The tarsal conjunctiva is thickened and has multiple follicles; in spite of congestion and edema of the lid, the discharge is scanty and watery. There is no involvement of the cornea. The ipsilateral preauricular glands are enlarged, which are neither painful nor fixed.

†*Kaposi sarcoma:* Kaposi sarcoma, which is highly malignant and was earlier thought to be rare, since AIDS became rampant, the incidence of this malady has increased manyfold. It is seen mostly in immune-compromised individuals; the most common immune-deficient status is infection by HIV. The incidence is also high in patients who have underground renal transplants. It is mostly seen in males. The male-to-female ratio is 15:1. In cases of HIV infection, the development of Kaposi sarcoma is a bad omen. The HIV-infected person rarely lives more than 2 years after the manifestation of the tumor. It is a systemic, multicentric tumor that first develops in the limbs; it may have visceral involvement as well. One-third of the patients with Kaposi sarcoma develop the tumor in the conjunctiva. In conjunctiva, there may be a single or multiple lesions of different shapes and sizes; the appearance may vary from flat plaque to nodule; and the color varies from purple to dark red. In children, it is far more aggressive than in adults. In spite of its being fatal, it progresses slowly and is painless. A favorable point in the growth is that the growth regresses with systemic treatment of HIV; otherwise, it may be excised or treated with cryo or radiation.

- *Watering:* Watering in simple conjunctival disease is mild and not too copious. Watering disproportionate to signs means corneal involvement, which is common in viral conjunctivitis. Watering of the eye with discharge is called blennorrhoea.
- *Gritty sensation:* This is common in all viral conjunctivitis.
- *Stickiness:* Stickiness of the lids is common in mucopurulent and purulent conjunctivitis, mostly seen in children; the lids get stuck together after sleep and need to be separated mechanically with a moistened swab.
- *Itching:* Itching is a prominent symptom that makes the patient seek medical help. It may be mild or severe. It is more severe in children; all exogenous allergic conjunctivitis causes itching. It is most marked in spring catarrh. Endogenous allergens do not cause itching.
- Abnormal mass on the conjunctiva
- Dry white spot on the conjunctiva (see Bitot's spot)
- Abnormal color of the conjunctiva
- Bleeding from conjunctiva
- Parasites are visible on the conjunctiva.

Infection and Inflammation of Conjunctivitis in Children

They form a group of disorders that may be infective or allergic and are empirically called conjunctivitis.

Conjunctivitis is the most common ocular disease in children. It may be seen in a wide range of ages, from neonates to teens. It is seen the world over, more common in developing countries, in malnourished children of both sexes with poor ambient hygiene. Its incidence among girls is higher than among boys. It is generally bilateral. In developed countries, allergies supersede infections. Conjunctivitis in children can be mild, moderate, or severe. The mild form is self-limited, nonvision-threatening, and easy to treat. The severe forms are blinding and may be fatal. The examples are gonococcal, pneumococcal, and diphtheritic. The causes of conjunctivitis can be divided into:

- *Microbial:*
  - Bacterial
  - Viral
  - Chlamydial
- *Allergic:*
  - Exogenous
  - Endogenous
- *Iatrogenic:*
  - Local drugs
  - Systemic drugs
  - Contact lens
  - Miscellaneous

> The most common offender in underdeveloped countries is the use of folk medicine of uncertain composition and effectiveness. In modern medicine, $AgNO_3$ used to be the most common form of iatrogenic conjunctivitis.

As per onset, conjunctivitis can be:

- *Hyperacute:* Gonococcal, pneumococcal, and diphtheritic
- *Acute:* Above organism and many other bacteria and viruses
- *Chronic:* Bacterial, viral, and chlamydial
- Recurrent conjunctivitis of any origin lasting for >4 weeks due to noncompliance with treatment or treatment by subclinical dose is known as recurrence conjunctivitis.

Hyperacute Conjunctivitis

The most common example of hyperacute conjunctivitis is ophthalmia neonatorum.

Ophthalmia neonatorum: Any conjunctivitis developing within 1 month of birth is called ophthalmia neonatorum. It can be microbial or nonmicrobial; the microbes could be bacteria, viruses, or chlamydia. The nonmicrobial causes are chemical and iatrogenic; later, they are mostly in the form of folk medicine.

Flowchart 12.1 depicts various etiological types of ophthalmia neonatorum.

Organisms that produce ophthalmia neonatorum are given in **Box 12.1**.

Gonococcal Ophthalmia Neonatorum

Out of all the bacterial ophthalmia neonatorum, gonococcal ophthalmia is the most serious; it is a fast-developing conjunctivitis that is potentially blinding and occasionally has widespread systemic manifestations that can be fatal. Fortunately, the disease is fully preventable with a simple and cheap prophylaxis. It is an acquired infection. The newborn gets the infection during birth from the birth canal of the infected mother. Children delivered by cesarean section do not develop gonococcal ophthalmia neonatorum. A newborn may develop conjunctivitis during home delivery by an untrained midwife due to a lack of asepsis.

Flowchart 12.1: Various etiological types of ophthalmia neonatorum.

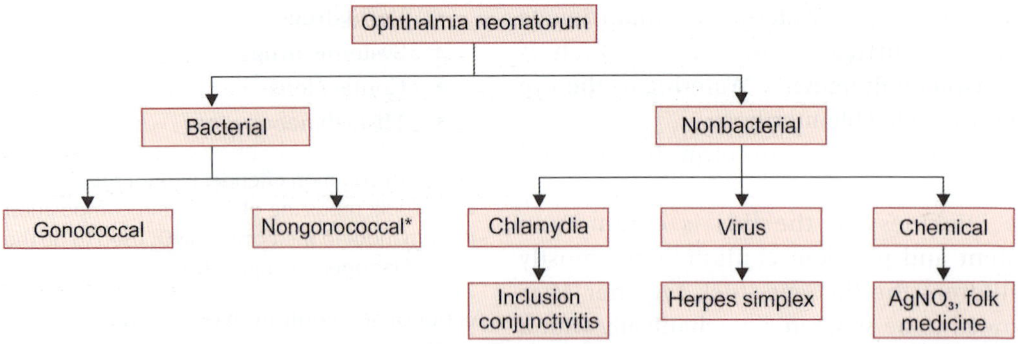

**Nongonococcal:* Previously, only gonococci were supposed to be the microorganisms to cause ophthalmia neonatorum. Presently, with the decline in maternal gonococcal infection, the gonococcus has mostly been replaced by other organisms to cause ophthalmia neonatum. Organisms that are commonly isolated are *Staphylococcus, Streptococcus, Pneumococcus, Haemophilus, Pseudomonas*, and *Acinetobacter*.

BOX 12.1: List of organisms that cause ophthalmia neonatorum, barring the last; which is metal.

- *N. gonococcus*
- *Neisseria meningitidis*
- *Staphylococcus aureus*
- *Streptococcus*
- *Pneumococcus*
- *Haemophilus*
- *Pseudomonas aeruginosa*
- Chlamydia
- Virus
- Silver nitrate

The incubation period is short, i.e., 1–3 days; it is bilateral; it may be missed initially because the neonate keeps the lids closed for an average of 18 hours, obscuring the redness. The condition is worse in premature and underweight neonates. The absence of immunity, lack of tears, and absence of lymphoid tissue in the conjunctiva of the neonate, along with the inherent narrow interpalpebral appearance, make the situation worse.

The condition becomes evident by the second day with swelling of the lids and the outpouring of conjunctival discharge, which is watery to begin with. Within hours, the discharge turns serous, only to be purulent in the next few hours. Gonococcal ophthalmia neonatorum produces the most copious discharge; the lids may get glued together, the swollen lids obliterate the interpalpebral aperture, and it may require a lid retractor to separate the lids. Wiping the discharge reveals an edematous, severely red conjunctiva. There may be pseudomembrane formation. In spite of severe purulent conjunctivitis, there is no lymphadenopathy.

The cornea is always at risk of being involved because gonococcus can penetrate intact corneal epithelium. Any part of the cornea may be involved as a gonococcal ulcer. That may perforate. Central perforation is more common. That may lead to sloughing of the cornea, terminating in an anterior staphyloma or a small central perforation. A central perforation heals by producing a central leucoma. This is invariably accompanied by an anterior polar cataract.

Central corneal leukoma, along with anterior polar cataract, reduces vision drastically. Diminished vision in neonate preludes nystagmus that lasts for the rest of the life.

An adult with bilateral central leucoma, anterior polar cataract, and nystagmus has definitely suffered from ophthalmia neonatorum.

The natural history of an untreated case of gonococcal ophthalmia neonatorum is given here:

- The condition becomes visible within the second to third day.
- The lids are soft and can be separated with ease.
- The conjunctiva is congested.
- There is no follicular reaction.
- By the fourth day, the lids are swollen enough that they are difficult to separate; this is associated with copious purulent discharge.
- The acute stage continues for 10–15 days; by this time, the lids become soft and can be separated without difficulty, and the discharge becomes less.
- The conjunctiva may be thrown into folds.
- The pseudomembrane disappears.
- In 6–8 weeks, the conjunctiva becomes normal.

Complication

The complications can be ocular or systemic.

- The ocular complications are mostly corneal. They are:
  - Small central corneal ulcer—central perforation—central leucoma—anterior polar cataract—nystagmus
  - Large sloughing ulcer—endophthalmitis—panophthalmitis—anterior staphyloma—nystagmus in a blind eye
- The systemic complications are:
  - Pneumonitis in 10–20% of cases
  - Meningitis
  - Osteomyelitis

The systemic complications may be concurrent with ocular complications or may follow. The systemic complications may prove fatal.

Diagnosis

The diagnosis of gonococcal ophthalmia neonatorum is easy. A newborn delivered vaginally develops bilateral purulent conjunctivitis with swollen lids, which is, for all practical purposes, a case of gonococcal ophthalmia neonatorum. The diagnosis is confirmed by a positive smear stained by Gram's stain or Giemsa stain.

> The smear should be taken prior to starting the antibiotic; otherwise, the results will invariably be negative. The gonococci are gram-negative bean-shaped intracellular organisms.

> The organisms other than gonococcus that pass through intact corneal epithelium are *N. meningitidis*, *Pneumococcus*, *H. influenzae*, *Corynebacterium diphtheriae*, and *Listeria*.

Differential diagnosis: The differential diagnosis of gonococcal ophthalmia neonatorum encompasses all conjunctivitis developing within 30 days of birth. They are collectively called nongonococcal ophthalmia neonatorum.

Flowchart 12.2 depicts the difference.

Out of all microbial ophthalmia neonatorum, gonococcal infection is most important due to its propensity to involve the cornea and being potentially life threatening. Nongonococcal ophthalmia neonatorum is milder than gonococcal, with a variable incubation period. Cornea is not involved except in pneumococcal infection. The type of organism is confirmed by smears and culture. The infection is seldom from the birth canal; it generally spreads from other infants in the nursery or due to a lack of asepsis among the paramedical staff handling the newborn. The prophylaxis and management are similar to those of gonococcal ophthalmia neonatorum.

Nonbacterial Ophthalmia Neonatorum

The nonbacterial causes of ophthalmia neonatorum are:

- Chlamydial
- Viral
- Chemical

Flowchart 12.2: Comparison between gonococcal and nongonococcal ophthalmia neonatorum.

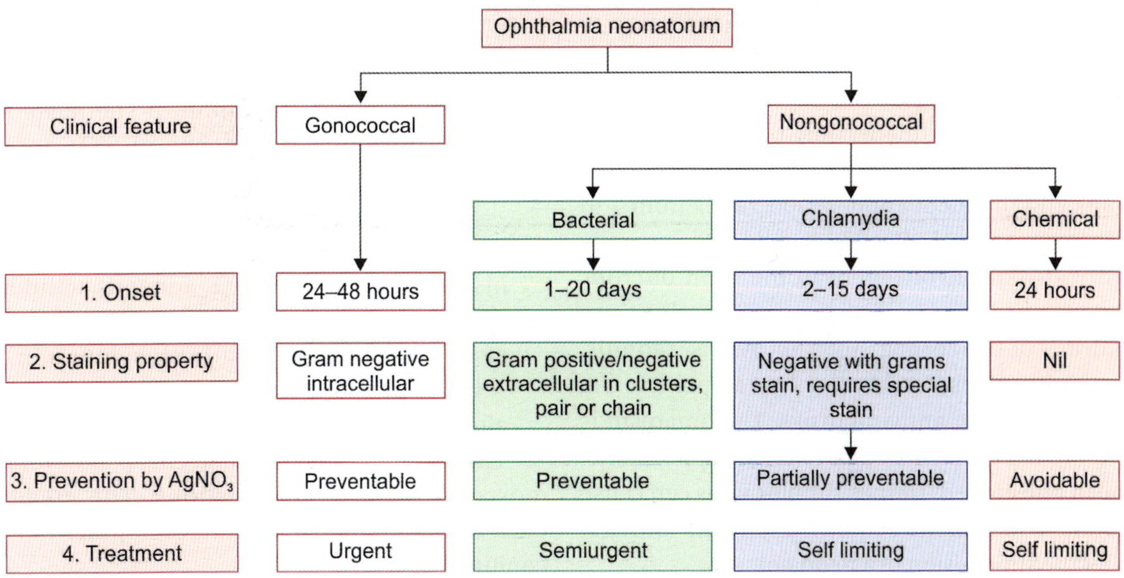

Chlamydial Ophthalmia Neonatorum

Chlamydial ophthalmia neonatorum is also known as inclusion conjunctivitis in newborns; with better health care, the incidence of gonococcal infection has been reduced dramatically. Chlamydial infection seems to have overtaken bacterial infection as the causative organism for ophthalmia neonatorum. In developed countries, genital chlamydial infection is an important cause of ophthalmia neonatorum, while gonococcus remains the most important cause in developing countries. Unlike its gonococcal counterpart, the incubation period is longer, taking 5–15 days for the infection to manifest. It is never as acute as gonococcal conjunctivitis; the lids are less swollen; the discharge is less copious and serous; the lids do not get stuck; and corneal involvement is just superficial keratopathy with micropannus. The cornea never perforates solely due to chlamydial infection; perforation is always secondary to bacterial infection by organisms that pass through intact corneal epithelium.

About 10–20% of neonates with chlamydial infections are likely to develop pneumonitis. The diagnosis of chlamydial infections is confirmed by the presence of cytoplasmic inclusion bodies in Giemsa stains. Crede's prophylaxis is less effective than in bacterial ophthalmia. Crede's method was the mainstay of prophylaxis in ophthalmia neonatorum, which has been replaced by povidone iodine 2.5%. Povidone is claimed to be better than Crede's method in all bacterial ophthalmia.

Infants with pneumonitis are better treated by a neonatologist. The inclusion of conjunctivitis, in spite of treatment, is known to linger for months. Children >1 month can be treated with azithromycin suspension (20 mg/kg). The local treatment consists of erythromycin 0.5%, three times a day; erythromycin is not available as eye drops and the incubation period varies from 7 to 14 days. The conjunctival infection is mild and generally associated with skin involvement in the form of crops of vesicles on the lid skin. Other manifestations are microdendrites of the cornea, anterior uveitis, retinitis, and optic neuritis. Conjunctivitis does not respond to the usual antibacterial and antiviral drugs. The organism is resistant to Crede's prophylaxis, and the role of povidone, too, has been questioned. Herpes simplex virus can cause fatal systemic involvement, requiring systemic antiviral drugs under the supervision of a neonatologist.

Chemical Ophthalmia Neonatorum

Chemical ophthalmia neonatorum is an iatrogenic conjunctivitis. Crede's prophylaxis has been used for more than one and a half centuries with satisfactory results. It is a paradox that Crede's prophylaxis, which is meant to prevent ophthalmia, can cause chemical conjunctivitis within 24 hours of instillation in many children. Chemical conjunctivitis is the mildest of all other ophthalmia neonatorums and is self-limited. With the advent of effective chemoprophylaxis, the Crede's method has been given up and replaced by povidone 2.5% in single drop in each eye soon after birth. This has proved to be better than $AgNO_{3,}$ as povidone is not known to cause chemical conjunctivitis.

Management of Bacterial Ophthalmia Neonatorum

Treatment of bacterial ophthalmia in newborns differs from nonbacterial treatment. However, prophylaxis in all ophthalmia except chemical is the same. It has been noted above that bacterial ophthalmia in newborns can be divided into two groups, i.e., more serious gonococcal and less serious nongonococcal. Both types are acquired from infected birth canals. The management can be divided into two parts, i.e., prophylaxis and actual treatment.

- *Prophylaxis:* Prophylaxis begins with suspecting gonococcal infection in the mother based on a history of sexually transmitted diseases (STDs) and an antenatal clinical examination of the mother. If any of them are positive, the mother should receive a full course of antigonococcal treatment weeks before delivery.
- *The second part is:*
    - Prevention of ophthalmia before it sets in
    - Treatment of the mother if she has a history of STD or clinical evidence of STD. Infants born to such mothers should also get a full dose of antigonococcal chemotherapy.
- *Crede's prophylaxis:* This consists of the compulsory instillation of a 1% $AgNO_3$ aqueous solution in each eye. It was mandatory to discard the $AgNO_3$ solution after 1 week and store a fresh solution in the dark. A bottle at room temperature, at least the solution after evaporation, becomes concentrated.

The method was simple and cheap and would prevent most of the bacterial infections. The greatest drawback of the method was the development of chemical conjunctivitis.

- *Povidone:* Povidone is an effective and affordable prophylaxis method. It consists of 1 drop of 2.5% povidone instilled in each eye soon after birth. This is more effective than $AgNO_3$ and is not known to cause chemical conjunctivitis. The other advantage is that it is commercially available and does not need to be prepared in a pharmacy. It is also kept in a dark bottle and stored at room temperature.
- In the absence of povidone, some antibiotics can be used; the most common is erythromycin. Erythromycin is not available in drop form; it is to be used as an ointment. Other broad-spectrum antibiotics, such as tobramycin or garamycin, can also be used.
- A combination of povidone drops and erythromycin ointment is claimed to be the best option.

Treatment of Established Gonococcal Ophthalmia Neonatorum

- Isolate the neonate from other healthy children.
- Clean the discharge with a wet swab; if necessary, lid retractors should be used to separate the swollen lids.
- Put 0.5% erythromycin or 1% tetracycline in the ointment.
- Crystalline penicillin drops, which were the mainstay of treatment earlier, are no longer in vogue.
- Repeat the erythromycin/tetracycline ointment every 8 hours.
- The other alternative is to use a 0.3% tobramycin drop every 5 minutes for 6 times, followed by every 10 minutes for 6 times, and then every hour for 6 times. Frequent use of an aqueous solution has the added advantage of lavaging the conjunctival sac. The acute stage will subside in 8 hours.
- Systemic treatment of gonococcal ophthalmia neonatorum consists of a single dose of ceftriaxone (125 mg intramuscular) or kanamycin (75 mg) with local gentamicin eye drops.
- All cases of gonococcal conjunctivitis are likely to have other STDs, including HIV. 30% of cases of gonococcal ophthalmia neonatorum have chlamydial infection as well, requiring separate management.

Table 12.7 depicts the salient features of different types of ophthalmia neonatorum.

Membranous Conjunctivitis

In contrast to ophthalmia neonatorum, membranous conjunctivitis does not develop within the first month. It develops between 1 and 10 years. Like gonococcal ophthalmia, it is also sight- and life-threatening unless treated well. It is fully preventable by systemic immunization. The cause of ophthalmia neonatorum is gonococcus, and that of membranous conjunctivitis is diphtheria bacilli.

Corynebacterium diphtheriae is a nonmotile, noncapsulated, club-shaped, gram-positive bacillus that produces a fatal toxin. The disease is fully preventable by vaccination.

The list of organisms that produce membranous conjunctivitis is long, as shown in **Box 12.2**. Diphtheria tops the list and is the most important of all. The last three are noninfective.

Diphtheritic Conjunctivitis

This is an important cause of hyperacute conjunctivitis seen in nonimmunized children in virulent form and milder form in immunized children between 1 and 10 years, with acute onset, bilateral, beginning as nonspecific bacterial conjunctivitis with fibrinous exudate developing on and in the conjunctival epithelium, resulting in the formation of a true membrane. A true membrane may be preceded by a pseudomembrane.

The child is acutely ill, toxic with fever, and cough due to involvement of the throat.

TABLE 12.7: Clinical features of various types of ophthalmia neonatorum, both gonococcal and nongonococcoal.

Type	*Causative factor*	*Source*	*Prophylaxis*	*Treatment*
Chemical	$AgNO_3$ drop	Container	Avoid AgNO3	Self-limiting
Gonococcal	Gonococcus	Infected birth canal	Povidone and erythromycin	Urgent
Nongonococcal bacterial	Both Gram-positive and Gram-negative, cocci/bacilli	Infected birth canal and failure of asepses	Povidone erythromycin	Semi urgent
Chlamydia	Chlamydia trachomatis	Infected birth canal	Povidone has a limited role	No specific treatment
Herpes simplex	HSV 2	Birth canal	Povidone has a limited role	No specific treatment

BOX 12.2: A list of conditions responsible for membrane formation in conjunctiva (micro-organismal and nonorganismal).

Membranous/pseudomembranous conjunctivitis
- *Corynebacterium diphtheriae*
- *Streptococcus*
- *Staphylococcus aureus*
- Gonococci
- Koch weeks bacillus
- Epidemic keratoconjunctivitis
- Primary herpes simplex
- Cicatricial pemphigoid
- Erythema multiforme
- Spring catarrh

The ocular condition is divided into the following stages:
- Stage of infiltration
- Stage of suppuration
- Stage of cicatrization
- Stage of corneal involvement
- Stage of systemic involvement

Stage of Infiltration

In this stage, the lids are tender, swollen, and brawny, making it difficult to evert. The conjunctiva is congested with copious watery discharge. The inflamed conjunctiva is covered with a patchy pseudomembrane, which is soon converted into a true membrane. At this stage, no attempt should be made to remove the membrane because it will leave a bleeding, raw area. The membrane is generally localized in the fornices and palpebral conjunctiva; in severe cases, it may extend over the bulbar conjunctiva, which heralds corneal involvement. The preauricular lymph glands are enlarged.

Stage of Suppuration

The lid becomes soft and less edematous, reducing pain and tenderness. The discharge is converted into a purulent discharge. The membrane separates to slough off, leaving a raw surface. At this stage, the cornea may suffer from a lack of blood supply, predisposing it to ulceration. A raw surface is left following the sloughing of the membrane, which may later cause adhesion between two conjunctival surfaces.

Stage of Cicatrization

The epithelium from the periphery may grow and cover the raw surface; this prevents the formation of adhesion and fibrosis between two surfaces. If the two raw surfaces come into contact with each other, a symblepharon will ensue. The manifestations of adhesion and cicatrization are trichiasis, entropion, and ocular surface disorders.

Stage of Corneal Involvement

The two predisposing factors for corneal involvement are:
1. Ability of the bacilli to pass through the tact corneal epithelium
2. Wide-spread thrombosis of perilimbal blood vessels is cutting off blood supply to the cornea. The combination of the above two factors is a formidable situation, preluding a large, sloughing corneal ulcer.

Stage of Systemic Involvement

The systemic involvement is due to the toxin liberated by the organism. They can be:
- Extraocular muscle palsy
- *Internal ophthalmoplegia:* This is generally permanent, and in later life, patients may be exposed to a number of unnecessary investigations if a history of diphtheria in childhood is not obtained. Such a condition may be confused with Addis pupils or glaucoma.
- Diphtheritic myocarditis and pneumonia can both be fatal, either separately or in combination.

Treatment

Diphtheria is fully preventable by diphtheria, pertussis, and tetanus (DPT) vaccination in 1st year. The child is protected by maternal immunity for up to 2 years; hence, infection by diphtheria before 1 year is uncommon. If the mother lacks immunity, the child can get diphtheria even before. Though DPT gives sufficient immunity to ward off systemic infection, an adult may develop a milder form of conjunctivitis.

All cases of conjunctivitis with membrane or pseudomembrane should be treated as diphtheritic unless proved otherwise.

Diphtheria produces a potent exotoxin, which is the cause of fatality rather than the organism. The toxin gets fixed to the tissue. It cannot be neutralized by antibiotics. It is only neutralized by antitoxin that is administered parentally and, to a lesser extent, by local instillation. The role of local antitoxin is debated. Parental antitoxin should be administered in consultation with pediatrician.

Diphtheria bacilli are sensitive to many local and systemic antibiotics, ranging from penicillin onward.

They do not respond to sulfa and trimethoprim. The most commonly used systemic antibiotics are penicillin G and erythromycin. Penicillin is administered at a dose of 6,00,000 IU/BD for 10 days. The dose of erythromycin is 25–50 mg/kg for 10 days. The role of local and systemic antibiotics in diphtheritic conjunctivitis is twofold, i.e., they reduce the number of bacteria.

This is based on the principle "The lesser the number of organisms, the lesser the production of exotoxin."

Diphtheritic infection is invariably associated with a mixed infection by pneumococci and staphylococci, which by themselves worsen the clinical course. The use of local and systemic antibiotics helps in controlling secondary invaders.

Atropine is mandatory in corneal involvement. It is safer to use 1% atropine sulfate as an ointment rather than drops to reduce the side effects of atropine.

In case the child is sensitive to antitoxins, they should be replaced by human diphtheria immunoglobulin. The child should be isolated during treatment. The child is better quarantined until conjunctival smears are positive.

Table 12.8 shows a comparison between the two common vision and life-threatening conjunctivitis of childhood.

Other Infective Conjunctivitis in Children

Infective conjunctivitis in children can be acute or chronic. The former is more common. They are generally bilateral and are seen more in malnourished children living in unhygienic environments. They are contagious; they start in one eye and spread to the other eye. The infection spreads by fomites, droplets, and infection from the nasopharynx and ear; it may be in small epidemics; the disease per se is nonvision-threatening and self-healing without leaving any scars. However, some of them may become chronic; such cases require investigation to pinpoint the causes. The cases that merit investigation are those that do not respond to standard antibacterial treatment.

Acute infective conjunctivitis in children is generally mucopurulent in nature and develops over days, in contrast to conjunctivitis in neonates, which is generally hyperacute.

Acute infective conjunctivitis in children is caused by: Bacteria, viruses, and chlamydia. In order of frequency, fungi and parasites do not cause acute infective conjunctivitis. Both cocci and bacilli, irrespective of Gram-staining properties, cause mucopurulent conjunctivitis; cocci are more likely to cause acute conjunctivitis.

TABLE 12.8: Difference between gonococcal and diphtheritic conjunctivitis in children.

Gonococcal ophthalmia neonatorum	***Diphtheritic conjunctivitis***
Microbiology: Gonococci are strictly human, gram-negative intracellular paired organisms that produce endotoxins and require enriched media to grow	*Corynebacterium diphtheria* can be pathogenic or saprophytic. Gram-positive bacilli that produce exotoxins grow on many media
Source of infection: The birth canal of the infected mother	From other patients or carriers
Mode of inoculation: Direct spread from mothers, genital tracts	Droplet
Age of onset: 2–3 days after birth	1–10 years of age
Prevention: Prophylaxis by antibiotic ointment, povidone $AgNO_3$	Vaccination in the first year of life
Laterality: Bilateral	Bilateral
Lids: Swollen	Brawny swelling
Conjunctiva: Hyperemic and chemosed	Hyperemic
Membrane: Occasionally pseudomembrane	True membrane
Discharge: Purulent	Serous
Corneal involvement: Common	Common
Systemic involvement: Possible	Possible
Treatment: Local drops and ointment are rarely systemic antibiotics	Local antibiotic drops, local antidiphtheria serum, and systemic antibiotics

TABLE 12.9: Organisms responsible for nongonococcal conjunctivitis in children.

Organism	Conjunctival involvement	Other ocular involvement	Systemic involvement	Treatment
Streptococci	Acute bilateral, mucopurulent conjunctivitis, pseudomembrane formation, and ophthalmia neonatorum	Keratitis and orbital cellulitis	Pneumonitis and otitis media	Antibiotic drops and systemic antibiotics for systemic infection
Staphylococci	Similar to above with chemosis and papillary reaction	Keratitis	Same as above	Same as above
Pneumococci	Acute bilateral mucopurulent conjunctivitis with petechial hemorrhage, and pseudomembrane formation	Serpiginous ulcer, hypopyon dacryocystitis, anterior uveitis, and perforation	Life-threatening pneumonia	Antibiotics local and systemic
Gonococci	Ophthalmia neonatorum in newborns and conjunctivitis in older children similar to adults*	Central perforation	Pneumonitis, meningitis, and osteomyelitis	Antibiotic, local and systemic
Acinetobacter	Hyperacute conjunctivitis	Superficial punctate keratitis and central corneal ulcer	Pneumonitis	Local and systemic antibiotic. The organism is resistant to penicillin
Haemophilus influenzae	Ophthalmia neonatorum and acute mucopurulent conjunctivitis	Central corneal ulcer	Multiorgan involvement	Antibiotic drops, i.e., fluoroquinolones, aminoglycosides, polymaxin B, and gentamicin
Pseudomonas	Acute mucopurulent conjunctivitis requiring urgent attention	Sloughing cornea ulcer	Multiorgan involvement	Gentamicin

**Gonococcal conjunctivitis in older children* is seen in children following child abuse or sexual assault in precocious adolescents. It is generally unilateral and is associated with profuse purulent discharge, severe conjunctival hyperemia, marked inflammatory swelling of the lids, and corneal ulcers. The treatment of choice is a single intramuscular injection of ceftriaxone as per the weight of the patient. Children weighing <50 kg, get 125 mg of ceftriaxone and erythromycin 0.5% ointment four times a day, with atropine ointment if the cornea is involved.

The common cocci responsible are:

- *Gram positive: Staphylococcus aureus, Streptococcus pyogenes*, and *Streptococcus pneumoniae*
- *Gram negative:* Gonococci

Common bacilli responsible are gram-negative, i.e., *Haemophilus influenzae, Moraxella catarrhalis, Pseudomonas aeruginosa*, and *E. coli*.

Table 12.9 depicts bacterial conjunctivitis in children other than ophthalmia neonatorum.

Viral Conjunctivitis in Children

There are many viruses that infect conjunctiva in children; most of them involve conjunctiva only; only a few involve the cornea as well, causing keratoconjunctivitis. Some of the viruses that inflict conjunctiva may also have systemic involvement.

Both DNA and RNA viruses are known to cause conjunctivitis of various severity; some are very mild, others are severe to very severe, and some of them are associated with subconjunctival hemorrhage ranging from petechiae to large hemorrhage involving the whole of the bulbar conjunctiva. Only a few can be prevented by vaccines; most of the viruses do not impart immunity. The viruses do not respond to antibiotics. There are no effective antiviral drugs that can be used for viral conjunctivitis.

The common viruses that cause conjunctivitis are:

- *DNA viruses:*
  - Adenoviruses
  - *Herpes:*
    - Herpes simplex
    - Herpes zoster ophthalmicus
    - Varicella zoster
  - Molluscum
  - Vaccinia
  - Smallpox

- *RNA viruses:*
  - *Picornaviruses:*
    - Enteroviruses (acute hemorrhagic conjunctivitis)
    - Rhinoviruses
- Mumps
- Rubella

Adenovirus Conjunctivitis

Adenoviruses are the most frequent virus to inflict conjunctiva in children. There are about 40 serotypes, and not all of them cause conjunctivitis. The common serotypes responsible are 3, 7, 8, 19, and 37. None of them impart lasting immunity; there are no vaccines against them.

The two common conjunctival infections by adenovirus are:

1. Pharyngoconjunctival fever
2. Epidemic keratoconjunctivitis

Though the term epidemic is prefixed to the second type only, the first is also seen in epidemics. Both types may have systemic involvement.

Corneal involvement is common in both types, less so in pharyngoconjunctival fever.

Pharyngoconjunctival Fever

Common serotypes to cause pharyngoconjunctival fever are serotypes 3 and 7; the other types may occasionally be responsible.

The disease is seen in children and young adults, but not in neonates. The most common systemic association is upper respiratory infection, i.e., pharyngitis. It may be considered to be a syndrome consisting of bilateral conjunctivitis, fever, and pharyngitis with enlargement of preauricular lymph nodes. The conjunctiva is congested with follicles in both tarsal conjunctivae. The infection starts in one eye, with the other eye following soon. The discharge is watery; the presence of mucopurulent discharge is a sign of bacterial infections. The cornea is involved in about 30% of eyes. The keratitis is short-lived. The disease is spread by droplets, with an incubation period of 4–15 days. Pharyngitis may precede or follow conjunctivitis. In severe form, there may be petechiae on the conjunctiva. The conjunctivitis dies down in about a fortnight. There are no known locally acting antiviral drugs against the virus. However, vidarabine has been used orally to treat systemic involvement with an unequivocal result. Broad-spectrum antibiotics are used empirically to ward off secondary bacterial infection. Especially, if the corneae are involved. Many of the clinicians consider them to have a placebo effect and prefer lubricant, ketorolac, diclofenac, and similar drugs to dampen ocular discomfort.

Epidemic Keratoconjunctivitis

This disorder has some common features with pharyngoconjunctival fever and hemorrhagic conjunctivitis, minus fever and pharyngitis. Corneal involvement is a more or rather most common feature of epidemic keratoconjunctivitis.

The most frequently occurring adenoviruses to cause epidemic keratoconjunctivitis belong to serotypes 8, 19, and 3. Other serotypes also cause the same less often. The incubation period is 5–15 days; the transmission is by contact, i.e., eye-figure-eye or fomites. It is common for it to occur following ocular examination by tonometer, speculum, and lid retractors. It generally does not spread through droplets. It is not transmitted by merely looking at an inflamed eye. It has an acute onset. The child generally complains of a sandy foreign body in one eye. That has severe conjunctival congestion spreading from the fornix toward the limbus and tarsal conjunctiva. The conjunctiva has a mixture of both follicles and papillae. The other eye soon gets involved. The discharge is watery to begin with. Some patients may complain of unexplained itching, the discharge soon becomes mucoid and mucopurulent due to the added bacterial infection; there may be petechial hemorrhages. The lids are edematous. The lid margins get stuck if the lids are kept closed for a few hours; rarely, pseudomembrane may develop. The presence of photophobia is an indication of corneal involvement. The course of events is longer than in pharyngoconjunctival fever. The acute phase subsides in about a fortnight. The termination may assume any of the following:

- Subside without corneal involvement
- Subside with residual keratitis
- Appearance of subepithelial infiltration
- Initially, i.e., for the first 7 days, the corneal involvement is limited to the superficial epithelium that gives a positive fluorescein stain. This is followed by focal epithelial keratitis, which also gives a positive stain that lasts for about a month. Along with focal keratitis, the most troublesome changes are seen under the epithelium, i.e., nonstaining subepithelial infiltrates that are scattered all over the cornea. They keep

changing their positions and numbers. Infiltration in front of the pupil causes blurring of vision and scattering of light without photophobia or watering. These opacities are known to linger for months or years and may be mistaken for corneal dystrophy.

Management

- Cold compress
- Separating the lids and preventing their sticking is best achieved by putting an antibiotic ointment three times a day.
- There is no antiviral drug that is effective against adenovirus.
- Antibiotic drops are given only to prevent and treat associated bacterial infections.
- Nonspecific drugs such as silver nitrate 1% drop two times a day and betadine 2.5% solution given every 2 hours too have been claimed to be effective.
- Artificial tears in gel form, applied four times a day, alleviate gritty sensations.
- Olopatadine 0.2% once a day reduces itching if present.
- Nonsteroidal anti-inflammatory drops give much-needed relief from dull aches.
- Local steroids are indicated only in cases of non-staining subepithelial infiltration. The steroids should be tapered as per the protocol of the institution, both in frequency and strength.
- Cycloplegics are recommended in associated anterior uveitis.

Acute Hemorrhagic Conjunctivitis

This type of acute bilateral conjunctivitis is seen in epidemics. Sometimes, it is difficult to differentiate between epidemic keratoconjunctivitis and pharyngoconjunctival fever. It is caused by enterovirus type 70, with an incubation period of <1–2 days. It is commonly seen in crowded localities, i.e., cinema halls, malls, public transport systems, and educational institutions. It spreads by droplets and fomites. It starts in one eye first then the other eye gets involved. The symptoms are similar to other hyper-acute viral conjunctivitis, i.e., redness, watering, and foreign body sensation; subconjunctival hemorrhage is a constant feature imparting the name to the disease. The management is similar to the above acute viral conjunctivitis.

Table 12.10 shows comparison between various types of epidemic viral conjunctivitis.

TABLE 12.10: Comparison between various types of epidemic viral conjunctivitis.

Clinical feature	*Epidemic keratoconjunctivitis*	*Pharyngoconjunctival fever*	*Epidemic hemorrhagic conjunctivitis*
Virus	Adenovirus 8 and 10	Adenovirus 3, 4, and 7	Enterovirus 70 and Coxsackie virus
Age	Mostly children and young adults	Children and young adults	All
Sex	Equal in both	Equal in both	Equal in both
Onset	Acute	Acute	Hyper acute
Nature of occurrence	Epidemic	Epidemic	Epidemic passing into pandemic
Incubation period	4–8 days	6–10 days	1–2 days
Spread	Fomites, by discharge	Droplets and fomites	Fomites
Lid edema	Moderate	Mild-to-moderate	Marked
Preauricular lymph glands	Generally enlarged	Enlarged	Not enlarged
Discharge	Watery	Watery	Watery
Subconjunctival hemorrhage	Mild, mostly in tarsal conjunctiva	Rare	*Constant feature:* Severe begins as petechial becomes large and lingers for days
Follicular reaction	++	++	+

Contd...

Contd...

Clinical feature	*Epidemic keratoconjunctivitis*	*Pharyngoconjunctival fever*	*Epidemic hemorrhagic conjunctivitis*
Fever	±	Constant feature ranges between 101°F and 104°F	Nil
Pharyngitis	Absent	+++	Nil
Corneal involvement	*Constants*: Late onset lasts longer	±	Occasionally, transient
Duration	Conjunctivitis subsides in 7–10 days: Corneal changes persist	Corneal changes last for a few days	Rarely, when present lasts for 5–7 days
Role of antiviral drug	Nil	Nil	Nil
Immunity	Nil	Nil	Nil

Herpes Conjunctivitis in Children

Both herpes simplex and zoster can involve conjunctiva in children. Infection by herpes zoster is less common in children compared to adults. In contrast, chicken pox is likely to be a more common cause of conjunctivitis than zoster, though both are caused by varicella.

Herpes simplex is always associated with some conjunctival catarrh.

Herpes simplex conjunctivitis is an acute episode that may be confused with simple catarrhal conjunctivitis unless clusters of vesicles on the lids are discovered. It is a primary type of conjunctivitis caused by a type 1 virus, unlike secondary conjunctivitis, which is in fact reactivation of a previous primary infection and seen in adults and is variably associated with corneal involvement.

Rarely, conjunctivitis in children can be caused by the type 2 herpes simplex virus.

Herpes simplex conjunctivitis in children can be divided into three age groups:

1. Among neonates
2. Between 6 months and 6 years
3. In teen age

1. More frequent neonatal herpes simplex conjunctivitis can be divided into:
   a. Ophthalmia neonatorum
   b. Rare congenital

   The second is associated with severe systemic involvement that may be fatal; however, it is often missed, leading to catastrophe. Ophthalmia neonatorum due to the herpes simplex virus is caused by type 2 viruses during passage through the infected birth canal.
2. Children under 6 years get infected by adults.
3. In teens, it is transmitted by kissing an infected person and is rarely sexually transmitted.

Clinical Features

The common features of herpes simplex conjunctivitis are similar in all three groups above. They involve not only the conjunctiva but also the skin and cornea. The incidence of corneal involvement increases with age. Herpes simplex conjunctivitis is generally unilateral, with an incubation period of 1–2 weeks. The eyes are congested, and follicular reactions develop only after the lymphoid tissue has developed in the conjunctiva, which takes about three months; hence, follicles are seen only after 3 months of age. Rarely, pseudomembrane may develop on the tarsal conjunctiva. Lacrimation and photophobia herald corneal involvement. The corneal involvement starts as small, discrete epithelial lesions that join to form dendritic ulcers. The skin lesions are small vesicles over the lid, lid margin, and forehead. The vesicles, unlike zoster infections, may spill over the midline. The condition is self-limited and dies down in 2–3 weeks.

Herpes Zoster Conjunctivitis

This is always associated with herpes zoster ophthalmicus, which is less common in children. Herpes zoster ophthalmia is caused by the varicella zoster virus, which incidentally also causes chicken pox in children. Chickenpox is far more common than herpes zoster ophthalmicus in children. Conversely, zoster ophthalmicus is more prevalent in adults. Isolated herpes zoster conjunctivitis without involvement of the trigeminal nerve has not been reported.

Conjunctivitis precedes vesicle formation; the vesicle involving conjunctiva may be limited to the lid margin. Less common are actual vesicles on the conjunctiva. There may be pseudomembrane formation.

Molluscum Conjunctivitis

Molluscum conjunctivitis is caused by Molluscum contagiosum, a DNA poxvirus. It causes unilateral chronic conjunctivitis following the development of molluscum lesions on the lid margin and parts of the body. The typical skin lesion consists of a translucent, sessile, painless, slow-progressing nodule with umblication; the lesion contains a cheesy material that can be obtained by simple puncture. It contains the virus. The lesion spreads through close body contact. It may be sexually transmitted; the incidence is showing an upward swing due to the increase in the number of immunodeficient persons of all ages. Molluscum causes peripheral superficial keratitis at the lower part of the conjunctiva. Conjunctivitis in an immune-competent person is self-limiting. The lesion on the lid margin requires separate management. The common method to treat a lid lesion is to puncture the nodule and cauterize the interior with tincture iodine or a weak solution of carbolic acid.

The commonly used investigations in various conjunctivitis are:

- Smear for Grams and Giemsa stain for organisms
- Smear for cytology
- Culture of the organism and sensitivity to anti-infective drugs
- Stain for inclusion bodies

Gram stain gives the following information:

- Gram positive/negative
- Cocci/bacilli
- Intracellular/extracellular

The Giemsa stain shows viral cytoplasm or intracellular bodies and bacterial morphology.

Stains used in examinations of conjunctival smears are:

- Gram stain
- *Giemsa stain:* Cell morphology, cytoplasm, and intracellular inclusion bodies. Characteristics of epithelial cells and types of inflammatory cells.
- *Hansel stain:* Hansel stain is used to identify bacterial and identification of eosinophil reactions.

Table 12.11 shows cell types and their probable cause on the stained specimen.

Table 12.12 shows the summary cytological results.

TABLE 12.11: Cell types seen in stained slide.

Cell type	*Probable cause*
Polymorphs	Bacterial infections
Polymorph + lymphocytes	Inclusion conjunctivitis
Poly +, lymph +, and macrophage	Trachoma
Lymphocytic	Viral infection and drug toxicity
Eosinophilic	Allergic conjunctivitis
Epithelial cells	*Cytoplasm inclusion body:* • Basophilic—chlamydia • Eosinophilic—poxvirus • Pink intranuclear inclusion body-Herpes–simplex and zoster

TABLE 12.12: Cytological characteristics of various cells and diseases caused by them.

	Probable cause			
Cell type	*Bacteria*	*Virus*	*Allergic*	*Chlamydia*
Polymorph neutrophil	++	±	Nil	Nil
Eosinophil	–	–	++	±
Lymphocyte	–	+	–	+
Plasma cell	–	–	–	+
Inclusion body	–	+	–	++
Organism	+++	+	–	±

Commonly used media to grow organisms are:

- Blood agar
- Chocolate agar
- Brain-heart infusion
- Lowenstein–Jensen
- Thayer–Martin
- Sabouraud
- Loeffler's

Table 12.13 Results of various culture media for bacteria and fungi and their optimum temperature for good results.

Chlamydial Conjunctivitis in Children

Chlamydia is a group of microorganisms which have been placed between the smallest bacteria and largest virus. They were in the past known as bedsonia. Chlamydia inherits the property of both bacteria and viruses.

TABLE 12.13: Use of various types of media in bacterial and fungal infection.

Culture	*Bacteria*	*Fungi*
Blood agar	Good result and 37°C	Good result at room temperature, nonspecific
Chocolate agar	Good result at room temperature, best for hemophilus, gonococci, and meningococci	No growth
Brain heart infusion	All bacteria grow at 37°C	Fair at room temperature nonspecific
Lowenstein-Jensen	Many weeks at room temperature for *Mycobacterium tuberculosis* and *Mycobacterium leprae*	Nil
Thayer martin	Gonococci and meningococci at room temperature	Nil
Loeffler's medial	Corynebacterium	Nil
Sabouraud	Not used	Specific for fungi that may be broth or agar give good result

The characteristics that are similar among them are:

- They are walled cells.
- They divide by binary fission.
- They contain both DNA and RNA.
- They have ribosomes.
- They contain active enzymes similar to bacteria.
- They are susceptible to antimicrobial.
- They can be cultured on special media.
- They are nearer to gram-negative bacteria.
- They are intracellular parasites.

The following properties bring chlamydia nearer to viruses:

- They are filterable.
- They are not visible on a light microscope without a special stain.
- They are better visualized in immunofluorescence.
- They are visible on the specular microscope.
- They do not grow on cell-free media.
- They cannot be cultured on the usual media used to grow bacteria.
- They form inclusion bodies.
- They have two stages, i.e., infective and noninfective.

Chlamydia has the following species of ocular importance:

- *Chlamydia trachomatis*
- *Chlamydia lymphogranuloma venereum*
- *Chlamydia psittacosis*
- *Chlamydia pneumoniae*

> The first three are acronymed as PLT organisms, where P stands for psittacosis, L for lymphogranuloma venereum, and T for trachoma.

> - Only the last two, i.e., trachoma and lymphogranuloma venereum, are of ophthalmic interest.
> - Trachoma is of more public health interest than lymphogranuloma venereum.

The chlamydial infection by *C. trachomatis* is called trachoma. *C. trachoma* is:

- Exclusively human parasites
- An obligate parasite
- It is intracellular.
- It is gram-negative.
- Aerobic
- Requires growing cells to live
- They stain better by Giemsa stain
- Other special stains are Castaneda, Macchiavello, and simple chemicals such as Lugol's iodine.
- 200 μ in diameter

Chlamydia trachomatis has two forms:

- Elementary body
- Reticulate or initial body

The former is responsible for infection, is metabolically inert with a rigid cell wall, and is called Halberstaedter Prowazek Greeff bodies.

The reticulate bodies have fragile cell bodies that help them replicate.

Natural History of C. trachomatis Infections

The extracellular infective elementary body gets attached to the epithelial host cell. The host cell invaginates to engulf the elementary body to make it intracellular **(Fig. 12.24)**. Once inside the host cell, the elementary body is endocytosed, containing the reticulate body.

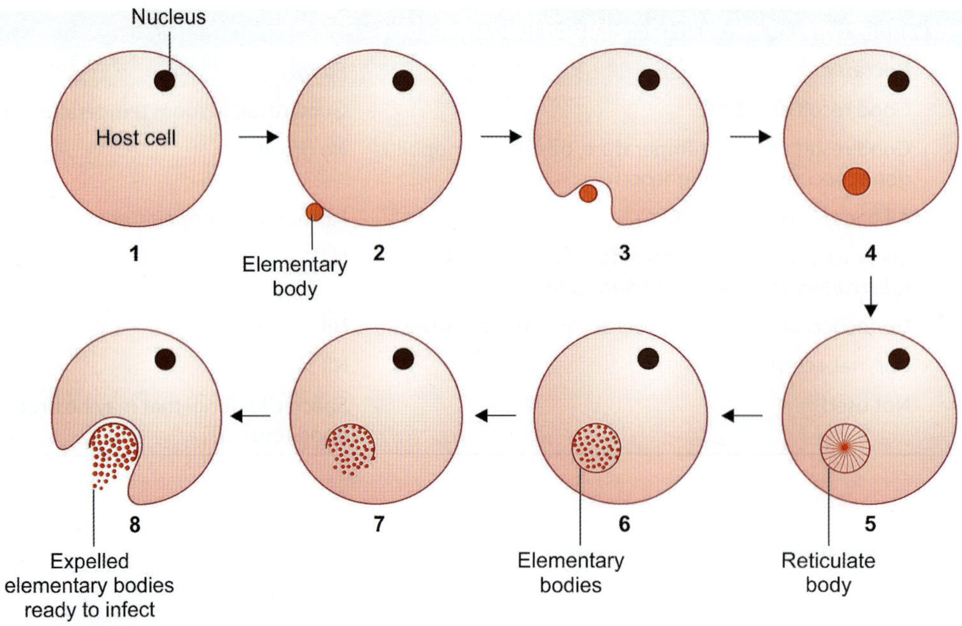

Fig. 12.24: Natural History of *C. trachomatis*. (1) Host epithelial cell showing nucleus; (2) Elementary body attached to the host cell; (3) The host cell engulfs the elementary body; (4) Elementary body in the host cell; (5) The elementary body is converted to a reticulate body; (6) The reticulate body is converted into an elementary body; (7) The elementary bodies are released into the host cell; (8) The host cell expels the elementary bodies to invade a healthy host cell.

The elementary body is converted into a reticulate body that matures and bursts, releasing elementary bodies about 100–500 in numbers.

C. trachoma has many types of serovars, i.e., A, B, Ba, C, D, and K. The A, B, Ba, and C are responsible for trachoma and inclusion conjunctivitis and are called TRIC organisms, where TR represents trachoma and IC represents inclusion conjunctivitis. D to K are responsible for paratrachoma, i.e., oculogenital trachoma.

Flowchart 12.3 shows serovars (serotypes) of chlamydia and their manifestation.

Trachoma in Children

Trachoma is a chronic keratoconjunctivitis with an acute onset in childhood. The common age to contract the disease is between 3 and 10 years **(Flowchart 12.4)**. A trachoma-free child outside this age group may get infected by trachoma if he comes to the endemic area or comes into contact with a person suffering from infective trachoma. Childhood trachoma per se is not blinding but infectious. It only becomes blinding if superimposed with bacterial infections (blinding trachoma).

Untreated adult trachoma is potentially blinding. Acute trachoma in children is often self-limiting. Those children who are not cured spontaneously pass into the stage of blinding (cicatricial) complications. It takes about two decades to develop cicatricial changes serious enough to cause blindness.

Flowchart 12.4 shows the age-wise distribution of trachoma.

Trachoma is widely distributed all over the world; no race is immune, no genetic link has been established, and its preponderance is more in tropical and subtropical countries with hot, dry, and dusty weather. Tropical countries with high rainfall and high humidity show less prevalence. Though it is seen the world over, there are endemic areas where the prevalence is higher. The common factors responsible in these endemic areas that predispose to primary infection are: childhood, economically backwardness, poor hygiene, a lack of running water, the habit of open-air defecation, an excess fly population,* malnutrition, a lack of social awareness, and illiteracy. The availability of running water, flush latrines, and a reduction in fly population greatly reduces

**Excess fly population:* All flies are known to be vectors in trachoma. A fly, *Musca sorbens*, also known as eye seeking fly, is responsible for the maximum spread. This particular fly invades infected conjunctiva and nasal discharge and is considered to be the main vector in the transmission of trachoma in 90% of cases in endemic areas.

Flowchart 12.3: Different types of chlamydia and their ocular manifestation.

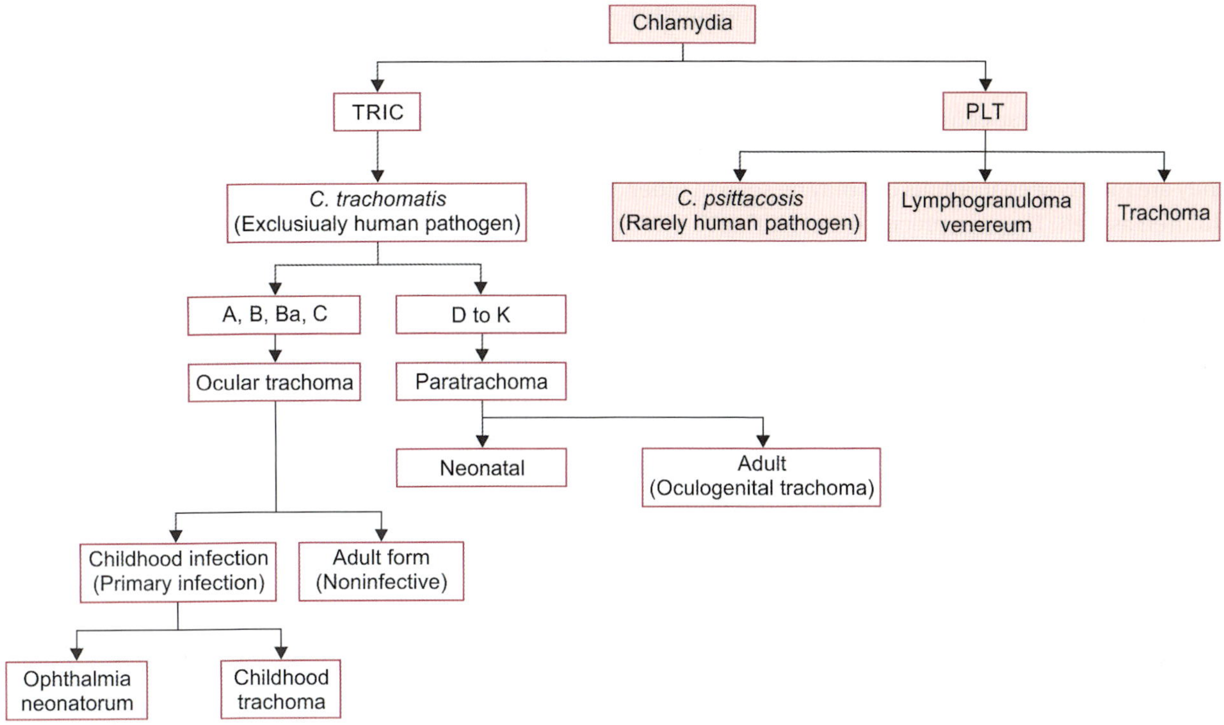

Flowchart 12.4: Age-wise distribution of trachoma.

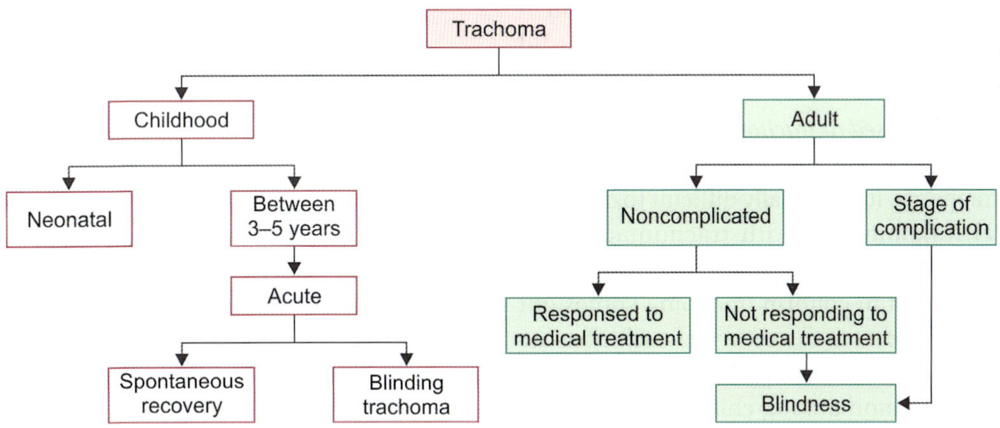

the prevalence of trachoma in children. It is equally common among boys and girls; however, in adults, it is more prevalent among women compared to men.

It is difficult to distinguish it from the house fly *Musca domestica*, which is not known to be a trachoma vector.

The disease in children is self-limited so long as it is not complicated by secondary bacterial infection. It is not possible to distinguish pure trachoma from mild bacterial conjunctivitis, and the mild form is called trachoma dubium.

Signs of Childhood Trachoma

The signs can be conjunctival, corneal, or on the lid.

The conjunctival signs can be:

- *Congestion:* Congestion is pan conjunctival, more marked in tarsal conjunctiva and fornices.

- *Follicles:* Trachoma follicles have the appearance of wet semolina, frequenting the upper tarsal conjunctiva and upper fornix more often than other parts of the conjunctiva, still less common on the plica semilunaris and caruncle. Bulbar conjunctiva is least effected; the follicles at the limbus are called Herbert's follicles. They are mostly seen in adults but may be seen in older children as well. They are precursors of Herbert's pits*; pathognomonic of advanced trachoma.
- *Leber cells:* Leber cells are microscopic bodies seen in stained slides under a light microscope. A typical Leber's cell consists of the central part of blood vessels; the central part is necrosed over a period of time. The Leber cells are specific to trachoma and absent in other forms of follicular conjunctivitis.
- *Papillae:* Papillae are less frequent in trachoma in comparison to spring catarrh.
- *Conjunctival scar:* It is a hallmark of adult trachoma and is absent in children.

The corneal signs: The corneal signs are rare in childhood trachoma. There may be minimal superficial vascularization; no pannus is seen in childhood trachoma. Secondary bacterial infection may cause superficial keratitis that may be converted into frank corneal ulcer.

The lid changes: Lid changes due to trachoma are absent in childhood trachoma except for moderate edema of the lid due to a super-added secondary infection.

Some nonspecific terms used in trachoma (at all ages):

- *Trachoma dubium:* During the initial stages of childhood trachoma, it is clinically difficult to correlate conjunctival inflammation with trachoma; it may only be confused with mild bacterial conjunctivitis unless a specific test to confirm trachoma comes out to be positive. It is better to treat every case of subacute conjunctivitis as trachoma in endemic areas. In the past, it was so common among children in endemic areas that it was called a family disease.
- *Trachoma pur:* Uncomplicated trachoma in childhood without secondary infection is called trachoma pur; there are few or minimal signs of trachoma. There is hardly any discharge.
- *Blinding trachoma:*
  - Heavy infections by virulent bacteria in the trachomatous eye, generally in a malnourished child, are called blinding trachoma, for which trachoma cannot be directly held responsible.
  - Blindness in trachoma in adults is caused by cicatricial changes in the upper lid and marked vascularization of the cornea. It takes 15–20 years for cicatricial changes to occur to cause corneal opacity. The lid changes and vascularization do not respond to medical treatment.
- *Para trachoma:* In contrast to trachoma, which is an exclusively ocular disorder caused by C trachoma A, B, Ba, and C, paratrachoma is caused by C trachoma D to K. It has two forms. The first is in neonates, causing mild ophthalmia neonatorum. The second is oculogenital; neither of the two causes blindness; however, in adults, trachoma and paratrachoma may coexist. Paratrachoma is amenable to medical treatment.

Grading of Trachoma

No distinction has been made between stages of trachoma in childhood and adulthood. Some changes are seen exclusively in children and absent in adults, and vice versa.

Various grades include:

- *As per age:* Childhood trachoma/adult trachoma
- *As per prognosis, the Jones classification of 1974:*
  - Blinding trachoma: In children to adults
  - Nonblinding trachoma
  - Paratrachoma
- *As per changes in conjunctiva:* MacCallan's classification (1908)
- As per blepharopathy and keratopathy (WHO 1987)
- As per WHO guidelines for treatment

MacCallan's classification:
This is the oldest grading system that evolved in 1903 and has been widely used for clinical purposes since then. It has been replaced by better grading.

Stage	Clinical impression
Stage I	Incipient trachoma
Stage II • IIA • IIB	 Marked follicular reaction Marked papillary reaction
Stage III	Stage of cicatrization with follicles and papillae
Stage IV	Stage of healed complication

Herbert's pits: Herbert's pits are diagnostic of adult trachoma; they are in fact a regressed form of Herbert papillae. They are round depressions at the limbus. They are not seen in children.

Macallan concentrated more on conjunctival changes, i.e., follicles and papillae, without considering blepharopathy, i.e., tarsal scaring, trichiasis, entropion, and keratopathy, as well as primary and secondary vascularization due to lid changes, which are the main causes of blindness due to trachoma.

In 1987, WHO came out with a better classification.

WHO classification 1987:

Grade	Clinical feature
Tr. 0	No trachoma
Tr. D	Trachoma dubium, early trachoma without enough signs
Tr. I	Immature follicle on upper tarsus with minimal corneal changes
Tr. II	Mature follicles with papillary hypertrophy, early pannus, and Herbert's pits at limbus
Tr. III	Tarsal conjunctival scaring, along with changes in stage I and II
Tr. IV	Extensive scarring of tarsal conjunctiva absent inflammatory signs. This stage is noninfective.

Earlier Jones (1974) has put forward a classification differentiating blinding and nonblinding trachoma **(Table 12.14)**.

WHO further gave a new classification **(Table 12.15)**.

- The last three grades, i.e., TS, TT, and CO, are not seen in children; TS and TT are potentially blinding. The stages TS, TT, and CO are noninfective but blinding
- TF and TI are more infectious and are managed by local antibiotic drops
- TT does not respond to medical treatment; it requires surgical correction of the lid margin
- CO vascularization subsides following surgical correction of the lid margin, leaving corneal opacity that requires keratoplasty

FISTO

The above grade is acronymed as FISTO, where

F—Follicle

I—Inflammation

S—Scaring

T—Trachomatous trichiasis

O—Opacity (cornea)

Corneal Changes in Trachoma

Corneal changes are the main cause of diminished vision in trachoma. They may be minimal in childhood that inflict corneal epithelium. The other causes of corneal changes are scarring of the lids and lid margin, more marked in the upper lid and seen in adults.

TABLE 12.14: Differentiating blinding and nonblinding trachoma.

Type	Causative strain	Clinical feature
Blinding trachoma	*C. trachoma* A, B, Ba and C in endemic area	Prominent secondary bacterial infection, highly contagious
Nonblinding	*C. trachoma* A, B, Ba and C in hypoendemic area	Without secondary infection less contagious than above
Para trachoma	*C. trachoma* D to K	Oculogenital in adult and ophthalmia neonatorum infants

TABLE 12.15: WHO classification of trachoma.

Grade	Pathology	Part involved	Signs	Age group
TF	Trachomatous inflammation	Tarsal conjunctival epithelium	Five or more follicles in tarsal conjunctiva	Children
T1	Pronounced trachomatous inflammations	Tarsal conjunctival epithelium	Follicle ++ thick tarsal conjunctiva obscured tarsal glands	Children
TS	Inflammatory reaction starts subsiding, scars become obvious	Tarsal conjunctiva and tarsal plate	Scar on tarsus	Adult
TT	Scaring	Lashes	Trichiasis corneal vascularization	Adult
CO	Scaring of corneal surface	Cornea	Corneal vascularization, corneal opacity of various grades causing diminished vision	Adult

The corneal changes in trachoma are:

- *Punctate keratitis,* which may be epithelial or subepithelial in the form of punctate keratitis, subepithelial, or punctate keratitis, produces larger lesions than superficial ones.
- *Vascularization* of the cornea is always superficial, in spite of its prolonged nature. It manifests as an invasion of the corneal epithelium by conjunctival vessels, accompanied by infiltration and epithelial keratopathy. Initially, the vessels lie between the epithelium and Bowman's membrane. Over years, the Bowman's membrane is destroyed. The severity of vascularization depends on duration; longer the duration, the more vascularization occurs. The corneal vascularization does not invade the stroma. The vascularization of the cornea is called pannus. Trachomatous pannus is mostly seen in the upper part. A fully developed trachomatous pannus is visible under oblique illumination without magnification. Early pannus is visible on slit lamp examination, which includes cellular infiltration accompanied by vascularization.

  Trachomatous pannus is divided into two types, i.e., progressive and regressive. In progressive pannus, cellular infiltration is extant ahead of the terminal end of new blood vessels. In contrast to this, the terminal branches leave the infiltration behind the progressing terminal.
- *Limbal changes:* The limbal changes consist of hyperemia, edema, follicle formation, and Herbert's pits; the last is not seen in children.

Diagnosis of trachoma in children: Diagnosis of trachoma in adults is easier than in children. As per WHO guidelines, any conjunctivitis with any of the following two is considered diagnostic:

- Follicle in the tarsal conjunctiva/limbus
- Epithelial keratitis
- Trachomatous pannus

This is not applicable to children because the disease does not reach the fibrotic and vasculogenic stages, which take 15–20 years following childhood trachoma. The paradox is that trachoma in children may be self-limited without going to the stage of complication.

The signs of nonblinding trachoma are:

- Mild conjunctival congestion
- Follicles in upper tarsal conjunctiva
- Superficial keratitis
- No papillae
- No itching

> All cases of bilateral conjunctivitis in endemic areas in children should be considered trachoma unless proved otherwise.

The disease is confirmed by:

- Giemsa staining of conjunctival scraping for:
  - Intracellular cytoplasmic inclusion body
  - Capping of nuclei of epithelial cells
  - Leber's cells
- Microimmunofluorescence test
- Polymerase chain reaction (PCR)
- Detecting chlamydial DNA
- Fluorescent monoclonal antibody detection.

All the tests are available only in higher centers and expensive; hence, more attention should be paid to clinical signs and symptoms.

Differential Diagnosis

Differential diagnosis consists of nonblinding conjunctival inflammation such as:

- Chronic folliculosis
- Follicular conjunctivitis
- Chronic viral conjunctivitis
- Spring catarrh

Management

Management consists of:

- Prophylaxis
- Therapeutics

Prophylaxis: Prophylaxis consists of:

- *Awareness:* Persons in endemic areas should be made aware of the fact that childhood trachoma that looks so benign, if not treated in childhood, will culminate in blindness.
- *Reduction in vector population: C. trachomatis* is shed in stool, where it is transmitted to the eyes by vectors *M. domestica* and *M. sorbens*, which later comprise only 10% of the fly population but are responsible for 90% of transmission. The best solution would be to eliminate flying, which is impossible. The next step is to stop open-air defecation. Which is practical if the community has sufficient running water and a number of flush latrines.
- *Personal cleanliness:* In the form of face and hand wash.

- *Chemoprophylaxis: C. trachoma* is sensitive to many broad-spectrum antibiotics and sulphonamide, which can be administered orally or locally. Antimicrobials take a long time to reach the core of *C. trachoma*; hence, the antimicrobials are to be given for at least 3 weeks to be effective and repeated if needed.

WHO recommends:

- *Oral tetracycline:* 1.00–1.5 g/day as per the weight of the child for 3 weeks. It is not recommended for children under 8 years of age.
- Erythromycin, or triple sulfa, is given in three divided doses for 3 weeks, as per the weight of the child.
- Single dose of azithromycin (20 mg/kg) as a single dose
- *Local antibiotics:* 1% tetracycline ointment TDS, 1% oxytetracycline TDS, chloramphenicol 1% drops or ointment TDS, erythromycin 0.5% TDS, ciprofloxacin 0.3% drops TDS, and rifampin eye drops. The antibiotics are administered for 3 months.

Therapeutic

- *Nonblinding trachoma:*
  - 20% sulfacetamide drop three times a day
  - Add any of the antibiotic ointments at bedtime.
  - Both of the above regimes should be continued at least for 3 months at a stretch.
- *Blinding trachoma:*
  - Treat secondary infections by appropriate antibiotics as per protocol of the institute
  - Add atropine if the cornea is involved.
  - Put the child on antitrachoma therapy for 3 months, both systemic and local.
  - Correct a vitamin A deficiency.
  - Deworm the child.

To eradicate trachoma globally (GET), WHO has devised a strategy acronymed *SAFE,* where:

S—stands for surgery
A—stands for antibiotic
F—stands for facewash
E—stands for environment

Surgery is not applicable for children because they do not have any lid deformities. Antibiotics, face washing, and improvements in environment are sufficient for children.

Miscellaneous Infective and Inflammatory Conditions of Conjunctiva in Children

The condition can be divided into the following categories:

- Uncertain etiology
- Definite etiology

Uncertain Etiology

They are infrequent, and most of them are not curable but treatable. They are:

- Conjunctival folliculosis
- Erythema multiforme
- Stevens–Jonson syndrome
- Iatrogenic conjunctivitis
- Ligneous conjunctivitis

Definite Etiology

- Granuloma of conjunctiva
- Cysts of conjunctiva
- Benign tumors of the conjunctiva
- Myiasis of conjunctiva

Folliculosis: This is not true conjunctivitis. It is a state of lymphoid hyperplasia of unknown origin. The condition is observed during routine examination of the conjunctiva. It is noninfective, nonallergic, and bilateral. The follicles are not as large as infective conjunctivitis; they are smaller than the papillae of spring catarrh, seen mostly in the lower fornix or distal part of the tarsal conjunctiva. Bulbar conjunctiva and cornea are not involved. The condition is benign and self-limited. The importance of the condition lies in the fact that it is often mistaken for either trachoma or tarsal spring catarrh, and the child is unnecessarily treated for the same.

Erythema multiforme: It is a disease with pronounced systemic and ocular involvement. The cause of the disorder is not well understood. Half of the eyes with involvement may terminate in blindness and may be fatal with systemic involvement. Previously, the condition was thought to be allergic. The absence of itching, papillae formation, follicular hypertrophy, and nodules without association with atopy removes it from the list of allergic conjunctivitis; presently, it is thought to be an autoimmune disorder. Erythema multiforme may develop at any age. However, it is more common in children and young adults. The systemic involvement consists of skin and mucous membrane lesions. Though erythema multiforme is entirely different from Stevens-Johnson syndrome, some clinicians still believe Stevens-Johnson syndrome is a severe form of erythema multiforme.

Stevens-Jonson syndrome: This is a serious multifactorial, multiorgan disorder that may be seen in all ages; however, children and young adults are more prone. Ocular involvement may be extensive enough to cause blindness, and systemic affliction may prove to be fatal. Out of all the etiological factors that have been blamed for Stevens–Johnson syndrome, the most outstanding group consists of drugs used to treat serious conditions; indiscriminate use of them for minor ailments may also result in the disease. The drugs are available over the counter; it may take many days to weeks for the drugs to cause disorders, even after the disease for which they were used has been cured. However, sometimes, the first dose may precipitate the disorder as seriously as following prolonged and multiple doses.

The common drugs are:
Sulfa, including acetazolamide and its derivatives, many antibiotics, especially the penicillin group of drugs, analgesics, hypnotics, and folk medicines, constitute the long list of offending drugs. Some of the infections, such as both types of herpes simplex and mycoplasmal respiratory infection, have been blamed often. In some instances, no definite cause can be attributed, and autoimmunity is held responsible. The disease is better put into two clinical categories, though they have a common pathological background.

The groups are:

- Systemic
- Ocular lesion

Systemic: The systemic consists of a prodroma and an actual disease. The prodromal stage may be passed as a common cold or nonspecific fever.

The mucocutaneous stage consists of macules on the dorsum of the hands and feet and the exterior surface of forearms and legs. Soon, the macules are converted to papules and vesicles. All the mucous membranes are predisposed to the disorder. The mucocutaneous involvement lasts for 1–2 weeks; healing takes <1 week.

Ocular lesion: The disorder may involve the skin of the lid, conjunctiva, and cornea in various combinations. The conjunctival lesion begins as mucopurulent conjunctivitis that may be passed as of no significance until it becomes purulent and develops a pseudo- or true membrane. The conjunctival vessels are associated with vasculitis, leading to thrombosis and necrosis. The necrosed conjunctiva sloughs to leave raw areas that may result in symblepharon of various degrees.

Even without sloughing, the conjunctiva heals through fibrosis, leading to trichiasis, entropion, and obliteration of the lid glands and ducts of the lacrimal gland.

Obliteration of lacrimal ducts, ducts of meibomian glands, and loss of goblet cells lead to severe dry eye. The symblepharon may be small or total.

Management: No specific treatment is available for the condition. Early diagnosis is the most important part of management. Local and systemic steroids may be able to minimize vasculitis. Frequent and copious use of lubricant gel may lessen the chances of symblepharon, and a soft contact lens may be used for the same. The cases are best treated by dermatologists and internists.

Iatrogenic conjunctivitis in children: These are mostly drug-induced and can be acute following a single application or chronic and mild following prolonged use of drugs. The drugs can be grouped into two categories: Those that have definite therapeutic value and those that have doubtful or no therapeutic use drugs. The latter includes mostly home medicine or folk medicine. The drugs in the first category are atropine, homatropine, pilocarpine, Alphagan, latanoprost, sulfacetamide, and penicillin.

The conjunctivitis is generally associated with hyperemia of the lid margin and excoriation angle. The most common feature is follicular hypertrophy with itching, redness, and watering. The treatment is to remove the offending drug; this is generally sufficient. Instilling steroid drops provides prompt relief.

Ligneous conjunctivitis: This is a rare chromic conjunctivitis in children; it may be seen in neonates, less commonly in adults; girls are more effected; it is generally bilateral and may be asymmetric; it does not involve the cornea; its main features are localized to the tarsal conjunctiva, causing wood-like hardening of the tarsal plate. Membrane formation is common; the membrane is mistaken for diphtheritic conjunctivitis. Rarely, granuloma may develop at the outer angle. It may be confused with Stevens–Johnson syndrome. There is no satisfactory treatment. Antibiotic drops and a weak solution of steroids prevent secondary infections and reduce inflammation. Lubricants in gel form offer some relief.

Oculomyiasis

Myiasis is a term used to describe larval infection by various larvae of flies belonging to the order Diptera. The larvae are generally referred to as maggots that infect both humans and animals. The maggots are obligate parasites **(Figs. 12.25 and 12.26)**.

The common flies that cause the infestation are the hornet fly, sheep botfly, and screwworm. Besides these, there are many flies of the order Diptera that, too, have been reported to cause ocular myiasis. Myiasis is known to infect skin, all mucous membranes, and unattended wounds. Myiasis is generally seen in extremely poor, malnourished people, drug addicts, persons suffering from leprosy, bed sores, etc. All flies do not cause myiasis. Rarely, it can be seen in a healthy individual without injury or diabetes. It is seen at all ages.

Ocular myiasis accounts for only 5% of systemic myiasis. Ocular myiasis has been divided into orbital, extraocular, intraocular, and a combination of ocular and adnexal myiasis; to this may be added paraorbital and intracranial myiasis.

To begin with, there may be a single larva producing minimal clinical features. This is generally followed by a sudden increase in the number of maggots in the wound. The maggots reach the ocular and paraocular structures via the conjunctiva; this occurs following the deposition of eggs in the conjunctiva or a paraorbital wound. The maggots have been found in eviscerated sockets and phthisis bulbi. They are common in unattended malignancies.

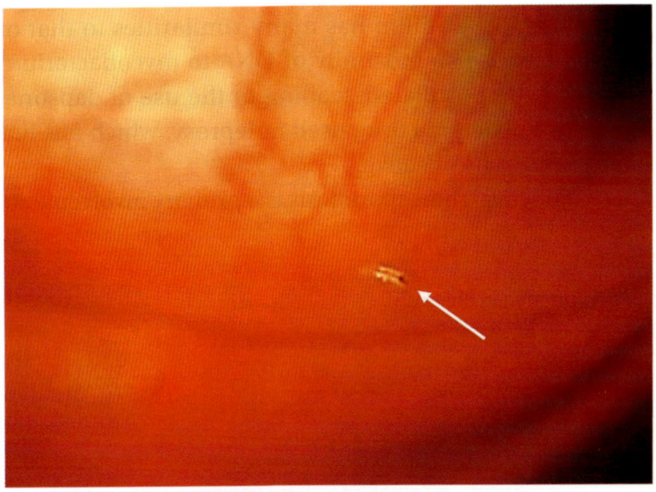

Fig. 12.25: Live maggot in lower fornix.

The most common and earliest presentation mimics localized conjunctival congestion, which soon becomes edematous with discharge of varied natures. At this stage, careful inspection may reveal a single large and a few smaller maggots under the translucent conjunctiva. In a few hours, they may cause rent in the conjunctiva and come to the surface. Some of them may go deep enough to become orbital; only a few may erode the sclera and become intraocular, causing disastrous endophthalmitis.

From the orbit, it may reach the paraorbital sinuses or even the brain. Another route for the maggot to reach the orbit is from the infected nasopharynx.

The diagnosis of the condition with wriggling maggots is not difficult. At this stage, they may be picked up and examined under a microscope to identify and classify them.

Management

The management comprises:

- Physically removing as many maggots as possible after anesthetizing the conjunctiva with a copious amount of 4% xylocaine
- Cleaning and dressing the wound with antiseptics and antibiotics
- Previously, hydrogen peroxide, turpentine, and mild carbolic solutions were used to flush out the maggots.
- The present-day treatment is to administer an ivermectin tablet at a dose of 200 μg/kg. Ivermectin can also be used as a local 1% ointment.

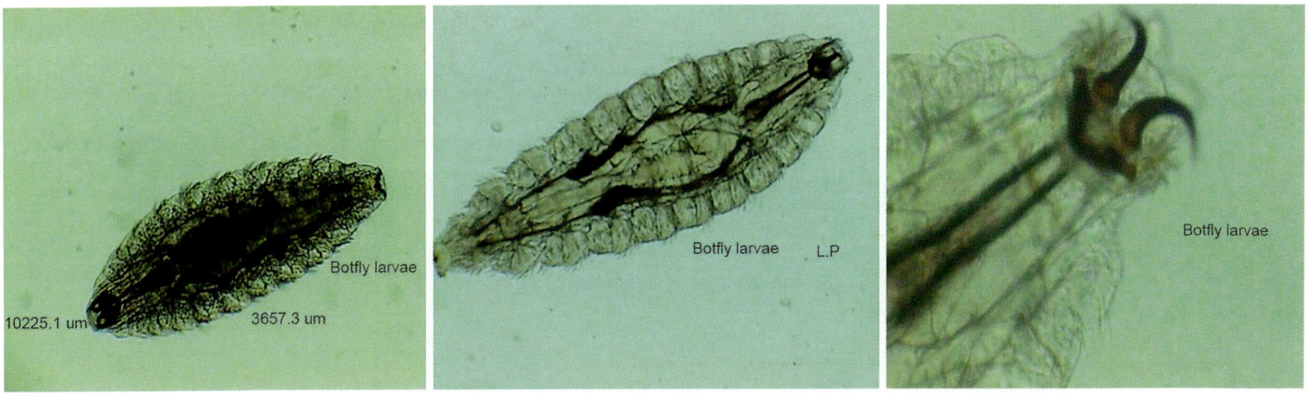

Fig. 12.26: The same under the microscope.
Courtesy: Dr Satish Bataliya and Dr Sharad Jain.

Growths of Conjunctiva in Children

Tumors of the conjunctiva are rare in children and, when present, are benign. Most of them are acquired. In adults, conjunctiva may get involved due to the extension of growth from the lids. The conjunctival growths in children may be solid or cystic.

Flowchart 12.5 depicts a rough classification of new growths of conjunctiva in children.

Burst Chalazion

They are infrequent under 5 years. They occur in lids only in long-standing chalazion without going into cystic change or having been operated on; they do not develop following spontaneous regression either. They develop when the conjunctiva over the chalazion in the tarsal plate ruptures, causing the material to drain, followed by granulation tissue. The burst chalazion is without pain or lymphadenopathy. The growth is sessile. They are not known to become malignant in children. In contrast to repeated chalazia in adults, where they have a propensity to turn malignant, the burst chalazion is almost symptomless except for a visible, smooth swelling on the skin of the lid over the original chalazion. The growth may compress the globe and cause astigmatism that passes off with the removal of the growth. The treatment of a burst chalazion is the same as an ordinary chalazion, i.e., incision, drainage, and curettage.

Rhinosporidiosis of Conjunctiva (Conjunctivo-Sporidiosis)

Oculorhinosporidiosis has been discussed in a previous chapter; the following is a recapitulation of the same with special reference to conjunctival involvement.

Rhinosporidiosis is a chronic granulomatous disease of mostly mucous membranes caused by the organism *Rhinosporidium seeberi*; the taxonomy of the organism is yet to be decided precisely.

Formerly, it was thought to be a fungus; presently, it is considered to be a protists eukaryotic parasite, a mesomycetozoea.

After extensive laboratory tests, it was found that the DNA of rhinosporidium has many similarities to that of cyanobacteria. The proximity of DNA to mycobacterium has also been postulated, leading to the use of dapsone, an antimycobacterial drug used in leprosy, which has not been found to be effective.

Conjunctival rhinosporidiosis is a primary involvement.

Flowchart 12.5: New growths of conjunctiva in children.

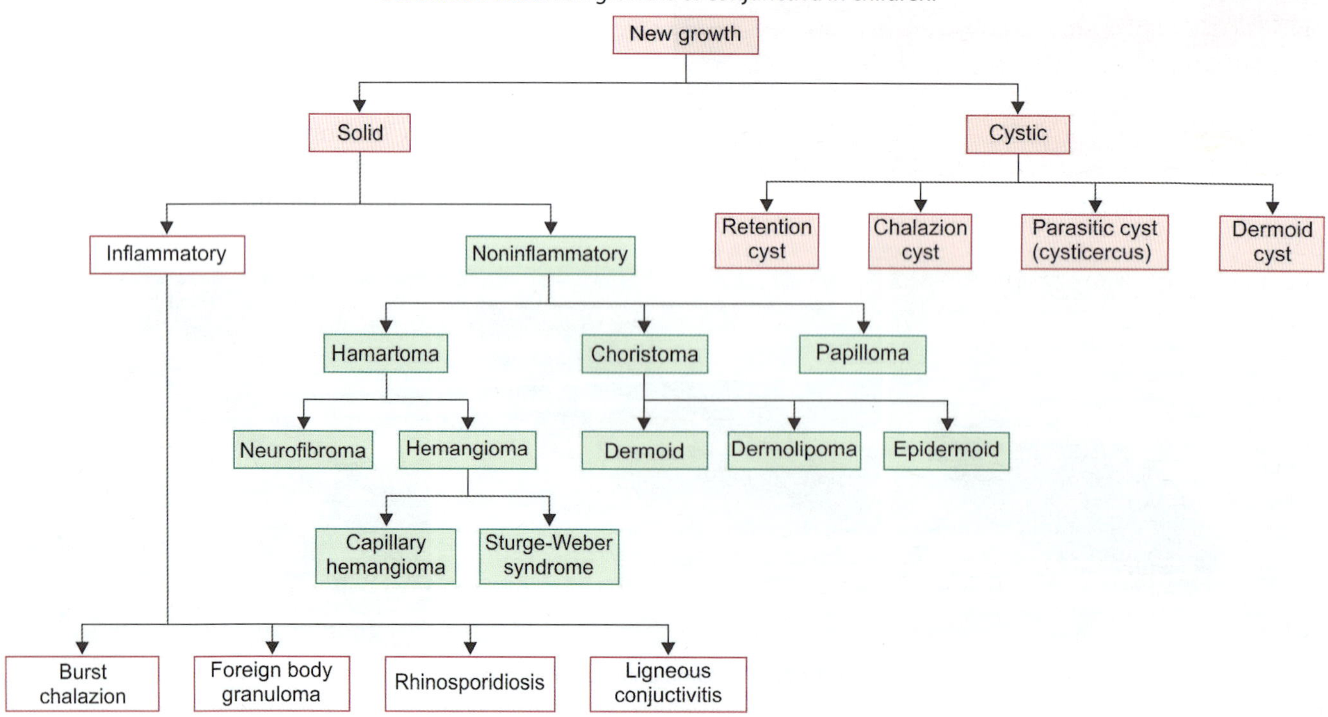

Simultaneous involvement of the sac is not associated with primary conjunctival involvement. The growth in conjunctiva is always solitary and unilateral, without any predilection for side. All the parts of the conjunctiva, i.e., the tarsal, fornix, and bulbar conjunctiva, are involved. Involvement of the bulbar conjunctiva is the least frequent. A typical conjunctival lesion is slowly progressive, painless, and bright red colored. That is not felt by the child until it becomes visible. The surface of the growth is rough and sprinkled with white dots that represent sporangia.

The growths in fornices are pedunculated and flat, with crenated edges that bleed not only on manipulation but spontaneously as well. The growths on the tarsal conjunctiva are flat and sessile. Involvement of the two tarsal conjunctiva is equal in frequency. The simultaneous involvement of both tarsal conjunctivas is not known. The growth on the limbus and bulbar conjunctiva is less common, they are rounded and sessile.

Rhinosporidiosis of conjunctiva per se does not cause conjunctivitis. Conjunctivitis is secondary to a superimposed bacterial infection. Rhinosporidial lesions are not influenced by the HIV status of the patients.

Symptoms

A visible red growth in the interpalpebral conjunctiva is the most common symptom. Other symptoms are bleeding from the conjunctiva and lacrimation. Conjunctival growth per se does not prelude lacrimation. This occurs only if the growth from the upper lid rubs against the cornea.

Diagnosis

Diagnosis in an endemic area is simple and easy. The conditions that are confused are:

Burst chalazion, foreign body granuloma, hemangioma, and papilloma. Conversely, these conditions can be confused with rhinosporidiosis.

Management

There is no drug that is effective against rhinosporidiosis. Recently, ivermectin in doses of 200 μg/kg orally in a single dose has been used without constant good results.

The best treatment for conjunctival rhinosporidiosis is complete removal under local anesthesia. The resultant bleeding stops even without ligation; the growth is not known to occur either at the original site or anywhere on the conjunctiva, in spite of the patient living in the same endemic area.

Allergic Conjunctivitis

Allergic conjunctivitis is very common all over the world at all ages. Its prevalence among children is more frequent in developed countries where infectious conjunctivitis has been eliminated to a great extent. The most common cause of conjunctivitis is allergic, while in underdeveloped countries, infectious conjunctivitis still outnumbers allergic conjunctivitis. Allergic conjunctivitis is more commonly subacute in children. The signs and symptoms are variable; they may be mild enough to be ignored or troublesome enough to make the child skip school and the adult abstain from work. Most allergic conjunctivitis is self-limiting, lasting from a few hours to many years. Allergic conjunctivitis generally involves both the eyes, which may not be symmetrical or simultaneous. None of the allergic conjunctivitis is blinding; it does not cause systemic disorders; however, allergic pulmonary and dermatological features are more frequent with allergic conjunctivitis. Allergic conjunctivitis per se is not curable but manageable. The allergens causing conjunctivitis are broadly divided into two groups, i.e., external and internal allergens.

SUGGESTED READING

1. Cady LD. Study of trachoma dubium. AJO. 1958;45(1):41-3.
2. Eerson PM, Baily RL, Mahdi OS, Wairaven GE, and Lindsay SW. Transmission and Ecology of Fly M. Sorbens, a putative vector of trachoma. Trans R Soc Trop Med Hyg. 2000;94(1):28-32.
3. Gupta PC, Ram J, Faisal TT, Agarwal A, Khurana S, Prasad A. Ocular myiasis. J Oph Vis Res. 2018;13 (3):361-2.
4. Kalamkar C, Radke N, Mukherjee A. Orbital myiasis in eviscerated socket and review of literature, BMJ Case Rep. 2016:bcr2016215361.
5. Khurana S, Beswal MA, Bhatti H. Ophthalmomyiasis. Indian J Med Micro. 2010;28(3):257-61.
6. Kuriakose E. Oculosporidiosis Rhinosporidiosis of the Eye. BJO. 1963;47(6):346.
7. MacCallan AF. Epidemiology of trachoma. BJO. 1931;15:360.
8. Misra N, Gogri P, Misra S, Singh A, Ingale A. Ivermectin treatment for massive orbital myiasis in an empty socket with concomitant scalp pediculosis, Australas Med J. 2013;6(10):504-6.
9. Misra S, Misra N. In: Nagarkar NM, Mehta R (Eds). Clinical Presentation: Ophthalmological Spectrum in Rhinosporidiosis. Singapore: Springer Nature Pvt Ltd; 2022.

10. Mukherjee PK, Jain PC, Mishra R. Exanthemata, a causative factor of chronic dacryocystitis in children. IJO. 1969;17(1):27.
11. Naranayan S, Jay Prakash K. Incidence of ocular myiasis due to infection with larvae of oestrus ovis. IJO. 1991;39:176-9.
12. Pavan-Langston D. Cornea and External Diseases in the Manual of Ocular Diagnosis and Therapy. Wolters Kluwer (India); 2008.
13. Puthran N, Hegde V, Anupama B, Andrew S. Ivermectin treatment for massive orbital myiasis in an empty socket with concomitant scalp pediculosis. Indian J Ophthalmol. 2012;60(3):225-7.
14. Samaddar R, Sen M. Rhinosporidiosis in Bankura. Indian J Pathol Microbiol. 1990;33(2):129-36.
15. Sharma VK, Gupta PC, Ram J. Trachoma, and Herberts Pit. QJM. 2019;112(6):457.
16. Sivaramasubramanyam P, Sadanand AV. Oculo myiasis. BJO.1968;52(1):64-5.
17. Sudarshan V, Goel N, Gahine R, Krishnani C. Rhinosporidiosis in Raipur, Chhattisgarh: A report of 462 cases. Indian J Pathol Microbiol. 2007;50(4):718-21.
18. Thylefors B, Dawson CR, Jones BR, West SK, Taylor HR. Simple system for the assessment of trachoma and its complications. Bull WHO. 1987;65(4):477-83.

CHAPTER

13 Xerophthalmia

The term xerophthalmia encompasses all the ocular changes brought about by a deficiency of vitamin A. The sole cause of which is hypovitaminosis A. Hypovitaminosis A is broadly divided into two parts, i.e., systemic and ocular. Systemic involvement precedes ocular involvement; it is not possible to have ocular manifestation without systemic avitaminosis, which sets in when the serum level of vitamin A falls below the optimal level of 50 IU. The systemic involvements per se are not vision-threatening; they are precursors of xerophthalmia. The systemic manifestations are metaplasia and keratinization of the skin and respiratory epithelia. It also causes degenerative changes in medullated nerve fiber.

The ocular manifestations are collectively known as xerophthalmia, which has two components, i.e.,

1. Photochemical changes in rods.
2. Epithelial metaplasia of conjunctiva and cornea.

Cones are not effected in xerophthalmia.

PHOTOCHEMISTRY OF SCOTOPIC VISION (NIGHT VISION)

The retinal periphery is densely endowed with rods and a few cones. Rods are responsible for night vision. The rods are present in the periphery of the retina, in contrast to the cones that are densely packed in the macula and are responsible for photopic (day vision) and only a few rods.

The rods contain a pigment called visual purple, or rhodopsin. Rhodopsin can absorb up to 500 nm of light. Rhodopsin is joined with the aldehyde of vitamin A. When rods are photo extractor, the aldehyde in vitamin A is changed to a substance called all trans-retinal. The conversion of 11-cis-retinal to all trans-retinal has many stages. The reaction is reversible in dim light. Rhodopsin has many components, i.e., bathorhodopsin, lumirhodopsin, and metarhodopsin 1 and 2. The ability to see in dim light is brought about by photodecomposition and its regeneration into vitamin A. The conversion of 11-cis-retinal to all trans retinal is brought about by light. In the presence of light, the magenta-colored rhodopsin is bleached. All trans-retinal is converted to 11-cis retina in the retinal pigment epithelium and transported to rods.

11-cis-retinal joined the opsin to the rhodopsin. Regeneration of rhodopsin is not photo-dependent. Thus, the absence of a retina leads to disruption of night vision.

Xerophthalmia is preceded by systemic involvement that does not need to pass through the milder stages of night blindness/Bitot's spots.

The terms xerophthalmia broadly mean dry, while ophthalmia is a combination of ill-defined conditions that represent many unrelated conditions, i.e., ophthalmia neonatorum (acute conjunctivitis in newborns), Egyptian ophthalmia (trachoma), and other conjunctivitis.

XEROPHTHALMIA

Xerophthalmia manifests when the daily supply of vitamin A falls below the optimal level of 50 IU (700–900 μg; 1 IU = 0.3 μg of retinol or 0.6 μg of β-carotene).

In nature, vitamin A is available for oral use. A systemic route is required only as a therapeutic measure, as an injection in an emergency. The injections may either be water-soluble or in oil; the latter is no longer in vogue. Water-soluble injection is available as 50,000 IU in 1 mL. The requirement of vitamin A in an infant is five times greater than that of an adult, who requires only 12 μg per kg of body weight, while an infant requires 65 μg per kg, which is roughly 7,500 IU. Vitamin A is dispensed either in IU or in micrograms (retinol). The main source of vitamin A for an infant is the mother's milk, provided the mother is not malnourished or suffering from avitaminosis. Vitamin A exists as retinol, retinal (retinaldehyde), and retinoic acid in the body. Vitamin A (retinol) is a fat-soluble vitamin that is stored mostly in the liver and in small quantities in fat following oral consumption or injection. The source of vitamin A can be a vegetable or an animal. All varieties of vegetables, pulses, cereals, and nuts contain vitamin A in small quantities. The leafy green vegetables and yellow-red fruits, too, are rich in vitamin A. Red palm oil is the richest source of vitamin A. Dairy products, animal protein, fish, and eggs are high in vitamin A. The natural source of vitamin A is called pro or previtamin A. They need to be broken down to retinol for utilization in the small intestine.

The vitamin A present in vegetables as B-keratin or carotenoids, which has only one-sixth the activity of retinol. Hence, it has to be consumed in large quantities over a long period, so it cannot be relied on as an urgent remedy for keratomalacia or advanced xerophthalmia. They are best considered to be food supplements.

> Vitamin A in megadoses, both single and divided, is capable of causing toxicity. Another fat-soluble vitamin known to cause toxicity is vitamin D. Incidentally, a megadose of vitamin A antagonizes vitamin D. Vitamin A in large doses is also detrimental to serum zinc. Other fat-soluble vitamins, i.e., vitamin E and K, are not directly involved in a child's metabolism.

Deficiency of vitamin A is brought about mostly due to insufficient dietary supply, increased requirements, as in measles and other infectious diseases, which increase requirements by many fold. Worm infestations are considered to be a high risk factor. The next cause is poor utilization, as in diarrhea. It is common to have more than one of the above factors acting at a given time. Vitamin A deficiency is rarely isolated; it is almost always associated with calorie-energy malnutrition and a poor supply of trace elements, especially zinc.

Xerophthalmia is seen mostly in underdeveloped countries. The introduction of vitamin A supplementation in large doses in the national programs of various countries has considerably reduced the incidence of xerophthalmia. In these countries, vitamin A deficiency still remains a major cause of childhood blindness and death, in spite of national programs.

Xerophthalmia is a disorder of childhood. It is not seen in the first year of life if the infant is breast-fed and the mother is not malnourished. The most common age when a child is most likely to develop xerophthalmia is between 2 and 5 years, equally in both sexes; both eyes are involved simultaneously. It generally develops gradually. However, an attack of measles or severe gastroenteritis may precipitate an acute attack with a fast-developing catastrophe of keratomalacia in children already in the subclinical stage.

Symptoms

Diminished Night Vision (Nyctalopia)

The main symptom to attract attention is ever-increasing night blindness. To begin with, the child seems to bump against obstacles in a dimly lit room, gradually worsening to total incapacitation. In this stage, the child cannot locate his food kept in front of him in dim light. The child has to be helped to move out of the room to urinate or defecate. He seems to be as normal as the sunrise. He has no difficulty with photopic vision, unless he has causes other than vitamin A deficiency as well. The condition is known by many local terms; one of them is chicken blindness. The chicken and birds belonging to the family of chickens have either no or very poor night vision because they have no or scanty rods in the retina. In contrast, the birds of the owl family have well-developed rods, so they have sharp night vision and poor day vision.

Conjunctival Changes

Night blindness is followed or accompanied by xerosis of the conjunctiva and Bitot's spot. Parents and Anganwadi workers, as well as ASHA workers (accredited social health activists), may not be able to discern early xerosis. The earliest signs of xerosis are vertical wrinkles in the bulbar conjunctiva on the temporal side and in the interpalpebral aperture. The normal conjunctiva is wet and glossy and is not thrown in vertical folds when looking towards the temporal side, which is evident in prexerotic conjunctiva **(Fig. 13.1)**.

Xerosis is caused by metaplasia of the conjunctival epithelium that leads to the destruction of goblet cells, which are the main source of mucin in the tear film;

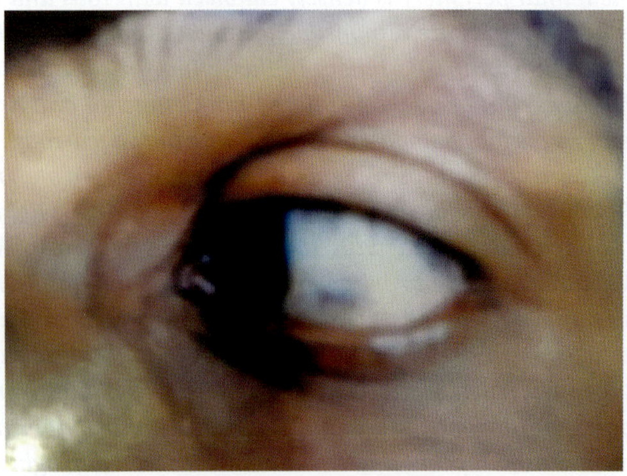

Fig. 13.1: Xerosis conjunctiva.

thus, a state of mucin deficiency ocular surface disorder results in xerophthalmia. Why xerosis develops only in the interpalpebral aperture is not well understood.

The possibilities are:

- The temperature of the conjunctiva in the interpalpebral aperture is lower than under the lids.
- Ultraviolet rays in sunlight are detrimental to conjunctival epithelium in the absence of mucin and at a lowered temperature.
- Corynebacterium, a saprophyte, is often isolated from xerotic conjunctiva; the organism produces gas in the presence of light that gives a foamy appearance to the Bitot spot.

The parents may be able to spot fully developed xerosis. This brings the child for medical consultation. The Bitot's spots slowly grow as marble-white, foamy, elevated single spots in the bulbar conjunctiva, mostly on the temporal side. The marble-white area is triangular in shape with its base toward the limbus, a little away from the limbus; the surface lacks the smoothness of normal conjunctiva, occasionally they may be linear or circular; shape and size do not have any clinical significance. The foam can be wiped off, only to appear in a few hours. Normal conjunctiva does not stain with kajal (kohl) and surma, but a Bitot's spot stains black with them; this is yet another point that draws parents' attention. The Bitot's spot does not stain with any vital stain either. The Bitot's spot is nontender, nonpainful, and moves with conjunctiva. The raised area is made up of desquamated, keratinized epithelial cells.

It takes a few days to weeks to disappear with a therapeutic dose of vitamin A, in contrast to lesions that are due to causes other than vitamin A deficiency. The therapeutic dose of a single injection of vitamin A is 50–100 thousand IU.

Corneal Changes in Xerophthalmia

Corneal changes are concurrent with changes in conjunctiva. It is presumed that changes in the cornea are actually continuations of conjunctival changes.

The corneal changes comprise of:

- Dry spots with decreased tear film breakup time.
- Punctate keratopathy on the periphery, commonly in the lower nasal quadrant.
- Once the epithelium has been involved, the next structure to be involved is the stroma that results in the following types of corneal ulcers:
    - Small circular ulcer on the periphery.
    - Large circular punched-out ulcer in the center, surrounded by an edematous cornea.
    - Involvement of the whole of the cornea.

Fortunately, the ulcer, if treated with a parenteral megadose of water soluble vitamin A, can be prevented from perforating. Otherwise, the central ulcer is known to perforate within 1–2 days.

Once the perforation has occurred the eye may end in—central adherent leukoma → large leukoma → partial anterior staphyloma → large anterior staphyloma → total staphyloma → blindness.

The corneal ulcer due to xerophthalmia develops in the stage of keratomalacia, where the cornea becomes soft and seems virtually to melt. The ulcer is sterile, with no or little congestion without hypopyon. Hypopyon develops following a superimposed secondary infection that is common in malnourished children. A perforation with hypopyon may end in endophthalmitis and panophthalmitis.

Classification of Xerophthalmia

From time to time, various classifications have been put forward for xerophthalmia; to grade it in clinical practice to treat and predict the prognosis.

The following are some of them:

Earliest classification (1965)

- Prexerosis
- Xerosis
- Conjunctival xerosis
- Corneal xerosis—Keratomalacia—perforation—sequelae of perforation—blindness.

The classification put forward by the World Health Organization (WHO) (1976) was based on clinical signs that were put in two broad groups:

1. Primary signs
2. Secondary sings

Primary Signs

- X 1A—conjunctival xerosis only
- X 1B—conjunctival xerosis with Bitot's spot
- X 2—corneal xerosis
- X 3A—corneal xerosis with ulcer
- X 3B—keratomalacia

Secondary Signs

- X N—night blindness
- X F—xerophthalmic fundus
- X S—xerophthalmic scar

Note: X stands for xerosis. These signs are more descriptive than diagnostic.

WHO 1982 modified the ocular sings as:
- X N—night blindness
- X 1A—conjunctival xerosis
- X 1B—Bitot's spot
- X 2—corneal xerosis
- X 3A—keratomalacia/corneal ulcer involving less than one-third of the cornea.
- X 3B—same as above, with more than one-third involvement of the cornea.
- X S—xerophthalmic-related corneal scar
- X F—xerophthalmic fundus

A still better classification was suggested in 1991, which is as follows:
- X N—night blindness
- X CJ—conjunctival xerosis
- X B—Bitot's spot
- X U/K—xerosis with corneal ulcers or keratomalacia may perforate.

Note: Keratomalacia is defined as the drying and clouding of the cornea due to vitamin A deficiency and insufficient protein and calories.

Symptoms of Xerophthalmia

Symptoms may be broadly divided into:
- Systemic
- Ocular

Systemic

The systemic symptoms are related to dryness of the skin, recurrent respiratory tract infections, diarrhea, and poor development. The systemic symptoms may be subtle and may not be correlated to xerophthalmia until night blindness sets in.

Ocular Symptom

Ocular symptoms of xerophthalmia can be related to changes in any of the following in isolation or combination:
1. Conjunctiva
2. Cornea
3. Retina
    i. Night blindness
    ii. Changes in fundus

Any of 1 and 2 may precede the other, or both may run concurrently. There are instances where corneal and conjunctival symptoms have preceded night blindness as per the WHO classification, though the reverse is true.

> Xerophthalmia with night blindness means a severe vitamin A deficiency requiring urgent treatment.

Differential Diagnosis

The diagnosis of xerophthalmia is not difficult. The conditions that may pose problems are:
1. Xerosis of conjunctiva due to causes other than vitamin A deficiency.
2. Tapetoretinal degeneration is causing night blindness.

Retinitis pigmentosa, a common cause of night blindness after 10 years, is not related to vitamin A deficiency but is a commonly mistaken diagnosis of xerophthalmia. Which can be solved by a simple therapeutic trial with the administration of water-soluble vitamin A at a dose of 100,000 IU, following which night blindness due to vitamin A deficiency improves within 48 hours. But it has no effect on night blindness due to retinitis pigmentosa.

Management

> Xerophthalmia is fully preventable. It is treatable before keratomalacia sets in.

The management can be divided two parts:
1. Prophylaxis
2. Therapeutic

Prophylaxis

An infant born to a mother without clinical or subclinical vitamin A deficiency and protein caloric malnutrition is unlikely to develop xerophthalmia. This is a Utopian condition that rarely exists in under developed countries which harbor maximum number of xerophthalmic mother and children.

The prophylactic steps are:
- All children irrespective of their vitamin A status should be on pro vitamin A rich diet and sufficient calories.
- All expectant mothers should have sufficient vitamin A in their diet before and after delivery besides usual iron, folic acid calcium, and sufficient protein and calories along with zinc.
- All mother soon after childbirth should receive an additional dose of 100,000 IU of vitamin A orally.
- All children up to at least age of 2 years should be breast fed with usual solid food.
- All children should be covered by national immunization program.

- All children should get additional oral dose of 100,000 IU of vitamin A along with measles vaccine.
- All children suffering from measles should get a shot of therapeutic dose of injectable vitamin A as part of management of measles.
- WHO recommended universal schedule of vitamin A prophylaxis is as tabulated in **Table 13.1**.

Modified schedule of WHO 1992 for children is as tabulated in **Table 13.2**.

Therapeutic

The following is the recommendation for therapeutic management of xerophthalmia from X N–X 3B. Oral therapy is sufficient unless the child has repeated vomiting or severe diarrhea, where an intramuscular injection is needed.

The schedule recommended by the WHO is:

1. Immediately on diagnosis in a xerophthalmic child above 1 year: 200,000 IU orally or 100,000 IU by injection.
2. The next day, repeat the aforementioned dose.
3. 1 month later, as aforementioned.

TABLE 13.1: World Health Organization (WHO) recommended universal schedule of vitamin A prophylaxis.

S. No.	*Age*	*Dose*
1.	Infant <6 months without breastfeeding	50,000 IU orally
2.	6–12 months	100,000 IU orally every 6 months
3.	Older than 12 months	As above
4.	Children weighing <8 kg	As above
5.	1–6 years	200,000 IU every 6 months
6.	Lactating mother	200,000 IU on delivery

TABLE 13.2: Modified schedule of World Health Organization (WHO) 1992 for children.

S. No.	*Age*	*Dose*
1.	9 months	100,000 IU along with measles vaccine
2.	18 months	200,000 IU along with booster dose of DPT and oral polio vaccine
3.	24 months	200,000 IU orally, every 6 months up to age of 5 years amounting to 9 doses

(DPT: tetanus-diphtheria-acellular pertussis vaccine)

Note: Children under 1 year and under 8 kg in weight should get half the aforementioned dose.

LOCAL TREATMENT

- Xerosis, Bitot's spot, and night blindness do not respond to any local therapy, including local retinol drops.
- Care should be taken to prevent bacterial infections.
- Lubricants are not recommended because of their cost and their doubtful efficacy.
- Once the cornea is involved, it should be treated as any fulminating corneal ulcer, i.e., with atropine ointment, broad-spectrum antibiotics, and dorzolamide drops to keep the intraocular tension.

ANCILLARY TREATMENT

All children, irrespective of vitamin A status, should be:

- Encouraged to get enrolled in school.
  - Where they get a midday meal that will look after their calorie, vitamin, and mineral requirements. The children in Anganwadi get regular vitamin doses as per the national program.
  - Dewormed regularly.
  - The children getting megadoses of vitamin A should get an adequate amount of vitamin D and zinc.
  - Children with central corneal opacity may be considered for keratoplasty later.
  - Rehabilitation

SUGGESTED READING

1. McLaren DS, Kraemer K. Manual on vitamin A deficiency disorder, 3rd edition. Basel, Sight and Life Press; 2012.
2. Nema N, Nigam R. Vitamin A deficiency in eyes in systemic disorder, 1st edition, New Delhi: Wiley India; 2015.
3. Salmon JF. Keratomalacia. In: Salmon JF (Ed). Kanski's Clinical Ophthalmology, 9th edition (International). New Delhi: Elsevier; 2020.
4. Singh KJ. Modified classification of xerophthalmia. Indian J Opthalmol. 1991;39(3):105-7.
5. Sommer A. Field guide to detection and control of xerophthalmia, 2nd edition. Geneva: WHO; 1982.
6. Tandon R. Keratomalacia. In: Tandon R (Ed). AIOS Ready Reckoner in Ophthalmology, 2nd edition. New Delhi: Jaypee Brothers; 2017. pp. 20-1.
7. WHO technical report series no. 590. WHO Technical Report Series; 1976. pp. 17-18.
8. WHO technical report series no. 671. WHO Technical Report Series. 1982;13.

CHAPTER 14

Allergy and Autoimmunity in Pediatric Ophthalmology

Allergy is a common cause of ocular malady and morbidity. Next to infection, allergy itself does not cause infection; it causes inflammation, which can be modified by superimposed infection by microbes. Microbes themselves are known to initiate allergies. Beside microbes, some organic chemical substances, mainly proteins, can also cause allergies. In contrast to this, autoimmunity is always caused by an antigen against own body of the subject; it is a systemic immune response of the body to its own tissue.

ALLERGY

Allergy (hypersensitivity) is defined as an altered inflammatory reaction to the reintroduction of an allergen in already sensitized tissue. It is an antigen antibody reaction different from idiosyncrasy and toxic reactions. Allergy is greatly influenced by heredity. Allergy can be of acute or delayed onset. In other terms, allergy is enhanced immune resection due to any mechanism involving an outside allergen.

Some terms are used in the study of allergies are given in the following text.

ALLERGENS

They are the substances that trigger allergies. They are mostly protein-rich in nature. The immune system recognizes them as foreign and dangerous to the body. To overcome this, the immune system reacts by producing antibodies. The most common antibody involved in protecting the body is immunoglobulin E (IgE) in nature. This process initiates allergic symptoms. That may be local or widespread; it may be mild enough to ignore or serious enough to be fatal.

Common allergens include:

- Dust
- Drugs
- Foods
- Pollen
- Fungal spores
- Insect and mite feces
- Insect bites and stings
- Animal proteins
- Animal dander

ATOPY

The term atopy is often used interchangeably with allergy. In fact, in the presence of atopy, the immune system of the body is more sensitive to common allergic factors that may have been inhaled or swallowed because the body has a stronger reaction to these allergens than to their absence.

Types of Allergy

Allergy can be acute or delayed. Immediate allergy takes place within seconds of exposure to the same antigen that has sensitized the person earlier. The examples are—hay fever, urticaria, anaphylaxis,* and Arthus phenomenon.† The vascular endothelium is the main site of action.

**Anaphylaxis:* This is a hyperacute allergic reaction that may manifest within seconds to minutes following exposure to an allergen that may be as common as food or a drug. Some of the common antibiotics, when injected, may cause it immediately following the injection; even a test dose may precipitate it. The common clinical features of anaphylaxis are:

Shock, fall in blood pressure, breathlessness, edema of the respiratory epithelium, feeble pulse, skin rash, and sudden collapse. It can be fatal.

†*Arthus phenomena:* This is a severe local reaction at the site of the introduction of an antigen in a previously sensitized person. It is equivalent to a type 3 allergy.

Delayed allergy takes hours to days to manifest following exposure to a specific antigen, which is invariably a microbial protein. In contrast to the immediate reaction, which primarily affects the vascular endothelium, the delayed reaction involves lymphoid tissue primarily. It does not produce circulating antibodies. The other sources of delayed hypersensitivity are contact antigens.

ANTIGEN

Antigen is a substance that finds its way into the body to start antibodies to fight disease. It is a protein on the surface of a cell that can differentiate the cells as self or nonself and produce antibodies. Antigens present in the body are called autoantigens.*

Immunization

Immunization, commonly known as vaccination, is a method to protect a person against diseases. The vaccination creates a status that otherwise would have been produced by a disease, commonly bacterial or viral, without the person actually getting them. Immunization can be active or passive. It can be against a single disease or multiple diseases.

Active Immunization

Active immunization stimulates the immune system to produce antibodies against a particular infectious agent.

There are two main types of active immunization. They are:

1. Live-attenuated vaccine
2. Inactivated

Passive Immunization (Passive Immunity)

This is produced by introducing preformed antibodies in an unprotected individual. It is generally acquired but can happen in utero; the newborn may also acquire it through mother's milk.

TOXOID

When a toxin meant to cause severe diseases such as tetanus or diphtheria is either inactivated or its toxicity is reduced, retaining its immunological properties is called a toxoid. The toxin concerned is generally an exotoxin. The toxicity is reduced either chemically or by heat. The toxins are secreted by bacteria; though toxoid is an altered form of toxoid, they are not produced by microorganisms (bacteria). The toxoid gives longer immunity and rarely causes adverse reactions following injection. The common examples are diphtheria and tetanus vaccines/toxoid.

Vaccines

Vaccines, when administered, cause a protective immune response either by a live attenuated or killed microbes. The vaccines retain the ability to incite the formation of antitoxin that are themselves antibodies directed against the microbial toxin. The list of vaccines used in public health is long. The commonly used vaccines of ocular importance are:

- Chickenpox (*Varicella*)
- Diphtheria
- Measles
- Meningococcal
- Mumps
- Pneumococcal
- Rubella (German measles)
- Shingles (Herpes Zoster)
- Tetanus (Lockjaw)
- Whooping cough (pertussis)

Classification of Allergy (Hypersensitivity)

The most accepted classification of hypersensitivity is given by Gell and Coombs.

They have put hypersensitivity into following types:

- *Type 1:* Immediate
- *Type 2:* Cytotoxic

**Autoantigen:* Autoantigens are antigens present in the body that can start antibody formation in the body. That have manufacture them they are also called self-antigens. They are present in proteins, their compounds, deoxyribonucleic acid (DNA), and ribonucleic acid (RNA). They produce autoimmune diseases.†

†*Autoimmune disease:* The normal immune system protects the body against invading microbes. When the body with an intact immune system recognizes these bodies, it releases antibodies to fight them. In cases of autoimmune disease, the immune system fights against normally present tissues. Some of the common examples of autoimmune diseases are:

There are many autoimmune disorders that affect the eyes.

- Rheumatoid arthritis (RA)
- Multiple sclerosis (MS)
- Thyroid diseases
- Behçet's disease. This rare autoimmune disorder is a leading cause of blindness in some developing countries.
- Reiter's syndrome.
- Sjögren syndrome

- *Type 3:* Immune complex mediated hypersensitivity.
- *Type 4:* Delayed cell mediated
- *Type 5:* A recently added types by Rajan.

Clinical Features of Various Types of Allergy

Type 1 (Immediate)

When already sensitized cells come in contact with a specific antigen; a chain of reactions starts that includes the attachment of IgE to mast cells, which triggers degranulation of mast cells and the release of chemical modulators. To this are added chemo tactics—stimulating factors, i.e., histamine, and prostaglandin, resulting in the release of inflammatory cells, causing allergic disorders. In cases of allergic conjunctivitis, the usual path is as follows:

Allergen → Dissolved in tear film → Allergen + IgE antibody → Mast cell degranulation → Release of chemical mediator → Clinical presentation.

Type 2 (Delayed)

It is an antibody reaction where IgG and IgM act against antigen present in cell wall causing cell damage, examples are cicatricial pemphigoid and Mooren's Ulcer.

Type 3 (Delayed)

It involves the interaction of IgG, IgM, and IgA with antigens. It forms an immune system. The examples are Stevens-Johnson syndrome, immune corneal ring, and marginal corneal infiltrate.

Type 4 (Cell-mediated)

The cell mediation is through T lymphocytes and not antibodies; hence, it is called cell-mediated hypersensitivity. It is a delayed hypersensitivity. Examples include phlycten, corneal allograft rejection, and contact dermatitis.

Allergic Disorder of Eye

Allergic disorders of the external eyes are confined to the ocular surface and the epithelium of the skin of the lids. The surface epithelia involved in allergic disorders are the conjunctival corneal epithelium. The allergic disorders are multifactorial, with common complaints of itching, redness, chemosis, watering, mucoid-to-ropy discharge, and running of the nose.

The allergic involvement of external eyes is very common; about one-fifth of the population in various age groups suffer from allergic conjunctivitis at some point in their lives. They are seen in all races and both sexes. Some of the disorders may show a particular preponderance in some races with geographical and weather variation; they are more common in childhood and adolescence and are generally bilateral and symmetrical. May be acute or chronic. The chronic cases can be persistent, long-term, or recurrent, some of the conditions are self-limiting and may pass off as the child ages with extensive or little treatment (spring catarrhal).

The allergic diseases have two phases, i.e., the initial phase consisting of acute onset, and the other that follows is a chronic phase. In the first phase, there is the release of antigen-mediated granules and the release of histamine and histamine-like substances.

In the second phase, there is the release of proinflammatory mediators and immune cells.

The allergic manifestation of the external eyes can be any of the following, either alone or in combination:

- Conjunctivitis
- Keratoconjunctivitis
- Keratopathy
- Blepharoconjunctivitis
- Blepharodermatitis

Most of the allergic conditions are nonvision-threatening; however, some can be potentially incapacitating. They are not curable, but most of them are manageable. The management may be as short as a few hours, i.e., acute allergic conjunctivitis, to years, as in vernal conjunctivitis. Some of the allergic conjunctivitis patients have a positive family history. They may be associated with atopia, both in parents or members of the family.

They are influenced by race, age, sex, weather, family history, and varied allergens. An allergen that causes a severe reaction in one person may have no effect on another person.

Out of four types of allergies, type 1 and type 4 are more common than types 2 and 3 to cause allergic diseases of the outer eye.

In spite of their being so common, there is no satisfactory categorization of allergic diseases of the ocular surface. The most suitable classification used is given by Gell and Coombs, which gives clinical features of various allergic ocular diseases.

Gell and Coombs divided allergy into four types with distinct features that have been discussed earlier.

ALLERGIC CONJUNCTIVITIS

Allergic manifestations of conjunctiva are very common; they constitute the largest group of external ocular diseases next only to infection in children. They have been blamed for being an important cause of absenteeism from school among children.

The allergic conditions that inflict conjunctiva are topographically divided into four groups.

1. Conjunctival
2. Limbal
3. Keratoconjunctival
4. Keratopathy

The allergic conditions are:

- *Seasonal:* Acute and chronic; the first example is hay fever conjunctivitis. An example of the second is perennial allergic conjunctivitis
- Vernal conjunctivitis (spring catarrh)
- Atopic conjunctivitis
- Giant papillary conjunctivitis (GPC)
- Cicatricial pemphigoid
- Stevens–Johnson syndrome
- Chronic graft versus host disease

The other classification is based on the types of hypersensitivities that have been mentioned earlier. It has been observed that most of the allergic conjunctivitis is nonvision-threatening, but the reverse is also possible.

Table 14.1 *mentions the various nonvision-threatening allergic conjunctivitis.*

The vision-threatening allergic conjunctivitis are:
Severe vernal keratoconjunctivitis (VKC), atopic keratoconjunctivitis, Stevens–Johnson syndrome, and cicatricial conjunctivitis.

TABLE 14.1: Nonvision-threatening allergic conjunctivitis.

Conjunctivitis	*Age*	*Type of allergy*
Seasonal conjunctivitis	All ages	Type 1
Perennial allergic conjunctivitis	All ages	Type 1
Giant papillary conjunctivitis	Adults	Types 1 and 4
Phlycten	Children and adolescents	Type 4
Vernal keratoconjunctivitis	Children and adolescents	Type 1

Acute Allergic Conjunctivitis in Children

Acute allergic conjunctivitis constitutes about 75% of all allergic conjunctivitis at all ages. The terms acute seasonal conjunctivitis and hay fever conjunctivitis are used interchangeably. The condition is seen worldwide in all races and both sexes. It is generally bilateral; occasionally, the patient may present with unilateral involvement with a history of atopy in the family. The causative factor is a concentrated amount of external allergen floating in the air. The allergen gets mixed with tears to activate the mast cells.

The common allergens blamed are pollen, mites, animal dander, and aeroallergens. Many times, it is not possible to identify the offending allergen. The condition is benign, nonvision-threatening, short-lived, and self-limiting. The first episode is pretty frightening; the patient gets accustomed to subsequent episodes. The child may even learn to identify and avoid the allergen.

The episodes are acute in onset and consist of a foreign body sensation with copious watering but little itching. Running of the nose is common. Conjunctiva initially becomes glossy, followed by chemosis.

The chemosis may force the swollen conjunctiva through the interpalpebral fissure and overhang the cornea from all sides. The cornea itself is not affected.

Though the condition is self-limiting, a drop of a water soluble steroid is often sufficient to ameliorate the condition. Other drugs used are local vasoconstrictors and local antihistamines.

Perennial Allergic Conjunctivitis

These are chronic forms of seasonal allergic conjunctivitis, less common in children. The causative factors are persistent allergens to which the child is exposed. It lasts throughout the year and is confused with chronic bacterial, chlamydial conjunctivitis, or ocular surface disorders. It shows exacerbations and remissions. The etiopathogenesis of perennial allergic conjunctivitis is similar to seasonal allergic conjunctivitis; both are caused by the degranulation of mast cells, which results in the release of prostaglandin, histamine, leukotrienes, cytokines, and many more chemicals.

The condition is generally bilateral, giving a chronically red eye, mild-to-moderate persistent itching without ropy discharge that is characteristic of VKC. There may be excoriation of the canthi. The cornea remains unaffected, as do other ocular surfaces.

Management is frustrating. No specific treatment is available; the condition is mostly self-limiting; a change of residence or workplace may bring dramatic relief, recurrences are common. The best solution is to identify the allergen and avoid it, which is easier said than done; desensitization is of limited value. The present practice is to use antihistamine drops and lubricants many times a day for a long time. Steroids are best avoided.

The mainstay of treatment is the following, either alone or in combination:

Local Antihistamine Drugs

H1 antagonists' drugs that are used to treat allergic conjunctivitis are: promethazine, pheniramine, pyrilamine maleate, antazoline, levocabastine, and olopatadine. Fexofenadine, levocitrizine, and desloratadine—the last three—are not available as drops; they are used orally. Three commonly used H1 inhibitors are levocabastine, olopatadine, and bepotastine. Besilate levocabastine 0.05% drops is a second-generation H1 histamine inhibitor that is available without an added decongestant effect. It is a fast-acting drug with a prolonged effect. It is more effective than mast cell stabilizer alone; however, it is also available in combination with mast cell inhibitors with the presumption that they will enhance each other. It is used four times a day.

Olopatadine

The most commonly used drug in this group is olopatadine; given as 0.1% drops two times a day or 0.2% drops in the morning. In recalcitrant cases, olopatadine may be used in concentrations as high as 0.7%. The higher doses are used as prophylaxes. It is a selective H1 inhibitor with the added advantage of a mast cell-stabilizing effect.

Mast cell stabilizer: These drugs prevent the degranulation of mast cells, thus preventing the release of histamine and allied substances. They are neither antihistamines nor vasoconstrictors; they are available as 2% and 4% drops known as sodium cromoglycate and disodium cromoglycate. Other mast cell stabilizers available are:

- *Lodoxamide:* It is a strong mast cell stabilizer, far more than the former two. It is available as a lodoxamide tromethamine suspension (0.1%) to be used three times a day.
- *Nedocromil:* This is a less commonly used mast cell stabilizer available as a 2% solution to be used three times a day.

Local decongestants: They have no effect on hypersensitivity; they lack mast cell stabilizing properties and the properties of antihistamines. They cause immediate vasoconstriction, giving the false impression of a white eye, which is of short duration and is in fact flowed by rebound dilatation of vessels.

Steroids: Local steroids are usually not required; they are used to give prompt relief more for social requirements than therapeutic regions.

Lubricants have no therapeutic value in combating allergies; all they do is smoothen the ocular surface. Children rarely require them.

Nonsteroidal anti-inflammatory drugs (NSAIDs) are mostly used as systemic analgesics and anti-inflammatory drugs. They do not have any antihistamine effect; they are used to relieve mild-to-moderate itching alone or with antihistamines and to substitute a steroid when contraindicated, most commonly used NSAID is ketorolac 0.4%.

VERNAL CONJUNCTIVITIS (SPRING CATARRH)

This is a common allergic conjunctivitis, neither restricted to the spring season (vernal) nor a catarrh in its true sense. It is seen throughout the year in susceptible children the world over with acute exacerbations, remission, and a protracted course. The acute symptom depends on the quantity and type of allergen in the ambient atmosphere. It is worsened with the release of pollen at the end of winter and beginning of summer, thus called spring catarrh. However, besides pollen, other aeroallergens, i.e., dust, animal dander, mites, and fabric too can cause vernal conjunctivitis; it waxes and wanes with change of season or change of habitation. Exacerbations may be worse than the original attack. The condition may have a positive family history of allergic disorders and may be present in siblings. It is a type 1 hypersensitivity that is cell-mediated; TH2 cells have constantly been thought to be the key factors. Besides the cells, IgE and IgG too play an important role; there is a fivefold rise of histamine in tears during an attack.

It is the most common type of allergic conjunctivitis in children; the allergen being exogenous, the disorder is bilateral, and it may start in one eye. When bilateral, it may be asymmetric; spring catarrhs of early onset and prolonged course are more likely to be symmetric. It is more common in boys; girls are not immune.

80% of children are under 10 years of age when presenting for their first consultation. The most common age group to be inflicted is between 5 and 10 years. However, it has been seen in children as young as one year old. The severity and recurrence gradually wanes as the child reaches teens. Surprisingly, the incidence is equalized among boys and girls as their age.

The disease can be put into two broad age groups on the basis of age of onset.

- A more common variety in prepubescents. It is called type 1.
- A less common postpuberty variety called type 2 is seen equally in both sexes; the type 1 group has an average duration of 5–6 years, while type 2 has a shorter period of more intense suffering of 1–2 years. Some authorities consider the type 2 variety to be a modified form of atopic conjunctivitis.

There may be a history of frank spring catarrh in one of the parents. The involvement of the father is more common; less common is the involvement of siblings. It is more common to have a history of atopia in the family.

Topographically, spring catarrh can be:

- Conjunctival
- Limbal
- Corneal (Rare)
- Mixed (1+2)

Clinical Features

Symptom

The most common symptom for which a child is brought to an ophthalmic clinic is itching in both eyes. In the initial days, the itching is mild and tolerable; gradually, its intensity increases. One eye may itch more than the other initially. Later, both eyes become equally itchy. Itching is associated with redness of the eyes; redness increases following itching.

The vicious cycle goes on, causing social embracement for the child and worry for the parents.

> The child rubs the yes because they itch; they itch because the child wants to rub.

The itching is limited to waking hours more in bright light, the child is never awakened due to itching; however, he finds it difficult to open the eye after sleep, which is referred to as morning misery, which is an active state of spring catarrh with severe blepharospasm and ropy discharge, leaving the child miserable on awaking. The lids do not get stuck, as in bacterial conjunctivitis. Itching is associated with ropy discharge; the child learns to pull the ropy discharge only to get another crop of similar discharges. The child, in an attempt to remove the discharge, may injure the bulbar conjunctiva, worsening already present hyperemia. The tears are alkaline in nature, hence the excoriation of both canthi.

The lids, due to the weight of the tarsal papillae, develop mild pseudoptosis that gives a sleepy appearance **(Fig. 14.1)**.

The skin over the lids has a darker hue than normal, which is a matter of concern among girls.

Signs

The signs of conjunctival spring catarrh depend on the part of the conjunctiva involved. The most common part to be involved is the upper tarsal conjunctiva, followed by the limbus and lower tarsal conjunctiva; the fornices and bulbar conjunctiva are not involved much. Unfortunately, the term limbal spring catarrh is often used as a synonym for bulbar conjunctivitis. The classical lesion of spring catarrh is a papilla.

The papillae of spring catarrh are spread all over the tarsal conjunctiva irregularly; they first appear on the upper tarsal border and gradually spread toward the lashes without involving the lid margin. The papillae are polygonal structures with a flat surface; flatting is more evident at places where they are compressed between the tarsus and the globe; hence, the papillae on the lateral edges are not flat but pointed. Papillae are never round-topped, in contrast to follicles.

A typical papilla has a tuft of conjunctival vessels covered by conjunctival epithelium without lymphoid tissue **(Fig. 14.2)**.

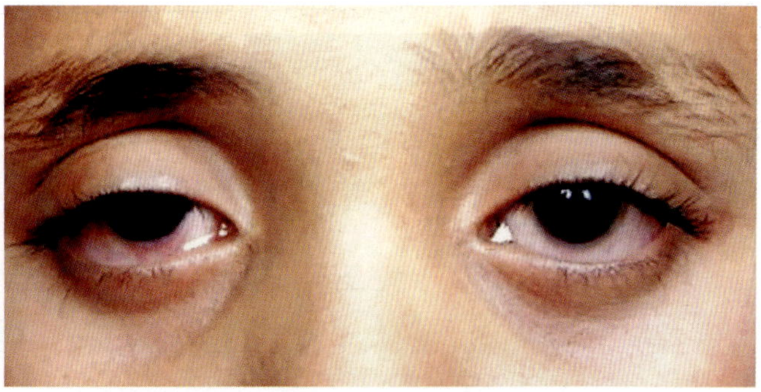

Fig. 14.1: Bilateral moderate ptosis due to spring catarrh.

This is in contrast to this—the central core of the follicle is lymphoid tissue covered by epithelium without vessels, and the conjunctival vessels skirt the follicle on their outer surface.

The size of the papillae of the spring catarrh varies from <1 mm to 3–4 mm. Papillae larger than 3.00 mm are called giant papillae and are seen in severe untreated spring catarrh and GPC **(Fig. 14.3)**. The papillae of VKC have been put into four grades according to their size.

Grades of Papillae in Spring Catarrh

- 0—no papillary reaction
- 1—few papillae (0.2 mm)
- 2—papillae^{++} (0.3–1.0 mm)
- 3—papillae larger than 1.0 mm all over the tarsal conjunctiva or all-round cornea.
- 4—papillae >3.00 mm

A lid can have papillae of varied sizes; generally, the smaller occupy the central part of the tarsal conjunctiva. The larger papillae assume a cobblestone appearance.

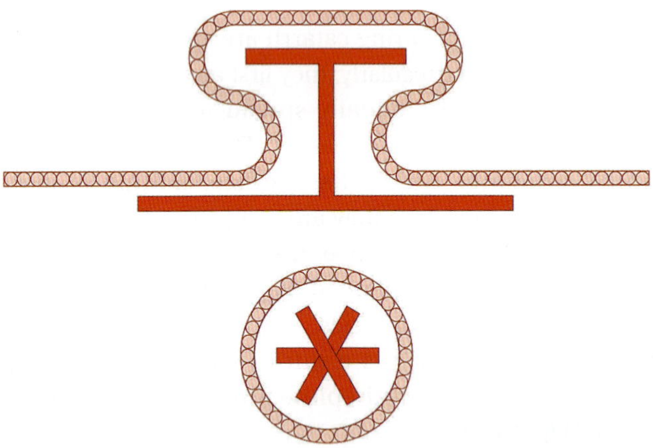

Fig. 14.2: Structure of a typical papilla of spring catarrh.

The papillae do not coalesce with each other; there is a gap between adjacent papillae. The coble stone papillae invariably contain ropy discharge that can be pulled out without much effort. The child learns to pull them out only to get another crop of stringy discharge. The flat-topped papillae with white ropy discharge in the crevices have been given the condition name "milk spilled over coble stone." The superficial surface is slimy due to a thin layer of mucus that forms a pseudomembrane. The pseudomembrane gives a velvety appearance, often referred to as the Maxwell–Lyons sign. Though the membrane is loose occasionally, it can be deep, causing scarring and extending into the fornix.

The spring catarrh is a self-limiting disease; hence, the papillae may regress even without treatment, either due to a change in weather or the absence of allergens. The papillae automatically regress and disappear as the child reaches adulthood without leaving any scars. Which is characteristic of trachoma and cicatricial conjunctivitis, both not seen in children.

Limbal form of Spring Catarrh

This can be an independent entity or associated with the tarsal form. The combination of the two is commonly referred to as a mixed type. Both share the same etiology of type 1 hypersensitivity to exogenous allergens. Occasionally, the presence of atopy, either in the child or parents, is possible. The isolated tarsal form is not sight-treating, while the limbal form may cause a diminution of vision. The causes of this are pannus formation, ocular surface defects, and astigmatism. The limbal form is more common in persons of Asian and African origin.

The lesion develops more commonly on the upper pole, followed by the temporal, nasal, and lower poles in succession; it may not always encircle the cornea **(Fig. 14.4)**.

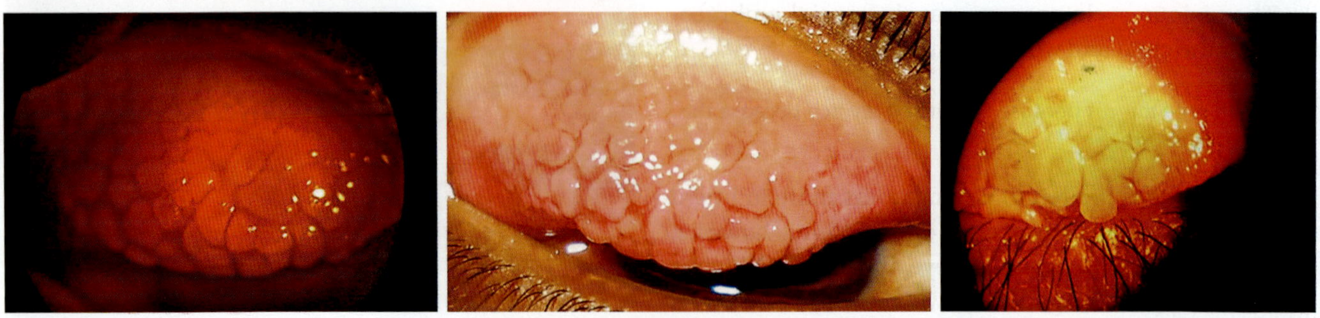

Fig. 14.3: Papillae of various sizes in spring catarrh.

The lesions differ in appearance from tarsal forms, which are flat-topped; in contrast to limbal lesions, which are rounded and confluent, consisting of more eosinophils and fewer vessels, they do not assume cobble stone appearance, may cause superficial pannus and peripheral corneal opacification called pseudogerontoxon, pseudo arcus, or cupid bow. It does not form a complete circle but is segmental. It is due to a lipid deposit in the cornea. It is known to wax and wane; the other condition where such lesions are seen is atopic conjunctivitis.

In the long run, they degenerate to produce Trantas-Homer spots if not treated **(Fig. 14.5)**.

Trantas spots: Develop mostly at the upper limbus as white raised dots formed by the accumulation of degenerated epithelial cells and eosinophils. Limbal stem cell deficiency is supposed to be the main factor causing them; stem cell deficiency is also thought to be responsible for pannus formation and even responsible for frank superficial vascularization. The Trantas spots are short-lived and self-limited. They are not seen in tarsal form; the limbal spring catarrh has a more prolonged course and is more likely to develop corneal complications.

Corneal Involvement in Vernal Catarrh

Involvement of the cornea is an extension of the limbal form of long standing. Besides the usual symptoms of conjunctival vernal catarrh, it is associated with out-of-proportion lacrimation. In contrast to conjunctival lesions, corneal lesions are associated with photophobia, foreign body sensations, and blurring of vision.

The probable causes of diminished distant vision in vernal catarrh are—irregular myopic astigmatism, mild-to-moderate keratoconus, superficial vascularization, Shield ulcer,* and corneal plaque.†

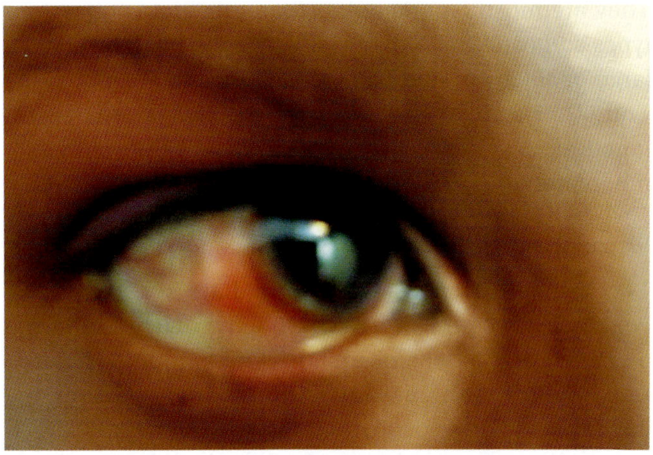

Fig. 14.4: Limbal lesion in spring catarrh.

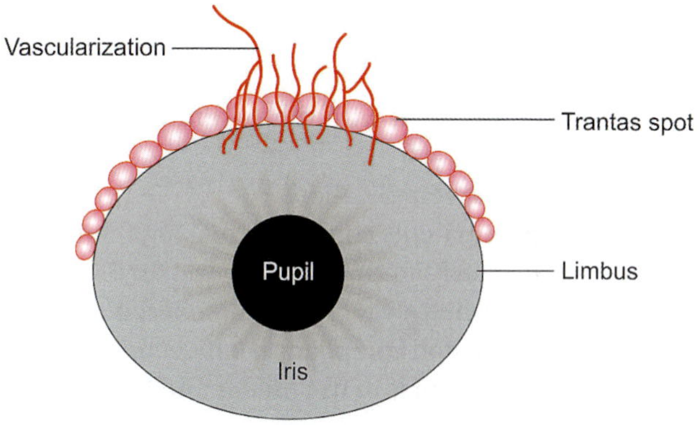

Fig. 14.5: Trantas spots.

**Shield ulcers* are rare occurrences seen in long standing untreated spring catarrh in late teens and early adulthood. Commonly situated between the upper border of the pupil and the upper limbus, it has an irregular geographical shape caused by the de-epithelization of the cornea by tarsal papillae and toxic substances released from the inflammatory modulators. They are noninfective breaches in the corneal epithelium; they occur in about 3% of cases. Shield ulcers are preceded by superficial punctate keratitis that leads to a break in the corneal epithelium.

The shield ulcer has been clinically divided into three grades. The first consists of irregular edges with a clear base; the second grade is the accumulation of inflammatory cells on the base, making it translucent or opaque; and the third grade is the development of a plaque.

The ulcer may require adding topical cyclosporine (0.05%) as drops four hourly daily along with treatment with steroids and artificial tears. It takes about 3 weeks to be effective; the healed ulcer leaves a superficial opacity, hampering vision.

†*Corneal plaque:* Plaque formation in spring catarrh is rarer than Shield ulcers. They comprise of thickened mucus deposited on the superficial punctate keratitis. They are white in color, raised on the surface without vascularization, not staining with fluorescein, and may be single or multiple. The plaque can be removed by spatula or even picked up by forceps, leaving a raw area. That is treated either by bandage contact lenses or a more common pad and bandage. The treatment consists of prevention through the use of steroids and lubricants. Once the plaque has developed, it does not respond to steroid alone; it requires the addition of acetylcysteine in 10–20% drops, 1–4 times daily. This does not dissolve the plaque but loosens the adherence of the plaque to the epithelium. The conditions other than spring catarrh that can cause corneal plaque are herpes zoster, keratoconjunctivitis, sicca, recurrent corneal erosion, and Sjogren syndrome, none of which are seen in children.

A summary of corneal involvement is:

- Pannus in the upper cornea.
- Superficial punctate infiltration is the earliest and most common corneal involvement due to the release of inflammatory substances. It is seen in 3–10% of cases.
- Microerosion
- Shield ulcer (ulcerative VKC)
- Plaque formation
- Keratoconus

This is a rare complication of vernal conjunctivitis, the exact cause of which is evasive. The most common argument put forward is disruption of corneal collagen due to repeated rubbing, causing microtrauma. This theory does not seem to be very convincing. The condition may be genetically predisposed.

Management of Spring Catarrh

Spring catarrh is a self-limiting disorder of childhood and adolescence. It cannot be cured. The aim of management consists of:

- The management of spring catarrh is very personalized.
- Counseling the parents.
- Alleviation of acute symptoms of itching and watering.
- Delay recurrence.
- Give maximum relief with the minimum amount of medication.
- Avoid iatrogenic complications.

Counseling for parents consists of making them aware that the disease is self-limiting and may last for 5–10 years, yet it cannot be wished away. The treatment requires their utmost cooperation and compliance. It must be impressed upon them that the aim is to use milder and less dramatic innocuous drugs rather than strong drugs like steroids that give prompt relief. The child in teens prefers to use steroids for dramatic relief from symptoms and social embarrassment. It may be impressed that steroids are potentially dangerous if used indiscriminately for long periods of time, which may lead to a gross loss of vision in the form of steroid-induced cataracts, glaucoma, and microbial keratitis. The worst offender being herpes simplex. A combination of cataracts and glaucoma is the most undesirable situation.

The various modalities are:

- Physical
    - *Cold compress:* The action of cold compress is not well understood, but most probably the vasoconstriction induced by cold helps in lowering the concentration of modulator. Cold may be applied three times a day, eye drops kept in the refrigerator are claimed to be more effective.
    - *Dark glasses:* Dark glasses help in reducing glare and photophobia.
- Therapeutic
    - Lubricant
    - Vasoconstrictor
    - Antihistamine—short-acting/long-acting
    - Local
    - Systemic
    - Mast cell stabilizer
    - Steroids—local/systemic
    - Nonsteroidal anti-inflammatory
- *Surgical:* Surgical methods have little use.

A short description of therapeutic agents used in the management of spring catarrh is given in the following text.

Lubricants

Lubricants are neither antipruritic nor anti-inflammatory. They are mostly marketed as tear substitutes of various types and combinations. They form a barrier between the large papillae and the pain-sensitive corneal epithelium. The other actions of lubricants are lavage of the conjunctival sac, diluting and removing histamine, and other modulators.

Vasoconstrictors

The vasoconstrictors cause immediate constriction of conjunctival vessels, giving a false sense of well-being and a cosmetically better look of short duration. Unfortunately, this is followed by vasodilatation, which worsens the appearance. All vasoconstrictions are adrenaline derivatives; adrenaline, being a physiological antagonist of histamine, causes vasoconstriction and has a mild antipruritic effect.

Antihistamine

Antihistamines used in ophthalmology are H1 blockers; however, now H2 inhibitors are being used concurrently with the presumption that they enhance each other's action by modulating cell growth and cell migration. H2 inhibitors are not available as local drops.

The antihistamine can be used either locally or systemically. The local drops are more frequently used due to more efficiency and ease of application. The systemic drugs can be used either orally or parenterally. The antihistamines are divided into three generations according to their efficiency and lack of side effects.

The first-generation drugs can either be long- or short-acting. *They are:*

- Brompheniramine
- Chlorpheniramine
- Dimenhydrinate
- Diphenhydramine
- Doxylamine
- Pheniramine maleate

All of them are not available as local drops; most of them are used either orally or by injection to combat systemic allergies. They are mild hypnotics that reduce vomiting and motion sickness. They have mild parasympatholytic action, hence causing dryness of the mouth.

The lists of second-generation antihistamines are:

- Cetirizine
- Fexofenadine
- Ketotifen
- Azelastine
- Acrivastine
- Astemizole
- Ebastine
- Mizolastine
- Terfenadine

Many of them are not available as local drops; their advantage over the first generation is their lack of sedation, parasympatholytic action, and long duration.

The lists of third-generation antihistamines are:

- Levocetirizine (Xyzal)
- Fexofenadine (Allegra)
- Desloratadine (Clarinex)
- Olopatadine
- Bepotastine

The newer antihistamines are:

Olopatadine, ketotifen, azelastine, epinastine, and bepotastine are the newer antihistamines out of them. Olopatadine is the most widely used antihistamine for allergic conjunctivitis. It is available as a clear solution in strengths of 0.1%, 0.2%, and 0.7%. It is a selective H1 receptor-blocking antihistamine without parasympatholytic action; hence, it does not cause mydriasis or dryness of the mouth. In addition to its antihistamine action, it is a mast cell stabilizer, preventing histamine release. It can be used during the active stage of spring catarrh and as a prophylactic agent in between. 0.1% is used twice a day, while 0.2 and 0.7% are used once a day. It is not used by children under 2 years of age.

Oral antihistamine: The role of oral antihistamines in the management of allergic conjunctivitis has been debated for a long time. The local antihistamines produce faster results as compared to systemic drugs; the oral tablets/syrups take more time to be effective and produce unwanted side effects such as dryness of the mouth, dryness of the conjunctiva, and sedation. Oral histamine, when used along with topical drops, enhances the effect of local drops. Out of all the systemic antihistamines, desloratadine and levocetirizine are more suitable. The oral antihistamines should be administered with usual precaution. They are known to potentiate the action of other antiallergic medicines such as mast cell stabilizers and steroids.

Mast Cell Stabilizer

They are collectively called cromones. The sensitized conjunctiva is rich in mast cells. The cromones prevent the influx of calcium. Thus inhibiting degranulation of the mast cells that inhibit the release of histamine and other chemical modulators. Their action is potentiated by local antihistamines. Some of the antihistamines have mast cell-stabilizing effects as well. The commonly used mast cell stabilizers are sodium cromoglycate, which is available as a 4% clear solution to be used 2–4 times a day, and nedocromil sodium, which is available as a 2% clear solution. The third mast cell stabilizer has a 2% disodium cromoglycate action, which is similar to sodium cromoglycate. Lodoxamide tromethamine is available as a 0.1% solution; it is far more potent than sodium cromoglycate.

Dual-action mast cell stabilizers have both antihistamine and antidegranulation effects; they are olopatadine, epinastine, and azelastine.

Nonsteroidal Anti-inflammatory Drugs

For systemic use, these drugs are used either orally or as injections for relief of pain and inflammation. They act as antiprostaglandin substances by inhibiting cyclooxygenase and lipoxygenase. They have less antipruritic action than antihistamine; they are available as local drops. The commonly used NSAIDs for allergic conjunctivitis are:

- Ketorolac 0.5% drops
- Diclofenac 0.1%
- Pranoprofen 0.1%
- Indomethacin 1%
- Flurbiprofen 0.03% and piroxicam 1%

NSAIDs are less effective than steroids; all of them are known to produce local burning, hence not as popular as antihistamines and steroids.

Steroid

Steroids are potent anti-inflammatory and antiallergic agents. They are available as local drops, subconjunctival injection oral tablets, and intramuscular injection. They are used to manage all types of allergic conjunctivitis, most commonly as local drops or ointments. The drops can either be a clear solution or a suspension. The suspensions have the disadvantage that the crystals in suspension get entangled with the papillae and act as foreign bodies, increasing inflammation. The drops are used at a frequency of as little as once a day to six times a day during waking hours; ointments are used at night. A stronger concentration should be used in exacerbations or when a lower strength in frequent doses is not effective. It is better to start with the weakest steroid in the lowest concentration at the least frequent doses and gradually increase the frequency. Stronger steroids are used only when this regime fails. The strong steroids used are dexamethasone, betamethasone, prednisone, and prednisolone. A common practice is to start with the steroid with the lowest constriction that gives the best result, add olopatadine BD to it, and gradually taper the steroid. When the best result is achieved, the steroids are discontinued, and olopatadine after 10 days. 0.1% olopatadine is replaced by 0.2% once a day and continues for 3 months in recalcitrant cases. 0.7% may be used for a shorter period.

Commonly used steroids are:

- Betamethasone sodium phosphate: 0.1%
- Dexamethasone sodium phosphate: 0.05–0.1%
- Prednisolone acetate: 1%
- Loteprednol etabonate: 0.2–0.5%
- Fluorometholone acetate suspension: 0.1% and 0.25%
- Rimexolone suspension: 1%
- Difluprednate emulsion: 0.05%
- Medrysone suspension: 1%.

Medrysone is hydroxymethylprogesterone. It is a synthetic glucocorticosteroid. Its structure is akin to progesterone without progesterone-like action.

Immunomodulator

Immunomodulation is defined as a change in the body's immune system by agents that increase or decrease its function. The drugs that bring about immunomodulation are known as immunomodulators or immunosuppressants. They are calcium inhibitors. Common immunomodulators used to treat allergic conjunctivitis are aspirin, cyclosporine, tacrolimus, and low-dose mitomycin. Cyclosporine and tacrolimus are the most commonly used immunomodulators, mitomycin and aspirin have not shown encouraging results.

Cyclosporine is the most use full drugs against T cell dependent immune mechanism. It is a natural product and a calcium inhibitor. It is available as a solution in strengths ranging from 0.05–2%. The other use of cyclosporine is to increase tear production in ocular surface disorders.

Tacrolimus

This is an immunosuppressant and immunomodulator; it is in fact a macrolide of fungus origin meant as an anti-rejection drug in organ transplants. It inhibits histamine release. It is 100 times more potent than cyclosporine in preventing histamine. It can be used with cyclosporine. It is available as 0.02%, 0.03%, and 0.1% ointments. It causes burning in the eyes initially, which passes off in due course. Besides allergic conjunctivitis, it is used in autoimmune diseases not responding to steroids, i.e., dry eye syndrome, scleritis, Mooren's ulcer, cicatricial conjunctivitis, and atopic conjunctivitis.

Allergic Manifestations of Conjunctiva in Adults

Seasonal and perennial allergic conjunctivitis are seen in all ages except extremes. Vernal conjunctivitis is exclusively seen in children between 3 and 10 years; becoming rare after puberty. Allergic conjunctivitis developing after puberty is less frequent, moderate in nature, lasting for 3–4 years, and difficult to treat, without family and personal history of atopy. *The other postpediatric allergic conjunctivitis are:*

- Atopic conjunctivitis
- Giant papillary conjunctivitis
- Cicatricial conjunctivitis

ATOPIC CONJUNCTIVITIS

Atopic conjunctivitis is far less common than VKC, more symptomatic with protracted course that may last for decades. It is rare before 20 years but has been reported in late teens as well. It is more common in males, bilateral, with frequent involvement of lids and paraorbital skin with other evidences of atopia in the patients, as well as positive family history. The most common associated atopic disease is atopic dermatitis. The patients are more prone to suffer from chronic allergic rhinitis and bronchial asthma. The common site of allergic dermatitis is lateral skin folds of neck, antecubital, and popliteal fossa. The condition is caused due to type 1 and type 4 hypersensitivities; the symptoms are similar to VKC but less pronounced. The common symptom are itching of the eyes, chromic redness, watering and ropy discharge similar to VKC dark hyperpigmentation of lids, sleepy eyes thickening of lid margin, staphylococcal anterior blepharitis, excoriation of skin at canthi, papillary hyper trophy, the papillae are smaller than seen in VKC they are more in lower lid.

The cornea shows gelatinous thickening, Trantas spot may be present. On long run super facial vascularization and peripheral ulcer may develop. The person is prone to develop atopic cataract.

Overall prognosis is less favorable than VKC. The treatment is more frustrating than VKC that consists of oral long-acting histamine, mast cell stabilizer and low dose nonglaucoma producing steroids. Immunosuppressive drugs such as cyclosporine and tacrolimus ointment are claimed to give good result. Oral steroid, cyclosporine, and tacrolimus may be started in consultation with dermatologist. Lubricants give frequently relief from ocular surface disorder.

Table 14.2 *shows comparison between VKC and atopic conjunctivitis.*

TABLE 14.2: Comparison between vernal keratoconjunctivitis (VKC) and atopic conjunctivitis.

Feature	*VKC*	*Atopic conjunctivitis*
Etiology	Types 1 and 4 hypersensitivity	Types 1 and 4 hypersensitivity
Atopia	May be present	Prominent feature
Laterality	Bilateral	Bilateral
Age	3–5 years	Above 20 years
Sex	More common in boys	More common in males
Seasonal variation	Rule	Year round
Itching	Severe	Mild
Blepharitis	Nil	Common
Hyperpigmentation of lid skin	Mild	Prominent
Papillae	Big, more in upper lid	Small, more in lower lid
Eczema lid	Absent	Common
Limbal involvement	Common	Less frequent
Trantas spot	Common	Less common
Shield ulcer	Common	Absent
Cataracts	Steroid induced	Atopic, may become worse with long-term use of steroid
Glaucoma	Steroid induced	Steroid induced
Conjunctival scaring	Absent	Common
Keratoconus	Less common	More
Association of herpes simplex	Nil	Possible

GIANT PAPILLARY CONJUNCTIVITIS

It is an iatrogenic allergic conjunctivitis due to the persistent presence of an allergen in the conjunctiva, which is a foreign body placed in the conjunctival sec for therapeutic purposes like contact lenses, monofilament sutures, etc.

The allergy is a reversible, delayed hypersensitivities reaction. The common foreign bodies that cause GPC are contact lenses, exposed monofilament sutures, artificial eyes, orbital prosthesis, scleral shells, scleral buckles, and stumps of cyanoacrylate adhesive. Even filtering blebs and limbal dermoids have been blamed.

Most of the time, it is not the substance of the foreign body but the protein present in them that acts as an allergen. All contact lenses can cause GPC, but ultra-thin, large soft contact lenses with low water content are more likely to cause GPC.

The exact cause of GPC secondary to contact lens is not well understood. *The various hypothesis are:*

Repeated trauma, antigen present in the roughened contact lens, allergy to contact lens material, deposit on the lens, poor lens hygiene, contact lenses left in the eye for a long time, sleeping with contact lens, lenses with a large diameter are more likely to cause GPC. Rigid lenses cause less GPC. GPC is not associated with atopy, family history is often absent.

The clinical features can be divided into two parts:

1. Milder prepapillary stage
2. Severe papillary hypertrophy stage

Prepapillary Stage

The earliest symptom is persistent itching even after the contact lens has been removed, mucoid discharge at both the canthi on awaking, and diminished vision by 1–2 lines.

Late symptoms include diminished vision even with contact lenses that had best corrected vision in the past; patients become aware of the presence of contact lenses, ropy mucus discharge; itching; and mild congestion of the conjunctiva. The conjunctiva is still transparent.

Papillary Hypertrophy Stage

Papillae develop in the upper tarsal conjunctiva; initially, they are small and indistinct from the papillae of VKC, gradually increasing in number and size. The lower tarsal conjunctiva is rarely effected. The conjunctiva is thickened and loses transparency. The epithelium over the flattened papillae breaks down and produces conjunctival ulcers that stain with fluorescein and rose Bengal, ropy discharge, thickening and hardening of the upper tarsus, pseudoptosis, sleepy appearance, gelatinous, limbal nodules, and superficial punctate keratitis. Absence of keratoconus is in contrast to VKC and atopic conjunctivitis. The condition may be bilateral. The condition has a protracted course unless the offending antigen is removed.

Management

The condition is better managed than VKC and atopic conjunctivitis.

The first step in the case of contact lens users is to remove the lens and fall back to spectacle correction; this simple step will alleviate most of the symptoms. Adding mast cell stabilizers and steroids gives prompt relief.

Once the symptoms have subsided, the contact lens may be started with proper lens hygiene. If needed, a different type of lens may be used.

The monofilament sutures, sclera implants, and other prosthesis may be removed to get prompt relief.

CICATRICIAL CONJUNCTIVITIS

They are a group of autoimmune bilateral diseases of conjunctiva seen in the fifth to sixth decade, except for drug-induced disease. The drug-induced disease may develop at any age. Cicatricial conjunctivitis is common in females; it may be localized to the eyes only or may have involvement of other mucosal surfaces and skins. A fully developed disease is potentially blinding. Traditionally, it has been divided into two broad groups, i.e., primary and secondary. Both types can be caused due either type 2 or type 3 hypersensitivity.

The conditions are best managed by internist and dermatologist. Ophthalmologist role is limited to preventing symblepharon, ocular surface disorder, and secondary xerosis of conjunctiva and cornea, secondary infection.

Table 14.3 shows comparison between conjunctivitis caused by various allergen their clinical feature and management in all ages.

PHLYCTEN

Phlycten is a common keratoconjunctival disorder in childhood. It is more common than other allergic keratoconjunctivitis. The main difference is in the nature of the allergen. In allergic keratoconjunctivitis, the causative allergen is exogenous and inert. In phlyctenular keratoconjunctivitis, the allergen is endogenous and microbial. In the past, tubercular protein was the most blamed antigen. Tubercular protein remains an important antigen in developing countries. The incidence of phlycten has not diminished much in developed countries where childhood tuberculosis has been mostly eradicated; this leads to a search for other organisms that may also share the blame.

Many organisms were investigated as causative factors; staphylococcal infection has pushed tubercular protein to the back seat. The other microbes that are now a days suspected to causing phlyctenular disease are *Streptococcus*, *Gonococcus*, *Haemophilus*, *Chlamydia*, coccidioidomycosis, and lymphogranuloma venereum.

In fact, any organism that can activate an immune reaction to an already sensitized conjunctiva will result in phlyctenular disease. The role of intestinal parasites is being given more importance presently. Other microbes and agents blamed for causing the disease are *Propionibacterium* acnes and human immunodeficiency virus (HIV).

The sensitization in the case of phlycten is a delayed hypersensitivity of type 4.

Phlyctenular disease is commonly seen between the ages of 3–10 years. Its incidence falls sharply after 7 years. Though it is a disease of childhood, rarely it can be seen in adults as well. In contrast to spring catarrh, which is more common in boys, phlyctenulosis is more common in girls. It is more common among undernourished children

TABLE 14.3: Clinical features of the different allergens causing conjunctivitis and their management.

Clinical condition	***Age***	***Sex***	***Onset***	***Season***	***Allergen***	***Symptoms***	***Therapy***	
							Definitive	***Preventive***
Acute allergic	All	Both	Hyper acute	All	Many	Foreign body (FB) sensation, watering, chemosis	Weak steroid solution	Avoid allergen
Seasonal allergic	All	Both	Subacute	Particular season	Variable	Hyperemia conjunctiva, mild itching	Mast cell stabilizer, steroid, or oral long-acting antihistamine	Nil
Spring catarrh	3–5 years	More in boys	Variable	Summer	Many	Intense itching, watering	Strong steroid for a few days, followed by a weak solution for months, and mast cell stabilizer	Nil
Atopic conjunctivitis	Any	Both	Chronic	Not specific	Not specific	Symptoms similar to recurrent spring catarrh	Weak solution steroid and mast cell stabilizer	Nil
Giant papillary hypertrophy	Any, more in adult of both sexes	Both	Chronic	Any	Contact lens, contact lens preservative, monofilament suture	Pseudoptosis, minimum itching, foreign body sensation, persistent redness	Change the contact lens and contact lens preservative; remove the offending foreign body	Remove contact lens

who have not been properly immunized and is known to be heavily infested by intestinal parasites. The phlycten can be unilateral or bilateral, simultaneous, or the other eye may be involved later. The bilateral cases are more severe than the unilateral ones.

The phlycten can be confined to the conjunctiva only or may involve the cornea as well, either as an extension from the limbus or, rarely, as a primary lesion. Out of all the lesions, limbal involvement is the most common and symptomatic, though it develops at the corneoscleral junction and does not involve the sclera **(Fig. 14.6)**.

Conjunctival phlycten can develop anywhere on the conjunctiva; a phlycten on the bulbar conjunctiva develops as localized congestion away from the limbus, more frequently on the lateral side; in a few days, at the center of congestion, the actual phlycten develops as a pinpoint nodule that enlarges to become a blister like nodule. It enlarges till it is about a millimeter or two in diameter with a smooth surface; in a few days, the surface ulcerates to form a crater. This stage lasts for another 2–3 days, then fades away without any scars. The phlycten on the bulbar conjunctiva is seen more than felt. It is painless and nontender. Initially, bulbar phlycten in teens may be confused with episcleritis. No organism has ever been isolated from a phlycten.

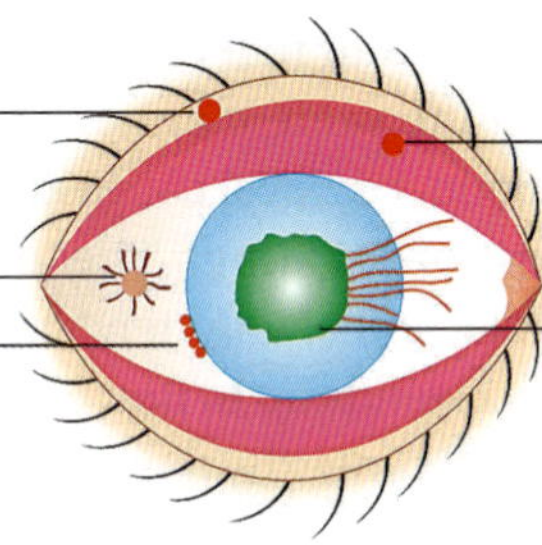

Fig. 14.6: Phlycten at various locations.

Phlycten on the tarsal conjunctiva is far less common and behaves like phlycten on the bulbar conjunctiva. A tarsal phlycten may rub on the cornea, and the patient may have a foreign body sensation. Phlycten on inter-marginal strip is the least common.

> Phlycten, in spite of being allergic, does not cause itching per se.

Limbal Phlycten

This is the most common form of phlyctenulosis and the most symptomatic. The clinical course of a limbal phlycten is the same as that of a bulbar phlycten, until it reaches the cornea. A limbal phlycten may be single or multiple; when more than one, they may be separate and independent of each other or may be confluent, forming a crescent of multiple phlyctens like sausage. Limbal phlycten may develop anywhere on the circumference of the cornea; its most common location is the lower limbus. The presence of multiple phlycten of various sizes is called miliary form, while a large ulcerative form is called necrotizing. Acute bacterial conjunctivitis is frequent with phlyctenular disease. It may precede phlycten or be concurrent. However, bacterial conjunctivitis never causes phlycten; at the most, it may be blamed as the cause of lowered resistance to herald hypersensitivities.

If a phlycten develops on the cornea or a limbal phlycten encroaches the cornea, it becomes more symptomatic than bulbar. So long as it does not cross over to the cornea, its presentation is similar to that of conjunctival phlycten.

Once a phlycten extends into the cornea, it becomes symptomatic, which consists of foreign body sensations, copious watering, localized redness, photophobia, and blepharospasm. In fact, phlyctenular keratoconjunctivitis produces the most severe blepharospasm in children; it is surpassed only by interstitial keratitis. The blepharospasm of phlyctenulosis may be so severe that it may require the use of local anesthetic agents in both eyes to open the eyes. A limbal phlycten sits astride the limbus, half on the conjunctiva and half on the cornea. A limbal phlycten behaves in the same manner as a conjunctival phlycten in its evolution, i.e., local congestion-development of phlycten-ulceration-healing. The only difference between the two is that limbal phlycten leaves a permanent opacity. The opacity extends up to Bowman's membranes. It is dome-shaped with convexity toward the pupil.

Corneal Phlycten

Cornea is mostly involved due to the extension of limbal phlycten toward the center of the cornea, or rarely as primary phlycten.

Corneal phlycten may be mistaken for peripheral corneal infiltrate; the differences between the two are that marginal ulcers are rare in children and always have a strip of clear cornea between the limbus and the lesion.

The phlyctenulosis of the cornea may result from a single limbal phlycten or multiple phlyctens. They take two forms, i.e.,

1. Diffuse infiltrative
2. Ulcerative

1. *Diffuse infiltrative:* Less common of the two. It is seen in the primary form of phlyctenular keratitis at the center of the cornea with moderate to heavy superficial vascularization, marked photophobia, and diminished vision.
2. *Ulcerative:* There are two forms, i.e., (i) Fascicular, (ii) Scrofulous.
   - *Fascicular* ulcers are exclusively seen in phlyctenular keratitis. It is not to be confused with pneumococcal keratitis, which is invariably associated with hypopyon. Fascicular ulcers are even devoid of anterior chamber reactions. The typical fascicular ulcer is generally single, a large ulcer that does not perforate, in contrast to the pneumococcal ulcer. It stains and leaves macular opacity after healing. It is an extension of the limbal phlycten and has a tendency to move centrally, accompanied by a leash of superficial vessels that develop in an epithelial furrow. An active fascicular ulcer is associated with severe photophobia and blepharospasm. The position where the fascicular ulcer will stop is uncertain. It may cross the pupil, causing diminished vision. Once the ulcer stops moving, it starts healing. A healed ulcer leaves a macular opacity, trailed by a linear opacity extending from the healed ulcer to the limbus. It represents the atrophied leash of blood vessels.
   - A scrofulous ulcer is a superficial, marginal ulcer similar to a catarrhal ulcer. The ulcer is formed by the breakdown of micro phlyctens inside the limbus; it heals spontaneously and is less frequent than fascicular ulcers.

Flowchart 14.1 depicts various types of phlycten.

Differential Diagnosis

- A limbal phlycten is not difficult to diagnose due to its clinical features of nodule/nodules at the limbus with marked photophobia and blepharospasm. All blepharospasm in children be suspected to be phlyctenular unless proved otherwise.
  Other causes of blepharospasm in children are:
  - Corneal abrasion
  - Corneal ulcer
  - Embedded foreign body in either in cornea or tarsal conjunctiva
  - Buphthalmos
  - Interstitial keratitis
  - Acute anterior uveitis
- Absences of itching differentiated it from spring catarrh.

Flowchart 14.1: Types of phlycten.

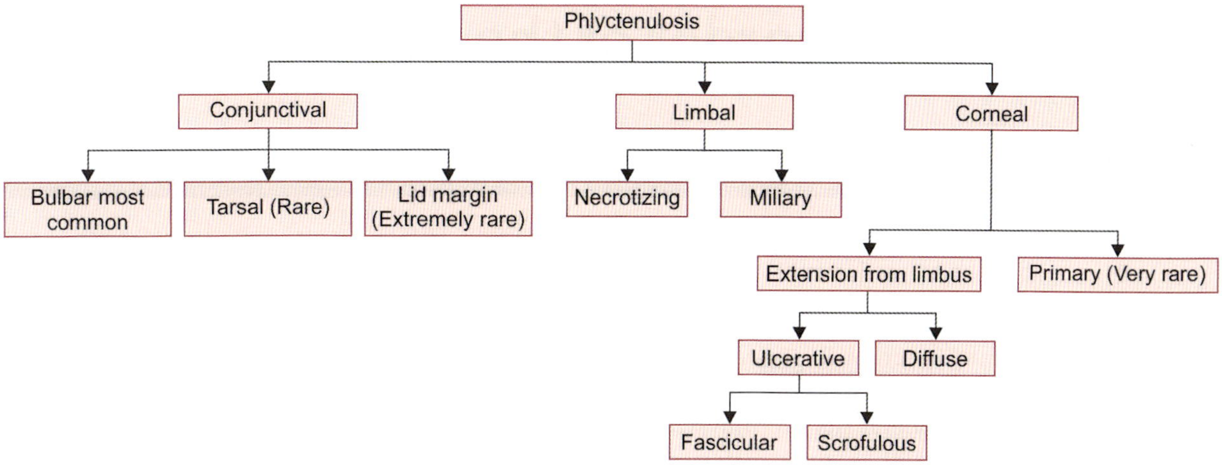

- Bulbar phlycten should be differentiated from episcleritis. Episcleritis is not seen under 10 years. Episcleritis does not move with conjunctiva.
- Tarsal phlycten and phlycten of lid margin required high degree of suspicion. A therapeutic trial with local steroids will alleviate these two.
- Corneal phlycten
    - Fascicular ulcer need to be differentiated form ulcus serpens; a pneumococcal infection of cornea that is always associated with severe anterior chamber reaction and hypopyon.
    - Peripheral phlyctenular infiltrates must be differentiated from catarrhal infiltrations, which are again rare in children.

Investigations

All children with phlycten in developing countries should be investigation for:

- Tuberculosis—by X-ray, chest, ESR, MT.
- Worm infection
- Protein caloric deficiency
- Immunization status

Management

- All types of phlyctens are self-limited.
- Phlycten are known to recur after treatment

- If the child is found to have tuberculosis, he should be treated in consultation with pediatricians.
- All children should be dewormed under the national program of deworming.
- Associated anterior blepharitis should be treated concurrently with phlycten, as should accompanying conjunctivitis. Children under 7 years old should be given oral erythromycin in consultation with pediatrician. Children above 7 are put on oral doxycycline 50 mg once a day for 15 days.
- All phlycten respond dramatically to steroid drops; this leads to the abrupt stopping of steroid, which is not desirable; steroid should be tapped as per protocol.
- Fascicular ulcers too respond to steroids without harm.
- All children with phlyctenulosis should get an additional dose of vitamin A.

SUGGESTED READING

1. Das S. Shield ulcer—a very rare presentation. Kerala Jr. Ophthalmology. 2017;29:244-7.
2. Dhawan M, Tania Hans, Sing B. Rebapide 2% ophthalmic suspension for treatment of allergic keratoconjunctivitis. Delhi Jr. Ophthalmology. 2006.
3. Khan MD, Kundi N, Saeed N, Gulab A, Nazeer AR. Incidence of Keratoconus in Spring Catarrh. Br J Ophthalmol. 1988;72(1):41-3.
4. Kumari R, Saha BC, Sinha BP, Mohan N. Tacrolimus versus cyclosporine: comparative evaluation as a first-line drug in vernal keratoconjunctivitis. Nepal Jr. Ophthalmol. 2017;9:128-35.
5. Rajan TV. The Gell-Coombs classification of hypersensitivity reactions: interpretation. Trends Immunol. 2003;24(7):376-9.
6. Singhal D, Sahay P, Maharan PK, Sharma N, Tityal JS. Vernal keratoconjunctivitis. Surv Ophthalmology. 2019; 64(3):289-311.

CHAPTER 15

Disorder of the Cornea in Children

The anteriormost transparent part of the globe is the cornea; its most important function is optical, with a maximum diopter. The other function is protective; it constitutes one-third of the globe. It sits over the scleral opening like a watch glass with convexity forward. The cornea is more curved than the sclera, with a curvature of 7.8 mm against a scleral curvature of 11.5 mm, giving it a bulging look. The junction of the cornea and sclera is the limbus of the eye. The apex of the curved cornea is 2.7 mm from the limbal plane; its area is 1.3 cm^2. Neither the diameter nor the curvatures of the cornea are equal in all meridians. Its horizontal diameter is 11.6 mm and its vertical diameter is 10.6 mm; this anomaly makes the cornea horizontally oval. The cause of this difference is brought about by the constant pressure exerted by the lids on the globe. This difference in curvature makes the vertical meridian more myopic, and the posterior surface of the cornea is more curved. This makes the central cornea thinnest; if the two corneal surfaces were equal, the two surfaces would have been parallel. The corneal thickness in the center is 0.5–0.6 mm and 0.6–0.8 mm on the periphery. The thin central cornea makes it more venerable for perforation. The central 3.00 mm in front of the pupil is the optical zone, which is almost spherical. Corneal diameters >12.7 mm and <10.00 mm are considered abnormal. The former is called megalocornea, and the latter is called microcornea. The cornea of a newborn is flatter than that of an adult; it is slightly more curved on the periphery as compared to adults.

The corneal diameter of the newborn is also less than the adult diameter, with an average diameter of 10.00 mm, which rapidly reaches adult size by 1 year. The interpalpebral aperture of a newborn being narrower than that of an infant, and the cornea of a newborn seems to be larger. The cornea of a newborn is slightly hazy; the haze clears within a few days; persistent haze is pathological.

The cornea comprises the following layers, which are not of equal thickness, diameter, or development. They are the epithelium, Bowman's membrane, stroma, Descemet's membrane, and endothelium. To this, a new layer has been added called Dua's membrane, which is an ultrathin layer of uncertain origin and composition. It lies anterior to the Descemet's membrane, with an average thickness of 10 μm. It is made up of collagen types 1 and 6, with abundant elastin that is far more abundant than anywhere in the cornea.

EPITHELIUM

This is the anteriormost layer of the cornea that develops from the surface ectoderm and is continuous with the conjunctival epithelium, receiving nutrition from the conjunctiva. This continuity makes the cornea vulnerable to infections from the conjunctiva. The anterior surface of the corneal epithelium is endowed with microvilli to anchor the tear film to the corneal surface. The epithelium is relatively impermeable to water-soluble substances; the other function of the epithelium is to ward off many microorganisms. The anterior surface of the corneal epithelium is endowed with microvilli to anchor the tear film to the corneal surface that cannot invade the corneal substance until the epithelium is intact. Some organisms that can evade this protective mechanism are *Gonococcus meningococcus*, *Corynebacterium diphtheriae*, *Shigella*, and *Listeria*. The corneal epithelium can be rubbed off with ease; it is very active mitotically, hence wounds of the corneal epithelium heal faster than other layers.

BOWMAN'S MEMBRANE

Bowman's membrane is formed by condensation of the anterior layer of the stroma. Its diameter is shorter than the diameter of other layers by 1.00 mm all-round. This is because its development is completed before the other layers develop. Bowman's membrane is easily destroyed and does not regenerate once destroyed. It does not mingle either with the conjunctiva or sclera, in contrast to other layers except the endothelium, which is a continuation of the uveal endothelium.

STROMA

The stroma of the cornea forms the largest bulk of the cornea, constituting 90% of the corneal substance. Its regeneration is followed by opacification.

DESCEMET'S MEMBRANE

The Descemet's membrane is the basal layer of the corneal endothelium; it is thinner in children as compared to adults. Its thickness increases with age; it can stand considerable external force and raised intraocular pressure; and it is relatively resistant to infections.

ENDOTHELIUM

The corneal endothelium is continuous with the iris endothelium; it is highly active metabolically. It is responsible for maintaining deturgescence of the cornea, which keeps the cornea transparent. Disruption of the corneal endothelium results in edema of the cornea. The causes that harm the endothelium are trauma, infection, inflammation, toxin, intracameral drugs, and dystrophies.

The nerve supply of the cornea is trigeminal via the ciliary nerve; the fibers reach the stroma from the sclera and conjunctiva. The cornea is very sensitive to pain; all sensations such as touch, temperature, and pressure are translated to pain. The corneal pain caused by external factors can be relieved by local anesthetic agents, but pain secondary to inflammation and raised intraocular tension is not abolished by local anesthetic agents.

The cornea, due to its high rate of metabolism, requires a constant supply of oxygen and nutrition. The oxygen dissolved in tear film is the main source. The tear also supplies other nutrition to the cornea. The oxygen supply is diminished when the lids are closed during sleep; the other source of oxygen is from the capillaries of the tarsal conjunctiva. The next sources of nutrition to the cornea are the limbal blood vessels, which are just sufficient for peripheral 1.00 mm; nutrition to the endothelium comes from aqueous in the anterior chambers.

The two functions of the cornea are:

1. Optical, for which the cornea should be transparent with a regular surface.
2. Protective function is provided by the toughness of the cornea, which is as strong as the sclera.

Corneal transparency is maintained by the following factors, which act in combination:

They are:

- Anatomical
- Optical
- Deturgescence
- Intraocular pressure

Anatomical

The cornea is devoid of any blood vessels, the nerve fibers are transparent, there are no pigments, the epithelium is multilayered, the cells are arranged in a regular fashion, and so are the fibers of the stroma. The Descemet's and Bowman's membranes are acellular, and the endothelium is single-layered with high metabolism.

The epithelial cells, in spite of long exposure to atmospheric air, remain nonkeratinized in normal conditions.

Optical

The cornea attributes the maximum diopter to the overall refractive power of the eye; the anterior surface is more important than the posterior surface because of the difference in refractive indices of the air and cornea. The refractive index of air is one, while that of the cornea is 1.38 μ, as against the refractive index of $n \approx 1.33$ *of aqueous*. The anterior surface of the cornea is not as smooth as it seems to be. Its irregularity is compensated by the tear film.

Deturgescence

To maintain transparency, the cornea needs to be in a state of relative deturgescence, or loss of deturgescence, is the cause of loss of transparency, which is brought about by the accumulation of fluid in the corneal substance. The relative dehydration is due to the active transfer of fluid from the stroma to the epithelium by way of the endothelial pump system in the stroma. Loss of endothelial cells due to any cause allows fluid to reach the stroma, causing edema and a loss of transparency.

Intraocular Pressure

Normal intraocular pressure is essential for the transparency of the cornea. A prolonged or sudden rise in intraocular pressure causes derangement of the endothelial pump system, causing edema of the stroma, which in turn passes the fluid into the epithelium, which may be thrown into bullae formation.

CHILDHOOD CORNEAL DISORDERS

Corneal disorders in children are frequent; many of them are preventable; others are treatable, remaining neither preventable nor treatable. Corneal disorders in children may be of short duration or may be permanent. Corneal disorders are some of the major causes of blindness in all ages. They may be uniocular or may involve both eyes simultaneously or separately. When bilateral, they need not be symmetric or concurrent; the cornea may be involved alone or with maladies of other structures of the eye or its adnexa. Systemic disorders may have a bearing on corneal disorders. Corneal disorders may be acute, chronic, symptomatic, or asymptomatic. Chronic, slowly progressive lesions are generally not painful. The corneal lesions may or may not be associated with pain or redness.

The corneal disorders in children are:

- Congenital anomalies
- Trauma
- Infection
- Inflammation
- Nutritional
- Degeneration
- Dystrophies
- Malignancies of the cornea are not known.
- Growth from conjunctiva at the limbus may invade the cornea; like limbal dermoid, premalignant lesions of conjunctiva may invade the cornea in adults.

The clinical features of corneal disorders in all ages may be any of the following, singly or in various combinations:

The common symptoms can be divided into two groups, i.e., active or dormant. *The symptoms of active lesions are:*

- Foreign body sensation
- Pain in the eye
- Lacrimation
- Photophobia
- Redness
  - Generalized
  - Localized (Circum ciliary)
- Diminished vision
- Visible opacity of the cornea

The symptoms of dormant lesions are:

- Diminished vision
- Visible corneal opacity
- Distortion of the cornea
- Squint
- Nystagmus

ETIOPATHOLOGY AND CLINICAL PRESENTATION OF CORNEAL DISORDERS

Corneal morbidities in children are similar to those seen in adults, with minor variation, i.e., phlycten, fascicular ulcer, interstitial keratitis, and keratomalacia, which are seen in children only.

The pathological presentation of corneal disorders can be:

- Morphological
  - Shape
  - Size
  - Curvature
  - Thickness
- Transparency
  - Opacity
  - Edema
  - Vascularization
  - Deposits
    - Anterior surface (see in the following text)
    - Posterior surface [KPs, red blood cells (RBCs), and malignant cells]
- Irregularity of the surface
- Loss of brightness—cloudy cornea
- Loss of sensation
- Vascularization
  - Superficial
  - Deep
- Associated with uveitis
- Raised intraocular pressure

Morphological Changes

Shape

A normal cornea on casual glance looks circular, which on careful examination will reveal that it is shorter in vertical meridian than horizontal. This is confirmed when measured by a corneal calliper, which may be mechanical or digital **(Fig. 15.1)**. In infants, it should be measured under short-term general anesthesia, along with the measurement of intraocular tension in suspected glaucoma. In school-going children, it can be measured

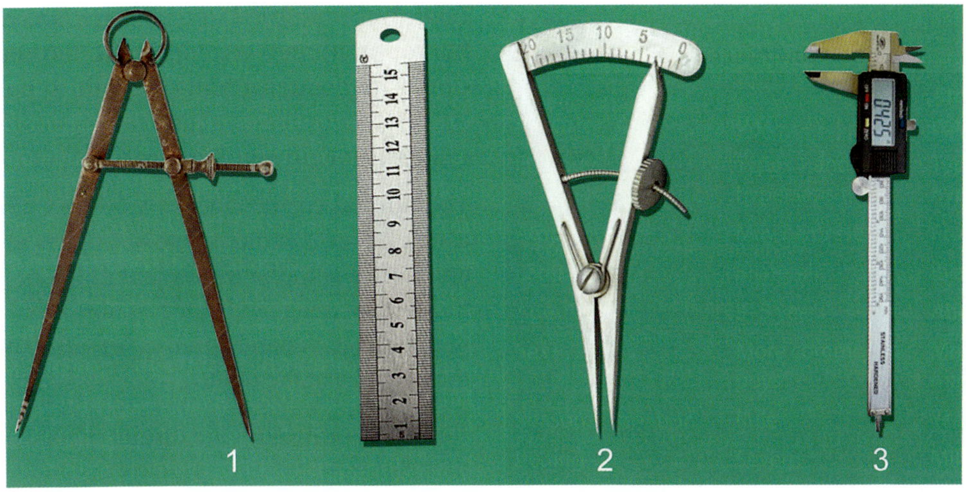

Fig. 15.1: Two types of corneal callipers. (1: Old type of calliper, which requires a separate scale to major. 2 and 3: self-recording corneal calliper)

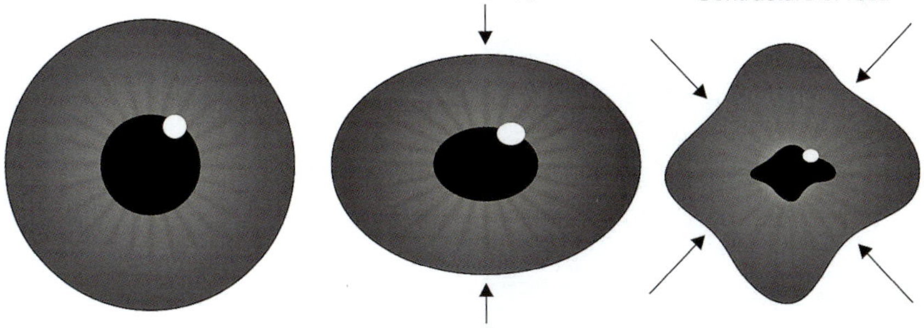

Fig. 15.2: Showing changes in shape, size, and curvature of the cornea in soft eyes. (1. Normal eye with a circular cornea and a central circular pupil. 2. Soft eye with a horizontally oval cornea and pupil. 3. Phthisis bulbi with quadrilateral globe, cornea, and pupil)

under topical anesthesia with little persuasion. The cornea becomes horizontally oval or quadrilateral in the phthisis bulbi and perforates the globe due to the pressure of the lids **(Fig. 15.2)**.

Figure 15.1 are examples of various types of corneal callipers.

The shape of the cornea becomes irregular due to growth at the limbus, i.e., papillae of the spring catarrh, limbal dermoid, corneal phlycten, intraepithelial epithelioma, and pterygium. The last two are not seen in children.

Size of Cornea

The average diameter of the cornea of a full-term normal baby is 10.00 mm, which assumes an adult size of 11.5 mm by 1–2 years. Too small or too large a cornea can be made out of simple oblique illumination. Measurement with a corneal calliper gives precise measurement. A cornea with an average diameter <10.00 mm is called a micro cornea; a microcornea in a microphthalmic eye may be as small as 2–3 mm **(Fig. 15.3)**. A cornea larger than 13.00 mm is called a megalocornea. A buphthalmic eye may be as large as 17–18 mm in diameter **(Fig. 15.4)**.

Change in Corneal Curvature

Corneal curvature is best and most precisely measured on a keratometer. A keratoscope gives a rough idea of changed curvature. Corneal curvature can be made out by looking from the temporal side while the child looks at a distant object. It is only natural that AC will deepen if the corneal curvature is increased, provided all other causes of deep anterior chamber have been excluded. A child with a grossly increased corneal curvature,

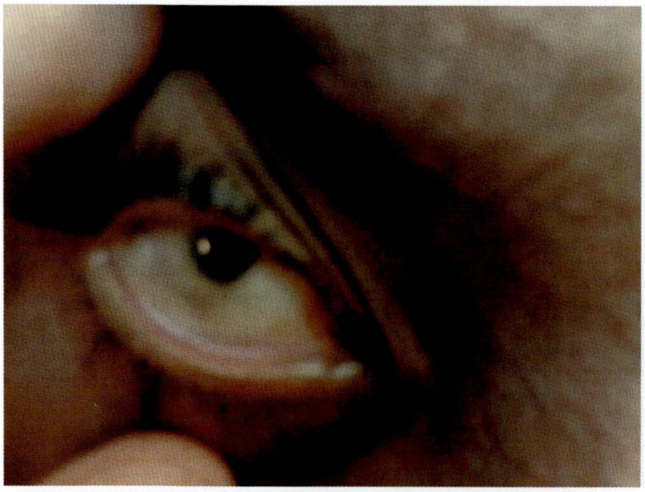

Fig. 15.3: Microcornea in microphthalmos.

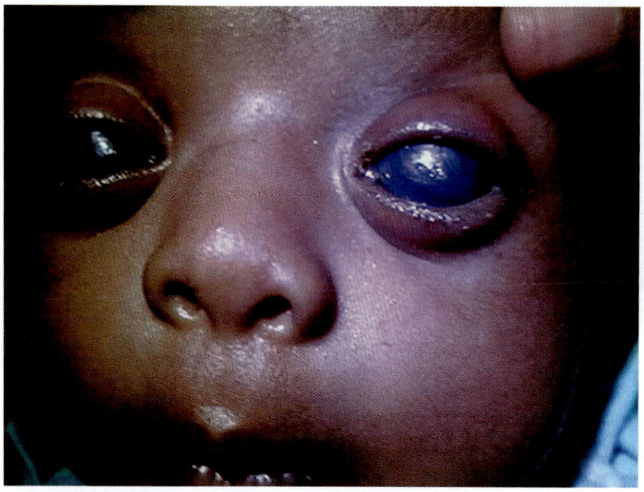

Fig. 15.4: Large cornea in buphthalmos.
Courtesy: Dr ML Garg.

when looking down the cornea, produces a dent in the lower lid called Munson's sign. Another sign that denotes increased corneal curvature is Rizzuti Benedict's sign.

Accurate measurement of corneal curvature is done by keratoscope, keratometer, photo keratometer, ultrasonography (USG), computed tomography (CT), and optical coherence tomography (OCT).

The most common cause of increased corneal curvature is keratoconus. Other causes are buphthalmos and keratoglobus. An irregular increase is seen in partial corneal staphyloma, and the lower part of the cornea bulges in pellucid degeneration (not seen in children; it develops in the third decade).

Causes of diminished corneal curvatures are: Microphthalmos, microcornea, cornea plana, sclerocornea, perforated globe, and phthisis bulbi.

Change in Corneal Surface

The normal cornea acts as a convex mirror that creates a small, erect virtual image of objects without distortion and moves with the movement of the object; distortion of the corneal image indicates an abnormal surface. The size of the image depends on the curvature of the cornea and the distance of the object.

> More is the curvature and greater the distance smaller is the image.

The normal cornea is covered by tear film and does not stain with any stain; it is only the tear film that stains, which is soon washed away. This property of staining of precorneal tear film is utilized in applanation tonometry, contact lens fitting, and noting tear break-up time. The corneal surface is very sensitive to pain; however, some irregularities are associated with diminished sensation.

Gross irregularities can be seen on oblique illumination; finer irregularities are seen on the window reflex, Placido's disc, keratoscope, keratometer, and computerized corneal topography.

The irregularities can be of partial thickness or may involve the whole depth of the substance.

The partial thickness irregularities are: Bullous keratopathy, superficial corneal opacity, deposits on the cornea, i.e., foreign bodies, band keratopathy, corneal plaque, radial keratotomy (RK), dermoid, phlycten, papillae of the spring catarrh, and pterygium (not seen in children).

Full-thickness irregularities are: Keratoconus, keratectasia, adherent leukoma, corneal staphyloma, intercalary staphyloma, and keratoplasty.

Changes of Corneal Brightness

Normal cornea should be bright and transparent a lusterless cornea is always associated with diminished vision. Loss of brightness may be short lived or permanent. Most common cause of lusterless of cornea is xerosis of cornea, other causes are—corneal ulcer, corneal opacity, superficial and deep vascularization, bullous keratitis, band keratopathy, stromal edema, corneal dystrophy degenerations, and deposits.

Change in Corneal Thickness

Cornea is not uniformly thick. It is thicker at the periphery and thinnest at the center. Which makes it more liable to be perforated in the center. The change in thickness can be uniform or localized. Increased thickness is less common than thinning of the cornea.

The most common cause of increased thickness is stromal edema. Stromal thickening is brought about by the loss of corneal deturgescence secondary to damage to the endothelium. Defective epithelium per se does not cause stromal edema as long as the Bowman's membrane is intact. Corneal dystrophies are other causes of increased corneal thickness.

The causes of decreased thickness are keratoconus and buphthalmos. As the thickness of the cornea is reduced in a corneal ulcer, it has a greater tendency to perforate. When it does not perforate, the intraocular pressure forces the thin cornea to bulge forward, resulting in descemetocele. Corneal thickness is measured by pachymeter, CT, and OCT.

Change in Corneal Transparency

The cornea, being part of optical media, must be transparent for good vision, loss of transparency of the central cornea is more deleterious than peripheral.

The common causes of loss of transparency are:

- Congenital
- Acquired

The cornea at birth is slightly hazy. The haze passes in a few days. If the haze persists, the cause should be explored, which may be:

- Birth trauma
- Buphthalmos
- Intrauterine infection
- Mucopolysaccharides
- Anterior chamber dysgenesis
- Limbal dermoid
- Congenital dystrophies
- Sclerocornea

The acquired causes are: corneal ulcers and their sequels; superficial and deep keratitis; corneal vascularization; adherence of the iris to the cornea; deposits on the cornea; epithelial down growth; corneal edema; bullous keratitis; corneal dystrophies; degenerations of the pterygium; and dermoid.

Vascularization of Cornea

The absence of vessels in the cornea plays an important role in maintaining corneal transparency, which is of utmost importance to its optical function. Cornea has fine vessels on the extreme periphery that do not encroach beyond 1.00 mm all-round on the periphery. The encroachment of vessels on the cornea is prevented by the compactness of the stroma and the antivascular factors present in the cornea. Once vascularization starts, it cannot be stopped by the administration of antivascular factors. The vessels once developed never disappear completely; they leave obliterated channels as ghost vessels, which are devoid of blood and remain visible on high-power slit lamps.

The factors that encourage corneal vascularization are:

- Trauma
  - Mechanical
  - Chemical
  - Unattended foreign body in the cornea
  - Lid deformity
  - Keratoplasty
- Infection
  - Trachoma (Superficial)
  - Syphilis (Deep)
  - Chronic blepharoconjunctivitis (superficial)
- Inflammation
  - Interstitial keratitis
- Allergy
  - Phlycten
  - Spring catarrh
- Hypovitaminosis B
- Ocular surface disorder
- Hypoxia
- Degeneration
- Keratoconus
- Mechanical (contact lens)

The above factors may act alone or in various combinations.

Corneal vascularization can be grouped into the following categories:

- Depth in cornea **(Fig. 15.5)**
  - Superficial (epithelial)
  - Deep
    - Stromal (interstitial)
    - Inter lamellar
    - Retro corneal

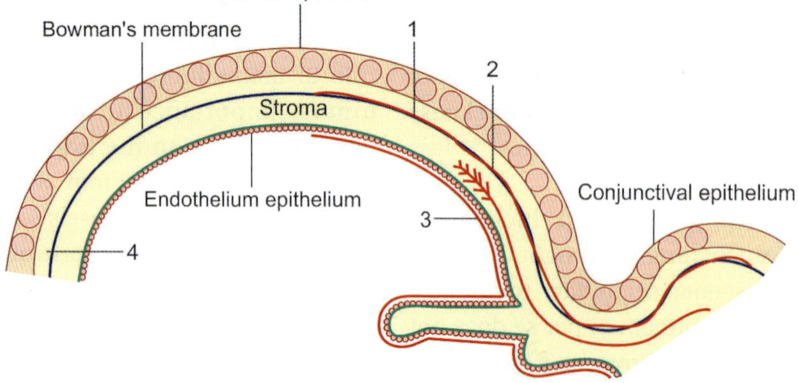

Fig. 15.5: Depth of two types of corneal vascularization.

- Extant from limbus
  - Micro pannus
  - Macro pannus
- Associated with conjunctival vascularization

Corneal Pannus

Corneal pannus is fibrovascular inflammation of the layers of the cornea. It is the ingrowth of fibrovascular tissue from the conjunctiva into the limbus. Encroachment happens between the epithelium and Bowman's membrane, resulting in the separation of the two that may sometimes destroy the latter.

The pannus develops in the upper part of the cornea, mostly; however, in severe cases, the whole cornea may be involved. The surface over the pannus looks rough and raised due to the encroachment of conjunctival vessels, which are tortuous and may anastomose with each other. The most common cause of superficial vascularization is trachoma. The other causes are acne, rosacea, eczema, alkali burn, phlycten, spring catarrh, toxins, and chronic blepharitis. The pannus formation is a protective process. It can be sectorial or large enough to cover the whole circumference. It generally involves the upper cornea. Pannus in the lower cornea is rare. The pathology of pannus formation is subepithelial.

According to activity, pannus can be progressive or regressive.

Progressive pannus is that superficial vascularization of the cornea in which infiltration extends beyond the end of blood vessels, denoting active inflammation. In contrast to this, in a regressive pannus, the encroaching blood vessels leave the infiltration behind **(Fig. 15.6)**.

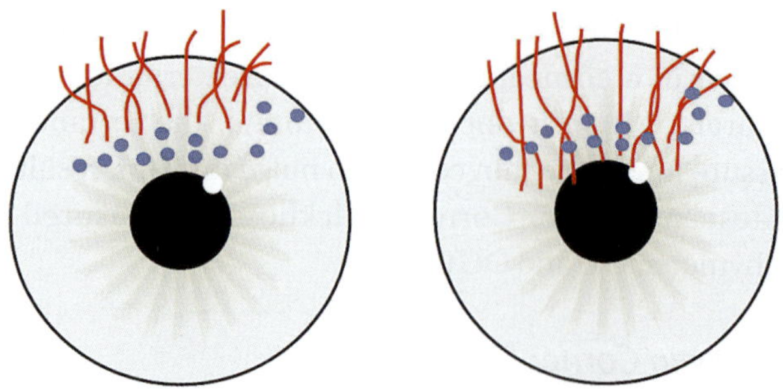

Fig. 15.6: Two types of corneal pannus.

TABLE 15.1: Classification of pannus.

Name	*Description*
1. Pannus crassus	Highly vascular, thick, and opaque
2. Pannus phlyctenulosis	Pannus is associated with phlycten
3. Pannus siccus	Poorly vascularized, dry appearances are seen in xerophthalmia
4. Pannus tenuis	Translucent, thin, and less vascular

Pannus per se does not require any specific treatment; treatment of the cause may enhance the regression of pannus. Applications of cryotherapy, heat cautery, or laser therapy have been used to treat heavy vascularization.

As per appearance pannus has been divided into classes as given in **Table 15.1**.

The above division is descriptive, more of academic interest than clinical. In a more practical division, the pannus has been broadly divided into two groups, i.e., the micro- and macro-pannus.

The *micropannus* occupies only 1 mm of the normal limbus; it is very common in noninfectious conditions

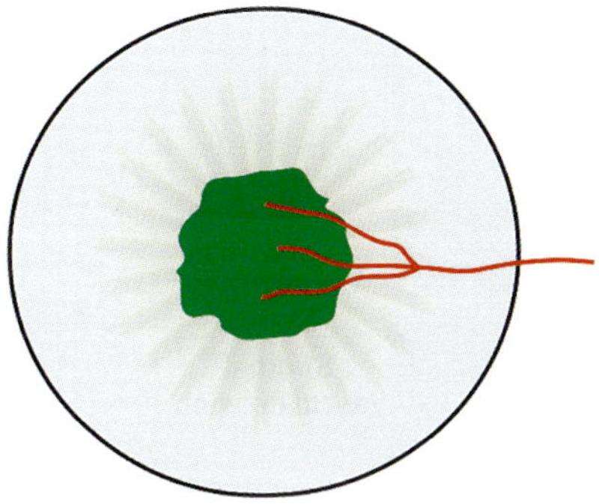

Fig. 15.7: Fascicular ulcer showing larger superficial vascularization and positive staining.

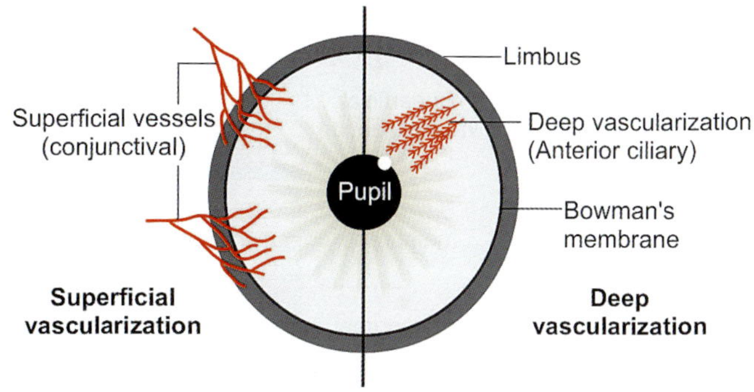

Fig. 15.8: Difference between superficial and deep vascularization of cornea.

like contact lens use. The other conditions are early stages of trachoma, spring catarrh, small phlycten, chronic blepharitis, and ocular surface disorder.

The *macropannus*, or gross pannus, is visible in diffuse illumination on oblique illumination without magnification; it extends beyond 2 mm of the limbus. The common causes are advanced trachoma, leprosy, phlyctenulosis, ill-fitting contact lenses, blepharo-conjunctivitis, severe riboflavin deficiency, herpetic keratitis, graft rejection, and fascicular ulcer.

Fascicular ulcers are seen in rosacea keratitis and phlyctenular keratitis. It is a superficial, large ulcer that is fed by 1–2 large tortuous vessels, visible without magnification. Extending from the conjunctiva to the ulcer. The ulcer has a tendency to creep from the periphery to the center **(Fig. 15.7)**.

Deep Vascularization of Cornea

Deep vascularizations of the cornea are far less common than superficial vascularization. They are caused by growth from anterior ciliary arteries at the level of the stroma without involving the epithelium or Bowman's membrane.

The characteristics are:

- They do not develop before 3–4 years of age.
- It may be unilateral or bilateral; some of the eyes have unilateral involvement and remain unilateral.
- When bilateral, they may be simultaneous or develop with a gap of a few weeks to months, symmetric or asymmetric, and one eye may be more involved than the other.
- The vessels enter the cornea under the Bowman's membrane; hence, when seen obliquely, there is a gap of about 1.00 mm between the visible vessels and the limbus **(Fig. 15.8)**.
- *The vessels are:*
  - Straight
  - Parallel to each other.
  - Branch at acute angle (Bottle brush).
  - They are sectorial in distribution.
  - The vessels remains in the same plan.
  - They impart pink color to the cornea called Hutchinson's salmon patch.
  - In severe cases may be accompanied by raised superficial vessels that have an epaulet appearance.
- The cornea has a ground-glass appearance.
- When inflammation subsides the vessels are reduced to empty white tubes that are called ghost vessels which last for rest of life.
- They are always associated with anterior uveitis.
- Cause of deep corneal vascularization consists of all conditions grouped under term of interstitial keratitis, which may extend from periphery or be central. The causes are congenital syphilis, tuberculosis (adult), leprosy (adult), mucus plaque, and herpes simplex in second decade.
- The superficial corneal vessels continue with conjunctival vessels.
- Deep vascularization in the stroma from anterior ciliary vessels.
- Retro corneal—extension from uveal neovascularization.
- Intracorneal vascularization—superficial vessels finding way into corneal subsequent to lamellar injury **(Fig. 15.9)**.

Retro Corneal Vascularization

They are rare in children. In children, the main cause is mechanical trauma, either accidental or surgical, which are—penetrating injury at the limbus, conjunctival downgrowth following a limbal-based conjunctival flap

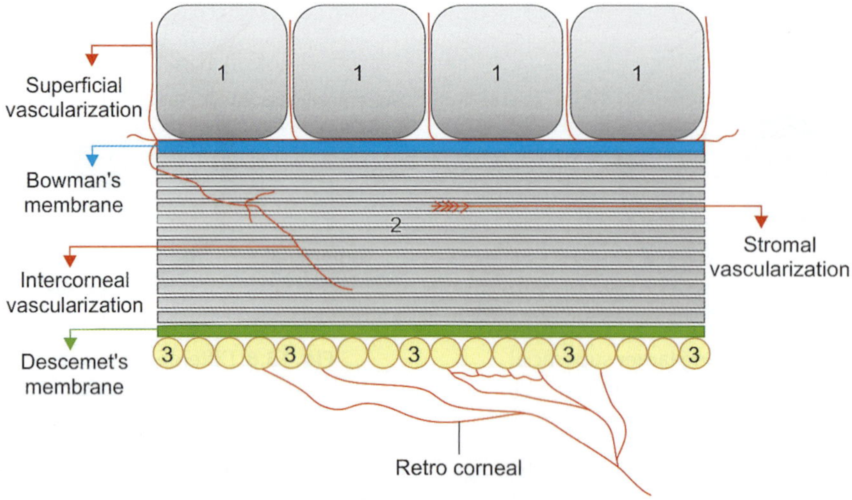

Fig. 15.9: Details of corneal vascularization. (1. Corneal epithelium; 2. Corneal stroma; 3. Endothelium)

that gets access to the anterior chamber, and penetrating keratoplasty. It can also happen in neovascularization of the iris.

Intercorneal Vascularization

This is the rarest form of corneal vascularization at all ages. It happens when conjunctival vessels grow under a partial-thickness corneal wound, whether accidental or surgical, i.e., a lamellar wound or keratoplasty.

Other clinical feature of corneal disorder are:

- Epithelial
  - Loss of sensation
  - Staining
  - Deposit
  - Xerosis
  - Encroachment
- Descemet's membrane
  - Rupture in Descemet's membrane
  - Folds in Descemet's membrane
  - Split in Descemet's membrane
- Endothelium
  - Keratic precipitate

Loss of Corneal Sensation

Cornea is very sensitive to touch, temperature, pressure, and changes in pH. Cornea, when subjected to any of the aforementioned, develops pain. Sensation is an essential protective feature of the cornea. Corneal sensation may be marginally dampened or totally absent **(Fig. 15.10)**.

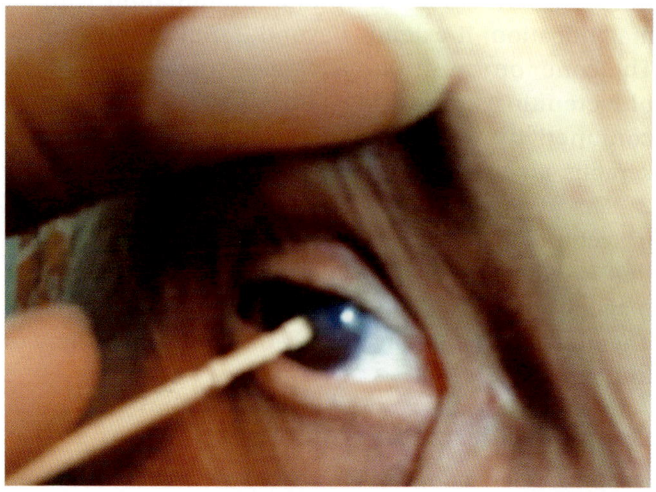

Fig. 15.10: Totally absent corneal sensation in a case of postherpetic neuralgia.

Examination of corneal sensation is of great ophthalmic and neurological importance.

> There is no condition where corneal sensation is enhanced.

The common causes of diminished corneal sensations are:

- Recent use of local anesthetic drops
- Prolonged use of a contact lens
- Corneal infections
  - Herpes simplex
  - Herpes zoster
  - Leprosy

- Neurological
  - Trigeminal neuralgia
  - Postherpetic neuralgia
  - Cerebral pontine angle tumor
- Corneal degeneration
- Deposit on cornea*
- Corneal scar
  - Corneal edema
  - Repair of a corneal wound
  - Keratoplasty
  - Recent peritomy
  - Large limbal section
  - Buphthalmos
  - Absolute glaucoma
  - Xerotic cornea

The superficial foreign bodies are generally referred to as corneal foreign bodies and classified as superficial and deep. They are always acquired and can be removed with ease, while true deposits are mostly systemic.

- Xerosis of the cornea
- Staining of the cornea

Encroachment on Cornea

The most common cause is pterygium, which is not seen in children; pseudopterygium is more common in children; dermoid; fascicular ulcer; phlyctenulosis; large papillae of the limbal spring catarrh; and over-filtering bleb are some of the other causes.

The following are various types of dermoids **(Figs. 15.11A and B)**.

Corneal Dystrophies in Children

They are congenital, may be obvious at birth or manifest later, are generally bilateral, symmetric or asymmetric, hereditary, slowly progressive, independent of systemic disease, and mostly central. The corneal dystrophic have been put into two broad categories:

1. Where the gene has been mapped.
2. Where the gene has not been mapped well.

Topographically, it may be:

- Epithelial
- Subepithelial

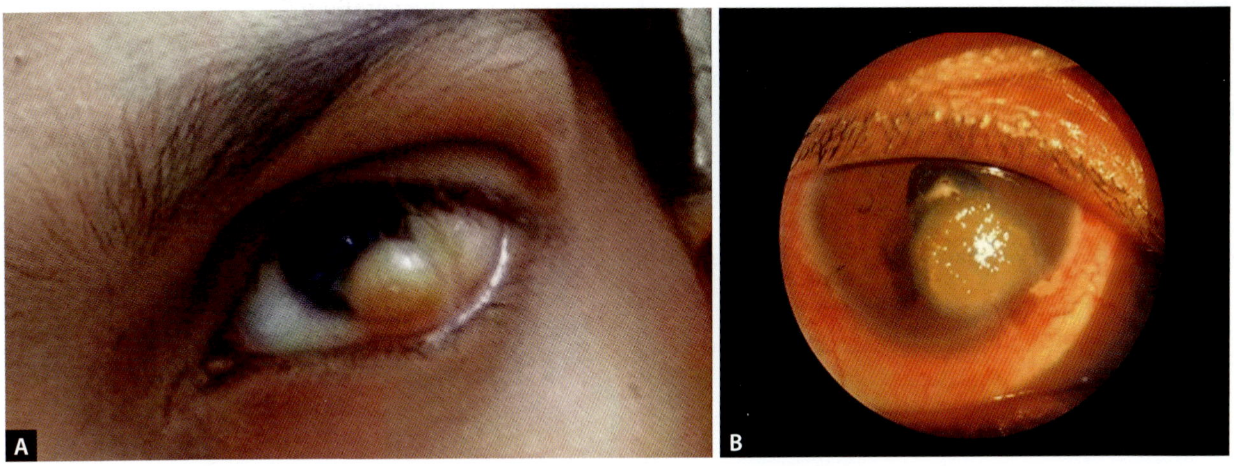

Figs. 15.11A and B: Corneal opacity (dermoid).
Courtesy: Dr Nupur Chakarwarty.

**Deposits on Cornea:* Deposits on the cornea can be superficial or deep. They can be organic or inorganic. The inorganic deposits are mostly metals, the most common metal found on the cornea is iron. The deposits of iron, according to their location, have been put in the following groups:

Iron containing corneal opacities:

Name		*Topography*
Ferry's	-	Border of trabeculectomy
Fleischer	-	Base of keratoconus
Stokers	-	Pterygium head
Hudson-Stahli	-	Lower one-third of corneal

Note: Kayser Fleischer ring is a nonferrous deposit. It is due to intraocular copper deposited under the Descemet's membrane on the periphery; it is a golden brown ring. Calcium is deposited in the epithelium and superficial stroma in band keratopathy.

- Combined epithelial and subepithelial
- Combined epithelial and stromal
- Stromal
- Endothelial

Most of the corneal dystrophies are autosomal dominant, starting in childhood and becoming obvious by adolescence, progressively worsening as age increases, with no vascularization or inflammatory signs. Corneal dystrophies per se are rarely diagnosed under 5, though they may begin even at an earlier age.

The following is a list of dystrophies that manifest in childhood and their topographical distribution. The following **Flowchart 15.1** shows the distribution of corneal dystrophies as per depth of involvement.

Table 15.2 shows differentiating features of various types of corneal dystrophies in children.

Clinical Description in Short of Anterior Corneal Dystrophies in Children

Meesmann's dystrophy (hereditary juvenile epithelial dystrophy): This is a hereditary autosomal dominant disorder seen under 4 years and is generally asymptomatic. The lesions are seen as microvesicles in the deeper layers of epithelium on retro illumination. Corneal sensation on the exposed part of the cornea is diminished. The progression is slow. In cases of unmanageable diminished vision, lamellar keratoplasty may be tried; there is generally an abnormal tear film secondary to microvesicles; irregular astigmatism is common if corneal erosion occurs; and it may be managed by a bandage contact lens.

Stocker and Holt (hereditary epithelial dystrophy): It shares hereditary features of the previous condition, i.e., it is an autosomal dominant trait that causes so much confusion in diagnosis that some clinicians consider it nothing but a variation of Meesmann's dystrophy.

It begins in infancy with a mild-to-moderate loss of vision, depending on the amount of opacification of the cornea. That may just be a slight haze to complete opacification; irregular astigmatism is common, as is diminished corneal sensation. Treatment depends on the severity of the loss of vision. Severe loss of vision requires lamellar keratoplasty; corneal erosion is treated by excimer laser.

Reis Buckler's dystrophy: This is an autosomal dominant condition involving Bowmen's membranes. *Common age of onset:* 3–5 years with severe progressive loss of vision and diminished corneal sensation. Corneal erosion is frequent, and the condition may end up with permanent central corneal opacity, for which keratoplasty is required. Corneal erosion and irregular astigmatism are managed by bandage contact lenses and soft contact lenses, respectively.

Flowchart 15.1: Characteristic features of anterior, stromal, and posterior dystrophies.

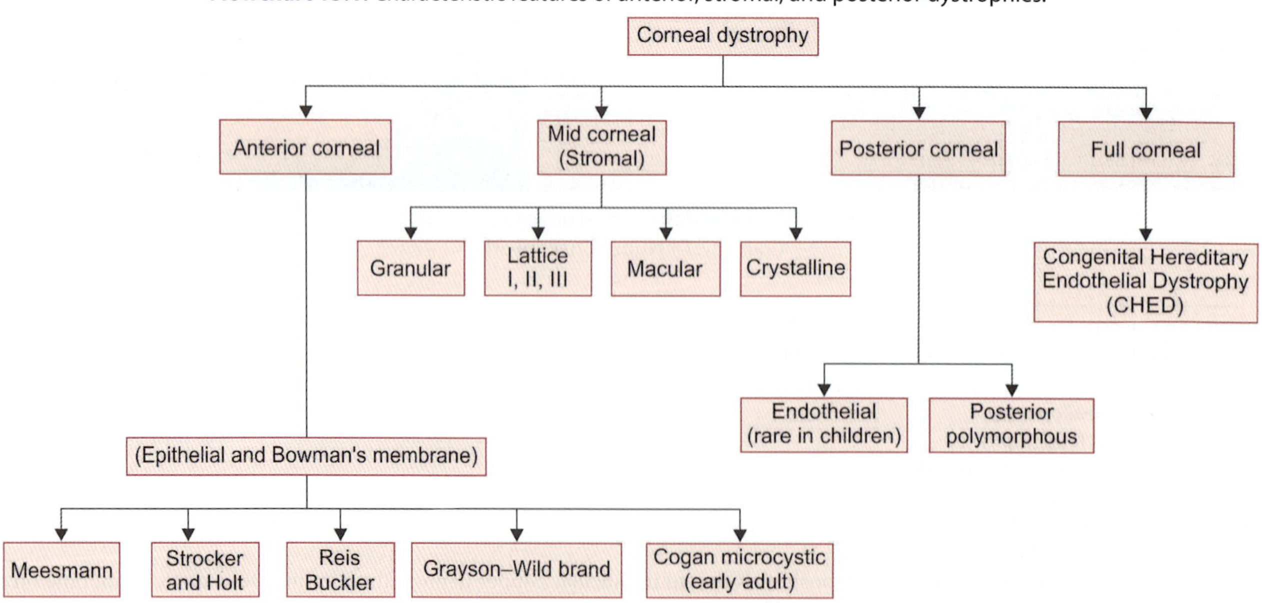

TABLE 15.2: Features of various types of corneal dystrophies in children.

Name	Age of onset	Heredity	Visual loss	Corneal sensation	Erosion	Complication	Treatment
Anterior dystrophy							
Meesmann's	3–4 years	Autosomal dominant	Mild-to-moderate	Slight reduction	± ±	Nil	Not required. Bandage contact lens may help in erosion
Stocker–Holt	Infancy	Autosomal dominant	Mild-to-severe	Reduced	± ±	Irregular astigmatism	Lamellar keratoplasty, bandage contact lens
Reis–Buckler	3–4 years	Autosomal dominant	Severe 6/60 or less	Reduced	Recurrent	Corneal opacity	Pad and bandage, contact lens, penetrating keratoplasty
Grayson–Wilbrandt	10 years	Autosomal dominant	Gradual loss	Normal	± ±	Nil	Contact lens
Stromal dystrophy							
Groenouw's I Lattice	10 years	Autosomal dominant	Moderate	Reduced	+ +	Corneal opacity	Penetrating keratoplasty
Groenouw's II macular	<10 years	Recessive	Severe	± ±	± ±	Corneal opacity	Penetrating keratoplasty
Granular	10 years	Autosomal dominant	Mild	Normal	+ +	Corneal vascularization Nil	Nil
Schnyder infancy	Infancy	Autosomal dominant	Mild	Normal	Nil	Nil	Nil
Posterior dystrophy							
Posterior polymorphous corneal dystrophy	Congenital	Autosomal dominant/ recessive	Mild	Normal	Nil	May develop glaucoma, endothelial decompensation	Symptomatic

Grayson-Wilbrandt (hereditary anterior membrane dystrophy): This is not seen before 10 years, is autosomal dominant in nature with normal corneal sensation without corneal erosion, loss of vision is moderate and gradual, and biomicroscopy may show prominent corneal nerves that are thicker than normal. The condition may require keratoplasty.

Biber-Haab (Stromal dystrophy): This is a type of stromal dystrophy of autosomal dominant nature manifesting at the end of the first decade to begin with and does not interfere with vision. Diminished vision develops gradually over years due to slow-progressing opacity that extends from limbus to limbus. Corneal erosion is common, causing watering and a foreign body sensation that brings the child for consultation and is found to have the dystrophy. Corneal erosion is treated by lubricants and bandage contact lenses; otherwise, simple patching may give much-needed relief from watering and foreign body sensations. Other treatments include penetrating keratoplasty and excimer lasers.

Groenouw Type I dystrophy (granular corneal dystrophy): The condition gets its name from the white, granular appearance of the cornea. It is an autosomal disorder that starts in the first decade in the center of the cornea and has white dots with clear stroma in between. Initially, the condition is asymptomatic; the diminution of vision is slow and moderate; by the fourth decade, the person develops symptoms of photophobia, lacrimation, foreign body sensation, and reduced uncorrectable vision; corneal sensation remains normal. Children require no specific treatment; keratoplasty may be required in adults.

Groenouw Type II dystrophy: The most outstanding feature of the condition lies in its hereditary pattern, which is autosomal recessive, in contrast to autosomal dominant in most of the other dystrophies. The condition is first noticed at 5 years of age with white opacity in the mid-cornea that may spread toward the periphery and may involve the endothelium. As age advances, the condition becomes worse with ever-increasing erosion that requires management by lubricant and bandage contact lenses. The ultimate treatment is penetrating keratoplasty, before which contact lenses may be used to improve vision as best as possible.

Clinical features of cornea degenerations are:

- Acquired
- Nonhereditary
- May be peripheral spreading towards center
- Follow—trauma
- Inflammation of the cornea or uvea may be associated with systemic disease.

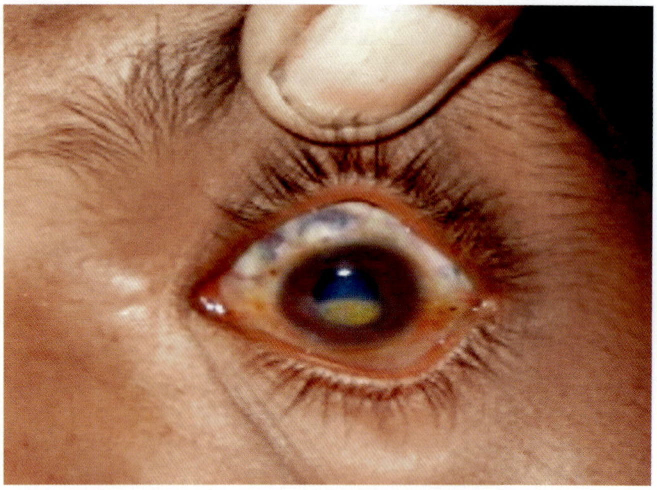

Fig. 15.12: Band keratopathy in an eye suffering from uveitis since childhood.

CORNEAL DEGENERATION

- Age-related
  - Nonpathological may have a genetic predisposition
  - Bilateral
  - Do not interfere with vision
- Pathological
  - Primary—rare
    The causes are—hypercalcemia, hyperparathyroidism, chronic renal failure, and sarcoid.
  - Secondary
    - Band keratopathy*
    - Fatty degeneration
    - Peripheral—Terrien pellucid (not seen in children)
    - Salzmann nodular degeneration, deposition of hyaline matter in front of Bowman's membrane, and epithelium were seen in long standing untreated phlycten in the second decade.

Treatment

The treatment consists of frequently using lubricants to treat residual uveitis. If these fail, the most commonly used treatment is debridement of the band. This is an office procedure done under local anesthesia and performed with magnification. The procedure consists of anesthetizing the eye with a local anesthetic agent

---

Secondary band keratopathy:* This is an acquired deposition of calcium in the corneal epithelium, Bowman's membrane, and superficial stroma. Depending on the involvement of basement membrane bands, keratopathy has been divided into two types: epithelial and stroma. The condition is slowly progressing and may lead to a gross loss of vision. It may be unilateral if the causative factor is unilateral, as seen following trauma. Mostly accidental; surgical trauma too has been reported to be the contributing factor, so has been the intraocular injection of silicon oil following extensive repair of the globe injury. Bilateral cases are seen in long standing anterior uveitis and congenital glaucoma. They are common in phthisis bulbae. The symptoms of band keratopathy are varied; they generally have a history of chronic anterior uveitis, untreated congenital glaucoma, or trauma. The main symptom is gradually diminishing uncorrectable vision with watering on examination; the eye has signs of previous inflammation. The lesion consists of a spindle-shaped opacity in the intermarginal strip in front of the pupil. It starts 1.00 mm inside the limbus on each end as a vertical line from which the main opacity spreads toward the center, rarely meeting each other **(Fig. 15.12). The opacity shows deposits of calcium that is generally subepithelial; protrusion of the calcium deposits over the epithelium is common and is the cause of foreign body sensation. The opacity may show multiple circular vesicles in the substance of the band. The band does neither stain nor is vascularized, the sensation over the band is diminished.

Edema of the cornea: To maintain the clarity of the cornea, it should be in a stage of compactness, which is brought about by the active detergence of the stroma, i.e., less permeable to fluid than the endothelium. Fluid laden with nutrition from aqueous solutions is passed to the stroma in a controlled amount due to the presence of a mechanism called optimal stromal swelling pressure. Normally, intact endothelium sends back sodium in the aqueous solution, which is hampered following an insult to the endothelium that may be traumatizing, inflammatory, or chemical. Once sodium finds its way into the stroma, the stroma imbibes fluid and gets swollen. The swollen stroma is less transparent than a normal stroma. This disturbs the arrangement of the corneal collagen fibers, causing scarring of the stroma and reducing transparency. The epithelium that gets nutrition from tear film plays little role in the production of stromal edema but is secondarily involved if water flows from behind, resulting in bullae formation on the epithelial surface.

and scraping the calcium deposits with a Bard Parker knife. Washing the debris and rubbing the raw area with ethylene diamine tetra-acetic acid (EDTA) 3% solution. The eye is bandaged after installing cycloplegics and antibiotics. The procedure needs to be repeated and is not very effective. The most effective treatment is keratoplasty. The results of which, too, do not vary unceasingly. Bandage contact lenses give temporary relief.

The causes of corneal edema are:

- *Trauma to endothelium:* Injury to the endothelium is more deleterious than injury to the epithelium in causing corneal edema. The Bowman's and Descemet's membranes are not capable of swelling. Because they are homogeneous and do not contain either cells or fibrocytes in the stroma. The common injuries inflicted on the endothelium are:
  - Intraocular lens (IOL) manipulation, anterior chamber IOL (AC-IOL), glaucoma valve, penetrating keratoplasty, and suture passing through the endothelium.
- *Epithelial trauma:* Secondary to ill-fitting contact lenses, the removal of foreign bodies, and chemical injury.
- *Aphakia:* Aphakia and pseudophakia are both major causes of corneal edema.
  - The foremost cause is the presence of a large amount of vitreous in AC following intracapsular lens extraction.
  - Too much manipulation of IOL is a major factor. The second cause during IOL surgery is the use of a large volume of fluid. The third cause is the accidental direction of the fluid toward the endothelium, which damages it.
  - Anterior chamber and iris fixed IOL. Used to be an important contributory factor in the production of corneal edema in the long run in the past.

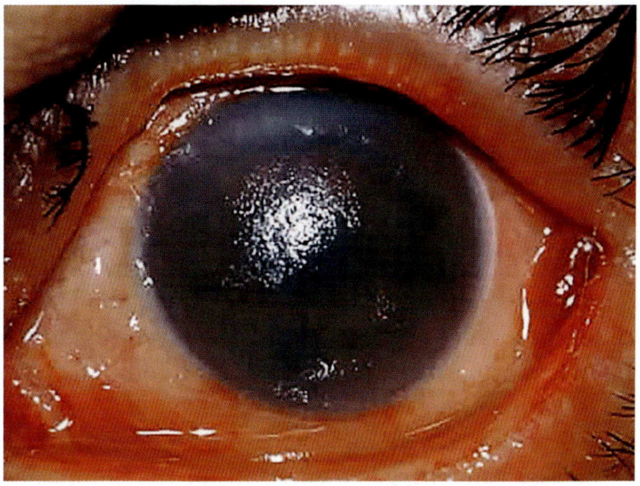

Fig. 15.13: Generalized corneal edema.

- Silicone oil in AC
- Rupture of the Descemet's membrane in long standing buphthalmos.
- Keratoconus—acute hydrops
- Chronic uveitis
- Corneal staphyloma
- Corneal hypoxia
- Disciform keratitis.
- Fuchs dystrophy*
- Iridocorneal endothelial syndrome (ICE)†
- Congenital hereditary endothelial dystrophy

Corneal edema can be localized or generalized **(Fig. 15.13)**, central cornea is more frequently involved than the periphery.

Treatment

There is no medical treatment; hypertonic solutions have been empirically used without much efficacy. The best results are achieved by doing lamellar keratoplasty;

**Fuchs dystrophy:* It is an acquired bilateral condition seen after the fourth decade. The incidence rises with age and is common in both sexes. It is a chronic disorder due to the accumulation of aqueous in the stroma, causing swelling of the stroma and leading to glair diminished vision, watering, and pain in the eye. It has been classified into four stages, which are:

- Stage 1, usually asymptomatic. Thickened Descemet's membrane.
- Stage 2, painless; the vision may be diminished upon awakening, which clears in a few hours.
- Stage 3, painful, marked edema of the stroma with severe loss of vision.
- Stage 4, pain becomes less, but vision is greatly lost due to subepithelial scarring and deep corneal opacity.

†*Iridocorneal endothelial syndrome:* It is an infrequent condition with uncertain etiology characterized by proliferation and migration and endothelial cells into the iris and angle of the anterior chamber, resulting in angle-closure glaucoma, corneal edema, and atrophy of the iris. Some clinicians attribute it to a virus infection, especially to herpes simplex. ICE is not a single entity but comprises three syndromes, namely essential iris atrophy, Chandler syndrome, and Cogan-Reese syndrome.

better results have been achieved by still advanced keratoplasty in the form of Descemet's membrane endothelial keratoplasty (DMEK). The condition becomes worse following lens extraction and a glaucoma valve implant.

BULLOUS KERATOPATHY

This is a noninflammatory, recurrent, and painful condition of the cornea due to the accumulation of fluid under the epithelium secondary to overhydration of the stroma, mostly due to pathology in the endothelium. The symptoms consist of a gritty sensation that becomes painful to causes watering. The vision is subnormal due to the associated irregular astigmatism. The diminished vision is more marked on awakening; the movement of the lids on the bullae causes a foreign body sensation; rupture of the bullae precipitates more pain. The number of bullae varies from single to multiple, scattered all over the cornea. Sliding of the epithelium, which is essential for repair of epithelial defects, is disturbed by ruptured bullae. The bullae may be infected and cause hypopyon. Sometimes, the hypopyon may be sterile.

Management

Management is frustrating. The best way is to avoid the conditions that damage the endothelium, i.e.,

- During phacoemulsification, there is too much viscoelastic in AC.
- Avoid mechanical damage to the endothelium by—instruments, IOL, or the inadvertent passing of full-thickness corneal suture fluid directed toward the endothelium.
- Vitreous loss
- Failure to manage vitreous loss
- Raised intraocular pressure

The actual treatment is symptomatic and consists of:

- Dehydrating the epithelium by hyperosmotic eye drops, i.e., 5% NaCl or glycerin drops.
- The use of a hair dryer to blow hot air to the eyes has been reported to give temporary relief.
- Use of a bandage contact lens.
- Keratoplasty
    - Penetrating keratoplasty
    - Posterior lamellar keratoplasty
- Conjunctival flap
- Amniotic membrane graft
- Tarsorrhaphy

LOSS OF CORNEAL TRANSPARENCY

The most common cause of loss of transparency in the cornea is corneal opacity, where normal transparent keratocytes, which are arranged in regular fashions, are replaced by irregularly arranged opaque fibrocytes with or without incarceration of the uvea. They may be vascularized.

The opacities may be unilateral or bilateral; when bilateral, they may be simultaneous or may appear at different times. The causes of bilateral opacity may be different in two eyes. The opacities may cover the whole cornea or may be partial in thickness or area; their number, shape, size, and depth vary as per causative factor and duration; most of them are permanent; a few are known to disappear with treatments; according to the thickness of the opacity, they are categorized as nebula, macula, and leukoma; whenever there is evidence of iris attachment to the opacity, it is designated as leukoma adherent **(Fig. 15.14)**.

The corneal opacities may be part of corneal ectasia, iris adherence, vascularization, and stromal edema. The sensation over the opacity is either absent or reduced. They do not stain. Central corneal opacities not only cause uncorrectable diminished vision, they also cause scattering of light. Opacity in different combinations causes amblyopia squint. Bilateral corneal opacities developing in infancy may cause nystagmus. The causes of corneal opacity vary with age; some of them may be congenital and are permanent.

The following **Table 15.3** shows a list of corneal opacities as per age.

Causes of bilateral corneal opacity in children are **(Fig. 15.15)**:

- Congenital—sclerocornea, dermoid, anterior chamber dysgenesis

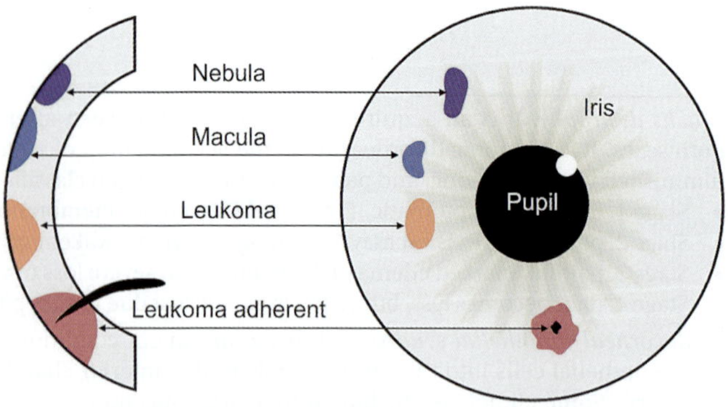

Fig. 15.14: Various grades of corneal opacity.

- Trauma—cracker (frequent)
  - Chemical (rare)
  - Folk medicine

TABLE 15.3: Corneal opacities in children.

Sr. no.	Age	Cause
1.	Newborn	Congenital, trauma, and buphthalmos
2.	Neonates	Poorly managed ophthalmia neonatorum
3.	1st year	Malnourished child, comatose child
4.	Preschool	Unmanaged above conditions include xerophthalmia, bacterial corneal ulcers, trauma, and interstitial keratitis
5.	5 years and above	All unattended causes To them, the following may be added • Phlyctenular keratoconjunctivitis • Spring catarrh • Corneal dystrophies • Keratoconus • Band keratopathy • Multiple foreign bodies iatrogenic

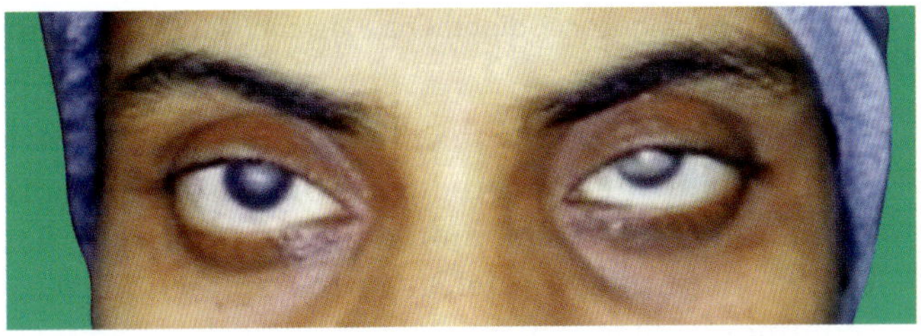

Fig. 15.15: Bilateral corneal opacity since childhood.

- Infection—Untreated ophthalmia neonatorum (central leukoma, anterior polar cataract and nystagmus)
  - Smallpox (Was most common cause of bilateral corneal opacity and staphyloma before smallpox was eradicated in year 1980).
- Inflammation—interstitial keratitis
- Allergic—phlycten, spring catarrh
- Degeneration—band keratopathy
- Nutritional—xerophthalmia, (reversible in early stage) keratomalacia
- Deposits

INFECTION AND INFLAMMATION OF CORNEA IN CHILDREN

Both conditions are grouped under the term keratitis. A group of disorders that cannot be attributed to the above conditions are put under the loose term of keratopathy, i.e., band keratopathy. It is better to divide keratitis into two broad categories: infective and noninfective keratitis. The other alternative is to divide keratitis according to whether both conditions are grouped under the term keratitis according to the depth of the lesion, i.e., superficial, deep, and mixed. Keratitis, when confined to the epithelium, Bowman's membrane, and anterior stroma, is called superficial keratitis, an example of which is a microbial corneal ulcer.

The following **Flowchart 15.2** shows the broad division of keratitis.

Flowchart 15.2: Division of keratitis.

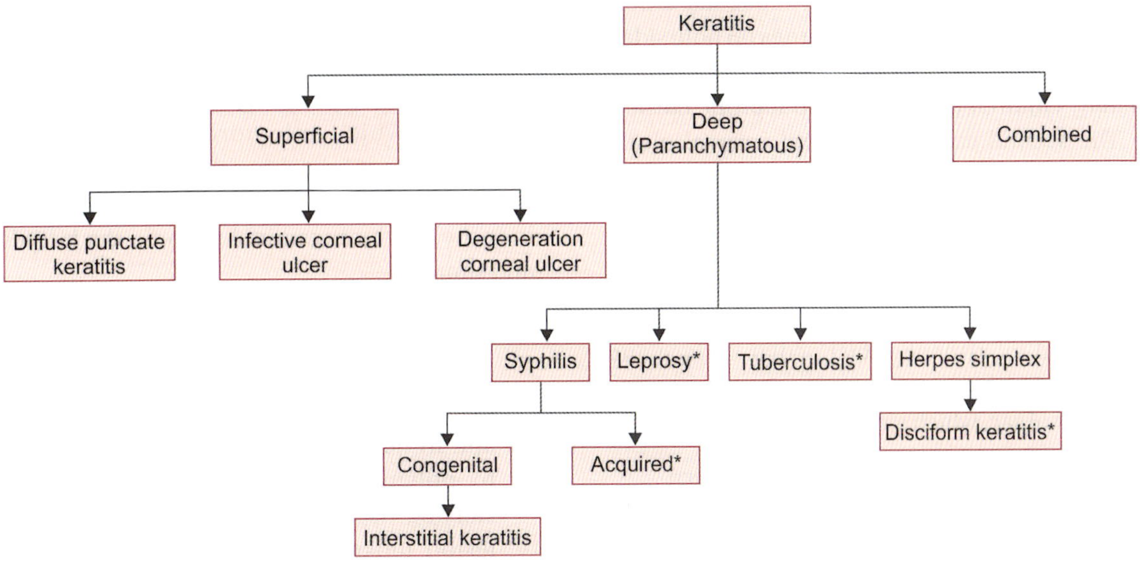

*Not seen in children.

CORNEAL ULCER IN CHILDREN (SUPERFICIAL SUPPURATIVE KERATITIS)

Clinically, a corneal ulcer is a breach in the epithelium superadded by ulcer producing factors that can be microbial or nonmicrobial with molecular death of the epithelium or superficial stroma. A breach in continuity of epithelium without molecular death is called corneal abrasion, which may or may not stain and is self-limiting unless infected. The larger the abrasion, the more are for it to get infected. The abrasion stains bright green with fluorescein. A deep ulcer of >24 hours duration is more likely to involve stroma; stromal involvement is associated with anterior chamber reactions.

The invasion of the cornea by microorganisms following a breach in the epithelium is varied. The organism can be bacterial, both cocci and bacilli, gram-positive and gram-negative, viruses, fungi, and rarely parasites; the only unicellular parasite known to cause corneal ulcers is *Acanthamoeba*. Bacilli are the most common microorganisms to cause corneal ulcers in all ages; both gram-positive and gram-negative bacilli have their equal share in causing suppurative corneal ulcer, which is generally acute in nature; fungi take longer time after breach to develop ulcers; and viruses are not known to produce suppurative keratitis.

General Consideration (in All Ages)

- *Corneal ulcers*, seen in all ages from neonates to ripe old age in both sexes all over the world, are more common in the third to fifth decade, generally uniocular unless there is permanent exposure of the cornea on both sides, as in leprosy, which is worsened by a lack of sensation. Fortunately, children do not develop leprotic corneal ulcers. The second cause of bilateral corneal ulcers is immune compromise. The other causes are blast injury, malnutrition, vitamin A deficiency, ophthalmia neonatorum, and folk medicines.
- *Loss of protective mechanisms*: Corneas are well protected by normal blink reflex, Bell's phenomenon, defensive head movement, intact ocular surface and tear film, and the absence of pathogenic organisms in the conjunctival sac, which gives additional protection.

The following conditions predispose to corneal ulcers:

- *Lid:*
  - Coloboma: congenital/acquired
  - Lagophthalmos
  - Trichiasis
  - Distichiasis
  - Entropion
  - Ectropion
  - Blepharo conjunctivitis
- *Orbit:* Proptosis
- *Sac:* Chronic dacryocystitis
- *Tear:* Ocular surface disorder
- *Others:* Keratomalacia, ill-fitting contact lenses, prolonged use of local anesthetic agents, antibiotics, steroids, raised intraocular tension, and corneal edema.

> - Central corneal ulcers are mostly infective.
> - Peripheral ulcers are noninfective, i.e., autoimmune, allergic, or degenerative (not seen in children).

Natural History of Corneal Ulcer

- *Microbial assault on the cornea*

  Normal corneal epithelium is resistant to most of the microorganisms except:

  > Gonococci, meningococci, diphtheria, *Haemophilus Listeria*, and *Acanthamoeba*.

  The organisms can overcome the protective barrier of the epithelium by producing protease. The most common way for microorganisms to get into the cornea is through a defect in the epithelium, i.e., commonly mechanical, less frequently chemical. Ocular surface defects and epithelial bullae predispose to corneal ulcers. The mechanical trauma may be trivial—a small spot, liner abrasion, or loss of epithelium on a large area. Absences of sensation, as in leprosy, and trigeminal neuralgia too have their share in producing corneal ulcers. The other route via which microorganisms can reach the cornea without breaching the epithelium is from the infected conjunctiva. The third route is through branches of the trigeminal nerve in the herpes zoster and simplex.
- *Evolution of corneal ulcer*
  - Once the organisms find their way into the epithelium, they start multiplying, producing toxin that facilitates spread both on the surface and in depth. This is associated with infiltration by polymorph nuclear cells and lymphocytes, causing tissue necrosis and cellular death. The lesion looks initially as a tiny white spot with edematous epithelium over it. This is followed by

actual ulcer formation that stains with fluorescein; a proper antibiotic at this stage will abort further development of an ulcer.

- The development of the ulcer proper is heralded by necrosis of the epithelium, which is shed off with stromal infiltration and the formation of a well-formed ulcer crater with a clear-cut edge and a floor.
- In the initial stages, the Bowman's membrane offers mild resistance, but gives way on long run, never to regenerate.
- This facilitates the seepage of toxin in the anterior chamber, producing anterior chamber reaction that may culminate in hypopyon if the organism is virulent or the inoculum is large. Predisposing factors mentioned earlier facilitate in spread of corneal ulcers.
- Anterior chamber reaction denotes anterior uveal involvement that is reflected as pain, photophobia, and circumciliary congestion.
- The Descemet's membrane is tougher than both Bowman's membrane and stroma. It withstands microbial and toxic onslaughts for quite some time. Initially giving a chance to heal, if this fails, the Descemet's membrane protrudes through, the rent in the stroma forming a translucent, shining bulge called a descemetocele or keratocele. This happens even with normal intraocular pressure **(Fig. 15.16)**.
- Once the Descemet's membrane fails to withstand normal IOP, it gives way; this is worsened by raised intraocular pressure, leading to a state of much dreaded perforation **(Fig. 15.16)**.

- *Fate of a perforated corneal ulcer*

The most common site for a corneal ulcer to perforate is the vortex of the cornea, as it is the thinnest and weakest part of the cornea; however, peripheral perforations are not an exception.

As the cornea perforates, aqueous leaks out of the eye, causing an instantaneous softening of the eyeball and flattening of the cornea.

As the aqueous escapes, the iris-lens complex moves forward, and the iris plugs the perforation unless the iris is atropinized because atropinized pupil does not move fast enough to plug the perforation.

The lens that has moved forward may touch the cornea, and if left for long, develop an anterior polar cataract, as happens in perforation in the ophthalmia neonatorum. In cases of large coloboma of the iris, either congenital or acquired, the iris fails to plug the perforation in the same way as atropinized pupil. Perforations of the periphery are rare, mostly seen in traumatic and degenerative ulcers; the latter are not seen in children.

If the perforation is large, as happens in sloughing corneal ulcers, the lens along with the vitreous may be expelled, and the eye goes into phthisis.

In large perforations, the iris and cornea are replaced by fibroblasts, which bridge the gap in an irregular fashion with uneven thickness. The newly formed pseudo cornea may remain flat or bulge as an irregular protrusion, forming an anterior staphyloma, which may be total or partial.

> Staphyloma is defined as ectatic cicatrization of the outer coat of the eyeball with uveal incarceration. When the cornea is involved, it is called anterior staphyloma, which can be total or partial.

Regression of Corneal Ulcer

The natural defense mechanism, which is enhanced by timely treatment, initiates healing of corneal ulcers that end in the formation of various degrees of corneal opacities, depending on the depth of the ulcer, i.e., nebula, macula, leukoma, and leukoma adherent **(Fig. 15.14)**, where the iris is incarcerated in the scar or there is evidence that the iris was in touch with the opacity in the past. A nebular opacity involves only the epithelium and superficial stroma. It is hardly visible in oblique illumination and is best seen on a slit lamp. In spite of its translucency, it can interfere with vision when central. A macular opacity is more visible than a nebula and involves the epithelium and most or the stroma, visible on simple oblique illumination, causing more damage to vision.

Leukoma is the densest opacity of the cornea visible in diffuse illumination. It generally involves all the layers of the cornea, with or without incarceration of the iris. Corneal opacities do not stain; the sensation is dulled over the opacity **(Fig. 15.14)**. The number may vary from single to many, may even involve the whole cornea. Rarely, there may be vascularization of the opacity. There is no medical treatment for corneal opacity; the only treatment available is keratoplasty.

Nonregression of Corneal Ulcer

Small superficial corneal ulcers may regress and heal even without treatment, leaving the corneal opacity of the nebula or, at the most, the macula.

Deep ulcers do not heal without treatment, and in spite of the best treatment, all ulcers may progress relentlessly,

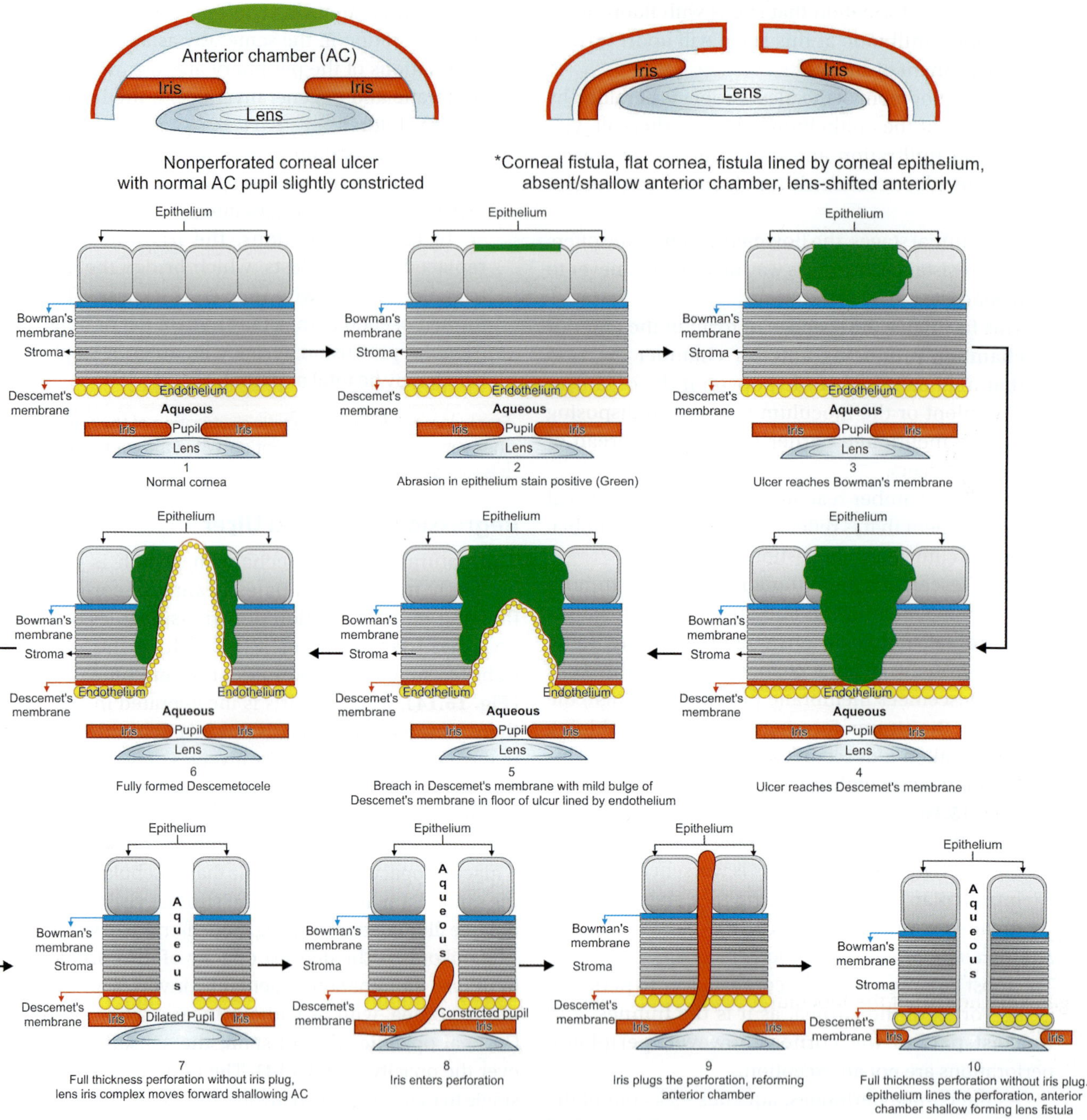

Fig. 15.16: Diagrammatic representation of natural history of corneal ulcer.

Corneal fistula:* The corneal fistula is the aftermath of the perforation of a corneal ulcer, where the iris fails to plug the defect. Resulting in continuous flow of aqueous, leading to softening of the eye, flattening of the cornea, wrinkles in the cornea, absence or persistent shallowing of the anterior chamber, and shifting of the lens iris complex forward. The two delayed features are the downgrowth of corneal epithelium in the fistula, which may extend to the endothelium. The second feature is the formation of peripheral anterior synechiae. The conditions carry a poor prognosis; application of adhesive glue is not always successful; logically penetrating keratoplasty should be the best option, which again carries a poor result **(Fig. 15.16).

Flowchart 15.3: Fate of a corneal ulcer.

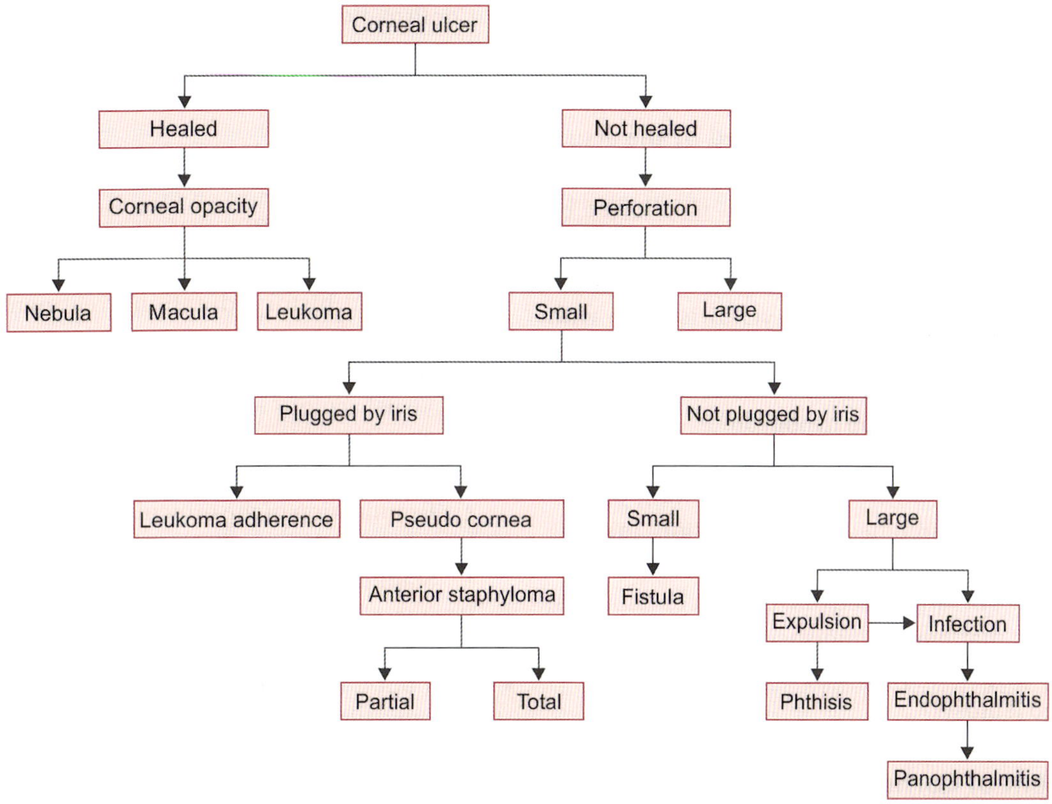

both in depth and on the surface. A virulent corneal ulcer may involve the sclera as well.

The **Flowchart 15.3** shows the fate of a corneal ulcer.

Clinical Features of Corneal Ulcers in Children

The presentation of a corneal ulcer is the same for all ages. They are varied as per severity, duration, and treatment received. The severity depends on the virulence of the organism, the size of the inoculums, and the multiplicity of microorganisms. Polymicrobial infections are more difficult to manage.

- *Symptoms*
  - *Pain*: Mildest symptom is a foreign body sensation with watering followed by redness and pain due to involvement of the anterior uvea. All organisms do not cause equally severe pain—pneumonia, *Pseudomonas*, and *Koch-Weeks* organisms produce more pain than other organisms; the ulcers that are not painful are leprosy (not seen in children), herpes simplex, and herpes zoster, due to inherent anesthesia. Late onset of pain and unexplained pain mean a rise in intraocular pressure.
  - *Blepharospasm:* Blepharospasm is a more marked and early manifestation in children; this is generally associated with watering.
  - *Lacrimation:* Both blepharospasm and lacrimation are caused by spasms of the ciliary body; the instillation of strong cycloplegia gives prompt relief.
  - *Photophobia:* Photophobia, like blepharospasm, is more marked in children than in adults. It is always associated with blepharospasm and lacrimation; it is abolished temporarily by the instillation of a local anesthetic agent.
  - *Redness:* Redness of the eye is due to:
    - Circumciliary congestion
    - Associated conjunctivitis
    - Absence of conjunctival congestion in corneal ulcers is unlikely.
  - *Diminished vision:* Visual acuity depends on the position of the corneal ulcer; an ulcer with surrounding infiltration causes more visual loss; central ulcers are responsible for more visual loss; and visual loss is enhanced by associated anterior uveitis and glaucoma.

Signs of Corneal Ulcer

The signs of corneal ulcers are as varied as the symptoms. The ulcer starts as a small gray spot surrounded by a zone of infiltration. To begin with, there is no ulcer creator, and the lesion does not stain. This is followed by the actual development of a corneal ulcer. The lesion rapidly spreads all round surrounded by infiltration. This is followed by the development of the ulcer creator. At this stage, the ulcer takes up stain. The ulcer stains bright green, and the surrounding infiltration taking yellowish hue with fluorescein **(Figs. 15.17A to C)**. A slit-lamp examination shows an anterior chamber reaction. An ulcer with a virulent organism may develop hypopyon.

With the involvement of the uvea, the child complains of pain not so much in the eye but radiating on the ipsilateral head with circumcorneal congestion. Initially, the corneal sensation is present at places away from the ulcer, only to get abolished as the ulcer sloughs. The conditions that have diminished or absent corneal sensation are herpes simplex, herpes zoster, postherpetic neuralgia, and leprosy.

Management of Corneal Ulcer

Each ulcer poses a different problem and each clinician has his protocol to treat.

> Corneal ulcers in children must be considered an ophthalmic emergency.

All the protocols are based on the following parameters:

- Confirmation of an ulcer
- Detection of specific microorganisms responsible.
- Specific treatment
- Ancillary treatment
- Postulcer management

Confirmation of Ulcer

- The presence of an ulcer and its stage are confirmed by detailed history, duration, treatment taken, and staining.
- The clinical examination should include:
  - Visual acuity
  - Slit lamp examination
  - Corneal sensation
  - Examination of the orbicularis
  - Regurgitation test
  - Staining
- Positive staining will confirm the presence of a corneal ulcer.
- Find out if the ulcer is infective or noninfective. The infective ulcers are caused by bacteria, viruses, fungi, and parasites. Out of them, bacteria top the list, both cocci and bacilli; gram-negative and gram-positive cause corneal ulcers. Infection with more than one organism is very common.

Viral ulcers may have a protracted course; they are not fulminating unless secondarily infected by bacteria or fungi.

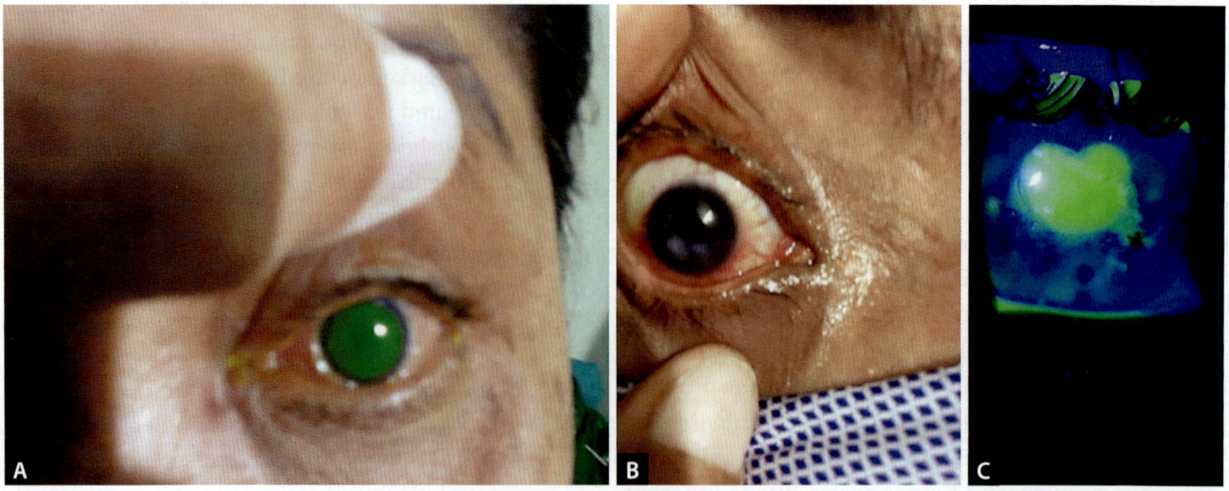

Figs. 15.17A to C: Staining of corneal ulcer by fluorescein: (A) Generalized; (B) Localized; (C) Fluorescein stain under cobalt blue light.

Fungal ulcers begin with a slow rate of expansion unless they are secondarily infected. It is rare for a virus to infect a bacterial or fungal ulcer; the reverse is more common.

Specific Microorganism Responsible

The organisms responsible for ulcers can be roughly identified by their clinical appearance. The best example is a dendritic corneal ulcer. The bacteria and fungi are identified by examination of scraping, staining, and culture. Viruses are difficult to stain and culture.

Characteristics of Bacterial Ulcers

- Bacteria are most common organisms to cause corneal ulcers.
- In most instances, barring gonococci, meningococci, diphtheria, *Haemophilus*, and *Listeria*, corneal ulcers require a breach in the epithelium. All pus-forming bacteria cause acute ulceration.
- Bacterial ulcers are mostly central.
- Most of the single-organismal ulcers respond to broad spectrum antibiotics better.
- Systemic antibiotics are not required to treat bacterial corneal ulcers.
- Most of the bacteria produce an anterior chamber reaction and hypopyon when the organism is virulent.
- The bacterial ulcers have a centrifugal spread.
- They may be very painful.
- They stain brightly with fluorescein unless sloughed.
- Sloughed ulcers require a pool staining agent without staining the ulcer.
- Sensation over the cornea outside the ulcer is generally normal.
- Bacterial ulcers are often associated with mucopurulent conjunctivitis.
- Scrapping from the untreated ulcer demonstrates the presence, type, and staining nature of the organism and are subjected to culture, and sensitivity to antibiotics.
- The culture of the bacteria should be the first examination before starting antibiotics.

Characteristics of Viral Corneal Ulcer

There are >100 viruses that inflict mankind out of which only a few involve the eyes. Both deoxyribonucleic acid (DNA) and ribonucleic acid (RNA) viruses cause ocular lesions. All the viruses that invade conjunctive infect the cornea due to the continuity of the conjunctival epithelium with the corneal epithelium. This is worsened by the fact that the periphery of the cornea shares a blood supply with the conjunctiva.

All viruses are nonsuppurative; they involve only the superficial cornea; most of them are difficult to treat; recurrence is common; and all of them cause diminished corneal sensation. Out of all the viruses that involved the eye, the following viruses are more common to cause ulcers than the others: Herpes simplex type 1 and 2, and Herpes zoster. Primary herpes simplex is a disease of infants and children. Other virus that occasionally causes superficial keratitis is molluscum.

Characteristics of Fungal Corneal Ulcer

- Fungal ulcers take a week to 15 days to develop following injury by organic matter, vegetable matter, or animal matter.
- An ulcer developing quickly following an injury is most probably not fungal.
- Prophylactic use of antifungal drugs has hardly any effect on corneal ulcers.
- The fungal ulcers are central and spread centrifugally, may spread to the sclera.
- The ulcer forms a thick epithelial plaque that breaks down as the ulcer deepens.
- A fungal ulcer is always associated with a severe anterior chamber reaction with the formation of a thick, organized, fluffy, almost immobile hypopyon that is yellowish gray in color.

Characteristics of Noninfective Corneal Ulcer

Noninfective corneal ulcers are often referred to as sterile ulcers, they are better called keratitis rather than ulcers; they are less frequent than infective ulcers and are often missed; they do not response to antibiotics but give better results with steroids.

- They are generally peripheral.
- They are bilateral, need not be symmetric, and there may be a gap between the development of an ulcer between the first and second eyes.
- There is minimal circumciliary congestion.
- There is no anterior chamber reaction, hence no hypopyon.
- Corneal sensation is retained.
- The causes are allergies, autoimmune disorders, and toxins.

Characteristics of Central Corneal Ulcers

- They are infective.
- May be superficial or deep.
- Stain brightly.
- Predisposed to perforation.
- May spread to the periphery.
- The association of hypopyon is common.
- It may be caused by bacteria, viruses, fungi, and *Acanthamoeba*.
- Cause a disproportionate loss of vision.
- Healed ulcers leave opacity that causes amblyopia, squints, and sometimes nystagmus.

Characteristics of Peripheral Corneal Ulcers

- They are also referred to as marginal corneal ulcers.
- They are less common than central ulcers.
- They have a chronic course.
- They are milder than central ulcers.
- They are rare in children.
- They generally do not perforate because the periphery of the cornea has more blood supply, and the periphery is the thickest part of the cornea.
- They do not incite an anterior chamber reaction.
- They are noninfective.
- Most of them respond to mild steroids.
- *The causes of peripheral corneal ulcers are:*
    - Extension of conjunctival disease
    - Phlycten
    - Spring catarrh
    - Rosacea
    - Staphylococcal blepharitis
    - Mooren's ulcer (not seen in children)
- Peripheral corneal ulcers stain poorly.
- They rarely cause diminished vision, except for irregular astigmatism caused by the lesion.
- Occasionally, they may be numerous enough to encircle the periphery and form a girdle.

Predisposing Factors in Formation of Corneal Ulcers

- Trauma
    - Accidental, exposure to repeated trauma, i.e., particles from grinders and welding (not seen in children).
    - Surgical—failure of antisepsis and asepsis during corneal surgeries.
        - Keratoplasty
        - Refractive surgeries
        - Removal of a suture
        - Removal of foreign bodies
- Iatrogenic
    - Contact lens
    - Contact lens solution
    - Contaminated drops/instrument
- Failure of defense mechanisms
    - Lagophthalmos
    - Coloboma lid
    - Trichiasis (not seen in children)
    - Entropion (not seen in children)
    - Ectropion (not seen in children)
    - Proptosis
- Constant source of microbes—chronic dacryocystitis
- Loss of sensation
- Ocular surface disorder
- Keratomalacia
- Corneal anesthesia
- Bullous keratitis
- Malnutrition
- Raised intraocular pressure (IOP)
- Immunosuppression
    - Local—indiscriminate use of steroids
    - Systemic
        - Immunosuppression drugs
        - Human immunodeficiency virus (HIV) infection
        - Herpes simplex
        - Herpes zoster
- Diabetes—diabetes is not a problem per se in children but, a child suffering from type 1 diabetes is always in danger of developing an ocular infection, and the cornea is no exception.

Recognization of Causative Factor in Infective Corneal Ulcer

- *History:* The history of trauma by organic matter in recent the past goes in favor of fungal corneal ulcers.
- Clinical examination

> All corneal ulcers not responding to usual treatment should undergo examination of the microbes responsible for ulcer.

- Staining
- Microbial evaluation
- Examination of corneal scrap
- Corneal swab is not a preferred examination

Flowchart 15.4: Various stains used for specific bacterial ulcers.

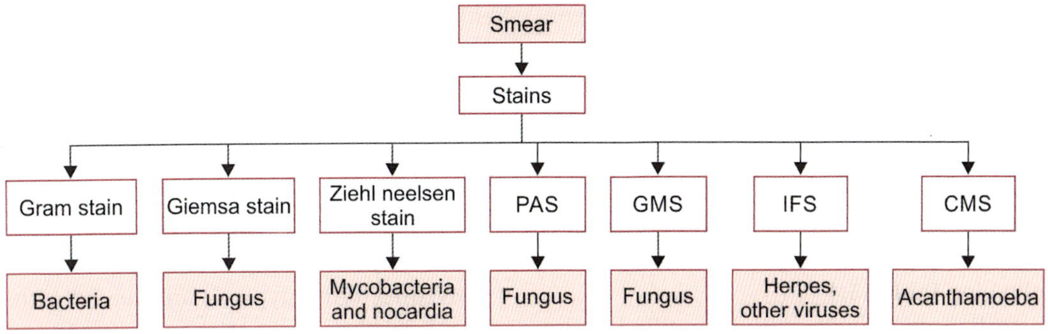

(CWS: calcofluor white stain; GMS: Grocott–Gomori methenamine-silver stain; IFS: immunofluorescence stain; PAS: periodic acid Schiff stain)

Flowchart 15.5: Various media used to culture corneal pathogen.

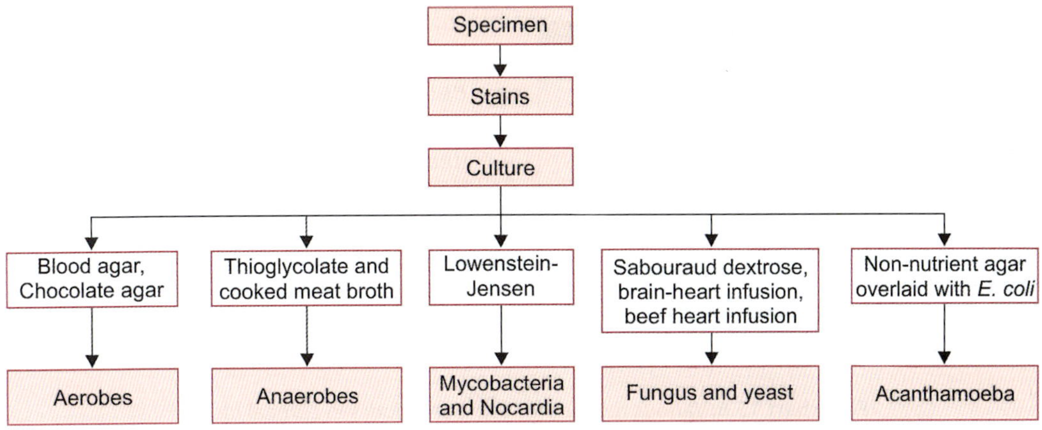

- Gram stains to find out
  - If the ulcer is uni- or poly- organismal.
  - Gram positive/negative
  - Cocci/bacilli/mixed
- *Other stains:* There is a long list of special stains for specific organisms. The common stains are Giemsa and calcofluor white stain; potassium hydroxide (KOH), which is not a stain, is used to screen fungus, modified Ziehl–Neelsen stain is used for mycobacteria.
- Culture—aerobic/nonaerobic
- Sensitivity

Flowchart 15.4 shows the variety of stains used in identifying organisms in corneal ulcers.

Flowchart 15.5 shows summary of various media to identify organisms in corneal ulcer.

Outline of Management of Corneal Ulcers (in All Ages)

Treatment of corneal ulcers in children does not differ from that of adults; it can be divided into:

- Specific
  - Antimicrobial
    - Simple drops
    - Fortified drops
    - Subconjunctival injection
    - Systemic
- Cycloplegics
  - Long acting
  - Short acting
- Supportive
  - Pad and bandage
  - Analgesic
  - Ocular hypotensive—(when required)
  - Cauterization
  - Soft contact lenses

Some of the clinical appearance would give a rough idea of what could be the causative organism, i.e., bacteria, virus, or fungus.

Viral and fungal ulcers have a characteristic clinical presentation and are less frequent than bacterial ulcers.

Hence, it is advisable to start antibacterial drugs in all cases empirically until the organisms have been identified by smear. A smear should be taken before starting antibiotics. The best empirical regime is to start a broad-spectrum antibiotic that is effective against both gram-positive and gram-negative cocci and bacilli; this should be of suitable strength and frequency. At this stage, it is better not to use a combination of antibiotics. The commonly used antibiotics and their strengths are given in the following **Table 15.4**.

Any of the earlier mentioned drops is instilled in the lower fornix only one drop at a time, hourly for the first day, during waking hours, and ointment of the same is applied at night; if necessary, a pad can be applied at night. Instilling more than one drop at a time has no therapeutic advantage. Because the second drop is not retained and spills over.

TABLE 15.4: Commonly used antibiotics and their strengths.

Antibiotic	*Strength*
Gentamicin	0.3%
Ciprofloxacin	0.3%
Ofloxacin	0.3%
Tobramycin	0.3%
Chloramphenicol	0.3%
Erythromycin	0.5%

The commonly followed protocol for the use of antibiotic drops to treat corneal ulcers is given in the following **Flowchart 15.6.**

- *Methicillin-resistant organisms are best treated with vancomycin 500 mg/mL.
- Mycobacteria (atypical) are treated with amikacin 2% and clarithromycin 1%.
- *Nocardia* responds to amikacin and trimethoprim-sulfamethoxazole.
- *Klebsiella, Proteus, Enterobacter,* and *Escherichia coli* can be treated with fortified gentamicin or tobramycin.
- *Pseudomonas* corneal ulcer responds poorly to all antibiotic drops. Commonly used antibiotic drops to treat *Pseudomonas* corneal ulcers are aminoglycosides, fluoroquinolones, and chloromycetin.

Sometimes, a combination of two or more antibiotics is instilled to widen the spectrum of each component without antagonizing each other.

Flowchart 15.6: Various regimes for using antibiotics in corneal ulcers.

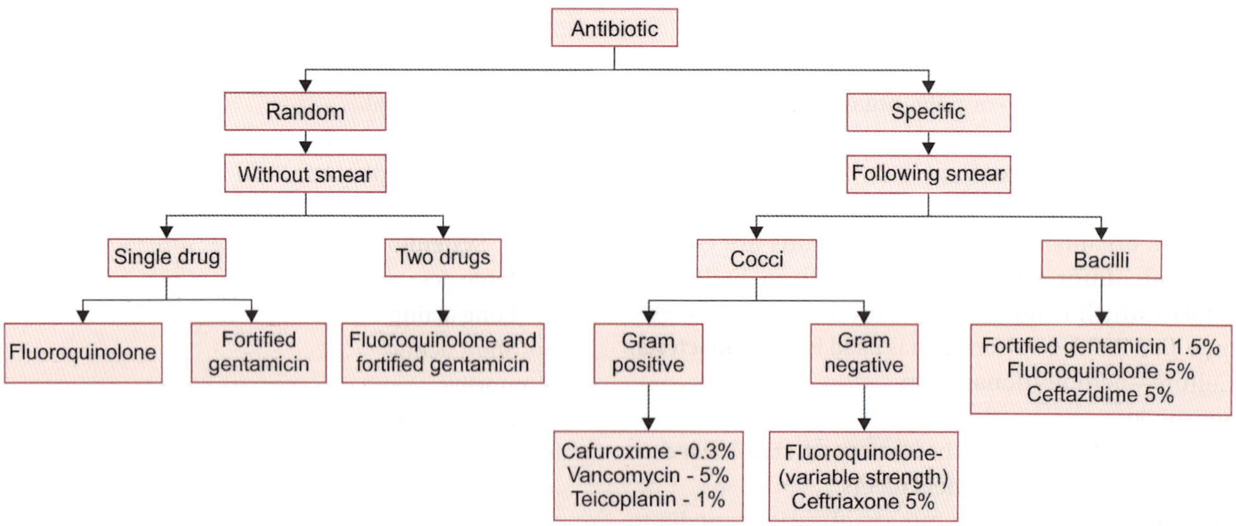

*Methicillin-resistant strains: Resistance to methicillin is increasing.

The organisms are:

- Staphylococci
- Streptococci
- *Clostridium*
- *Corynebacterium*

The common combinations available are:

- Neomycin 0.3%, polymaxin 10,000 units, and bacitracin 500 units.
- Neomycin 0.3% with chloromycetin.

In the past, when ordinary antibiotics were found to be ineffective, subconjunctival antibiotics were administered. All locally-acting antibiotics can be used as subconjunctival injections. Administering a subconjunctival infection to a child is not an easy task.

This brought fortified drops in vogue.

The common antibiotics used as fortified drops are:

- Gentamicin 15 mg/mL
- Cefazolin, cephalosporins, cefuroxime, or ceftazidime 50 mg/mL
- Tobramycin, 15 mg/mL
- Ciprofloxacin, 3 mg/mL
- Norfloxacin, 3 mg/mL
- The second line of drugs used are vancomycin and amikacin.

How to Prepare Fortified Drops

- They are not available commercially.
- They are prepared at hospital pharmacies.
- They cannot be preserved for >48 hours.
- To prepare fortified drops of gentamicin, 2.00 mL of injectable gentamicin that contains 40.00 mg/mL is added to 5.00 mL of commercially available 0.3% gentamicin eye drops.
- To prepare fortified drops of cefazolin, cephalosporins, cefuroxime, or ceftazidime, 500 mg of injectable antibiotic is added to 2.5 mL of sterile injectable water, which is then added to 7.5 mL of artificial tear. This gives a concentration of 50 mg/mL with a strength of 5.0%. This can be used for 3–4 days if kept in the refrigerator.
- To prepare a fortified drop of vancomycin—draw 2.00 mL of artificial tear from a 10.00 mL container, add this to 500 mg of powder, shake with draw the solution, and add to remaining 8.00 mL of artificial tear.
- To prepare a fortified drop of amikacin, add 250 mg of amikacin to 8.00 mL of artificial tear.

The advantages of ophthalmic ointments are:

- They form a protective layer on the cornea, facilitating healing.
- They act as lubricants.
- They are slowly absorbed and drained, maintaining high concentrations in the conjunctival sac.
- Prevent the sticking of lid margins.

Commonly used antibiotics as subconjunctival injections are:

- *Crystalline penicillin:* 1 million units/mL
- *Gentamicin:* 20–40 mg/mL
- *Tobramycin:* 20–40 mg/mL
- Other antibiotics used subconjunctivally are amikacin and vancomycin.

The subconjunctival injections are given a few millimeters away from the limbus, injection at the limbus is painful and uncomfortable. The subconjunctival injections reach therapeutic levels in a short time and are eliminated equally fast. They are generally administered once a day, followed by local instillation of the drop.

The subconjunctivally given antibiotic reaches the aqueous via:

- Conjunctiva to corneal epithelium
- Stroma
- Transscleral

> Oral antibiotics have no added advantage over local instillation or subconjunctival injection because most of them do not cross the blood-aqueous barrier.

Corneal ulcers secondary to contact lenses are caused by:

- Any bacteria—the common organisms that cause contact lens-related corneal ulcers are *Pseudomonas aeruginosa*, *Staphylococcus*, *Streptococcus*, and *Serratia*.
- Viruses do not produce lens-related corneal ulcers.
- Fungi are superadded to bacterial ulcers.
- *Acanthamoeba*, a parasite, has emerged as the main causative organism to cause contact lens-related corneal ulcers.

> Ring shaped ulcers are caused by—*Bacillus* species, *Pseudomonas*, *Proteus*, *Streptococcus*, and *Listeria*.

Nonantibiotic treatment of corneal ulcers are:

- Removal of discharge
- Cycloplegics
- Pad and bandage
- Bandage contact lenses
- Cauterization of ulcers
- *Ocular hypotensive:* Systemic and/or local drops
- Paracentesis

Removal of Discharge

Discharge should be removed before starting antibiotics by sterile wet swab to reduce the bulk of microorganisms in the conjunctiva; secondly, it reduces the chances of gluing the lids.

> Irrigation of the conjunctival sac does not have any advantage; moreover, it washes away protective lysozyme from the conjunctival sac.

Cycloplegia

Cycloplegic, when put in the conjunctival sac, passes through the substance of the cornea to reach the aqueous; some of it gets absorbed through the conjunctiva and nasolacrimal duct to reach the throat, from where it gets absorbed in the systemic circulation.

Cycloplegics have no action on the cornea; they are neither antibiotics, analgesics, nor anti-inflammatory drugs. They lack anesthetic properties. The main function of cycloplegics in corneal ulcers is to prevent and/or treat associated anterior uveitis, which causes tenderness, pain, photophobia, and lacrimation. Cycloplegics prevent the formation of posterior synechiae and break those already present. The use of cycloplegics gives prompt relief from pain. In cases of stromal involvement and hypopyon, atropine is the best cycloplegic. In children, atropine should be used with usual precaution.

> Mydriatic without cycloplegic action have no role in treatment of corneal ulcer.

Pad and Bandage

In the past, bandaging an eye with a corneal ulcer over a pad was a routine protocol worldwide. Pads and bandages prevent movement of the lid over the ulcer. Moving lids rub over the ulcer and destabilize the freshly laid epithelium. Pads and bandages reduced this, but not the movement of the globe underneath. The disadvantage of bandaging is that it raises the temperature in the eye under the lids, encouraging microbial growth. Hence, bandaging of the eye with copious discharge is better avoided. Moreover, frequent instillation of antibiotics is hampered by bandaging. A presently frequent antibiotic drop in the effected eye is considered to be an alternate.

Bandage Contact Lens

Bandage contact lenses are a better option without hampering frequent instillation of drugs.

Cauterization

Cauterization of ulcers has little role in present-day management of corneal ulcers. In the past, cauterization was done either by chemicals or physical methods. The commonly used chemical to cauterize the ulcer was a weak solution of carbolic acid or an alcoholic solution of iodine. The physical methods consisted mainly of heat through a cautery.

Paracentesis

In rare instances of large hypopyons not responding to usual antibiotics, cycloplegia paracentesis may be tried to drain the pus. In addition to this, paracentesis lowers intraocular pressure, which reduces the risk of perforation. The paracentesis port can be used to give intracameral injection* of antibiotics if needed. Paracentesis should be performed under surgical antisepsis and asepsis.

Keratoplasty

Keratoplasty is replacing an opaque cornea with a transparent cornea from a donor eye (no eyes are removed from living persons). Vision improves only in cases of loss of vision due to corneal lesions. Keratoplasty as per depth is divided into two main groups, i.e., superficial (lamellar) and deep (penetrating). Lamellar keratoplasty is done for pathology in the superficial layers between the epithelium and the superficial stroma. Generally, they are large. Easy to perform, less postoperative complications because the Descemet's membrane and endothelium are not disturbed, with the least chances of rejection and the least postoperative astigmatism. The indications for lamellar grafts are: superficial corneal opacities, whether congenital or acquired, may be infectious or noninfectious. They are congenital opacity degenerations such as band

---

**Intracameral injection:* Intracameral injection delivers water soluble drugs in the anterior chamber to deliver drugs in the appropriate strength and quantity to bypass the ocular barriers. This gives a high concentration of antibiotics to give prompt results. Intracameral antibiotics should be given at a specifically prescribed concentration to avoid damage to the corneal endothelium. Besides antibiotics, anesthetic agent mydriatic and miotic too can be given when needed (not in corneal ulcers).

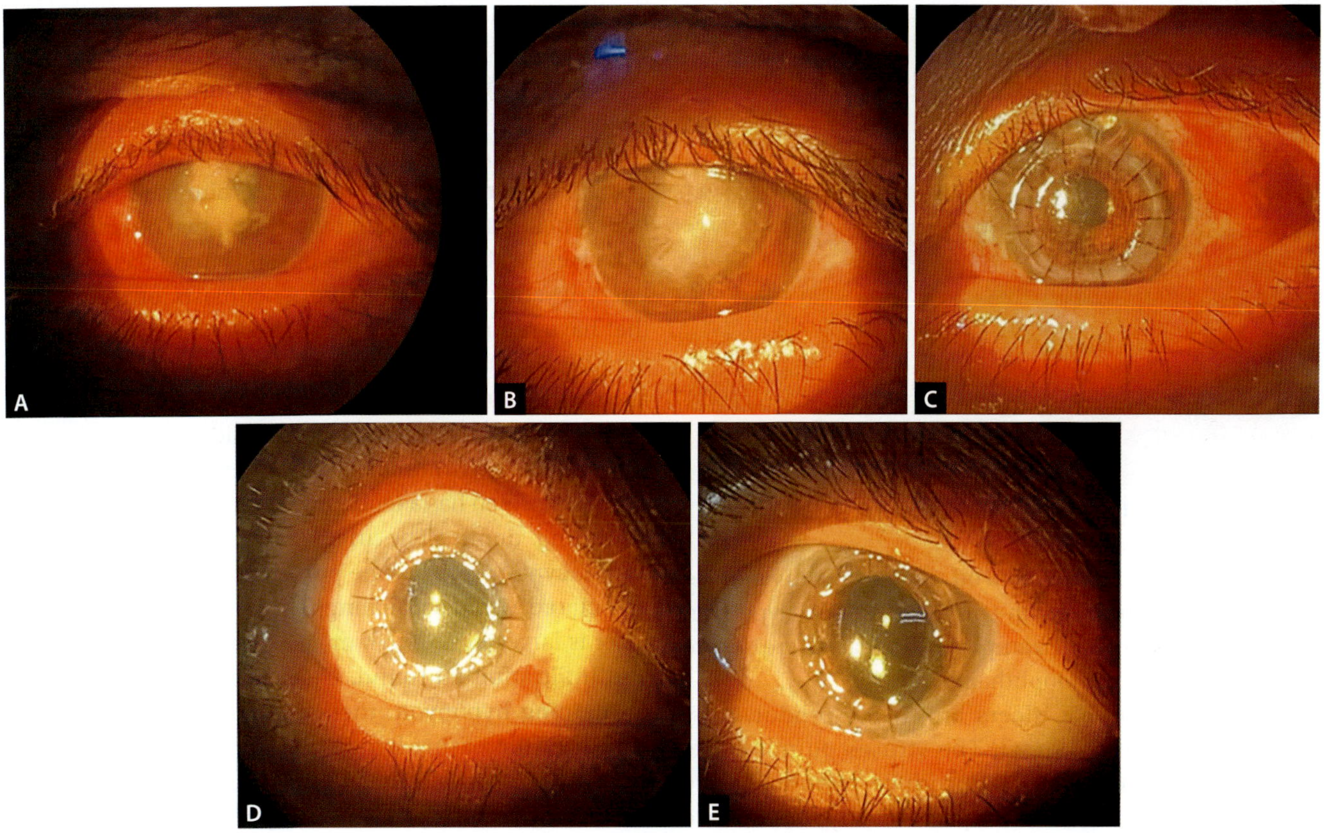

Figs. 15.18A to E: Keratoplasty in—(A) Central corneal ulcer; (B) Same ulcer not responding to treatment; (C) Result in penetrating graft in the in the immediate postoperative period; (D) After 24 hours; and (E) After 7 days.

keratopathy, bullous keratopathy, keratoconus, postlasik opacities, and superficial corneal vascularization. The penetrating keratoplasty replaces corneal pathology from the epithelium to the endothelium. They are generally smaller than lamellar graphs. The chances of rejection and postoperative astigmatism are more. The indications of penetrating keratoplasty are full-thickness corneal opacities, corneal ulcers not responding to usual medical therapy, full-thickness degeneration and dystrophies, reoperation following initial failed keratoplasty, keratoconus, and keratectasia.

Donated eyes, if not used within a few hours, are preserved in eye banks, which are highly specialized, highly sophisticated facilities. Available in all tertiary eye hospitals. All keratoplasty should be done under an operating microscope with ten zero sutures. Keratoplasty done in advanced hospitals has very rewarding results.

The following **Figures 15.18A to E** show keratoplasty done on a progressive corneal ulcer in a patient in their teens.

Complications of Corneal Ulcer

- Immediate—hypopyon **(Fig. 15.19)**
- Delayed
  - Descemetocele
  - Perforation
  - Adherent leukoma
  - Corneal ectasia
- Late
  - Corneal opacity
  - Vascularization

Hypopyon Corneal Ulcer

Hypopyon is defined as the accumulation of pus in the anterior chamber, of various shades of white or yellowish white, rarely blood-tinged or green **(Fig. 15.19)**. All white matters in the anterior chambers are not true hypopyons. The causes of hypopyon can be infective or noninfective. The later are grouped under the term pseudo hypopyon. The causes of this are lens matter,

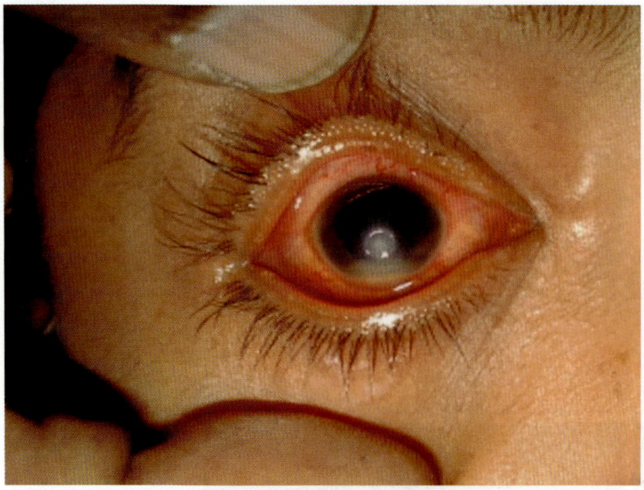

Fig. 15.19: Hypopyon corneal ulcer.

malignant cells, and silicon oil. The other division of hypopyon is hypopyon with corneal ulcer and hypopyon without corneal ulcer. Examples of the latter are severe anterior uveitis and endophthalmitis.

Hypopyon corneal ulcers are ulcers produced by virulent bacteria and fungi. The viruses do not cause hypopyon. All bacteria can produce hypopyon; the most common bacteria to produce hypopyon are pneumococci, *Pseudomonas*, staphylococci, streptococci, gonococci, and *Moraxella*. Out of these, pneumococci and *Pseudomonas* are more divesting. Pneumococci are so common causes that pneumococcal corneal ulcers are taken as types specific to hypopyon corneal ulcers. All bacterial corneal ulcers with hypopyon are suspected to be pneumococcal unless proved otherwise. The typical pneumococcal ulcer is called ulcus serpens because of its serpiginous character.

ULCUS SERPENS

The term ulcus serpens is commonly used for corneal ulcers caused by *Pneumococcus*. The ulcer is acute and fast growing. The diagnosis is based on the characteristics of a pneumococcal corneal ulcer, i.e., a central, fast growing ulcer with rapidly developing hypopyon. The most common source of the organism is chronic dacryocystitis, making it mandatory to examine the sac in all cases of acute corneal ulcers. Pneumococci do not exclude other pyogenic organisms from the list of hypopyon corneal ulcers.

Pneumococcal corneal ulcers are always associated with anterior uveitis. The inflammation in such cases is not only microbial but also due to the toxin produced by it. The clinical features of ulcus serpens do not differ much from other bacterial ulcers; the only difference is in the severity of the ulcer, which is surpassed by *Pseudomonas* only. Surprisingly, in spite of the fast growth of ulcers with severe uveitis, the pain is less than expected, which delays the initiation of specific treatment.

The ulcer may start even after a minute of scratching the cornea. The ulcers can be put into two broad groups, i.e., ulcers with chronic dacryocystitis and ulcers without dacryocystitis. The latter group consists of those eyes that have reduced corneal sensation from things such as keratomalacia, postherpetic anesthesia, lagophthalmos, and contact lens use. Occasionally, associated otitis media may be a factor other than dacryocystitis.

Following a trauma, a small central corneal ulcer develops, which has a tendency to spread in all directions, including depth. The ulcus serpens has a peculiar tendency to spread in one particular direction, which is associated with the healing of the opposite edge. The ulcer is large, with slough on the floor, edematous edges, and infiltration all round. Ulcer is associated with fast developing hypopyon; there is severe anterior uveitis with ever-increasing hypopyon, resulting in secondary glaucoma, a not-welcome factor, along with the destruction of Descemet's membrane heralds perforation.

Management of Ulcus Serpens (Pneumococcal Corneal Ulcer)

- A pneumococcal corneal ulcer is an ophthalmic emergency.
- All fast-growing, large corneal ulcers with large hypopyons should be considered pneumococcal and managed as such until a definite bacterial result has been reached.
- It is better to hospitalize the child with a pneumococcal corneal ulcer. The child should undergo a pediatric check to exclude systemic pneumococcal involvement.
- *Atropinization:* Atropine should be used as per the protocol of the institution. Atropine in children should be in the form of an ointment rather than a drop. The strength of atropine should not exceed 1% and not used >2 times a day in children.
- *Fortified antibiotic:* Each institute has its own protocol for the use of fortified antibiotic drops. The common protocol is to use fortified gentamicin drops to begin with empirically until the result of sensitivity is available. If the organism is not found to be sensitive to gentamicin, it is better to switch over to the other antibiotic drops to which the isolated organism is sensitive.

The fortified drop is put in the conjunctiva sac every 5 minutes, six times. This is followed by instillation every 10 minutes six times, then every 15 minutes for another six times, and then every hour. At night, gentamicin ointment is used.

- Observe for progress of the ulcer and hypopyon. Generally, frequent fortified drops give results as good as subconjunctival injections.
- If the hypopyon does not respond, a subconjunctival injection of gentamicin is considered.
- Put the child on β blockers/local carbonic anhydrase inhibitors in consultation with the pediatrician to keep IOP low.
- Systemic antibiotics do not seem to have any role in the management of corneal ulcers per se.

Complication

All hypopyon corneal ulcers are fraught with the danger of perforation and its sequel.

Successfully treated corneal ulcers with or without hypopyon will develop central corneal opacity with the course of events, i.e.,

- Various grades of opacity
- Adherent leukoma
- Descemetocele
- Pseudo cornea
- Anterior staphyloma

Descemetocele (Keratocele) (Fig. 15.20)

This is one of the complications that, if not managed well, results in corneal perforation. It involves the bulging of intact Descemet's membrane through a deep corneal ulcer where the epithelium, Bowman's membrane, and stroma have been destroyed. It can happen with normal intraocular tension; a rise in intraocular pressure causes an increment of descemetocele, both in depth and size. It is commonly seen in virulent corneal ulcers. The descemetocele looks like a drop of clear fluid surrounded by a sloughing corneal ulcer. It most often happens in the center of the cornea. It is usually painful initially due to the rubbing of the lids over the descemetocele. The pain becomes less as the ulcer sloughs. Descemetocele is an ophthalmic emergency. Generally, by the time descemetocele develops, vision is greatly reduced. Perforation is precipitated by a sudden rise in intraocular pressure, trauma direct to the cornea, or trauma indirect due to a sudden rise in intrathoracic pressure, as in prolonged coughing and sneezing. The management is frustrating. The aim of the treatment is to prevent perforation along with the intense management of corneal ulcers. The first step is to reduce intraocular tension with local and systemic carbonic anhydrase inhibitors or local β blocker drops. The first aid is to patch the eye with a pad and bandage following the instillation of atropine, a broad-spectrum antibiotic, and local antiglaucoma drops. The treatment in the specialized center is soft bandage lens and cyanoacrylate glue over the impending descemetocele. Tetracycline is given empirically in all sloughing corneal ulcers with the assumption that, besides its antibiotic property, it has an anticollagenase effect that prevents further worsening. The surgical management consists of guarded paracentesis, an amniotic membrane graft, and a conjunctival flap (Gundersen flap). The last resort is to do a large, penetrating keratoplasty. The prognosis, in spite of all efforts, is frustrating. The end result is perforation, which may lead to adherent leukoma, partial or total corneal staphyloma, or corneal fistula. Endophthalmitis following perforation is a common complication.

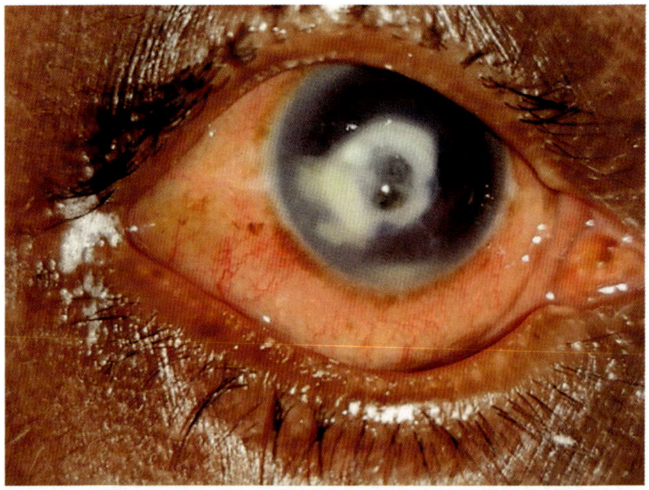

Fig. 15.20: Descemetocele in advanced corneal ulcer with hypopyon.

Other Hypopyon Corneal Ulcers

Bacteria are the most common microorganisms to produce hypopyon corneal ulcers. All pus-forming bacteria, i.e., cocci and bacilli, both gram-positive and gram-negative, can cause hypopyon corneal ulcers with varied severity. Common bacteria that cause hypopyon corneal ulcers are pneumococci, *Pseudomonas*, staphylococci, gonococci, and *Moraxella*. Other bacteria known to cause hypopyon are *Bacillus cereus*, *Clostridium*, *Escherichia coli*, *Haemophilus influenzae*, and Propionibacterium acnes.

Next group of organisms to produce hypopyon corneal ulcers are fungi. The common fungi that cause corneal ulcers are *Aspergillus*, *Fusarium*, *Alternaria*, Cephalosporium, and *Curvularia*. All of them are filamentous fungi, and out of them, the most common fungus to cause corneal ulcers is *Aspergillus*. Other fungi that produce corneal ulcers are *Candida* and *Cryptococcus*.

Besides bacteria and fungi, the organism that causes hypopyon corneal ulcers is a parasite called *Acanthamoeba*. Viruses do not produce hypopyon.

SPECIFIC BACTERIAL ULCERS

The list of bacteria that cause corneal ulcers is many, some mild, others with disastrous results. Most of them are common; a few are less frequent. The clinical picture and management differ on the basis of their staining characteristics, i.e., gram positive or negative. The following is a list of them **(Table 15.5)**.

The following **Table 15.6** shows first-line antibiotic therapy for bacterial corneal ulcers.

The following **Table 15.7** gives the clinical features of specific bacterial corneal ulcers.

TABLE 15.5: Classification of bacteria causing corneal ulcer.

Bacteria	
Gram positive	***Gram negative***
Staphylococcus epidermidis	*Pseudomonas aeruginosa*
S. aureus	*H. influenza*
Streptococcus Pneumoniae	*Neisseria gonococcus*
Bacillus	*Proteus* *Klebsiella* *Moraxella*

TABLE 15.6: The choice of antibiotic against different types of bacteria.

Staining	***Initial antibiotic***
Gram-positive cocci	Gentamicin, tobramycin, and cefazolin
Gram-negative cocci	Cefazolin
Gram-positive bacilli	Penicillin, tobramycin, and gentamicin
Gram-negative bacilli	Gentamicin, tobramycin
No organism	Ciprofloxacin, cefazolin

TABLE 15.7: Clinical features of specific bacterial corneal ulcers.

Causative organism	***Clinical feature***
Staphylococcus (*S. epidermidis and S. aureus*)	Central, round/oval in the compromised cornea; a clear cut border may be shallow; a prominent anterior chamber reaction may be hypopyon
Streptococcus (*S. pneumoniae*)	Central, early involvement of stroma, irregular undermined edge, fast-growing intense anterior chamber reaction, and fast-growing hypopyon, serpiginous, folds in Descemet's membrane
Bacillus cereous	Mostly post-traumatic following contamination, very fast-growing severe pain, marked conjunctival reaction, edematous lid, may develop ring ulcer
Gonococcus	Can penetrate intact epithelial cells, starting as acute conjunctivitis with profuse purulent discharge. Intense infiltration of the cornea, central corneal ulcer, early central perforation
Pseudomonas	Rapid-growing, central, or peripheral ulcers may be post-traumatic and are frequently seen in contact lens wearers. Their spread is due to the production of protease and perforation, and greenish hypopyon endothelial plaque is common
Moraxella	Chronic slow-growing peripherals in compromised corneas in immunocompromised persons, debilitated persons, infiltrate++, and overhanging edges take many days to perforate
Proteus	Fast-growing corneal ulcer. Corneal abscess, folds in Descemet's membrane hypopyon, and perforation
Escherichia coli	*Less common:* Elderly patient, prominent anterior chamber (AC) reaction, hypopyon hyphema, gas in AC
Haemophilus influenzae (*Koch–Weeks* bacilli)	Marked conjunctivitis, central corneal ulcer, hypopyon, rarely perforate

MYCOTIC (FUNGAL) CORNEAL ULCER

Fungal corneal ulcers are less frequent than bacterial corneal ulcers in general; they are still rare in children unless the child is immunocompromised due to systemic or local causes. The local causes that predispose to fungal keratitis in children are the injudicious use of antibiotics and steroids; other causes are lagophthalmos, keratomalacia, malnutrition, lid deformity, and proptosis.

The prerequisite for a fungal corneal ulcer to develop is trauma. Some fungi have been claimed to produce ulcers without trauma even.

The trauma is generally organic; injuries caused by vegetables such as plant leaves, twigs, and thorns are very common and cause corneal ulcers. Injuries from animal tails or nails are frequent. Occasionally, field soil and organic manure may be the cause. It takes 15 days for an ulcer to develop following an injury to organic material.

> A fast-growing ulcer following an organic injury need not always be fungal.

A fungal ulcer is an indolent ulcer developing slowly with prominent ciliary congestion and the usual lacrimation and photophobia.

Characteristics of Fungal Ulcer

- History of:
  - Injury by organic matter
  - Not responding to usual antibiotic drops
  - Indiscriminate use of steroids
  - Suggestions of immune compromises
- Appearances **(Figs. 15.21A and B)**
  - Prominent circumciliary congestion
  - Central, slow-growing ulcer:
    - Large
    - Elevated rolled margin
    - Gray, white, and dry-looking
    - Subepithelial infiltration round the ulcer
    - Immune ring beyond the infiltration
    - Satellite lesion
    - Endothelial plaque
    - Large, immobile yellow hypopyon
- Chances of perforation are less than in a bacterial ulcer unless a secondary infection sets in and there is a rise in intraocular pressure.
- Corneal vascularization
- Severe iridocyclitis
- Secondary glaucoma (frequent)

Investigations

- All large hypopyon corneal ulcers not responding to usual antibiotic therapy should undergo the following microbial workup to find out if the fungus is yeast or filamentous.
  - Demonstration of fungal hyphae—scrap from the ulcer is added to a 10% KOH solution and seen under a light microscope. The presence of hyphae denotes a fungal infection but fails to identify the fungus; no stain is required in this test.
  - Lactophenol cotton blue stain—this test stains molds and yeast; pale to dark blue.

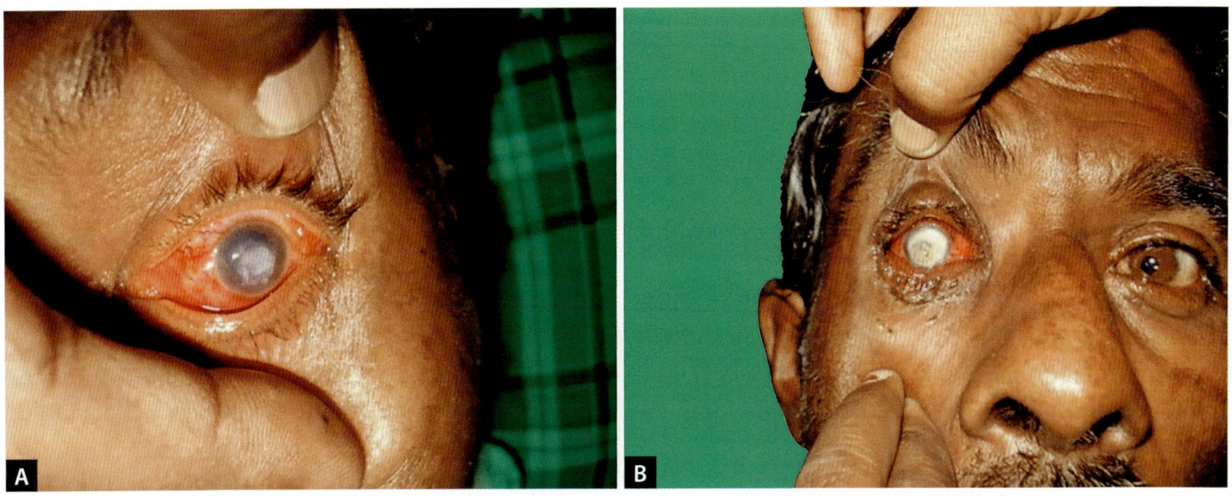

Figs. 15.21A and B: Fungal corneal ulcer—early and late stages in a farmer.

  - Indian ink is used to stain *Cryptococcus*. It is a negative stain that does not stain the fungus; the fungus stands out prominently against the background.
  - Calcofluor white is added to KOH, and the slide examined under a fluorescent microscope.
  - Giemsa stain
  - Periodic acid Schiff (PAS) stain
  - Methenamine silver stain
- *Culture of fungi:* Fungi are difficult to culture; they take a long time to yield results. They cannot be used to find sensitivity. Commonly used cultural media are:
  - Sabouraud dextrose medium may be with or without added antibiotic. Antibiotics are added to suppress bacterial contamination.
  - Sabouraud, dextrose, and agar broth
  - Blood agar
  - Brain-heart infusion
  - Corn meal agar
  - Potato dextrose agar

Management of Mycotic Corneal Ulcers

The management of mycotic corneal ulcers is difficult and time consuming. Even the best treatment fails to give a clear cornea. The corneal opacities following fungal infections are generally large, deep, and dense.

Unsatisfactory results in treatment can be attributed to:

- Late initiation of antifungal treatment
- Use of the wrong antifungal drug.
- Use of antifungal drugs in subtherapeutic strength, frequency, and duration.
- Poor penetration of antifungal drugs through the cornea to reach the aqueous.
- Superadded bacterial infection
- Secondary glaucoma

Antifungal drugs to treat corneal ulcers can be divided into two broad groups:

- Those against filamentous fungi and those against nonfilamentous fungi.
- Drugs used against filamentous fungi include natamycin 5% as the first line. The second line consists of miconazole (imidazole), ketoconazole (1–5%), and amphotericin B (0.2–0.5%). Nonfilamentous fungi are best treated with amphotericin B.

All antifungal drugs are only fungistatic.

Viral Corneal Ulcer

Almost all viruses can cause superficial keratitis and corneal ulcers, the viruses that cause keratitis are mostly DNA viruses.

They are:

- *Human herpes virus:* Herpes simplex
- Varicella-Zoster virus, Herpes zoster, and chickenpox
- *Cytomegalovirus*
- Epstein–Barr virus
- Adenovirus

One thing common about the viruses mentioned earlier is that all of them cause systemic diseases of various seriousness. The most common virus to cause corneal pathology is herpes simplex.

Herpes Simplex Corneal Ulcer

Over the last few decades, the incidence of herpes simplex viral infections of the eye and its adnexa has shown an upward swing. Cornea, too, has its share in this increment. Making herpes simplex keratitis a major corneal morbidity. The incidence of herpes simplex corneal involvement is less reported in underdeveloped countries where bacterial keratitis outnumbers them.

The disease is self-limiting in immunocompetent persons, including children, immune compromise may be local or systemic. Herpetic keratitis can be primary or recurrent. Primary keratitis has a higher chance of being self-limited. There may be a gap of a few months to years between the apparent cure and the next attack, which is referred to as recurrent herpetic keratitis. The recurrence can neither be predicted nor prevented.

There is no preventive vaccine against herpes simplex infection.

The herpes simplex virus has traditionally been divided into two types, i.e., type 1 and type 2. The division is arbitrary. Type 1 is said to involve the body above the waist; naturally, this is the type that infects the eyes and their adnexa. The type 2 infection is localized to the body under the waist, mostly the genitals. It rarely infects the eyes, but the possibilities cannot be excluded. Both types involve the skin, mucous membrane, mucocutaneous junction, conjunctiva, and cornea. The corneal involvement is invariably associated with anterior uveitis.

Herpes simplex infection can be congenital or acquired. The former is associated with multiple congenital malformations, including ocular. The acquired infection, as per age, can be:

- Neonatal
- Childhood
- Adolescent

Clinically, herpes simplex infection is divided into two groups as per mode of acquiring the infection. They are primary and recurrent.

Primary Herpes Simplex Infection

Primary herpes simplex infection occurs in those persons who have not been exposed to herpes simplex in the past. About 90% of the population becomes seropositive in the first two decades and is not likely to get primary herpes simplex disease, systemic or ocular, but remains at risk of recurrent disease. Children are most vulnerable to getting a primary herpes infection.

Children suffering from herpes simplex infections are put into the following clinical groups:

- As a rule, children under 6 months are protected by their mother's immunity.
- A small percentage of infants get infected during passage from their mother's infected birth canal, which may prove fatal.
- Herpes simplex conjunctivitis is the most common condition of nongonococcal ophthalmia neonatorum.
- By 6 months, immunity passed to the fetus weans off, and the child becomes prone to herpes simplex infection. The common age group to get an infection comprises children between 6 months and 10 years.
- The children in this group get infections from older children or adults from lesions in their lips, lids, or even their genitals.
- The third age group to get infected is teens.
- The primary herpes simplexes infections are self-limited, often missed, and are precursors of recurrent disease.
- The eye and its adnexa are involved in the following ways in primary lesions:
    - *Lids:* Vesicles and blepharitis
    - *Conjunctiva:* Nongonococcal ophthalmia neonatorum, follicular conjunctivitis, pseudomembranous conjunctivitis
    - *Cornea:* Micro dendrite, dendritic keratitis
    - *Uvea:* Anterior uveitis

Recurrent Herpes Simplex Keratitis

Out of all the recurrent herpes simplex diseases of the eyes, keratitis is the most important and difficult to manage. The patients are seropositive for the virus but lack antibodies against the herpes simplex virus. The patients have been exposed to the primary herpes simplex in the past, of which they patients is unaware. Following primary infection, the virus reaches the trigeminal ganglion and remains dormant, only to be activated due to a fall in immunity—local or systemic, trivial trauma to the eye, stress, or a physiological condition such as menstruation, fever, or allergy. The lesions develop in the skin, lips, angle of the mouth, and cornea.

Corneal Lesions in Recurrent Herpes Simplex

The corneal lesions can be:

- Epithelial
- Stromal
- Endothelial
- Combination

Epithelial lesions are the most common and earliest to manifest; they may even pass off without involving the stroma. The common epithelial lesions are:

- Micro- or macro-dendritic ulcers
- Geographic (amoeboid) ulcers
- Keratitis meta-herpetic
- Less common lesions are:
    - Blotch epithelial lesions
    - Satellite epithelial lesions
    - Filamentary keratitis

The aforementioned may precede a dendritic ulcer or may be present along with it.

Dendritic Ulcers

Dendritic ulcers are a type-specific form of herpes simplex keratitis. However, such epithelial defects may be seen in herpes zoster ophthalmicus and mild trauma due to faulty contact lens fitting and Thygeson keratitis.* Dendrite ulcers are unilateral and can start at all ages after 6 months of age. The epithelial defects start as minute central specks that get converted to a micro dendrite that is converted to a regular dendritic ulcer. The dendritic

**Thygeson keratitis:* It is a superficial punctate keratitis with an insidious onset and a chronic and recurrent course. The lesions are small, raised oval intraepithelial spots with a whitish-gray color covering the whole of the epithelial surface in both eyes. The diagnosis is based on the exclusion of other causes of superficial punctate keratitis. The most widely used drug is a weak solution of water-soluble steroid drops.

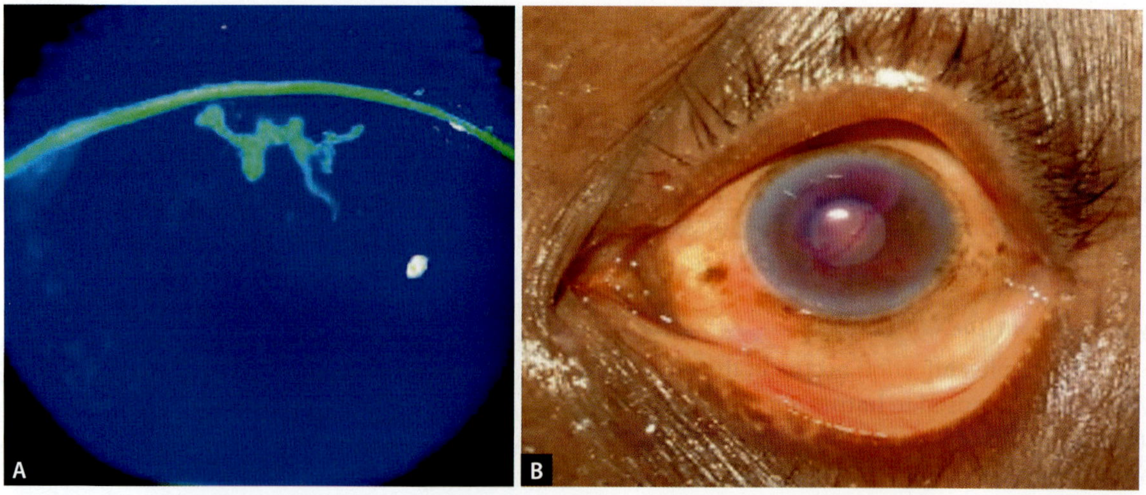

Figs. 15.22A and B: Dendritic ulcer staining with fluorescein (under a cobalt blue filter) and Rose Bengal (under white light).

ulcers are single; they commonly start in the center, rarely in the periphery; extension from the center to the periphery is possible.

The dendritic ulcer has the peculiar look of a twig of a plant with terminal branching; the branches invariably end with a rounded bud. The ulcer creeps in one direction at the same time as the distant end heals by epithelial slide. The bed of the ulcer stains bright green with fluorescein and periphery by Rose Bengal **(Figs. 15.22A and B)**.

The ulcer is most of the time confined to the epithelium without any anterior chamber reaction, and no hypopyon is formed. The presence of hypopyon is suggestive of a secondary bacterial infection.

The corneal sensation is dull, explaining the absence of pain. The absence of pain does not prevent lacrimation; the ulcer may be associated with conjunctivitis and circumciliary congestion without ciliary tenderness.

Occasionally, opacities develop under dendritic ulcers; they are called ghost images; their shapes are duplications of epithelial defects and do not require separate treatment; and antiviral drugs are known to worsen them. They may remain for years to come. Herpes simplex keratitis being uniocular, all eyes with watering of short duration should be stained with fluorescein and examined under a cobalt blue filter with high magnification. Of course, other causes of watering, like foreign bodies in the tarsus or even the cornea, should be excluded.

Amoeboid (Geographic) Ulcer

A dendritic ulcer should heal in a fortnight without treatment and within a week with treatment. If such healing does not take place, the treatment should be altered by changing the antiviral drug. The nonhealing dendritic ulcer keeps increasing not only in the long axis but also in all directions, changing the dendritic ulcer to a wider ulcer that may be 4–5 mm in dimension and deep enough to reach the stroma. Due to its irregular shape, it is called a geographic ulcer. The cause of the uncontrolled spread is attributed to compromised immunity in the peripheral cornea and the use of steroids indiscriminately. The geographic ulcer does not respond well to idoxuridine drops, which are used for dendritic ulcers; other antiviral drugs give better results.

Metaherpetic Keratitis

These are caused by retarded healing at the level of the basement membrane during the treatment of dendritic and amoeboid ulcers. There is no viral component that can be thought to be the cause. Most probably, they are due to damage to the nerve endings. By nature, they are slow to progress, have little inflammatory reaction, and are difficult to treat. Treatment is prolonged and consists of antiviral local drops and ointment for a long time. In the absence of corneal sensation, the role of bandage lenses has been questioned, and some clinicians insist on prolonged pads and bandages instead.

Stromal Involvement

Stromal involvement is a major contributing factor in causing diminished vision. The stromal involvement is preceded by dendritic and geographic ulcers. It takes multiple attacks of epithelial ulcers to herald stromal involvement; it starts in the center and spreads toward the periphery, not reaching the limbus.

Based on the clinical presentation, stromal involvement can either be:

- Necrotizing
- Non-necrotizing

Necrotizing stromal ulcer: Necrotizing stromal involvement is an infective process that requires active replication of the virus, causing active stromal infiltration and resulting in subepithelial cheesy material in the stroma, causing anterior uveitis with keratic precipitate without hypopyon. Vascularization is frequent and scaring. Stromal necrosis may perforate when severe and uncontrolled.

Non-necrotizing stromal ulcer: Non-necrotizing stromal involvement is an immune reaction generally associated with decompensated immunity, both local and systemic. The precipitating factors are:

- Chemical cauterization
- Too much use of idoxuridine

Though it is categorized as stromal involvement, it is in fact an involvement of both epithelium and endothelium as well.

Endothelial

Endothelial involvement in herpes keratitis is a dysfunction of endothelial cells that leads to initial hydration of the stroma, followed by edema, which results in opacification of the stroma. The causes of endotheliitis are direct invasion by viruses or due to anterior chamber reactions.

Thus, the composite picture comprise of:

- Epithelial edema
- Stromal thickening
- Folds in the Descemet's membrane
- Anterior uveitis
- Raised IOP
- Peripheral ring opacity

Complications of Herpes Simplex Keratitis

- Most troublesome complication is recurrence that may happen even following successful treatment of keratitis.
- Persistant central corneal opacity
- Anterior uveitis
- Secondary glaucoma
- Deep vascularization
- Trophic ulcer
- Complicated cataract
- Persistent hypoesthesia of the cornea
- Scleritis
- Perforation

Management of Herpetic Keratitis

The following is the most common protocol for managing herpes simplex keratitis.

- There is no immunization against herpes simples.
- The disease is long-drawn and recurrent.
- The eyes are prone to secondary infection, overshadowing the viral component.
- The viruses are eliminated mostly by local antiherpes drugs.
- Systemic antiviral drugs are rarely required.
- Associated uveitis and secondary glaucoma are red flags that require concurrent management.
- Steroids per se are contraindicated, except in selected cases. That too in the weakest possible strength.
- Special attention is given to hypoesthesia of the cornea.
- Chemical cauterization has little role to play in the present scenario.
- Only a few cases may benefit from therapeutic keratoplasty.

> Corneas from persons with a past history of herpes simplex keratitis are not used for keratoplasty.

The treatment can be divided into:

- Medical
  - Antiviral chemotherapy
  - Broad-spectrum antibiotics
  - Cycloplegic drugs
  - Antiglaucoma drugs
  - Steroids
- Ancillary
  - Debridement
  - Lubricants
- Surgical
  - Tissue adhesive
  - Keratoplasty

Medical

Antiviral Chemotherapy

The commonly used antiviral drugs are given in **Table 15.8**.

TABLE 15.8: Various types of antiviral drugs used in herpetic keratitis.

Drug	Analog of	Dose	Mode of action
Idoxuridine	Thymidine	0.1% hourly and 0.5% ointment at night	Works on epithelial lesions, does not penetrate the stroma, is insoluble in water, causes epithelial toxin, and hypersensitivity to the drugs is common
Trifluridine	Thymidine	1% solution TDS	It inhibits deoxyribonucleic acid (DNA), acts against primary and recurrence-effective stromal keratitis, and has no cross-resistance
Vidarabine	Adenosine	3% ophthalmic ointment 5 times a day for 5 days	Effective on epithelial keratitis
Acyclovir	Guanosine	3% ointment 5 times a day for 7 days	Stops viral replication, effective against types 1 and 2, primary and recurrence, and effective against epithelial and stromal lesions
Famciclovir	Prodrug of acyclovir	Oral tablet: 250 mg TDS for 7 days	Same as above

Broad-spectrum Antibiotics

There are no antibiotics that are effective against the herpes simplex virus. The antibiotics are administered to prevent and treat secondary bacterial infections. This is more important due to:

- Presence of a breach in the epithelium in the form the ulcer.
- Diminished sensation

Cycloplegic Drugs

Cycloplegic drugs are neither chemotherapeutic agents nor local analgesics. They do not prevent virus multiplication. Their main role is the management of associated anterior uveitis, which is inevitable with stromal and endothelial involvement.

The commonly used cycloplegics are: atropine sulfate 0.5–1% ointment or drops. It is better to avoid atropine under 10 years. The best protocol is to use atropine 1% ointment only once and replace it with homatropine hydrobromide 2% solution two times a day, subsequently. cyclopentolate, a common cycloplegic, is not used because it is suspected to reactivate uveitis. Hence, the best alternative to atropine remains homatropine.

Except atropine no cycloplegic is available in ointment form.

Pure mydriatics, i.e., epinephrine and its derivatives, have no role in corneal ulcers.

Antiglaucoma Drugs

Glaucoma associated with herpes simplex keratitis is always secondary to anterior uveitis. It has to be anticipated that it will be mandatory to record intraocular tension regularly, preferably by no-touch applanation tonometers. The drugs of choice are β blockers and local carbonic anhydrase inhibitors as drops. Latanoprost, its analogues, and miotics are contraindicated.

Steroids

Steroids in all forms are contraindicated in the presence of epithelial breaks. They are given stromal involvement, which is also their weakest possible strength.

Ancillary Treatment

Debridement and cauterizations, which were only available as treatment for epithelium involvement before antiviral chemotherapies became available, are no more in vogue. Lubricants help in healing epithelial defects.

Surgical

- *Tissue adhesive:* Tissue adhesives are used to prevent impending perforation and seal small perforations.
- *Keratoplasty:* Keratoplasty has no role in the presence of an active lesion. They are best suited for the management of residual corneal opacity. The donor material has a chance of getting involved even after a successful graft.

Treatment of Specific Lesions

Primary Lesions

A correct diagnosis of a primary lesion is of utmost importance. It requires a high degree of suspicion. Once the diagnosis is confirmed, the eye should be treated like a dendritic ulcer, keeping in mind that the condition is self-limited. The presence of blepharitis and blepharoconjunctivitis may point toward the presence of corneal involvement. Neonatal herpes simplex can be fatal and is best managed by a neonatologist.

A child with primary herpes simplex, after an apparent cure, goes into a state of latency where the virus reaches the trigeminal ganglion and lurks, only to be activated following a fall in local and systemic immunity. The latent period between primary and recurrent disease is anybody's guess; it varies from a few months to years. There is no preventive method to stop recurrence, which may be epithelial, stromal, or endothelial.

Dendritic Lesions

The dendritic lesions respond to local instillation of antiviral drugs, i.e., idoxuridine, vidarabine, trifluridine, and acyclovir. The last two are better than the former two, due to their epithelial toxicity.

Geographic Lesions

Geographic or amoeboid ulcers are a larger and wider form of dendritic ulcers, epithelial and natural; hence, management is the same as that of a dendritic defect, in addition to debridement of the edges followed by antiviral drops. Indolent ulcers may develop following too much use of antiviral drugs for too many days. They are better managed by reducing the frequency of antiviral drugs. Lubricants can be used as often as 4–6 times a day to encourage healing. Patching of the eye helps the epithelial slide over the ulcer to facilitate healing.

Stromal Lesions

Stromal involvement may be any of the following:

- Disciform keratitis without necrosis
- Necrotizing stromal keratitis

> Management of disciform keratitis involves judicious use of steroids under the umbrella of antiviral drugs, with usual monitoring of intraocular pressure and anterior uveitis.

Following is a chart showing the natural history of herpes simplex keratitis.

Self-limiting primary infections → seropositivity → latency → trigger → small central superficial ulcer → micro dendrite → dendritic ulcer → geographic ulcer → marginal keratitis → healing of epithelial defect → stromal involvement → indolent ulcer → disciform keratitis → non necrotizing/necrotizing keratitis → endotheliitis.

HERPES ZOSTER CORNEAL INVOLVEMENT

Herpes zoster infection in children is less common; hence, corneal involvement is less frequent than in herpes simplex. Half of the children suffering from herpes zoster ophthalmicus have ocular involvement, in the form of lesions on the skin of the lids, forehead, conjunctiva, sclera, and cornea, besides the uvea, trabecular meshwork, extraocular muscles, and damage to cranial nerves.

The corneal involvements can be:

- Epithelial
- Stromal
- Neural

The common corneal involvements are micro dendritic or fully developed dendritic ulcers that stain better with Rose Bengal; they are transient, self-limited, and do not go to the geographic ulcer stage.

Stromal keratitis is nonstaining, central, may be vascularized, generally associated with anterior uveitis. The neural corneal changes are—neurotropic keratitis,* recurrent epithelial defect, erosion, vascularization, and secondary bacterial involvement.

- Deep keratitis may be associated with episcleritis, and rarely, scleritis.
- Secondary glaucoma is common.

The management of herpes zoster keratopathy in children does not differ from that in adults. It is basically divided into two parts: systemic and local. The epithelial defects are self-limited and transient, best treated by acyclovir ophthalmic ointment three times a day along with cycloplegic.

Corneal involvement with no epithelial defects is treated with local steroid titration as per need; this should also look after anterior uveitis as well. Secondary glaucoma is treated by β blockers and local carbonic anhydrase inhibitors.

Systemic antiviral drugs have a limited role in keratopathy.

Neurotropic keratitis: In the past, this was referred to as neuroparalytic keratitis. This is an example of degenerative keratopathy associated with loss of corneal sensation. Which result in a breach in the epithelium and delayed healing, leading to corneal ulceration, which may lead to corneal melting and ultimately perforation.

EPSTEIN–BARR VIRUS KERATITIS

This virus belongs to the group of herpes viruses, also referred to as human herpes viruses. It is almost universal; all persons are infected by this virus some time or other in their lives; the most common involvement is called infective mononucleosis.

The corneal involvement causes dendritic ulcers and stromal keratitis. The stromal involvements are basically subepithelial infiltrates that are non-necrotizing; in the long run, the cornea may be vascularized, the keratopathy is self-limited and heals without any treatment; antiviral drugs have a limited role to play, use of steroids too has not been proven to be of much benefit; and the lesions are generally confused as herpes simplex keratitis.

PARASITIC KERATITIS

The two parasites that cause keratitis are *Acanthamoeba* and microsporidia, a fungal parasite that has traditionally been considered to be a protozoa.

Acanthamoeba Keratitis

Until the seventh decade of the last century, *Acanthamoeba* was considered to be a nonocular pathogen. Since then, it has been found to be a major cause of central corneal ulcers, which are most of the time missed. The diagnosis is by exclusion, preceded by a high degree of suspicion. Its treatment is a challenge that carries a bad prognosis; since then, it has been found to be a major cause of central corneal ulcers, which are most of the time missed. A corneal ulcer is a cause of eye loss.

Acanthamoeba is a free-living parasite present in air, soil, and water at a temperature that ranges from subzero to boiling point. Many species are commensals of the mouth and throat. Many persons who have suffered from an *Acanthamoeba* infection without obvious clinical features are known to develop immunity against it. The incidence of *Acanthamoeba* infection is pretty high among immune-compromised person suffering from HIV or non-HIV syndromes. The organism is a unicellular protozoa belonging to the family Acanthamoebidae and the genus *Acanthamoeba* with two forms, i.e., a motile trophozoite and a cystic form. The cysts are resistant to treatment. It is not uncommon to see both coexisting at some point. There are many species of *Acanthamoeba* out of which only *Acanthamoeba* Culbertsoni is known to inflict eyes; that too the ocular surface, i.e., conjunctiva and cornea only; no intraocular involvement has been reported, in severe infections, episclera and sclera may be involved.

Both stages are visible under a light microscope, a confocal microscope, and a phase contrast microscope. They are seen in KOH solution as reflectile bodies. To examine them under a light microscope, they are stained with hematoxylin and eosin. Other stains that make them visible are Gram stain, Giemsa stain, and calcofluor white; the last requires a fluorescent microscope.

The organism is difficult to culture; it is cultured aerobically in nutrient-rich blood and chocolate agar overlayed with dead *E. coli* and *Klebsiella*.

The infection is seen world over in physically active persons of both sexes. The organism finds access to the eye both by droplets or contaminated water at any temperature, contaminated soil, and dust. The two sources of water that are commonly blamed are water from swimming pools and contact lens solutions. The organisms in water are not killed by the usual chlorination; hence, they may even be found in piped drinking water.

The next source of contamination is contaminated contact lenses, contact lens cleaning solutions, both commercial/homemade, and contact lens storing fluid. The soft contact lenses have a propensity to cause infection.

Scratches by the finger nails too have been blamed; immunocompromised persons of any age are at a higher risk. The exact incubation period is debatable. Like most corneal ulcers, a breach in the epithelium is a prerequisite. However, it is claimed that organisms can pass through intact corneal epithelium as well.

Out of nonimmune-compromised conditions, trachoma seems to make persons more predisposed.

The condition is mostly unilateral; bilateral involvement is rare. When present, it may prove to be a disaster because, initially, the disease is diagnosed and treated as either a bacterial or fungal ulcer in vain.

Clinical features depend on the severity and extent of the corneal ulcer. In the initial stage, it may be as innocuous as a simple central corneal ulcer with the usual foreign body sensations of watering, redness, and photophobia. A history of injury by soil, dust, or vegetables may wrongly lead to the diagnosis of a fungal ulcer.

Pseudo dendrites, punctate keratitis, and stromal infiltration with unexplained pain should arouse suspicion of *Acanthamoeba* keratopathy and be investigated as such. Treatment at this stage may save the cornea.

The second stage is the extension of keratitis, both in depth and area. With severe pain due to the involvement of corneal nerves. Scattered stromal infiltrations may form a ring all-round or may be in the form of a satellite lesion, again diverting the treatment in favor of fungus keratitis. The third stage consists of associated scleritis, sclerouveitis, and secondary glaucoma.

Treatment

Treatment is difficult; the most common cause of failure is to reach the correct diagnosis at the optimal time. It is never a first diagnosis; it is mostly a diagnosis of exclusion. The ulcers are generally treated for too long, with disastrous results as bacterial corneal ulcers; still worse is their being diagnosed and treated as fungus ulcers.

The points that mislead to the diagnosis of fungal keratitis are:

- History of injury by organic matter.
- Organisms are visible in the KOH solution and mistaken for fungi.
- Presence of satellite lesions.
- Not responding to broad-spectrum antibiotics.

Management

Management of an *Acanthamoeba* corneal ulcer is one of the most frustrating experiences, even for trained keratologists. It is long-drawn, with a high incidence of recurrence not only in the host cornea but also in the recipient cornea in the case of keratoplasty. Severe pain in the initial stage is an indication of failure.

The management consists of:

- Detailed history of contact lens use, its type, duration, and method of cleaning and disinfecting. Storage fluids, too, are equally contributing factors. Homemade fluids are more likely to be predisposing factors.
- *Exclude:* Immunosuppression (HIV), organ transplants, and autoimmune diseases.
- Drugs recommended for treatment include many belonging to diverse therapeutic groups and therapeutic uses.

> Antiamebic drugs for intestinal amebiasis have no role to play in the management of *Acanthamoeba* keratitis.

> The most important nonmedical act is to stop using contact lenses.

The common protocol of treatment for Acanthamoeba keratitis consists of the following steps:

- A nonhealing bacterial/fungal keratitis that does not respond to treatment should be considered an *Acanthamoeba* keratitis.
- That requires a high degree of suspicion.
- A high degree of suspicion requires:
    - Clinical examination of the cornea by confocal microscope and phase contrast microscope.
    - Examination of scraped material in KOH solution. The organisms look like refractile bodies in KOH solution.
    - The presence of the organism is confirmed by Gram, Giemsa stain, and calcofluor white. The last requires a fluorescent microscope.
    - Corneal biopsy
- Usual treatment with cycloplegic and broad-spectrum antibiotics; the latter has no effect on *Acanthamoeba* corneal ulcer; it is given empirically to treat and prevent secondary infections.
- Local antiglaucoma drugs.
- Steroids have hardly any effect on *Acanthamoeba*, they are best avoided.
- Antiacanthemic drugs:
    - *Biguanides:* In a dose of 0.02% solution every hour for the initial 3–4 days, followed by every 2 hours for the next fortnight, and observe progress.
    - Diamidine
- Propamidine 0.1%
- Hexamidine 0.1%

  The above drugs are instilled twice an hour for the first 2 days, followed by six times a day.
    - Neomycin is a locally acting antibiotic generally used in combination with polymyxin and bacitracin. In kerato *Acanthamoeba*, it is used as 5.0 mg/mL drops used every 2 hours.
    - Antifungal drugs too have been tried, but not with equal success rates. They can be used as local drops or orally, along with anti-*Acanthamoeba* drugs.
    - Penetrating keratoplasty often fails in most cases.

MICROSPORIDIAL KERATITIS

Microsporidial keratitis, which was unknown a few decades ago, is emerging as a clinical menace to the cornea, similar to that of *Acanthamoeba*; both of them are often missed during primary diagnosis. Both are difficult to cultivate and eradicate. The organism is an obligate intracellular fungal parasite with a true nucleus minus mitochondria. The organism has three stages, i.e., infective, proliferative, and spore. Spore is the infective stage. The organism requires a high degree of suspicion, especially in corneal involvement. It stains with Gram stain Periodic acid-Schiff (PAS) and Gomori methenamine silver stain. The organism has both systemic as well as ocular manifestations. The ocular manifestations are chronic conjunctivo, keratitis, and acute ulcerative keratitis. One of the causes of its frequent ocular involvement is a rise in immune suppression. The keratitis can be unilateral or bilateral, mostly epithelial; however, the possibility of stromal and uveal involvement cannot be ruled out. The corneal lesion starts with erosion of the epithelium, which is best visualized under a confocal microscope. The epithelial changes may be confused with herpes simplex keratitis. The other finding is intraepithelial opacity. Unlike *Acanthamoeba* keratitis, it has no relation to contact lens use.

There is no specific treatment; the cases are initially managed as bacterial, viral, or fungal keratitis. The treatment consists of the usual cycloplegic broad spectrum antibiotic, which later has no therapeutic value in combating microsporidial keratitis. It is given empirically to ward off secondary infections. However, fumagillin, which is antimicrobial, is used hourly for the first two days and then reduced to four times a day until a satisfactory result is obtained. Oral albendazole, given along with fumagillin, is supposed to enhance the effect of the later.

Surgical treatment consists of full-thickness keratoplasty. The recipient cornea is always fraught with the chance of getting infected and rejected.

Management of Nonhealing Corneal Ulcers

The following factors contribute to the nonhealing of corneal ulcers:

- Missing the exact type of microbe.
- Use of the wrong antimicrobial drugs.
- Antimicrobials are used in subtherapeutic doses, i.e., strength, frequency, and duration.
- Loss of protective mechanisms in the eye, i.e., lid deformity, loss of sensation, lagophthalmos, and proptosis.
- Uncontrolled glaucoma
- Uncontrolled diabetes
- Malnutrition
- Indiscriminate use of steroids
- Immunocompromised status

The management consists of:

- Search for causes preventing healing.
- Remove such factors.
- Recognizing the organism.
- Identify the best antimicrobial and use it in its proper strength, frequency, and duration.
- Use of cycloplegic
- Repeated debridement and cauterization
- Keeping intraocular tension low
- Conjunctival autograft
- Amniotic membrane graft
- Penetrating keratoplasty

DEEP KERATITIS IN CHILDREN

Deep keratitis is also known as parenchymatous or interstitial keratitis. It is a nonulcerative keratopathy that is far less common than ulcerative keratopathy (corneal ulcer).

It can be diffuse or central; later, it is called disciform keratitis, which is more commonly seen in adults, the most common cause of which is herpes simplex.

INTERSTITIAL KERATITIS IN CHILDREN

The typical parenchymatous keratitis in children is generally referred to as interstitial keratitis (IK). The main cause of this is congenital syphilis, which manifests after 3 years of age. The most common age group to be involved is between 5 and 10 years; boys and girls are equally effected. The disease has an acute onset with a long course, beginning in one eye, followed by the other eye. It is a self-limited condition that may resolve without treatment, even leaving a hazy cornea that has a telltale story in the form of obliterated vessels, giving a permanently hazy cornea. The condition is becoming less frequent following the advent of antisyphilitic chemotherapy, frequent use of steroids, and the recognition of the disease in expectant mothers.

The primary lesion is in the stroma; the epithelium and endothelium are involved late. Anterior uveitis is early and prominent, which is so profound that one of the theories of the disease is that it is the uveitis that precedes corneal involvement. The controversy arises because of two opposite findings, i.e., treponema has been isolated from a fetus born to a syphilitic mother without evidence of ocular involvement. Conversely, treponema has not been demonstrated in corneas inflicted by interstitial keratitis. Most probably, the disease is a sensitive reaction to treponema in an already sensitized fetus.

Interstitial keratitis is supposed to be the counterpart of neurosyphilis in adults; hence, it takes a minimum of 3 years to manifest.

Clinical Picture

The clinical picture of interstitial keratitis in children is divided into the following stages:

- Progressive
- Florid
- Regressive

Progressive

The progressive stage lasts for 2–3 weeks, with symptoms common to any keratitis or foreign body in the cornea with features of lacrimation, photophobia, and blepharospasm. The eye has prominent circumciliary congestion and a hazy cornea that may be confused with congenital glaucoma. The haze starts from the periphery toward the center; the vessels grow in the stroma, and new vessels sprout in the stroma with signs of acute iridocyclitis; occasionally, the peripheral choroid may also be involved. The signs of anterior uveitis are often missed due to the presence of corneal hazes.

Florid Stage

The florid stage follows the progressive stage and lasts for 2–3 months with maximum clinical features. The cornea develops extensive deep vascularization giving the cornea a red hue. The red hue imparts a-peculiar color called salmon red; color, the causes of hazy corneas are many, found extending from epithelium to endothelium with abundant keratic precipitates. The cornea ultimately passes into a stage of ground glass. The changes are best appreciated on high power of the slit lamp. They are bedewing of epithelium, cellular infiltration along newly formed vessels in front of the Descemet's membrane, which itself is wrinkled. Bowman's membrane is wavy. At this point of deep vascularization of the stroma, the epithelium also gets vascularized on the periphery in a ring shape called an epaulet.

Regressive Stage

It takes 1–2 months for the condition to start regressing. The process of regression continues for the next 2–3 years; the regression starts from the center. Once the inflammation subsides and the vessels regress, the vision gradually improves with diminished lacrimation and photophobia. The obliterated vessels are left as white streaks; they are referred to as ghost vessels. In the long run, band keratopathy may develop and the corneal thickness may be reduced.

Systemic Signs of Congenital Syphilis

The following signs point toward the possibility of congenital syphilis in a case of interstitial keratitis in a child:

- Hutchinson's teeth*
- Permanent deafness
- Frontal eminence
- Saddle-shaped nose bridge
- Rhagades at the angle of the mouth
- Anterior bowing of the shin
- Clutton's joint†

Retardant physical and mental development with cardiovascular disorders.

> Interstitial keratitis, Hutchinson's teeth and deafness constitute Hutchinson's triad almost a sure clue toward interstitial keratitis in children.

Differential Diagnosis

Differential diagnoses are few; they consist of congenital hazy cornea, buphthalmos, and extensive phlyctenulosis. In fact, in all cases of severe blepharospasm in a child between 5 and 10 years old, interstitial keratitis should be considered as a possible cause and investigated.

Diagnosis

Diagnosis is clinically straight forward if Hutchinson's triad is noticed in a child with blepharospasm, photophobia, and lacrimation, supported by other signs of congenital syphilis, i.e., saddle nose, frontal bossing, in a child born to a mother with syphilis. The investigations

---

**Hutchinson's teeth:* Hutchinson's teeth are major signs of congenital syphilis. The teeth are smaller than normal, and the space between two teeth is greater than expected, with a notch at their biting edge.

†*Clutton's joints:* Clutton's joints are seen in children suffering from congenital swelling of both knees equally due to synovitis and the accumulation of fluid. It lasts up to 1 year.

to clinch the diagnosis are positive serological tests in mother and child. Examination of cerebrospinal fluid (CSF) for reactive venereal disease research laboratory (VDRL) and elevated protein in CSF.

Treatment

- Systemic antisyphilitic treatments have no effect on interstitial keratitis, yet it is mandatory to give full antisyphilitic treatment to ward off future chances of cardiovascular and neurovascular complications.
- Interstitial keratitis is a self-limiting disease that starts improving within 2–3 months. During the period of recovery, the severe lacrimation, photophobia, and blepharospasm gradually lessen, making the child more comfortable. The treatment is directed to give relief to the child and enhance recovery.
- The sheet anchor of treatment consists of:
  - Use of steroids for corneal conditions that shorten the symptoms to a few weeks. To begin with, strong steroids are instilled every 2 hours for the first 2–3 days. Instillation of a few drops makes the child extremely relieved. The steroids are tapered in frequency and strength as per the protocol of the institute; they should be continued for months to years in minimum strength and frequency. Once the acute phase has subsided, a depot steroid may be used. While the child is on steroid, the cornea should be examined; at least it develops, steroid induces a corneal ulcer, and intraocular tension should be recorded frequently.
  - Treatment of associated uveitis by strong cycloplegics and steroids.

Other causes of interstitial keratitis (at all ages) are:

- Acquired syphilis
- Tuberculosis
- Leprosy
- Leptospirosis
- Brucellosis
- Lyme disease
- Herpes simplex

SUGGESTED READING

1. Athmanathan S, Garg P, Rao Gullapalli N. Ophthalmic antiviral chemotherapy: an overview. Indian J Ophthalmol. 1997;45:203-10.
2. Banumathy SP. Development of the cornea and sclera in anatomy of the eye. Arvind Eye Hospital, Madurai. p. 165.
3. Basak SK. In: Ramamurthy D, Biswas P (Eds). Cornea and external diseases in AIOS ready reckoner in ophthalmology, 2nd edition. New Delhi: Jaypee Brothers; 2017.
4. Chandratreya MP, Mudduluru D, Venugopal A, Varghese AK, Ghorpade AS. A study on childhood microbial keratitis in South India. Indian J Ophthalmol. 2023;71(3):841-5.
5. Dart JKG, Saw VPJ, Kilvington S. Clinical features of acanthamoeba keratits. Community Eye Health. 1995;8:1.
6. Duke Elder S. System of Ophthalmology, Vol. 3, Part 1, 137, 1st edition. London: Henry Kimpton; 1963.
7. Duke Elder S. System of Ophthalmology, Vol. 3, Part 2, 1st edition. London: Henry Kimpton; 1963. pp. 164-9.
8. Dwivedi D, Sonamani N, Anamika Dwivedi. In: Nema HV, Venkatesh P, Sharma YR, Nema N (Eds). Acanthamoeba in Eye in Systemic Disorder, 1st edition. New Delhi: Wiley India Pvt Ltd.; 2015. p. 177.
9. Edelhauser HF, Geroski DH, Ubels JL. In: Smolin G, Thoft RA (Eds). Corneal transparency in the cornea, 3rd edition. Philadelphia: Lippincot, William & Wilkins; 1994. pp. 28-32.
10. Garg P, Rao GN. Corneal ulcer: diagnosis and management. Community Eye Health. 1999;12(30):21-3.
11. Gupta AK, Krishna V. Corneal topography and wave front sensing in clinical ophthalmology. In: Gupta AK, Krishna V (Eds). Contemporary Perspectives, 9th edition. New Delhi: Jaypee Brothers; 2011. pp. 3-23.
12. Jain MR. Keratomycosis and antifungal drugs in diagnosis and management of ocular inflammation, 2nd edition. New Delhi: Jaypee Brothers; 1990. pp. 28-32.
13. Merrill L, Stass-Isern, David L, Zwick. In: Cibis GW, Tongue AC, Merrill L (Eds). Diagnostic techniques in ocular infectious disease in decision making in pediatric ophthalmology, 5th edition, year book. St. Louis, USA: Mosby; 1996. p. 288.
14. Merrill L, Stass-Isern, David L, Zwick. In: Cibis GW, Tongue AC, Merrill L (Eds). Smears, stains, and rapid diagnostic tests, year book, 5th edition. St. Louis, USA: Mosby; 1996. p. 292.
15. Mukherjee PK, Bandyopadhyay P. Infectious diseases of the eye, 1st edition. New Delhi: Wolters Kluwer; 2010.
16. Mukherjee PK, Preeti Bandyopadhyay. In: Nema HV, Venkatesh P, Sharma YR, Nema N (Eds). Ocular involvement in systemic bacterial diseases in the eye in systemic disorders, 1st edition. New Delhi: Wiley India Pvt Ltd.; 2015. pp. 85-97.
17. Mukherjee PK. Clinical examination in ophthalmology, 2nd edition. New Delhi: Elsevier; 2016.
18. Mukherjee PK. Ocular Microbiology, 1st edition. New Delhi: Jaypee Brothers; 2010.
19. Mukherjee PK. Pediatric Ophthalmology, 1st edition. New Delhi: New Age International; 2005.
20. Nema HV. Cornea, and limbus in anatomy of the eye and its adnexa, 2nd edition. New Delhi: Jaypee Brothers; 1991. pp. 3-9.

21. Rajalalcshmi PC, Lalitha P. Normal ocular flora in Ocular Microbiology, 1st edition. Madurai: Arvind Eye Hospital; 1999. pp. 3-5.
22. Rajalaxmi C, Lalitha P. Ocular mycology in ocular microbiology, 1st edition. Madurai: Arvind Eye Hospital; 1999. pp. 71-7.
23. Ran NA. Laboratory approach to rapid diagnosis of ocular infection and prospects for the future. J Ophthalmol. 1989;107:283-91.
24. Rauz S, Kolli S. Cornea in the Oxford Handbook of Ophthalmology, 4th edition. London: Oxford University Press; 2018. pp. 241-97.
25. Rizutti AB. Diagnostic illumination test for keratoconus. American Jr. Oph. 1970;70(1):141-3.
26. Saini JS, Jain A. In: Saxena (Ed). Cornea and external diseases in clinical ophthalmology, 1st edition. New Delhi: Jaypee Brothers; 2003. pp. 1-82.
27. Sengupta S, Sudharshan S, Biswas J. In: Nema HV, Venkatesh P, Sharma YR, Nema N (Eds). Interstitial keratitis in eye in systemic disorders, 1st edition. New Delhi: Wiley India Pvt. Ltd.; 2015. p. 135.
28. Sharma S, Garg P, Rao GN. Patient characteristics, diagnosis, and treatment of non-contact lens-related Acanthamoeba keratitis. Br J Ophthalmol. 2000;84(10):1103-8.
29. Sharma S, Silverberg M, Mehta P, Gopinathan U, Agrawal V, Naduvilath TJ. Early diagnosis of mycotic keratitis: predictive value of potassium hydroxide preparation. Indian J Ophthalmol. 1998;46(1):31-5.
30. Sharma S, Srinivasan M, George C. Diagnosis of Acanthamoeba Keratitis. Indian J Ophthalmol. 1990;38: 50-6.
31. Singh S, Sachdeva MPS. Acanthamoeba keratitis. BMJ. 1994;309(6949):273.
32. Smith GT, Dart JK. In: Jackson TL (Ed). Cornea in Moorfields manual of ophthalmology, 2nd edition. New Delhi: Jaypee Brothers; 2020. pp. 173-253.
33. Sridhar MS. Diagnosis and management of microbial keratitis, CME Series, 11. New Delhi: All India Ophthalmological Society; 2005.
34. Sridhar U, Gupta AK. Microbial keratitis: A guide to diagnosis and management in clinical ophthalmology. In: Gupta AK, Krishna V (Eds). Contemporary Perspectives, 9th edition. New Delhi: Jaypee Brothers; 2011. pp. 170-80.
35. Srinivasan M, Gonzales CA, George C, Cevallos V, Mascarenhas JM, Asokan B, et al. Epidemiology and etiological diagnosis of corneal ulceration in Madurai, South India. Br J Ophthalmol. 1997;81(11);965-97.
36. Stuphin JE. In: Fraunfelder FT, Roy FH (Eds). Acanthamebiasis in current ocular therapy, 5th edition. Philadelphia: Lippincot Williams and Wilkins; 2000. pp. 89-90.
37. Suresh PS, Tullo AB. Herpes simplex keratitis. Indian J Ophthalmol. 1999;47(3):155-65.
38. Thomas PA, Kuriakose T, Kirupashanker MP, Maharajan VS. Use of lactophenol cotton blue mount of corneal scrapping as an aid to the diagnosis of mycotic keratitis. Diag Microbiol Infect Dis. 1991;14(3):219-24.
39. Tuft SJ, Moodaley LC, Gregory WM. Prognostic factors for progression of keratoconus. Ophthalmology. 1994; 101(3):439-47.
40. Vajpayce RB, Angra SK, Sandramoulis, Honavar SG, Chabra VK. Laboratory diagnosis of keratomycosis, comparative evaluation of direct microscopy ant culture results. Annl. Oph. 1993;25:68-71.
41. Vengayil S, Panda A, Satpathy G, Nayak N, Ghose S, Patanaik D, et al. Polymerase chain reaction-guided diagnosis of mycotic keratitis: a prospective evaluation of its efficacy and limitations. Invest Ophthalmol Vis Sci. 2009;50(1):152-6.
42. Wilhelmus KR. In: Smolin G, Thoft RA (Eds). Acanthamoeba keratitis in the cornea, 3rd edition. Philadelphia: Lippincot Williams and Wilkins; 1994. pp. 262-6.

CHAPTER

16 Disorders of the Sclera in Children

Scleral disorders are relatively rare at all ages, but they are still rarer under 20.

The sclera is the outer coat of the eyeball, constituting almost 85% of the total surface, and is opaque; the rest of the globe is formed by a transparent cornea. It is stronger than the cornea when considered to be a protective part; it does not have any optical function, while the cornea is predominantly optical in function. Besides being protective, the other functions of the sclera are to anchor extraocular muscles, keep the interior of the eyeball dark, and let intraocular blood vessels and nerves pass through the sclera without supplying blood to it, making it avascular all over except 1 mm round the cornea at the limbus. Its sensations are duller than those of the cornea, retaining a moderate pain sensation. The sclera maintains the shape of the eyeball.

A fully developed sclera constitutes a hollow sphere of 22 mm in diameter with two openings, one large anterior and one small posterior. The first is referred to as the anterior scleral, while the later is called the posterior scleral foramen. The anterior foramen makes the limbus and has a diameter of 11.00 mm; the posterior foramen is 2.00 mm in diameter and transmits the optic nerve along with its covering and blood vessels. The posterior foramen is covered by a thin fibrous sheet of tissue with perforation in it; called lamina cribrosa, it is not flat but is depressed backward. Nothing passes through the lamina cribrosa; the exact purpose of the foramen is not well understood. The lamina is not as rigid as the wall of the sclera; it bulges forward in papilledema and bends back in glaucoma.

The foramina other than the two mentioned earlier are meant for the transmission of:

- Long and short ciliary vessels and nerves
- Exit of venae vorticosae
- Passage of anterior ciliary vessels.
- These foramina are situated round the entry of the optic nerve, in two groups as per their distance from the optic nerve. The long and short ciliary nerves and vessels pass through them.
- These apertures are situated more anteriorly, four in number, 4–7 mm behind the equator.
- Through the anterior aperture, pass the anterior ciliary arteries. They enter the sclera just in front of the insertion of the recti, and the anterior ciliary veins make their way through these openings **(Fig. 16.1)**.

The color of the adult sclera is marble white; it has a blue tinge at birth, which changes to white by 1 year. The anterior part of the sclera is visible round the cornea in the interpalpebral aperture and is referred to as the

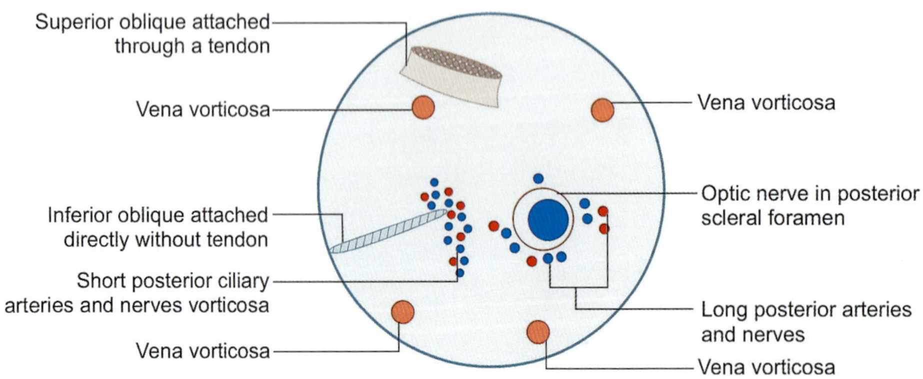

Fig. 16.1: Structures at the posterior sclera.

white of the eye in contrast to the cornea iris complex, which is called the black of the eye. The sclera is covered by transparent bulbar conjunctiva. The conjunctiva can be moved over the sclera and lifted up with ease. The second structure that covers the sclera is Tenon's capsule, which extends from the optic nerve to the limbus, not reaching the corneal margin; it terminates about 1–2 mm away from the limbus. The Tenon's capsule encompasses the globe snugly, with a potential space between the two. The sub-Tenon's space is used to place sub-Tenon drugs. The potential space is traversed by fine fibrils that enhance the attachment of the Tenon's capsule to the sclera. Posteriorly, the Tenon's capsule terminates round the optic nerve, merging with its covering. The sclera is not uniformly thick throughout; it is thicker at the limbus and round the optic nerve; it is 1 mm round the optic nerve and 0.75 mm round the limbus; and it is thinnest at the insertion of the recti.

ATTACHMENT OF EXTRAOCULAR MUSCLES

No Extraocular Muscle Originates from the Sclera

The attachment of the extraocular muscles to the sclera has a great bearing on the movement of the globe. Knowledge of the position of attachments is of great importance in squint surgery. The attachment of extraocular muscles to the sclera can be put into two groups: those attached anterior to the equator and those attached behind the equator **(Fig. 16.2)**.

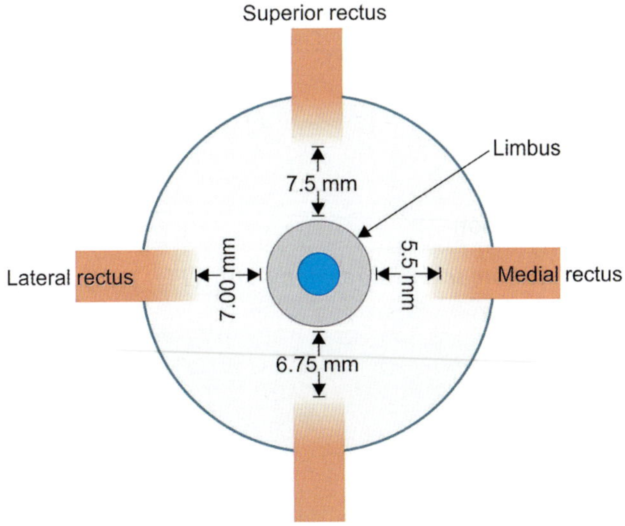

Fig. 16.2: Attachment recti anterior to equator.

The first group consists of four recti; the second group consists of two obliques. During squint surgery, the distance of attachment is measured in millimeters from the limbus, which is not equal for all muscles. The distance of insertion of the obliques from the limbus is far more that of the recti. The width of attachment of individual muscles is variable. The inferior oblique is the only muscle that attaches itself directly to the sclera. The other extraocular muscles are attached by various lengths of tendons. The sclera is thinnest at the insertion of the muscles; the muscles blend intimately with the sclera; hence, precaution must be taken while detaching muscles in squint surgery to avoid inadvertently nicking the sclera.

Anatomically Weak Spots in Sclera (Fig. 16.3)

The weak spots on the sclera are:

- Thin sclera at attachment of recti muscles.
- Thinned sclera following trauma and inflammation.
- The third group consists of various foramina through which the vessels and nerves pass.
- The other weak spots are:
  - Corneoscleral junction
  - Equator
  - Sclera over the ciliary body
  - Posterior pole

Development and Congenital Anomalies of Sclera

The sclera is fully mesodermal; it develops from the para-axial mesenchyme round the developing optic nerve, which has two parts: the anterior and posterior parts. The anterior part grows earlier and faster than its posterior counterpart. The anterior part of mesoderm not only gives rise to sclera but also to the attachment of recti that grow backward. In the initial stage, the limbus is far posterior to its final position on the developing ciliary body. The developing mesoderm reaches the future posterior pole by the 3rd month to grow round the developing optic nerve and give rise to the lamina cribrosa. The scleral spur, which is located relatively anteriorly, becomes evident by the 16th week; by the 20th week, the sclera is almost fully developed.

Disorder of Sclera

Disorders of the sclera can be:

- Congenital
- Acquired

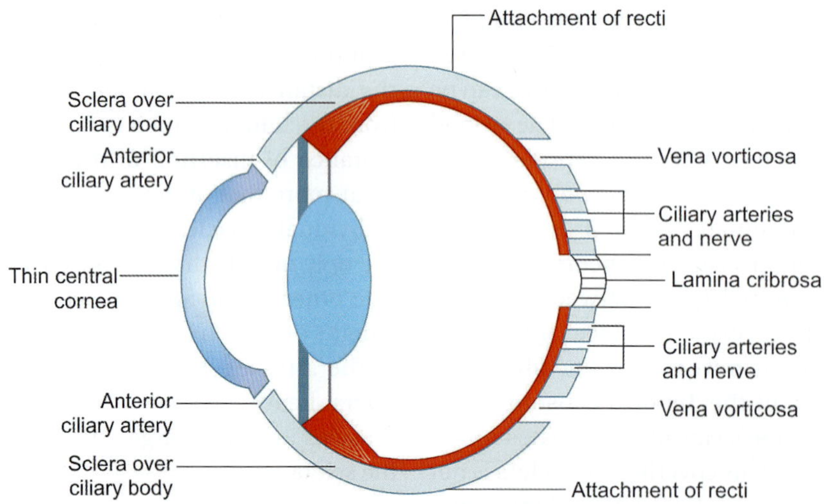

Fig. 16.3: Weak spots on the sclera and cornea.

Congenital

The congenital anomalies may be any of the following in isolation or in combination; most of the congenital anomalies of the sclera are bilateral and mostly symmetric.

They are caused by:

- Failure of the development of the optic cup.
- Retarded growth of the optic cup.
- Failure of mesoderm round the optic vesicle.

There are four types of common congenital anomalies:

1. Colobomas are generally associated with colobomas of the uvea.
2. Small eyeballs
   i. Anophthalmos
   ii. Microphthalmos
   iii. Nanophthalmos
3. Large eyeballs, congenital scleral ectasia
   i. Posterior staphyloma
   ii. Idiopathic scleral staphyloma
4. Other congenital anomalies of the sclera are:
   i. Blue sclera
   ii. Scleral melanosis
   iii. Intrascleral nerve loop
   iv. Sclerocornea

   Anomalies 1, 2, and 3 do not effect vision.

Acquired

The acquired disorders are:

- Ectasia
- Inflammation
- Trauma
- Infection (rare)

SCLERAL ECTASIA

The ectasia of the sclera are types of staphylomas involving the sclera.

> A staphyloma is defined as—ectatic cicatrization of outer coat of the eyeball with the uvea incarcerated.

The basic mechanisms of scleral staphyloma are the thinning and disorganization of scleral fibers with raised intraocular pressure; it may happen even with normal intraocular tension, depending on the thinning of the sclera.

The staphylomas can involve:

- Cornea only
  - Partial
  - Complete
- Sclera only
- Combination

As per location, scleral staphylomas are ***(Fig. 16.4)****:*

- Intercalary
- Ciliary
- Equatorial
- Posterior
- Combination

As per duration:

- Congenital
- Acquired

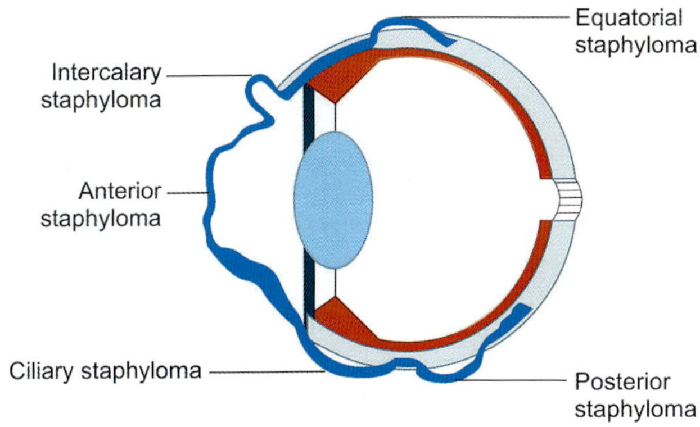

Fig. 16.4: Various types of corneoscleral staphylomas.

Flowchart 16.1: Types of staphylomas.

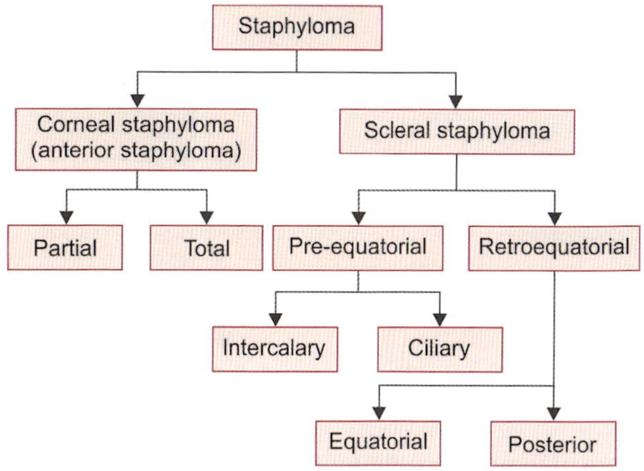

TABLE 16.1: Staphylomas and their predisposing factors.

S. No.	*Staphyloma*	*Outer coat involved*	*Anatomical defect*	*Uvea involved*
1.	Corneal	Center of the cornea	Thin central cornea	Iris
2.	Intercalary	Limbus	Entry of anterior ciliary vessels	Root of the iris
3.	Ciliary	Anterior sclera	Nonspecific	Ciliary body
4.	Equatorial	Equator of the sclera	The thinnest part of the sclera	Choroid
5.	Posterior	Posterior pole	Congenital weak	Choroid

Congenital Scleral Staphyloma

About 6% of eyes have some degree of ectasia; all of them are hidden either under the extraocular muscle or in a deeper situation behind the equator. They are symptomless, becoming evident at the time of either squint or retinal detachment surgery. Some authors also put posterior staphyloma in the category of congenital anomalies. Topographically, congenital staphylomas are equatorial or posterior.

Acquired Staphyloma of Sclera

Predisposing factors for producing scleral staphylomas are:

- Anatomical
  - Natural perforation passes through the following vessels and nerves:
    - Anterior ciliary arteries
    - Long and short ciliary arteries and nerves
    - Vertex vein
  - Lamina cribrosa
- Pathological
  - Buphthalmos—primary or secondary
  - Trauma
  - Severe scleritis
  - Necrotizing scleritis
  - Scleromalacia

  The last three are not seen in children.
- Infection—oculosporidiosis in endemic areas.

Flowchart 16.1 shows various types of staphylomas of the eye.

The relationship of staphylomas to the predisposing factors is shown in **Table 16.1**.

PATHOGENESIS OF VARIOUS TYPES OF SCLERAL STAPHYLOMA

Intercalary Staphyloma

Intercalary staphyloma generally develops at the upper limbus, mostly following a limbal incision for classical lens extraction with an incarcerated root of the iris.

Ciliary Staphyloma

The prerequisite for ciliary staphyloma is thinning of the sclera due to stretching, as seen in buphthalmos or following scleritis, scleromalacia, and oculosporidiosis. In 5-6% of cases, no cause can be found. The effect of

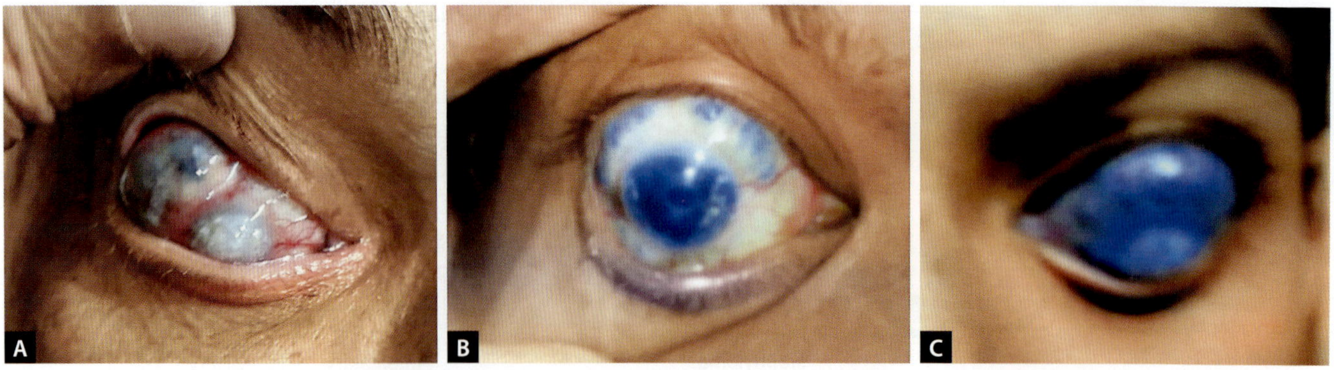

Figs. 16.5A to C: Extensive ciliary staphylomas and annular staphyloma since childhood.

intraocular pressure depends on the thickness of the sclera. A very thin sclera may bulge even in the presence of normal intraocular pressure; a relatively thick sclera may stand even with a high intraocular pressure (IOP) **(Figs. 16.5A to C)**.

The number of ciliary staphylomas varies from 1 to >1 in various places of various sizes; however, they may be numerous enough to encircle the limbus, causing an annular staphyloma. Generally, these eyes are painful without vision.

Equatorial Staphyloma

The most common cause of equatorial staphylomas is congenital idiopathic weakness. They amount to 6–7% of all staphylomas. Unlike intercalary and ciliary staphylomas, they are not visible and were discovered during squint and retinal detachment surgery.

Posterior Staphyloma

Posterior staphylomas, found exclusively in pathological myopia, may produce a slight bulging of the involved eye. On retinoscopy, a posterior staphyloma gives two readings, one at the rim of the staphyloma and the other at the bottom of the staphyloma. The difference between the two readings gives the depth of the staphyloma, i.e., measured by adding minus lenses to the initial reading. The staphylomas may be large enough to engulf the optic nerve. The posterior staphylomas are best visualized on indirect ophthalmoscopy. They are confirmed by ultrasonography (USG), computed tomography (CT), magnetic resonance imaging (MRI), and optical coherence tomography (OCT). The best results are seen by wide-field OCT and 3D MRI. Like all staphylomas, posterior staphylomas, too, do not respond well to treatment. Posterior scleral support has been tried without much success.

Symptoms

- Small staphylomas under the extraocular muscles and very posteriorly placed may be asymptomatic and go undetected unless the extraocular muscle is detached for any reason.
- Anteriorly placed congenital staphylomas are visible as black, lobulated protrusions under the conjunctiva, which is generally attached to the staphyloma.
- The presence of irregular astigmatism is common with intercalary and ciliary staphylomas.
- High myopia is the rule in posterior staphyloma.
- Visual loss depends on the position and size of the staphyloma.
- Unmanageable glaucoma is a common feature.

INFECTION OF SCLERA IN CHILDREN

Avascularity and the absence of epithelium exposed to the exterior make the sclera immune to infections. However, a severe infection of the peripheral cornea may spill over to the sclera at the limbus. An infected penetrating wound or an infected foreign body may cause a scleral abscess.

INFLAMMATION OF SCLERA

Inflammations of the substance of the sclera, which are referred to as scleritis, are not seen in children. Older children in late teens may suffer from episcleritis, i.e., an inflammation of the superficial sclera. It is mostly an autoimmune disease seen in rheumatoid arthritis; in many cases, no cause can be pinpointed. Episcleritis is a self-limited condition that is often mistaken for phlycten. The main differentiating points are that episcleritis is seen in late teens away from the limbus, is more diffuse than phlycten, may be tender, and does not involve the cornea. The common factor among the two is their positive response to local steroids, both of which are known to recur.

Other congenital anomalies of the sclera are:

Blue Sclera

A fully developed sclera is marble white with streaks of blood vessels traversing the surface and occasionally associated with melanosis without any bulge. In contrast to this, the thin sclera of newborns is more translucent, with a blue tinge imparted by the underlying choroid. Within 1 year, the sclera of an infant gets the white color of the adult sclera. Sometimes, the sclera remains bluish throughout life without clinical significance.

The systemic conditions associated with blue sclera are:

- Osteogenesis imperfect (blue sclera-brittle bone syndrome)
- Ehlers–Danlos syndrome (adults)
- The two local conditions with a black tinge are buphthalmos and microphthalmos.

Scleral Melanosis

Scleral melanosis is not uncommon in children; it may be present at birth or may make its presence felt in the first year and progress until the end of the first decade to become stationary. It is basically melanocytic hyperpigmentation. Generally bilateral, it is asymptomatic and does not involve vision. It may be associated with melanosis of the conjunctiva. The conjunctiva can be moved freely over pigmentation. A differential diagnosis consists of conjunctival nevi and acquired melanosis. It does not require any treatment **(Fig. 16.6)**.

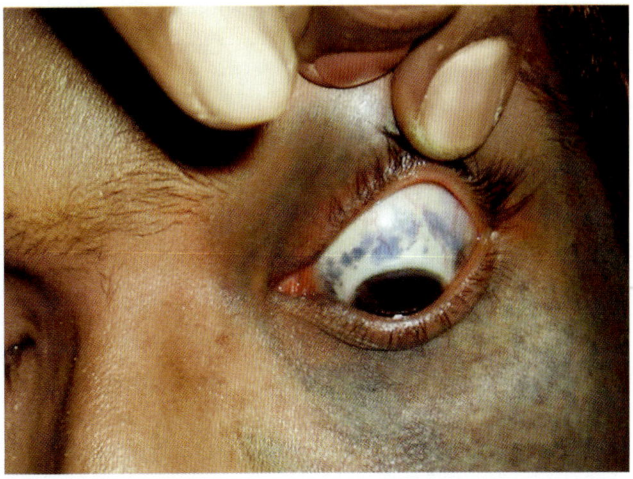

Fig. 16.6: Scleral melanosis along with melanosis of the skin.

Intrascleral Nerve Loop

The nerves and vessels destined for the uvea traverse through the substance of the sclera without serving it. In rare instances, a small bunch of long ciliary nerves change their intrascleral course to appear on the surface of the sclera under the transparent conjunctiva as small nodules, generally on the nasal side. The cause of the condition is not known. It does not require treatment.

Sclerocornea

The normal sclera stops at the limbus, leaving a transparent cornea. On rare instances, the sclera engulfs the cornea from periphery, converting the transparent cornea as opaque as the sclera. The corneoscleral step at the limbus is obliterated, and the cornea is generally flat.

SUGGESTED READING

1. Misra S, Misra N. In: Nagarkar NM, Mehta R (Eds). Clinical presentation with scleral involvement in ocular rhinosporidiosis in clinical presentation, ophthalmological spectrum in rhinosporidiosis, 1st edition. Singapore: Springer Nature; 2022. pp. 41-57.
2. Mukherjee PK. Disorders of the sclera in pediatric ophthalmology, 1st edition. New Delhi: New Age International; 2005. pp. 720-4.
3. Mukherjee PK. Examination of the sclera in clinical examination in ophthalmology, 2nd edition. New Delhi: Elsevier; 2016. pp. 139-42.
4. Mukherjee PK. Fraun Felder FT, Roy FH (Eds). Rhinosporidiosis in current ocular therapy, 5th edition. Philadelphia: WB Saunders Company; 2000. pp. 66-7.
5. Mukherjee PK. In: Bandyopadhyay P (Ed). Infectious Diseases of the Eye, 1st edition. New Delhi: Wolters Kluwer; 2010.
6. Murray PI, Pavesio CE, Denniston AKO. Sclera in Oxford handbook of ophthalmology, 4th edition. Oxford, UK: Oxford University Press; 2018.
7. Nema HV, Singh VP, Nema N. Development of the eye and its adnexa, 2nd edition. New Delhi: Jaypee Brothers; 1991. pp. 10-12.
8. Pandey N. In: Nema HV, Venkatesh P, Sharma YR, Nema N (Eds). Rhinosporidiosis in the eye in systemic disorders, 1st edition. New Delhi: Wiley India; 2015. pp. 153-5.
9. Riordan-Eva P. In: Vaughan D, Asbury T, Riordan-Eva P (Eds). Anatomy & embryology of the eye in general ophthalmology, 15th edition. Stamford, Connecticut: Appleton & Lange; 1999.
10. Scheie HG, Albert DM. Sclera in the textbook of ophthalmology, 9th edition. Philadelphia: WB Saunders Company; 1977.

CHAPTER

17 Disorder of Uvea in Children

The uvea is middle, vascular pigmented layer of the inner coat of the eye, sandwiched between the retina and sclera. It consists of the iris, ciliary body, and choroid. Each part has a specific function. The iris divides the aqueous chamber into two unequal parts, the anterior and posterior chambers, each communicating with each other through a central circular aperture called the pupil. Which circulate aqueous from the posterior to the anterior chamber. The pupil also acts as a diaphragm, which regulates the entry of light. The iris is vascular and pigmented. It is the only uveal part that hangs parallel to the corneal plane. The iris has an uneven surface, that gives it a rugged appearance. The iris is divided into two parts, the pupillary and ciliary. The ciliary body is highly vascular, rich in plane muscle, and pigmented. The function of it is the accommodation and production of aqueous. The aqueous solution is secreted from the epithelium of the ciliary body. The iris is attached to its body anteriorly, and the posterior end tapers to merge with the choroid. The junction is called ora serrata, which is poor in blood supply. The choroid is the largest part of the uvea, extending from the ora to the edge of the optic nerve. Unlike the other two parts of the uvea, it is devoid of musculature. It is highly vascular and pigmented. The main function of the choroid is to supply nutrition to the overlying retina. The other functions are to keep the inner side of the globe dark, regulate the temperature, and participate in the uveoscleral outflow of aqueous.

The disorders of the uvea can be:

- Congenital
- *Acquired:*
    - Infection
    - Inflammation
    - Trauma
    - Degeneration and dystrophy
    - New growth

The congenital conditions have been discussed in Chapter 3. The infection and inflammation collectively are called uveitis. Degeneration and dystrophies are rare in children. The new growths of the choroid are not seen in children. The new growth of the iris and ciliary body is rare in children.

UVEITIS IN CHILDREN

For the purposes of diagnosis and management, the condition is divided in various ways. The most common division is as per the part of the uvea involved **(Table 17.1)**. It is topographically divided into the following groups:

All the above can be acute or chronic. Some are self-limiting and prone to recurrence; a few of them are short-lasting; the chronic have a protracted course. Uveitis can be congenital or acquired, infective or non-infective. Infective uveitis can be caused by a purulent organism. The purulent uveitis is panophthalmitis and

TABLE 17.1: Disorders based on the part of uvea involved.

Part of uvea involves	*Disorder*
Iris	Iritis
Ciliary body	Cyclitis
Iris and ciliary body	Iridocyclitis
Choroid: • Posterior: – Central (macular) – Juxtapapillary: - Disseminated - Diffuse	Choroiditis
• Peripheral	Pars planitis
Choroid and retina	Chorioretinitis
All parts of the retina	Panuveitis
Uvea, retina, and vitreous	Endophthalmitis
All coats of the eye with vitreous and periocular tissue	Panophthalmitis
Cornea and anterior uvea	Keratouveitis
Sclera and uvea	Sclerouveitis

endophthalmitis following perforating injury, accidental or surgical, with or without retained intraocular foreign body.

The child is neither a compressed man nor a pediatric eye; it is a miniature adult eye. This is true for childhood uveitis, which is not a milder form of adult uveitis.

Childhood uveitis differs from adult uveitis in clinical presentation and management in various parameters.

CLASSIFICATION OF UVEITIS (IN ALL AGES)

Due to the diverse clinical features and etiology, there is no classification that encompasses all types of uveitis.

The various classifications used are given below:

- *Chronological:*
  - Congenital
  - Acquired
- *Topographical:*
  - Anterior
  - Intermediate (pars planitis/chronic cyclitis/hyalitis/peripheral retinitis)
  - Posterior uveitis
  - Panuveitis

  Table 17.2 describes the distribution of uveitis as per location in the first two decades.
- *Etiological:*
  - *Infective:*
    - Nonpurulent organism
    - Purulent organism
  - Noninfective
    - Autoimmune
    - Traumatic
    - Nonspecific:
      - Fuchs heterochromic uveitis
      - Still's disease (JRA)
      - Behçet's disease
      - Reiter's disease
      - Sympathetic uveitis
      - Sarcoid (black girls, white boys uveitis)

TABLE 17.2: Distribution of uveitis as per location.

Anterior	*Posterior*	*Both*
AIDS	AIDS	AIDS
Ankylosing spondylitis	Fungus	Behçet's disease
Behçet's disease	Behçet's disease	Herpes simplex
Herpes simplex	Cysticercosis	Herpes zoster
Herpes zoster	Cytomegalovirus	Pars planitis
Idiopathic	Toxocariasis	Rubella
Sarcoidosis	Toxoplasmosis	Toxoplasmosis
Tuberculosis	Tuberculosis	Sympathetic ophthalmia
Gonococcal		Vogt–Koyanagi–Harada disease (VKH)
Leptospirosis		

The microbes that cause uveitis are:

- *Bacteria:*
  - *Tuberculosis*
  - *Leprosy (not seen in children)*
  - *Syphilis*
  - *Streptococcus*
  - *Gonococcus—leptospirosis*
- *Virus:*
  - *Herpes simplex*
  - *Herpes zoster*
  - *Rubella*
  - *Cytomegalovirus*
- *Post viral, chickenpox, mumps, and measles*
- *Protozoa—toxoplasmosis*
- *Helminths—toxocara*
- *Fungus (rare)*
- *Pathological*:*
  - Granulomatous
  - *Nongranulomatous:*
    - Acute
    - Chronic
  - Undetermined

**Pathological:* Since Woods classified uveitis into two groups, a debate has been going on over the last half century regarding its validity in clinical practice in the present scenario. Wood (1961) postulated that uveitis of all types could be put in two groups based on clinical features of keratic precipitates (KPs) and cells in AC, i.e., granulomatous and nongranulomatous uveitis. Fine KPs were supposed to be characteristic of nongranulomatous uveitis, and large mutton-fat KPs, Busacca nodules, and choroidal granuloma were hallmarks of granulomatous uveitis. He thought that chronic infectious diseases produced granulomatous uveitis and that nongranulomatous diseases were noninfectious. However, in the long run, this theory was not substantiated histopathologically. Some of the diseases that were supposed to be granulomatous clinically proved otherwise, and vice versa. Some cases did not fit in either; the best examples are lens-induced uveitis, peripheral uveitis, and sarcoid.

TABLE 17.3: Classification of disorders into granulomatous and nongranulomatous.

Granulomatous	*Nongranulomatous*
Tuberculosis	Seronegative arthritis
Herpes	Trauma
Vogt–Koyanagi–Harada syndrome	Behçet's disease
Sympathetic ophthalmia	Fuchs uveitis
Lens-induced uveitis	Lens-induced uveitis
Toxoplasmosis	Tuberculosis
Sarcoidosis	Syphilis
	Sarcoidosis
	Leptospirosis
	Leprosy

- *Laterality:*
  - *Unilateral:*
    - Viral keratouveitis
    - Sarcoid
  - *Bilateral:*
    - Sympathetic ophthalmia
    - Vogt–Koyanagi–Harada syndrome
    - Behçet's syndrome
  - *Either:*
    - Sarcoid
    - Toxoplasmosis
    - Tuberculosis

Table 17.3 describes conditions belonging to each group in all ages.

From the above table, it will be seen that some of the conditions are seen in both groups: tuberculosis, sarcoidosis, and lens-induced uveitis.

Wood further divided nongranulomatous uveitis into two classes, i.e., acute self-limiting and chronic recurrent.

Nongranulomatous

This is more common under 20 years of age with an acute onset that is painful, which brings the child for consultation. The condition is mostly uniocular in the beginning, only to involve the other eye over weeks or months, and rarely simultaneously. The condition in the majority of cases is self-limiting, with few recurrences; an attack generally lasts for 4–6 weeks even without treatment. It is cured earlier than granulomatous.

On examination, there is marked circumciliary congestion and marked ciliary tenderness. The anterior segment is more frequently involved than the posterior, which is more frequently affected by granulomatous uveitis.

The most striking feature is the anterior chamber reaction with cells and flair. KPs are numerous, small, and fine. There may be fibrinous exudation and hypopyon. The pupil is constricted and may not respond to light due to the multiple small synechiae that are easy to break. In long-term and recurrent attacks, peripheral synechiae may develop.

Nodules on the iris are less common; the vitreous, choroid, and retina are generally not involved. The loss of vision is minimal in the early stages and may worsen with recurrence.

Granulomatous Uveitis

This is generally a chronic inflammation that inflicts all the three parts of uvea with preponderance of choroidal involvement. It is more frequently bilateral. There may be actual invasion of uvea by organism in microbial uveitis, causing proliferation of tissues. The proliferation is directly proportionate to virulence of organism; weighed against immunity. The incident is generally slow to develop without pain. The KPs are large mutton fat in appearance, even visible without magnification on oblique illumination. The anterior chamber reaction is relatively less with fewer cells than in granulomatous uveitis. The posterior synechiae are thicker, broader, and stronger than in nongranulomatous uveitis, they are difficult to break, peripheral anterior synechiae are more common, nodules on iris are frequent. The vision is generally reduced due to involvement of posterior pole.

As per description given above, it will show that there is no clear-cut line of demarcation between the two clinically. The matter can be settled only on histopathological examination. The examples are as follows:

- Occasionally an acute noninfectious anterior uveitis may present with large mutton-fat KPs.
- Chronic recurrent anterior uveitis of noninfectious origin may be as indolent as granulomatous uveitis.
- Uveitis due to leptospirosis presents as nongranulomatous which in fact should present as granulomatous.
- Lens-induced uveitis due to its noninfectious origin should present as nongranulomatous uveitis but looks granulomatous clinically.
- Sympathetic uveitis that presents as granulomatous lesions with epithelial cells and giant cells should present as nongranulomatous due to its allergic origin.

TABLE 17.4: Difference between nongranulomatous and granulomatous disorders.

Nongranulomatous		Granulomatous
Onset	Acute	Insidious
Pain	Marked	None or minimal
Photophobia	Marked	Slight
Blurred vision	Moderate	Marked
Circumcorneal flush	Marked	Slight
Keratic precipitates	Fine, white	Large, gray (mutton fat)
Pupil	Small and irregular	Small and irregular (variable)
Posterior synechiae	Common	Frequent due to anterior uveal involvement
Iris nodules	None	Sometimes
Site	Anterior	Anterior, posterior, or diffuse (Pan)
Course	Acute	Chronic
Recurrence	Common	Sometimes

- Similarly, sarcoid which should present as nongranulomatous uveitis presents as granulomatous uveitis with nodules formation.

The difference between the two is summarized in **Table 17.4**.

CLINICAL TERMS AND THEIR FEATURES AS USED IN UVEITIS

- *Ciliary tenderness* is the sensation of pain on the application of pressure on the globe through the lids due to inflammation of the ciliary body. Tenderness is at its maximum near the limbus and diminishes toward the periphery. Ciliary tenderness is not found in posterior uveitis. It should not be confused with the tenderness of the lid.
- *Circumciliary flush (congestion):* Redness of conjunctiva round the limbus, maximum at limbus, fading toward periphery, caused due to dilatation of anterior ciliary vessels. Does not disappear following instillation of weak vasoconstrictor, absent in posterior uveitis, should be differentiated from conjunctival congestion.
- *Keratic precipitates:* Deposits of inflammatory cells, i.e., epithelioid cells, macrophages, RBC, and iris pigment on the edematous corneal endothelium are called KPs. The KPs are divided into various categories as per size, shape, and color and named accordingly. Deposition of KPs is mostly a passive process, where the circulating particles, due to the relatively lower temperature of the cornea, get passively deposited on the swollen endothelium in a triangular fashion due to gravity. The apex of the triangle is toward the center of the pupil. In rare instances, the swollen endothelia engulf the particles like macrophages. The large KPs are visible in bright pinpoint light, even with little or no magnification. The large KPs are more likely to be distributed in a triangular fashion, while the small are evenly spread all over the endothelium. The fine deposit virtually dusts the endothelium like powder. As per size, shape, and color, the KPs are large, medium, fine, pigmented, circular, or crenated. The largest KPs are called mutton-fat KPs*.
- *Anterior chamber reaction:* Normal aqueous is an optically clear, freely circulating fluid in the anterior chamber. The circulation is due to a convection current. In inflammation of the anterior uvea, there is a reactionary dilatation of blood vessels in the iris and ciliary body, resulting in the pouring of protein-rich, denser fluid. The normal aqueous is nonparticulate, hence a beam of light does not show any suspended material; the abnormal aqueous is particulate, with suspended inflammatory cells, protein particles, RBC, and other cells that stand out as shining motile bodies in bright light, causing the positive Tyndall effect†, best seen on a narrow beam of 3 mm × 1 mm with maximum illumination and high magnification.

**Mutton-fat KPs:* These are large in size and small in number. Their size may be as large as 1 mm × 1 mm; they have a pale color that imparts the name mutton-fat KPs to the deposit and have a greasy lardaceous appearance. Most of the time, their presence points to the nature of inflammation. They are more common in granulomatous uveitis. However, their presence in nongranulomatous uveitis is not exceptional. They are also seen in recurrent uveitis of both types, fade away with the ebbing of inflammation, and may last for a few weeks after the inflammation has subsided. In the long run, they are hyalinized with a crenated border and pale center. The common causes of mutton-fat KPs are tuberculosis and sympathetic ophthalmia. Red-tinged KPs are seen in herpes simplex and herpes zoster uveitis.

Endothelial dusting is caused by minute KPs in acute nongranulomatous anterior uveitis. The KPs are not to be confused with other nonuveitic pigmentations of the cornea.

†*Tyndall effect* is the scattering of a beam of light when passed through a turbid solution. The colloidal particles suspended in the solution prevent light to passing and stand out as bright spots.

While examining the aqueous on the narrow beam of the slit lamp, the following are noted:

- Flare
- Cells
- Exude
- Pus (hypopyon)
- Blood (hyphema)
- Nodule

- *Flare* is the turbidity of intraocular fluid caused by a disturbed aqueous-uveal barrier. Protein particles in aqueous solutions cause them to lose their clarity. The suspended particles in the path of bright light stand out as minute, shining bodies against the dark iris. This phenomenon is called aqueous flare, or simply as flare. To examine the flare, it is better not to dilate the pupil. To appreciate flare, a bright beam of white light is focused on the iris at an angle of 45°. The beam should be circular with 2.00 mm diameter. High magnification is essential for the best result. The degree of obscuration of iris details denotes the haziness of aqueous. Clearly visible details mean less flare, and failure to see iris details denotes maximum density. The denser the flare, the greater the inflammation. Flare is not always a sign of active uveitis.

  As per Hogan's dictum of 1959 and Standardization of Uveitis Nomenclature (SUN), the flare is graded as follows:

Grade of flare	Visibility of the iris and lens
0	No flare. Iris and lens structures are visible in detail
1^+	Mild flare. The iris structure is still visible
2^+	Moderate flare. Smudged lens and iris structure
3^+	Marked flare. Iris and lens details are partly obscured
4^+	Coagulated aqueous. Lens and iris are not visible

- *Cells in aqueous:* Normal aqueous is devoid of any type of cell; the presence of cells is an indication of inflammation of the anterior uvea, especially ciliary body. The cells originate in the anterior uveal vasculature. More are the cells, more is the inflammation. The cells are examined with an undilated pupil under the bright light of a slit lamp with maximum magnification in a beam of 3 mm × 1 mm. The cells should actually be counted in each field. The following chart is based on Hogan's observation of 1959:

Cells per field	Grade
No cells	0
1–2 cells	Require searching for cells in various fields, all fields may not have cells
3–7 cells	1^+
15–20 cells	2^+
20–50 cells	3^+
More than 50	4^+

  Points to remember about cells in AC:
  - Phenylephrine releases pigment cells in AC that may be confused with inflammatory cells.
  - Cells in AC reflect active inflammation of the anterior uvea.
  - The cells arise from the uvea and are not aqueous.
  - The size of cells varies from submicroscopic to grossly visible under moderate magnification.
  - The large cells are either macrophages or lymphocytes.
  - White cells are a sign of inflammation.
  - Pigmented cells are not always inflammatory.
  - Cell density less than +1 may not indicate active inflammation.

- *Exude in AC:* In severe inflammation, the flare and cells get enmeshed to form sheets of fibrin, dense enough to obscure the details of the iris and lens pattern. The presence of such sheets is called plastic iritis.
- *Pus (hypopyon):* Pus in the anterior chamber is called *hypopyon*. In cases of severe AC reactions, there is an outpouring of WBC resulting in actual pus formation; the hypopyon itself is sterile. The characteristics of hypopyon are:
  - It settles down at the most dependent part of AC, i.e., the bottom of AC, if the head is erect.
  - If the hypopyon is fluid enough, it changes its position according to the position of the head.
  - The color of hypopyon is white. It may be tinged red in the case of a perforating injury to the limbus. The two organisms that cause blood tinged hypopyon are herpes simplex and zoster.
  - Dirty, yellow-tinged, immobile hypopyon is suggestive of fungus infection.
  - The hypopyon is measured in millimeters from the limbus to the upper border of the hypopyon.
  - The upper border is horizontal.
  - White matter, except pus in AC, is called pseudo-hypopyon.

Any white matter in AC is to be considered as pus unless proved otherwise.

- The substances that are mistaken for pus are cortical matter, the nucleus of a ruptured lens, malignant cells, parasites, and silicone oil **(Fig. 17.1)**.
- A white matter in the upper part of the anterior chamber is called inverse hypopyon; this is caused by the migration of silicone oil from the posterior chamber. This has a horizontal lower border.

- *Blood (hyphema):* The presence of blood in AC is called hyphema; it is rare in uveitis. It can be seen in acute as well as chronic uveitis. The causes can be herpes simplex, herpes zoster, gonococcus, trauma in the eye with uveitis, or chronic uveitis with neovascularization of the iris.
- *Iris nodule:* There are no nodules on the normal iris surface. The presence of nodules indicates iris disease. They may be inflammatory or noninflammatory. The common inflammatory causes are tuberculosis, leprosy, and syphilis. The noninflammatory causes are sarcoid (Berlin's nodule), neurofibromatosis (Lisch nodule), parasitic cyst, congenital cyst, and secondary infiltration (see below).
- *Changes in the iris:* It is obvious that the iris will show pathological features when inflamed. The iris changes in uveitis are:
  - Loss of pattern
  - Miosis
  - Adhesion
  - Nodule

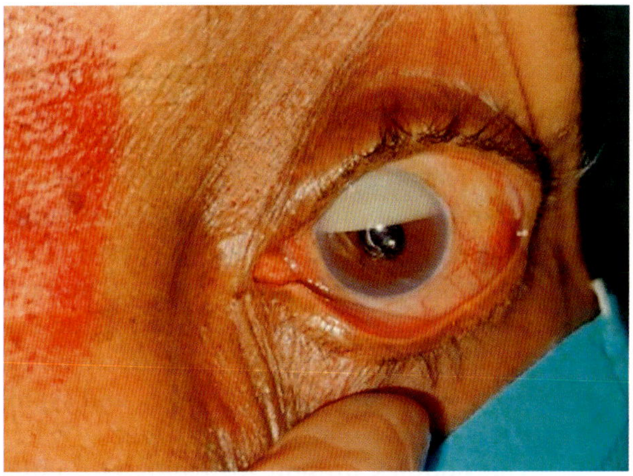

Fig. 17.1: Silicone oil in anterior chamber in an adult.

- *Loss of pattern:* The anterior surface of a healthy iris is rough and devoid of blood vessels, except for a few days following normal birth. The roughness of the iris is due to collarettes, crypts, and furrows; they are nonpathological. The collarettes divide the iris into two parts, i.e., the inner pupillary zone and the outer ciliary zone. Arrays of furrows radiating from the center to the periphery are present all round the pupillary zone. Beside these furrows, there are a number of pits in the ciliary zone; they are called crypts. The furrows and crypts give the iris ruggedness, which is lost in the edema of the iris stroma. The cause of the loss of ruggedness, which is referred to as iris patterns, is the accumulation of fluid in the iris stroma. This hampers the movement of the iris over the lens, and the iris may develop adhesion in the center, periphery, or both. The pattern is lost in the early stages of inflammation of the iris. In the long run, the edema is replaced by scattered areas of atrophy. Atrophic patches are common in herpes infections.
- *Miosis:* Normal iris moves smoothly over the anterior lens capsule without impeding the flow of aqueous. As the iris gets fluid-laden in acute iritis, it becomes heavy and sticky, and the edge of the swollen iris moves toward the center, reducing the diameter of the pupil. This miosis is worsened by the overaction of constrictor pupillae. The miosis of iritis should be differentiated from congenital or physiological microcoria, ingestion, and instillation of parasympathetic drugs.
- *Adhesion:* The heavy, sticky, fluid-laden posterior surface of the iris develops adhesion to the lens. These adhesions are called posterior synechiae*. To begin with, the adhesions are few, small, and break with mydriatic easily; as the disease progresses, they become larger, wider, and more difficult to break. Still later, the whole of the pupillary border gets glued to the lens with miosis

Posterior synechiae:* This is defined as postinflammatory adhesion between the posterior surface of the edematous iris and the anterior lens capsule, posterior chamber intraocular lens (IOL), after cataract, and vitreous following intracapsular lens extraction/dislocation of the lens **(Fig. 17.2).

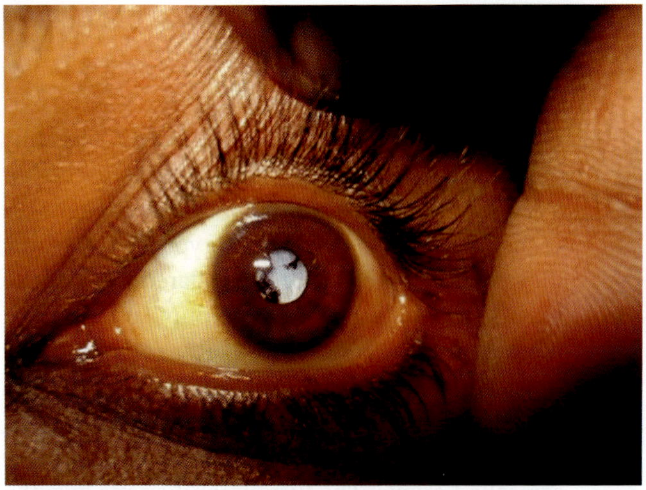

Fig. 17.2: Multiple posterior synechiae in chronic uveitis with complicated cataract.
Courtesy: Professor Nidhi Pandey.

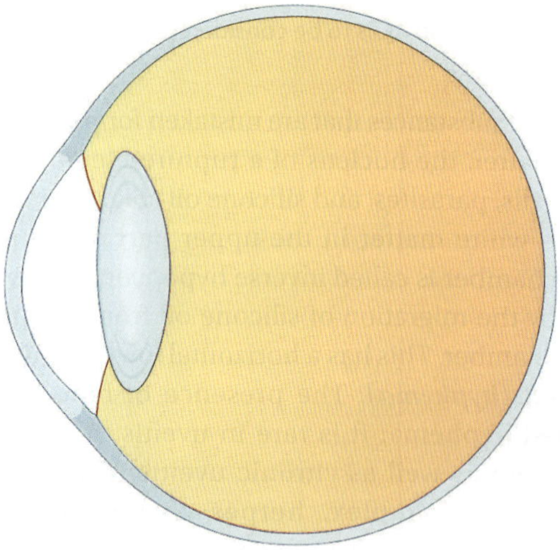

Fig. 17.3: Iris bombe.

and irregularities. A sheet of exudate may cover the small pupil; this along with synechiae all round separates the anterior chamber from the posterior chamber. The exudate is called the occlusio pupil, while the ring synechiae are called the seclusio pupillae. The peripheral counterpart of posterior synechiae is peripheral anterior synechiae* which are adhesions between the posterior surface of the cornea and the anterior surface of the iris.

Iris bombe: This is the bulging of the central part of the iris in the case of total posterior synechiae. The AC is deep in the center and shallowest at the top of the bulge. If the peripheral part of the iris touches the peripheral cornea, it obliterates the angle of the anterior chamber, forming a new angle called the pseudo-angle of the anterior chamber.

Both ring synechiae and pseudo-angle are contributing to the rise of intraocular pressure in anterior uveitis **(Fig. 17.3)**.

The other causes of pseudo-angle are congenital deformity of the angle, dysgenesis of the angle, persistent hypotony, chronic narrow-angle glaucoma, and neovascularization of the angle.

Festooned pupil: This happens when the pupil fails to dilate equally all around. The strong posterior synechiae resist breaking in spite of powerful mydriatic. The pupil has a flower petal appearance **(Fig. 17.4)**.

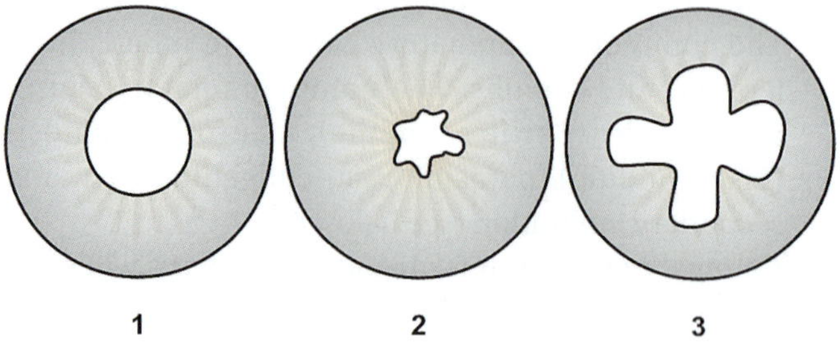

Fig. 17.4: Constricted and atropinized pupils in anterior uveitis. (1) Normal central circular pupil; (2) Centrally constricted irregular pupil in iritis; (3) Festooned pupil following instillation of atropine.

- *Nodule:* There is no nodule on the normal iris surface. The presence of nodules is an indication of inflammation of the iris. The noninflammatory causes of nodules on the iris consist of Lisch nodules in neurofibromatosis, secondaries, Berlin's nodules in sarcoid, and parasitic cysts. The inflammatory conditions that cause nodules on the iris are tuberculosis, leprosy, and syphilis. They are not seen under 20 years of age.

The nodules present in uveitis are nothing but cellular aggregates in relation to the iris surface. According to topography, they are called

**Peripheral anterior synechiae:* Anterior synechiae are defined as adhesion between the anterior surface of the iris and the posterior surface of the cornea, which can be central or peripheral.

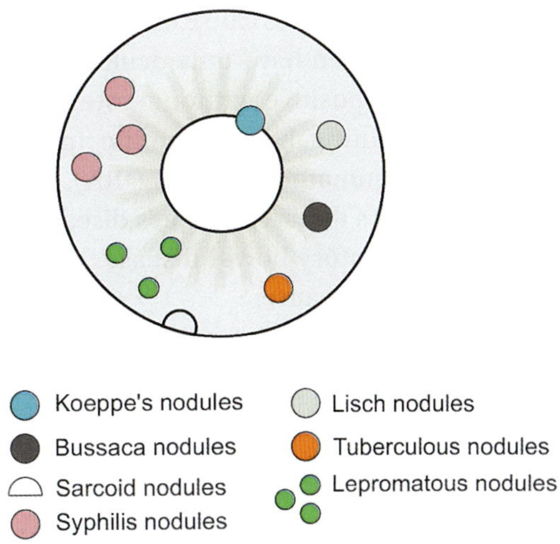

Fig. 17.5: Various types of nodules on the iris in both types of uveitis.

Koeppe's nodules* when present at the pupillary margin. Busacca nodules† are present on the iris away from the margin but not in the angle. The Berlin's nodules (sarcoid) are present at an angle **(Fig. 17.5)**.

- *Lenticular changes:* In the early stages, the lens remains clear except for marks of iris adhesion on the anterior lens capsule as black spots. These black spots are arranged in a circular fashion round the anterior pole of the lens. Corresponding to the original site of adhesion, the size of the pigment depends on the width of the synechiae. The spots remain visible for months even after the pupil has been dilated fully and the inflammation subsided. They are not to be confused with remnants of persistent pupillary membrane and Vossius ring‡ following blunt injury to the globe. The persistent pupillary membrane originates from the anterior surface of the iris, while posterior synechiae develop from the back of the iris. If the pigments are not cleared, they give rise to anterior capsular opacities. This happens more in broad adhesion; recurrent uveitis heralds the development of posterior subcapsular opacity that has polychromatic lustre on the slit lamp. In fibrinous anterior uveitis, an opaque membrane develops on the posterior surface of the lens and is called the posterior cyclitic membrane, this is the posterior counterpart of the occlusio pupillae.
- *Changes in vitreous:* Vitreous, due to its close proximity to the uvea all-round, drowns in inflammatory changes of the uvea. The vitreal changes are similar to change in aqueous, comprising cells, coagulated exudates, and fibrin. Anterior uveitis causes the pouring of cells in the anterior vitreous, leaving the posterior vitreous clear. Anterior cells are more marked in cyclitis than in iritis. The cells in the anterior vitreous are seen best in the bright beam of the slit lamp, while those in the posterior vitreous are visible with +76 to +90 D.
  Hogan's classification of vitreous haze is given in **Table 17.5**.

TABLE 17.5: Hogan's classification of vitreous haze.

Sr. no.	*Density of opacity*	*Grade*
1.	No opacity	0
2.	Few scattered large cells; the details of the retina are well visualized	+1
3.	Fundus slightly obscured	+2
4.	Marked obscuration of the retina	+3
5.	Retina is not visible	+4

In cases of cyclitis, the number of cells per field is more than in the anterior chamber.

- *Change in fundus:* The fundus should be examined on every visit with a direct and indirect ophthalmoscope. The macula is best seen at +90 D. Macular edema is more common in pars planitis but may be present in all types of acute and chronic uveitis.
  - *Early changes:* The fundal glow may be dulled due to haze in the media spanning between the cornea

**Koeppe's nodules:* Koeppe's nodules are thought to be ectodermal in origin, the iris equivalent of mutton-fat KPs. They are composed of epithelial and giant cells surrounded by lymphocytes; they are seen both in granulomatous and nongranulomatous uveitis. They may project into the pupil from the pupillary border. They are self-limiting and disappear in a few days; their disappearance is enhanced with the use of steroids. They are replaced by posterior synechiae on disappearance.

†*Busacca nodules:* The Busacca nodules are presumed to be mesodermal in nature. They are present between the pupillary border and the angle; they are mostly seen in granulomatous uveitis. It takes a few weeks to months for them to disappear with prolonged steroid instillation.

‡*Vossius ring:* Vossius ring is the deposition of iris pigment on the anterior surface of the lens following blunt injuries. It is noninflammatory in nature. The ring consists of a circle of black pigment originating from the posterior surface of the iris, mostly consisting of iris pigment and epithelial cells. The condition is often mistaken as remnants of ring synechiae. It does not require any treatment.

and vitreous in various combinations. The haze may be due to corneal edema, KPs, flare, or fibrinous exudate in front of the pupil, which is generally small and irregular, making it more difficult to see the fundus.
- *Delayed changes:* Occlusio pupillae and vitreous haze
- *Late changes:* Late changes consist of band keratopathy, a small irregular rigid pupil, posterior subcapsular opacity, posterior cyclitic membrane, and a complicated cataract.

- *Changes in macula:* Changes in macula are best seen with a +90 D lens. Acute anterior uveitis seldom involves the macula; however, cystoid macular edema (CME) is not an exception that is mostly self-limiting; macular edema is more pronounced in intermediate uveitis.

SPECIFIC TYPES OF UVEITIS IN CHILDREN

It is logical to presume that childhood uveitis does not differ from adult uveitis. It is true as far as etiopathology is concerned; clinically, uveitis in children differs in many ways. *They are:*

- Childhood uveitis is not only more challenging to diagnose but also more difficult to treat as compared to adult uveitis.
- Children suffer from uveitis in all anatomical locations, i.e., anterior, intermediate, and posterior uveitis.
- Anterior and intermediate uveitis are more common than posterior uveitis.
- Intermediate uveitis is as common as anterior uveitis and is frequently missed in children.
- Posterior uveitis in children is mostly infective and may be congenital or acquired (posterior choroiditis).
- Posterior uveitis is less common than adult uveitis.
- Only 10% of cases among uveitis seen at all ages belong to children.
- The incidence of pediatric uveitis is more in the latter half of the second decade than in the earlier years of the first decade.
- Girls show a slight preponderance; white uveitis is five times more common in girls.
- Panuveitis is less common in children; exceptions are sympathetic ophthalmia, Vogt-Koyanagi-Harada syndrome, and Behçet's disease.
- In 50% of cases, no definite cause can be pinpointed.
- About 30% of children have only ocular involvement and are HLA-B27 positive without systemic involvement; the remaining have systemic involvement from juvenile rheumatoid arthritis (JRA), ankylosing spondylitis, Reiter's disease, Behçet's disease, sarcoidosis, and inflammatory bowel disease. Out of them, JRA is most common cause.
- About 50% of cases are bilateral, which need not be symmetric or simultaneous.
- Band keratopathy is more common in children with uveitis.
- A child with uniocular uveitis may not complain unless it is acute.
- Pediatric uveitis ranges from mild self-limiting anterior uveitis to severe blinding endophthalmitis.
- Masquerading conditions like life-threatening retinoblastoma may be mistaken for severe panuveitis.
- Undetected uveitis leads to permanent diminished vision, causing amblyopia and/or squinting.
- About 25% have systemic involvement. Childhood uveitis may have varied systemic involvement.
- Childhood uveitis has a relatively poor prognosis.
- Systemic drugs should be used with usual caution in consultation with a pediatrician.

Childhood uveitis can be congenital or acquired. The former are silent and detected on routine examination. The conditions that may lead to the diagnosis of congenital uveitis are squint, amblyopia, nystagmus, and masquerade syndromes.

The common congenital uveitides are infective. They are transmitted mostly transplacentally: toxoplasma, rubella, cytomegalovirus, syphilis, herpes simplex, and HIV.

The acquired causes can be infective or noninfective. The most common infectious cause is tuberculosis. The incidence of tubercular intraocular involvement in children is lower as compared to adults.

Other causes of acquired infective uveitis are bacterial, viral, and parasitic.

The noninfective causes are:

- Autoimmune diseases
- Disorders of doubtful etiology
- Trauma
- Masquerade syndromes

Toxoplasmosis of the Uvea in Children

Congenital toxoplasmosis of the uvea is more common than acquired and is a self-limiting condition that either heals fully or remains dormant to be activated in adulthood. The fetus gets the infection from the mother in one of the following ways: transplacental, or from a dormant lesion in the uterus.

Toxoplasmosis has predilection for neural tissue; it involves the brain in the form of encephalitis and the retina in the form of retinitis, and surprisingly, it does not involve the optic nerve. In fact, the so-called choroiditis, which is most common ocular involvement, is retinochoroiditis, not the other way around. By the time, the infected fetus is born, the chorioretinitis is healed. As the anterior segment is not involved, the usual examination of the anterior segment does not reveal its presence.

The child may be brought with convulsion and ordered a fundus examination; the other presentation is infantile esotropia. On examination of the fundus, the child is found to have a large patch of retinochoroiditis on the macula that is the cause of diminished vision, squint, amblyopia, and occasional nystagmus. X-rays of the skull may show intracranial calcification.

> Three Cs of congenital toxoplasmosis are convulsion, calcification (intracranial), and choroiditis (central).

Besides, there is a patch of choroiditis over the macula. There may be juxtapapillary patches scattered away from the disk and macula, not causing diminished vision. A juxtapapillary choroiditis between the macula and the disk causes diminished vision as much as a macula patch.

The patches of choroiditis are generally bilateral oval larger than the disk, and mostly horizontally oval. There are two types of patches. The first and more common is a healed lesion caused due to infection contracted in the early months of pregnancy that is a central white area surrounded by clumps of black pigments. The blood vessels travel across the patch without any change, and the white colors in the center are due to exposed sclera following the destruction of the retina and choroid in the patch. The patch is surrounded by irregular clumps of choroidal pigment. The vitreous is not involved; there are no cells in the vitreous adjacent to or over the patch.

The second type of lesion is due to an infection contracted late in pregnancy. They are active lesions that present as fluffy edematous lesions with cells in the adjacent vitreous, without pigments on the periphery.

The child with ocular toxoplasmosis may have only ocular lesions that are benign, barring diminished vision and its consequences, like nystagmus. Unilateral cases are more likely to have squints and amblyopia (most common squint is esotropia). The other possibility is that the child has a combination of ocular and systemic involvement. The most common symptom of systemic involvement is convulsion. This makes it mandatory for every child with convulsion to undergo an X-ray to exclude intracranial calcification and fundus examination for evidence of an active or dormant patch of central choroiditis.

The child may have microcephaly and mental retardation. A lesion may have the deceptive appearance of an apparently healed lesion. Some eyes have recurrence after 5–6 years; recurrence is more common among girls. The recurrence starts as an acute lesion with greater involvement of the vitreous; the whole of the vitreous is studded with cells and debris, giving it a translucent appearance and smudging the lesion. The smudged appearance has been called head light in fog; the other common features of recurrence are—posterior vitreous detachment, papillitis, and vasculitis.

The complications of congenital toxoplasmosis can be divided into two parts:

1. Due to healed chorioretinitis, which causes diminished distant vision, squint amblyopia, and nystagmus.
2. Due to recurrence, they are similar to acquired lesions; the complications are generalized uveitis, complicated cataracts, various types of glaucoma, exudative retinal detachment, vitreous hemorrhage, and neovascularization.

The differential diagnosis of congenital toxoplasmosis uveitis is limited to congenital coloboma of the macula.

The acquired lesions must be differentiated from—herpes simplex and rubella chorioretinitis, tubercular choroiditis, miliary tubercle of choroid cytomegalovirus infection, and retinoblastoma.

Diagnosis

> A condition that merits differentiation is active or regressed retinoblastoma that shows intraocular calcification in 75% of cases.

Diagnosis of congenital toxoplasmosis chorioretinitis is not difficult if the child is brought with systemic signs of—convulsion, retarded growth, mental retardation, and squint, making it mandatory to get an X-ray of the skull for intracranial calcification and fundus evaluation for a patch of macular choroiditis.

The TORCH test* is a nonspecific test that represents many diseases and is the most common test ordered to screen for congenital toxoplasmosis.

The other tests for congenital toxoplasmosis are serological tests:

- Serum, antiplasma, and antibody
- ELISA†
- Polymerase chain reaction (PCR‡)
- Immunoglobulin IgG and IgM

IgG may be positive without ocular involvement. Positive IgM is a strong indication of recent ocular and systemic infections.

Treatment

- There is no prophylaxis against toxoplasmosis.
- A healed patch of macular lesions does not require any treatment.
- All that is needed is a correction of the squint for cosmetic reasons.
- Amblyopia may not respond to usual treatment.
- A child with a healed lesion should be watched for recurrence.
- Treatment of active lesions consists of:
    - Chemotherapy by sulfadiazine, pyrimethamine alone or in combination with sulfate. Other drugs used are clindamycin and tetracycline.
    - Chemotherapy along with steroids
    - Photocoagulation of peripheral lesions
    - Usual treatment of uveitis

Rubella Uveitis in Children

Acquired rubella does not involve the eyes. Its systemic features are so mild that they are ignored and taken as an upper respiratory infection.

If the mother acquires the disease in the first trimester, the fetus is at risk of developing ocular as well as systemic disease. The systemic features may be life-threatening. Ocular lesions consist of—rubella, cataracts, glaucoma, and microphthalmos; they are so overwhelming that they overshadow the milder uveal involvement, which consists of nonprogressive chorioretinitis that has the appearance of salt pepper chorioretinitis, which requires differentiation from syphilitic chorioretinitis and retinitis pigmentosa (retinitis pigmentosa manifests after the first decade). Rubella chorioretinitis is peripheral; hence, it does not interfere with central vision and does not require any specific treatment.

Acquired Uveitis in Children

Like uveitis in all ages, the causes of uveitis in children too cannot be pin-pointed in all cases.

The causes that can be pin-pointed are divided into the following groups:

- Noninfective
- Infective
- Masquerades

The noninfective causes are:

- Juvenile rheumatoid arthritis
- Ankylosing spondylitis (not seen before the second decade)
- Reiter's syndrome (rare in children)
- Still's diseases
- Behçet's diseases
- Sympathetic ophthalmia
- Vogt–Koyanagi–Harada syndrome (not seen before the second decade)
- Fuchs heterochromic iridocyclitis (rare in children)
- Lens-induced uveitis
- Posner–Schlossman syndrome (unilateral, also known as glaucoma cyclitic uveitis)

**TORCH test:* The word TORCH is an acronym for a group of tests used to exclude various infections in the mother and the newborn. The test is nonspecific. The letters stand for:
T—Toxoplasmosis
O—Others (which include many infective agents, mainly congenital syphilis)
R—Rubella
C—Cytomegalovirus
H—Herpes simplex

More specific is an X-ray of the skull. A small, calcified lesion that is not delineated on an X-ray becomes obvious on CT and MRI.

†*ELISA:* ELISA is an acronym for enzyme-linked immunoassay; it is used to detect antibodies in the blood.

‡*PCR:* PCR is an acronym for polymerase chain reaction; it detects specific genetic material of a given organism, mostly viruses. It is useful in detecting the presence of viruses during active infections. It may be positive even after the infections have been treated.

- Kawasaki disease (systemic vasculitis in children)
- Pars planitis

Infective uveitis in children is:

- Tuberculosis
- Syphilis
- Rubella
- Herpes simplex
- Herpes zoster
- AIDS
- Cytomegalovirus
- Toxocariasis (nematode)
- Toxoplasmosis (protozoa)

Masquerade syndrome causes uveitis in children.

These from a group of conditions that mimic uveitis in spite of their not being, so some of them are life-threatening malignancies.

They are:

- Retinoblastoma
- Leukemia
- Medulloepithelioma
- Lymphoma
- Reticulum cell sarcoma (not seen in children)
- Malignant melanoma (not seen in children)
- Juvenile xanthogranuloma
- Intraocular foreign bodies
- Retinal detachment

Out of the long list, retinoblastoma is the most important clinical entity that requires proper evaluation and management due to its propensity to be fatal.

Features of posterior uveitis in children:

- *Age:* **Table 17.6** depicts the age-wise distribution of posterior uveitis in children.
- *Side:* Unilateral choroiditis is more likely to be caused by toxoplasmosis, toxocariasis, or endogenous bacterial infections like tuberculosis.
- *Vision:* Reduced vision with or without squints should always arouse chances of central toxoplasmosis.
- *Afferent pupil:* This denotes widespread chorioretinitis and optic nerve involvement.
- *Pain:* Generally, there is no pain in posterior uveitis.
- *Anterior segment involvement in posterior uveitis:* Anterior segment involvement is most likely to be absent unless the lesion is widespread, as seen in endogenous endophthalmitis, Vogt–Koyanagi–Harada syndrome, sympathetic ophthalmia, tuberculosis, sarcoidosis, and Behçet's disease. Anterior segment involvement may be serious enough to cause hypopyon. A combination of anterior segment reaction with posterior segment involvement is better labeled as panuveitis. The anterior segment involvement that is present with posterior choroiditis is generally granulomatous.
- *Involvement of vitreous:* Vitritis is frequent in bacterial endophthalmitis and toxoplasmosis.

TABLE 17.6: Age-wise distribution of posterior uveitis.

Age	*Type*
Congenital	Toxoplasmosis, rubella, cytomegalovirus, syphilis, and herpes simplex
Under 3 years	All congenital causes may present for the first time in this age group due to squint, amblyopia, and nystagmus. Other causes are toxocariasis and masquerading syndromes, especially retinoblastoma
Above 3 years	All the above plus acquired toxoplasmosis, toxocariasis, tuberculosis, syphilis, sympathetic ophthalmia, Vogt–Koyanagi–Harada syndrome, Behçet's syndrome, and sarcoidosis

Uveitis in Children due to Connective Tissue Involvement

Connective tissue disorders are a group of autoimmune diseases that can involve the eye between 5 years to old age. These may be acute, chronic, or recurrent. Recurrence may be in the same eye or may involve the other eye simultaneously or separately. May alternate between the two.

The most common systemic manifestation is arthritis, which may be mono or polyarthritis, pauciarticular (less than four joints), or (more than five joints). Some children may not have joint involvement at the time of ocular involvement, especially in JRA. Most common ocular involvement of the uvea is uveitis, which is more common in the anterior uvea than the posterior.

The connective tissue disorders that are responsible for uveal involvement are:

- Juvenile rheumatoid arthritis, also known as juvenile idiopathic arthritis (JIA), the terms are often used as synonyms.
- Ankylosing spondylitis
- Reiter's disease (inflammatory arthritis is due to infection in another part of the body; the triad of the condition is arthritis, conjunctivitis/uveitis, and urethritis

- Relapsing polychondritis (anterior uveitis, episcleritis, and peripheral ulcerative keratitis)
- Other conditions that are associated with uveitis (in all ages) are:
  - Psoriatic arthritis
  - Sarcoidosis
  - Still's disease (fever, rash, and joint pain)

Other noninfective causes of uveitis (in all ages) are:

- Idiopathic anterior uveitis
- Sympathetic uveitis
- Vogt–Koyanagi–Harada disease
- Behçet's disease (generalized vasculitis)
- Fuchs heterochromic iridocyclitis (unilateral iridocyclitis, cataract)
- Posner–Schlossman syndrome (glaucomatocyclitic crisis, acute unilateral uveitis)
- Kawasaki disease (<5 years, generalized vasculitis)

UVEITIS IN JUVENILE RHEUMATOID ARTHRITIS OR IDIOPATHIC RHEUMATOID ARTHRITIS

Juvenile rheumatoid arthritis is a common cause of uveitis in children under 16 years old. It is defined as "arthritis of at least 6 weeks' duration without any identifiable cause of joint involvement in pediatric age group".

It is more common in girls; if it involves more than one joint but less than four joints at a time, it is called pauciarticular (oligoarticular). Involvement of five or more joints, without wrist involvement, is called polyarticular. The patients have antinuclear antibodies and are HLA-B27 positive without rheumatoid factor. Uveitis may develop years after the first episode of arthritis; however, early involvement is not uncommon. Ocular disorders may linger even after joint involvements have resolved.

The uveitis is generally nongranulomatous, involving the anterior segment. Polyarticular diseases, which comprise about half the cases in children, have only a 5% chance of developing iridocyclitis. Uveitis is maximum in pauciarticular that comprises 40% of all arthritis in children. The incident of iridocyclitis in this group is at its maximum, i.e., 75–95%. The incidence of iridocyclitis is minimal in Still's disease, which accounts for 10% of arthritis but only 1% of uveitis. Pauciarticular arthritis can be divided into two broad *groups according to the serology test:*

1. Positive antinuclear antibody
2. Positive HLA-B27

The first is most likely to present with chronic iridocyclitis. The second presents as acute or recurrent uveitis. It is not unusual for a child to be brought with diminished vision to have asymptomatic advanced anterior uveitis that has not received any treatment. The disease is bilateral but not symmetric.

Presenting features of uveitis in JRA:

- It is rarely seen in children <5 years and above 16 years.
- There is a female preponderance.
- The disease is mostly bilateral.
- It can present as acute and symptomatic.
- Acute symptomatic cases have a better prognosis because they draw attention earlier and are treated better.
- The more dangerous group consists of children with gradual but smoldering iritis called silent or white iritis.
- 25% of cases are potentially blinding.
- Children under 5 years of age with pauciarticular and positive ANA are at higher risk of sight-threatening complications. They must have an ocular examination every 3 months during the 1st year of presentation and then every 6 months for the next 5 years, and every year until 16 years.
- ANA-positive children with polyarticular involvement should have ocular examinations twice a year for 5 years.
- Children with oligoarticular and ANA-negative conditions should have an ocular evaluation every year.

Clinical Presentation in Juvenile Rheumatoid Arthritis Uveitis

The cases may be divided into the following main groups:

- Presenting as idiopathic anterior uveitis
- Presenting as white iritis
- Presenting in the stage of complication

- *The first has the usual features of acute iritis:*
  - Dull pain in the eye
  - Ciliary tenderness
  - Circumciliary congestion
  - Cells and flare in AC
  - Constricted irregular pupil that dilates with usual cycloplegic with ease
  - Small posterior synechiae are common.
  - Frequent hypopyon
  - Clear lens and vitreous

- Variable vision ranges from 6/9 to 6/18.
- Responding well to steroids
- Recurrence is common.

- *White iritis:* This is a common mode of presentation of JRA iridocyclitis in children; the incidence is far more common among girls, it is generally unilateral and so slow and almost symptomless that it goes undetected till it has reached an irreversible state of complication.
- On examination in the stage of complication, the cornea shows evidence of early band keratopathy*, small KPs, cells, and flare, a small pupil of variable size with multiple posterior synechiae, a cycloplegic-resistant pupil, a complicated cataract, and secondary glaucoma.

Symptoms

Band keratopathy is relatively asymptomatic; observant parents may notice the white band against the black iris and bring the child for consultation.

The loss of vision due to the band is gradual and painless. Once the bands cover the pupil, the vision is greatly reduced. The eye may occasionally be blind, not due to the band but to the underlying pathology, i.e., phthisis. Watering and foreign body sensations develop when the calcium crystals protrude through the epithelium.

Management

Treatment of band keratopathy is difficult; small peripheral bands do not require any treatment; there is no way to stop the progression of band keratopathy. The best treatment is a lamellar corneal graft. The use of EDTA has not proved to be very effective.

Complications of Anterior Uveitis in Juvenile Rheumatoid Arthritis

The most common complication of an untreated or partially treated eye is amblyopia because many eyes may suffer from white iritis and the child does not complain of it.

Management of amblyopia by itself in children above 8 years of age is difficult, still all antiamblyopic measures should be given trial.

The other frequent complication is a complicated cataract that can be unilateral or bilateral; when bilateral, it is generally not equal in two eyes. Cataract itself may be the cause of diminished vision or may worsen the vision caused by uveitis. The cataract may have normal

---

**Band keratopathy:* Band keratopathy develops in two forms in children and young adults: primary and secondary. The first is less common without other morbidities, most probably a type of dystrophy. The secondary type is degeneration, seen in children and young adults with other ocular morbidities.

The ocular disorders that predispose to band keratopathy are—chronic anterior uveitis, especially JRA uveitis; rheumatoid uveitis; panuveitis; microphthalmos, the absolute stage of juvenile glaucoma; penetrating injury; keratoplasty; anterior segment ischemia, silicone oil, sodium, *hyaluronate*, and chondroitin sulfate in AC, besides a horde of congenital anomalies of the anterior segment. The condition can be unilateral or bilateral but not symmetric; it is a chronic, slowly progressing degenerative condition never seen in the acute stage of primary disease, developing months to years after the primary disorder has died down.

The condition has acquired its name due to its band shape; it is in fact a spindle-shaped opacity with truncated ends. The band develops in the interpalpebral aperture in the Bowman's membrane and anterior stroma, initially leaving the epithelium intact. The band develops in two parts, i.e., one on the medial and the other on the lateral end of the cornea, 1 mm inside the limbus, as a sharp vertical line from the periphery. The edge toward the pupil is irregular and serrated. The two ends progress slowly toward the pupil to merge with each other in the center of the cornea. The area of the band in front of the pupil is wider than on the periphery.

The opacity is formed due to the deposition of extracellular, noncrystalline salts of calcium carbonate and phosphate. The exact source of the salt is not known. The patients with band keratopathy have normal serum calcium; surprisingly, the corneal endothelium that is continuous with the uveal endothelium is not affected, nor is the epithelium. In the long run, some of the calcium crystals protrude through the epithelium, causing foreign body sensation and watering, in otherwise asymptomatic eyes. The vision remains normal as long as the band does not cover the pupil; the band is white in color with a rough texture, retaining touch sensation; there are few irregular vacuoles in the substance of the band that represent the corneal nerve endings; the holes do not stain with fluorescein that gets pooled in the craters, giving a false impression of staining; and the condition may be mistaken for infective keratitis.

The exact cause of the disorder is disputed. There are many unanswered riddles, i.e., source of calcium, specific salt of calcium, selective involvement of Bowman's membrane, sparing of endothelium, minimal involvement of epithelium, and predilection for exposed cornea in the interpalpebral aperture.

There is unanimity in the opinion that it is degeneration. The various theories put forward are that it is influenced by actinic rays, which influence the chemical composition of the tear and corneal epithelium, which has low carbon dioxide and low pH. The corneal hemidesmosome acts as a scaffold over which calcium from the tear is deposited. As children are more likely to mobilize calcium, they are more likely to develop the condition. The condition, in spite of being chronic, does not develop vascularization.

intraocular tension or may be associated with glaucoma or even hypotony. The involvement of the cataract may be minimal without reducing vision, or it may be extensive enough to reduce vision to the perception of light. In all such cases, the projection of light should be tested to exclude peripheral involvement. This test is not accurate enough for the diagnosis of all peripheral lesions. In cases of opaque media, such lesions are better delineated by ultrasound (USG) and optical coherence tomography (OCT).

The treatment of an operable cataract is nothing shorter than phacoemulsification with PC IOL. A quiet eye is a prerequisite for lens extraction. The eye should be noncongested without flare for a minimum of 3 months before the surgery. The eye after surgery should be under strong cycloplegic therapy for about a month, along with intense local steroid therapy for at least 3 months.

UVEITIS IN ANKYLOSING SPONDYLITIS

Ankylosing spondylitis is yet another autoimmune arthropathy that affects adults more than children. Uveitis, when present, is equally common in both age groups. In adults, the spine is more involved, while in children, the lower peripheral joints are more involved than the joints of the hands. 80% of children with ankylosing spondylitis are HLA-B27 positive. 25% of children with ankylosing spondylitis are at risk of developing anterior uveitis, 50% of children who are HLA-B27 positive with uveitis either have ankylosing spondylitis or will develop it.

Uveitis in ankylosing spondylitis is nongranulomatous, anterior uveitis that is generally unilateral and acute, with a high propensity to recurrence in 80% of eyes, the other eye following suit. The first attack of anterior uveitis generally lasts for 4–6 weeks in spite of treatment; recurrence is common and may happen as often as every month or as delayed as 1 year.

The clinical presentation is similar to anterior uveitis in JRA. Hypopyon is common. Complications like cataract, band keratopathy, and CME are less common, but glaucoma is as common as anterior uveitis in JRA.

Diagnosis

Male children in the second decade with unilateral, acute iritis, pain in peripheral joints, and positive HLA-B27 are more likely to be suffering from ankylosing spondylitis. Rather than JRA, X-rays of the sacroiliac joint may show evidence of sacroiliitis.

Differential diagnosis and management are similar to anterior uveitis in JRA.

UVEITIS IN CHILDHOOD: REITER'S DISEASE

Reiter's disease (syndrome) is also known as reactive arthritis. It affects adults more than children, producing unilateral, nongranulomatous anterior uveitis. Previously, it was thought to be a triad of conjunctivitis (red eye), arthritis, and urethritis. Now, it is clear that the redness of the eye that was attributed to conjunctivitis is not simple conjunctivitis but a combination of conjunctivitis, peripheral keratitis, and iritis, where conjunctivitis has less clinical significance than the other two. Out of the remaining two, iritis is clinically more significant. The pathology is supposed to be a reactive reaction to an infection away from the primary site of infection. The two other disorders caused following reactivations are urethritis/cervicitis by nongonococcal organisms. Dysentery is yet another neglected cause. The genital lesions are mostly due to chlamydia and dysentery caused by *Shigella* and *Salmonella*.

75% of cases are HLA-B27 positive and are likely to develop red eye, out of which 10–15% will develop anterior uveitis. Children with Reiter's disease are rheumatoid factor-negative. Postvenereal form develops in adolescent males, while postdysentery form develops more frequently in girls.

The ocular features are bilateral mucopurulent conjunctivitis, acute anterior uveitis, superficial punctate corneal infiltrates, and subepithelial infiltrates in the cornea.

Extraocular features are—oligoarthritis of large joints of the lower limbs, plantar fasciitis; oral aphthous ulcer; nongonococcal urethritis/cervicitis/balanitis; and dysentery.

Treatment

- Conjunctivitis is self-limiting.
- Anterior uveitis is treated by the usual treatment of anterior uveitis, i.e., cycloplegics and steroids.
- Nonocular symptoms are best treated by an internist, rheumatologist, or gynecologist.

KAWASAKI SYNDROME

This is a rare but potential life-threatening acute vasculitis. The ocular components are anterior uveitis, disk edema, dilated retinal vessels, and conjunctivitis in children.

The systemic features are fever, rash, desquamation of the skin of the limbs, enlarged lymph nodes in the neck, pharyngitis, and glossitis. Uveitis is most marked in the 1st week. The cases are best managed by pediatrician, ophthalmologist looking after uveitis.

INTERMEDIATE UVEITIS SYNDROME

This is a conglomeration of some conditions with overlapping, diverse clinical features, all of which are chronic inflammations, mostly of the vitreous. According to the SUN, the main site of inflammation is in vitro (hyalitis). The other conditions included are pars planitis and posterior cyclitis, making it a triad of hyalitis, pars planitis, and posterior cyclitis. Some cases are self-limiting; few have serious consequences, like peripheral periphlebitis, neovascularization, the development of vitreoretinal bands, retinal holes, posterior vitreous detachment, vitreous hemorrhage rarely retinal detachment, and cataracts. Frequent and prominent complications are CME and disk edema.

The cases can be broadly divided into two major categories:

1. Idiopathic
2. Infective

The former is more common than the second. The organisms that have been blamed as infective agents are—tuberculosis, syphilis, leptospirosis, Lyme (*Borrelia burgdorferi*), toxoplasma, and toxocara. The nonorganismal causes are sarcoidosis, multiple sclerosis, inflammatory bowel disease, and intraocular lymphoma.

Clinical Features

The disorder is seen mostly in children above 8 years of age and adolescents. It is a chronic bilateral disease; when bilateral, it is neither symmetric nor concurrent. Equally among boys and girls with varied presentations. The various modes of presentation are based on visual status.

They are:

- *Asymptomatic:* The child, especially with uniocular involvement, may not be aware of it and may not complain; the disorder is detected on routine school screening. The vision of such children may be 6/12 or 6/9. On close questioning, they may say that they see black spots in front of the eye. In such children, vision remains stationary, and the disease may resolve without treatment. On the other end of the spectrum, in the same age group, are the children who have a silent but far advanced disease with posterior subcapsular/posterior cortical cataracts, even band keratopathy. This makes it mandatory for the other eye to be examined minutely with an indirect ophthalmoscope and three mirror gonioscopes for died down disease or the beginning of the disease.
- *Cases with loss of vision:* On examination by indirect ophthalmoscope, three mirror gonioscopes, +90D, fluorescein angiography, and OCT may show the following:
  - Snowball and snow banking on the retinal periphery, especially in the lower temporal quadrant.
  - Periphlebitis
  - Neovascularization
  - Vitreous hemorrhage
  - Inflammatory choroidal and retinal detachment
  - Cyclitic membrane
  - Macular edema
- *Examination of the anterior segment shows:*
  - Few KPs
  - Cells in AC
  - Fine, easily breakable posterior synechiae
  - KPs and cells without posterior synechiae
  - Absence of synechiae is so common that in the past, the presence of adhesion was thought to go against the diagnosis of intermediate uveitis, and the child was thought to be suffering from JRA anterior uveitis.
- *Fundus examination:*
  - The most important findings are seen in the vitreous; they are:
    - Snowballs on the periphery
    - Peripheral vitritis
    - Vitreous hemorrhage
    - Vitreous bands
  - The next area to shows changes are in the macula:
    - Simple macular edema that may be confused with central serous retinopathy.
    - Cystoid macular edema
    - Macular hole (rare)

Course of the disease:

- The asymptomatic case has spontaneous regression.
- Others may have diminished vision, the causes of which are:
  - *In the posterior pole:* Macular edema, peripapillary edema, and papillitis

- *Round the pars plana:* Snowballs, snow banking or peripheral vessels, neovascularization, and periphlebitis
- *Ciliary body:* Cyclitis membrane
- *Lens:* Postsubcapsular and posterior cortical cataracts, worsened by prolonged use of steroids
- *Cornea:* Peripheral corneal edema, early band keratopathy
- *Glaucoma:* Secondary and steroid-induced
- Squint and amblyopia

Differential Diagnosis

Asymptomatic intermediate uveitis is difficult to diagnose in the first instance. Complaints of floaters in a patient between 5 and 15 are highly suggestive.

The common conditions that should be differentiated from pars planitis are idiopathic anterior uveitis, white iritis, JRA anterior uveitis, infective uveitis, masquerade syndromes, sarcoidosis, and small intraocular foreign bodies on the periphery.

Investigation

- Investigation should be directed to exclude systemic causes; failing to find systemic causes may be detrimental to the ultimate result of treatment.
- The local examinations; those are mandatory.
  - Slit lamp biomicroscopy
  - Indirect ophthalmoscopy with indention
  - Examination with +90 D
  - Three mirror gonioscopies
  - Fundus fluorescein examination
  - Ultrasonography
  - OCT

Management

Out of all uveitis in children, intermediate uveitis is the most confusing. It may be:

- Mild, nonprogressive, and self-healing
- Smoldering vision is threatening.
- Present for the for the first time in an advanced stage with cataract, CME, and vitreous hemorrhage.
- May be idiopathic or:
  - Secondary to systemic disease
  - Idiopathic associated with systemic diseases

Mild, nonprogressing self-healing cases are best left alone with regular checkups; in contrast to these, vision-threatening cases should be treated as emergencies. Vision 6/12 or less is considered to be the cutoff level at which treatment should be started.

Cases secondary to systemic diseases are divided into two parts.

The first is the management of a primary systemic condition in consultation with a pediatrician or internist; the second part is the management of ocular manifestation as per the protocol given below in **Flowchart 17.1**.

Note: The management schedule is very personal and depends on the protocol followed and the stage of the disease.

Cycloplegic: Strong, long-acting drugs like atropine are seldom required. Short-acting cycloplegics like home atropine, tropicamide, and cyclopentolate given two times a day for a fortnight are sufficient; the above drugs are mydriatic as well; hence, separate pure mydriatics like phenylephrine are not needed.

Flowchart 17.1: Protocol for the management of intermediate uveitis.

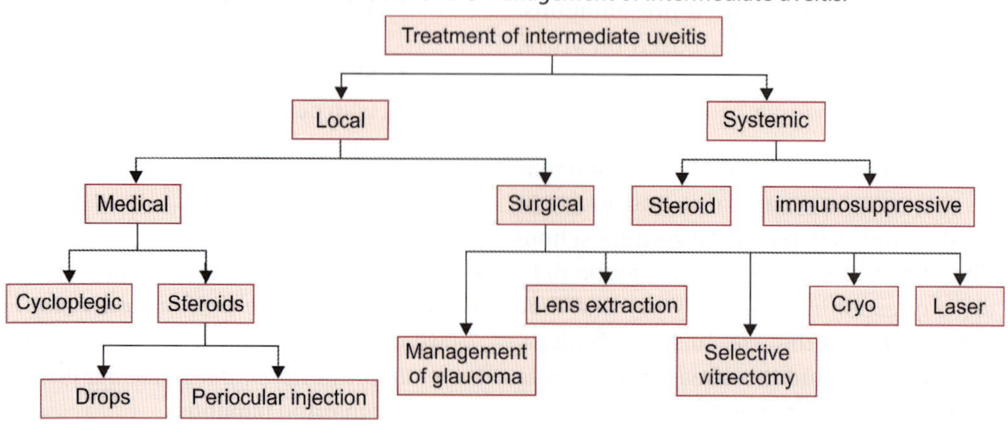

Steroid:

Steroids can be given in three forms, i.e.:

1. Local drops and ointment
2. *Periocular injection:*
   - Clear solution
   - Depot
3. Systemic

> *Steroids should be used.*
> Soon enough, strong enough, frequent enough, long enough, and sufficient enough.

Local steroid drops: Initially, strong steroid drops like dexamethasone or betamethasone are preferred; once vision has improved and progress arrested, weaker drugs like loteprednol, fluorometholone, and methylpre-dnisolone should replace them. All steroids should be tapered as per the personal preference of the treating ophthalmologist.

Systemic steroid: They are rarely required.

Periocular injection: Any injectable steroid can be used, but long-acting depots like triamcinolone acetonide and methylprednisolone are preferred. The route of choice of periocular injection is the anterior sub-Tenon's.

Immunosuppressive drugs: Commonly used immuno-suppressants used are methotrexate, azathioprine, cyclosporine (cyclosporine is also available as drops), and mycophenolate mofetil.

Other methods used are:

- Cryotherapy in neovascularization
- Lasers are used for neovascularization and vasculitis.

Surgery: The disease itself is not amenable to surgery. Surgery is directed toward changes in the vitreous, cataracts, and glaucoma.

The vitreous changes that require surgical interventions are—nonresolving vitreous hemorrhage and large vitreous opacities. The retinal detachment may require detachment surgery.

Corticosteroids are the first choice of treatment; this is followed by cryotherapy and vitrectomy. Immunosuppressants are considered to be last resort in cases where steroids are contraindicated or not effective in the standard dose schedule. The protocol used differs from widely used Kaplan four-step protocols. The Kaplan protocol consists of the use of topical and periocular injections as the first step; if this fails, systemic steroids are added; in the third step, immunosuppressants are used either alone or along with steroids. This is followed by a therapeutic vitrectomy. Before planning a vitrectomy, steroids and immunosuppressants should be given a chance.

SYMPATHETIC OPHTHALMIA

The incidence of this bilateral vision-depriving disease has become rarer over the last three decades. In the past, it was thought to be inevitable in 0.1% of all penetrating injuries to the eyes. The incidence has fallen greatly with better understanding of the disease and better management. It is less common in developed countries; in developing countries, it is more prevalent in rural populations than in urban populations. No race is immune; dark persons seemed to be more predisposed. Both sexes are likely to be affected equally; however, it is more common in boys, not due to any immunity to girls but due to the simple fact that boys are more exposed to ocular trauma, which is seen in all ages but present in more severe from in young male adults.

The clinical picture is typical: there is a history of penetrating injury in one eye within 5 mm of the limbus. The injury is mostly accidental, but it can be surgical as well. The common surgical procedures that cause sympathetic ophthalmia are: 0.01% of vitrectomies may end up in sympathetic ophthalmia; all intra-ocular surgeries can cause sympathetic ophthalmia. Iris inclusion surgeries were the worst offenders, followed by lens extraction, needling, and phacoemulsification. Following injury, there is a week to a fortnight of window period when there are no signs of inflammation in either eye, barring those that cannot be correlated to the injury.

The injured eye is traditionally called the exciting eye, and the other eye that develops ophthalmitis is called sympathizing eye.

> All patients with unilateral penetrating injury do not develop sympathetic ophthalmia in the contralateral eye.

All children with ocular injuries will not develop sympathetic ophthalmia, only those children who are specifically predisposed will develop sympathetic ophthalmia. The absence of intraocular lymphatics seemed to play an important role.

Eyes with prolapsed uvea are more prone to developing sympathetic uveitis. The disorder is basically a bilateral chronic granulomatous panuveitis with acute exacerbation and remission that generally starts in the anterior uvea of exciting eye, spreading to the posterior uvea. It may include the optic nerve. The reverse is also possible, i.e., the lesion starting as choroiditis and creeping to the anterior uvea.

The lesion in the sympathetic eye is the same as in the excited eye. The better eye gets involved after some times, the time lapse between the trauma and the development of uveitis can be as short as a few weeks or may be as delayed as five to six decades.

The first symptom of sympathetic ophthalmitis is photophobia, followed by watering and redness. Difficulty in reading at pre-presbyopic age is a common feature due to a loss of accommodation. The distant vision initially is not reduced much. The signs are similar to those seen in acute granulomatous anterior uveitis, which spreads to the involved posterior uvea. If not treated at this stage, the eye goes into a stage of complications and blindness.

The first sign of sympathetic ophthalmia is cells in retrolenticular space, even before the eye develops circumciliary congestion; the anterior chamber shows 2+ to 3+ cells, hypopyon is rare.

> It is a paradox that the originally injured eye may recover from the onslaught and have better vision than the sympathizing eye.

The cornea is studded with KPs of various sizes, ranging from fine dusty to large mutton-fat KPs.

The iris is generally thickened. In fact, the whole of the uvea is thickened, with the choroid being the most edematous. The pupil is miotic, immobile, and irregular with multiple broad posterior synechiae; the iris may develop both Koeppe's and Busacca nodules. The posterior segment involvements, besides thickened choroid, are posterior vitritis, vitreous cells, macular edema, and papillitis.

Surprisingly, the retinal and choriocapillaris are not affected. The choroid develops deep yellow nodules called Dalen Fuchs nodules; they are conglomerates of lymphocytes and epithelioid cells, accompanied with retinal pigment epithelium. Fluorescein angiography may show a few hyperfluorescent spots. However, occasionally, there may be hypofluorescence. The eyes are generally soft and may, in the long run, pass into secondary glaucoma. The common complications are complicated cataracts, secondary glaucoma, band keratopathy, retinal detachment, phthisis, and bilateral blindness.

The etiopathogenesis is not well understood. The recent theory is that it is an autoimmune disorder due to exposure to previously immune-privileged ocular antigens from trauma, with a subsequent bilateral autoimmune response to uveal pigment.

Diagnosis

The diagnosis is simple, with a positive history of penetrating injury in a male under 30 years of age. The history of injury should be elicited with the utmost care in all young males with bilateral asymmetric chronic uveitis. The other conditions that have a similar presentation are—lens-induced uveitis, Vogt–Koyanagi–Harada syndrome, and Harada syndrome.

Management

- Management of an injured eye with salvageable vision. All eyes with penetrating injuries, especially within 5.00 mm of the limbus and uveal prolapse, should be meticulously repaired, followed by a subconjunctival injection of a water-soluble steroid, and the eye bandaged with atropine. The bandage is removed after 24 hours, and the patient is put on atropine drops 2 times of day and a strong steroid every hour. Steroid drops are tapered following any intraocular surgery. The other eye is kept under surveillance for evidence of uveitis for the next few months to years for uveitis. Slight evidence of uveitis should be treated with mild cycloplegics and steroids. Treatment started at this stage mitigates the possibility of severe complications.

> The first symptom of involvement of the other eye is photophobia, and the sign is retrolental cells.

- Management of eye without salvageable vision. There is no option but to sacrifice the eye by enucleation.

> Evisceration is contraindicated.

Enucleation should be undertaken within a fortnight of injury. Removal of the eye thereafter does not have any therapeutic benefit because the other eye is already sensitized to liberated antigen from the injured eye, which may be uveal pigment.

Enucleation after the other eye has developed sympathetic ophthalmia too does not have any beneficial role. In such an eventuality, both eyes should be treated vigorously with atropine and local and systemic steroids for many months or years.

If systemic steroids fail to give the expected result or are contraindicated, an appropriate immunosuppressant may be required. Initially, immunosuppressants should run concurrently with steroid, and steroid gradually tapered.

Vogt–Koyanagi–Harada Disease

This multisystemic disease is rare under 10 years of age; it shares the same pathology as that of sympathetic ophthalmia, i.e., an autoimmune, T cell-mediated disease, both of which cause chronic granulomatous uveitis. The main difference is the absence of ocular injury in Vogt–Koyanagi–Harada syndrome and prominent extra-ocular features.

The extraocular lesions are:

- *Skin:* Vitiligo, poliosis, and alopecia
- *Auditory:* Hyperacusis, tinnitus, and hypoacusis that may end in deafness.
- *Vestibular:* Vertigo
- *CNS:* Multiple cranial nerve palsy, sterile meningitis, and encephalitis
- Though there is no ocular injury as in sympathetic ophthalmia, there may be a history of skin injury that is presumed to liberate antigen in melanocytes; it is associated with HLA-DR-4.

It is generally seen in the third decade, may be seen in persons in late teens, is more common in females, and dark-colored persons are more prone to developing the malady.

The disease has the following stages:

- *Prodromal:* Consisting of mild symptoms of headache, brow ache, neck stiffness, and vertigo
- *Systemic involvement:*
  - Cutaneous
  - Neurologically, in addition to the lesions described above, they may consist of encephalopathy, myopathy, and changes in the CSF.
  - Auditory self-limited tinnitus and vertigo
- *Ocular involvement:*
  - *Anterior segment changes consist of:*
    - Symptoms of photophobia include lacrimation, redness, dull ocular pain, diminished near and distant vision.
    - Signs of granulomatous anterior uveitis
    - Signs of posterior uveitis—multiple exudative patches of choroiditis, self-limiting exudative retinal detachment papillitis, macular edema, and choroidal thickening, which are visible on ultrasonography

Fundus fluorescein angiography: Fundus fluorescein angiography shows delayed choroidal filling, multiple small areas of leak, large areas of hyperfluorescence, pooling of stain in subretinal fluid, and optic nerve staining.

Optical coherence tomography—shows thickening of the choroid and macula.

Treatment

Treatment is basically medical; before the ocular signs develop, the patients are generally seen and managed by an internist and an ENT (ear–nose–throat) specialist. Once the ocular signs develop, the treatment is similar to sympathetic ophthalmia, i.e., local prolonged cycloplegia, initially with atropine followed by short-acting cycloplegia, intense steroid drops, or periocular injections. Most of the cases require immunosuppressants along with systemic steroids.

Lens-induced Uveitis

So long as the lens is inside an intact capsule, it does neither produce an antigen nor a chemical reaction. Once the lens matter comes out of the sanctuary of capsule, it produces an antigen antibody reaction.

The various modes by which the lens proteins come out are:

- A penetrating injury that may be accidental or surgical.
- Lens protein is leaking from an intact capsule. There are two situations where this can happen, i.e., a blunt injury producing a cataract that goes to the stage of hypermaturity and liquefaction. The liquid protein passes through the capsule, mixing with the aqueous.

The resulting reaction is types 2 hypersensitivity:

Blunt injury to lens → traumatic cataract → mature cataract → hypermaturity → liquefaction of cortex → leak of cortical matter → antigen antibody reaction → panuveitis.

The second type of reaction is endophthalmitis phacoanaphylactic.

The process is similar to pathogenesis of sympathetic ophthalmia, i.e., injury → panuveitis in injured eye → subsidence of uveitis in injured eye → latent period → panuveitis in the other eye.

Management

It consists of the complete removal of lens matter in the first eye before the other eye develops uveitis. Treat both the eyes with strong cycloplegics and steroids for long-term and usual management of aphakia in children.

BEHÇET'S SYNDROME

This is a rare, multisystemic disorder seen mostly in far eastern countries in adults. However, older children too are known to be affected. The exact cause in not well known. The patients may be HLA-B51 positive. The two prominent systemic features are genital and oral; besides them, the patient may have joint involvement, meningitis, and encephalitis.

The common ocular involvement is anterior uveitis with prominent hypopyon. Posterior segment involvements are macular edema, retinal vasculitis, exudates, and hemorrhage in the retina.

Treatment

Systemic and mucocutaneous lesions are treated by internists and involve the administration of oral steroids in high doses or immune suppressants. Incidentally, systemic management alleviates the ocular conditions as well.

The local treatment consists of prolonged cycloplegia and local steroids.

SARCOID UVEITIS IN CHILDREN

Sarcoid is a chromic, multisystemic T-cell-mediated disease that can involve all organs, including the eyes. It is commonly seen in adults. The incidence increases with age. However, it has been noticed in children with confirmed histopathology reports. It is more common in colored races. Dark girls are more likely to be affected than white boys.

In the eyes, it produces panuveitis, which can be both granulomatous and nongranulomatous. It may start as an acute episode with an exacerbation of a chronic lesion. It is generally bilateral but not symmetric. Isolated ocular lesions are unknown. Besides the uvea, other parts of the eye and its adnexa are frequently involved, including swelling of the parotid and lacrimal glands, nodules on the lid skin, and nodules in the lower fornix. The lid and conjunctival nodules are most suitable for histopathological examination. Histopathology of such specimens shows a noncaseating granuloma, no organism has been detected in the granuloma. Another histopathological finding is vasculitis.

The uveal lesions are—fine to large KPs; posterior synechiae; nodules on the iris that may be small enough to be seen only on high power; and large nodules visible on ordinary oblique illumination. The large KPs may clog the angle.

The posterior segment involvements are—vitreous cells and flares; dense vitreous strands; or white mass on the pars plana. There may be a white material round the retinal arteries called candle wax drip.

Diagnosis

Diagnosis is difficult. It is by exclusion that the eye should by routinely examined in all persons presumed to be suffering from sarcoidosis.

The common diagnostic systemic investigations are:

- Raised serum calcium
- Reversal of the serum albumin–globulin ratio
- Generalized lymphadenopathy
- X-rays of the chest show a hilar lesion.
- X-rays of terminal phalanges show changes.

Management

The treatment is mainly directed at systemic lesions. The ocular treatment is as for usual uveitis, i.e., cycloplegics, frequent steroid initially followed by low-loss steroid for months to years, keeping IOP low by β-blockers.

FUCHS' HETEROCHROMIC IRITIS

Previously, Fuchs' heterochromic iritis was thought to be a disorder confined to adults that accounted for 2% of all cases of adult uveitis. Now it is known that it does occur in children as young as 5 years old. The cause of nondetection in children lies in the fact that it is unilateral in 90% of cases, producing hardly any symptom. The condition in children is picked up in routine school checkups where the two eyes show a difference in color.

> The brown eye looks less brown, and the blue eye becomes more blue.

If the child presents with heterochromia and diminished vision, the most frequent cause of diminished vision is posterior subcapsular opacity secondary to uveitis. The eyes do not develop band keratopathy, in spite of its long duration.

The KPs are small stellate dots sprinkled all over the endothelium with thin iris stroma.

> Posterior synechiae are absent.

The vitreous may show cells, debris, and strands. There is no unanimity regarding the cause of the disease.

Abiotrophy, inflammation, and trauma have been blamed from time to time without conclusive evidence.

The cases are treated with a weak solution of steroids; cycloplegics are not required.

ENDOPHTHALMITIS

Endophthalmitis is one of the potential causes of permanent loss of vision in all ages, with far-reaching socioeconomic implications.

Endophthalmitis is defined as panuveitis with superadded vitritis; obviously, the retina is not spared. This, in short, is inflammation of all intraocular contents except the lens. It is also known as suppurative panuveitis.

Broadly, it is divided into two categories on the basis of etiology, i.e., infectious and noninfectious. The former is more common. In the case of infective endophthalmitis, the infection reaches the eye either from outside the coats of the eye or through hematological spread from a distant origin. The former is called exogenous endophthalmitis, and the latter is endogenous endophthalmitis. Numerically, endogenous endophthalmitis is less common. The organisms responsible for endophthalmitis are mostly bacteria, followed by fungi, and least by parasites, i.e., toxocara; some authors disagree regarding parasites as causative factors. Both gram-positive and gram-negative organisms are responsible for endophthalmitis. Gram-negative bacilli are more virulent and carry a poor prognosis. Viruses are not known to cause endophthalmitis. The course of disease depends on virulence, size of inoculums, local and systemic immunity, and preventive measures taken. The severity, besides the above factors, depends on the duration of onset; the shorter the duration, the greater the severity.

According to severity, endophthalmitis can be hyperacute, acute, chronic, delayed, or relapsed.

Exogenous Endophthalmitis

It is the most common form of endophthalmitis encountered in clinical practice. It follows a full-thickness perforating wound that carries an infective organism with it. The trauma can be accidental or deliberate (surgical); the latter is called postoperative endophthalmitis. Other causes of exogenous endophthalmitis are perforating corneal ulcers, corneal fistula epithelial downgrowth, infected filtering blebs, scleromalacia, and perforated corneal staphyloma. The accidental wound may be the route of entry for a retained, infected foreign body.

Postoperative Endophthalmitis

Postoperative endophthalmitis is the most unwelcome episode in clinical practice. With a better understanding of the prevention of intraoperative infection, its rate of occurrence has come down drastically. The common surgeries that are associated with postoperative endophthalmitis are—lens extraction of any type with or without an intraocular implant; and all surgeries where there is communication between the intraocular content and the ambient atmosphere. Such surgeries are prone to postoperative endophthalmitis. To this list may be added various irrigating fluids and viscoelastics.

The other invasive procedures known to cause postoperative endophthalmitis can range from as minor as stitch removal and paracentesis to as major as fishing out a dropped nucleus. The others in the long list are—needling, capsulotomy, postoperative manipulation of the IOL, IOL exchange, iridotomy, iris inclusion surgeries, penetrating keratoplasty, vitrectomy, accidental perforation of the globe during squint and retinal surgery, and yttrium aluminum garnet (YAG) laser capsulotomy. It is a paradox that vitrectomy, which requires a longer time to perform with a larger quantity of fluid to circulate inside the globe, has a lesser frequency than other intraocular surgeries. The hypothesis put forward is that a large volume of fluid helps a larger amount of organisms be flushed out before they colonize and multiply.

As per severity, postoperative endophthalmitis can be hyperacute, acute, chronic, or delayed. A fulminating endophthalmitis developing following uneventful cataract surgery within 4 hours is called hyperacute; the chances of it going downhill are higher.

Endophthalmitis developing after 48 hours and before 4 days is designated as acute. Infection developing after 4 days is called chronic. Bleb-related endophthalmitis is put in the category of delayed endophthalmitis.

Hyperacute postoperative endophthalmitis is caused by most virulent organisms, like *Pseudomonas aeruginosa*, many *Bacillus* species, gram-positive coagulase negative staphylococci, *Staphylococcus* epidermidis, and aureus.

Low-virulence organisms like *Propionibacterium acnes* and fungi cause chronic endophthalmitis.

Toxic Anterior Segment Syndrome

Toxic anterior segment syndrome (TASS) is a hyperacute, noninfective postoperative endophthalmitis where sterile microparticles gain access to the anterior segment, causing toxic damage to the intraocular tissue. The other possible causes of the unfortunate malady are—bacterial endotoxin, abnormally incompatible pH and osmolarity of the irrigating solution, drugs added to the viscoelastic and irrigating solutions, denaturing of the viscoelastic, and lastly, inadequate sepsis.

The condition develops within 12–24 hours post-operatively with prominent corneal signs of severe corneal edema all over and a moderate to intense anterior chamber reaction, i.e., flare, cells, fibrin, and hypopyon, which is generally small. The pupil may be semi-dilated and fixed, independent of preoperative cycloplegia. There is unexpectedly low vision. In spite of the classical features of TASS described above, all such cases should be thought to be due to acute microbial endophthalmitis unless proved otherwise.

The best diagnostic test is the examination of aqueous for an organism that is confirmed by culture and PCR. The best management is cycloplegia, subconjunctival injection of vancomycin/amikacin, frequent instillation of steroids, and constant monitoring. Relative afferent pupillary defect (RAPD) and inaccurate projections are red flags.

Clinical Features of Postoperative Endophthalmitis

The symptoms depend on severity and onset; the shorter the onset, the more severe the infection. Hyperacute endophthalmitis becomes obvious within 24 hours. The symptoms consist of a disproportionate fall in expected vision, edema of the lids, chemosis of the conjunctiva, watery to thick conjunctival discharge, hazy cornea, intense anterior chamber reaction, even hypopyon, exudative membrane over the IOL/lens, retrolenticular, and retro-IOL cells. Cells in the anterior vitreous: in severe cases, an anterior vitreous abscess may obscure the fundus glow.

Chronic and Delayed Postoperative Endophthalmitis

The pathology involved is similar to that seen in acute postoperative endophthalmitis; the only difference is the duration of onset and the nature of the organism. The common organism remains *Staphylococcus* epidermidis and coagulase-negative cocci of low virulence. Streptococci are more frequent causative organisms in children, in contrast to staphylococci, which are more common in adults. *Propionibacterium acnes*, an anaerobic gram-positive commensal, is being reported more frequently than before.

An uneventful phacoemulsification with or without IOL should be almost symptomless without congestion, watering, or pain after 4–5 days under usual steroid and cycloplegia. If the child has persistent pain, photophobia, lacrimation, redness, and vision less than expected, chronic postoperative endophthalmitis should be the first condition to be excluded.

On examination, the eye has prominent circumcorneal congestion and visible dilated episcleral vessels; the cornea may show some edema with large KPs, +2 to +3 flare and cells; a few fibrinous strands; and the pupil is not dilating well with usual cycloplegic. Exudate in the pupillary area or on the IOL, retro-IOL space, and anterior face of the vitreous. Retinoscopy glow is absent or faint. A white plaque on the posterior capsule is a red flag.

Such eyes should be examined with a slit lamp, a direct and indirect ophthalmoscope, a gonioscope for small hypopyons, and a B scan if the media is hazy.

An uncomfortable child with unexpected reduced vision is an ominous sign. Loss of fundal glow and flare-up of inflammation under steroid point toward chronic postoperative endophthalmitis in an otherwise uneventful surgery. There may be an abscess formation in the vitreous. The extent of which can be best seen on a B-scan, the periphery of the fundus, can be best assessed by an indirect ophthalmoscope. The fundus, when visible, shows retinal vasculitis, hemorrhage, and exudate.

Post-traumatic Endophthalmitis

If postoperative endophthalmitis is excluded, accidental injuries are the most frequent cause of exogenous endophthalmitis. Blunt injuries do not cause endophthalmitis. To produce post-traumatic endophthalmitis, a penetrating wound is essential. If it is hidden, it should be searched. A soft, disorganized eye is a sure sign of a penetrating injury. About 5% of eyes sustaining penetrating injuries with or without retained foreign bodies are likely to develop post-traumatic endophthalmitis. Post-traumatic endophthalmitis is more common in boys and rural populations. The pathogenesis of post-traumatic endophthalmitis is similar to that of postoperative endophthalmitis. It is associated with a visible injury to the cornea, corneoscleral, or sclera, all of which can be with or without uvea incarcerated in the wound. It is not rare to find a foreign body entangled in the wound.

Like postoperative endophthalmitis, post-traumatic endophthalmitis can be hyperacute, acute, or chronic. The presentation depends on the virulence of the organism, the size of the inoculums, the immune status of the child, and the immune status of the eye. Generally, accidental wounds are contaminated by multiple organisms. Viruses are not known to produce endophthalmitis; fungi produce late and delayed post-traumatic endophthalmitis. *Bacillus cereus* is the most virulent organism responsible for post-traumatic endophthalmitis. Most of the time, post-traumatic endophthalmitis is uniocular.

The diagnosis of post-traumatic endophthalmitis is straightforward with a positive history of trauma. The presentation is similar to postsurgical endophthalmitis; the common differences are a disorganized soft globe with a visible site of trauma and occasional incarceration of intraocular structures.

Diminished vision RAPD, absence of vision, restricted movements, and proptosis are bad signs that point toward impending pan-ophthalmitis in all exogenous endophthalmitis.

Investigation: All eyes with trauma should undergo X-rays orbit both the AP and lateral views. B-scan USG is useful to find out the position of the lens, the extent of vitreous involvement, the intraocular foreign body, and retinal detachment.

Management: The management of all exogenous endophthalmitis is identical, may it be postoperative or traumatic. The most crucial being time lapse between surgery/trauma and the onset of endophthalmitis. In all cases, an X-ray and, if possible, B-scan imaging should be done to exclude intraocular foreign bodies. If pus is found to trickle through the wound, it should be subjected to staining, culture, and sensitivity tests. Until the results are available, the wound is washed with a fortified antibiotic solution that looks after gram-negative and gram-positive cocci and bacilli. The same antibiotic is given as a subconjunctival injection. This should be followed by the repair of the wound and the release of the intraocular tissue from the wound. Abscission of prolapsed iris is better than an attempt to reposit it. Cutting the choroid and ciliary body is fraught with severe bleeding unless rows of diathermy burns can be put round the wound. It is common practice to give amikacin 400 μg in 0.1 mL or vancomycin 1 mg in 0.1 mL intravitreal. The rest of the treatment is similar to the management of postoperative endophthalmitis, including vitrectomy.

Bleb-related Endophthalmitis

Endophthalmitis secondary to infection of the filtering bleb following trabeculectomy is less common than endophthalmitis, which used to happen when iris inclusion and corneoscleral (Eliot) trephining were in fashion. The pathology common to all types of bleb-related endophthalmitis is the entry of pathological organisms into the vitreous.

The natural history as follows:

Postoperative conjunctivitis → Blebitis → Infection reaching under sclerotomy → Infection passing to the sclerectomy → Vitritis → Endophthalmitis

It can happen within a few days due to an intraoperative infection, or it may be delayed for months or years. The term blebitis is generally used to denote an indolent infection of tissues between the conjunctiva and superficial scleral flap by low-virulence bacteria. The most common cause of bleb in any eye is trabeculectomy, but it may happen inadvertently after a limbal incision in classical lens extraction of bygone days or in small incision cataract extraction, and rarely following an accidental penetrating wound at the limbus.

Predisposing factors in bleb-related endophthalmitis are:

- Chronic conjunctivitis
- Blepharitis
- Dacryocystitis
- Blebitis
- Juvenile glaucoma (the exact cause of this predisposition is not known)
- Thin bleb
- Leaking bleb
- Bleb at a place other than the superior limbus
- Use of antimetabolites
- Use of a contact lens in an eye that has undergone filtering surgery too soon

Clinical features:

- *Symptoms:*
    - Redness is localized or generalized
    - Dull to severe ache
    - Visible, swollen bleb
    - Reduced vision
    - Fluctuating vision
    - Symptoms of full-blown postoperative endophthalmitis

- *Sings:*
  - *Acute:*
    - Variable vision
    - Conjunctivitis
    - Swollen bleb
    - Visible exudate in the thin bleb
    - Exudate round the iridectomy
    - Micro-hypopyon
  - *Chronic:*
    - Localized conjunctival congestion round the bleb
    - May have a positive Seidel sign
    - Reduced corneal curvature
    - Shallow AC
    - Micro-to-frank hypopyon
    - Cell in retrolental space
    - Localized anterior vitreous abscess
    - Soft eye

Treatment of Postsurgical Endophthalmitis

In postsurgery endophthalmitis, local antibiotics have a doubtful role, yet they are used as standbys before subconjunctival or intravitreal injections are ready. They are instilled as frequently as every 5 minutes for the first hour. In blebitis, local, fortified, broad-spectrum antibiotic drops have given encouraging results.

The common fortified antibiotic drops used are:

- Gentamicin (40 mg of injectable drug added to 5 mL of eye drop)
- Vancomycin (25–50 mg/mL)
- Tobramycin (14 mg/mL)
- Cefazolin (50 mg/mL)

The above drops can be used separately or in combination:

- The initial regimen of instillation of drops varies from institute to institute; the commonly used regimen is to put one drop every 5 minutes six times, followed by one drop every 30 minutes for the next 20 hours.
- Subconjunctival injections are given twice a day.
- Usual cycloplegics and steroids drop locally
- In frank endophthalmitis, intravitreal antibiotics are mandatory.
- If intravitreal injection of antibiotics fails, vitrectomy is inevitable.

Endogenous Uveitis (Metastatic Uveitis)

This condition is less common than post-traumatic and postoperative endophthalmitis. Its early diagnosis is imperative for children. It is potentially blinding. In one-fourth of cases, it is bilateral. The ocular condition is invariably overshadowed by more obvious systemic infections. It is equally seen among boys and girls. Its incidence is higher in underdeveloped countries. It is indolent to begin with. The predisposing factors are malnutrition and chronic systemic infections of one or many organs. Immune-compromised children are more at risk. The immune-compromised conditions that have been found to be associated with metastatic endophthalmitis are—children on immunosuppressive drugs used in organ transplants; various types of leukemias and lymphomas. Other causes are congenital and acquired HIV infections. They are more common with prolonged and extensive abdominal surgery and subacute bacterial endocarditis. They are caused by myriads of organisms, common among which are fungi, followed by bacteria and parasites (rare). The most common fungus is candida, and common bacteria are streptococci, staphylococci, pneumococci, and *Pseudomonas*.

As the conditions are hematogenous metastasis, it is more likely to involve the choroid than the anterior uvea. The lesion soon spreads to the retina and vitreous to form a vitreous abscess. The anterior verity directly infects the anterior vitreous. Once the vitreous abscess is formed, the infection soon spreads all over to mimic a picture akin to postoperative endophthalmitis. If not managed at this stage, it may pass into stage of panophthalmitis.

Clinical Picture

- The clinical picture is invariably overshadowed by a more serious systemic condition. The patient is referred to an ophthalmologist as a child with redness of the eyes. On examination, it turns out to be metastatic endophthalmitis.
- It may present as uveitis with or without hypopyon.
- It may present as a white reflex in the pupillary area.
- There may be an absence of retinal glow.

Investigation

The eye should be examined with a slit lamp; a plus ninety lens will outline the posterior vitreous abscess and may circumviate small mid-vitreous abscess to expose the retina and optic nerve. B-scan ultrasonography shows the position of the lesion in relation to the equator.

Management

Management is similar to endogenous uveitis, i.e., strong cycloplegic, periocular, and frequent local steroid management of raised intraocular tension. Systemic antibiotics have a doubtful role in endogenous endophthalmitis. Intravenous broad-spectrum antibiotics have a definite role to play. The overall prognosis is grave. The condition may benefit from vitrectomy and intravitreal antibiotic injections.

Panophthalmitis (Purulent Uveitis)

The condition is the severest form of all uveitis; it is the end result of untreated endophthalmitis, which is a blinding disease. All the efforts to salvage vision are futile. It is caused by virulent pus-forming bacteria; pneumococci are the most common organism, followed by staphylococci, streptococci, *Bacillus cereus*, *Pseudomonas*, and *Escherichia coli*. Fungus endophthalmitis does not end up in panophthalmitis unless a pus-producing organism has been introduced into an already infected eye inadvertently by way of intravitreal injection. Viruses do not cause panophthalmitis. It is seen in all ages. In children, the most common cause is a penetrating injury with or without a retained intraocular foreign body, followed by a perforated corneal ulcer. Intraocular surgeries have their own share. The conditions start as endophthalmitis, which, if not controlled, spreads to all the intraocular structures with blood supply. The lens is not involved but may extrude through the perforation **(Fig. 17.6)**.

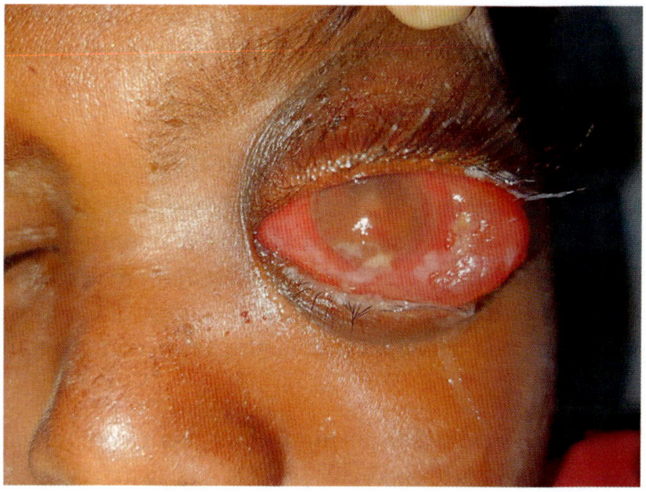

Fig. 17.6: Panophthalmitis in a child following a penetrating injury.
Courtesy: Professor Nidhi Pandey.

The vitreous is converted into a veritable bag of pus. The inflammatory cells and organisms permeate through the sclera, not affecting it much. All the peribulbar structures, i.e., Tenon's capsule, episcleral, extraocular muscles, nerves, and blood vessels, get inflamed in severe infection, and a peribulbar abscess may form, causing exophthalmos and loss of motility. The conjunctiva is congested, and the cornea, if not perforated already, becomes hazy, followed by the formation of a sloughing ulcer, which eventually perforates, causing extrusion of the lens, part of the uvea, and pus.

Clinical Picture

The clinical picture depends on severity and duration. In children, it is preceded by fever, headache, vomiting, and, over and above the features of systemic disease that the child already has, a penetrating wound from organic matter is more likely to present within 2–3 days. Postoperative endophthalmitis may take weeks to months to pass on to panophthalmitis. The initial presentation is akin to severe endophthalmitis. In cases of fully developed panophthalmitis, the child is ill and irritable, with pain radiating from the distribution of the fifth nerve.

The lids are swollen. The eye is moderately proptosed, the conjunctiva is congested and chemosed, the cornea is generally hazy, and a sloughing ulcer may perforate. As the ulcer perforates part of the uvea prolapse, the eyeball loses its normal tension and structure following perforation. There is doubtful perception or no perception of light when light is present, and the eye has RAPD. Loss of movement of the globe is a red flag.

> In a case of endophthalmitis (RAPD), losses of vision and absences or movements are some signs of impending panophthalmitis.

Management

Once panophthalmitis has set in, vision becomes unsalvageable. Any amount of antibiotics, local or systemic, and steroids are of no use. The only treatment left is to eviscerate the eye to relieve pain and improve appearance. In children, evisceration should be done under general anesthesia. It is better to put an acryl sphere in the scleral shell following evisceration to facilitate the fitting of an artificial eye later. If an eye with panophthalmitis is not eviscerated, in the long run, it gets auto-eviscerated and passes into phthisis.

All the eviscerated material should be subjected to histopathological examination to exclude the possibility of the eye harboring retinoblastoma.

Fungal Endophthalmitis in Children

Many fungi are known to produce endophthalmitis; out of about fifteen fungi reported to cause endophthalmitis, the following three are common—*Candida, Aspergillus,* and *Histoplasma*. Out of the three, *Candida* is the most common, and *Histoplasma* is the least common in children.

There are some predisposing factors that cause fungal endophthalmitis in children:

- Prematurity
- Prolonged stay in the neonatal nursery
- Undetected type 1 diabetes
- Septicemia
- Prolonged systemic antibiotics
- Immunosuppression
- Postorgan transplant status
- Indwelling catheter
- Penetrating injury (surgeonal/accidental)
- Juvenile drug addiction

Candia Endophthalmitis

Candida albicans, a yeast, is a commensal on the skin, oral mucosa, and vagina.

It causes endophthalmitis in two ways:

1. Exogenous by way of a surgical or accidental wound
2. Endogenous

Fungal endophthalmitis has more signs than symptoms.

The symptoms are less pronounced than those of other known fungal endophthalmitis, depending on the initial location of the lesion, i.e., anterior/posterior. The anterior involvement is more common in exogenous endophthalmitis due to the anteriorly placed point of entry. Lesions in the posterior segment start more frequently in endogenous endophthalmitis. There may be diminished vision if the macula is involved. The other symptom is floaters.

Frequent signs are iridocyclitis with thick yellowish, slow-moving hypopyon. In exogenous endophthalmitis, the unexpected rise of intraocular tension is a frequent cause of pain.

Other signs are: In the early stage, the vitreous may be hazy without exudate, as time passes, the vitreous develops fluffy exudate near the point of entry of the organism, with string-like opacities. Gradually, the whole of the vitreous gets involved, invading the uvea, retina, and optic nerve. Endogenous endophthalmitis is generally bilateral.

Diagnosis is by exclusion. The features that help in diagnosis are—positive predisposing factors; history of penetrating injury by organic matter; thick yellowish hypopyon; and fluffy or string-like exudates in vitreous.

The investigations to confirm are:

- Anterior chamber and vitreous tap for smear and culture; the stains used are Grocott methenamine silver and PAS
- Vitreous biopsy
- Culture of aspirated matter for fungus
- Polymerase chain reaction (PCR) detects the fungal genome and is faster than culture, which may take days to weeks. The medium used for the culture of fungus is Sabouraud medium.

Treatment

The definitive treatment is pars plana vitrectomy with intravitreal antifungal drugs.

- Commonly used intravitreal antifungal drugs are—amphotericin B 5–10 μg/0.1 mL; and voriconazole 50 μg/0.1 mL.
- Local antifungal drugs have no role.
- Oral antifungal drugs may be given as supplements with intravenous antifungal drugs.
- Oral antifungal drugs have no role.

TOXOCARIASIS

Toxocara infection is the most common zoonotic ocular disease due to nematodes in children all over the world. It is seen in two forms, i.e., systemic and ocular; in fact, ocular infection is a late extension of systemic infection. The average age of systemic involvement is 3 years. It can be seen in children between 18 months and 3 years.

It is caused by *ascaris toxocara canis*, which is a round worm (*Ascaris*) in dogs of all ages but is more frequent in puppies.

The puppies get infected in two ways:

1. Ingestion of ova, which is more common.
2. Transplacental from an infected gravid bitch reaching the gut of the puppy. Once in the gut, the ova are transformed into larva.

Dogs are the definitive host; humans are not natural hosts; they may be considered accidental hosts. The worm develops into third-stage larvae in humans but does not lay eggs. This is the cause of the absence of ova in the human stool. The life cycle of the worm is different in humans and dogs.

- The canine cycle of a gravid bitch differs from the life cycle of male dogs and nonpregnant bitches. The pregnant bitches already harbor the parasite in the form of encysted larvae. The encysted larvae migrate into the developing embryo through placental circulation. In this way, the puppy, when born, is already infected by third-stage larva; this may be considered to be a congenital transmission of zoonotic disease in puppies.
- In adult dogs and nongravid bitches, the ova develop in third-stage larvae in the intestine. The infection reaches the dog's stomach in two ways: direct ingestion of food contaminated by ova and ingestion of larvae in half-cooked meat.
- The third-stage larvae are released into the gastrointestinal tract, penetrate the wall of the gut, and reach systemic circulation. After some months, the third-stage larvae get encysted and lie dormant.
- In humans, the life cycle is similar to that of an adult dog.
- Once the organism reaches the systemic circulation, it spreads to distant organs like the brain, eyes, liver, lung, and subcutaneous tissue. The encysted organism in these organs forms a granuloma, which is the main presenting feature of the disease.
- Less common way of circulation of the organism is:

  Lungs → Trachea → Esophagus → Gastrointestinal tract
- The eggs can survive in the soil for years without hatching.

> - The eggs hatch only in the intestines of either humans or dogs.
> - The larvae do not grow to become mature worms.
> - As they do not return to the gut, they are not excreted in human feces.

Systemic Involvement

Systemic involvement of toxocara infection can be divided into two categories: the first is visceral larval migrans and the other is distant spread, including eyes. Organs other than the eyes that are involved are the lungs, liver, brain, and muscles. Some authors do not agree with this classification and divide toxocariasis into two groups, i.e., intestinal and extraintestinal. They put visceral larval migrans, ocular toxocariasis, and involvement of other organs in the second group.

Visceral Larval Migrans

This is seen in children under 3 years of age. It is not accompanied by ocular involvement, which is sometimes referred to as ophthalmic larval migrans. Visceral larval migrans is a mild, self-limiting disease that presents as malaise followed by fever. The child may be irritable, with cough, pneumonia, hepatosplenomegaly, cutaneous lesion, leukocytosis, and eosinophilia. Positive ELISA test in titer of 1:32. The stool is free of ova, larvae, or cysts.

Ocular Toxocariasis

It is a uniocular condition, most of the time asymptomatic. The child does not complain, and the parents are unaware of the condition unless the child presents with squints and rarely nystagmus or a white reflex in the pupillary area. The white reflex may unnerve the parents, as they think that the child has a cataract. Less common is the discovery of a posterior polar lesion on ophthalmoscopy ordered for some unrelated condition. Still less common is an eye with signs of chronic endophthalmitis. Eyes without uveitis are white, nontender, with only a few cells in the aqueous and a mild flare.

Ocular toxocariasis has a variable mode of presentation depending on the part of the eye involved. The most common lesion is a solitary posterior granuloma.

The various presentations are:

- Diffuse, chronic endophthalmitis with acute exacerbations is seen between 2 and 10 years of age. The child is brought with diminished vision or squint. The eye is noncongested with active or healed anterior uveitis, vitritis, macular edema, and snow. On a long run, the eye may develop multiple complications, like posterior cyclitic membrane, exudative retinal detachment, complicated cataracts, glaucoma, or even hypotony.
- *Posterior polar involvement:* The posterior polar involvement consists of isolated granulomas that may be smaller than disk diameter or may be 2–3 DD large.

  The color of the granuloma is yellowish-white. It may be visible as a white glow on retinoscopy or may present as a white reflex in the pupil. The vision is reduced. It is seen that between 5 and 15 years may be associated with a vitreous band.

- *Peripheral granuloma:* This is seen even in adults; the other common age of presentation is 5–6 years, frequently asymptomatic, and discovered on routing indirect ophthalmoscopy.
- Pars planitis, optic neuritis, anterior uveitis, and chorioretinitis

Diagnosis

The diagnosis of ocular toxocariasis is by exclusion. All the unilateral intraocular white masses in the white eye of a child should be presumed to be toxocara granuloma/silent retinoblastoma. Possibilities of later should be investigated as urgent. History of pica and contact with puppies are not reliable features; peripheral blood smears show eosinophilia most of the time. Imaging of the eye by X-ray, CT, MRI, and USG does not show calcification. The most useful investigation is ELISA. Reading 1:8 is diagnostic. ELISA of aqueous or vitreous is more accurate.

Differential Diagnosis

The most important condition that should be differentiated from posterior pole granuloma is retinoblastoma, a common cause of white reflex in the pupillary area in children of the corresponding age. A retinoblastoma may be bilateral, which is unheard of in toxocariasis. Another point of differentiation is intralesional calcification, which is invariably present in retinoblastoma but never in toxocariasis. The ELISA test is negative in retinoblastoma as well as in eosinophilia.

Other conditions that should be differentiated are retinopathy of prematurity, persistent hyperplastic primary vitreous, Coats disease, and chronic endophthalmitis.

Management

Presentation treatment is so bizarre that there is no specific treatment except awareness about its possibility. The best way to avoid the condition is to avoid possible contaminated food and undercooked meat. The role of routinely deworming a child does not seem to be effective.

The most effective preventive method is universal deworming of dogs/bitches of all ages. The puppies should be dewormed more frequently than adults.

Medical Treatment

Children suffer from polyhelminthic disorder, for which a universal deworming drive is available. This covers toxocariasis as well. Even with all scepticism, it is worth giving it a try. The only disadvantage of using anthelmintics is the death of the worm, which may initiate severe intraocular inflammation. The way to prevent this is to administer anthelmintics under the cover of steroids. That does not seem to be logical. In ocular toxocariasis, steroids can be used alone, without anthelmintics, orally, or as a periocular injection. Anterior segment inflammation following the death of an intraocular worm is managed by usual strong cycloplegia and frequent steroids.

Surgery

Once retinoblastoma has been excluded, vitrectomy seems to be a viable alternate to medical treatment. The advantage of vitrectomy is that it not only removes the mass in toto but also allows the cutting of vitreous bands. The removed tissue can be histopathologically examined for conformation.

AIDS (HIV-1)-RELATED UVEITIS IN CHILDREN

Before discussing uveal involvement in AIDS, it is imperative to know about the disease in shorts.

Acquired immunodeficiency syndrome, which is acronymed as AIDS.

AIDS is a chronic, multisystemic viral disease caused by a virus called human immunodeficiency virus type 1. It is an RNA virus that uses host cells to manufacture DNA for multiplication. The virus has affinity for T helper lymphocytes, i.e., CD4; the viruses invade the CD4 cells to destroy them; this leads to severe immune deficiency, paving the way for many organisms that may be infective or commensal. These dormant cells, which would have been dormant for life, become active and produce uncommon and unsuspected systemic and local diseases. These opportunistic organisms can be viruses, bacteria, fungus and protozoa. The common viruses seen in AIDS patients are—herpes zoster, herpes simplex, cytomegaloviruses, Epstein–Barr virus, adenovirus, and Molluscum contagiosum viruses. The two common protozoa that are seen in AIDS are toxoplasma and pneumocystis carinii.

Half of the persons infected with HIV do not transmit the disease for quite some time. 90% will develop AIDS, which is uniformly fatal if not treated. 75% of AIDS patients will develop ocular manifestations. Many uncommon malignancies have their origins in HIV-1, the most common being Kaposi sarcoma.

The HIV-1 virus can be isolated from all ocular fluids, like tears, aqueous, and vitreous.

Ocular manifestation is never in isolation; it is always associated with the involvement of other organs. Ocular involvement due to AIDS can be put into two groups, i.e., intraocular and extraocular. Sometimes, it may become periocular. Intraocular involvement in the form of chorioretinitis is more common than extraocular lesions. The eyes are involved in two forms, i.e., the HIV-1 virus itself and AIDS-related complications.

In children, HIV-1 infection can either be congenital or acquired. Congenital infection is transplacental transmission from an infected mother.

The acquired form may be perinatal or postnatal. In the former, the child gets infected from the infected birth canal. The two common sources of acquired infections are—accidental transfusion of infected blood to a child who requires frequent transfusion, i.e., thalassemia, hemophilia, and other bleeding disorders, through infected needles and surgical instruments. The most unwanted but preventable cause is intravenous self-administered drugs in juvenile drug addicts.

Ocular involvement is time-related; hence, they are not seen under 10 except in congenital form. The intraocular lesions can be divided into two types, i.e., anterior segment and posterior segment involvement. Both types are caused by either the HIV-1 virus itself or due to activation of an opportunistic organism. The anterior lesions are benign conditions like follicular conjunctivitis, superficial punctate keratitis, pseudodendritic, corneal ulcer, and ulcerative geographic ulcers. The anterior uvea may develop nongranulomatous iritis or iridocyclitis. The malignant lesion is Kaposi sarcoma.

Kaposi Sarcoma

A few decades ago, Kaposi sarcoma was considered to be a rare disease of old age involving mostly the lower limbs. Its incidence has risen manyfold with an increase in AIDS patients of all ages. It is a fatal disease, and there is no definite anticancer drug that is effective against it. A patient with Kaposi sarcoma lives <3 years from the date of its appearance.

The exact cause of Kaposi sarcoma is not known, but it is more common in some races. It is more frequently seen in dark races, more in males, the ratio of men to women is 15:1. About 20–30% of patients with Kaposi sarcoma of organs other than the ocular adnexa have a chance of developing the tumor in the lids and conjunctiva. No intraocular involvement has been reported. Involvement of the conjunctiva and lids is an indication of a shortened life. The ocular involvement has an indolent course. Many times, repeated infection by opportunistic organisms like pneumocystis*, candida, and cytomegalovirus may precede the development of Kaposi's sarcoma. The lesion is multicentric. It is a vascular tumor developing from the endothelium. It involves the lid more frequently than the conjunctiva. The conjunctival lesion is a soft, purple-colored tumor.

Diagnosis

Diagnosis of Kaposi sarcoma is not difficult in a known case of AIDS. About 15–20% of AIDS patients develop Kaposi sarcoma. Besides AIDS, it is seen frequently in immune-suppressed individuals, like those with organ transplants or those who require frequent transfusions.

Otherwise diagnosis is by exclusion. The conditions that require to be differentiated are pyogenic granuloma, foreign body granuloma, and cavernous hemangioma.

Treatment

Treatment by chemotherapy, radiation, or cryo has limited value in eradication. Any treatment employed for Kaposi's sarcoma should be taken under the cover of systemic treatment for AIDS.

Posterior Segment Involvement in AIDS

- Retinal cotton wool spots caused by microinfarction of the nerve fiber layer
- Retinal vasculitis—mostly perivasculitis
- Intraretinal hemorrhages
- Maculopathy
- Choroidal granuloma (mycobacterial)
- Chorioretinitis

**Pneumocystis* was previously called Pneumocystis carinii and was a protozoa. Presently, it is called Pneumocystis jirovecii and is considered to be a fungus. This is based on nucleic acid and biochemical analysis. It is a fatal disease in immunocompromised persons, and in spite of its being a fungus, it responds to systemic chemotherapy with a simple drug like trimethoprim-sulfamethoxazole. The other drug used is aerosolized pentamidine.

Diagnosis

The diagnosis is confirmed by:

- Positive ELISA and western blot
- CD4 cell count <200 cells/mm^2
- Presence of systemic infection by opportunistic organisms
- Presence of Kaposi sarcoma

Management

The cases should best be treated by person specially trained to manage AIDS. Ocular treatment is palliative.

MASQUERADE SYNDROMES OF THE UVEA IN CHILDREN

There are some conditions that may be benign or malignant but present as uveitis, in spite of their not being so. They are initially managed as uveitis, many a time with disastrous results, especially when the offending disorder is malignant like retinoblastoma or leukemia.

Masquerading syndromes are seen under 15 years of age in both sexes in all races the world over. They prove to be fatal more often in underdeveloped nations, not because they have not been suspected but due to a lack of advanced diagnostic methods. Most of them are proven cases of malignancy; others may be locally invasive.

The former group is headed by retinoblastoma, followed by myelogenous leukemia. Intraocular foreign bodies and intraocular granulomas are two non-neoplastic conditions that may be mistaken for uveitis. All of them cause KPs, flares, cells in the anterior chamber and vitreous, even synechiae, hypopyons, or pseudohypopyons.

Diagnosis is by exclusion; all such cases should be subjected to an X-ray orbit, CT, MRI, USG, and peripheral blood smear examination.

NEW GROWTH OF THE UVEA IN CHILDREN

New growths of uvea under 20 years are rare but not an exception. They can be benign or malignant. Malignant new growth, like malignant melanoma of the choroid, is a disease of the fourth decade and above. The benign tumors can be inflammatory or noninflammatory. The inflammatory conditions are nodules on the iris and a foreign body granuloma. The benign tumors of the uvea in children are hemangioma neurofibroma (Lisch nodules*), nevi of the iris, and juvenile xanthogranuloma[†]. The locally malignant tumor medulloepithelioma is seen in the ciliary body and is commonly referred to as diktyoma[‡].

SUGGESTED READING

1. Chawla R, Kapoor M, Mehta A, Tripathy K, Vohra R, Venkatesh P. Sympathetic Ophthalmia: Experience from a Tertiary Care Center in Northern India. J Ophthalmic. 2018;13(4):439-46.
2. Coles RS. Uveitis. In: Sorsby A (Ed). Modern Ophthalmology, 1st edition. London: Butterworth; 1964. Volume 4. pp. 636-86.

**Lisch nodule:* Lisch nodules seen in neurofibroma type 1 are dome-shaped lesions on the iris surface, the color of which varies according to the presence of pigment in them. The most common color is yellowish brown. They vary in number, position, and size, ranging between 1 and 2 mm. They may be single or multiple. They do not require any specific treatment.

[†]*Juvenile xanthogranuloma:* It is a rare dermatological disorder with uveal involvement. It is a type of histiocytosis. Surprisingly, 10% of cases of neurofibromatosis type 1 involving the iris may develop xanthogranuloma. In children, it is a cause of unsuspected spontaneous, nontraumatic, self-limiting recurrent hyphema. Of all the parts of the uvea involved, the iris is affected most. The none uveal structure to be involved is the optic nerve, which culminates in diminished vision. The incidence of ocular involvement is <0.4%; however, cutaneous involvement is seen in almost 40% of cases with ocular involvement.

The condition is seen in an infant as young as 1 year. The most common complication is the transient rise of intraocular tension that is self-limiting. The management consists of local steroid drops and β-blockers if tension is high. It does not generally recur.

[‡]*Diktyoma:* It is the second most primary intraocular tumor in children.

Diktyoma (medulloepithelioma or teratoneuroma) arises from the primitive medullary epithelium of the ciliary body, which is derived from the angle of the embryonic medullary epithelium lining the optic vesicle, which is non pigmented, simulating the embryonic retina. Making it a congenital condition that may not be evident at birth. It becomes evident by 4 years of age and another 1–2 years to be diagnosed. It has been reported to arise from the retina, iris, and optic nerve as well. It is nonhereditary. It may be asymptomatic when small, hidden behind the iris, or present as a pale white growth encroaching on the pupillary area when the pupil is dilated. It is a slow-progressing, locally malignant condition. An undiagnosed tumor may grow slowly and be visible in the nondilated pupil as well. It is well delineated in USG. It does not get calcified. Large growths are known to cause neovascularization of the angle and secondary glaucoma. The management consists of cryotherapy, plaque radiotherapy, and external beam radiation. Local resection along with adjacent iris may be sufficient in the early stages. Large tumors not responding to the above methods may require enucleation. It rarely metastasizes; recurrence following resection is possible.

3. Cunningham ET, Crawford JB. Uveal tract and Sclera. In: Vaughan D, Asbury T, Riordan EP (Eds). General Ophthalmology, 15th edition. New York: Appleton and Lange; 1999. pp. 143-58.
4. Dutta Majumdar P, Biwas J. Paediatric uveitis: an up-to-date. Oman J Ophthalmol. 2017;6(3):140-50.
5. Garg SP, Venkatesh P, Lalit V; All India Ophthalmological Society. Uveitis: Approach to Diagnosis and Management in CME Series No. 6. [online] Available from https://www.aios.org/cme/cmeseries6.pdf. [Last accessed March, 2025]
6. Gupta SK. Diktyoma. Indian J Ophthalmol. 1981;29(1):51-4.
7. Kadayifcilar S, Eldern B, Turner B. Uveitis in childhood. J Paediatr Strabismus. 2003;40:335-40.
8. Kalidasan CS. Diktyoma of ciliary body. Indian J Ophthalmol. 1975;23(2):13-4.
9. Maleki A, Anesi SD, Look-Why S, Manhapra A, Stephen FC. Pediatric uveitis: A comprehensive review. Surv Ophthalmol. 2022;67(2):510-29.
10. Rathiman SR, Sudhir B. Intermediate Uveitis. In: Ramamurthy D, Biswas P (Eds). AIOS Ready Reckoner in Ophthalmology, 2nd edition. New Delhi: Jaypee Brothers Medical Publisher; 2019.
11. Rathinam SR, Babu M. Algorithmic Approach in the Diagnosis of Uveitis. Indian J Ophthalmol. 2013;61(6):255-62.
12. Rathinam SR. (2010). Uveitis made simple workup and management. [online] Available from https://www.aios.org/cme/cmeseries20.pdf. [Last accessed March, 2025]
13. Shanmugalingam S. (2016). An unusual case of silicone oil in the anterior chamber simulating intraocular implant. [online] Available from https://www.eyenews.uk.com/education/case-reports/post/an-unusual-case-of-silicone-oil-in-the-anterior-chamber-simulating-intraocular-implant. [Last accessed March, 2025]
14. Sharma P. Uvea and Its Disease. In: Agarwal LP (Ed). Essentials of Ophthalmology, 1st edition. New Delhi: Modern Publishers; 2000. pp. 156-75.
15. Sinha R, Naithani P, Garg SP, Newer investigation and management guidelines in uveitis. IJO. 2010;55(1):88-91.
16. Stephen FC. Paediatric uveitis, July 2017, ocular immunology, and uveitis.
17. Tugal-Tutkun I. Pediatric Uveitis. J Ophthalmic Vis Res. 2011;6(4):259-69.
18. Wood AC. Endogenous inflammation of the uveal tract, 1st edition. Baltimore: Williams & Wilkins; 1961. pp. 22-3.

CHAPTER

18 Disorders of the Vitreous in Children

In the past, the vitreous was not given much importance in clinical ophthalmology; its main functions were attributed to its clarity, which was of optical importance only. With the advent of better understanding, it is now placed on the same level as the retina and lens.

The vitreous is the largest intraocular structure that is a semisolid transparent gel, filing the vitreous cavity extending from the posterior lens capsule to the optic nerve. It is surrounded by the posterior lens capsule, zonules, ciliary epithelium, and the internal limiting membrane of the retina. The retinal vessels come into close contact with the outer surface of the vitreous without access to the vitreous body in a normal eye. In adults, it measures 4 cc in volume; its volume depends on the size of the globe. Its refractive power is 1.336. The main functions of the vitreous, besides their optical purposes, are: Keeping the retina in place, supporting and stabilizing the lens, and being loosely attached to the retina without any potential space in between. However, when this proximity is disturbed, the vitreous gets separated from the retina; this mostly happens in the posterior pole and is called posterior vitreous detachment; anterior detachment is less common.

The various physiological attachments of the vitreous are:

- Vitreous base
- Round the fovea
- Round the optic nerve
- Round the blood vessels
- Posterior lens capsule

They are shown in **Figure 18.1**.

- *Vitreous base:* The vitreous base is an ill-defined area along the ora serrata; at this place, the attachment of the normal vitreous is strongest. The vitreous base straddles the ora serrata, extending 2.00 mm on each side of the ora, encircling the inner surface of the globe. The vitreous base is also attached to the ciliary epithelium; the attachment lasts for the rest of life. It is most commonly detached following trauma, pulling the pigment epithelium and blood vessels along with it.
- *Round the fovea:* The attachment around the fovea is the smallest and weakest of all attachments, hence, commonly disrupted in posterior vitreous detachment.
- *Round the optic nerve:* This is very strong in comparison to other attachments; it is all round the periphery of the disc margin with a narrow space at the apex of the disc.
- *Round the blood vessels:* The hyaloid vascular attachment in the normal eye has been questioned, and when present, it is thought to be pathological; the attachments are weak.
- *Posterior lens capsule:* Developmentally, the primary vitreous develops from the ectodermal cells shared with the developing lens capsule. Hence, there is a strong bond between the posterior lens capsule and the primary vitreous, which remains intact even when the vitreous is fully developed. This bond remains strong until 25 years of age, making it difficult to remove the lens in toto surgically, making intracapsular lens extraction under 25 years of age an

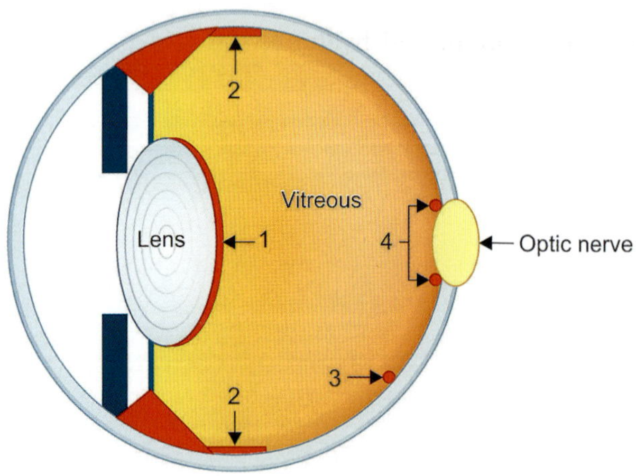

Fig. 18.1: Attachment of vitreous in a child's eye.

absolute contraindication. After 25 years, the adhesion becomes loose and is lost by the 6th decade.

The pathological adhesions are mostly vitreoretinal, found in the chorioretinal scars, peripheral pigment clumps, posterior border of lattice degeneration, borders of ruptured choroid and coloboma of choroid, and peripheral retinal vessel sites of retinal periphlebitis.

APPLIED ANATOMY OF VITREOUS

The shape and volume of the vitreous body depend on the size and shape of the globe. It is smaller in microphthalmos and nanophthalmos and larger in buphthalmos. The vitreous, once lost, is not capable of regeneration, in such a situation, it is replaced by the aqueous. There is no way to expand the vitreous volume; in contrast to this, its volume can be reduced by expressing its water content, either by administering oral hypertonic fluids like oral glycerin, intravenous mannitol, or carbonic anhydrase inhibitors. The other physical method to reduce the volume is to apply uniform, intermittent pressure over the globe. This not only reduces the volume of the vitreous but also reduces intraocular pressure sufficiently.

The vitreous does not have a true capsule-like lens. The vitreous is denser on the periphery all-round due to its abundant collagen content and is referred to as its cortex. The remaining part is considered to be its nucleus. The vitreous does not contain any nerves; hence, it is devoid of sensation. The absence of blood vessels makes it immune to infection and inflammation; it gets infected only when organisms find their way into the vitreous body by inoculation, either during surgery or penetrating injury. In spite of its being avascular, it is a rich medium for microorganisms to grow.

The vitreous is 98–99% water, with some solids like collagen, protein, and hyaluronic acid dissolved in it. The ascorbic acid content of the vitreous is higher than that of plasma. It also contains sodium, potassium, chloride, and phosphate. There are about 50 enzymes vitreous; the actual function of these chemicals is not well established except for collagen, which can bind with water, 200 times more than its weight. This is the basis of its hydrogel status, which has a very high viscosity.

DETAILS OF DEVELOPMENT OF VITREOUS

The development of vitreous, in short, has been discussed in Chapter 2. The following is a more elaborate description of the same:

The vitreous makes its presence felt as early as 13 mm of embryo. Its development has been divided into three stages, which are:

- Primary vitreous
- Secondary vitreous
- Tertiary vitreous

- *Primary vitreous:* The primary vitreous is first to appear between the developing lens and retina. During this period, cells from the lens and retina contribute to its development, where retinal cells dominate over their lenticular counterparts. The lenticular cells, following the formation of the lens capsule, lose contact with the primary vitreous. The retinal cells do not stop contributing to the formation of the primary vitreous. The development of tunica vasculosa lentis is an important contribution to the formation of not only the vitreous but also the lens. The tunica adds the mesodermal part of the primary vitreous, which pushes the ectodermal component of the developing vitreous. The hyaloid, which is a branch of the primitive dorsal ophthalmic artery, enters the optic cup through the fetal fissure. To join the developing tunica vasculosa lentis, the hyaloid artery has a short presence in the eye. It starts disappearing by the 65.00 mm stage and is completely absorbed at birth. From the proximal parts of the disappearing hyaloid artery sprouts the future central retinal artery.
- *Secondary vitreous:* The secondary vitreous represents the future mature vitreous; it is a combination of ectoderm and mesenchyme. We have noted that at 13 mm, the capsule of the lens develops to exclude the surface ectoderm of the lens from the formation of the vitreous further, but the neuroectoderm of the optic cup continues to contribute to the development of the secondary vitreous until the 65–70 mm stage. The secondary vitreous contains primitive tissue called hyalocytes, which are derived from the primary vitreous. At this stage, the tunica vasculosa lentis and hyaloid artery start to atrophy. The secondary vitreous ultimately replaces the primary vitreous and the tunica vasculosa lentis, leaving a narrow space in the central core of the secondary vitreous called the Cloquet canal.
- *Tertiary vitreous:* The tertiary vitreous is not really a part of the mature vitreous. It differs from the development of the primary and secondary vitreous as it is secreted by the ciliary epithelium without any optical properties. Its main function is to keep the lens in

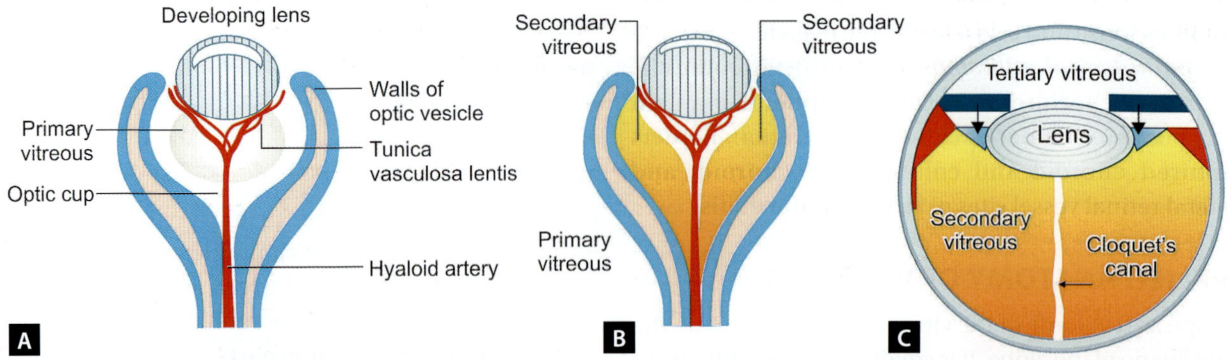

Figs. 18.2A to C: Development of vitreous. (A) The primary vitreous in relation to the developing lens and hyaloid artery—the secondary vitreous has not yet materialized; (B) Secondary vitreous, obliterating the primary vitreous; and (C) Secondary vitreous completely replaces the primary vitreous and hyaloid systems of the artery, barring the Colloquies canal and tertiary vitreous.

position and help with accommodation in the form of the suspensory ligament (zonule) of the lens. It occupies a triangular space between the developing lens and ciliary body, and as the eye develops, it enlarges in size, pulling the ciliary body away from the lens. This is the space where the zonules develop. The fibers divide into two groups. The first part is just behind the iris, attached to the anterior periphery of the lens capsule. The second part runs parallel to the developing anterior vitreous membrane and gets attached to the posterior lens capsule **(Figs. 18.2A to C)**.

CONGENITAL ANOMALIES OF THE VITREOUS

The vitreous being the largest intraocular structure, it is logical to presume that it will have a proportionately large number of congenital anomalies, yet it has a lesser number of congenital anomalies. They may be as small as vitreous floaters or may be extensive enough to replace the whole vitreous with mesodermal tissue, mostly fibrovascular in nature. The congenital anomalies mostly involve mesodermal tissues; they may involve the hyaloid vascular system without hyperplastic changes in the vitreous or may be associated with hyperplastic changes in the vitreous. The anomalies of the hyaloid vascular system are:

- The hyaloid artery from the apex of the disc to the back of the lens remains visible in segments as an attenuated tract occasionally containing blood. This is the rarest of all the congenital anomalies of the hyaloid vascular system.
- The anterior end of the artery remains attached to the posterior lens capsule as a free-floating stalk when the rest of the hyaloid vessels get atrophied.
- A part of tunica vasculosa lentis fails to disappear and persists as a small gray speck on the posterior pole of the lens; this spot is called Mittendorf's dot and is visible on oblique illumination and distance direct ophthalmoscopy. It is best seen on a slit lamp. It is generally asymptomatic, rarely reducing central vision.
- The posterior end of the hyaloid artery remains attached to the optic nerve head and is called Bergmeister's papilla. The papilla is made of a central core of blood vessels surrounded by glial tissue. The condition is symptomatic and diagnosed on routine fundus examinations; when large, it may be mistaken for growth of the optic disc.

PERSISTENT HYPERPLASTIC PRIMARY VITREOUS (SEE CHAPTER 3)

Symptoms of Disorders of the Vitreous

The primary disorders of the vitreous are rare in children when compared to adults. The two functions of the vitreous are optical and stabilizing the retina and lens; the symptoms are optical and retinal. Secondarily, the vitreous may be invaded by structures surrounding it. The most common example is invasion of the vitreous by retinal blood vessels or infection spreading from the uveoretinal complex, ending in mild vitritis to severe endophthalmitis. The most common symptoms of vitreous disorders are vitreous floaters. The other symptoms are photopsia, Weiss ring*, erythropsia, diminished vision, and sudden painless loss of vision. The symptoms, when due to local causes, are unilateral; otherwise, they are bilateral.

Signs of Vitreous Disorders

Vitreous opacities: The vitreous opacities are the most common disorders of the vitreous and may be pinpoint or extensive. They are of various shapes and sizes, ranging from single dots to scattered dots or strings. It is not unusual to have them in large sheets. When motile, they are called floaters; otherwise, they may be fixed in a certain gaze. They may change their position in different movements, may be felt all through the waking hours, and may be more visible after sleep. They may settle down and not be felt with a straight gaze. They are not seen when the lids are closed or in darkness, in contrast to photopsia, which is better felt in closed eyes and dark ambient.

The vitreous opacities can either be primary due to changes in the vitreous or secondary to pathology in the retinouveo complex or optic nerve. The primary changes in vitro are as follows:

Muscae Volitantes

These opacities are so common that they are considered to be physiological. They are common in moderate myopia; the patient becomes aware of them in the late years of the first decade. They are generally unilateral and not associated with visual loss.

They are perceived either as scattered dots or as dots in a string. They are best seen against a light-colored background, such as the sky or light-colored wall. They neither have pathological significance nor do they require any treatment.

The sudden onset of a shower of vitreous floaters should not be taken lightly. All such eyes should be examined with an indirect ophthalmoscope, as it may be the beginning of pars planitis, retinal breakage, or inflammation of the uvea. They represent degenerative changes in the vitreous.

Vitreous Degeneration

Vitreous is a semisolid gel that does not show any movement or ripple within its body unless it is liquefied. Vitreous in a child's eye is more firm and solid than vitreous in the senile group.

The liquefaction of the vitreous is known as synchysis. It is a common feature of old age. In children, liquefaction is seen in high myopia and trauma with or without a retained foreign body. It is also seen following vitreous hemorrhage, endophthalmitis, and severe posterior uveitis. The vitreous loses its semisolid nature and becomes watery in consistency.

It may be so fluid as to flow out during intracapsular lens extraction in age-related cataracts. The liquefaction invariably leads to syneresis or the collapse of the vitreous. Liquefied vitreous does not require any specific treatment.

Synchysis Scintillans

Synchysis scintillans is a different kind of vitreous liquefaction seen in younger patients, and it is bilateral without much complaint. The patient may not be aware of its presence. There is the deposition of cholesterol crystals in the vitreous. The crystals are suspended in the vitreous. They may remain hidden at the bottom of the vitreous and become visible with the movement of the eye, like a golden shower. Sometimes they are visible under oblique illumination in clear media. They are best seen with a slit lamp. They are also visible with a direct ophthalmoscope. On retinoscopy, they may be visible as cloudy dots. Synchysis scintillans persists lifelong and does not require any treatment. They are not to be confused with asteroid hyalitis, which is seen in elderly males. They are accumulations of calcium soaps and are fixed bodies with minimum movement.

Vitreous Detachment

Normal vitreous has firm attachment to the retina, ora serrate, and optic disc. This keeps the retina snug with the choroid; the vitreous detachment is always pathological. The prerequisite for vitreous detachment is its liquefaction. The detachment of the vitreous is common after the sixth decade and is considered to be precursor of retinal detachment; it may happen in the early decades following blunt trauma. Vitreous detachment is far less common in children, but not an exception. The factors that cause

**Weiss ring* is actually not a developmental anomaly. It is defined as a circular peripapillary optical structure visible in the vitreous following the detachment of the vitreous from the optic nerve head. It is associated with floaters in the field and flashes of light. It is not to be confused with posterior vitreous detachment, which is far more common than the Weiss ring.

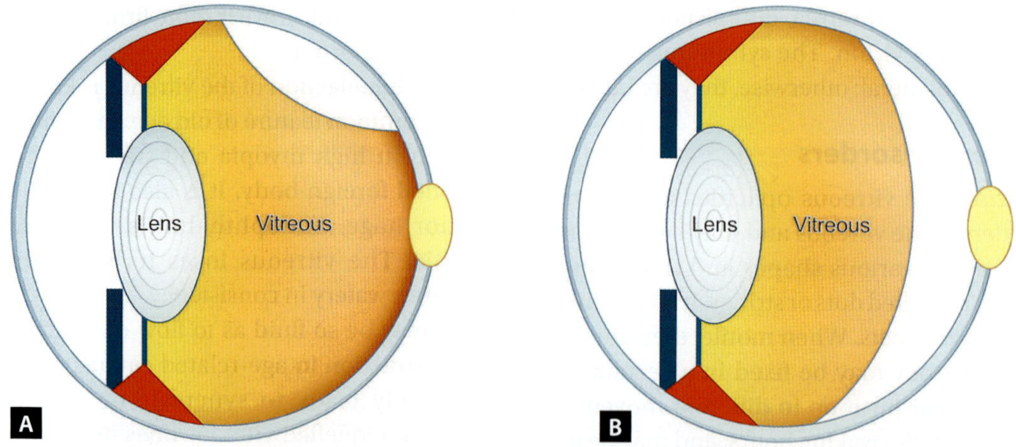

Figs. 18.3A and B: Various types of vitreous detachment. (A) Small posterior detachment and (B) Extensive posterior detachment.

vitreous detachments in children are high myopia, chronic uveitis, blunt or penetrating injury to the globe, occasionally vitreous hemorrhage, and pull-on capsule hyaloid attachment, which may also cause vitreous to lose its moorings. The vitreous detachment in all ages is divided into two broad groups, i.e., the more common posterior vitreous detachment and the less common anterior detachment **(Figs. 18.3A and B)**.

The former can be:

- Small peripheral with a tendency to increase.
- Central conical large detachment happens when the vitreous remains attached to the disc and base, detaching from the internal limiting layer of the retina all-round.
- *Globular detachment:* This is the most extensive detachment of the vitreous when the vitreous loses its attachment to the optic nerve and the internal limiting membrane retains its attachment at the base.

The posterior detachment can either be simple, i.e., it retains the spherical shape of the posterior surface, or it is called collapsed detachment when the posterior border of the vitreous loses its rounded shape and seems to hang from the base.

The posterior detachment may be asymptomatic and found during routing indirect ophthalmoscopy, examination by plus 70 lenses, or ultrasonography. The symptoms, when present, may be flashes of light and Weiss rings.

Anterior Vitreous Detachment

The whole of the anterior vitreous is separated from the zonule and base, pushing the vitreous back. It can occasionally be localized to zonules or less.

Infection of the vitreous can be either as mild as localized vitritis or extensive endophthalmitis, i.e., generally associated with retinouveitis, which has been discussed in detail earlier.

SUGGESTED READING

1. Gerstenblith TA, Rabinowitz MP (Eds). Posterior vitreous detachment. Wills Eye Manual, 6th edition. Philadelphia: Wolters Kluwer; 2012.
2. Mukherjee PK. Disorder of the retina and vitreous. In: Pediatric Ophthalmology, 1st Edition. New Delhi: New Age International (P) Ltd; 2005.
3. Mukherjee PK. Examination of vitreous. In: Clinical Examination in Ophthalmology. Gurugram, Haryana: Elsevier; 2016. pp. 358-63.
4. Murray PI, Pavesio CE, Denniston AKO. Posterior vitreous detachment. In: Oxford Handbook of Ophthalmology, 4th edition. Oxford, UK: Oxford University Press; 2018. p. 530.
5. Nema HV, Nema N, Singh VP. The Vitreous. Anatomy of the Eye and its Adnexa, 2nd edition. New Delhi: Jaypee Brothers Medical Publishers (P) Ltd; 1991.
6. Pahwa JM, Billore OP. Anatomy of the Vitreous, 1st edition. New Delhi: IBH Publishing Company; 1985. pp. 1-9.
7. Tasman W. Disease of the retina and vitreous. In: Harley RD (Ed). Pediatric Ophthalmology, Vol. 1. Philadelphia: WB Sanders Company; 1983. pp. 599-602.

CHAPTER

19 Disorders of Lens in Children

The lens is responsible for about one-third of the dioptric power of the normal adult eye. It is a crystal-clear disc-shaped structure suspended by the zonules from the ciliary body behind the iris, in front of the vitreous **(Fig. 19.1)**.

The area of the vitreous just behind the lens has a small depression called the patellar fossa, in which the posterior surface of the lens rests. There is strong adhesion between the posterior surface of the lens and the anterior surface of the vitreous. In children, this bond is so strong that the lens cannot be extracted from the eye without pulling the vitreous with it or rupturing the lens capsule. This adhesion gradually weakens as a person ages and completely disappears in the sixth decade.

The lens is a disc-shaped structure, thicker at the center that looks circular when seen from the front or back and elliptical when looked from the side **(Figs. 19.2A and B)**.

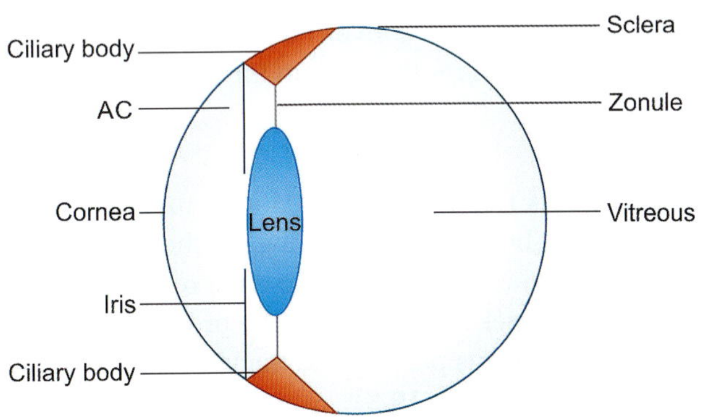

Fig. 19.1: The position of the lens in relation to the rest of the globe. (AC: anterior chamber)

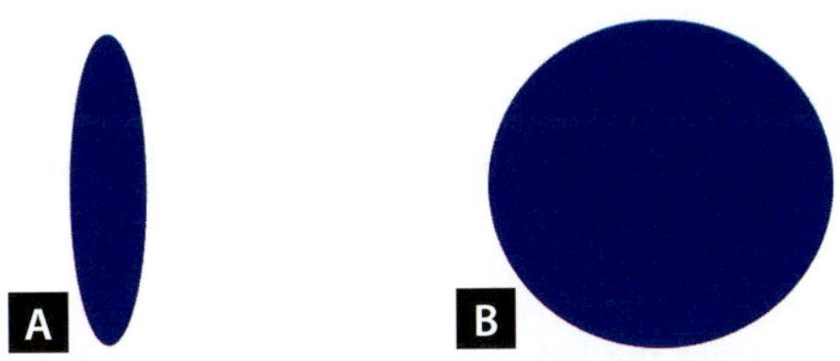

Figs. 19.2A and B: Appearance of lens from (A) side and (B) front and back.

In adults, its diameter is 9–10 mm in all meridians, with a central thickness of 4.5 mm. The lens in utero is spherical up to 6 months of gestation, after which it starts flattening. The thickness of the lens gradually tapers on the periphery; the two surfaces of the lens meet in a rounded manner; this is called the equator of the lens. The curvature of the two surfaces is not equal. The anterior surface is flatter; the posterior surface is more curved **(Fig. 19.3)**.

The radii of curvature of two surfaces are 10 mm and 6 mm, respectively. The curvature changes during accommodation when the posterior surface becomes more curved than the anterior surface. The equator has a smooth curve. The central most part of the anterior surface is called the anterior pole, while the corresponding posterior point is called the posterior pole **(Fig. 19.3)**.

The lens, zonules, and part of the ciliary body divide the eyeball into two unequal chambers: (1) One small aqueous chamber and (2) a large vitreous chamber.

The iris glides smoothly over the anterior lens capsule reflexly. The normal pupil is placed in front of the anterior

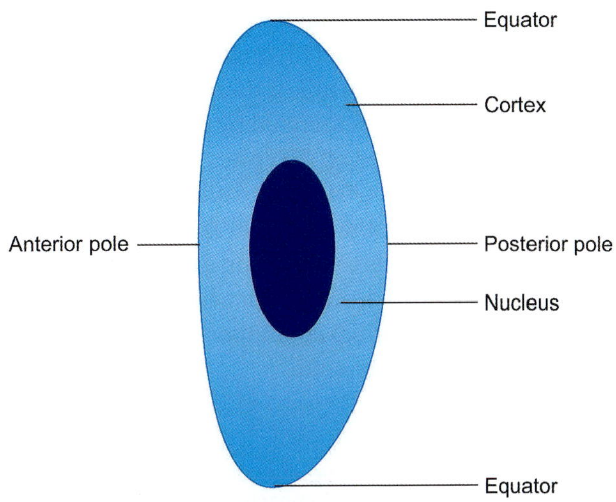

Fig. 19.3: Unequal curvature of the lens equator and poles.

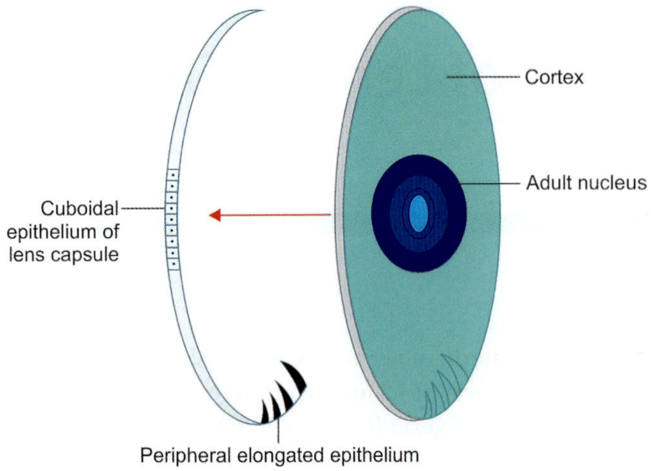

Fig. 19.4: Details of the capsule and various nuclei

pole of the lens, slightly down and medially. The lens has the following parts **(Fig. 19.4)**:

- Capsule
- Epithelium
- Lens fibers
  - Cortex
  - Nuclei
- Zonules

> The lens is virtually a mass of epithelium wrapped in a capsule and suspended by a zonule.

CAPSULE

Though the capsule envelops the rest of the lens from all sides, it is not a true membrane; it is a basement membrane of the epithelium. It is the thickest basement membrane in the body and is a homogenous transparent membrane of unequal thickness. It does not have any specific structure. It is thickest on the periphery (equator, 14 μ) and thinner on the poles. The posterior pole is thinner than the anterior pole (3 μ). The capsule is secreted by the epithelium. The capsule cannot be peeled off the cortex but can be stripped during *capsulorrhexis**. To the capsules are the zonules attached all round at the equator. The normal capsule does not allow aqueous to permeate into the substances; it also does not allow proteins from the lens to leak into the aqueous under normal conditions. The capsule, once destroyed, does not regenerate.

LENS EPITHELIUM

The lens epithelium is shown in **Figure 19.4**.

Only the anterior part of the lens under the capsule has epithelium. The epithelium is single-layered. It is cuboidal and short at the center and does not divide; it only elongates. The elongation is gradual; the longest cells are most peripheral at the equator, are columnar, and divide vigorously. The epithelial cells keep on increasing in size and number to form new lens fibers. This process goes on unhindered throughout life; hence, the size and weight of the normal lens increase with age; there is no posterior epithelial layer under the posterior capsule.

LENS FIBERS

The fibers of the lens constitute the main bulk of the lens. They can be divided into two groups without any clear-cut margin of demarcation.

They are: (1) Cortex and (2) nucleus. The cortex occupies the larger part in young persons, but its volume gets reduced as a person ages when the nucleus becomes larger than in younger persons. The cortex is loose and the nucleus is compact; the peripheral epithelial cells at the equator divide and elongate. The elongated part of the epithelium does not have nuclei. They form new lens fibers, which are collectively called the cortex. As new cortical fibers are laid down, the old fibers get compressed and pushed centrally to be converted into a denser nucleus. This process continues throughout life.

NUCLEUS

The nucleus is not a well-defined structure, it does not have a specific border and is nothing but the condensation of cortical fibers. The earliest presence of the nucleus is felt in the 7th week of conception. According to the age of formation of various parts of the nucleus, they are called by different terms **(Fig. 19.5)**.

- Embryonic
- Fetal
- Infantile
- Adult

The embryonic nucleus is the earliest condensation of the fibers that corresponds to the first 3 months of

---

**Capsulorrhexis* is a surgical procedure of capsulotomy where the capsule is peeled from the lens capsule from the cortex generally in a continuous curvilinear fashion in phacoemulsification of the cortex. The most common is capsulorrhexis of the anterior lens capsule in children; the posterior capsule is also rhexied during intraocular lens (IOL) surgery.

gestation, formed by the elongation of primary lens fibers that originate in the posterior wall of the lens vesicle. Any pathological change at this stage will cause the smallest and most central congenital opacity.

The fetal nucleus develops through the deposition of lens fibers over the embryonic nucleus. The period of this development lasts from 3 months of gestation until birth. The fibers meet at the center in the peculiar fashion of letter Y, one each in the anterior part and the other in the posterior part. The posterior Y is placed upside down. The anterior Y is erect. Pathological changes during this period will result in a central opacity that is larger than embryonic opacity but does not extend to the periphery. The fibers of the nucleus laid down before and after the start of the pathological changes in the fetal nucleus remain clear.

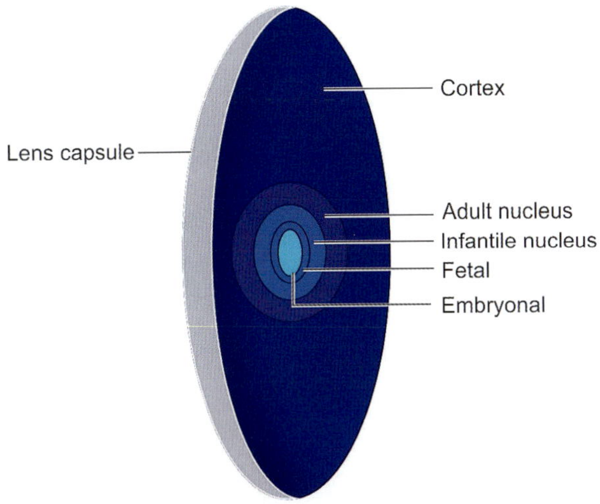

Fig. 19.5: Details of various nuclei in relation to the cortex.

The infantile nucleus corresponds to the fibers laid down from the last week of gestation to puberty.

The adult nucleus is laid down after puberty and continues throughout life, forming the main bulk of the nucleus

ZONULES

The zonules are structureless, transparent sheets of fibers that arise from the ciliary body and get attached to the equator of the lens. Their function is to keep the lens in place and allow the effect of the contraction of the ciliary muscles to be transmitted to the lens during accommodation. They are divided into three groups according to the location of their attachment, i.e., (1) preequatorial, (2) equatorial, and (3) retroequatorial. The preequatorial fibers extend farthest on the anterior lens capsule, making them vulnerable to damage during capsulorrhexis.

DEVELOPMENT OF LENS

The following is a summary of the development of lenses:

- The lens starts developing in very early fetal life. It is fully ectodermal in origin. The development of the lens cannot be comprehended without understanding the development of the optic vesicle and subsequent changes around it **(Fig. 19.6)**.
- Two diverticula develop on the lateral side of the cephalic end of the forebrain.
- Each diverticulum extends laterally toward the surface ectoderm.

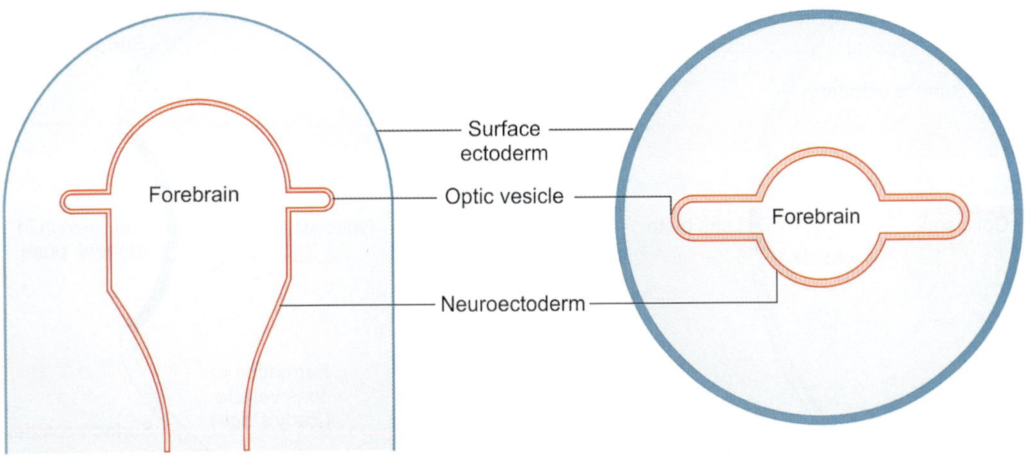

Fig. 19.6: Development of the optic vesicle in relation to the surface ectoderm from the forebrain.

- The distal end of each diverticulum enlarges to form a primary optic vesicle **(Figs. 19.7 to 19.9)**.
- At about 4–5 mm in the stage of development, the vortex of the primary vesicle touches the inner side of the surface ectoderm.
- The contact of primary optic vesicle and the surface ectoderm heralds the actual development of the lens by formation of a lens plate (placode) by the thickened ectoderm **(Fig. 19.8)**.
- A depression develops in the middle of the lens placode and is termed a lens pit **(Fig. 19.10)**.
- Simultaneously, changes start in the primary optic vesicle. Soon after meeting the surface ectoderm, the tip of the primary optic vesicle retracts back and invaginates to form the secondary optic vesicle **(Fig. 19.10)**.
- In the meantime, the invaginated lens pit deepens, and its edges come together to form a hollow structure called a lens vesicle **(Fig. 19.11)**.
- The lens vesicle loses its contact with the surface ectoderm and migrates backward in the concavity of the optic curve.
- Going back to the stage of development of the lens vesicle, the following three changes are noticed:
  1. *Development of primary lens fibers:* The cells of the posterior wall of the lens vesicle enlarge in length and are called primary lens fibers. They become long enough to obliterate the cavity of the lens vesicle. The development of the primary lens fibers stops by the 3rd month of gestation. The primary lens fibers occupy the central most part of the lens; they are compressed to form the embryonic nucleus.

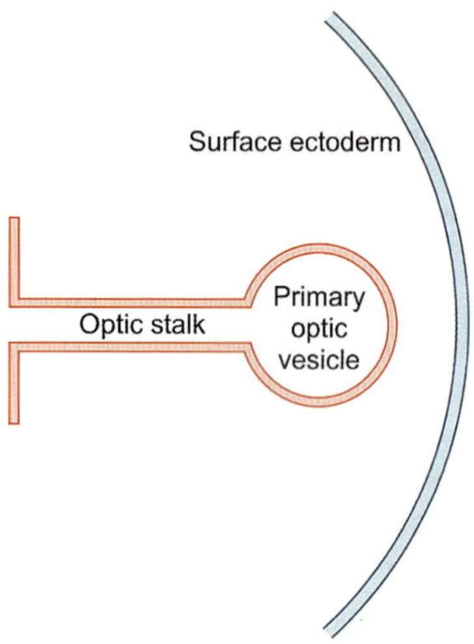

Fig. 19.7: Development of primary optic vesicle.

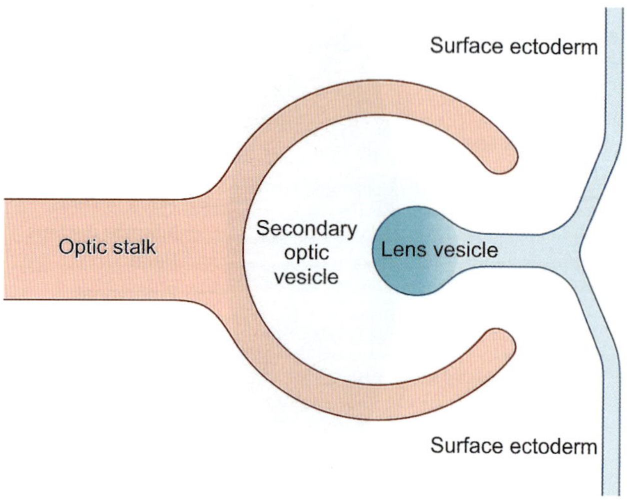

Fig. 19.9: Formation of secondary optic vesicles and lens vesicles.

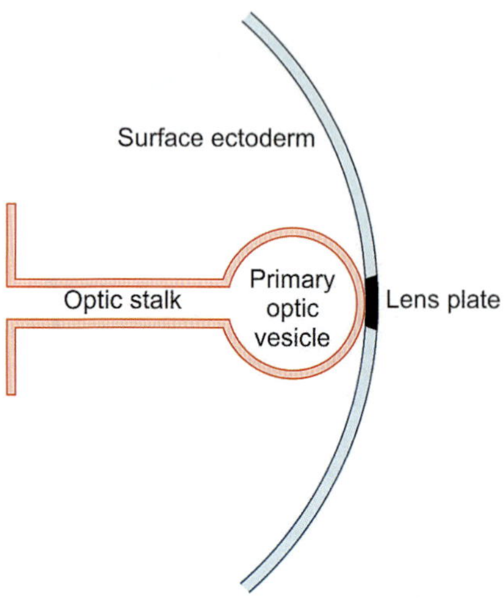

Fig. 19.8: Formation of lens plate.

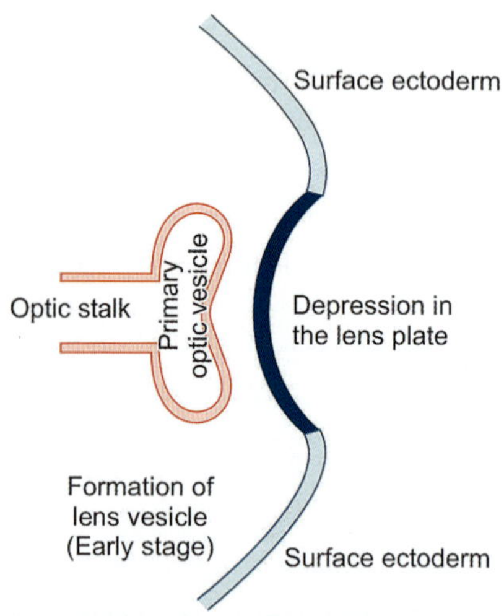

Fig. 19.10: Development of lens pit.

Any derangement in the development of primary lens fibers at this stage will result in dense central congenital cataracts **(Fig. 19.12)**.

2. *Development of secondary lens fibers:* In contrast to primary lens fibers, which develop from the posterior part of the lens vesicle, secondary fibers develop from anterior epithelial cells; in fact, they develop from the equatorial ends of the anterior epithelial cells. From the secondary lens fibers develop the fetal and infantile nuclei. The secondary lens fibers are laid down throughout life; the older fibers are pushed over the infantile nucleus to form the adult nucleus. The remaining part between the adult nucleus, the capsule posteriorly, and the epithelium anteriorly becomes the cortex of the lens.

   At birth, the lens is fully formed and functional. As compared to an adult lens, it is more spherical; its diameter is less than that of an adult lens, i.e., it is about 6 mm at birth.
3. *Development of zonules:* The zonules, or suspensory ligaments, of the lens have only one function, i.e., to keep the lens suspended and centered in the middle of the pupil; they do not have any visual function, and their other purpose is to transmit the effect of the ciliary contraction to the lens during accommodation. Developmentally, the zonules are considered to be tertiary vitreous. The zonules have both ectodermal and mesodermal origins.

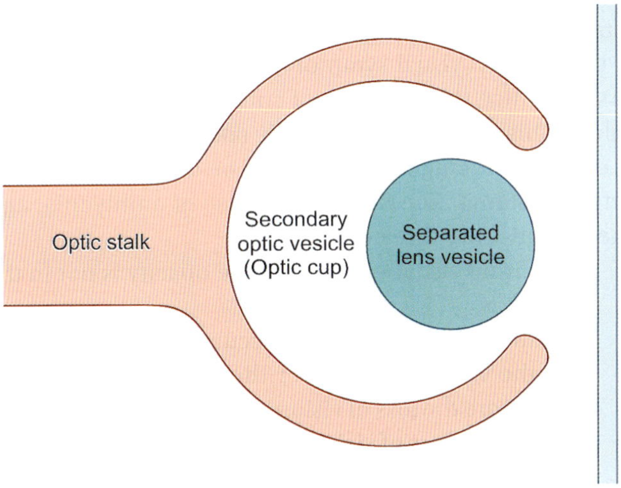

Fig. 19.11: Formation of lens vesicle.

PHYSIOLOGY OF LENS

The lens has only one function. Their purposes is to converge rays from far as well as near on the retina. The former is called distant vision and the latter is called near vision. For these two functions, the lens must remain clear and be able to change its curvature reflexively to increase its refractive status. This is called accommodation, which is partly lenticular and partly neurological. Both are complimentary to each other; however, there is no accommodation in the absence of a lens in the presence of a normal neurological path, as happens in aphakia and pseudophakia. Accommodation is associated with convergence and miosis. All three are synergistic. The lens does not play any role in convergence or miosis.

For clear vision and proper focusing, the lens should be transparent and pliable.

Transparency is maintained by:

- Anatomical factors
- Biochemical factors
- *The anatomical factors responsible for lens transparency are:*
  - Absence of blood vessels in the lens. The lens is avascular and remains so all through life. No blood vessels grow in the lens at anytime during life. This is in contrast to the development of vessels in other avascular structures, i.e., the cornea and vitreous, where vascularization is common following infection, inflammation, trauma, and metabolic disorders.
  - There are no nerve fibers in the lens.

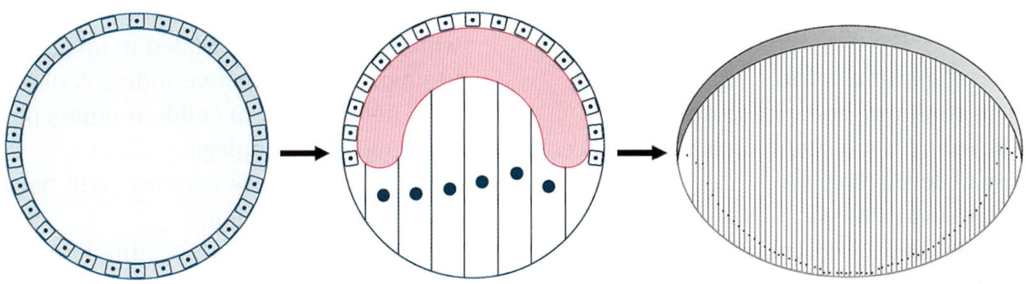

Fig. 19.12: Development of primary lens fibers.

    - The nuclei of the lens fibers are almost transparent and shifted on the periphery.
    - The lens fibers are compactly arranged without any space in between.
    - The lens capsule is semipermeable.
    - The lens is immersed in aqueous from which it gets its nutrition. The aqueous is rich in glucose with a low oxygen content.
    - The contact of aqueous is most marked with the anterior lens capsule.
    - Most of the transport of nutrition happens at the lens epithelium.
    - The normal lens neither allows aqueous to enter its substance nor allows the intracapsular content to leak into the aqueous. However, it allows nutrients to enter the lens and waste products to exit.
- *The biochemical factors responsible for lens transparency are:*
    - The lens is relatively dehydrated in normal life, its water content is 65%, and the rest is mostly protein.
    - Its oxygen content is also low; it is always in a state of relative hypoxia.
    - The lens requires a continuous supply of energy for active transport of:
        - Ions
        - Amino acids
    - The transport of ions takes place mostly in the lens epithelium.
    - The lens metabolism can be aerobic or anaerobic.
    - 80% of glucose is metabolized anaerobically.
    - The aerobic cycle is very small. It consists of a tricarboxylic cycle.
    - The anaerobic path is glycolytic path.
    - Glucose is converted to pentose and nicotinamide adenosine dinucleotide phosphate (NADPH).
    - Then, part of the glucose is reduced to sorbitol and gluconic acid.
    - The lens protein is mostly soluble and is called crystallins. They can be α, β, and γ in nature.
    - Any derangement in the above biochemical changes can lead to a loss of transparency in the lens.

Some peculiarities of the human lens:

- It continues to grow from gestation to death.
- It does not have any blood supply after birth; hence, it is not capable of developing:
    - Hemorrhage in it or bleed
    - It does not develop an infection.
    - It is not inflamed.
- It has no dystrophy.
- It does not develop any new growth.
- No secondaries are deposited in it.
- It is not capable of movement, but its curvature changes during accommodation.
- It does not have any nerve supply; so, it has no pain sensation.
- Its refractive index is 1.39, and its total power is +17 D.
- Its accommodating power varies between +16 D at birth and +1 D to +2 D at 50 years.
- Its capsule is the thickest basement membrane in the body.
- Size wise its protein concentration is highest in the body.
- The protein in a normal lens is soluble.
- The only pathological change seen in the lens is loss of its transparency. This is called a cataract.

Symptoms of Disorder of Lens (in All Ages)

The symptoms of disorders of the lens are:

- Visual
- Nonvisual

The only nonvisual symptoms with which a child is brought for examination are changes in the color of the lens, i.e., whiteness in the pupil. This loss of transparency is the cause of visual symptoms. The mother may be the first to notice the presence of congenital cataracts in an infant. This observation should be taken seriously because it can be as benign as a cataract or a malignancy, i.e., retinoblastoma. The first is the cause of amblyopia, and the second is life-threatening.

- There is no visual symptom if the opacity is not in the visual axis.
- Diminished distant vision occurs when the opacity is in the visual axis. Nearer the opacity to the nodal point, more the loss of vision. A posterior polar opacity causes more loss of vision than a nuclear opacity of the same size; an anterior polar opacity may not cause any loss of vision despite being on the visual axis unless the pupil constricts on it.
- Changes in near vision can be due to presbyopia, which is not directly related to opacity in the lens but to changes in refractive index. A near vision defect does not manifest in children unless produced by the instillation of cycloplegic.
- An eye with mature cataracts will have loss of both distant and near vision.
- Improvement in near vision happens in central nuclear sclerosis, which pushes the refraction toward

index myopia. So, the patient's presbyopic correction is neutralized, and the patient has better vision without near addition. This is called second sight.

- Central nuclear sclerosis also enhances myopic refraction. This causes diminished distant vision but can be corrected by minus lenses for some time.
- Diminished vision in bright light can happen in central nuclear, posterior capsular, and posterior polar cataracts as the pupil constricts in bright light and the opacity obstructs the available light. These patients have difficulty in night driving and vision in open spaces. They have better vision in twilight or when light falls on the object.
- *Everything looks in multiples:* This is also called uniocular diplopia. This is more marked in relatively bright objects on a dark background, like a crescent moon or streetlights.
- Colored halos are seen due to the accumulation of fluid in lens fibers in immature cataracts. This should be differentiated from colored halos or narrow-angled glaucoma.
- Pain, redness, and watering are absent in usual cataracts. The presence of any or all may cause the onset of secondary glaucoma or lens-induced uveitis, both of which are emergencies.

DISEASES OF LENS

It has been discussed earlier that the lens is not capable of getting infection, inflammation, neoplasm, or dystrophy. All the changes in the lens are physiochemical in the form of altered shape, size, position, and transparency. Out of these, loss of transparency is the most frequent and is called a cataract.

Thus, the disorders of lens in children can be:

- Congenital anomalies of the lens **(*See* Chapters 1 and 2)**
- Loss of accommodation (cycloplegia)
- Loss of transparency—cataracts—congenital and acquired
- *Effect of trauma:* Traumatic cataract.

CONGENITAL ANOMALIES OF TRANSPARENCY OF LENS

A congenital anomaly of the transparency of the lens is the most common disorder of the lens in children. It is more common than the morphological or topographic anomalies discussed earlier; loss of transparency of the lens is called a cataract. Opacities in the lens, i.e., capsular, cortical, or nuclear, are all referred to as cataracts. They may be as small as a single dot or may be multiple dots, and they may involve all the parts of the lens from capsule to capsule and center to equator all-round.

The opacities present at birth are called congenital and those appearing in the first year or later but not after puberty are called developmental.

Congenital cataracts may increase in size, except for opacities developing in embryonal and fetal nuclei. Fibers laid down after opacification of embryonal or fetal nuclei remain transparent. The opacities thus formed are not known to change in size; many times, it is difficult to differentiate between the two. About one-third of congenital and developmental cataracts are hereditary, 50% are sporadic in rest and no cause can be determined. **Flowchart 19.1** depicts an outline of the probable causes of congenital cataracts in children.

The causes can either be in the mother or in the fetus.

Flowchart 19.1: Maternal and fetal causes of congenital cataracts.

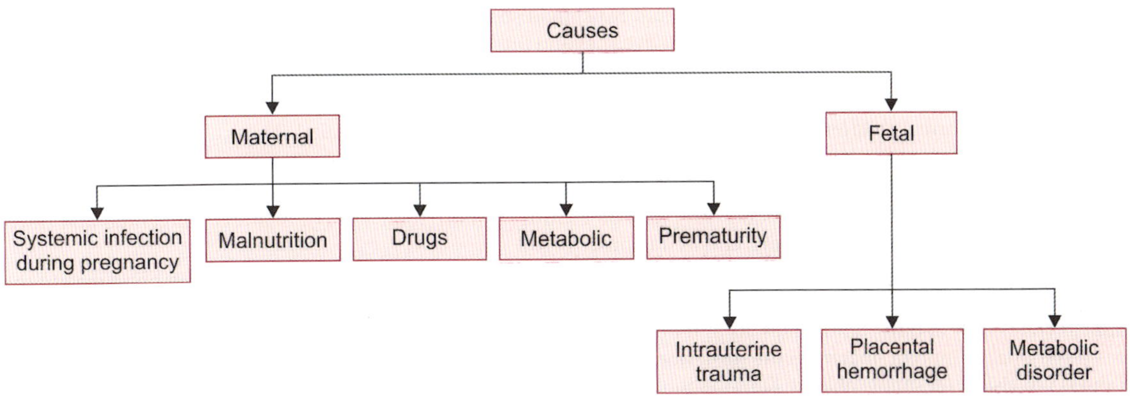

Flowchart 19.1 gives probable cause of true and developmental cataracts.

PREDISPOSING FACTORS

Genetics seems to have an important role. About 10–30% of the cases show hereditary tendencies. The congenital cataracts are mostly autosomal dominant. Many of the congenital cataracts can be traced to chromosomal anomalies.

Maternal factors play an important part in causing congenital cataracts.

They can be:

- *Maternal infection:*
  - *Viral:* Rubella, rubeola, cytomegalovirus, herpes simplex, and herpes zoster
  - *Bacterial:* Syphilis
  - *Parasitic:* Toxoplasmosis

  Out of all maternal infections, rubella is the most important infection because it not only causes bilateral cataracts but also multiocular and systemic congenital anomalies. The encouraging part of the disease is that it is fully preventable if the mother is immunized in her childhood. Maternal rubella contracted during the first trimester is most likely to cause congenital anomalies. This makes it mandatory for every female child to be immunized against rubella between 9 and 12 months.
- *Placental anomaly:* This leads to hypoxia in the developing fetus.
- *Maternal malnutrition:* Especially vitamin D deficiency.
- *Drugs:* Many drugs are best avoided during the first trimester.
- *Metabolic errors in mother:* There are many metabolic disorders that cause congenital cataracts. The main among them are galactosemia, hyperparathyroidism, hyperglycemia, and hypoglycemia. Out of these galactosemia* is most common metabolic disorder that causes congenital cataract, making urine examinations for reducing substances compulsory in all congenital and developmental cataracts.

Chromosomal anomalies that are associated with congenital cataracts are Down syndrome† and Edward syndrome§

Ocular anomalies associated with congenital and developmental cataracts are coloboma of the anterior uvea, coloboma of the lens, microspherophakia, lenticonus, ectopia lentis, Peters anomaly, and Rieger anomaly, and Mittendorf's dot.**

Figure 19.13 shows the topography of various congenital opacities of the lens.

Peculiarities of congenital cataract:

- Only a few of them are preventable (Rubella).
- The exact cause of congenital cataract is not well understood.
- In about half of the cases, no cause can be definitely attributed.

**Galactosemia* is an inborn error of galactose metabolism. The cataracts are not present at birth but become evident within a few months as oil droplet opacity in the fetal nucleus. It is common for babies to be fed milk products that contain disaccharides. These patients have a tendency for growth retardation, hepatic dysfunction, and mental retardation. Avoiding mammalian milk products reduces the chance of complications and retards the density of the cataract, but it does not cure the cataract fully.

†*Down syndrome:* It is also known as Trisomy 21 and is a chromosomal disorder seen in both boys and girls. In 95% of cases, it is sporadic and seems to be related to the age of the mother at the time of the child's birth. In the general population, it occurs in children born to mothers over 30 years of age. The incidence of the syndrome is 1 in 1,500 live births; that rises to 1 in 50 if the mother is in her late forties; it is more common in elderly primi. The child has a distinct facial appearance with a small head, a broad nose bridge, an epicanthic fold, and an upslant of the interpalpebral aperture. The systemic conditions consist of increased birth weight, hypotonia, mental and growth retardation, dysthyroid status, and cardiac anomalies. Recurrent systemic infection, short life span, and ocular feature are squint, high astigmatic error, poor accommodation, keratoconus, and Brushfield spot‡ on the iris. 15% of the children with Down syndrome have either congenital or developmental cataracts; if the child survives beyond the fourth decade, they may develop presenile cataracts.

‡*Brushfield spots on the iris:* These are small grey to frank white, small nodules of doubtful origin; some authors believe them to be collections of connective tissue, found on the anterior surface of the iris, arranged all around the pupillary border; they are harmless and nonspecific; rarely, they may be seen in normal children as well. They are more frequent in eyes with congenital cataracts than without.

§*Edward syndrome:* Ii is also known as trisomy 18, it is less common than Down syndrome. Children with Edward syndrome have a very short life span. Most of them die before 5 years. The facial appearance resembles that of Down syndrome. The common ocular manifestations consist of bilateral ptosis, epicanthic fold, pseudoesotropia, true esotropia (more than 40 PD), bilateral congenital and developmental cataracts, hypoplasia of the optic nerve, amblyopia, and nystagmus.

***Mittendorf's dot:* It is an embryological remnant of the hyaloid artery. The hyaloid artery extends from the optic disc to the posterior surface of the tunica vasculosa lentis, which is the source of nutrition to the developing lens up to the 60 mm stage. The tunica vasculosa should disappear completely at birth. Sometimes, its anterior part fails to disappear and remains attached to the posterior pole of the lens, which causes a stationary pinpoint opacity in the posterior pole, known as Mittendorf's dots **(Fig. 19.13)**. It generally does not interfere with vision and is not visible on simple oblique illumination. It becomes evident during routine retinoscopy or ophthalmoscopy. It does not require any treatment.

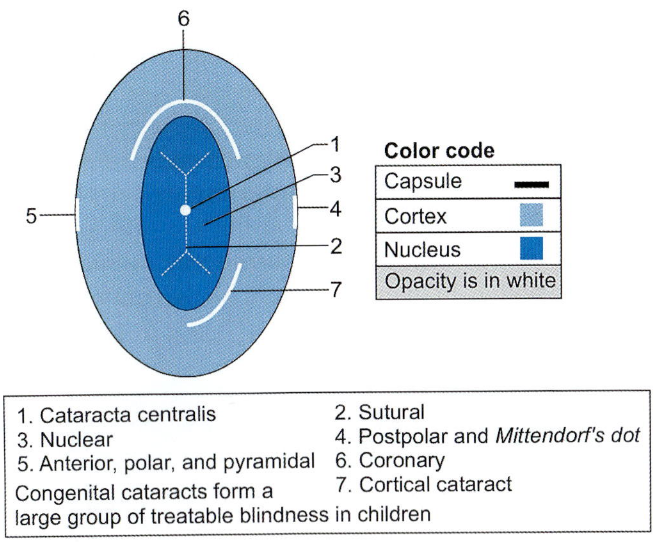

Fig. 19.13: Topography of some of the common congenital cataracts.

- Most probably, congenital cataracts are multifactorial in origin.
- Congenital cataracts may be present at birth or develop after birth.
- Any opacity present at birth is a true congenital cataract.
- A cataract developing between birth and puberty is called a developmental cataract.
- Many of the predisposing factors are common in both, except in traumatic and secondary cataracts. The predisposing factor may act singly or in combination.
- Congenital cataracts are treatable (surgery, optical).
- In some, progress can be arrested (galactosemia).
- There is no medical treatment for congenital cataract.
- About 10–30% are hereditary.
- The only symptom of congenital cataract is diminished vision.
- All cataracts do not reduce vision; only opacity in the visual axis causes diminished vision. Opacity near the nodal point causes more loss of vision; opacity in the anterior pole rarely causes diminished vision unless the pupil is a constrictor. Opacity larger than 3 mm on the posterior pole causes maximum loss of vision.
- Cataracts larger than pupils are visible on oblique illumination.
- Microsurgery, with or without IOL, is the definitive treatment of congenital and developmental cataracts.
- All tests required to confirm benignness of the white reflex in the pupillary area should be employed to exclude retinoblastoma.
- Only those that interfere with vision require treatment.
- They may be true congenital, i.e., present at birth. Opacities <7.5 mm are prenatal; opacities >7.5 mm are considered to be developmental.
- They can be capsular, cortical, or nuclear, separately or in combination.
- They can be bilateral, symmetric, or asymmetric.
- When unilateral, the other eye should be examined under full dilatation for subtle changes in the apparently normal eye.
- Uniocular congenital cataracts carry a poor prognosis.
- In 50% of the cases, no cause can be found.
- Causes can be in the mother or the fetus.
- Rubella cataracts can be fully prevented if the mother is immunized before pregnancy.
- Visually significant cataracts should be removed as early as possible.
- Unilateral visually significant cataract requires urgent intervention, i.e., it should be operated on within a few weeks of birth with the best optical correction.
- Bilateral dense cataracts require removal and visual correction within the first 6 weeks of birth.
- It is better not to operate both the eyes in same sitting.
- Rubella cataracts are highly prone to postoperative severe uveitis.
- Postoperative, vigorous antiuveitis treatment with cycloplegics and steroids for months is a must for all operated cases of congenital cataracts.
- 100% congenital cataracts will develop posterior capsular opacity unless posterior capsulorrhexis and anterior vitrectomy is done along with the primary procedure.
- The onset of nystagmus and amblyopia are bad omens.

CLASSIFICATION OF CONGENITAL CATARACT

Due to the wide fluctuation in parameters like etiology, location, density, and association with other ocular and systemic disorders, it is not possible to have a very satisfactory classification of congenital cataracts. The older classification was to divide them as capsular and lenticular, which did not take into consideration various types of nuclear opacities with or without cortical involvement **(Flowchart 19.2)**.

Flowchart 19.2 depicts types of congenital and developmental cataracts.

Congenital and developmental cataracts can be localized or generalized. **Flowchart 19.3** shows various possibilities.

A better option is to divide congenital cataracts as follows:

- Capsular:
  - Anterior capsular
  - Posterior capsular
- Cortical:
  - Coronary **(Fig. 19.14)**
  - Blue dot
  - Sutural
- Capsulocortical—reduplication cataract
- Nuclear:
  - Rubella
  - Galactosemia
  - Centralis pulverulenta
- Nucleocortical—lamellar

Flowchart 19.2: Types of congenital and developmental cataracts.

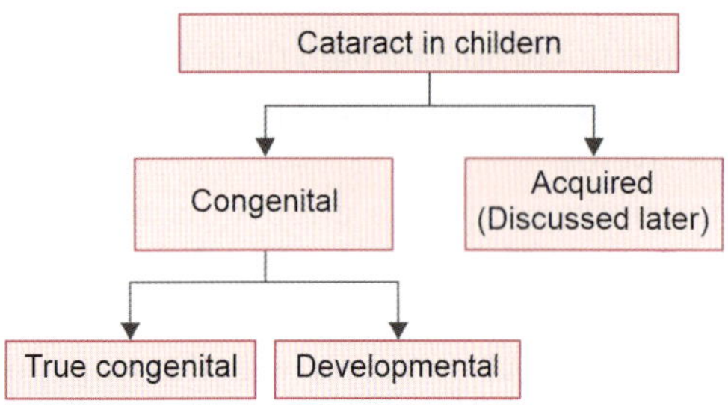

The other classification in vogue is:

- True congenital versus developmental cataract

A true congenital cataract is axial, situated either in the embryonic or fetal nucleus, and is <5.75 mm in diameter.

- *Depending on location:* Central versus peripheral—central opacities situated near the posterior pole are more symptomatic while peripheral cataracts not encroaching upon the visual axis may go unnoticed.

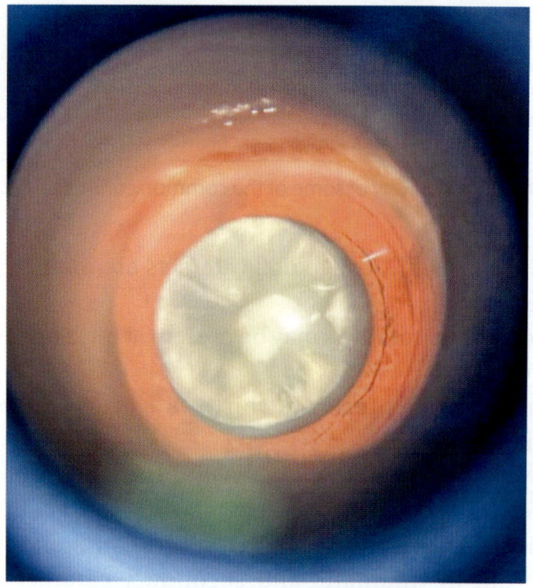

Fig. 19.14: Coronary cataract.
Courtesy: Dr Yamini and Dr Nidhi Pandey.

Flowchart 19.3: Expanded classification of congenital cataracts.

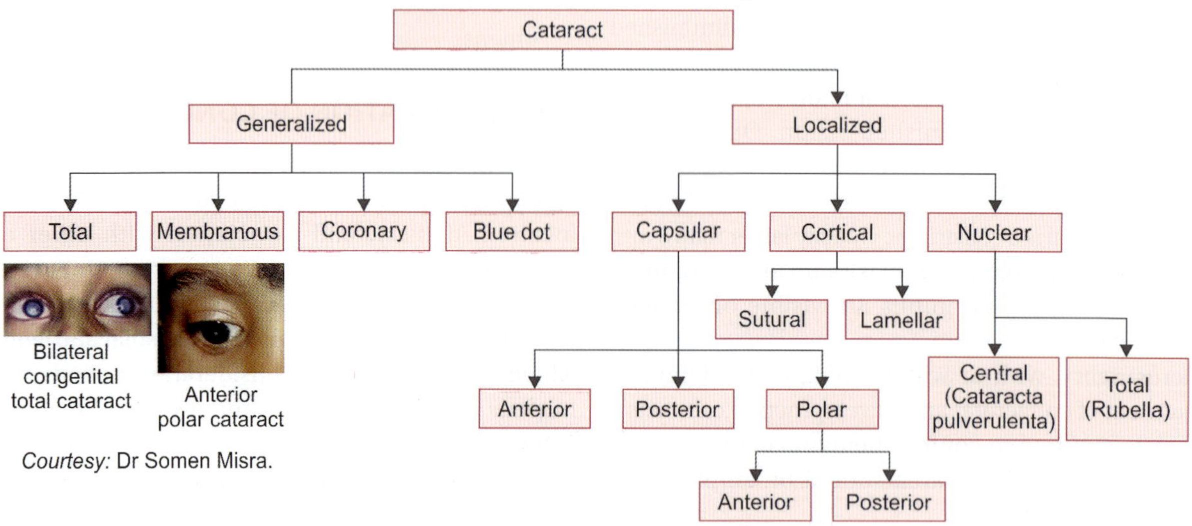

- *Complete versus partial:* Complete cataracts need surgical intervention within 2 months of birth.
- Associated with disorders:
  - Local congenital anomalies:
    - Uveal coloboma
    - Subluxation of lens
    - Microspherophakia
    - Coloboma of the lens
    - Persistent hyperplastic primary vitreous
  - Systemic anomalies:
    - Marfan syndrome
    - Marchesani syndrome
    - Homocystinuria
    - Peters anomaly
    - Reiger anomaly
    - Treacher Collins syndrome
    - Down syndrome
  - Metabolic disorders:
    - Galactosemia
    - Diabetes
    - Hypocalcemia

SYMPTOMS OF CATARACT IN CHILDREN

> Opacities situated at different depths, position, and densities have different presentation.

The common symptoms are:

- *Nil:* Opacities away from the visual axis are symptomless; hence, they may go unnoticed.
- *Symptomatic:*
  - *Visible opacity:* Opacity larger than a normal pupil attracts attention early. Opacities may be discovered during routine refraction and fundus examinations.
  - *Visual:* Opacities in the anteroposterior axis cause early and more visual loss. Out of all axial opacities, those in the posterior pole cause more loss of vision, in spite of their small size, because they are on or near the nodal point, followed by posterior subcapsular opacities. Vision with posterior polar cataract may improve by dilatation of the pupil, either physiological (i.e., twilight) or pharmacological (by use of mydriatic, posterior capsular opacities larger than posterior polar cataract), which too causes disproportionate loss of vision. Due to their large size, they do not gain vision by physiological dilatation but may gain vision following wide dilatation by strong mydriatic. Opacities away from the nodal point do not cause much loss of vision unless the pupil is small enough to be obscured by the opacities; scattered opacities like blue-dot cataracts do not interfere with vision and peripheral cortical cataracts may also not interfere with vision. They may be discovered in mydriasis.
  - *Complications of diminished vision:* Squint, amblyopia, and nystagmus in various combinations.
  - *Parents of infants* with a history of childhood cataracts in the family may bring the child suspecting that the child may have a cataract.

CLINICAL PRESENTATION OF SOME COMMON CONGENITAL CATARACTS

Anterior polar cataract: These are generally bilateral, situated on the anterior pole of the lens, in the middle of the pupil, are of pinhead size, and may require magnification and bright illumination to be visible. Otherwise, they may be in the form of a plaque; rarely, there are many plaques deposited over one another in the form of a cone. Such a condition is called a pyramidal cataract.

> Bilateral anterior polar cataract with nystagmus in a child is always due to bilateral perforation of the cornea following gonococcal ophthalmia neonatorum. As the opacity does not cause any visual symptoms, it does not require any treatment.

Simple (flat opacities): These are small opacities in the epithelium of the lens without encroaching on the cortex. The exact cause of the opacity is not well understood and may be associated with remnants of the central part of persistent pupillary membranes. May be small enough only to be picked up by the high power of the slit lamp. They are smaller than the constricted pupil and away from the nodal point. They do not interfere with vision and do not progress; hence, they do not require any treatment.

Pyramidal cataracts [projection in anterior chamber *(AC)]* ***(Fig. 19.15)****:* Due to their conical shape, they are called pyramidal. They are generally bilateral and symmetric, with a circular base at the anterior pole and a pointed apex in the AC. The exact cause is not known; it could be genetics (autosomal dominant). They are sometimes associated with reduplicated cataracts. Still, rarely, a third opacity larger than the second may also be found. That may have a circular opacity a little deeper; the size of the second opacity may be the same as the first or may be slightly larger. Occasionally, the two adjacent opacities

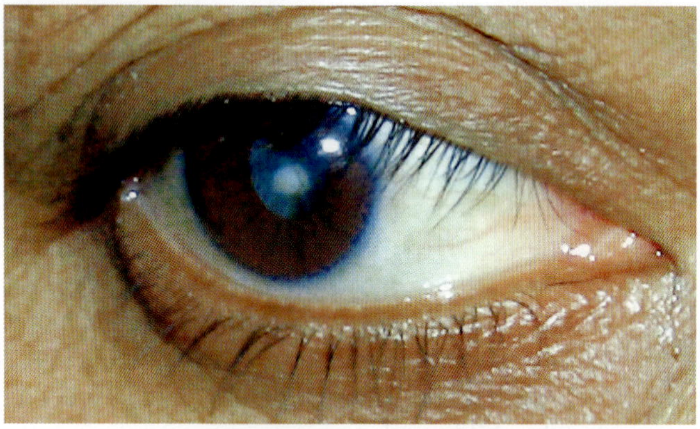

Fig. 19.15: Pyramidal cataract.

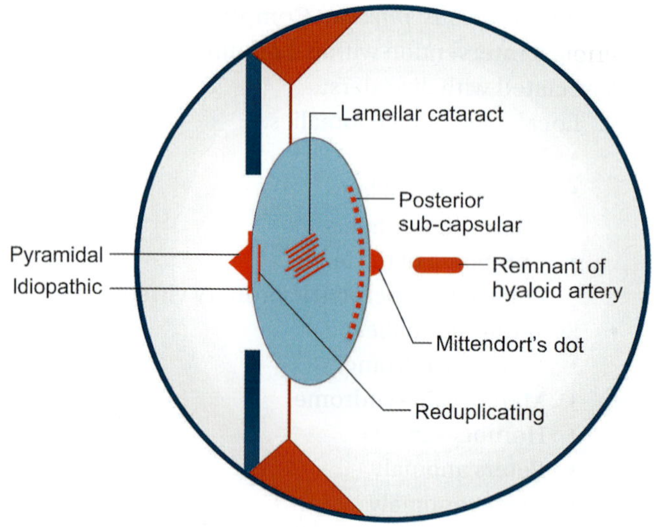

Fig. 19.16: Various lenticular and extra lenticular lesions that produce a black shadow on retinoscopy (keratoconus and posterior lenticonus have not been shown).

are joined by an isthmus. The projecting cone is composed of hyaline material. The pyramid may get dislocated in the AC and mistaken for a foreign body in the AC; this generally used to happen during needling, where the cortical matter got absorbed following needling but not the core of the pyramid, which required to be removed separately. The opacity does not diminish vision unless the pupil is constricted, which may hamper vision in bright light. The condition does not require any treatment unless the cortex behind it gets opacified. Children with pyramidal cataracts develop age-related cataracts earlier.

Another anterior polar cataract that is neither congenital nor developmental is a central opacity acquired following perforation of a central corneal ulcer in the first few days of birth due to mismanaged gonococcal ophthalmia neonatorum. Mechanisms of production of acquired anterior polar opacity are as follows: Small central perforation → leak of aqueous → collapse of AC occlusion of perforation → reformation of AC → central leukoma → anterior polar cataract. They are generally bilateral. The eyes soon develop nystagmus that lasts for life.

> The triad of bilateral central corneal opacity, bilateral anterior polar cataract, and nystagmus in an adults should always be considered to be sequel of gonococcal ophthalmia neonatorum.

POSTERIOR POLAR AND POSTERIOR SUBCAPSULAR OPACITY

Posterior polar and posterior subcapsular opacities are as common as their anterior counterparts. There are two types of posterior polar opacities: (1) Mittendorf's dot (described earlier) and (2) posterior capsular opacity.

All posterior polar cataracts produce black shadow in pink retinal glow on retinoscopy.

The following is a list of conditions that produced black shadow (cataractous as well as noncataractous in all ages).

*Conditions that produce black shadow in pink glow **(Fig. 19.16)**:*

- Anterior polar cataract
- Pyramidal cataract
- Reduplicating cataract
- Posterior polar cataract
- Posterior subcapsular cataract
- Mittendorf's dot
- Posterior lenticonus
- Remnant of hyaloid artery
- Apex of keratoconus
- Dens lamellar cataract
- Localized after cataract
- Central cataracta pulverulenta

POSTERIOR POLAR CATARACT

There are two forms; the first is not exactly due to an error in the development of the lens. It is due to the remnant of the anterior part of the hyaloid vessel attached to the posterior capsule. This is called Mittendorf's dot (described earlier). Sometimes a tag of vessels may be seen protruding in the vitreous. The second is a less common posterior polar cataract due to localized thickening of the posterior capsule.

Both the conditions are axial and on the nodal point, hence cause severe loss of vision. Unfortunately, such opacities are discovered late, causing nystagmus and squint. The most common mode of their discovery is routine retinoscopy/ophthalmoscopy in a child brought with nystagmus and squint, which are already too late to correct.

NUCLEOCORTICAL CATARACTS

Lamellar Cataract

Lamellar cataract is often referred to as zonular or perinuclear cataract as well.

This is a congenital lenticular opacity that involves only a particular zone of nucleus, laid down at a fixed period of gestation. Fiber developing before and after the episode remains clear. Earlier, it develops smaller and it is denser. This is the most common form of congenital cataract, accounting for half of all congenital cataracts. It is generally bilateral and may not be symmetric. It does not increase in size once formed. Most of the lamellar cataracts are hereditary; siblings too may have them in various shapes and densities. The opacity may be dense enough to be detected at birth. The most common presentation is diminished variable vision, which brings the child to examination. On examination, the distant vision is reduced, which does not improve with pinhole, may even diminish. Vision may improve with dilatation. There are no anomalies of the eye that may be correlated to the lamellar cataract; on retinoscopy, it stands out as a dork dot or a blotch in the middle of the pink glow **(Figs. 19.17 to 19.20)**.

On slit-lamp examination, the cataractous disc has a rough surface with variable transparency; the anterior surface often shows ridges radiating from the center to the edge of the circular opacity; the border of the opacity is not clear cut. From the periphery of the opacity, arise opaque spikes, radiating toward the periphery in variable numbers and are called riders.

Like other congenital cataracts, the cause of the defect is elusive. The most common factor may be its hereditary predisposition; the second factor may be vitamin D

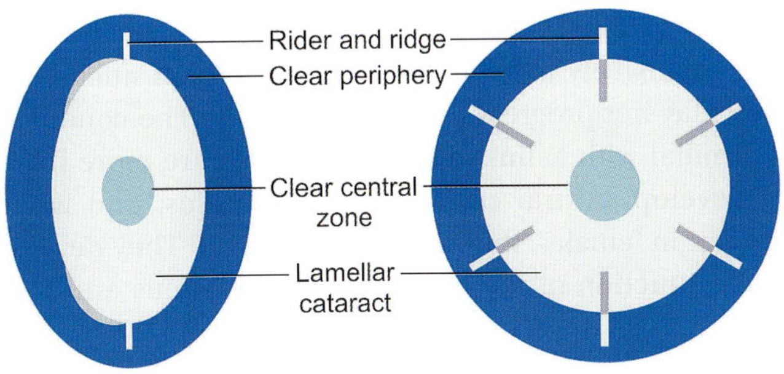

Fig. 19.17: Two views of lamellar cataract.

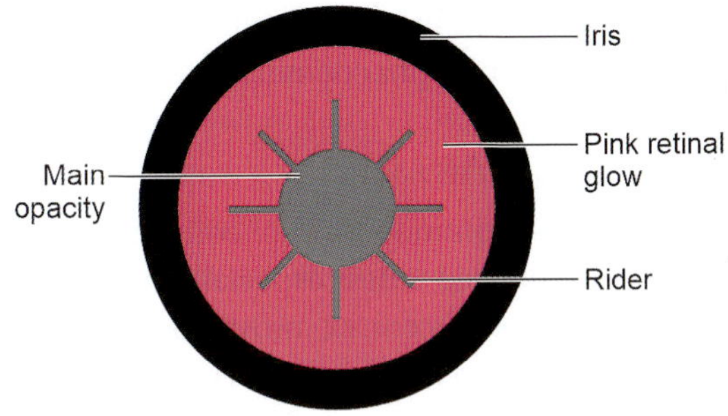

Fig. 19.18: Lamellar cataract in retroillumination.

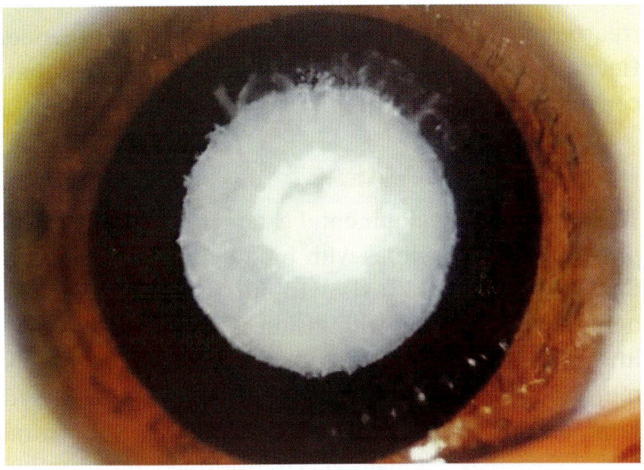

Fig. 19.19: Lamellar cataract.
Source: T Shiva Sankar (IJO 68-07-2020).
Courtesy: Dr Santosh G Honavar, editor, Indian Journal of Ophthalmology (IJO).

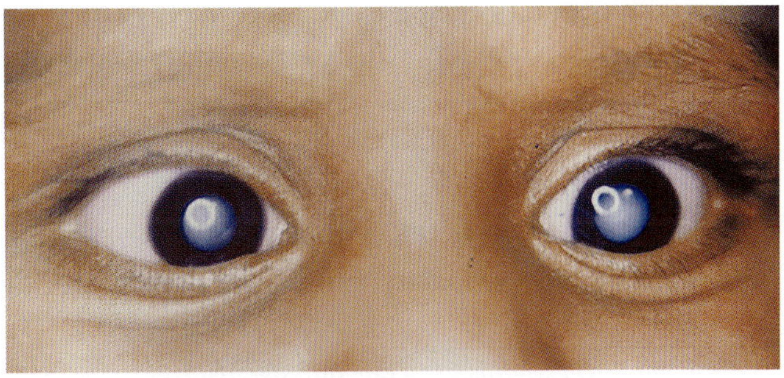

Fig. 19.20: Bilateral lamellar cataract.
Courtesy: Dr Somen Misra.

deficiency in the mother; and the third is maternal rubella during the first trimester. This is more logical because the development of opacity is concurrent with rubella. Unfortunately, this condition does not always give a positive TORCH [toxoplasmosis, rubella cytomegalovirus, herpes simplex, and human immunodeficiency virus (HIV)] result; generally, it is performed to exclude rubella (see rubella cataract below). The opacity manifests in the first 8 years of a child's life and requires early treatment. The definite treatment is phacoemulsification with IOL.

BLUE DOT CATARACT

These are the most common form of congenital opacities, but they are least noticed unless especially looked for. They are scattered all over the cortex, mostly on the periphery as tiny blue pin-point reflective dots. They are fixed in the cortex. The cause is not known. They are asymptomatic and diagnosed on routine slit-lamp examination, fundus examination, or retinoscopy. They do not require any treatment. They generally develop in adolescence. Hence, it is better to call them developmental rather than congenital.

CORONARY CATARACT

These are also developmental cataracts that manifest at puberty as opaque lines with broad club-shaped heads directed toward the axis without reaching the axis, hence not interfering with vision. They become visible in mydriasis and are seen as black lines against a pink retinoscopy glow. Technically, they may be considered forms of lamellar cataract involving the cortex. The central end of the streak gradually gets transformed into rounded clubs. The opacity due to their shape is called the corona. As they develop on the periphery and do not cause much visual disturbance, the patient may be unaware of their presence. The opacity becomes visible in mydriasis. Lenses with coronary cataracts are more likely to develop presenile cortical cataracts, which may hamper vision and need to be operated on.

CORALLIFORM CATARACT

These are relatively rare. They look like spikes radiating from a central dense opacity, mostly in anteroposterior direction. They look like lumps of coral. They have a strong autosomal dominant trait. They may reduce vision, requiring early management.

CATARACTA CENTRALIS PULVERULENTA (POWDERY CATARACT)

They are true congenital cataracts, developing during the first few weeks of the lens's development; hence, they are situated in the earliest nucleus, i.e., the embryonic nucleus, which is the smallest and most stationary. These are generally bilateral, manifesting as oval lumps of white powder granules. In spite of being central, loss of vision is not very marked.

TOTAL NUCLEAR CATARACT

Total nuclear cataracts may be considered a larger form of cataracta centralis pulverulenta. They too are bilaterally nonprogressive and generally involve not only the embryonic but also the fetal nucleus, and rarely, infantile nuclear. They cause diminished vision in bright light, causing great inconvenience to the child. Hence, it requires early management. The common causes of total congenital nuclear cataracts are rubella and galactosemia; they can be idiopathic as well.

CONGENITAL MEMBRANOUS CATARACT

This is a rare condition, often mistaken for congenital aphakia, which by itself is rarer. Due to some ill-understood causes, the developing cortex and nuclei get absorbed, leaving the posterior capsule, part of the anterior capsule, and a few strands of opaque lens fibers unabsorbed. Intra-uterine trauma has been attributed to a cause that has not been confirmed. It may be part of Hallermann–Streiff syndrome (HSS)*.

SUTURAL CATARACT

Sutural cataracts are congenital opacities of the lens that exclusively involve Y suture of the fetal nucleolus; they may not progress or progress slowly. The condition is familial with X-linked heritage; males are more likely to develop sutural cataracts than females, and when present in females, they are less significant. They develop at the junction of the closure of fetal nucleus and may

**Hallermann–Streiff syndrome* is a rare disorder that consists of malformations of the skull and face (craniofacial), sparse hair (hypotrichosis), eye abnormalities, dental defects, degenerative skin changes, and short stature. The ocular features are congenital cataract and congenital corneal opacity.

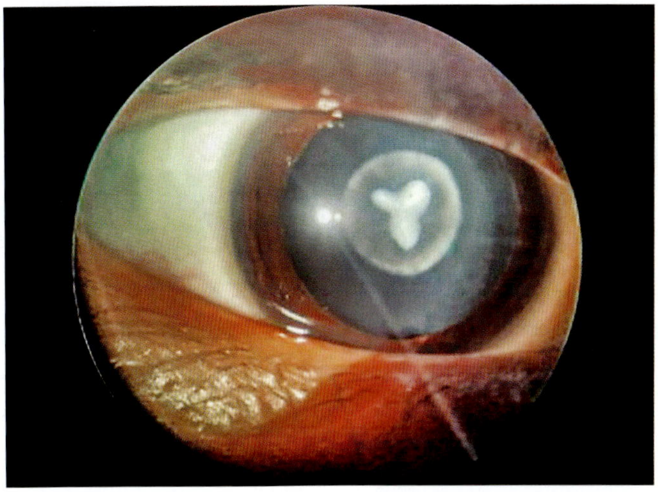

Fig. 19.21: Sutural cataract.
Courtesy: Dr Yamini and Dr Nidhi Pandey.

be anterior or posterior; sometimes both sutures are involved. The anterior suture has an appearance of alphabet Y, and the posterior suture is inverted Y as the opacity is stationary. Without causing diminished vision, it does not require any treatment except for the error of refraction **(Fig. 19.21)**.

RUBELLA CATARACT

The most common example of total congenital cataract is rubella cataract, due to an infection contracted in the first trimester. Its incidence may be as high as one-fifth of all congenital cataracts. The opacity starts in the earliest nucleus, i.e., the embryonal nucleus. Rubella acquired by the mother after the first trimester has far less chance of causing cataracts. In the first trimester, 50% of eyes will be affected, in the second trimester, it is 30%, and then the incident drops to 10–15%. Subsequent pregnancies are not affected by maternal rubella. The eyes are affected in the first trimester, but other organs are affected by rubella in different periods of gestation, independent of ocular involvement.

RUBELLA VIRUS

The rubella virus is a *ribonucleic acid (RNA)*-toga virus. As it is wrapped in a lipid covering, it is called a toga virus. The virus is a single-stranded virus and is teratogenic. The infection is seen worldwide, and the risk of contracting it lurks throughout the year for both sexes of all ages. The incidents are less in infants; the incidence declines after the fourth decade. Epidemics are known to have broken out among nonimmunized males as well. The disease is fully preventable by a vaccine given at 12 months and repeated when the children enter school, giving them lifelong immunity.

RUBELLA VACCINE

The vaccine is available in combination with measles and mumps under the national program of immunization. The vaccine imparts 90% immunity. The vaccine is ineffective once viremia has set in. All women planning pregnancy should be tested for rubella antibodies. Antibody-positive women can go for pregnancy; otherwise, they should get themselves vaccinated and wait for 3 months to plan a pregnancy. The vaccine is a live-disabled virus; hence, persons with congenital or acquired immunosuppression should not get the rubella vaccine. The rubella vaccine itself is toxic to the fetus; hence, it should not be administered to pregnant women. All children should be immunized at 12 months; this is followed by another booster shot on entering the school. Besides immunizing individual child, it imparts herd immunity to the population. Children of both the sexes should be immunized. Only immunizing girls has not been found to be an effective herd immunity tactic.

RUBELLA DISEASE IN WOMEN

The mother gets infection from not only frankly infected persons but also from asymptomatic carriers. The infection in the mother is self-limiting, lasting for <1 week. It is also known as 3-day measles or German measles. The incubation period ranges between 12 and 24 days. The infected mother is most contagious when the rashes are erupting; they are also contagious 1 week before and after the rashes develop. There is no drug that works against the rubella virus. The disease in the mother manifests as common cold with enlargement of the occipital lymph nodes.

The infection can be confirmed by:

- Presence of virus in saliva and blood
- Immunoglobulin G (IgG) is present in the blood in a rising titer at a gap of 2 weeks or the appearance of new IgM.

The commonly ordered *TORCH test* is a screening test not specific to rubella.

The term TORCH is an acronym for the following infections: Toxoplasmosis, rubella, cytomegalovirus, herpes simplex, and HIV.

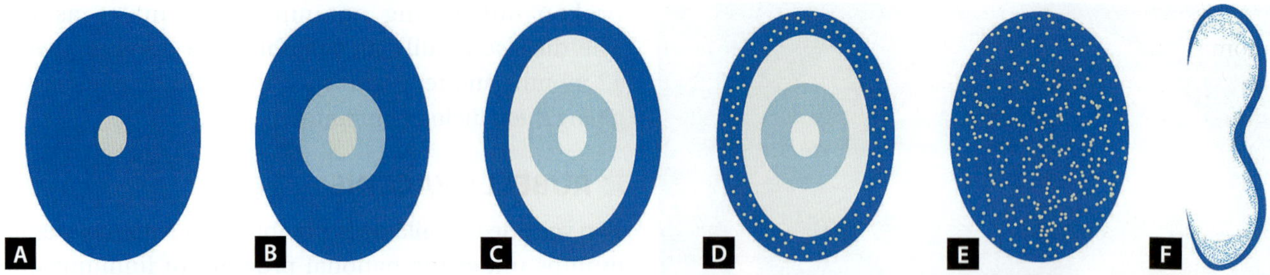

Figs. 19.22A to F: Various stages of rubella cataract. Involvement of: (A) Embryonal nucleus; (B) embryonal and fetal nucleus; (C) embryonal, fetal, and infantile nucleus; (D) involvement of embryonal, fetal, infantile nuclei and cortex; (E) liquefaction of cataract; and (F) membranous cataract.

The letter *O* in TORCH represents other diseases like syphilis and other viral infections.

The three organs most commonly involved in congenital malformations are: Eyes, ears, and heart. Other organs that may be involved are the skin and lymph nodes. It can cause: Pneumonitis, pancreatitis, panencephalitis, anemia, and thrombocytopenia.

The ocular involvements in congenital rubella are: Rubella cataract, aphakia, glaucoma, microphthalmos, rubella retinopathy, postoperative uveitis, transient corneal haze, squint, amblyopia, and nystagmus.

RUBELLA CATARACT

The rubella cataract starts in the first trimester as a small opacity in the embryonal nucleus and spreads to other nuclei and the cortex. The congenital rubella cataract is generally present at birth; it may remain stationary or increase in size and density. On rare occasions, the virus may remain dormant till birth with a clear lens and opacity developing weeks to months later again making it mandatory to exclude rubella in every case of congenital cataract.

The virus does not penetrate the lens capsule after 6 weeks of gestation; hence, the chances of infection reaching the lens are minimum thereafter. About half the fetuses of infected mothers are likely to develop congenital cataracts, mostly bilateral. The virus is known to survive in the lens for as long as 2–3 years after birth. The live virus in the lens may be liberated in aqueous following trauma, whether surgical or accidental, causing severe uveitis that should be anticipated and managed by vigorous and prolonged local steroids and strong cycloplegics. Failure to manage postoperative uveitis may result in permanent loss of the eye. Besides trauma, spontaneous leaks of cortical matter, along with viruses, are another cause of severe uveitis. After it leaks, the cataract is converted into a membranous cataract.

Figures 19.22A to F shows the natural history of the development of rubella cataracts.

Other ocular involvements in rubella are:

- *Glaucoma:* About 10% of eyes may have congenital or developmental glaucoma. It may or may not be associated with cataracts or microphthalmos. The etiopathology of congenital glaucoma in rubella is independent of cataract. The other causes of glaucoma in congenital rubella are intumescence of the lens, microphthalmos, viral uveitis, postoperative uveitis, and prolonged use of strong steroids and cycloplegic; all cases of congenital glaucoma should be investigated for the possibility of rubella as its cause.
- *Microphthalmos:* Microphthalmos is common in children affected by maternal rubella; it may be an isolated feature of associated with cataracts and glaucoma.
- *Retinopathy:* Retinopathy is frequently present in eyes affected by congenital rubella. It gives a pepper-salt appearance, like a mild form of retinitis pigmentosa, without diminished night vision. It is generally stationary and does not involve macula.
- Other ocular manifestations of maternal rubella are transient corneal haze, iris hypoplasia, squint, high error of refraction, nystagmus, and optic atrophy.
- *Rubella syndrome:* Rubella syndrome consists of the following triad: Ocular, auditory, and cardiac involvement. The auditory and cardiac involvements are independent of rubella cataract. However, it may exist with ocular involvement. The auditory defect is neurosensory due to a fault in organ of Corti. The cardiac involvement is present in 75% of cases with maternal rubella. The common cardiac anomalies

are patent ductus arteriosus, pulmonary artery anomaly, and ventricular septal defect. Less common systemic involvements are premature delivery, intrauterine growth retardation, underweight, anemia, thrombocytopenia, and hepatosplenomegaly.

Management of Rubella Cataracts

Rubella is a fully preventable systemic viral disease.

The ocular management consists of:

- Prophylaxis
- Management of cataracts, glaucoma, and postoperative uveitis
- Visual rehabilitation

These are described as follows:

- *Prophylaxis:* All children, irrespective of sex, should get a shot of MMR, i.e., measles, mumps, and rubella, at 12 months, and a booster shot, the booster commonly contains anti-Varicella factor also. The rubella vaccine itself is toxic to the developing fetus; hence, it is contraindicated in pregnancy.
- *Management of rubella cataracts:* Management of all congenital cataracts requires more expertise than adult cataracts. Rubella cataract is no exception. It has some peculiar features that require additional acumen due to the association of other ocular and systemic anomalies, poor anesthetic risk, and persistent postoperative inflammation.
    - *The ocular anomalies associated with rubella cataracts that require special attention are:* Microcornea, microphthalmos, shallow AC, poor mydriasis, membranous cataract, fluid cataract, and calcified anterior and posterior capsules. The association with glaucoma worsens the scenario. The presence of anomalies in the heart and lungs and their underweight make these infants prone to anesthetic and postanesthetic systemic complications. All bilateral cases should be operated on as soon as the child can undergo general anesthesia in two separate sittings.
    - *The parents should be counseled on the following points:*
        - Purpose of surgery
        - The requirement of prolonged mydriatic and steroid use may be for months to years following surgery.
        - Possibility of the development of glaucoma that may be both rubella- and/or steroid-induced
        - Chances of residual refraction following cataract surgery
        - 100% chance of posterior capsular opacity (PCO) that may require laser later.
    - The steps of surgery are the same as in any other congenital cataract. The pupil should be dilated with atropine; if required, a combination of two mydriatics may be used. The capsulorhexis should be generous, and as much as of the cortical matter should be removed. A posterior capsulotomy with an anterior vitrectomy is mandatory. Glaucoma, when present, requires separate medical and/or surgical management.
- *Visual rehabilitation:* (As per the requirements of the child, i.e., aphakia/pseudophakia.)

GALACTOSEMIC CATARACT

Galactosemic cataract is a rare inborn error of carbohydrate metabolism.

Galactose is a monosaccharide; it is an isomer of glucose. It gives a positive test for reducing substances in urine. Hence, all children with positive reducing substances in their urine should be investigated for galactosemia. Galactose is formed along with glucose by the hydrolysis of lactose. It is converted to glucose and stored as glycogen in the liver. Lactose, which is a milk sugar, plays an important role in its metabolism. It requires three specific enzymes in its metabolism: (1) Transferase, (2) galactokinase, and (3) epimerase.

The disorder is brought about by the absence of any of these enzymes; deficiency of transferase is the most common and that of epimerase is least. Accumulation of galactose in the serum leads to the metabolic disorder of galactosemia, an analog of diabetes, with normal glucose metabolism. Galactose is absorbed in the gut and converted to glucose and glycogen in the presence of lactose. In the absence of a specific enzyme, it is converted to galactitol or sugar alcohol, the toxic substance responsible for the clinical picture of galactosemia. Once galactitol rises beyond the threshold, the disorder sets in. Galactose, as a separate entity, is not available for consumption as it does not have any use in the body. In contrast to this, lactose is present in all mammalian milk, the exclusion of galactose from a child's feed reduces the signs and symptoms of galactosemia but does not eliminate it. Transferase deficiency is so common cause of galactosemia that it is called classical galactosemia. Only a few cases of epimerase deficiency have been reported so far.

Classical galactosemia has two components:

1. Systemic
2. Ocular

- The *systemic* changes are pretty serious and, if missed, may be life-threatening. The child fails to gain weight and has repeated unexplained diarrhea, vomiting, hepatosplenomegaly, jaundice, anemia, and aciduria.
- The ocular involvement is exclusively galactosemic cataract. 75% of infants with galactosemia have cataracts either at birth or become evident in the first few months. The galactosemic cataracts are bilateral and symmetric. They are central involving infantile nucleus; due to their peculiar shape, they are called oil droplet cataracts. The first change may occasionally be mistaken and posterior lenticonus, or zonular cataract with a clear cortex all around, soon, spills all over parts of the cortex, turning into a complete cataract. There are no congenital anomalies that can be attributed to galactosemia except cataracts.

Ocular management is intermingled with systemic management. Systemic management should get priority over ocular management. The surgery in galactosemic cataracts does not differ from other congenital cataracts.

Management of Galactosemia Cataract

The management is divided into two parts, i.e., the management of systemic galactosemia to save the life of the infant, followed by the management of cataracts. The first step is to recognize galactosemia by its signs and symptoms, confirmed by specific biochemical tests. Once galactosemia is diagnosed, the next step is stopping all mammalian milk products, including mother's milk and correcting fluid electrolyte imbalance. Substituting milk by soya may reverse or slow the lenticular changes, if opacity persists, the cataract should be removed by the usual microsurgical procedure.

The condition is confirmed by:

- All children born to galactosemic mothers should be screened for galactosemia.
- All neonates with unexplained diarrhea should have their urine examined for reducing substances.
- Once a reducing substance has been found, the urine should be examined specifically for galactose.
- Other tests available to confirm galactosemia are:
    - Estimation of urine and serum galactose
    - Presence of uridyltransferase in peripheral blood cells
    - Hepatic function test
    - Urine examination for amino acids

Galactokinase deficiency has no systemic involvement. The only positive finding is bilateral central developmental cataract, making it mandatory to examine all neonates with bilateral central cataracts for reducing substances in urine.

HYPOGLYCEMIC CATARACT

In some cases, there is a sudden fall in blood sugar in newborns. The most common is seen in children born to mothers with gestational diabetes without biochemical control. Such mothers produce sufficient insulin to keep raised blood sugar at bay. As soon as the child is born, the insulin present in the fetus becomes much higher than required, sending the child into a state of acute hypoglycemia. If this is not recognized and treated, it may prove fatal to the child. If the child survives, the child may develop opacities in the lens. The opacities are known to disappear with the correction of hypoglycemia. Repeated attacks of hypoglycemia have been blamed for causing lamellar cataracts by 1–2 years. Hypoglycemia is more common in premature infants. Deprivation of mother's milk in the first 48 hours and diarrhea in newborns are other contributory factors.

CONGENITAL DIABETES CATARACT

They are not really congenital; it is better to put them in the category of developmental cataracts. They have an acute onset; the cause is increased glucose in the lens. The accumulated glucose is converted into sugar alcohol, which is the chemical responsible for the opacification of lens fibers. As the sugar alcohol increases, the changed osmolarity of the lens attracts more water. This initially causes vacuoles in the cortex to get opacified. The opacities are initially scattered all over the cortex as dots of varied size and are called snowflakes. The snowflakes enlarge and increase in number so much so that in the next 2–3 days, the whole of the lens gets opacified.

In the stage of vacuole formation, the cataract is reversible if sugar is controlled. Once the lens proteins are coagulated, the chances of reversal are lost. Even with the best biochemical control.

RARE CATARACTS IN CHILDREN

Table 19.1 displays the less common types of cataracts in children.

TABLE 19.1: Less prevalent forms of cataracts in children.

Syndrome	*Lenticular finding*	*Nonlenticular finding*	*Systemic finding*
Lowe syndrome (oculocerebrorenal syndrome)	Bilateral central cataract, microphakia, ectopia lentis, and posterior lenticonus	Blue sclera, thin sclera, congenital glaucoma, anterior chamber dysgenesis, severe vision loss, and poor prognosis	Unknown enzyme deficiency, deficient amino acid metabolism, acidosis, mental retardation rickets, retarded growth, hypotony, short life span
Fabry syndrome	Star-shaped opacity in the posterior cortex	Vortex dystrophy of the cornea, conjunctival and retinal telangiectasia	Prominent skin lesion, recurrent fever, colic, no central nervous system change, lymph edema, renal failure
Wilson's syndrome	Anterior capsular* sunflower cataract	Kayser–Fleischer ring† of the cornea	Caused by faulty copper metabolism, chronic hepatic failure, hepatomegaly, and ataxia
Mannosidosis	Capsular opacities and cart-wheel opacities in the posterior capsule are best seen on retroillumination	Esotropia, anterior chamber, and malformation	Caused by deficiency of α mannosidase, hearing loss, splenomegaly, and congenital heart disease
Hypoparathyroidism	Bilateral punctate opacities and polychromic opacities in the cortex		Signs and symptoms of hypoparathyroidism

**Sunflower cataract (sunburst):* Sunflower cataract per se is not a congenital cataract. It is a developmental cataract due to the systemic toxicity of copper, as seen in Wilson's disease, brought about by a deficiency in copper-binding protein. The acquired form is caused by intraocular copper or copper-containing alloys. The foreign body need not always be in the lens; it can be lodged anywhere inside the eye. In both instances, the cataract is seen in the anterior subcapsular area as a disciform opacity that has a greenish-gray metallic tinge. With spoke-like cortical opacities, the cataract is called a sunflower cataract with yellowish petal-like riders. The condition is also referred to as chalcosis lentis.
†*Kayser–Fleischer ring:* This is another manifestation of copper toxicity, both local as well as systemic without involving the lens. It is the deposition of copper in the Descemet's membranes at the periphery. It starts at the upper part of the cornea and flush with the limbus.

ELSCHNIG PEARLS AND SOEMMERING RING

Elschnig pearls and soemmering ring are not congenital anomalies of the lens. They are, in fact, a postoperative status of less frequency, developing months to years after surgery.

Elschnig pearl: These are nonpreventable calcified after-cataracts that develop months to years following extracapsular cataract extraction in all ages, both in pseudophakic and aphakic eyes. They do not develop following intracapsular cataract extraction; paradoxically, they are seen in eyes with no or minimum postoperative inflammation. The pearls are formed due to the proliferation of remnants of cortical matter between the anterior and posterior capsules on the periphery. They resemble translucent fish spawn globules of varied size, and occasionally they may be present at the center of the pupil. They may be small enough to be hidden behind the iris and only visible following mydriasis; sometimes they may protrude through the undilated pupil; they are known both to progress and spontaneously regress; they may not cause any visual deficit; they are not known to cause glaucoma.

Soemmering ring: It is a harmless aftermath of extracapsular cataract extraction due to the accumulation of equatorial lens epithelium. The proliferating epithelial cells are caught between the posterior capsule and the edge of the anterior capsule. The cause of the adhesion is not well understood. The ring has an irregular doughnut appearance. It need not always be a complete ring. It may be in fragments. Its transparency ranges from cloudy to opaque. The ring may be thin enough not to be seen in a normal-sized pupil. To see such rings, the pupil needs full dilation. As the ring, with its opacity, is away from the visual axis, it does not hamper distance vision. Complete removal of cortical matter during surgery prevents the formation of the ring. The rings per se are harmless; they may rarely get dislocated in AC, which requires removal.

POSTERIOR CAPSULAR OPACITY

Posterior capsular opacity is a frequent sequel of extracapsular lens extraction both in aphakic and pseudophakic eyes; it may be seen in one-fifth of cases operated on in the general population. It is thought to have a genetic predisposition. The younger the patient, the higher the chances of PCO. In children under 10 years old, it may be as high as 100%.

It is said to be more commonly associated with degenerative conditions of the eyes. It is the thickening of the posterior capsule with cortical matter laid over it, may be very thin without causing any visual disturbance or may be thick enough to reduce vision to preoperative level. It takes 3–4 weeks to develop following posterior chamber intraocular lens (PCIOL) implantation. A visual acuity that was 6/6 drastically falls, requiring the patient to seek consultation. The patients have glare and/or scattered light as well. The PCO can be prevented by meticulous cleaning of cortical matter during the primary procedure and polishing of the posterior capsule. In children, it can be prevented by posterior capsulotomy along with anterior vitrectomy during primary procedure. The other method to minimize the incidence is the use of a biconvex IOL or a lens with posterior convexity, a heparin-coated IOL, or heparin used in irrigating fluid. Despite the best efforts, it may not be prevented in all cases. The posterior capsule may develop wrinkles, causing stretch lines in the posterior capsule.

Another complication is capsule contraction syndrome, caused due to contraction of the anterior capsular opening in eyes that have suffered from uveitis in the past.

The most dreaded complication is the entrapment of bacteria of low virulence, such as *Propionibacterium acnes* and *Staphylococcus epidermidis*, which may cause endophthalmitis when released in aqueous following a laser capsulotomy.

On rare occasions, laser capsulotomy may be followed by cystoid macular edema or worsening of cystoid macular edema, a transient rise of IOP, and rhegmatogenous retinal detachment. The management of PCO is laser capsulotomy that immediately restores vision. The recurrence of PCO following laser capsulotomy is rare.

AFTER-CATARACT

After-cataract is a more severe form of PCO. It used to be a frequent aftermath of needling in pre-microsurgical era. Its etiology and pathogenesis are similar to those of PCO.

It comprises of removal of as much cortical matter as possible and is the mainstay of its prevention following capsulotomy. Despite the best efforts, all cortical matter cannot be removed even by the best techniques of suction

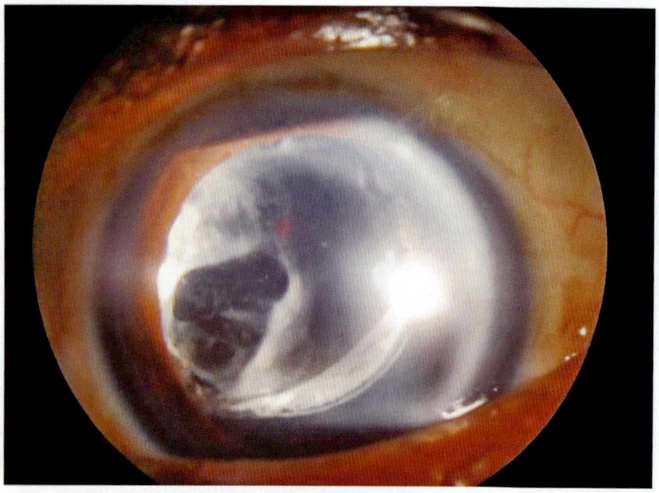

Fig. 19.23: Dense after-cataract.
Courtesy: Dr Santosh Patel.

and irrigation. The remnants of cortical matter get trapped between the edges of capsulotomy/capsulorhexis and posterior capsule and start proliferating into an opaque mass. More the cortical matter left, denser and larger the after-cataract. It may be as thin as to be seen on a slit lamp. In clinical practice, the thinnest after-cataract is called PCO. The opacity visible on oblique illumination is called *after-cataract* **(Fig. 19.23)**. Ordinarily, it takes weeks to months to develop. In a few cases, over months, it may develop Elschnig pearl or, still later, may develop Soemmering.

The incidence of after-cataract depends on the following factors:

- Almost all aphakic/pseudophakic children are likely to develop PCO after-cataract extraction.
- Most of the children will develop PCO after-cataract surgery within 1 year.
- The placement of IOL is also known to influence the formation of PCO.
- Preexisting uveitis increases the chances of PCO formation.
- The chances of PCO are more if postoperative inflammation if not managed well.
- It may be influenced by a genetic factor.

Symptoms of an after-cataract:

- After-cataract is more visible than PCO.
- Rapid fall of vision after full gain of vision.
- Gradual diminution of vision over months.
- Frequent changes in refraction.

Management of after-cataract: The incidence of after-cataract has become negligible in the microsurgical era of suction and irrigation. Nowadays, it is seen only in unattended traumatic cataracts following penetrating injuries. Thin after-cataracts can be managed by laser capsulotomies; thick after-cataracts require microsurgical irrigation and aspiration. After-cataract not managed before 8 years is mostly likely to cause intractable amblyopia and squint.

Differential Diagnosis of Congenital Cataract

The most important group of conditions constituting differential diagnosis is leukocoria, or white pupils, which consists of both benign as well as malignant conditions. The benign conditions are not life-threatening, but most of them are vision-threatening.

> On the top of the list of malignant conditions is retinoblastoma, which, if not treated in the initial stages is 100% fatal. Treated children have a normal life span.

The other causes are nonmalignant; they are:

- Inflammatory exudates in the pupil
- Posterior cyclitic membrane
- Large coloboma of choroid
- Retrolental fibroplasias
- Persistent hyperplastic primary vitreous
- Exudative retinopathy of Coats
- Toxocara endophthalmitis
- Endogenous endophthalmitis
- Congenital retinal folds

Complications of congenital cataract:

- Amblyopia
- Squint
- Nystagmus

Amblyopia in cases of congenital cataracts is of two types:

1. Due to the failure of the macula to develop during the first 2–3 months
2. Failure to restore normal refractive status
   a. Leaving an uncorrected aphakia
   b. Swinging toward myopia in pseudophakia

> Once nystagmus develops, it is too late to improve vision by any means.

MANAGEMENT OF CONGENITAL CATARACTS

The definite treatment of congenital cataract is surgical removal and visual rehabilitation of the resultant aphakia/pseudophakia.

The surgery should be done by a person who is:

- Well-versed with pediatric cataracts
- Well-versed in the use of operating microscopes
- No surgery should be attempted without operation microscope.
- There should be good, automated irrigation aspiration equipment available.
- The surgeon should have adequate knowledge of anterior vitrectomy.
- The surgeon should have sufficient knowledge of the use of viscoelastic substances.
- No surgery should be performed without viscoelastic substance.
- The surgeon should have adequate knowledge of power calculation of IOL.

> There is no medical treatment except in the case of galactosemia, where the process can be arrested by withholding mammalian milk and milk products from the child's diet.
>
> There is only one condition that can be prevented and it is rubella cataract by immunizing every girl against rubella in childhood.

Initially, the condition can be managed by dilating the pupil widely, provided the opacity is central with a clear periphery. This has a drawback of a loss of accommodation that may hamper child's education.

Prognostic factors in the management of congenital cataracts:

- *Density:* Faint, scattered cortical opacities require only a periodic checkup and no surgical intervention. All that is required is the correction of any errors of refraction, if present.
- *Position:*
  - Central posteriorly placed opacities require early surgery.
  - Peripherally- and anteriorly-placed opacities either require no treatment or late treatment.
  - Surgery in lamellar cataract, which is central, can be delayed for some time by keeping the pupil dilated. This prevents the development of amblyopia but creates a problem when the child starts going to school and finds it difficult to see near objects due

to a loss of accommodation. This is the stage when surgery with an IOL implant with near correction is the best option.

- *Bilaterality:* Bilateral dense opacities should be operated on within 6 weeks of birth to prevent stimulus deprivation and amblyopia. It is better to operate one eye first and the second eye in a few weeks.
- *Unilateral:* Dense central unilateral cataracts should be operated on within the first few days of birth. The visual prognosis in unilateral cataracts is always poor, despite early surgery.
- *Associated systemic infection:* Rubella cataract has the worst prognosis because of associated multiple systemic and ocular anomalies, severe post-operative uveitis, and glaucoma. Toxoplasmosis and *cytomegalovirus* also have a poor prognosis.
- *Associated ocular congenital anomalies:* Each may require a separate protocol of management besides the treatment of cataracts.

Unilateral congenital cataracts are sporadic, without family history. They may be missed more often than bilateral. They draw attention due to the squint, which is very common in unilateral cataracts. Generally, these eyes do not have evidence of intraocular inflammation. Trauma, frank or occult, is a very common cause of unilateral cataracts. In unilateral cases, the cause can be obvious in only 10% of cases. The lenses with dense opacity should be operated on soon. Unilateral congenital cataracts, despite the best surgical management, have a poorer result. They cause more amblyopia.

> The overall visual prognosis in congenital cataracts is never as satisfactory as that for adult cataracts.

The following investigations are required to select cases for surgery:

Clinical

Clinical examination begins with a history that includes a family history of cataracts in parent and sibling bilateral cases, which are more likely to be familial. The eyes of the blood relatives should be examined for signs of undetected opacities, aphakia, and pseudophakia. The mother should be asked if she has suffered from any exanthematous disease, drug use, or exposure to radiation in the first trimester. It should also be ascertained if the child was preterm. Premature children are more likely to have congenital or developmental cataracts. The parents may be able to say if the cataract was present at birth or developed after birth or have a history of trauma, especially in unilateral cases. The second important information is to find out if the condition is really unilateral or if the other eye too has opacity.

The common clinical features with which a child is brought for examinations are:

- Visible opacity in the lens, unilateral/bilateral
- Squint is common in unilateral congenital cataracts.
- Abnormal and uncontrolled movement of the eyes (nystagmus)
- Opacity in the lens is the most important cause of diminished vision, which results in squints and nystagmus, both carrying poor prognosis. Nystagmus, once developed, is the most important cause of poor vision, despite the best efforts. Squint is invariable esotropia and is associated with amblyopia.
- The parents may complain that the child bumps against obstacles while negotiating, and the child watches TV from a shorter distance than other children. The school-going child may not be able to read or write on the board.
- This makes the examination of vision the most important examination in a case of congenital/developmental cataracts.

Estimation of vision in the case of cataracts in a child

It is mandatory to record age-matched quantitative vision in each eye separately and exclude other causes of diminished distant vision by refraction and ophthalmoscopy.

Examination of vision is a time-consuming and daunting task. A newborn should be able to fix and follow. The fixation should be central, maintained, and steady.

Bright cornea, age-matched depth of AC, brisk pupillary reaction both direct and indirect, iris without coloboma or iridocorneal changes, and clear media denote fairly good vision but do not exclude errors of reflection and amblyopia. In children, Brückner's test is a handy test to exclude high errors of refraction, amblyopia, and leukocoria.

Measurement of Corneal Diameter

The corneal diameter should be examined from white to white, either by a mechanical caliper or digital. A diameter <9 mm carries a poor prognosis.

Biomicroscopy (Optical)

In children above 5 years of age, biomicroscopy can be done on the usual slit lamp with persuasion; younger children may be examined with a hand-held slit lamp or operation microscope if required under general anesthesia. Slit-lamp examination gives information regarding size, position, density, and location of opacity.

Ultrasonic Biomicroscopy

Ultrasonic biomicroscopy is as important as slit-lamp biomicroscopy. Ultrasound biomicroscopy (UBM) is a high-resolution ultrasound technique that uses 35–50 MHz to see the structure of the anterior segment with a resolution as good as or better than light microscopy. It is a noninvasive outdoor procedure that can be used in the presence of a cloudy cornea.

It is used to see the anterior segment and as the frequency increases, penetration is reduced. Ultrasonic biomicroscopy using 50 MHz has a penetration of 5 mm, in contrast to 4–5 centimeters using 7 MHz.

Ultrasonic biomicroscopy can be used for biometry, AC depth, position of the lens, thickness of the lens, and morphology of the lens such as plaque on the anterior capsule, posterior cortical opacity, posterior lenticonus, ectopia, iridodialysis, and cyclodialysis of foreign bodies in the anterior segment. It is also used for measurement of distance from angle to angle, sulcus to sulcus, and bag diameter.

Biometry

A scan is used to measure the axial length of the eye, which is an essential part of calculating the power of the IOL. An axial length <16 millimeters is a red flag. The measurement of axial length is also used post-operatively to monitor elongation of the globe, which is inevitable and causes a change in the refractive status of the eye over the years following the IOL implant.

> Every white reflex in the pupillary area is not a cataract.

Fundus Examination

Both eyes should be examined under complete cycloplegia by both direct and indirect ophthalmoscopes.

Examination of Intraocular Tension

Intraocular tension should be recorded in all cases of congenital or developmental cataracts and in all white reflexes in the pupillary area. It can be done by a Schiotz tonometer under general anesthesia under 10 years. Intraocular pressure (IOP) in children older than 10 years can be performed under topical anesthesia after they have been assured that the procedure is painless and harmless. No attempt should be made to record IOP in a struggling child, and the lid should be separated with figure of the examiner, avoiding pressure on the globe. In children, a Perkins hand-held tonometer may be used under general anesthesia. A noncontact tonometer is a better option; the tension should be regularly recorded following a successful IOL because postoperative rise of tension is a common feature.

Laboratory Tests in Cases of Congenital Cataracts

Most healthy children with operable cataracts do not require elaborate laboratory investigations, especially unilateral, familial, and traumatic cataracts, which hardly require any systemic examination except as ordered by anesthetic.

> The commonly followed rule of thumb is that in unilateral cataracts, there is something wrong with the eye, while bilateral cataracts have something wrong systemically.

The conditions that require systemic evaluation are:

- Bilateral cataract
- Lenticonus
- Membranous cataracts
- Suspected rubella cataracts
- Bilateral congenital ocular abnormality
- Systemic congenital anomalies
- Metabolic disorders

Biochemical: Urine examination should be done for reducing substances. If reducing substances are present, always suspect galactosemia unless excluded.

Serological tests: TORCH test.

Congenital cataracts in which surgery can be deferred are:

- Anterior capsular
- Nuclear cataracts that are smaller than 2 mm
- Lamellar cataracts
- Peripheral cortical cataract
- Scattered opacities

Anatomical peculiarities that have bearing on surgical procedures in cataract surgery.

TABLE 19.2: Comparison between a child's and adult's eyes.

Feature	Child eye	Adult eye
Volume	2.5 mL	7.1 mL
Axial length	17.00 mm	23.5–24 mm
Corneal diameter	10.00 mm	12.00 mm
AC depth	2.5 mm	3.2 mm
Pupil	1.5 mm	2.5 mm
Diameter of the lens	6.00 mm	9.3 mm
Shape of the lens	Spherical	Ellipsoid
Capsular bag	7.00 mm	9.00 mm
Refraction	+21 D (axial)	0.00 D (emmetropic)

(AC: anterior chamber)

Table 19.2 shows comparison between a child's and adult's eyes.

Other features of infantile eyes are:

- Ciliary body is smaller and cellular.
- Pars plana is near the limbus.
- Ora serrata does not develop well before 7 years.
- Ciliary processes are near the lens.
- Infantile eyes have low scleral rigidity.
- The anterior lens capsule is too elastic as compared to adults.
- Vitreous exerts more pressure.
- The eye may be maldeveloped, hence small.
- The eyes are more prone to develop postoperative uveitis.
- The eyes are highly prone to develop postoperative opacity in the visual axis.
- The eyes keep on increasing axial length post-operatively; hence, they are prone to myopic shift.

Intraocular Lens Power Calculation in Pediatric Cataracts

The aim of IOL in adults is to give 6/6 vision that should last for the rest of the life with good near vision with or without near correction. This is not possible in childhood cataracts because the eyes keep on increasing in length until 16 years of age, from 17 to 24 mm. This causes a myopic shift despite the well-calculated power of the IOL implanted in a child's eye, which requires frequent changes in refraction that are corrected either by a contact lens or spectacle. This can be minimized by leaving the eye undercorrected. The common practices are to undercorrect the eye by 10% between 2 and 8 years and by 20% under 2 years. The above estimates are true, following biometry.

TABLE 19.3: Undercorrection in relation to age.

Age of surgery	Desired refraction
1 year	+6 D
2 years	+5 D
3 years	+4 D
4 years	+3 D
5 years	+2 D
6 years	+1 D
7 years	+0 D
8 years and above	−1.00 D to −2.00 D

TABLE 19.4: Relationship between axial length and the recommended power of the intraocular lens (IOL).

Axial length	Suggested power
17 mm	28.0 D
18 mm	27.0 D
19 mm	26.0 D
20 mm	24.0 D
21 mm	22.0 D

The rule of thumb is that younger the child more should be under correction.

Table 19.3 gives a rough undercorrection in relation to age.

Table 19.4 gives a rough relationship between axial length and the recommended power of the IOL.

The principle of power calculation in children's eyes does not differ from that of adult eyes; both depend on axial length and corneal curvature. However, every institute and different surgeons have their favored method of IOL calculation. An ideal situation would be a customized IOL for each eye.

Simple needling and optical iridectomy are no more in vogue, so are anterior chamber (AC) and Iris Clip intraocular lens (IOL).

All surgeries for pediatric cataracts should be done under general anesthesia under an operating microscope with a viscoelastic substance. The simplest procedure is an anterior capsulotomy and irrigation aspiration. This leaves the eye aphakic, which is corrected by either contact lens spectacles or secondary IOL later.

Outline of Steps of Intraocular Lens in Pediatric Cataracts

1. The *first and most important* step before surgery is to counsel the parents and they should be informed:
    - Why the surgery is needed?
    - What will happen if the surgery is not done or postponed?
    - Prognosis
    - Possibility of repeat surgery, i.e., laser capsulotomy for PCO.
    - Change in refraction in the year to come.
    - Frequent change of glasses for distant vision.
    - Requirement of near correction.
    - Amblyopia and its management largely depend on the cooperation of parents.
    - Importance of compliance of antiamblyopic treatment.
    - Management of postoperative uveitis.
2. *Preoperative evaluation:* It has been noted that unilateral cataracts hardly require any preoperative evaluation unless desired by the anesthetist, in contrast to bilateral cataracts, which require a battery of investigations.
3. *Anesthesia:* All surgery should be done under general anesthesia administered by anesthetists well-versed in pediatric anesthesia.
4. *Preoperative preparation:*
    a. *Preoperative antibiotic drops:* The child should get prophylactic antibiotic drops of the surgeon's choice 4 times a day for 2 days prior to surgery. No systemic antibiotic is required unless asked for by pediatrician/anesthetist.
    b. *Mydriasis:* The pupil should be dilated as wide as possible with mydriasis cum cycloplegic of surgeon's choice. Atropine is rarely used nowadays but it should not be held back in the eyes with a very rigid pupil. Intraoperative miosis is managed by the method best suited for the patient and surgeon's choices.
    c. Ocular hypotensives are rarely required.
5. *The incision* should be 1.0–1.5 mm in a valvular fashion; it could be a clear cornea or scleral. Additional incisions are required for aspiration-irrigation. As the sclera is very elastic, all incisions should be sutured after the surgery is over.
6. *Viscoelastic and capsular stains:* The preferred viscoelastic for pediatric cataracts is 1.4% sodium hyaluronate, as this facilitates anterior capsulorrhexis, maintains the AC, and helps in managing low scleral irrigates. It also reduces vitreous pressure.
    a. The anterior capsule in pediatric cataracts differs from adult cataracts in its elasticity and tensile strength; this is more common in complete cataracts. Staining of the anterior capsule by 0.6% trypan blue is favored in total white cataracts.
7. *Capsulorrhexis:* The old practice of simple capsulotomy by knife has been replaced by capsulorrhexis. The preferred capsulorrhexis is manual continuous curvilinear capsulorrhexis (CCC). Due to the unusual elasticity and tensile strength of the anterior capsule in children, capsulorrhexis in children requires more dexterity; peripheral extension of capsulorrhexis is common in pediatric cataracts.
8. *Hydrodissection and hydrodelineation:* Successful capsulorrhexis, followed by the removal of the cortex and epithelial cells from the equator is the sheet anchor of cataract surgery in children. It will be recalled that there is no formed nucleus in children under ten. The hydrodissection should aim at maximum removable of lens cortexes and epithelial cells from the periphery of the lens; it may be done by single or multiple incisions. The choice of fluid for hydrodissection is a personal matter of choice for the surgeons; either ringer lactate or BSS can be used. The cortex is removed by manual phacoaspiration or automated irrigation aspiration. Membranous cataracts, which are common in rubella, may require phacoemulsification, so traumatic cataracts that have hardened due to calcium deposits are neglected.
9. *Posterior capsulorrhexis:* Opacities in the visual axis are very common. It used to be almost universal in cases where the posterior capsule was left untouched, fearing that the vitreous would find its way into the AC. This was found not to be true, and a posterior capsulorrhexis proved to be a boon. This was accompanied by an anterior vitrectomy as a primary procedure. Vitrectomy is more frequently performed before placing the IOL in the bag; however, vitrectomy can be performed after the IOL has been placed. Anterior vitrectomy can be performed either through a limbal or pars plana route.
10. *Placement of the intraocular lens:* The best results are obtained by putting the PCIOL in the bag. The most popular IOLs are polymethyl methacrylate (PMMA)

lenses. IOL in the bag has the advantage of better centering; the lens does not come in contact with the ciliary body. Once the lens has been implanted, all the viscoelastic substances are removed, and all incisions are closed with sutures.

Secondary Intraocular Lens Implants in Children

Primary PCIOL in a bag is the gold standard for pediatric cataracts. However, there are a few situations where a primary implant has not been attempted or an IOL could not be placed in place, leaving the eye aphakic.

The conditions are:

- Children under 2 years
- Large rent in the posterior capsule during primary surgery
- Vitreous in the posterior capsular rent
- Lensectomy in ectopia lentis
- Traumatic cataracts that have absorbed automatically or have extensive posterior capsular rupture
- Complicated cataracts in long-standing uveitis
- Pediatric vitreoretinal problems that have undergone pars plana vitrectomy.

Modalities available for secondary IOL implants:

- PCIOL in the bag, provided space is available between the anterior and posterior capsules
- PCIOL in sulcus
- Scleral-fixated IOL
- Angle-supported ACIOL
- Iris clips IOL

The last two have been given up in favor of the first four. The angle-supported ACIOL and iris clip IOL are prone to cause corneal decompensation.

Intraoperative complications in pediatric IOL surgery:

- Difficulty in capsulorrhexis
- Unwanted extension of capsulorrhexis on the periphery
- Dislocation of cataracts (rare)
- Intraoperative miosis*
- Increased intravitreal pressure
- Trauma to the corneal endothelium
- Fish mouthing of wound†
- Residual viscoelastic in the eye

Postoperative complications of pediatric IOL:

- Immediate
- Delayed
- Late

Immediate

The immediate complications are glaucoma and uveitis.

Glaucoma is seen in about 20% of cases. Glaucoma developing soon after surgery is caused by:

- Residual viscoelastic
- Pupillary block
- Shallow AC
- Formation of peripheral anterior synechiae

Glaucoma developing soon after surgery can be prevented by:

- Meticulous cleaning of viscoelastic
- Performing a peripheral iridectomy
- Water-tight closure of all wounds

Uveitis: Unattended uveitis is a major contributory factor in the nonimprovement of vision in pseudophakia. It can be exudative/fibrinous, or a combination. This is caused by an increased inflammatory uveal reaction, which is attributed to the higher vascularity of the infantile ciliary body, IOL in the sulcus irritating the ciliary body, and residual viscoelastic. It is best managed by its prevention. Once it has happened, it can be managed with intensive used of local steroids and judicious use of cycloplegic from the first day. Some authors use subconjunctival injections in appropriate doses of dexamethasone at the end of surgery, use heparin in irrigation fluid. Tissue plasminogen activator into AC is claimed to reduce incidents of postuveitis. Others depend on a liberal dose of steroids from the first postoperative day. Every institution has its own protocol to use steroids. In some cases, it may last for months in a minimum dose that gives maximum effects. Systemic steroids are

**Intraoperative miosis* is common in children; this can be reduced by maximum mydriasis with the use of a combination of phenyl epinephrine hydrochloride (2.5%), cyclopentolate (0.5%), and tropicamide (0.5%). Instillation of flurbiprofen (0.03%) two times a day for 2 days prior to surgery is claimed to help in maintaining intraoperative mydriasis. Some surgeons advocate using 0.3 mL of adrenaline (1:1,000) in 500 mL of irrigation solution. The anesthetic should be informed about the use of adrenaline during surgery.

†*Fish mouthing of wounds* is prevented by suturing all wounds by 10-0 nylon.

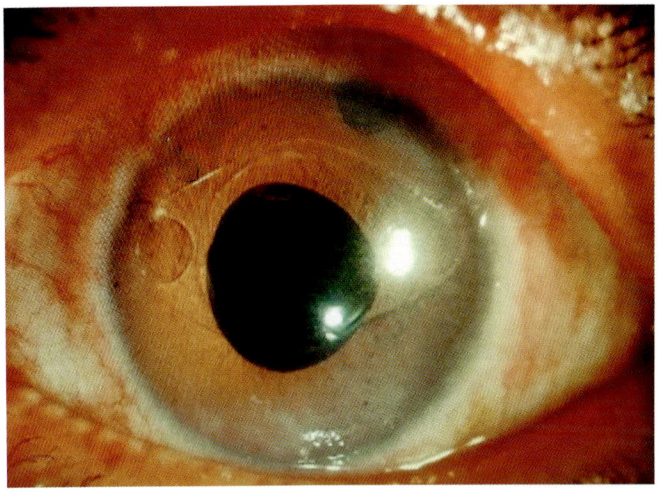

Fig. 19.24: Anterior chamber intraocular lens (ACIOL) with clear central pupil.
Courtesy: Dr Santosh Patel.

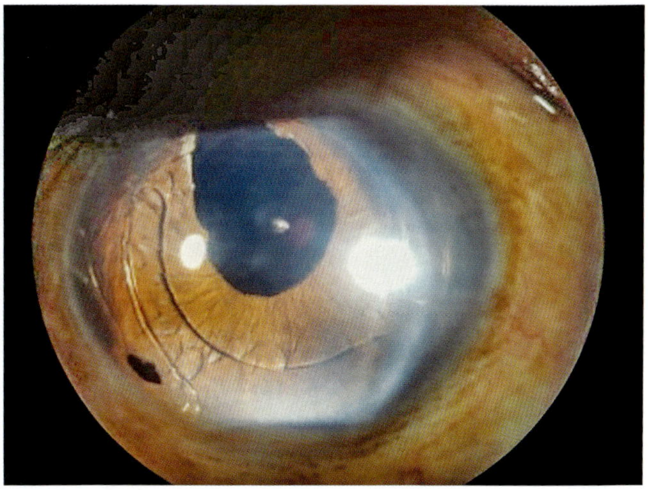

Fig. 19.25: Anterior chamber intraocular lens (ACIOL) with a shifted pupil.
Courtesy: Dr Santosh Patel.

rarely required. Generally, cycloplegics are used in BD doses. Atropine is rarely required; atropine should not be withheld when required.

Besides uveitis, one of the most important complications is pseudophakic glaucoma. This can be prevented by removing of all residual viscoelastic from AC and performing a peripheral iridectomy to prevent pupillary block. Pseudophakic glaucoma develops more commonly in infants. The incidence of pseudophakic glaucoma is directly related to the age of the child. It is less common in older children as compared to infants.

Delayed

The delayed complications are shown in **Figures 19.24 to 19.26**:

- PCO
- Pupillary capture
- Decentering of the lens
- Corneal decompensation

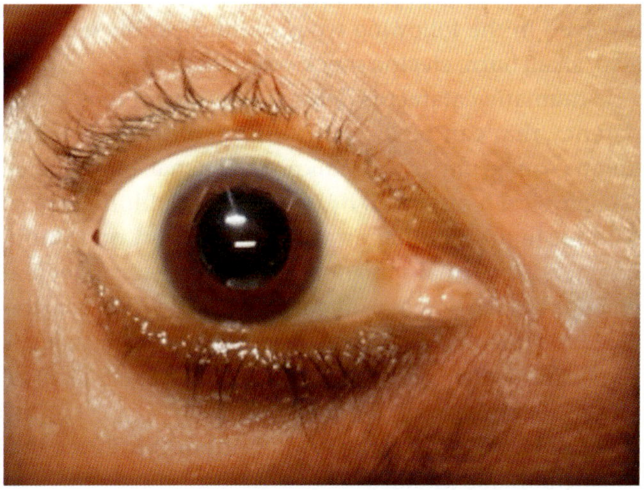

Fig. 19.26: Iris Clip intraocular lens (IOL) in place.
Courtesy: Dr Archana Kashyap.

Late

Late complications are:

- Amblyopia
- Myopic shift*
- Loss of accommodation
- Nonimprovement of vision
- Chronic glaucoma
- Secondary membrane formation
- Retinal detachment

**Myopic shift* is most probably related to the age of the operation. It is maximum under 1 year; at 2–3 years, it is about 4–5 diopters. It is reduced to 1.5 D between 8 and 9 years. The power of the lens should always be based on standard biometric procedures.

The power of the lens to be implanted should be 20% less than the calculated power of the IOL in children under 2 years and 10% less in children between 2 and 8 years. This roughly reduces myopic shift, i.e., postoperative myopia. This formula does not completely eliminate postoperative myopia. Residual myopia should be corrected by spectacle following retinoscopy and autorefractometry from time to time.

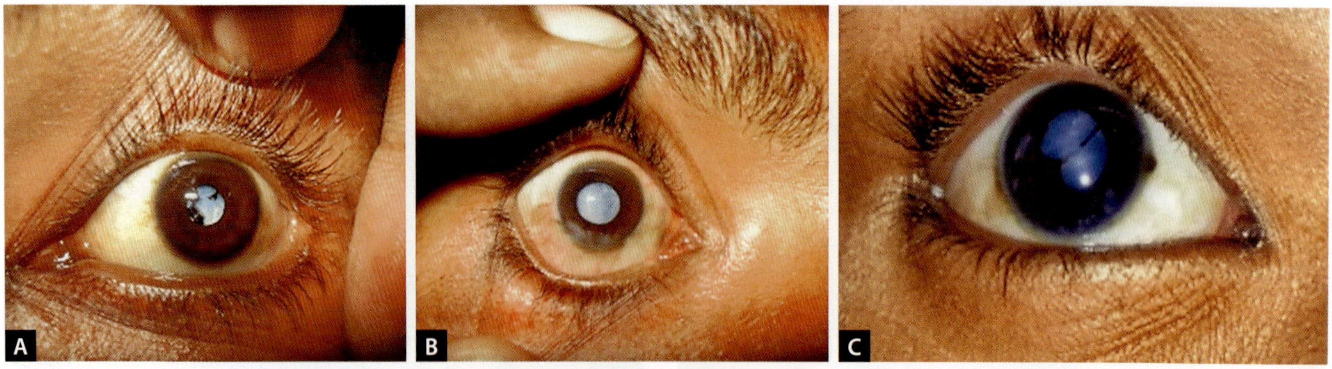

Figs. 19.27A to C: Various types of traumatic cataracts following a small penetrating injury.
Courtesy: Dr Santosh Patel.

TRAUMATIC CATARACT

Traumatic cataract is a very common cause of unilateral cataract. It may occur in any age and both sexes, with a preponderance in young adult males. Both the eyes are involved in the following types of injuries: Blast injury, acid/alkali burn, electric shock, and radiation.

Traumatic cataract is defined as a loss of lens transparency that can be directly attributed to trauma. The trauma can be physical, chemical, radiational, or electrical. The physical injuries can be penetrating or blunt, with or without injury to other structures, and with or without retained intraocular foreign bodies. Retained intraocular metallic foreign bodies can cause siderosis due to iron and chalcosis due to copper. The effect of trauma on the lens can be immediate or delayed. A traumatic cataract can be localized or generalized.

Mainly, there are two types of physical injuries that cause traumatic cataracts. *They are:*

1. Penetrating injuries.
2. Blunt injuries.

Penetrating Injuries

Penetrating injuries can be caused by small objects like pins, needles, large knives, shrapnels, and arrows that penetrate the lens capsule after passing through the cornea. Small, sharp objects may just prick the lens capsule; brittle things like thorns may break and remain embedded in the lens; and small particles flying at high speed may also get embedded in the lens or may pass through the whole lens to become intravitreal. Large penetrating wounds are invariably accompanied by uveal prolapse or disturbed vitreous. It can cause subluxation and dislocation of the lens. The end result of all penetrating injuries is loss of transparency, localized or total **(Figs. 19.27A to C)**.

Small, punctured wounds quickly get sealed, leaving a localized dot-like opacity that may not spread or may involve the whole lens soon. In such cases, the lens not only gets totally white but also swells to cause shallow AC, obstructs the pupil, and narrows the angle, causing secondary phacomorphic glaucoma with or without pupillary block. Sometimes, the swelling is so much that the cortical material protrudes not only through the rent but also passes in AC. In such cases, the opaque cortical material may fill the AC fully, settle down at the lower part of the AC, present as a pseudohypopyon, or block the angle. Most of the penetrating injuries to the lens are initially associated with softening of the eye, folds in the cornea, and AC of various depths. The tension gradually builds up following the healing of the corneal wound and may pass into a state of raised intraocular tension. The lens matter gradually gets absorbed. This happens more commonly in children who have not yet developed a fully formed nucleus. In children, the cortical material may get absorbed completely, leaving an after-cataract **(Figs. 19.28 to 19.30)**.

Blunt Injury

A blunt injury is a close globe injury either due to a contusion or a concussion. The former is more common.

- A forceful contusion can rupture the anterior lens capsule, the posterior lens capsule, dislocate, or subluxate the lens. A rupture in the lens capsule following a contusion behaves like a penetrating wound without a corneal wound, and the lens becomes opaque within hours.

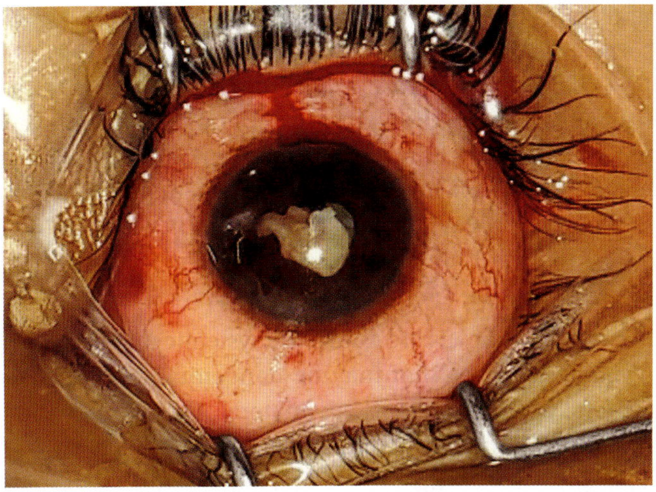

Fig. 19.28: Traumatic cataracts following corneoscleral injury.
Courtesy: Professor ML Garg.

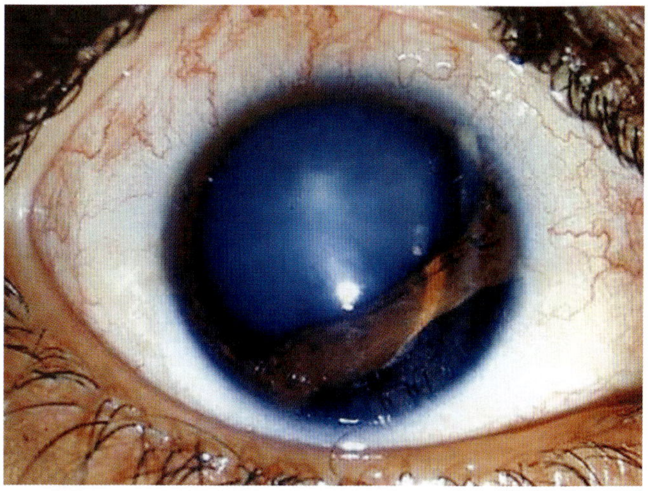

Fig. 19.29: Traumatic cataract with iridodialysis following blunt injury.
Courtesy: Dr Santosh Patel.

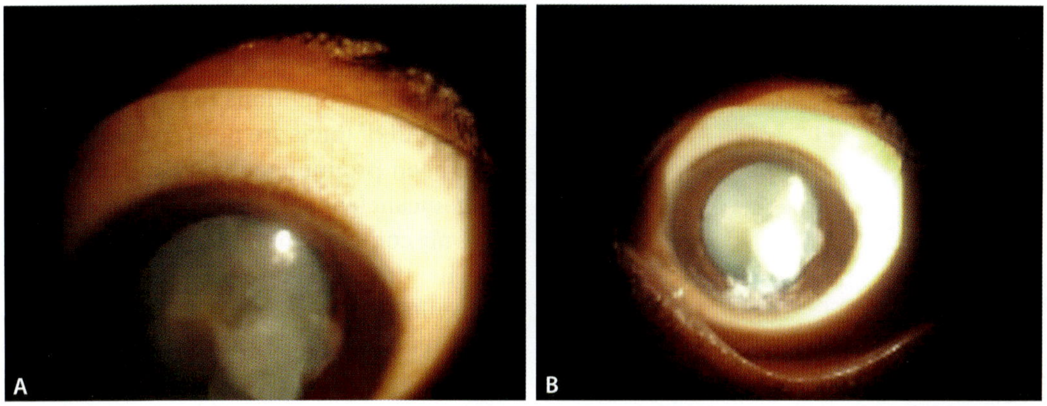

Figs. 19.30A and B: Traumatic cataracts with cortical material in anterior chamber (AC).
Courtesy: Dr Santosh Patel.

- If the force of the contusion is moderate, any of the following two or both may take place. The first is the Vossius ring* and the second is the rosette cataract.

ROSETTE CATARACT (PETALOID CATARACT)

In contrast to the Vossius ring, rosette cataracts develop in the posterior cortex in the axial region and are rarely seen in the anterior cortex as well. When present in the posterior cortex, they cause more visual loss. It develops in a few days to a few months following blunt close-globe injury and imbibement of aqueous, mostly through the posterior capsule.

Other causes of rosette cataract, besides closed globe injury, are radiation, electrocution, and chemical injury **(Fig. 19.31)**.

There are two types of rosette cataracts:

1. Typical early rosette cataract
2. Late rosette cataract

The former is more common. It develops as multiple opaque lines of different lengths radiating from a central

---

**Vossius ring:* This is an imprint of the posterior surface of the iris on the anterior lens capsule if the pupil is constricted during contusion due to the liberation of iris pigment that adheres to the lens capsule. This is a benign condition that, by itself, does not cause opacification of the lens capsule or require treatment. The condition is best seen after mydriasis and may be mistaken for postinflammatory iris pigment on the lens capsule. The ring lingers for weeks without causing any visual loss, only to fade away in a few months.

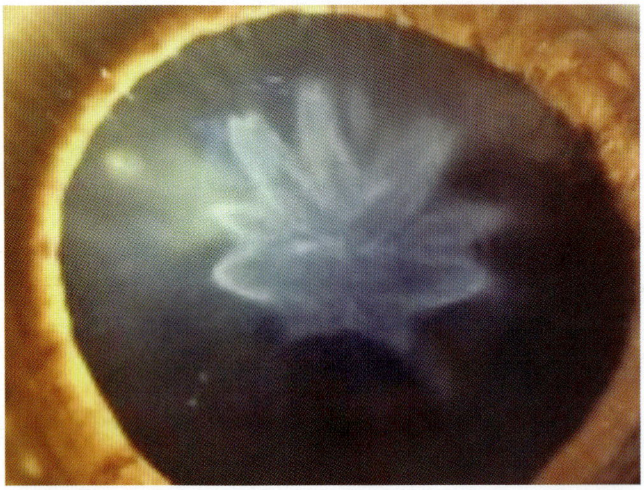

Fig. 19.31: Petaloid cataract.
Source: Gaurav Gupta and Jinagal J. IJO – 68; 1 - P2010-2020 with the permission of SG Honavar, editor, Indian Journal of Ophthalmology, IJO.

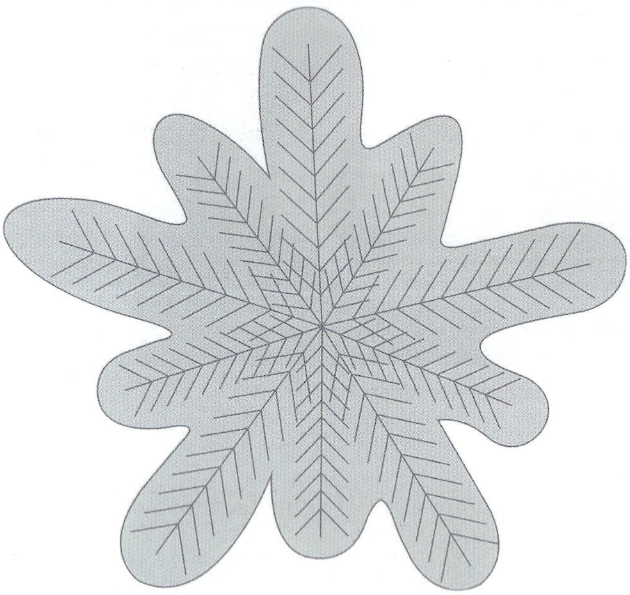

Fig. 19.32: Configuration of petaloid cataracts.

point. Each line has finer lines at an acute angle from the main stem, giving an overall picture of a diffused star. Generally, it remains stationary and is detected on routine examination of the media **(Fig. 19.32)**.

Rarely, it may gradually increase and get converted into a full-blown cataract over months.

LATE ROSETTE CATARACT

It develops 1–2 years following a blunt injury. It is smaller and more compact, but once developed, it follows a course similar to early rosette cataract and passes on to full-blown cortical cataract.

Other effects of blunt injury to the lens are anterior subcapsular vacuoles, anterior plaque, and delayed opacification without rosette cataract. This makes it mandatory to look for evidence of occult injury to the lens in cases of true uniocular cataract.

SECONDARY CATARACT IN CHILDREN

Secondary cataracts are due to the systemic manifestation of many diseases that may be congenital or acquired. Generally, these cataracts are bilateral. They are of varied morphology and location.

The systemic conditions producing secondary cataracts can be:

- Maternal infection
- Metabolic disorders
- Toxic
- Syndromes

The list of conditions that cause secondary cataracts is long. All of them are not very common. Many of them have been pronounced as systemic manifestations and insignificant lenticular involvement.

Only common conditions will be discussed here.

The three common maternal infections causing congenital cataracts are: (1) Rubella, (2) *cytomegalovirus*, and (3) toxoplasmosis. Out of these three, rubella is the most common cause of congenital cataracts with multiple ocular and systemic manifestations.

RUBELLA CATARACT

Discussed earlier in this Chapter.

STEROID-INDUCED CATARACT

Steroid-induced cataracts may be considered to be an acquired iatrogenic problem. The incidence of this condition is increasing due to the frequent use of strong steroids, especially following cataract surgery in children, keratoplasty, or granulomatous uveitis. A more common cause is the indiscriminate use of strong steroids for a long time in allergic conjunctivitis. This has turned into a major form of steroid-induced cataract in young patients and children. Both local and systemic steroids can cause cataracts. The exact cause of cataract formation due to steroids is not known. The exact salt, dose, frequency, strength, and duration of the steroid used in producing cataracts are also not understood. However, it is certain that prolonged, continuous use of strong steroids has more harmful effects than short-term, alternate-day use of weak steroid solutions. Genetics seems to play an important role in producing cataracts. Steroid-induced cataracts may be associated with steroid-induced glaucoma. The opacities are mostly posterior subcapsular in the axial region on the nodal point, causing much and early visual loss. The opacities have a disc-like appearance at the center. The density of the opacity gradually fades toward the periphery, not reaching the equator. In some cases, it may develop under the anterior capsule as well. The opacities are known to disappear following the elimination of steroids from the treatment or by reducing the frequency, strength, and duration. It is better to switch over to nonsteroidal drugs in place of steroids whenever possible. As a precaution, person of all ages under steroid for more than 3 weeks should have their lenses examined for under mydriasis with a slit lamp and get their intraocular tension checked regularly by an applanation tonometer.

SOME INTERESTING CATARACTS (IN ALL AGES)

- *Electrical cataract:* If a high-voltage electric current passes through the body of a person or someone is struck by lightning and survives, he may develop bilateral punctuate opacities in the lens that soon spread throughout the entire cortex to produce a complete cataract.
- *Blue-dot cataract:* Blue-dot cataracts are the most common form of congenital cataract. They are bluish-green opacities scattered all over the cortex or restricted to the peripheral cortex. They do not cause any symptoms. They are nonprogressive; hence, no treatment is required.
- *Sutural cataract:* They develop in the fetal nucleus, either in the anterior or posterior cortex. The simultaneous presence of anterior and posterior sutural cataracts is less frequent. The sutural cataracts have a peculiar configuration of the letter Y. They are nonprogressive, have sex X-linked inheritance, and boys have denser opacities. As the cataract does not have visual symptoms, it does not require any treatment.
- *Christmas tree cataract:* This is seen in myotonic dystrophy. The lenticular opacities are polychromatic dust or needle-like opacities in the posterior cortex in a Christmas tree fashion. The needles give a multicolored appearance on slit-lamp examination; they are not seen in children.
- *Cataract with polychromatic luster:* These are, in fact, complicated cataracts seen in chronic uveitis. The cataract in chronic uveitis may also have a breadcrumb appearance.
- *Sunflower cataract:* Sunflower cataracts are seen in eyes with retained intraocular copper foreign bodies, i.e., chalcosis. The cataract consists of central yellowish-brown petals that radiate toward the periphery.
- *Brown anterior subcapsular opacity:* This is associated with retained intraocular iron foreign bodies, i.e., siderosis. There is a discoloration of the iris, which looks greenish initially and turns brownish later. The cataract is due to the deposition of iron on the anterior epithelium and subcapsular zone as a ring. On long run, the whole of the lens gets opacified. It may be associated with pigmentary changes in the retina, causing acquired diminished night vision, not related to vitamin A deficiency.
- *Glass blower's cataract (exfoliation cataract):* They are seen following prolonged exposure to infrared rays over many years, mostly in glass blowers, gold smelters, iron smelters, and many other types of works that expose the lens to glowing heat. The lens shows true exfoliation in the form of capsular flakes that curl up, generally associated with disc-shaped posterior subcapsular opacity (not seen in children).

COMPLICATED CATARACT

Complicated cataracts can develop at any age following intraocular inflammation, trauma, or neoplasms. As it is secondary to other primary intraocular disorders, it is generally unilateral, slow-progressive, and generally overshadowed by the primary disease. It can be associated with age-related cataracts. It can advance the onset of age-related cataracts.

Common diseases that cause complicated cataracts are:

- *Inflammation of the uvea*—anterior uveitis and pan uveitis—causes more complicated cataracts than only choroiditis. Pars planitis is another cause of complicated cataracts.
- *Myopia:* Both simple and progressive myopia cause complicated cataracts. It is more common in the latter.

- *Retinal dystrophies* are commonly associated with complicated cataracts.
- *Retinal detachment:* Long-standing retinal detachment is generally associated with complicated cataracts.
- *Glaucoma:* Absolute glaucoma is a very common cause of complicated cataracts.
- *Steroids:* Prolonged local or systemic use of steroids is associated with various forms of cataracts.
- Intraocular tumors

Complicated cataracts generally develop in the posterior cortex as subcapsular diffuse opacity, which is denser at the posterior pole. The complicated cataracts progress slowly and are generally associated with complications of primary disease such as band keratopathy, pupillary membrane, peripheral anterior synechiae, patches of atrophy on the iris, irregular pupils, iris pigment on the lens, old keratic precipitates (KPs), and secondary glaucoma, all of which contribute to the nonimprovement of vision following successful IOL implantation. The cataract may show polychromatic luster and a breadcrumb appearance. In a long run, complicated cataracts spread to the whole of the lens, just like any age-related cataract.

In the case of a unilateral cataract, the possible causes in other eye should be excluded, and the patient should be informed about it and its prognosis.

Aphakia:
- The other name for the lens is Phakon (phacos).
- The eye with a lens inside is called the phakic eye.
- The eye without a lens is called aphakic.
- The eye without a natural lens but with an IOL is called pseudophakic.
- Clinically, aphakia means the absence of a lens, completely or partially, from the pupillary area.

Flowchart 19.4: Various possibilities of aphakia.

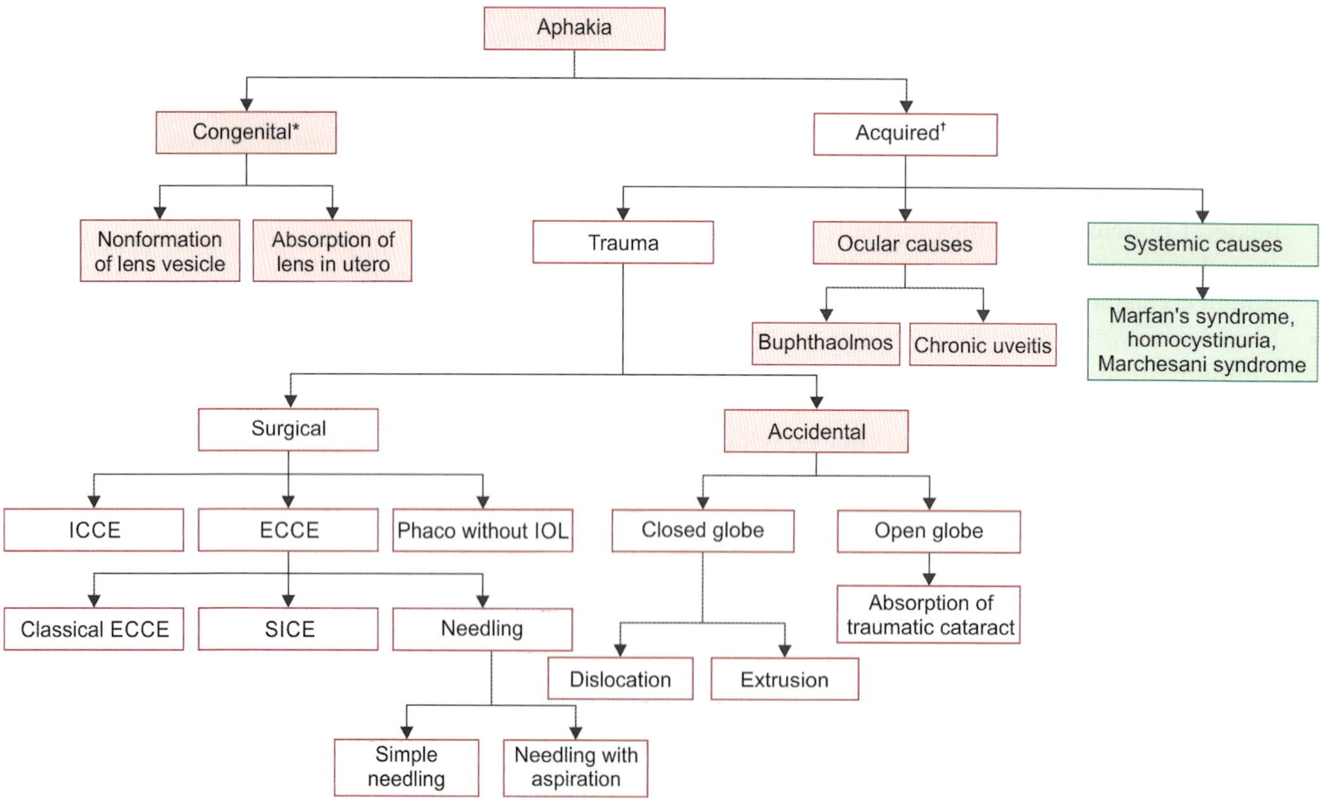

**Congenital aphakia* is extremely rare and may be associated with other congenital anomalies of the eye. It is said to be primary when the lens vesicle has not developed at all and secondary when a partially formed lens is absorbed in utero.

†*Acquired aphakia:* It is very common; the most common cause is surgical removal. This used to be 90% of all causes of aphakia. It has now been replaced by pseudophakia, which is in fact a form of aphakia where an artificial lens has been planted inside the eye in place of a natural lens.

(ECCE: extracapsular cataract extraction; IOL: intraocular lens; ICCE: intracapsular cataract extraction; SICE: small incision cataract surgery)

- Examples of the first are intracapsular removal of the lens, total dislocation of the lens in vitreous/AC, and extrusion of the lens through rent in the sclera (phacocele).
- Examples of the second are extracapsular lens extractions. (It leaves part of the anterior capsule, a complete posterior capsule, some cortical matter in the pupillary area, and the absorption of the lens following a traumatic cataract.).
- In pseudophakia, the IOL can be in the AC/PC; in the PC, it can be in the bag or in the sulcus. The former is the surgery of choice today.

CAUSES OF APHAKIA

The causes of aphakia are many. The most common being surgical extraction of the lens, and the rarest being congenital absence of the lens.

Flowchart 19.4 depicts various possibilities of aphakia in all ages.

SUGGESTED READING

1. Bhayana AA, Prasad P, Azad SV. Refractive errors and the red reflex: Bruckner test revisited. Indian J Ophthalmol. 2019;67(8):1381-2.
2. Eibschitz-Tsimhoni M, Archer SM, Del Monte MA. Intraocular lens power calculation in children. Surv Ophthalmol. 2007;52(5):474-82.
3. Ghauri AJ, Abbortt J, Butler L. Congenital cataract. In: Denniston AKO, Murray P (Eds). Oxford Handbook of Ophthalmology, 4th edition. Oxford UK: Oxford University Press; 2018.
4. Haargaard B, Wohlfahrt J, Fledelius HC, Rosenberg T, Melbye M. Incidence and cumulative risk of childhood cataract in a cohort of 2.6 million Danish children. Invest Ophthalmol Vis Sci. 2004;45(5):1316-20.
5. Heidary G, Kazlas M. The management of cataracts in infancy and childhood. In: Pavan-Langston D (Ed). Manual of Ocular Diagnosis and Therapy, 6th edition. Philadelphia: Lippincott Williams and Wilkins; 2008. p. 310.
6. Khokhar S, Agrawal S, Gupta S, Gogia V, Agrawal T. Epidemiology of traumatic lenticular subluxation in India. Int Ophthalmol. 2014;34(2):197-207.
7. Khokhar S, Agrawal T, Kumar G, Kushmesh R, Tejwani LK. Lenticular abnormalities in children. J Pediatr Ophthalmol Strabismus. 2012;49(1):32-7.
8. Khokhar SK, Dhull C (Eds). Essentials of Pediatric Cataract Surgery. Singapore: Springer Nature; 2022.
9. Khokhar SK, Pillay G, Dhull C, Agarwal E, Mahabir M, Aggarwal P. Pediatric cataract. Indian J Ophthalmol. 2017; 65(12):1340-9.
10. Kochgaway L. Pediatric cataract management. In: Ramamurthy D, Biswas P (Eds). AIOS Ready Reckoner in Ophthalmology, 2nd edition. New Delhi: Jaypee Brothers Medical Publishers (P) Ltd; 2017. pp. 709-11.
11. Lambert SR, Aakalu VK, Hutchinson AK, Pineles SL, Galvin JA, Heidary G. Intraocular lens implantation during early childhood: A report by the American Academy of Ophthalmology. 2019;126(10):1454-61.
12. Lambert SR. Treatment of congenital cataract. Br J Ophthalmol. 2004;88(7):854-5.
13. Liu Y, Chen W. Pediatric lens diseases. Singapore: Springer; 2017.
14. Mukherjee PK. Pediatric Ophthalmology, 1st edition. New Delhi: New Age International (P) Ltd; 2005.
15. Olitsky SE, Marsh JD. Abnormality of lens. In: Kliegman RM, St Geme JW (Eds). Nelson Textbook of Pediatrics, Vols. 1 and 2, 22nd edition. Amsterdam, Netherlands: Elsevier; 2024.
16. Ram J, Sukhija J. (2012). Pediatric cataract management. AIOS CME series (no. 26) [online] Available from https://www.aios.org/cme/cmeseries26.pdf [Last accessed March, 2025].
17. Ram J. Current surgical techniques for pediatric cataract surgery. In: Ready Reckoner Ophthalmology, 1st edition. New Delhi: Jaypee Brothers Medical Publishers (P) Ltd; 2010.
18. Sharma A, Basti S, Gupta S. Secondary capsule-supported intraocular lens implantation in children. J Cataract Refract Surg. 1997;23(Suppl 1):675-80.
19. Sharma A. Secondary IOL implantation in children. In: Ready Reckoner in Ophthalmology, 1st edition. New Delhi: Jaypee Brothers Medical Publishers (P) Ltd; 2010.
20. Singh D. Congenital and infantile cataracts. In: Current Ocular Therapy, 5th edition. Philadelphia: WB Saunders Company; 2000. pp. 538-41.
21. Singh D. India Ophthalmological Society. (1998). Pediatric cataract in the CME series. [online] Available from https://www.aios.org/cme/cmeseries1.pdf [Last accessed March, 2025].
22. Solebo AL, Russell-Eggitt I, Nischal KK, Moore AT, Cumberland P, Rahi JS; British Isles Congenital Cataract Interest Group. Cataract surgery and primary intraocular lens implantation in children < or = 2 years old in the UK and Ireland: Findings of national surveys. 2009;93(11): 1495-8.
23. The infant aphakia treatment study group; Lambert SR, Buckley EG, Drews-Botsch C, DuBois L, Hartmann EE, Lynn MJ, et al. A randomized clinical trial comparing cataract lens to intraocular lens correction of monocular aphakia during infancy: Grating acuity and adverse events at age 1 year. Arch Ophthalmol. 2010;128(7): 810-8.

CHAPTER

20 Disorder of Retina

The retina is the seat of vision, both central and peripheral. The central vision encompasses distant vision, fine vision, near vision, color vision, contrast, and spatial vision*. The peripheral vision consists of night vision, coarse vision, and the peripheral field.

Retina is considered to be a part of the central nervous system; it is out of the pouching of the brain. The retinal axons, originating from all over the retina, travel back to form the optic nerve. The retina is the most distal part of the visual path. The retina is the middle layer of the coats to the eye. It is sandwiched between the vitreous on the inner aspect, and the choroid lies on the outer side of the retina. The rest of the eye is constructed around the retina to house, protect, and nourish it. The retina moves along with the eyeball to increase its field. The optical system focuses both parallel rays arising from the far point and divergent rays from the near point on the fovea to give a sharp, inverted, miniature image of the object of interest. The inverted image is corrected by an electric impulse induced by an electrochemical process and transmitted to the visual cortex via a visual path. The normal retina is transparent with a pink tinge imparted by the underlying pigment epithelium and blood vessels.

PARTS OF THE RETINA

- Retina, for clinical convenience, has traditionally been divided into two broad parts without any definite anatomical demarcation, i.e., (1) the central retina and (2) the peripheral retina. The central retina roughly corresponds to the posterior pole of the globe, encompassing the macula and surrounding retina, lateral to the border of the optic disk; the rest of the retina is considered to be peripheral.

The foveal avascular zone (FAZ) is a region of 0.231–0.405 mm^2 within the fovea centralis at the center of the retina of the human eye that is devoid of retinal blood vessels **(Figs. 20.1 and 20.2)**. It is depicted on fluorescein angiography.

The central retina is rich in cones with fewer rods. The density of cones sharply falls from the center of the macula toward the periphery. The arrangement is reversed in the

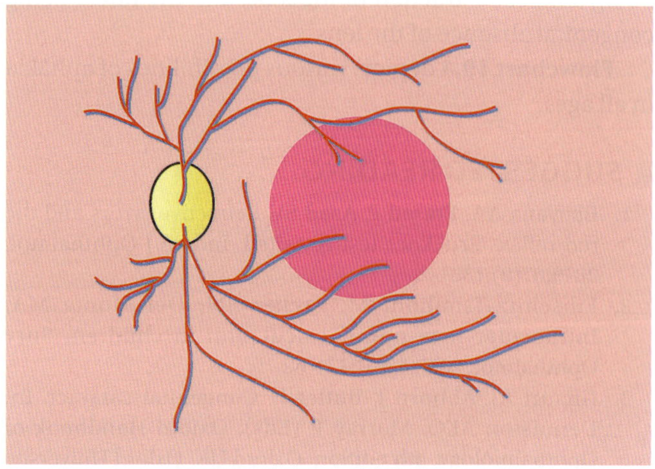

Fig. 20.1: Relative position and size of optic nerve and macula.

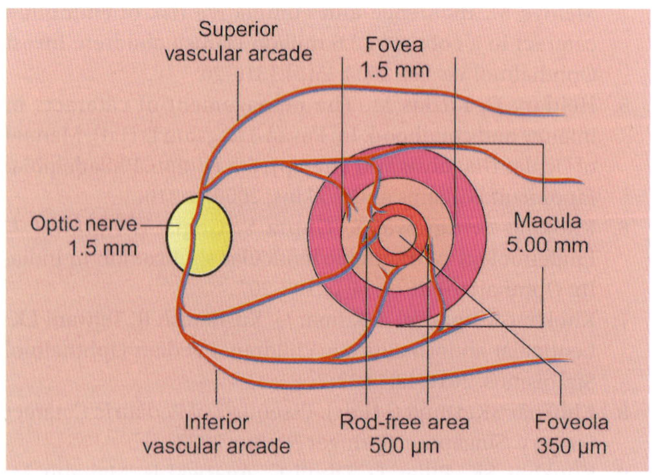

Fig. 20.2: Minute macular topography.

**Spatial vision* is a process to detect and differentiate sinusoidal patterns. It consists of contrast sensitivity; it is influenced by optical, retinal, neural, and adaptation by the eye.

periphery, with more rods and less cones. The central retina is meant for photopic vision (day vision). The periphery is meant for scotopic vision (night vision and fields of vision).

The central retina is endowed with distant vision, near vision (supplemented by accommodation), color vision, fine vision, and contrast. The vision falls precipitously from the center to the extreme periphery. The peripheral retina has no color vision.

- The other, more precise division is based on the embryology of the retina, i.e., the pigmentary retina and the neural retina. The former develops from the outer leaf of the optic cup and extends over the pigment epithelium of the ciliary body; it is single-layered. It does not participate in vision. The inner layer of the optic cup gives rise to multiple highly specialized layers of cells that actively participate in vision.
- The neural retina has nine layers. They are given as follows **(Fig. 20.3)**:
  1. Photoreceptors
  2. External limiting membrane
  3. Outer nuclear layer
  4. Outer plexiform layer
  5. Inner nuclear layer
  6. Inner plexiform layer
  7. Ganglion cell layer
  8. Nerve fiber layer
  9. Internal limiting layer
- Functionally, the neural layers are put into three groups given as follows:
  1. Visual cells (rods and cones)
  2. Bipolar cells
  3. Ganglion cells
- *Macula:* The shining spot seen during fundus examination and referred to as the foveal reflex is only a part of the macula called the fovea.

Macula, in fact, is a larger area at the posterior pole of the globe; it is many times larger than the disk. The center of the macula is two disk diameters away from the lateral margin of the disk, bisected by the horizontal raphe. It is 5.00 mm in diameter, in contrast to the diameter of the optic nerve, which is 1.5 mm in diameter. The area of the retina, referred to as the macula, is circular in shape and made up of many layers of ganglion cells. It is yellowish due to xanthophylls present in the area **(Fig. 20.4)**. On the basis of fluorescein angiography, it has been divided into the following parts: umbo, foveola, fovea, parafovea, and perifovea. A tiny part of the macula is umbo about its presence, which is doubted by many authors. It is a circular area of 0.33 mm in diameter around the center of the macula called the foveola that is surrounded by an avascular zone of 0.5 mm. The foveola is the most photosensitive part of the retina. It is a slightly depressed area in the macula and contains only cones and their nuclei. The second and third neurons are displaced circumferentially. The macula lacks the inner four layers, i.e., (1) nerve fiber layer, (2) ganglion cell layer, (3) inner plexiform layer, and (4) inner nuclear layer. The macula solely depends on the choriocapillaris for its blood supply. The above factors, along with the absence of blood vessels, make the fovea the thinnest part of the macula.

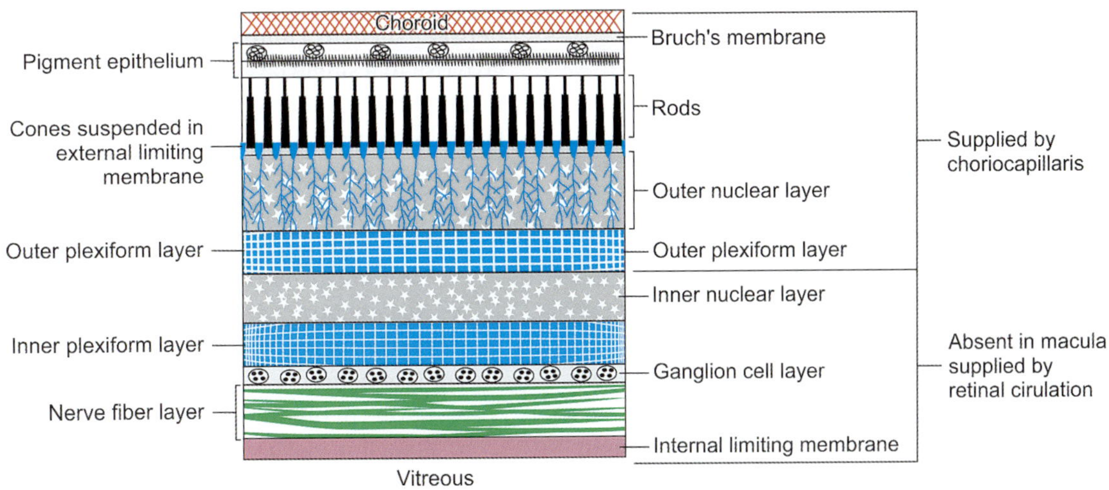

Fig. 20.3: Layers of the retina.

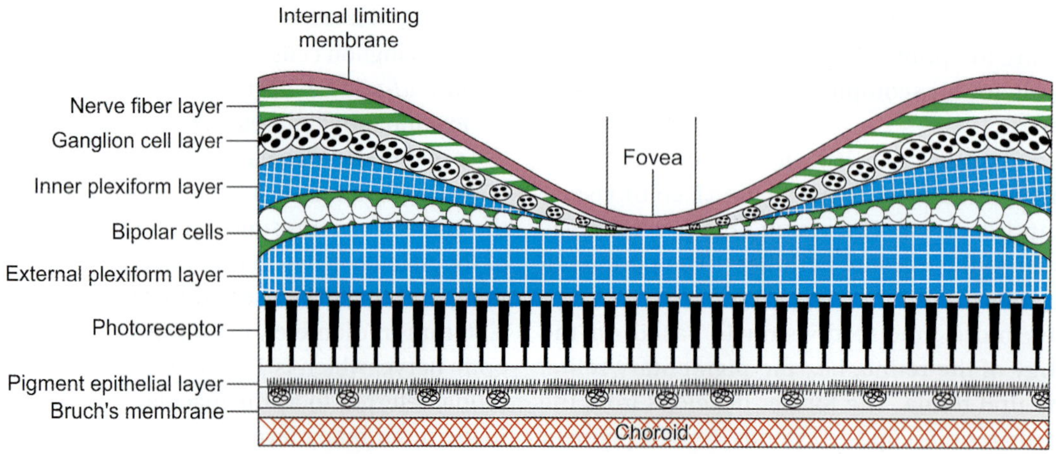

Fig. 20.4: Various parts of macula at fovea.

- *Fovea:* It is an oval depression with a rim, a slope, and a floor; it is less sensitive than the foveola; it comprises a circular area of 1.5 mm in diameter; the fovea is surrounded by a ring of 1.00 mm in width all round making the outer limit 2.5 mm; the rest of the macula constitutes the perifovea.
- *Foveal avascular zone:* The central 0.5 mm area of the macula is devoid of any blood vessels. That becomes apparent on fluorescein angiography and is called the avascular zone of the fovea.

The absence of blood vessels is explained by following:

- Retina gets its blood supply from two sources given as follows:
  1. Retinal circulation
  2. Choriocapillaris
- The cells up to the inner nuclear layers are supplied by retinal circulation.
- The remaining layers are supplied by choriocapillaris.
- As the inner half of the retinal layers are absent in fovea, the capillaries do not exist in this area.

Other properties of maculas are given as follows:

- The macula has the maximum number of cones and the least number of rods.
- The cones are tallest at the fovea.
- The cones are densely packed in the fovea.
- The cones are arranged vertically all over except for the foveola, where they are oblique.
- Each cone is connected to a single bipolar cell, which synapses with a single ganglion cell.
- The macular fibers enter the optic nerve on the lateral side in a straight line to occupy the central part of the optic nerve, accounting for 33% of all the fibers of the optic nerve.
- The insertion of the inferior oblique on the outer surface of the sclera marks the macula on the inner side.
- There are hardly any rods in the macula.
- The cones are covered directly by an internal limiting membrane.

LAYERS OF RETINA

- It has been noted earlier that the retina is ectodermal in nature except for the blood vessels that are mesodermal and developmentally independent of the retina; they are visible on the surface of the retina during fundus examination and give a pink glow on retinoscopy. They supply the inner layers of the retina.
- The optic cup has two layers with a potential space between them in a fully developed eye. The outer layers give rise to a single layer of retinal pigment epithelium firmly attached to the Bruch's membrane. The inner layer, in contrast, is nonpigmented and multilayered, collectively called the sensory retina **(Fig. 20.3)**.
- Histologically, the sensory retina has:
  - Two each of:
    - *Limiting membranes:* External and internal
    - *Nuclear layers:* Inner and outer
    - *Plexiform layers:* Inner and outer
  - One each of:
    - Layers of photoreceptors
    - Ganglion cell layer
    - Nerve fiber layer

DETAILS OF THE RETINAL LAYERS

Retinal Pigment Epithelium

This is the outermost layer of the retina that develops from the outer wall of the optic cup, is attached firmly to the Bruch's membrane without any potential space in between, and is continuous with the pigment epithelium of the ciliary body. The pigmented cells are cuboidal in shape; they do not divide, and their numbers too do not change. The microvilli in the pigmented cells act as anchors to the outer segment of photoreceptors. The base of the epithelium is crenated; the cells are rich in mitochondria. Color of the cells is imparted by the melanin present in them. The function of the layer is to enhance the efficiency of the cones. This is brought about by the absorption of scattered light. The pigments are absent in albinism. The pigment layer helps in the storage and transport of vitamin A. Another function of the pigment epithelium is to constitute the blood–retinal barrier.

Blood–retinal Barrier

The blood–retinal barrier is a physiological barrier that controls the passage of fluid to the retina. Only a few chemicals can pass through this protective barrier. It is two-layered: an outer layer and an inner layer.

The former is formed by the pigment epithelium, and the latter is formed by the tight endothelial cells in capillaries. The permeability of retinal blood vessels is different from that of blood vessels in other parts of the body. The passage of molecules from retinal capillaries to retinal cells is highly selective. This is possible due to the absence of an internal elastic layer and smooth muscles in the retinal capillaries. Only a basal layer covers the outer surface of the vessels.

The layers of the neural retina are given as follows:

- *Layer of photoreceptor:* The part of the retina that has the maximum number of cells is the layer of photoreceptors. The layer lies between the pigment layer and the outer plexiform layer. The cells of the photoreceptors, i.e., cones and rods, are not exclusively located in this space; they span between the outer plexiform layer and the microvilli of the retinal pigment epithelium layer. The body of the photoreceptors is closer to the retinal pigment epithelium than the outer plexiform layer.

  Structure of rods and cones: Each of these photoreceptors has a distinct function. The cones are meant for central photopic vision; the rods are concerned with peripheral scotopic vision. Though the rods and cones have different functions, locations, shapes, and sizes, they structurally share many common features. The rods are more numerous (120 million) and longer than the cones (6 million), and both the photoreceptors have an inner segment and an outer segment. The internal limiting membrane intervenes in between. Each photoreceptor has the following parts: cell body, nucleus, and cell processes.

  The long axis of the cells is at right angles to the surface of the retina. The rods have elongated bodies, and the cones have conical bodies. The apices of the outer segment of both are attached to the retinal pigment epithelium by microvilli. The nuclei of cones are larger than that of rods but paler; the synaptic ends of both cells are called spherules. Each cone is connected to a single bipolar cell, in contrast to rods, which are connected to more than one bipolar cell.
- *External limiting membrane:* This is a homogeneous sheet of plasma secreted by the photoreceptors and Müller cells.

  The external limiting membrane is stretched across the retina, from the optic nerve to the ora serrata. The photoreceptors seem to be suspended in it; the membrane divides the photoreceptors into two parts, i.e., (1) the inner segment and (2) the outer segment.
  1. *Outer nuclear layer:* The layer comprises the nuclei of the rods and cones. The nuclei of cones are nearer to the outer limiting membranes, which are connected to second-order neurons.
  2. *Outer plexiform layer:* The outer plexiform layer lies between the two nuclear layers, containing the synapses of photoreceptor cells, bipolar cells, and horizontal cells. This layer is least vascularized among other layers of the retina, hence prone to degenerative and metabolic disorders.
- *Inner nuclear layer:* This layer, besides bipolar and horizontal cells*, also contains amacrine cells† and Müller cells‡ supplied by the central retinal artery.

**Horizontal cells:* These cells lie within the inner nuclear layer along with amacrine cells and retinal interneurons. They act as modulators between photoreceptors and bipolar cells.

†*Amacrine cells:* These cells are scattered all over the retina; they do not have axons; they are found in the inner retina and join bipolar cells to the ganglion cells.

‡*Müller cells:* Müller cells are glial cells of the retina without any visual function; their function is similar to the function of astrocytes, oligodendrocytes, and ependymal cells of the central nervous system.

The astrocytes have an important role in retinal vascularization in the adult retina. They are situated in the nerve fibers and ganglion cell layer, or retina, amounting to 8–10 millions.

- *Inner plexiform layer:* This layer contains synapses of bipolar cells, ganglion cells, and amacrine cells, along with Müller cells.
- *Ganglion cell layer:* This layer contains the ganglion cells. It is not uniformly thick throughout the retina; it is thicker at the macula. There are about 1.2 million ganglion cells in each retina with axons. The axons of ganglion cells join to form the optic nerve; each ganglion cell is joined to four or five cones and many rods. The number of ganglion cells gradually gets reduced on the periphery. They are most numerous in the posterior pole.
- *Nerve fiber layer:* This layer contains mostly the axons of ganglion cells. The axons form the unmyelinated fibers of the optic nerve. The arrangement of nerve fibers in the retina is not regular; the fibers originating from the macula are called papillomacular fibers. They pass straight to the lateral side of the optic nerve. The fibers arising from the nasal side travel in a radial fashion, and the fibers from the rest of the retina sweep over and under the macula in a curve to reach the upper and lower poly of the disc respectively. Derangement in these fibers results in a specific field defect.

BLOOD SUPPLY TO THE RETINA

The retina, due to its high metabolic requirement, has a rich blood supply from two sources, comprising of:

1. *Retinal circulation:* Central retinal artery
2. *Uveal circulation (choriocapillaris):* Short posterior ciliary arteries

The blood supply is divided into two layers. The retinal circulation is responsible for blood supply on the inner side up to the outer plexiform layer. The choriocapillaris supplies the rest of the layers. The retinal circulation amounts to a small part of the circulation. The main supply comes from choriocapillaris.

CENTRAL RETINAL ARTERY

The central retinal artery arises from the first part of the ophthalmic artery at the orbital apex, with the following segments: orbital, intervaginal, intraneural, and intraocular. The orbital part runs anteriorly under the dural sheath of the optic nerve; until it reaches a point 10 mm posterior to the globe, then it takes an upward turn to pierce the covering of the optic nerve sheath to reach the subarachnoid space in a vertical course.

The intervaginal part is a small segment in the subarachnoid space. The intraneural part is a large segment that traverses through the center of the substance of the optic nerve up to the disk.

The central retinal artery proper is the part of the retinal artery that is visible on an ophthalmoscope. It supplies the optic nerve head and inner layers of the retina, ending as the artery of the retina. It gives the following branches in the substance of the optic nerve: pial, recurrent, and intraneural branches **(Figs. 20.5 and 20.6)**.

At the head of the optic nerve, the central retinal artery is divided into two branches, namely superior and inferior, each dividing into temporal and nasal branches. The four branches, thus, formed supply four quadrants of the corresponding quadrant of the retina separately; they do not anastomose with each other. The retinal arteries supply all of the retina except the avascular zone of the macula, which lies in superficial layers directly under the internal limiting membrane. The retinal system of arteries does not anastomose with choriocapillaris as well, which forms the larger system of vessels to supply the rest of the retina. The arterioles of the central retinal arteries are the end arteries.

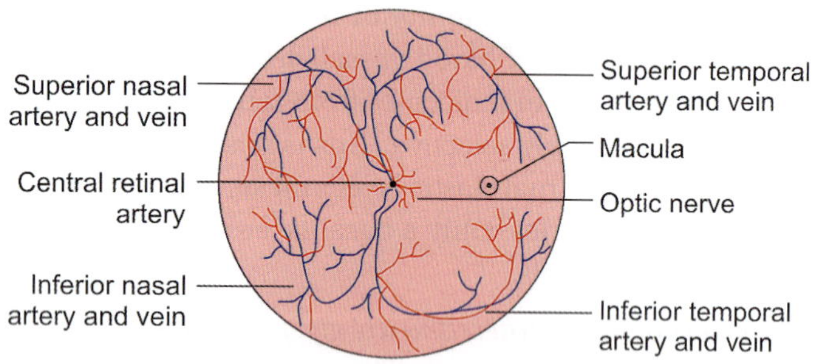

Fig. 20.5: Normal retinal vessels as seen by an indirect ophthalmoscope.

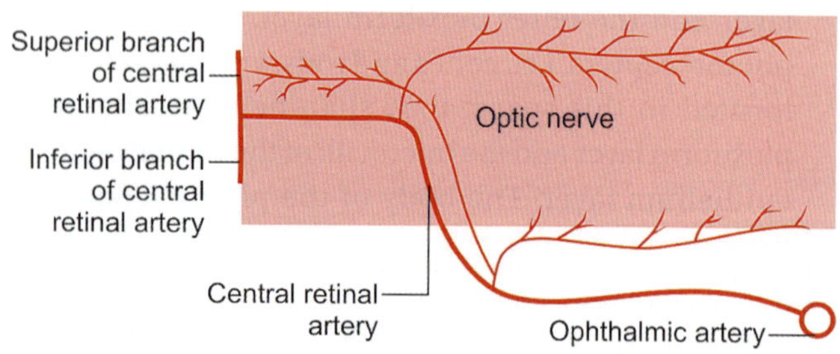

Fig. 20.6: Path of central retinal artery in the optic nerve and its oblique course in intervaginal.

CHORIOCAPILLARIS

A network of single layers of choroidal capillaries lying under the Bruch's membrane constitutes the choriocapillary complex, which supplies the outer layer of the retina. The choriocapillaris extends between the ora serrata and the border of the disk with a uniform density. Under the macula, they are more numerous, wider, and denser to meet the enhanced need of the macula, which does not have the support of the central retinal artery.

RETINAL VEINS

The retinal arteries are accompanied by retinal veins of the same name, i.e., the central retinal vein, superior and inferior retinal veins. The veins start on the periphery and end in the central retinal veins. That ultimately drains into the cavernous sinus and superior ophthalmic vein and less commonly into the inferior ophthalmic vein. The retinal veins are wider than the corresponding arteries; they lack the muscular coat of the arteries. The ratio of diameter between arteries and veins is 2:3. The veins are softer and have thinner walls than the arteries. The veins look darker than the arteries. Arteries generally pass over the veins; wherever they cross the veins, the arteries are placed over the veins. The arteries and veins share a common sheath at the arteriovenous crossing.

The central retinal vein, after passing through the lamina, continues backward along the artery, till 2.00 mm posterior to the entry of the artery, i.e., 12.00 mm from the back of the globe, and exits the nerve, traveling the intervaginal space obliquely, thus making its course longer in the intervaginal space, making it vulnerable to raised intravaginal pressure in the cerebrospinal fluid (CSF). This is most commonly held theory of the pathogenesis of papilledema.

EMBRYOLOGY OF THE RETINA

The embryology of the retina has been discussed earlier. The following is an abridged version of the same.

The presence of the retina becomes evident in very early stage of the development of the eye; this happens even before the neural tube closes at the 2.00-mm stage. The development of the retina is not uniform throughout its development. The development of the macula is a long-drawn process. As compared to the rest of the retina, the development of the macula spills over to neonatal age.

The retina develops from the optic cup. Both layers of the optic cup are involved in the development of the retina. The outer layer gives rise to a single layer of pigment epithelium; from the inner wall develop the other nine neural layers. Initially, there is a visible space between the two layers, which gradually shrinks to a potential space in the fully developed retina. This space is of utmost importance in the pathogenesis of retinal detachment. The neural layer has a propensity to separate and goes into a state of retinal separation.

Ora Serrata

The ora serrata is the serrated junction between the choroid and the ciliary body. It is the junction between the nonphotosensitive area of the retina and the photosensitive retina. It lies 5 mm anterior to the equator and is 2 mm wide, forming a confluence of a single-layered ciliary epithelium and a multilayered sensory retina. It is almost avascular and liable to separate from its mooring, causing retinal dialysis.

Sensory Retina

In the early stages of development, the sensory layer that arises from the inner layer of the optic cup is single-layered, from which develop the nine neural layers in three groups, i.e.:

1. Photoreceptors
2. Bipolar and ganglion cells
3. Axons of ganglion cells and nerve fibers

Development of Macula

The development of the macula is more complex than the development of the rest of the retina. The macula is the most sensitive part of the ocular system, though it is a part of the retina. Yet its development differs from that of the rest of the retina. The area in which the future macula will develop can be discerned at a very early stage. The development of macula goes into phases of accelerated growth and retardation. It progresses fast initially, only to slow down for some time and continue to grow fast thereafter. The growth lasts well into a few months in the postnatal period. The rest of the retina does not share this dormant period of macular growth. The retardation of macular growth corresponds to the period between 3 and 8 months. At 6 months of development, the macula is thicker than the rest of the retina and then starts thinning due to the migration of ganglion cells toward the periphery.

At birth, the ganglion cells present at the macula become single-layered.

CONGENITAL ANOMALIES OF THE RETINA

Retina, being the largest neural element concerned with vision, developing from two layers of the optic vesicle with a prolonged period of development, has many developmental anomalies that may be small enough to be insignificant to gross anomalies to cause extensive visual loss and configuration of the globe. The congenital disorders may be localized to the two layers of the retina or may involve other structures such as the uvea, vitreous, and optic nerve in various combinations. The anomalies are not only structural but may be biochemical as well, i.e., albinism and night blindness. Many of the congenital anomalies have genetic backgrounds. The congenital anomalies are mostly evident at birth and may remain stationary; others progress; a few of them with congenital backgrounds make their presence felt at later years, generally bilateral. The congenital anomalies are universal, with variable incidence in various races.

Classification of Congenital Anomalies of the Retina

Being multifactorial, it is not possible to have a single comprehensive classification that encompasses all the congenital anomalies of the retina.

The commonly used criteria to classify them are given as follows:

- Topography
- Appearance
- Physiological function
- Genetic predisposition

Out of them, the most practical classification is the topographical (anatomical) classification.

The anatomical anomalies are put into the following groups:

- Isolated anomalies of the retina:
    - Structures arising from the outer layer (retinal pigment epithelium)
    - Structures arising from the inner layers:
        - Anomalies of the peripheral retina
        - Anomalies of the central retina (macula)
        - Combination
- Congenital anomalies of retinal vessels
- Congenital anomalies of the optic nerve
- Congenital anomalies of the vitreous
- Combined vitreoretinal anomalies

Congenital Anomalies of Structures Arising from the Retinal Pigment Epithelium

Congenital anomalies of the retinal pigment epithelium are fewer than those arising from the sensory retina. As the layer involves the pigment of the retina, it results in an abnormality of pigmentation in the retina and its consequences. The congenital abnormality of the retinal pigment epithelium is not an anomaly of structures; it can be a postmaternal infection of rubella, syphilis, influenza, and other viral infections contracted by the mother in the first trimester. The condition consists of pepper-salt appearance of the fundus with normal blood vessels without optic neuritis. However, the optic disk may be paler than normal in such instances, without diminished night vision. The conditions are stationary and do not require treatment; they may be confused with more serious condition of retinitis pigmentosa.

More frequent and widely spread anomalies of pigmentation are albinism and its variations. It again does not have any structural anomalies; it is a metabolic disorder of the amino acid tyrosine, a precursor of melanin, the substance responsible for color of skin, hair, and eyes. Albinism is seen in all races with variable incidence. It has been reported to be as frequent as one in 20,000 live births, more common among dark races and equally common among boys and girls. With varying genetic preponderance, it could be autosomal dominant, autosomal recessive, or X-linked. In some instances, both parents with frank albinism or with some traits may have non-Albinotic children. This happens when one parent is a tyrosinase-negative albino and the other is tyrosinase-positive albino. Women are the carriers with minimal clinical features. It is present at birth and may be extensive enough to be noticed or mild enough to be missed. It is noticed early in dark races. Isolated involvement of the eyes is diagnosed on examination of the fundus later in life.

Albinism has been classified variously given as follows:

- Genetically, it is an autosomal condition that could either be dominant or recessive; other possibility is its being X-linked.
- According to appearance, depending on the involvement of three cardinal parts of the body,

i.e., the eye, skin, and hair, in isolation or in various combinations.

- Perfect, imperfect, and partial
- A better classification is:
    - Cutaneous
    - Oculocutaneous:
        - Tyrosinase positive
        - Tyrosinase negative
    - Ocular
    - Albinism is associated with other syndromes.

The color of eyes, hair, and skin depends on the presence of melanin in them. The basic pathology of albinism is a derangement of the production of melanin in these tissues. Melanin is produced in melanocytes, which are present in these tissues. Melanocytes are derived from the neural crest; the production of melanin involves interaction between tyrosine, an amino acid, and the enzyme tyrosinase.

Cutaneous Albinism

The skin in these children is light colored in patches and may be present at birth or develop later in life. The patches may involve the skin of the lids, lashes, and eyebrows without visual signs or symptoms; the condition should be differentiated from an unrelated condition of vitiligo.

Oculocutaneous Albinism

This is most common form of albinism and is called complete or perfect; there is no pigment in the skin, hair, or eyes, in contrast to imperfect albinism, where there is a deficiency of pigment in these places. Clinically, the condition falls into two broad groups, i.e., (1) tyrosinase positive and (2) tyrosinase negative.

The clinical features of oculocutaneous albinism consist of:

- *Skin:* Pale with freckles due to the absence of melanin
- *Eyes:*
    - Eyebrows are white and spare
    - Lashes are white (poliosis)
    - Conjunctiva is not congested but look so due to the paleness of the surrounding lids
    - Cornea, AC, and lens are normal.
    - The iris has prominent changes in the form of:
        - The iris is pale and bluish; due to the absence of pigment in the stroma, the iris looks translucent.
        - The pupil is central, circular, and brisk with normal size; it looks pink even in ambient light.
    - The vision is subnormal and variable, ranging from counting fingers to the loss of a few lines on the Snellen chart. Albinism does not cause a loss of light reflex or projection of light. The causes of diminished vision in albinism are:
        - Both types of errors of refraction are equally common, and astigmatism is frequent.
        - Hypoplasia of the macula
        - Nystagmus
        - Squint and amblyopia
    - There is no change in accommodation or convergence. The child keeps the book near the face to produce little magnification and turns the head to put the book in the null zone of the nystagmus. The child may develop head nodding.
    - The color vision and scotopic vision are normal; the child has better vision in the shade due to the translucency of the iris and the absence of pigment in the choroid.
    - *Fundus changes:*
        - Albinism per se is not cause of any opacity in the media.
        - The retinal and choroidal vessels stand out against the white sclera, resulting in a pale fundus.
        - There are no exudates or hemorrhage that can be attributed to albinism.
        - The optic nerve is pale; its borders cannot be defined, and its presence is denoted by the point where the retinal arteries exit.
    - *Neurological changes:*
        - These are rare and consist of abnormal crossing of temporal fibers in the chiasma.
        - Paresis of extraocular muscles
        - Deafness, mental retardation

Common syndromes associated with albinism are Chediak–Higashi syndrome* and Waardenburg syndrome†.

**Chediak–Higashi syndrome:* Chediak–Higashi syndrome is a rare, congenital, fatal disease associated with oculocutaneous albinism. It is an autosomal recessive disorder. Other features are mental retardation, hepatosplenomegaly, persistent lymphadenopathy, occasional lymphoma, and recurrent infections that may prove to be fatal.

†*Waardenburg syndrome:* The condition consists of localized hypopigmentation with less ocular features than systemic albinism. The changes consist of white forelock, heterochromia of the iris, poliosis of the lashes, long lashes, increased intercanthal distance, deformity of the lacrimal passage, and pseudo-/true squint.

Ocular Albinism

This condition is least common among albinism and involves only the eyes; the eyes look normal externally with nystagmus. The condition is diagnosed on a fundus examination that shows hypopigmented retina and choroid, resulting in a pale reflex on retinoscopy. Carrier females show less clinical features.

Management of Albinism

The child with albinism, besides having an ocular handicap, suffers from an array of social stigmas that may hamper the child's carriers. This stigma has profound socioeconomical ramifications, for which the cooperation of parents and teachers is essential, who should be made aware of the conditions and treat the affected child in par with normal children. They should be sent to school with normal children, unless the child is visually handicapped or mentally retarded.

The attending physician/ophthalmologist should try to salvage as much as possible by prescribing appropriate glasses, treat amblyopia, and squinting. The presence of nystagmus is a hindrance in restoring vision. The child should be encouraged to develop nonacademic skills such as music and dance whenever possible.

Ancillary methods are prescribing tinted glasses, use wide brimmed hats, and protect skin by full-sleeve shirts and trousers.

Other Congenital Anomalies of the Retinal Pigment Epithelium

The other anomaly is hypertrophy of the retinal pigment epithelium, which is reported less frequently in spite of its high prevalence. About 1% of the general population harbor this condition without being symptomatic. It is found in two forms, i.e., (1) typical and (2) atypical. The typical is more common, unilateral, generally solitary, rarely in clusters, without relation to any systemic conditions, and does not require further investigation. The condition has no genetic preponderance; the atypical forms are bilateral, with multiple lesions set apart, and oval, with a positive family history. Carcinoma of colon in late life is common.

Anomalies of Structures Developing from the Inner Layer of the Optic Cup

From the inner layer of the optic cup develop the nine sensory layers of the retina; hence, it is logical that they will be more numerous than anomalies of pigment epithelium. They are given as follows:

1. Retinal dystrophies
2. Retinal degeneration
3. Aplasia and dysplasia of the retina
4. Retinal folds
5. Retinal cysts
6. Congenital retinal detachment
7. Congenital retinoschisis

Retinal Dystrophies and Degenerations

In clinical oversight, the terms dystrophies and degenerations are used as interchangeable terms without being so. Unfortunately, there is no precise definition that separates the two.

The distinguishing features of each are given as follows:

- Dystrophies are abiotrophies
- Genetically determined
- Generally not evident at birth
- There is premature degradation of highly specialized cells.
- They are caused due to apoptosis (a state of programmed death of specialized cells).
- They are progressive
- Bilateral and symmetric
- Some of them have:
  - Faulty enzyme
  - Biochemical deficit
- They are not preventable.
- There is no treatment.
- Degenerations:
  - Acquired:
    - Infection
    - Inflammation
    - Trauma
  - Generally unilateral
  - Nonprogressive
  - Nonhereditary
  - Occasionally preventable

Classification of retinal dystrophies ***(Flowchart 20.1)****:* The condition can be given as follows:

- Localized to retinal only
- Associated with:
  - Dystrophies of Bruch's membrane
  - Vitreoretinal dystrophies
- The condition can be either peripheral or central (macular).

Flowchart 20.1: Classification of retinal dystrophies.

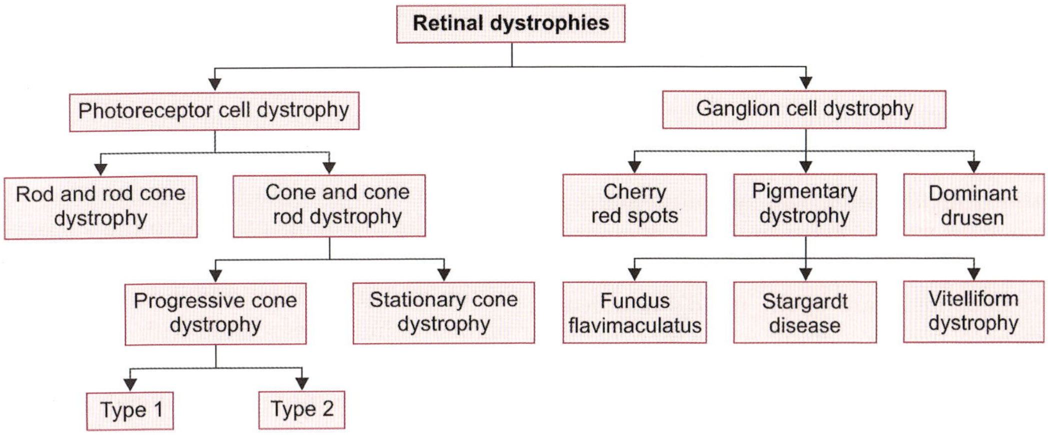

- The most useful classification of retinal dystrophies is on the basis of layers of retina.
- Other retinal dystrophies:
  - Bruch's membrane dystrophy:
    - Disciform macular dystrophy
    - Sorsby's dystrophy
  - Pigment epithelial dystrophy
  - Vitreoretinal dystrophies:
    - Juvenile retinoschisis
    - Wagner vitreoretinal dystrophy
    - Goldmann-Favre vitreoretinal dystrophy
    - Familial exudative vitreoretinal dystrophy

All the dystrophies mentioned above are not seen in children; only some are seen in the first decade. Out of all the conditions, photoreceptor dystrophies are the most common. They form a large group of peripheral dystrophies, which involve rods, mostly with minimum cone involvement and late onset. The conditions in this group are generally referred to as retinitis pigmentosa and its allied conditions.

Retinitis Pigmentosa

The term retinitis pigmentosa is not an appropriate in the true sense of clinical use because the condition is not an infectious state. It is better to call the condition as primary neurosensory dystrophy of the retina or simply as primary retinal dystrophy. As it is difficult to replace old terminologies, the condition remains to be called as retinitis pigmentosa. The better alternative would be to label it as pigmented retinopathy.

The conditions in this group are divided into two broad groups. The first is a more common typical form, and the second, less common, is referred to as an atypical form.

Flowchart 20.2 shows the division.

Flowchart 20.2: Primary neurosensory dystrophy of the retina (RP).

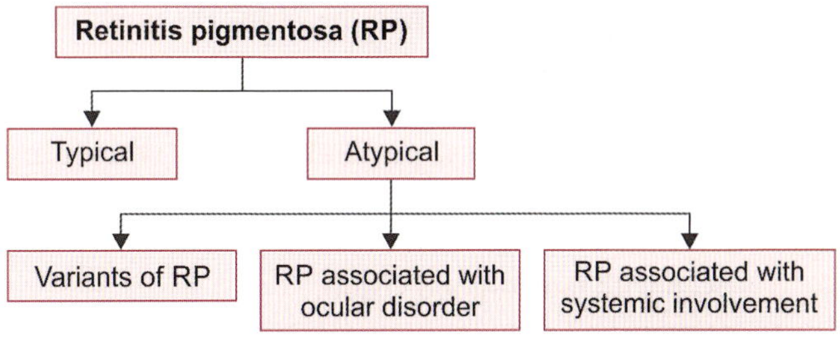

The term retinitis pigmentosa will be retained in the text for convenience.

Retinitis pigmentosa is the most common form of retinal dystrophies, with widespread distribution in all races, almost equal among boys and girls with a slight male preponderance. The cause attributed to this phenomenon is sex-linked inheritance. Though the disorder has a uniform distribution all over the world in all races, there seem to be some pockets of higher incidence among some societies and tribes where consanguinity is common.

The condition can be sporadic or hereditary. The former is also known as isolated or spontaneous, due to a mutation of a gene (there are about 20 genes responsible for the disorder). This group makes up for about one-third of cases. The hereditary type can either be autosomal or X-linked. The autosomal can both be recessive or dominant; all are not equally common in occurrence and prognosis. Out of the three, autosomal recessive is the most common, followed by autosomal dominant. The recessive is the mildest form; the sex-linked is the least common but most severe and rapidly progressive.

Clinical features of retinitis pigmentosa:

- *Symptoms:* The symptoms of retinitis pigmentosa are given as follows:
  - Diminished night vision
  - Diminished peripheral field
  - Diminished distant vision

  - *Diminished night vision:* The symptom starts in early teens in 90% of cases, but it is diagnosed in late 20s. By 10 years of age of the child, the parents become aware of the child's handicap. An early onset may be confused with a more benign condition of vitamin A deficiency and treated as such without success.
  - *Diminished peripheral field:* The child soon become aware of the fact that he has to move his head more to see the writing on the blackboard than his classmates and raise the chin. He may bump in others, finds it difficult to cross the road; this is worsened in dark ambient. The loss of peripheral vision is relentless, paralleling with worsening night blindness. By the fourth decade, he may be left with a tubular vision, making him incapacitated even with fair-to-good vision.
  - *Diminished distant vision:* Generally, children with retinitis pigmentosa have myopes; the myopia is axial that becomes worse with superadded index myopia of lenticular origin, which includes posterior subcapsular opacity and the development of presenile lenticular sclerosis. Macular changes are due to the involvement of cones. The macular changes comprise of cystoid macular edema, usual myopic changes, atrophic and cellophane maculopathy.

In the late stages, the optic nerve develops consecutive optic atrophy, where the color of the disk is waxy pale. If chronic glaucoma supervenes, it worsens the already constricted field.

The vision in the initial stages is within normal limits, which gradually diminishes over years but not terminating in total loss. The loss of central vision does not go parallel with diminished night vision or loss of field.

Signs of retinitis pigmentosa: Externally, the eyes of the child suffering from retinitis pigmentosa in early teens do not show any signs that may lead to a diagnosis of typical retinitis pigmentosa. The diagnostic signs lie in the fundus examination, both by direct and indirect ophthalmoscope.

> The triad of signs are bone spicule pigments, attenuated blood vessels, and a waxy pale disk.

Pigmentary changes in retinitis pigmentosa: The pigmentary changes do not develop abruptly. They follow a definite pattern of development and distribution. The source of their origin is the pigment epithelium, from where the pigments migrate to the surface of the retina along the course of blood vessels. The pigmentation starts in the mid-periphery, initially as mottling. The retinal pigmentation is associated with the translucency of the retina and increased visibility of the choriocapillaris, which become more pronounced with the passage of time. Clumps of pigments form cuff of pigment around the retinal veins and arteries. The pigments are irregular, star-shaped flat bodies resembling bone spicules. Bone spicules appearance is the most common form of their shape; there may be variation in shape and size. The pigments are anterior to the vessels; this is in contrast to choroidal dystrophies, where the round pigments lie under the vessels. The pigmentation starts in the mid-periphery on the lateral side, more often in the down-and-out quadrant. The predilection of the mid-periphery is attributed to the paucity of blood supply to the region. The pigmentation starts spreading both centripetally and centrifugally. They also spread superiorly and inferiorly, ultimately encircling the posterior pole. The posterior pole is left devoid of pigmentation for a long time. The outer edge of the ring may reach up to the peripheral retina. Occasionally, another ring of pigmentation may develop between the first and the optic nerve, with a gap in between the two **(Fig. 20.7)**.

> The macula gets pigmented only if the cones are involved. The pigmentation of the macula is not proportionate to night blindness or field loss.

Attenuation of blood vessels: The cause of attenuation of blood vessels is not well understood; the process is gradual in progression and involves both arteries and veins of all sizes. Attenuation of vessels generally precedes night blindness.

Optic atrophy: The disk looks waxy pale with obscuration of lamina without definite cupping; the margins are neither as sharp as in primary optic atrophy nor as smudged as in postneuritic/papilloedematous atrophy. There is no exudate or hemorrhage, either on the disk or retina.

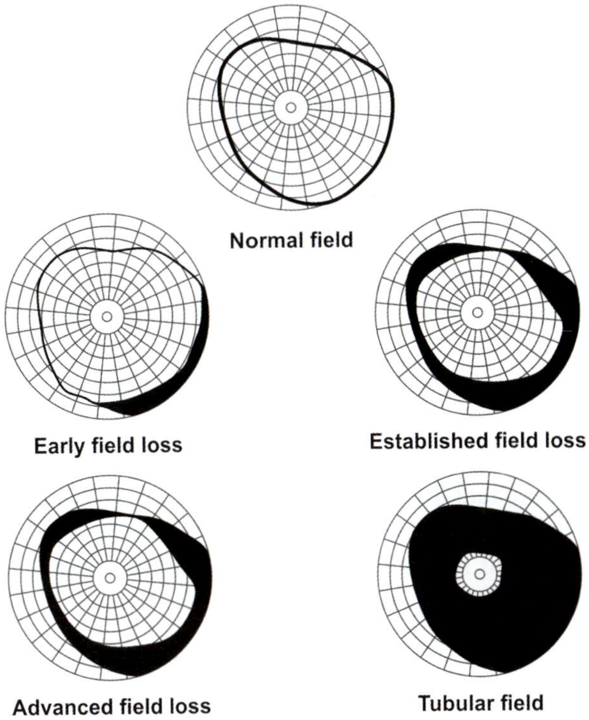

Fig. 20.7: Progression of field loss in retinitis pigmentosa.

Macular involvement: In the past, it was thought that retinitis pigmentosa is a disorder of rods; the macula that does not contain a sufficient number of rods was spared. With the advent of fluorescein angiography and optical coherence tomography (OCT), the hypothesis has taken a back seat, and frequent involvement of the macula is being reported that may be as minimal as a dull foveal reflex to cystoid macular edema. Involvement of the macula is a major cause of diminished central vision, color vision, and contrast.

Vitreous changes: Liquefaction and opacities in vitreous are very common in retinitis pigmentosa. The degree of vitreous degeneration is not proportionate to the clinical features of retinitis pigmentosa. Mostly blamed factor is degenerative myopia that is common in retinitis pigmentosa. The opacities increase with age. Retinitis pigmentosa is not a contributory factor in retinal detachment.

Error of refraction: Moderate-to-severe myopia is common in retinitis pigmentosa. Some of the cases do not improve with the best correction due to the involvement of the macula and associated lenticular changes.

Lenticular changes: Lenticular changes are late to develop in retinitis pigmentosa; hence, they are not encountered under 15 years of age. The opacity gradually increases, worsening the vision.

Glaucoma: Glaucoma secondary to retinitis pigmentosa is not seen under 15 years but is common in the third and fourth decades. Vision is worsened by already lost peripheral vision, macular lesions, and optic nerve changes.

Other ocular conditions associated with retinitis pigmentosa are keratoconus, squint, amblyopia, nystagmus, drusen, progressive external ophthalmoplegia, and subtle glioma of the disk.

Management of retinitis pigmentosa: There is no specific treatment for retinitis pigmentosa. A relentless search for the problem is going on the World over. The suggested methods are gene therapy (Luxturna*) in the early stages, implanted electric devices, neurotropic growth factor, and antiapoptotic factors, all of which are being suggested as cures.

Stem cells from the patient's body is yet another landmark in the management of retinitis pigmentosa.

The other modalities used to manage retinitis pigmentosa are optical and therapeutic; the optical options available are correction of axial myopia with appropriate changes, prescription of nanometer-controlled filtering lenses. Commonly used dark glasses worsen the condition. Low vision aids that magnify the images worsen the condition as part of the magnified image is covered by ever-progressing field loss. It is better to let the child be in school with normal vision. Children with macular involvement may be put in specialized institutions that deal with visually challenged children. The genetics of the condition should be explained to the parents and counseled to prevent consanguinity among the children.

Therapeutic methods used are supplementation with large doses of vitamin A as palmitate along with vitamin E. The use of vitamin E alone is said to be detrimental. Omege-3, along with vitamin A, is claimed to slow the progression of vision loss in retinitis pigmentosa.

**Luxturna:* It is administered as subretinal injection after vitrectomy. The drug works by supplying a copy of retinitis pigmentosa gene directly to the retina. The injected gene manufactures normal protein in affected retinal cells that convert light sensation to an electrical signal. It is prohibitively costly.

Atypical Retinitis Pigmentosa

This comprises a heterogeneous group of retinal dystrophies that do not have all the criteria of typical retinitis pigmentosa. It may only have one or two features and is commonly referred to as atypical retinitis pigmentosa. Some authors consider them as a variation of classical retinitis pigmentosa that will ultimately culminate in its typical form. The only common criterion between the two groups is diminished night vision.

Unilateral retinitis pigmentosa: This is an example where one eye has a triad of retinitis pigmentosa, i.e., diminished night vision, field loss, and consecutive optic atrophy. To this, it may be added the attenuation of blood vessels. The other eye on ophthalmoscopy does not show typical fundus changes of retinitis pigmentosa but has abnormal dark adaptation and subnormal electroretinogram (ERG). It is presumed that the unaffected eye will ultimately develop pigmentation with corresponding field changes.

Sector retinitis pigmentosa: In this rare condition, the fundus changes of retinitis pigmentosa are present in one sector of an eye in the mid-periphery, mostly the inferior quadrant. As a large part of the retina remains normal, there is no night blindness. The field defect is sectorial, corresponding to the area affected. However, since dark adaptation and ERG are subnormal, the condition does not progress and, hence, does not require any treatment.

Inverse retinitis pigmentosa (central retinitis pigmentosa): The only positive finding that puts this condition in the group of retinitis pigmentosa is subnormal ERG. Most of the authors considered it to be a cone dystrophy rather than a rod dystrophy; the only snag is the attenuation of vessels and the presence of typical pigmentation around the macula that spreads centrifugally. As the central retina is dominantly involved, it produces a central scotoma with diminished distant vision and color vision. The vision is reduced in bright light and marginally improved in dim light.

Retinitis pigmentosa sine pigmento: The condition has all the clinical features of typical retinitis pigmentosa without black pigments. It is claimed that the eyes develop pigmentation years after the first discovery of night blindness. Its progression is similar to that of its pigmented counterpart. It is to be differentiated from congenital night blindness that remains stationary throughout life. The condition may initially be confused with vitamin A deficiency and treated as such without-improvement.

Retinitis punctata albescens: This is yet another clinical paradox with the clinical features of typical retinitis pigmentosa, where black spidery pigments are replaced by multiple white dots all over the retina. Generally, it progresses as typical retinitis pigmentosa. Some stationary cases, too, have been reported. The condition may be confused with drusen of the retina.

Systemic Diseases Associated with Retinitis Pigmentosa

The systemic disorders that have some or all of the clinical features of retinitis pigmentosa are long. All are congenital, mostly hereditary, or with metabolic disorders.

Table 20.1 shows the involvement of the system with corresponding syndromes.

A short description of common syndromes that have retinal pigmentation (not always classical retinitis pigmentosa) is given as follows:

Laurence-Moon-Biedl-Bardet syndrome (obesity, polydactyly, and hypogonadal syndrome) **(Figs. 20.8 to 20.10)**.

The multiple systemic disorder is an autosomal recessive syndrome, may be seen in many members of the sibling, all not equally affected, and there may be some members who do not have all the components. It is seen in both sexes with a slight male preponderance; the condition can be noted at birth if the child has polydactyly, syndactyly, or evidence of hypogenitalism. The condition becomes obvious within a year, when it becomes evident that the child is overweight and mentally retarded. By 10 years, the diminished night vision becomes obvious;

TABLE 20.1: Systemic defects and their associated syndromes.

Systemic defects	*Syndrome*
Skeletal	Laurence–Moon–Biedl–Bardet syndrome and Marfan syndrome
Auditory	Refsum, Usher, and Cockayne syndromes
Renal	Cystinosis, cystinuria, and oxalosis
Striated muscle	Progressive external ophthalmoplegia and myotonic dystrophy
Metabolic	Mucopolysaccharidosis and lipidosis

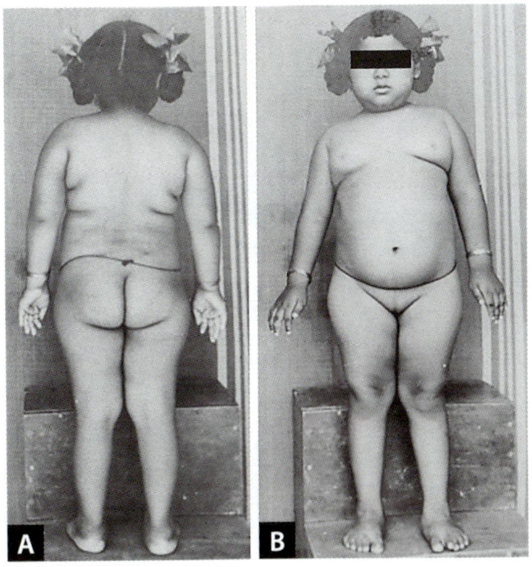

Figs. 20.8A and B: Laurence–Moon syndrome in a girl.

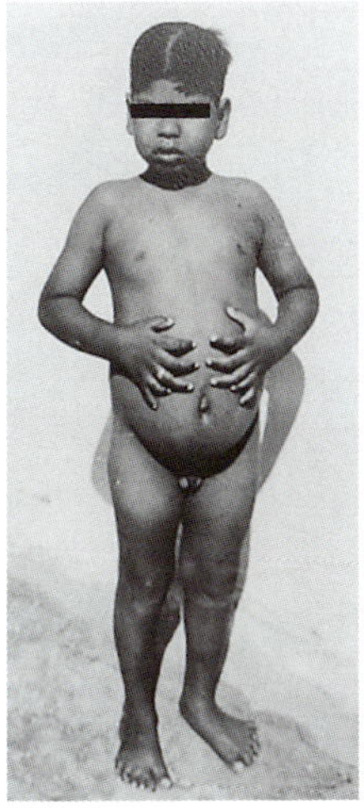

Fig. 20.10: Laurence–Moon syndrome in a boy.

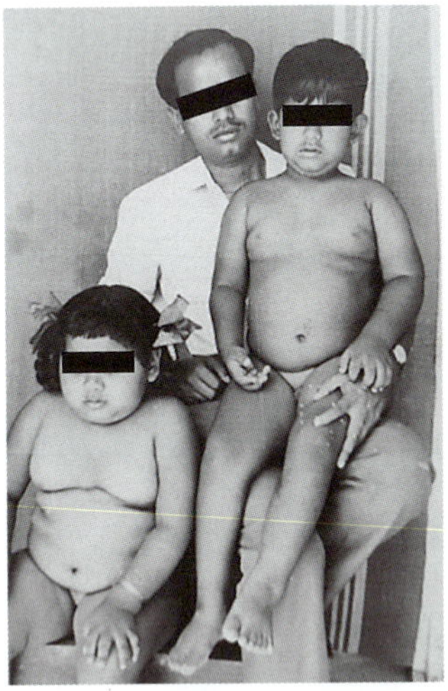

Fig. 20.9: Laurence–Moon syndrome in sibling father normal.

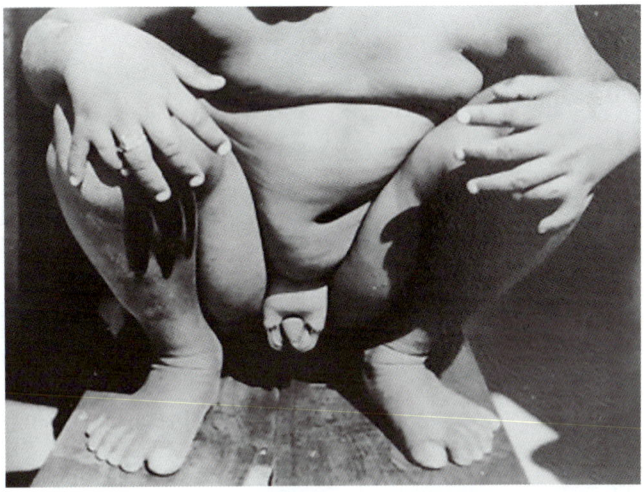

Fig. 20.11: Laurence–Moon syndrome, showing opacity, polydactyly, hypogonadism, and night blindness.

about 90% have features of typical retinitis pigmentosa. By 20 years, the child may start losing central vision due to the involvement of the macula and the onset of consecutive optic atrophy. Some children, instead of black pigments, have progressive albipunctatus changes where black spidery pigments are replaced by white spots. All children with polydactyly/syndactyly should be observed for unusual weight gain and screened for evidence of retinitis pigmentosa **(Figs. 20.11 to 20.14)**.

- *Refsum syndrome:* This is an autosomal recessive syndrome that is associated with multiple systemic anomalies. The most common among them, besides atypical retinitis pigmentosa, are peripheral neuropathies, ataxia, progressive hearing defects, and reduced corneal sensation. Less common are conduction defects of the heart that may prove to be fatal, alopecia, and ichthyosis. The ERG and dark adaptation are subnormal. The pigments are in clumps and look more like pepper and salt retina rather than typical bone spicule pigmentation of typical retinitis pigmentosa. The condition is attributed to a metabolic disorder of fatty acids or, to be more precise, phytanic acids. The chemical is found in both blood and urine. It is claimed that the progress of the disease can be reduced following dietary restriction of fatty acids. The disease starts in childhood with ocular, neurological, and subtle cardiac anomalies that progress to early death due to heart block.

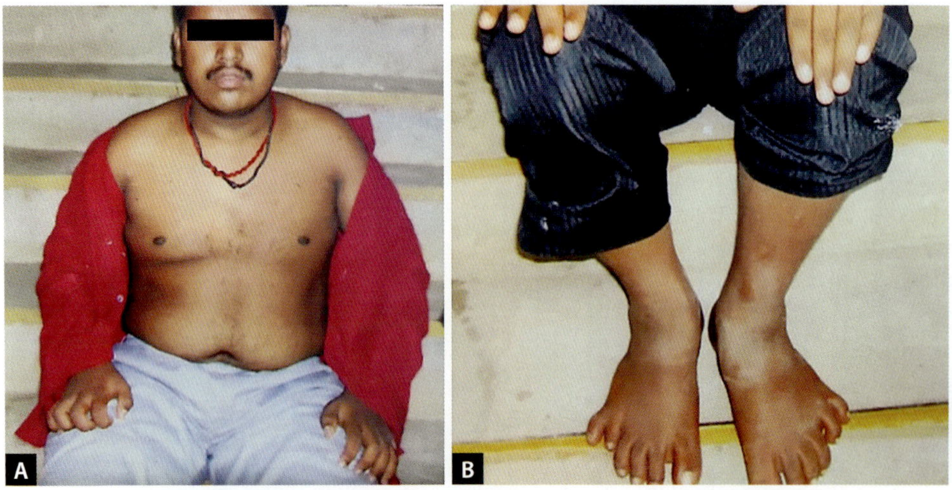

Figs. 20.12A and B: Laurence–Moon syndrome in male siblings.

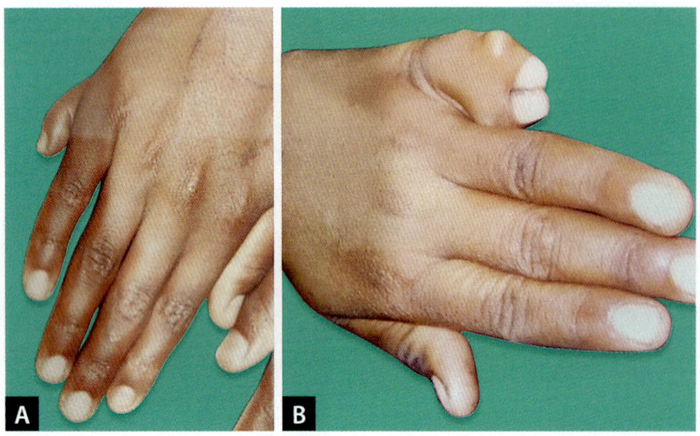

Figs. 20.13A and B: Polydactyly and syndactyly in otherwise normal children.

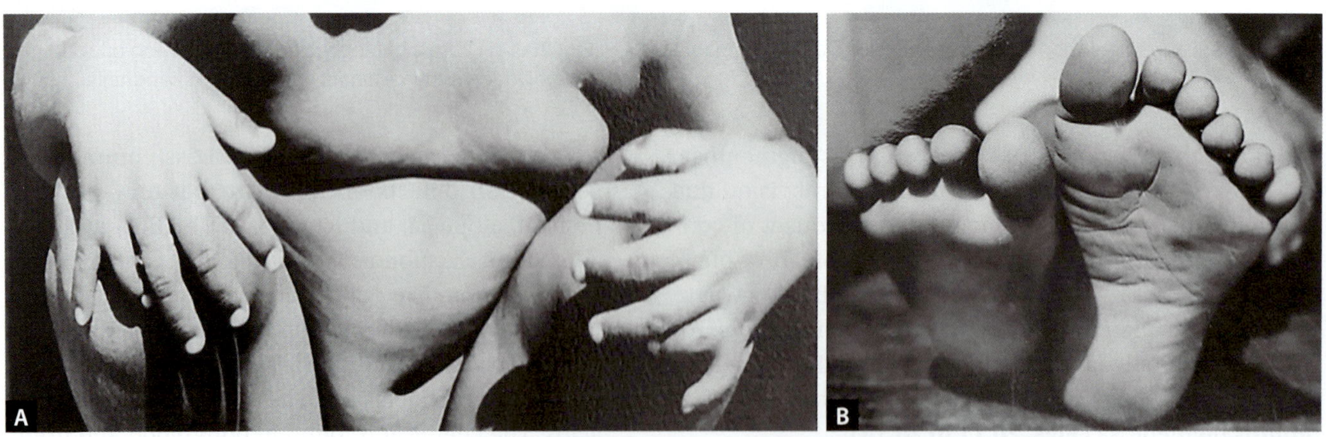

Figs. 20.14A and B: Polydactyly in a case of Laurence–Moon syndrome.

- *Usher syndrome:* This syndrome is an autosomal recessive disorder with neurosensory hearing defects and vestibular dysfunction, along with features of classical retinitis pigmentosa. The association of retinal pigmentation and neurosensory disorders of the ear is due to a fault in the embryology of the development of retinal pigments in the epithelium and the organ of Corti (the organ of Corti is an organ of the inner ear located within the cochlea that contributes to the faculty of hearing).

The auditory defects start early; the night blindness may be delayed by a decade and progress relentlessly; there may be involvement of the macula, worsening the vision. The peripheral field loss follows the pattern of typical retinitis pigmentosa. ERG and electrooculogram (EOG) are subnormal, as is the dark adaptation.

Other conditions of ophthalmic interest with hearing loss are Hallgren syndrome, Cockayne syndrome, and Refsum syndrome. Out of them, Hallgren syndrome is more frequent; it is an autosomal recessive trait with the involvement of the eyes and inner ear. Ataxia is a prominent feature (90%), followed by mental retardation in one-third of cases and nystagmus in 10%; neurosensory deafness is a major feature.

- *Cockayne syndrome:* The syndrome is an autosomal recessive that begins in infancy and progresses relentlessly. It is a rare syndrome with microcephaly—failure to thrive—that leads to short stature and retarded growth that may be a part of progeria (progeria is a genetic condition characterized by the dramatic, rapid appearance of aging that begins in childhood). The other features are deafness and mental retardation.
- *Pelizaeus-Merzbacher syndrome:* This condition differs from the other conditions mentioned above by being an X-linked trait. It may or may not have pigmentary changes with a predominantly neurological deficiency, unlike other syndromes, and may have diminished night vision. There is extensive demyelination of the brain that predisposes to neurological defects. The condition is noted in the first few months due to side-to-side oscillation of the head and nystagmus. Surprisingly, the condition stabilizes by 6 years and may have fairly good vision; the nystagmus is minimized by that time. The child may be mentally challenged.
- *Leber congenital amaurosis:* This is a rare condition present at birth with subnormal ERG and diminished night blindness. The condition is not to be confused with Leber hereditary optic neuropathy, which begins in the second decade with a normal retina.

Causes of Pigmentary Changes in the Retina Without Retinal Dystrophy

It is better to call them degeneration rather than dystrophies. They are given as follows:

- *Infection:* Congenital syphilis, rubella, influenza, and measles.
- *Drugs:* Many drugs taken for a long time cause pigmentary changes with an affinity for the retinal pigment epithelium.

  They are phenothiazines, chloroquine, hydroxychloroquine, mefloquine, quinine, ethambutol, indomethacin, and desferrioxamine.
- *Trauma:* Small laser and cryo spots.
- Congenital melanosis retinae

Summary of Causes of Diminished Night Vision in Children

- Vitamin A deficiency
- Rod and rod cone dystrophies:
  - Retinitis pigmentosa
  - Variations of retinitis pigmentosa:
    - Ocular:
      - Unilateral
      - Sector
      - Sine pigmento
      - Inverse retinitis pigmentosa
      - Congenital stationary night blindness:
        - With a normal fundus—autosomal dominant, recessive, X linked, and positive family history
        - Without normal fundus:
        - Oguchi disease*
        - Fundus albipunctatus†
    - Retinitis pigmentosa with systemic syndrome:
      - Laurence-Moon-Biedl-Bardet syndrome
      - Marfan syndrome
      - Refsum syndrome
      - Usher syndrome
      - Cockayne syndrome
    - Juvenile glaucoma
    - High myopia

**Oguchi disease:* The disorder is an autosomal recessive, nonprogressive night blindness with a positive Mizuo phenomenon, i.e., an abnormal golden yellow fundus glow on exposure to bright light. The glow gradually passes off when the eye is dark adapted. Dark adaptation itself is a delayed and abnormal ERG.

†Fundus albipunctatus: The condition is an autosomal recessive trait with stationary night blindness. The fundus is studded with tiny semolina white dots, mostly in the mid-periphery, leaving the macula unaffected.

Some Points to Keep in Mind when Diagnosing Peripheral Retinal Dystrophies

- *Night blindness:* Night blindness is the cornerstone of the diagnosis of peripheral retinal dystrophies. All cases either present with diminished night vision or may soon develop a night vision defect that becomes worse as time passes and is not corrected by any therapeutic methods such as the administration of a large dose of vitamin A.
- *Positive family history:* In all cases of diminished night vision not responding to the therapeutic trial with vitamin A, the first enquiry should be directed to the following questions if any of the following have a history of retinitis pigmentosa or its variants:
    - Parents, especially if there is consanguinity, even grandparents
    - Siblings
    - Blood relations
    - There are chances of other neurosensory defects among family members, i.e., deafness, ataxia, and mental retardation.
- *History of a field defect in the child:* The parents complain that the child bumps against the furniture and doors and finds difficulty getting down the stairs or picking up things that have fallen on the ground. Older children find it difficult to cross the road and drive.

Advanced loss of field can be detected even by a simple confrontation test.

- *Characteristics of field changes* ***(Fig. 20.6)****:*
    - Initially, the field changes correspond to the mid-periphery without central scotomas.
    - By the time the child is brought for consultation with vitamin A-resistant night blindness, the child already has advanced field change in the form of ring scotoma.
- *Dark adaptation:* The parents complain that the child takes a longer time to adjust to the ambient light in the room as he enters even a normally lighted room; the test is confirmed by an adaptometer.
- *Electroretinogram:* This investigation, when available, is a sensitive test that is always subnormal in pigmentary dystrophies of the retina. It may be positive even before diminished night vision and field defects have set in. It is most helpful in the diagnosis of sine pigmento and retinitis albipunctatus.
- *Electrooculogram:* This is a specialized investigation to note and assess the function of retinal pigment. It is subnormal in all pigmentary dystrophies of the retina.

Some Infrequent Retinal Dystrophies

The conditions are less common than primary retinal pigment dystrophies; they are hereditary, nonprogressive, and nontreatable. *They are given as follows.*

Congenital Stationary Night Blindness (Essential Night Blindness)

This is a rare hereditary disorder that runs in families. It can have any of the three inheritance patterns; the X-linked is more serious, and the main complaint is diminished nonprogressive night blindness. As it is a congenital disease with a normal fundus, the first mistaken diagnosis is vitamin A deficiency; the next common diagnosis is amblyopia.

Clinical features:

- The most outstanding symptom is night blindness of varied grades.
- Diminished distant vision: Generally mild to moderate; however, it may be high enough to cause nystagmus.
- Myopia is the most common type of refraction error that may be uncorrectable and a contributing factor to diminished distant vision.
- The fundus is essentially normal without attenuation of vessels or pigmentation. Only anomalies may be in the macula in the form of a dull foveal reflex.
- Color vision is normal.
- There are hardly any field changes, except that the patient may have a central scotoma.
- Electroretinogram, EOG, and dark adaptation—subnormal

Differential diagnosis: It consists of all causes of night blindness in children. They are given as follows:

- Vitamin A deficiency
- Atypical retinitis pigmentosa
- Stationary albipunctatus dystrophy
- Oguchi disease

Flecked Retina Syndromes

These are a group of retinal pigment dystrophies presenting as pigmentation of the macula and flecks on the retina. *The two main types are given as follows:*

1. Fundus flavimaculatus
2. Stargardt disease

Both are hereditary, with similar symptoms of diminished, noncorrectable distant vision, not culminating in legal blindness, bilateral, and progressive. The clinical features are so similar that some authors consider them as two stages of the same disorder, i.e., Stargardt disease being late and the more advanced stage of fundus flavimaculatus. The clinical difference that separates them is the presence of macular atrophy in the Stargardt disease.

Fundus flavimaculatus: The condition is a bilateral, symmetric autosomal recessive condition with flakes of acid mucopolysaccharide and lipofuscin in the retinal pigment epithelium around the macula. The flakes are scattered in small yellowish spots with irregular edges of different shapes, sizes, and numbers. In the long run, the flakes may get absorbed, leaving corresponding areas of atrophic patches on the retinal pigment epithelium, not involving the macula. The condition is diagnosed on routine fundus examinations because the child may be asymptomatic. Dark adaptations in the ERG and EOG are normal.

Stargardt disease: The condition is more common than fundus flavimaculatus. The patient with Stargardt disease (syndrome) is typically a young child between 10 and 15 years with a prior history of normal vision in both eyes in both sexes. The loss of vision is symmetric that ranges between 6/18 and 6/60 at the time of the first consultation. It is an abiotrophy considered to be a tapetoretinal dystrophy, and it is an autosomal recessive disorder mostly in children of consanguineous parents. Though the vision is subnormal; initially, the fundus looks normal, and the disorder may be mistaken as uncorrectable amblyopia or even malingering.

The child may complain of glare or photophobia. The child invariably has moderate uncorrectable myopia with red-green color deficiency; the color blindness is progressive and may terminate in total color blindness (achromatopsia), in which everything looks black and white or gray and white. The first fundus change is loss of foveal reflex with surrounding normal retina; the next visible change is bull's eye macula, which consists of a central oval area of normal retina surrounded by a ring of depigmented area surrounded by another ring of pigmentation. This ring is surrounded by small yellowish flakes deep in the macula; finally, the whole lesion enlarges to engulf a larger area involving the disk. The lesion not only spreads on the surface of the retina but also burrows deep into the retina. The development of optic atrophy and thinning of vessels is not uncommon. Both dark adaptation and ERG are normal, with abnormal EOG in late stages; the lesion initially produces central relative scotomas that soon become absolute.

There is no known treatment. In the initial stages, low-vision aids may help, but they lose their utility as the disorder progresses; at this stage, the child may be managed as visually challenged.

Dominant Drusen

The term is not to be confused with the drusen of the optic nerve; it involves the retinal pigment epithelium as well as Bruch's membrane. The condition is autosomal dominant. The age of presentation varies between the first and third decades and may not only be asymptomatic but also be missed on routine fundus examinations. The lesion begins as a small whitish dot at the posterior pole; involvement of the macula causes loss of central vision. The size of the dots is variable, scattered, or in clumps. The number and size of the dots increase with age; they may extend beyond the posterior pole and may even reach the periphery. By the sixth decade, they become confluent and form a small plaque on the macula. Serous detachment of the neuroepithelium is common. Subretinal neovascularization is also encountered at this age, with a tendency to bleed, resulting in a raised scar similar to age-related macular degeneration. The common symptoms are diminished central vision and metamorphosis; color vision, dark adaptation, ERG and peripheral fields are normal. Central and centrocecal scotomas with metamorphosis are associated with macular involvement.

Ganglion Cell Dystrophy

The true ganglion cell dystrophies of the retina are not primary disorders of the retina; they are secondary to a long list of systemic disturbances of many metabolic disorders of enzyme deficiency. They are hereditary in nature and divided into two groups, i.e.:

1. *Cherry-red spot:*
    a. Solely ocular (nondystrophic)
    b. Secondary to a disorder of metabolism and is dystrophic
2. Pigmentary disturbance—mostly ocular

Cherry-red Spots

They are nonspecific and nonhereditary. The phenomenon involves macula only with an edematous surrounding retina; it may be transient or long lasting **(Fig. 20.15)**.

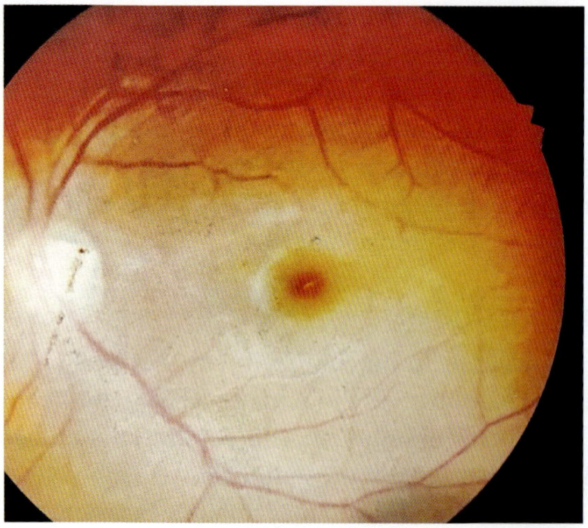

Fig. 20.15: A cherry-red spot.

They are given as follows:
- Commotio retinae
- Macular hole:
  - Traumatic
  - Idiopathic
  - Macular cyst
  - Central retinal artery obstruction

Out of the above list, only commotio retinae and traumatic cysts are seen in children.

Cherry-red spots of macula in children: The macula is highly vascular, and the blood supply is independent of retinal circulation originating from the choriocapillaris. Normally, the color of the macula does not differ from the surrounding retina. In the cherry-red spot, the macula stands out in the midst of a pale, almost white retina.

Commotio retinae (Berlin's edema): Commotio retinae is a manifestation of a direct blunt injury to the eye. It is not evident immediately following the injury. The child discovers diminished vision in the injured eye after a few hours or a few days. The loss of vision is generally not more than two to three lines on the Snellen chart that invariably deteriorates by pinhole. On retinoscopy, generally, there is mild-to-moderate hypermetropia, and, rarely, the red retinal glow is dulled. The diagnosis is confirmed by a fundus examination, which shows a gray, cloudy area covering the whole of the macula with a prominent red spot over the fovea. The whiteness is due to edema of the retina following concussion to the globe. The edema passes within a few days, restoring almost normal vision. In a few cases, the vision that has improved passes into a state of gradual reduction due to the unexplained deposition of pigments. The pigment has a tendency to increase, resulting in much reduction of central vision that may be permanent. Another serious sequel is the formation of a macular cyst. Years later, the cyst may rupture to form a macular hole.

The macular hole has a punched-out look; the shape is generally round but may be oval. The hole gives a bright red color that is more than the redness of commotio retinae. The hole is better seen by +90D on the slit lamp. It is best delineated on OCT. A still late complication may be retinal detachment.

The systemic causes that result in cherry-red spots are given as follows:
- Tay–Sachs familial idiocy that may be infantile or juvenile
- Niemann–Pick disease
- Sandhoff disease
- Gangliosidosis
- Sialidosis

All of them are hereditary, with a positive family history, starting in the first decade with variable bilateral visual loss and prominent systemic involvement.

Best Disease

This is a hereditary disease of autosomal dominant trait; the carriers are asymptomatic with a normal macula but an abnormal EOG. Hypermetropia is common that may lead to esotropia and amblyopia. The disease starts in childhood. The child may also be asymptomatic, even with an advanced disease. The diagnosis is straightforward. On ophthalmoscopic examination, a typical egg yolk appearance is seen on the macula. The EOG is abnormal with a near-normal ERG.

It is divided into two groups, i.e., (1) juvenile and (2) adult. On the basis of fundus findings, the condition has been classified as pre-vitelliform, vitelliform, stage of pseudohypopyon, vitelliruptive, and end stage. The previtelliform stage has a normal macula with a subnormal EOG; the last stage is the stage of scaring.

Retinal Degenerations

Retinal degenerations rarely manifests before the third decade, although they start earlier. The most common retinal degeneration seen under the second decade is lattice degeneration, followed by snail-track degeneration. Some authors presume that the latter is a precursor to lattice degeneration. The other rarer degeneration is retinoschisis.

Retinoschisis

Retinoschisis is different from retinal detachment. The two are often mistaken among them. Retinal detachment is a state of separation of the sensory retina from the pigment epithelium. In contrast to this, retinoschisis is split in the outer plexiform layer. Surprisingly, 5% of the general population has asymptomatic retinoschisis, mostly in the extreme inferotemporal retina. It is more common in hypermetropia. All retinoschisis is bilateral and does not need to be symmetric. Some authors put retinoschisis under peripheral retinal degeneration rather than dystrophy.

Figure 20.16 shows a composite picture of attachment and various types of retinal separation.

Retinoschisis can be put into two groups, i.e., (1) childhood and (2) adult (senile). Childhood retinoschisis can either be congenital or juvenile.

The congenital variety is present at birth; being asymptomatic is not diagnosed until fundus examination is undertaken for some unrelated conditions.

There may be a history of retinoschisis in one of the parents. It is generally inherited as an X-linked trait. The condition is mostly mistaken as shallow retinal detachment, and the child is managed for the mistaken diagnosis.

Juvenile (adult) retinoschisis: The clinical features are similar to congenital retinoschisis and are diagnosed by chance. The inheritance is the same as that of its congenital counterpart; in fact, many clinicians think that juvenile retinoschisis is not a separate entity but an advanced form of congenital retinoschisis.

The clinical pictures of retinoschisis are similar in all cases. They are diagnosed on fundus examination by an indirect ophthalmoscope supplemented by a panfundus lens and ultrasonography (USG) may help in clinching the diagnosis. The two layers of retinoschisis have different appearances. The inner layer has a smooth, noncorrugated surface, the color of which is paler than that of the surrounding normal retina and underlying outer layer. The inner layer is commonly sprinkled with snowflakes; the vessels retain their normal color and may have a silver wire appearance; there are no exudates, hemorrhages,

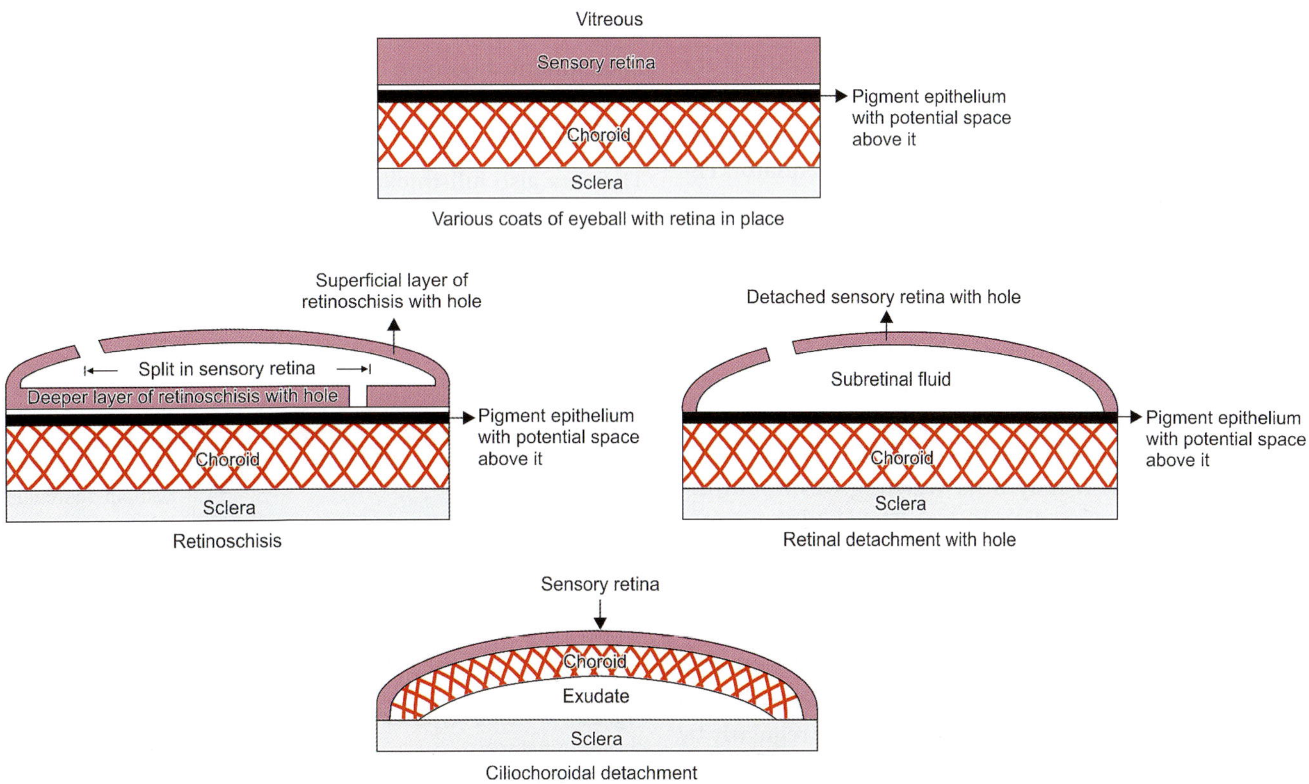

Fig. 20.16: Various types of retinal separation.

or traction bands; generally, there are no holes or tears; occasionally, a few circular degenerative holes may be seen. The outer layer does not show any evidence of fluid underneath.

All retinoschisis begins in the lower temporal extremity and does not cross the equator; the schisis spreads circumferentially and may even encircle the whole periphery. Spread to the macula is rare; when present, it is associated with visual symptoms.

Retinal detachment is rare; it happens only if both holes are full thickness. No treatment is warranted unless the macula is involved or retinal detachment has set in.

Lattice Degeneration

This is the most common retinal degeneration that sets in around 10 years and is fully developed by the end of the second decade. It is hereditary, equal in boys and girls, and slowly progressing; about 8–10% of children are asymptomatic, and the condition is discovered on routine fundus examination either for some unrelated condition or mild-to-moderate myopia. It is a common accompaniment of Marfan syndrome, Ehlers–Danlos syndrome, and Wagner syndrome. It generally begins in the lower temporal periphery in patches, and it is common to see various stages in the same eye. It is a precursor to rhegmatogenous retinal detachment in one-third of the cases.

On fundus examination by indirect ophthalmoscope, it is found in patches or singly parallel to the equator. The patches may unite to form a larger arc without encircling; there may be more than one row of degenerative patches parallel to each other with a gap in between. The degeneration does not extend to the posterior pole. The lattice degeneration may be associated with small holes, white pressure, snowflakes, and hypoplasia of the pigment epithelium. Some children may complain of floaters in one or both eyes or with flashes of light, which must be taken seriously as it may be a warning of impending rhegmatogenous retinal detachment. The condition per se does not require treatment, so long as it is asymptomatic. Some surgeons recommend prophylactic laser treatment for all areas of lattice degeneration. The eyes with flashes of light should be examined with scleral depression, and holes, when present, are better closed by laser. All eyes with lattice degeneration should be examined regularly by an indirect ophthalmoscope, and the result noted on the retinal chart.

Myopic Degeneration

Axial myopia of all types is prone to developing retinal degeneration. The incidence increases with an increase in myopia and age. The degenerative conditions are broadly divided into two groups, i.e., (1) central, involving the macula, and (2) peripheral retina. Peripheral degeneration is more common but less vision-threatening than central. The common peripheral degenerations are snail-track and lattice degeneration with or without holes; the latter carries a poorer prognosis. Myopic degeneration is a common contributory factor in producing retinal detachment in children.

Retinal Holes

About 3% of eyes have retinal holes that the person may not be aware of; they are more common in myopia of all grades; they are frequent with lattice degeneration, and holes generally develop adjacent to the lattice. A retinal hole is a full-thickness defect in the sensory retina, generally circular in shape and standing out as a bright red spot. There may be multiple holes in the same eye; the holes are not seen in clusters. The holes may be operculated or nonoperculated. The operculated holes are associated with vitreoretinal adhesion. All holes do not need treatment; only those that may precipitate rhegmatogenous detachment should be treated **(Fig. 20.17)**.

Retinal Tears

They are also full-thickness defects in the sensory retina, differing from retinal holes, which are circular in shape. The retinal tears are crescent or arrowhead shaped with

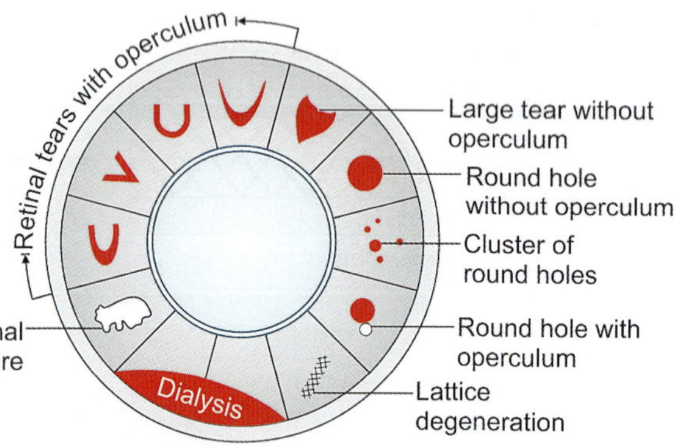

Fig. 20.17: Various types of retinal holes, lattice degeneration, and chorioretinal scars.

Source: Mukherjee PK. Ophthalmic Assistant. New Delhi: Jaypee Brothers Medical (P) Pvt. Ltd. 2013.

or without operculum. Most of the time on the periphery, generally single, there may rarely be multiples anywhere on the circumference. They are acquired mostly due to abnormal vitreous adhesion to the area with lattice degeneration; vitreous adhesion exerts traction to the apex to enlarge the tear, which ultimately ends in rhegmatogenous retinal detachment, more often than circular holes.

Retinal Dialysis

This is the most extreme form of separation of the sensory retina from the pigment epithelium; in fact, it is the disinsertion of the retina from the ora. This is a full-thickness circumferential separation at the ora. Blunt trauma in an otherwise normal eye is the most common causative factor in producing retinal dialysis. It is a shallow, crescent-shaped detachment with concavity toward the ora. It is independent of posterior vitreous detachment and may develop anywhere on the retinal periphery. The most common location being inferior temporal ora. The cause of the phenomenon is that the retina at the spot is most stretched and underdeveloped.

Retinal Detachment

The term retinal detachment, like much of the nomenclature in clinical practice, is a misnomer. The condition for which the term is used is not detachment of the retina, either from the choroid or from the vitreous. It is a separation of the sensory retina from the retinal pigment epithelium secondary to the accumulation of fluid in the potential space between the pigment epithelium and the sensory retina. A full-thickness defect in the sensory retina is mandatory for retinal detachment, which could either be rhegmatogenous or tractional.

Earlier, we have seen that the retina develops from two layers of the optic cup, with the pigment layer developing from the outer wall and remaining from the inner. The pigment epithelium is continuous as the ciliary epithelium, while the sensory retina stops at ora serrata. In the early stages of development, there is a gap between the two layers, which gradually shrinks and disappears at birth. The line of demarcation remains only as a potential space. The line of demarcation is a weak spot in the retina that carries the risk of opening up if something unusual gets access to the space, widening it with the accumulation of fluid and leading to the development of retinal detachment.

The factor that keeps the two layers attached is not clear.

The hypotheses put forward are given as follows:

- The cells of the pigment epithelium have microvilli on the inner surface that are attached to the outer end of the photoreceptor, the two forming a bond between them.
- The acid mucopolysaccharides present in the space act as a bonding substance that glues the two surfaces. The bond is not as firm as the pigment epithelium and Bruch's membrane; this predisposes separation between the pigment epithelium and sensory retina.
- The normal vitreous is a semisolid that exerts sufficient pressure on the retina from inside to keep the two layers together.
- Static state of normal vitreous
- Immobile retina
- Intraocular pressure
- Active metabolic transport between the pigment epithelium and retinal fluid
- Positive oncotic pressure gradient between subretinal space and choroid

The vitreous plays an important role in keeping the retina in place and preventing rhegmatogenous retinal detachment. The normal semisolid vitreous, in spite of its various anchors to the retina, does not exert any traction on the retina.

The places where the vitreous is anchored are given as follows:

- Ora serrata
- Round the optic disk
- At the fovea
- Along the major blood vessels
- Posterior surface of the lens **(Fig. 20.18)**

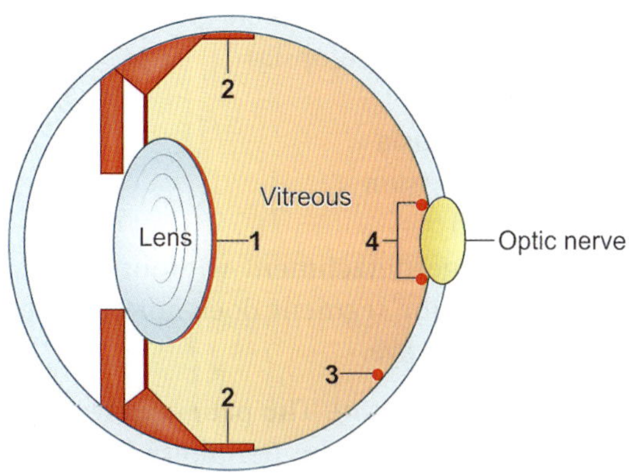

Fig. 20.18: Attachment of vitreous in a child's eye: (1) Retrolental, (2) ora serrata, (3) macula, and (4) edge of the optic nerve.

The abnormal attachments of the vitreous are at the chorioretinal scars and less commonly to the edges of peripheral degenerations and innocuous holes.

The local factors that contribute to retinal detachment, separately or in combinations, are given as follows:

- Retinal breaks:
  - Hole
  - Tear
  - Disinsertion
- Liquefaction of vitreous
- Traction on a weakened retina

Division of Retinal Detachment

Traditionally, retinal detachment has been divided into two groups.

They are given as follows:

1. Primary (simple, rhegmatogenous)
2. Secondary:
   a. Tractional
   b. Exudative
   c. Solid (tumor)

Symptoms of Retinal Detachment

The symptoms mostly depend on position and the extent of detachment. Detachments of the lower one-third are the least symptomatic. Conversely, detachment of the upper part causes early and pronounced symptoms. Involvements of the macula are acute enough to cause early symptoms.

- *Asymptomatic:* A detachment on the extreme periphery, especially in the lower part, may be without any symptoms. Even a large detachment in the lower third may go undetected.
- *Symptomatic:* The symptoms are given as follows:
  - Flashes of light (photopsia)
  - Floaters
  - Metamorphopsia
  - Diminished vision
  - Loss of field
  - Even a large detachment without involvement of the anterior segment does not cause pain or redness in the eye.

Flashes of light (photopsia): The patient may experience a bright flash of light on the periphery initially in the dark, but later, it persists even in normal light. It is caused by irritation of the retina and mostly subsides with the onset of detachment. It should be differentiated from flashes of light and auras of central nervous system origin.

Floaters: The floaters are generally due to RBC liberated from torn vessels at the site of the tear; the next common cause is liquefaction of the vitreous. They may initially be small pinhead-sized dots moving in space, may be in the form of string or in the form of a ring called the Weiss ring that denotes moderate posterior vitreous detachment. Sometimes, the opacities assume a cobweb configuration due to the condensation of collagen fibers in the collapsed vitreous. In the early stages, small floaters are mistaken as muscae, which are of no consequence but require evaluation.

Metamorphopsia: Metamorphopsia is less common in retinal detachment compared to acute lesions of the macula. The metamorphopsia of retinal detachment is due to the corrugation of the retinal surface.

Diminished vision: Sudden diminished vision is an ominous indication of macular involvement requiring urgent management. Diminished vision is faster in superior holes. Tear in the lower pole, even with a large disinsertion, causes less loss of vision and progresses slowly. The most common cause of diminished vision is macular involvement, followed by overhanging of the detached retina in front of the macula, and last, blood in front of the macula. Loss of projection of light indicates almost total detachment.

Field loss: A loss of field corresponds to the area detached. The patient experiences loss of field as a curtain coming down from above in detachment of the upper retina; lateral detachments cause field changes to develop from the sides.

In spite of tremendous loss of vision, retinal detachment per se is not painful.

Signs of Retinal Detachment

The signs are varied, with minimal external signs except pupillary defects and faulty projection in the advanced stage. The signs depend on the site of detachment, which is guided by position of the retinal tear, extent of detachment, and duration. Detachments of long standing have more signs.

The signs are put in two groups given as follows:

1. External
2. Fundus changes

1. *External:*
   a. The most prominent external signs of uncorrectable diminished vision in a noncongested, nontender eye. In cases of long-standing detachment, the vision may be as low as hand movement with faulty projections.
   b. Externally, the eye does not show any signs that may be correlated to retinal detachment except pupillary change.
   c. *Pupillary change:* Initially, in eyes with small detachments, the pupillary reaction remains normal; late and large detachments are associated with afferent pupil defects.
   d. Anterior chamber reactions are seen in the late stages of total detachment.
   e. Intraocular tension is low in advanced detachment.
   f. *Retinoscopy:*
      i. In mild-to-moderate cases, there is a hypermetropic shift in the form of an increase in hypermetropia and a decrease in myopia.
      ii. There may be gray reflex in the involvement of the posterior pole.
      iii. Occasionally, gray reflexes can be seen in the pupil, corresponding to detachment on the sides.
      iv. The absence of a retinal glow is a sign of total detachment.
2. *Fundus changes:* Fundus is best visualized by an indirect ophthalmoscope with scleral indentation under maximum cycloplegia. Good cycloplegia relieves intolerance of the bright light of an indirect ophthalmoscope. Direct ophthalmoscopy is limited to early screening; it fails to locate holes/tears in the periphery. Examination of the eye with rhegmatogenous retinal detachment of recent origin shows:
   a. The detached area looks pale in comparison to the nondetached retina, as raised, pale, corrugated surface. The cause of paleness is the absence of a choroidal hue. The blood vessels on a detached, pale retina look darker than on a nondetached retina. The detached retina may show undulation on movement. The height and extent of detachment do not change with the position of the head.
   b. *Retinal breaks:* No rhegmatogenous detachment is possible without a retinal break; hence, it is of utmost importance to find the breaks, their position and type, and draw them on the retinal chart. The presence of a break not only has a diagnostic value but also carries important therapeutic and prognostic values. The number of breaks may vary in number, shape, and size; they may be with or without operculum. A small hole in the upper periphery may cause a larger detachment compared to a large dialysis in the lower part.
   c. *Peripheral patches of degeneration and chorioretinal scars:* Many of the eyes with rhegmatogenous retinal detachment may have peripheral degeneration. Peripheral degeneration without holes is not harmful but requires to be kept under observation as it is prone to develop holes more frequently than areas without.
   d. *Vitreous changes:* The normal vitreous, which is semisolid, plays an important role in keeping the normal sensory retina snug with the pigment epithelium. Posterior vitreous detachment is invariably a predisposing factor in rhegmatogenous retinal detachment and is almost always present in rhegmatogenous retinal detachment. The anterior vitreous is not detached and does not play any part in rhegmatogenous retinal detachment. The vitreous may be attached to the operculum of a tear to exert a pull, precipitating detachment. The fluid vitreous finds access to the subretinal space through the hole. In long-standing cases, new vessels may be seen in the subhyaloid space.
   e. *Other findings:* Peripheral retinal degeneration and chorioretinal scars on the periphery.

Changes in Rhegmatogenous Retinal Detachment of Long Standing (More than a Month)

About a month following on set of detachments, the following features are added to the previously mentioned features:

- *High water mark:* Pigments deposited on the border of the detached retina; these pigments gradually fade, leaving their footprints on the border of detachment. They do not represent the edge of subretinal fluid; they are located behind the edge of subretinal fluid.
- *Retinal thinning:* They may be mistaken as retinoschisis.
- *Subretinal fibrosis:* These are the opaque fibrous bands that develop on the detached retina.
- *Intraretinal cysts:* They develop frequently in detachments of long duration, i.e., more than one year. The cysts disappear following surgical reattachment of the retina.

- *Total retinal detachment:* The whole of the retina is detached from the ora serrata, remaining attached to the optic nerve; the detached retina assumes an appearance of a funnel with an apex at the disk; there is no perception of light. The eye becomes soft, which is associated with features of chronic uveitis and complicated cataracts.

Fate of Untreated Rhegmatogenous Retinal Detachment

An unattended small hole at 12 o'clock may suddenly develop rhegmatogenous retinal detachment that progresses rapidly and may be aggressive enough to cause total detachment within a few days. In contrast to this, a large detachment at 6 o'clock may remain stationary for a long time due to the early formation of a line of demarcation. Such detachments are likely to have better chances of anatomical apposition and a guarded visual prognosis. Small localized detachments have been reported to get spontaneous reattachment. However, such situations are short-lived, and the retinal detachment recurs; a detachment with spontaneous attachment is most probably not rhegmatogenous. Most of the untreated, partially treated, or overtreated detachments develop either secondary glaucoma or hypotony following the development of chronic uveitis and complicated cataracts. In rare instances, hypotonic eyes may pass into a stage of phthisis.

Predisposing Factors in Rhegmatogenous Retinal Detachment

There is no single cause that can be attributed to being the sole reason to cause it; there are multiple factors that, in combination, cause rhegmatogenous retinal detachment. *They are given as follows:*

- *Male preponderance:* The reason behind this may be the vulnerability of men to trauma, a major single cause of detachment.
- *Family history:* Many members of the same family, especially the siblings, are found to suffer from retinal detachment, and there may be a history suggestive of retinal detachment among the parent and/or their siblings or among the blood relations. Most probably, many of them had myopia as a contributory factor.
- *Myopia:* Most people with moderate-to-high myopia have a tendency to suffer from retinal detachment, which is worsened by trauma, including surgical. Myopic aphakic and myopic pseudophakic eyes are more prone to detachment. Detachments in myopic eyes are more likely to be bilateral and more difficult to manage. The causes of the higher incidence of detachment in myopic eyes are influenced by the following factors—most of the time, they do not act singly, they invariably act in various combinations.
    - Myopic eyes have relatively lax adhesion between the pigment epithelium and sensory retina.
    - Myopic eyes are relatively longer than nonmyopic eyes, resulting in stretching and thinning of the retina that predisposes to tear formation.
    - Myopic eyes have an increased incidence of lattice degeneration.
    - There may be a common genetic predisposition between myopia and detachment.
    - Vitreous liquefaction and posterior vitreous detachments are more common in myopic eyes.
- *Trauma:* Both blunt and penetrating injuries hasten detachment, more so in myopic eyes. Blunt injuries cause more detachment than open globe injuries; generally, a blunt injury is followed by a tear that precipitates retinal detachment. The detachment may develop soon after a blunt injury or within a few days. All eyes with blunt injuries should be examined by an indirect ophthalmoscope for the possibility of peripheral holes. The common place for the development of holes is the periphery; rarely, they may develop behind the equator. All types of holes are possible; round holes are less common following blunt injuries. Dialysis following a blunt injury is frequent, and detachment following dialysis progresses faster than in a nontraumatized eye. Detachments following rents in the upper pole are the fastest to develop a detachment that progresses equally fast. The surgical traumas that produce detachment are aphakia, pseudophakia, and repeated needling, and even laser capsulotomy is blamed. Intracapsular lens extraction (no more in vogue and was not done in children) causes more detachment; they are generally associated with hole/holes at the upper part, which are generally round and difficult to locate. Pseudophakia does not bestow immunity against detachment; the incidence of post-surgical detachment is higher in children. Traumatic dislocation of the lens is also fraught with the possibility of retinal detachment, as is Marfan syndrome.

- *Inflammation:* Postinflammatory scars on peripheries are more likely to develop tears with the operculum that may end in detachment. Aphakic eyes with postinflammatory scars predispose to detachment more often.
- *Congenital anomalies:* The list of ocular congenital anomalies that predispose to detachment is long. Some of them are: uveal coloboma, persistent primary hyperplastic vitreous, and congenital pit of the optic nerve head. The edge of the uveal coloboma may act as a pseudo-ora-predisposing detachment. The congenital syndromes predisposing to detachments are Marfan syndrome, Ehlers–Danlos syndrome, Wagner syndrome, Pierre Robin syndrome, and Stickler syndrome.

Differential diagnosis: Moderate-to-advanced detachments are not difficult to diagnose. The history of floaters, flashes of light, and gray curtains in the field is strongly suggestive of retinal detachment. The presence of detachment may become evident on retinoscopy; the pink retinal glow is replaced by a dull gray glow. Shallow detachment in posterior pole generally reveals a hypermetropic shift. Examination of the fundus by direct ophthalmoscope may be sufficient to locate retinal detachment but not the cause that requires examination by indirect ophthalmoscope with +20 D, which will reveal even small holes on the periphery when seen with scleral indentation.

There are some conditions that come under the differential diagnosis of rhegmatogenous retinal detachment **(Fig. 20.19)**.

They have been put into two broad categories given as follows:

1. State of true detachment other than rhegmatogenous:
   a. Tractional retinal detachment
   b. Exudative retinal detachment
2. Pseudorhegmatogenous retinal detachment:
   a. Choroidal detachment
   b. Ciliochoroidal detachment
   c. Choroidal effusion syndrome
   d. Congenital and juvenile retinoschisis
   e. Large vitreous bands
   f. Lens dislocated in vitreous
   g. Parasitic cyst

Table 20.2 shows comparisons between various types of retinal detachments.

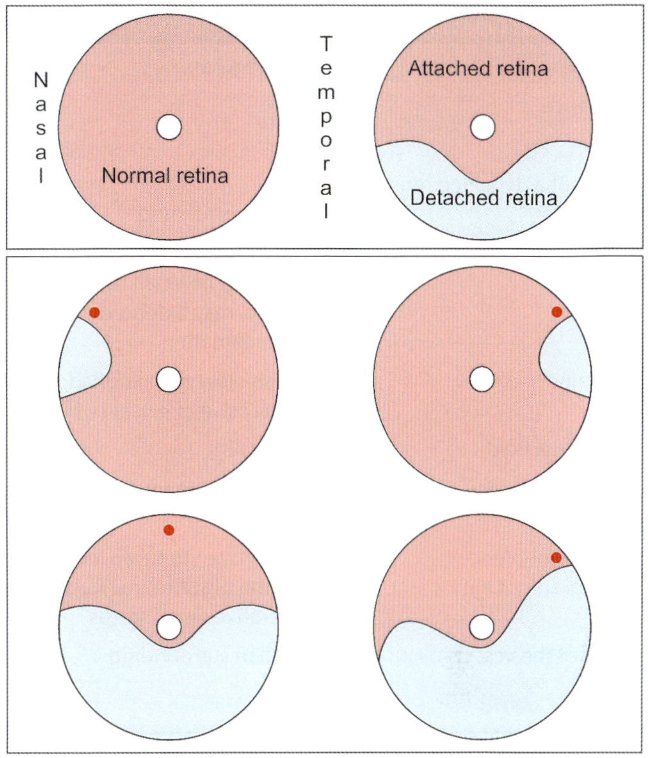

Fig. 20.19: Rough position of holes in relation to a detached retina.

Table 20.3 shows a comparison between rhegmatogenous retinal detachment and ciliochoroidal detachment.

Following imaging has a role in the differential diagnosis of various types of retinal detachment:

- Ultrasonography
- Computed tomography (CT)
- Optical coherence tomography
- X-rays have no role in the diagnosis of rhegmatogenous retinal detachment unless there is suspicion of an intraocular radiopaque foreign body.

Table 20.4 shows the principle of locating holes in rhegmatogenous retinal detachment **(Fig. 20.15)**.

Causes of Tractional Retinal Detachment in Children

- Retinopathy of prematurity
- Persistent primary hyperplastic vitreous
- Pars planitis
- Congenital toxoplasmosis
- Penetrating injury
- Incontinentia pigmenti
- Retinal degeneration

TABLE 20.2: Types of retinal detachments.

Features	*Rhegmatogenous*	*Traction*	*Exudative*
Incidence	Common	Common	Rare
Break	Essential	May not be present initially	Nil
Shape of a detached retina: • Surface • Border	 • Convex, corrugated • Convex	 • Concave/convex • Smooth concave	 • Convex, smooth • Convex
Size	Variable, may be small to begin with, may extend to total detachment	Generally smaller than rhegmatogenous, do not reach ora	Small, does not involve the whole retina
Elevation	May be shallow or ballooned, more extensive in upper part	Variable, generally low	It depends on the extent of subretinal lesion
Subretinal fluid	Does not shift	Does not shift	Always shifts
Ultrasonography	Outlines detachment but not the cause	Noncontributory	May show extent and cause
Optical coherence tomography (OCT)	OCT has proven to be an important tool to diagnose all types of retinal detachments. It enables the delineation of subretinal fluid and the position of the macula (off/on). It is useful in assessing pre- and postoperative visual status		
Color of the vessels	Darker than surrounding vessels	Darker than surrounding vessels	Darker than surrounding vessels, may have tufts of vessels on the apex of detached retina

TABLE 20.3: Comparison between rhegmatogenous retinal detachment and ciliochoroidal detachment.

Features	*Rhegmatogenous retinal detachment (RRD)*	*Ciliochoroidal retinal detachment (CRD)*
Predisposing factor	Myopia, aphakia, pseudophakia, trauma, and peripheral retinal degeneration—predisposed RRD	Uveitis, nanophthalmos, intraocular surgery, and hypotony are commonly associated with ciliochoroidal detachment
Topography	Between the sensory retina and the retinal pigment epithelium	Between the uvea and sclera
Location	Any part of the retina	Between the scleral spur and the vortex ampulla
Holes	Essential	Nonessential
Shape	Convex, funnel shape in total detachment	Convex, with four quadrilateral elevations separated by cleavage
Surface	Corrugated	Smooth
Color	White	Grayish black
Blood vessels	Dark	Normal
Nature of subretinal fluid	Mostly vitreous, may be blood	Transudate from the choroid
Anterior chamber	Normal	May be shallow
Ciliary body	Normal	Moved forward
Iris–lens diaphragm	Normal	Pushed forward
Intraocular pressure (IOP)	Normal or low	Very low
Recovery	Spontaneous recovery not possible	May resolve spontaneously
Surgery	Essential	Generally not required; it may improve with medical treatment of the underlying cause

TABLE 20.4: Principle of locating holes in rhegmatogenous retinal detachment.

Location of the detachment	*Most probable site of the hole*
Superionasal	Near the superior border of detachment
Superiotemporal	Near the superior border of the retinal detachment
Superior detachment on either side of vertical meridian	At 12 o'clock
Inferior detachment	On the side of higher fluid levels
Bullous inferior detachment	Above the midline

Nonrhegmatogenous Retinal Detachment

For a detachment to be labeled as rhegmatogenous, it is essential to have a break in the retina. In the absence of a rent, the condition is called nonrhegmatogenous. They are divided into the following broad groups:

- Tractional detachment
- Exudative detachment
- Solid detachment

The common features of nonrhegmatogenous retinal detachment are given as follows:

- Absence of break (primary cause of rhegmatogenous retinal detachment).
- Tractional detachment may develop a hole secondary to pull by a vitreous band or postinflammatory scar.
- Exudative detachments do not have breaks.
- The detached surface is smooth and concave and may be corrugated.
- Vitreous is not always liquefied.
- The presence of retinopathy is common in tractional detachment.
- The border of the detached area does not reach ora except in pars planitis.
- The detached retina is peaked at the site of traction.
- The treatment is directed toward relieving the traction through vitrectomy and fluid gas exchange.

Exudative retinal detachment: The overall incidence of exudative detachment is less in general and still less in children.

The causes of exudative retinal detachment are angiomatosis retinae, Coats' disease, retinoblastoma, pars planitis, and choroidal rupture.

Features of exudative retinal detachment:

- They are rare in children.
- Slowly progressive
- Generally unilateral
- May have signs of pars planitis or a history of blunt injury.
- The surface of a detached retina is convex, with convex boundaries.
- Neither holes nor traction bands are seen.
- The border of detachment does not reach ora serrata.
- The subretinal fluid shows signs of shifting.
- The elevation of detachment is moderate.
- Ultrasonography may reveal subretinal growth, over which the detached retina is stretched.
- There may be a tuft of blood vessels at the apex of the subretinal growth.

Prophylaxis for prevention of rhegmatogenous retinal detachment:

- All children born to any of the parents with a history of retinal detachment should be examined with an indirect ophthalmoscope under maximum cycloplegia every year.
- All children with moderate-to-severe myopia should be examined by an indirect ophthalmoscope for predisposing signs.
- All children with blunt injuries should undergo a comprehensive visual examination.
- If predisposing factors such as holes, degeneration, and patches of choroiditis are found, the children should be examined with an indirect ophthalmoscope twice a year.
- If indicated, the hole/holes should be closed by appropriate methods.
- There is no medical treatment to treat retinal detachment.
- Eyes with retinal detachment of recent origin should be treated as ophthalmic emergencies.
- Conditions that do not require prophylactic treatment are given as follows:
    - Hole surrounded by pigment all around
    - Small round holes near the ora serrata
    - Retinoschisis
    - Retina white without pressure

Specific Points Regarding Various Types of Breaks in Retina

- All holes do not cause retinal detachment and do not require treatment.
- All that is required is a regular, comprehensive retinal evaluation.

- The size of the break does not predict the extent of the ensuing detachment.
- Large breaks produce more detachment than small defects at the same location.
- Superior breaks produce early and more extensive detachment.
- Inferior breaks cause less and shallower detachment.
- Breaks behind the ora are more likely to cause detachment than breaks at the ora.
- Breaks with posterior vitreous detachment are more likely to cause detachment.
- Vitreous bands attached to the operculum are likely to increase the size of the break.
- Bands attached to the operculum produce more extensive detachment.

Management

- There is no medical treatment for rhegmatogenous or tractional detachment.
- Inflammatory exudative detachment may disappear with the management of inflammation.
- The principle of management of all retinal detachments with breaks is to locate the break/all the breaks and close the hole and all the holes by appropriate methods.
- The holes may be closed by trans-scleral cryo or intraocular laser with external plomb and encerclage with draining of subretinal fluid with internal tamponade.
- Use of air or gas to keep the retina snug with pigment epithelium
- Tractional detachment requires vitrectomy, cutting of the band, and treatment of the break, as in rhegmatogenous detachment.
- Exudative detachment requires management of the cause.

Functional Anomalies of the Retina of Congenital Origin

Besides congenital structural anomalies of the retina, there are some congenital disorders that hamper its function; all of them are rare, bilaterally symmetrical, stationary, and nontreatable.

They are given as follows:

- Congenital night blindness
- Congenital day blindness
- Congenital color blindness

- *Congenital night blindness:* The prominent features of congenital night blindness are given as follows:
  - Not responding to the administration of vitamin A.
  - Normal fundus
  - Retained central vision except due to myopia, which is frequent accompaniment.
  - Normal color vision
  - Normal field
  - Subnormal ERG and EOG
- *Congenital day blindness:* The prominent features of congenital day blindness are given as follows:
  - Diminished distant vision that diminishes in bright light and improves in dim light.
  - Partial color defect
  - Hereditary
  - Eyes are amblyopic
  - Nystagmus is common
- *Congenital color blindness:* The prominent features of congenital color blindness are given as follows:
  - All types and shades of color blindness are congenital
  - Total color blindness (achromatopsia) is extremely rare.
  - They are hereditary. Hereditary is variable.
  - May run in families
  - The incidence is as high as 7–8% among boys; girls are rarely afflicted.
  - There are no signs that may point toward the condition.
  - The condition per se does not cause any funds or field changes.
  - Electroretinogram and EOG are normal.
  - There is no treatment.

Congenital Anomalies of Retinal Vessels

They are so common, mild, and asymptomatic that they are generally ignored. They are given as follows:

- Topographically:
  - Abnormal division of central retinal artery
  - Abnormal course
  - Increased tortuosity
  - Malformed capillaries
- Extra vessels—cilioretinal vessels
- Telangiectasia

Commonly, the central retinal artery bifurcates into superior and inferior twigs at the head of the optic nerve; however, the division may develop behind the disk.

Rarely, there may be more than two twigs. The superior and inferior divisions after bifurcation divide into temporal and nasal branches; one of them may be absent.

Increased tortuosity is very common. They are of no clinical importance.

Cilioretinal Artery

The incidence of this anomaly is as high as 15–20% in the general population. It is hereditary in many cases, mostly uniocular. The term cilioretinal artery is not appropriate; the vessel is not a part of retinal circulation; it is part of ciliary circulation arising from the ophthalmic artery; it enters the eyeball on the lateral border of the optic nerve and traverses toward the macula, and it supplies the superficial layers of the retina between the disk and macula in a spindle-shaped area. The advantage of its presence is felt in obstruction of the central retinal artery, where the macula becomes ischemic with a cherry-red spot. The presence of a cilioretinal artery partially retains retinal blood supply to the macula; this retains central vision in central retinal obstruction. It is more common in hypermetropia.

Congenital Telangiectasia of Retinal Vessels

They have more clinical significance than other congenital anomalies of retinal vessels. They rarely occur in isolation. The common syndromes associated with them are given as follows:

- Von Hippel–Lindau (VHL) disease
- Sturge–Weber syndrome
- Wyburn–Mason syndrome
- Coats' disease

Congenital Anomalies of Retinal Vasculatures in the Second Decade

They are congenital but missed in childhood; they generally present as diminished vision or loss of vision in one eye or with a white reflex in the pupillary area.

They comprise the following disorders:

- Retinal telangiectasia
- Angiomatosis retinae
- Cavernous hemangioma of the retina
- Arteriovenous aneurysm

Retinal Telangiectasia

In this condition, the retinal vessels, mostly capillaries, are dilated in segments adjacent to the blood vessels, which leads to the leaking of blood, exudate, or both on a large scale. The examples are circinate retinopathy and macular star. The hemorrhage may seep into the vitreous, causing subhyaloid and intravitreal hemorrhage, predisposing vitreous bands. Most of the cases are bilateral, in contrast to Coats' disease* that is unilateral.

The condition has been put into the following stages:

- Stage of massive retinal and/or subretinal exudates without hemorrhages and apparently normal vessels.
- Stage of increased exudation with superadded retinal and subretinal hemorrhages in abnormal vessels.
- Stage of arteriovenous anastomosis with prominent vascular changes and massive exudation.
- Stages of complication consist of exudative retinal detachment, white reflex in the pupillary area, complicated cataracts, and glaucoma terminating in blindness.

The exact cause of the disorder is not known; there is no family history, and siblings are not affected.

Clinical features: Clinical features are varied depending on the stage of the disease at the time of the first consultation. It is divided into the following stages:

- Quiescent stage
- Stage of the white reflex
- Stage of complication
- Stages of blindness

- *Quiescent stage:* The child with unilateral involvement generally presents with uncorrectable diminished

**Coats' disease:* This is the most severe form of retinal telangiectasia, both congenital and acquired; the congenital verity is more common and seen under 15 years. The latter is rarer and seen in adults and thought to be a milder form, missed in childhood. Coats' disease is nonhereditary; 80% of patients are males; 90% are unilateral; commonly diagnosed in the second decade. It has even been reported at the age of 1 year. The child suffering from the disorder is otherwise healthy. In the early stages, it may be asymptomatic. Cases reporting late are generally in an advanced, nonsalvageable stage with a white reflex in the pupillary area, which may be thought to be retinoblastoma. Other modes of late presentation are complicated cataracts, secondary glaucoma, and squint. As one-tenth of the cases may be bilateral, it is mandatory to examine both eyes with an indirect ophthalmoscope. In spite of the other eye being asymptomatic, the other eye may have a milder form, which carries a better prognosis and should get precedence over the affected eye as far as treatment is concerned.

vision with or without a squint in the affected eye; otherwise, the condition is diagnosed on routine fundus examinations for an unrelated condition.

- *Stage of the white reflex:* This is the most frequent stage in which the child is brought for consultation, or the attending pediatrician wants to exclude more serious, life-threatening retinoblastoma.
- *Stage of complication:* The eye is congested and may have diminished vision, squint, may have cataract, secondary glaucoma, and found to have retinal detachment.
- *Stage of blindness:* Due to the above factors, the eye may be in a state of untreatable blindness; the eye may be congested, painful, and blind.

Signs

The signs are divided into the following categories:

- Eye without leukocoria
- Eyes with leukocoria
- Stage of complication

Eye without leukocoria: The child may be brought for a routine fundus examination, or the child reports with diminished vision and/or unilateral squint in a noncongested eye with a normal anterior segment.

Eye with leukocoria: This is the most common sign with which the child is brought by parents who think the child has a cataract or referred by a pediatrician who is justified to think that the child has retinoblastoma.

Stage of complication: The child reports with congested eye that may be painful, which on examination turns out to have raised intraocular pressure, an anterior chamber reaction, complicated cataracts of various grades, and retinal detachment. The eye is invariably blind.

In the early stages, the signs are confined to the posterior segment, which may have given as follows:

- *On retinoscopy:* The eye either has no glow or has a dull gray reflex instead of the usual pink glow.
- *Fundus examination:* Fundus examination holds the key to diagnosis in the form of the following:
    - Changes in vessels
    - Changes in retina
    - Combination of the above two.
    - Changes in retinal vessels:
        - The changes are seen both in arteries and veins of varied caliber.
        - The calibers of the vessels are irregular.
        - The vessels are tortuous.
        - Communication between arteries and veins
        - Neovascularization
    - *Changes in the retina:* The retinal changes are diagnostic. A coat has put them in two categories:
        1. Only retinal changes either on the surface as patches of exudate.
        2. With vascular involvement:
            a. It may be normal
            b. With minimal involvement that gets extensively involved, leading to Coats' stage two.

            Where lesions are prominent enough to be seen by an ophthalmoscope. It is better to examine the retina with an indirect ophthalmoscope.

        The changes are given as follows:
        - Yellowish white or greenish yellow, superficial deposition of cholesterol crystals on the retina.
        - Raised masses due to subretinal exudates.
        - Exudative retinal detachment, which may be localized or extensive, may be total even.
- The extensively detached retina may reach the posterior surface of the lens, which, if clear, gives a white reflex in the pupillary area and may rightly be thought to be retinoblastoma.
- There may be various grades of retinal hemorrhage.
- Retinal hemorrhage extending in vitreous.
- In the terminal stages, the eye goes into uveitis, secondary glaucoma, and complicated cataract.
- The unattended eye ultimately goes into a stage of painful blindness.

Investigations

Investigations are required to establish the diagnosis and differentiate it from other causes of leukocoria:

- X-rays and blood examinations are noncontributory.
- The most useful investigation is fundus fluorescein angiography (FFA) in clear media.
- Ultrasonography of the globe is conclusive in eyes both with clear as well as opaque media. The characteristic acoustic features are poorly mobile retinal detachment; dense, dispersed subretinal opacities; no solid mass or calcification.

- *Computed tomography (CT):* The most important role of CT in the diagnosis of Coats' disease is to exclude the possibility of retinoblastoma, which is outlined as a solid subretinal mass with calcification.
- *Magnetic resonance imaging (MRI):* The MRI picture does not differ from CT findings unless contrast resolution has been used that visualizes fainter enhancement. MRI is not suitable for visualizing intralesional calcification.
- *Optical coherence tomography:* The OCT can detect intraretinal edema, exudate, subretinal fluid, and subretinal growth.

The result of FFA depends on duration of the disease, stage of the disease, and type of disease. The frequent FFA results are given as follows:

- Vascular
- Retinal
- Combination
- The vascular changes are nonperfusion, capillary dropout, and leak.
- The retinal changes are increased tortuosity, beading, loops, neovascularization, bleeding, and multiple aneurysmal dilatations. These changes are visible on the fundus examination as well.

Differential Diagnosis of Coats' Disease

The list of conditions that constitute the differential diagnosis is long, headed by retinoblastoma, which is more common and fatal.

The features that point toward the possibility of Coats' disease are:

- The most important condition to be differentiated from Coats' disease is retinoblastoma.
- The characteristics of Coats' disease are given as follows:
    - Unilateral
    - Male preponderance in otherwise healthy children
    - Slow growing without family history
    - Without orbital invasion
    - No metastasis
    - Absent intraocular calcification
    - Computed tomography of the skull does not show intracranial calcification or angiomatosis
    - Late appearance of a white reflex in the pupillary area
    - Nonfatal
- The other conditions that need differentiation are given as follows:
    - Congenital cataract
    - Traumatic cataract
    - Persistent primary hyperplastic vitreous
    - Familial exudative vitreoretinopathy
    - Total retinal detachment
    - Intraocular toxocariasis

Angiomatosis Retinae (Von Hippel–Lindau Disease)

The condition is seen equally in boys and girls; it starts in the retinal periphery either as single or multiple lesions of microaneurysms in the capillaries, gradually developing into round, bright red nodules that increase in size to attain a size larger than the normal disk. The nodule has a feeding and a draining vessel; the former is an artery and latter a vein. In a normal retina, the arteries are thinner than the veins; in contrast to this, both attain the same caliber in angiomatosis. One-fourth of all cases have widespread systemic involvement that includes the central nervous system, lungs, liver, kidneys, pancreas, epididymis, and ovaries. The parts of the central nervous system involved are the cerebellum, medulla, pons, and spinal cord.

Hemangioblastoma is the most common cerebellar lesion. Infrequent systemic involvements are polycythemia, hypernephroma, and pheochromocytoma, the skin remains uninvolved. It is not possible to predict which child with angiomatosis retinae will go into systemic involvement; this makes it mandatory to seek neurological and systemic evaluation in all children with angiomatosis.

Ocular Involvements

Half of the children with VHL disease will have ocular involvement in the form of microaneurysms on the periphery that ultimately develop into a classical vascular nodule with a feeding and draining vessel.

Angiomatosis retinae come under the broad classification of phacomatosis, which are basically hamartomas. It is inherited as an autosomal dominant trait. The proteins in the vessels are inactivated by mutations in the tumor suppressor gene in the chromosome. This results in the overproduction of vascular endothelial growth factor (VEGF) in the eyes. The condition, in spite of its being nonhypoxic, produces VEGF, which is otherwise produced in hypoxic retinae.

Ocular manifestations are expected in roughly half of VHL patients. Retinal capillary hemangioblastomas (RCH) are the most commonly observed tumors in VHL.

A hemangioblastoma is a benign growth that arises from the endothelial cells of blood vessels.

They are often the initial manifestation of the disease. The treatment is directed toward ablation, surgical resection, and pharmacotherapy too, which have been tried to control the tumor without much success. Left untreated, the growth will often enlarge, emphasizing the importance of early diagnosis and treatment to preserve vision.

Complications of enlargement of peripheral mass or optic nerve involvement may be severe. A large mass may disrupt normal retinal architecture, eventually leading to exudative retinal detachment. Rarely, nonretinal manifestations, such as neovascularization of the iris or cornea, may progress to neovascular glaucoma and loss of vision. Ablative therapy of larger tumors carries increasing risks and offers limited success, often necessitating surgical resection. Coats' disease is sporadic without systemic involvement; this differentiates angiomatosis retinae from Coats' disease.

RETINAL HEMANGIOMAS

These are rare disorders of congenital origin and hereditary; they are less common than Coats' disease. The retinal hemangiomas are:

- Capillaries hemangiomas
- Cavernous hemangiomas
- Racemose hemangiomas

All of them are benign; the first two are hamartomas, and the third is not a true tumor but a congenital arteriovenous malformation. All of them have associated systemic involvement in various grades and combinations.

Capillary Hemangiomas

The capillary hemangiomas are put into two groups. They are given as follows:

1. Hemangiomas without systemic involvement
2. Hemangiomas with systemic involvement

The first not only involves the retina but also the optic nerve, and it may be found at any age but is more common in the second and third decades. The ocular features are the same as in the second group, in milder form.

The second type of hemangiomas is more extensive and is often misdiagnosed as Coats' disease, a nonhereditary unilateral condition seen in healthy males. The capillary hemangiomas are often thought to be precursors of angiomatosis retinae.

Retinal Cavernous Hemangiomas

These are less common than angiomatosis retinae. They are hamartomatous phakomas of the retina and optic nerve with skin involvement without the systemic features that are common in angiomatosis retinae. The condition is, most of the time, asymptomatic, not requiring any treatment. The condition is generally discovered or routine fundus examination. Some of the cases are stationary; others are progressive. The progression of the disease may stop at any stage. Spontaneous regression has been reported.

There is no medical or surgical treatment. The only treatments available are palliative. They are aimed at obliterating the affected vessels, which will automatically stop hemorrhage and exudation.

The two modes available are:

1. External application of cryo
2. Intraocular application of lasers, the preferred laser being an argon laser.

The vision does not improve immediately following either cryo or laser. It takes about 6–8 weeks for the vision to improve, not always to the normal level. Exudates require months to years to clear. Intravitreal anti-VEGF, too, has been tried with limited success.

Racemose Hemangioma of the Retina

They are basically congenital, nonhereditary, and sporadic arteriovenous communications without a gap between the two. They have ocular as well as systemic involvement; the systemic involvement is known as Wyburn–Mason syndrome. Though the common age of presentation is the third decade, yet it is not unusual to see cases in the first decade, seen equally in both sexes. Initially, the patient may be asymptomatic that develop ocular signs of diminished vision due to retinal exudation; the anterior segment is normal. The diagnostic features are found on fundus examination; they include dilatation and tortuosity of retinal vessels extending from the optic disk to the retinal periphery. The color and caliber of the arteries and veins are identical without any line of demarcation, frequently associated with retinal exudation and hemorrhage.

The condition can be differentiated from other angiomas by fluorescein angiography, which shows microaneurysms and capillary nonperfusion without leak. Some cases may show spontaneous regression. The involvement of the central nervous system is on the same side as the involved eye and generally involves the midbrain. The other involvement consists of facial bones.

Congenital Anomalies of the Macula

The two frequent congenital anomalies of macula are given as follows:

- Congenital coloboma
- Hypoplasia

Congenital Coloboma of the Macula

Coloboma of the macula is far less common than coloboma of the uvea. The etiopathogenesis of uveal coloboma is as simple as the failure of fetal fissure to close, which fails to explain the formation of macular coloboma, which is far away from the fetal fissure; hence, the closure of fetal fissure has no role in the formation of macular coloboma. The most widely prevalent theory is that macular colobomas are not truly developmental anomalies but are secondary to intrauterine infection in the early stages of development. The colobomas of the macula can be unilateral or bilateral, single or multiple of various sizes and shapes, the most common shape being horizontally oval. The size may vary from less than one disk diameter to many times larger than the disk. Horizontal alignment, or coloboma, goes against its being failure of the closure of fetal fissure that produces coloboma in the anteroposterior meridian in the lower surface, with a strong hereditary tendency. The colobomas of the macula have been put into two broad categories as per the presence of blood vessels and pigmentation given as follows:

- With abnormal retinal blood vessels
- With pigmentation/without pigmentation

Both types may exist in the same eye. Colobomas with abnormal vessels are less common; there may be anastomosis between the retinal and choroidal vessels that may invade the vitreous. The pigmented colobomas have piled up uveal pigment on their periphery, with retinal vessels passing over them. The choriocapillaris are absent at the floor of the coloboma.

The nonpigmented are not entirely devoid of pigment. The floor of the coloboma is white due to exposed sclera, the absence of uveal pigment, and choriocapillaris on the floor.

The floor of the coloboma may be ectatic. The coloboma may be associated with anomalies of the posterior pole in the form of the uveal, optic nerve, and coloboma of the globe. The common symptom of macular coloboma is a disproportionate loss of central vision. The children generally present with squint, amblyopia, and nystagmus. The most common disorder that should be differentiated from congenital coloboma of the macula is congenital toxoplasmosis, which gives positive TORCH results on a screening test. Confirmation of toxoplasmosis lies in the various serological tests available.

Hypoplasia of the Macula

This is often suspected to be an abortive form of coloboma of the macula. It could either be an isolated anomaly or be associated with albinism. The exact etiology remains obscure; the main complaint of the condition is uncorrectable diminished vision with its aftermath of squint, amblyopia, loss of color sensation, and nystagmus. The only sign is the absence of foveal reflex; the condition should be differentiated from other cone dystrophies.

METHODS EMPLOYED IN THE EVALUATION OF RETINA

The number of tests used to evaluate the retina is long; some are simple office procedures; while others are complicated and highly technical that require specialized expertise to decipher. Most of them are required to be performed in unison with multiple instruments.

The tests are given as follows:

- Routine office procedures
- Specialized procedures

Routine Office Procedures

- Record of vision
- Vision with a pinhole
- Best-corrected vision
- Color vision
- Field of vision:
    - Central (Amsler grid)
    - Peripheral:
        - Static
        - Dynamic

- Contrast*
- Photostress†
- Refraction
- Fundus examination:
    - Direct ophthalmoscopy
    - Indirect ophthalmoscopy
    - Examination with +90 D

Specialized Procedures

- Fundus fluorescein angiography
- Indocyanine green angiography
- Ultrasonography
- Optical coherence tomography
- Dark adaptometry
- *Electrophysiological test:*
    - Electroretinography
    - Electro-oculography
    - A visually evoked response
- *Imaging:*
    - X-ray
    - Computed tomography
    - Magnetic resonance imaging

CLINICAL FEATURES OF RETINAL DISORDERS

Symptoms

The symptoms of retinal disorders are never painful; they themselves do not cause an anterior segment reaction, redness of the eyes, ciliary tenderness, pain, or a rise in tension.

The common symptoms are given as follows:

- Vision:
    - Loss of vision:
        - It may be sudden or gradual
        - Retinal disorders do not cause diminished near vision
        - Uncorrectable, diminished vision
    - Floaters
    - Flashes of light
    - Obscuration of vision
    - Loss of field
    - Metamorphopsia
- Diminished night vision
- Diminished color vision

Signs

The signs of retinal disorder are restricted to the area behind the ora serrata; hence, they are devoid of features in the anterior segment except the white reflex in the pupillary area on oblique illumination and pupillary changes. Congenital disorders are associated with nystagmus. Squints are a common feature in children.

- The signs are best seen on a fundus examination.
- Retinoscopy may show either a pale reflex or an absent retinal glow.

The fundus should be examined both by direct and indirect ophthalmoscopes. A direct ophthalmoscopy is used as a screening procedure supplemented by an indirect ophthalmoscope that may require scleral indentation. Macula and disk are better examined by direct ophthalmoscope and slit lamp using either a Hruby lens or by +70 D to +90 D lens.

The signs are elicited by examining the retina under the following heads, depending on symptoms.

- *Scanning of the retina by direct ophthalmoscope.*
    - Examination of the macula
    - Examination of the periphery
    - Examination of the disk
    - Examination of the vitreous

An evaluation may require the use of various methods in combination.

The retina is scanned under the following heads:

- Color of the retina
- Retinal edema

**Contrast:* Contrast is tested on a specially designed optotypes Pelli–Robson chart or its modifications, where optotypes of the same size gradually fade from above to below. There are six rows of letters. Each row consists of eight letters. The chart measures the minimum contrast detectable for a specified size.

†*Photostress test:* This is a crude form to evaluate the dark adaptation of an eye. The principle is to make the visual pigments insensitive to ordinary light, resulting in a relative scotoma that fades in a few minutes, and the eye returns to pretest level. The time taken for the recovery roughly denotes adaptation time. The recovery time depends upon ability of the photoreceptors to synthesize visual pigment. The test has no utility in peripheral retinal lesions; it is best utilized as an office procedure to evaluate the macula to differentiate between macular and optic nerve disorders. The test is performed by noting the best-corrected vision. The eye is dazzled by the light of an indirect ophthalmoscope from a distance of 3 cm from the eye. After removing the sources of light, the patient is asked to read the best-corrected line. In normal eyes, it takes about half a minute to recover; in cases of macular disease, this is prolonged to over 1 minute.

- Retinal exudate
- Retinal hemorrhage
- Detachment
- Vascular changes
- An examination of the retina is not complete without an examination of the disk.

Color of the Retina

The normal retina is transparent; its pink color is imparted by choriocapillaris underneath, supplemented by xanthophylls. Generally, the choroidal vasculature is not visible on fundus examination except in a condition called tessellated fundus (tigroid fundus), where the choroidal vessels stand out prominently. It is often seen in myopia, but the phenomenon has no clinical significance.

Pallor of the Retina

Generalized pallor of the retina is seen in various forms of anemia and leukemia. In adults, severe pallor is seen in obstruction of the central retinal artery, obstruction of the branch causes pallor in the area supplied by it; other causes of pale retina are albinism, myopia, Waardenburg syndrome, and choroideremia.

Hyperemia of the Retina

Hyperemia of the retina can be arterial or venous; the latter is more common. The former is associated with dilatation of the arteries and increased tortuosity of the arterioles. It can be generalized of localized; it is seen in acute retinitis and uveitis. Venous congestion is passive in nature due to impeded venous flow. Common causes are papilledema, papillitis, leukemia, polycythemia, chronic heart failure, sickle cell retinopathy, cavernous sinus thrombosis, and central vein/branch vein obstruction.

Edema of the Retina

Retinal edema is a state of accumulation of fluid in the retina following breakdown of the blood–retinal barriers, either the outer or inner barrier, following an abnormality of any of the following:

- Increased permeability of capillaries
- Leaks of fluid from capillaries
- Breakdown of large protein molecules

The retinal edema is met in the posterior pole more commonly than other parts. Edema of the macula causes more symptoms than other locations in the posterior pole. Examples of the breakdown of the inner barrier are cystoid macular edema, commotio retinae, and vascular retinopathies. Central serous retinopathy is caused by the breakdown of the outer barrier. Common causes of retinal edema in children are retinitis, neuroretinitis, papillitis, chorioretinitis, retinopathies of childhood, and cystoid macular edema. Central serous retinopathy is a disorder of the late second and third decades that results due to localized circular edema of the macula.

Macular edema is considered to be clinically significant if it has the following features:

- Retinal edema is within 0.5 mm of the fovea.
- The area of edema has a diameter more than one disk diameter.
- Hard exudate within 0.5 mm of the fovea in an edematous retina.
- Thickening in the surrounding retina.
- Zone of thickening of one disk diameter.

The clinically significant macular edema is better visualized in red-free light than white light. It is best seen by a +90 D lens, and delineated by OCT.

The clinical features of macular edema are given as follows:

- Diminished central vision.
- Relative central scotomas.
- Acquired axial hypermetropia.
- Metamorphopsia.

In contrast to this peripheral area of retinal edema may go undetected, they produce corresponding field defects.

Cystoid Macular Edema

There are many causes of cystoid macular edema. All of them are not applicable to children. The most common cause in adults in the fifth decade or beyond used to be intracapsular cataract extraction. There are two possible causes of its production, i.e., the action of prostaglandins and damage to the capillary endothelium, resulting in the accumulation of fluid in the outer plexiform layer that has poor intercellular adhesion, which helps the formation of cysts in this layer. In spite of its predominant involvement of the macula, it may be asymptomatic to begin with, followed by metamorphopsia and central scotoma. On fundus examination, there is loss of foveal reflex, hard exudate, and deep hemorrhage. The unattended case may go into formation of a macular hole; the condition is best diagnosed by FFA. That shows a dye leak from the parafoveal vessels and from the disk. OCT is helpful in measuring the thickness of the affected macula.

The causes of cystoid macular edema are:
- Intracapsular cataract extraction
- Postcryo, postlaser status
- Intermediate uveitis
- Retinal telangiectasis
- Retinitis pigmentosa

Central Serous Retinopathy (Central Serous Chorioretinopathy)

This is a frequent disorder seen mostly in otherwise healthy males in their late teens and early adulthood with unilateral presentation. The other eye may get involved months after the first eye. In most instances where the disease is self-limiting, the presentation is typically unilateral, painless, and diminished vision in an apparently healthy male; women rarely suffer from the disorder. The common symptoms are metamorphopsia, a central circular gray to black spot in the central field with normal color sense. Brightness and contrast are occasionally diminished. In prepresbyopic persons, the condition may precipitate unilateral diminished near vision. Diminished vision, both far and near, will come back to an age-matched level with recovery.

On examination, the eye has the following features:
- Externally, the eye is normal.
- Normal pupillary light and near reflex.
- Diminished distant vision that may be as small as a loss of one to two lines on the Snellen chart.
- The vision may or may not improve with a pinhole.
- The vision comes to 6/6 by adding plus lenses that generally do not exceed more than 1–2 D sphere, which gradually decreases with the improvement of the condition.

The cause of the malady is not well established; the conditions are more common in persons with type 1 personality, and stress is also contributory. In women, pregnancy can precipitate the condition; many drugs, including high doses of steroids, too have been occasionally blamed. The condition is visualized in angiography with both fluorescein and indocyanine green; the latter is better. The changes are localized congestion of choriocapillaris, hyperpermeability of choriocapillaris, accumulation of fluid under the macula, detachment of retinal pigment epithelium, and defect in the blood-retinal barrier.

The condition is confirmed by the given points:
- Clear media
- Normal pupil
- Vision improving with plus lenses
- Normal disk and blood vessels
- Typical changes in macula consist of following points:
  - A circular swollen area larger than usual disk, edema not exceeding +2 D, round the fovea, absent foveal reflex.
  - A dark ring surrounds the circular, elevated retina around the macula.
  - No hemorrhage or exudate
  - The presence of pigment is suggestive of chronicity

Investigation: Generally, in a typical case, no investigation is required. In cases of nonimprovement of vision with plus lenses or no spontaneous recovery, the investigations ordered are:
- Fundus fluorescein angiography
- Indocyanine green angiography
- Optical coherence tomography
- *Fundus fluorescein angiography (FFA):* Fundus fluorescein angiography typically shows leakage and pooling that may be on the fovea or away from the fovea, generally above the fovea, as an ink blot or smokestack pattern.
- *Indocyanine green angiography:* Indocyanine green angiography shows a picture similar to that seen in fluorescein angiography with added multifocal hyperfluorescence. It also delineates occult choroidal neovascularization that is detrimental to visual improvement and requires additional management.
- *Optical coherence tomography:* Optical coherence tomography confirms the findings of FFA and indocyanine green fluorescence angiography (ICFA) and shows subtle findings such as small pigment epithelium defects and fibrinous subretinal fluid; it can be a helpful follow-up in chronic central serous retinopathy (CSR).

Differential Diagnosis

The common disorders that constitute a differential diagnosis of CSR are optic neuritis, papilledema, and optic nerve head pits.

Management

- *No treatment:* As the condition is self-limiting and the best vision is reached within a fortnight, no treatment is warranted. The patient should be counselled about possible recurrence, which may happen after a few weeks to months in the same eye or the contralateral.

The recurrences take a longer time to reach the previous vision. Recurrences require FFA, ICFA, and OCT to establish the cause.

- *Argon laser:* Argon laser treatment is indicated if the swelling persists for >4–6 weeks or if patients require early restoration of normal vision. Different institutions follow different protocols. Each lesion requires different management.
- *Photodynamic therapy (PDT)**:* This is used less frequently in severe diseases that do not respond to usual laser therapy.
- *Medical treatment:* There is no specific medical therapy. In the past, steroids were used without much effect. Antidepressants and anxiolytics may be required.

Retinal Exudate

The presence of exudates on the retina, superficial or deep, always reflects pathology. They are generally bilateral, and simultaneous but not symmetric and fade or disappear with treatment of primary causative factors; they themselves do not require any treatment. Exudate may be localized or scattered more frequently in the posterior pole; do not cause diminished vision unless on the macula.

As per ophthalmoscopic appearance, the exudates are as follows:

- Soft exudate
- Hard exudate

- *Soft exudates* are acute in nature due to deranged axoplasmic flow, resulting in the collection of axoplasmic debris in the nerve fiber layer. Due to their location in relation to layers of the sensory retina, they are also called superficial exudates. The exudates are basically vascular in nature. The pathogenesis consists of sudden local constriction of vessels, causing ischemia/anoxia in the nerve fiber layer. The soft exudates are white in color, in patches with irregular shapes and irregular margins, with a feathery look that imparts the name cotton wool exudate. The exudates are not seen above the vessels, do not coalesce to form large plaques, and disappear with or without treatment in 1–2 months. Common conditions with soft exudates are retinitis, severe anemia, dysproteinemia, collagen diseases, leukemia, papillitis, papilledema, septicemia, and hypertensive retinitis. A common cause of soft exudate in adults is not seen in children.
- *Hard exudates* are seen less commonly in children. In adults, the leading cause is diabetic retinopathy. The hard exudates are supposed to be vascular in origin, to which exudation is superadded. Sometimes, exudation is more prominent than its vascular counterpart; in contrast to soft exudates, which are seen in the nerve fiber layer, hard exudates develop in deeper neurosensory. Later, which is more compact than the nerve fiber layer. This compactness is supposed to be the cause of their circular shape.

The pathogenesis of hard exudates is given as follows:
Defective oxidation → Neural degeneration → Products of degeneration → Exudation → Deep (hard) exudates

The hard exudates are made up of albumin, hyaline, cholesterol, and calcium. The hard exudates are round, discrete bodies with clear-cut edges; their sizes range from pinhead to many times larger, seen on the periphery, under the vessels. The white color of the exudates is attributed to their calcium and lipid content. They are responsible for macular star[†] and circinate retinopathy[‡], which are never acute, take months to develop, and many months to years to disappear without leaving a scar. A combination of both types of exudates is a common feature in advanced retinopathies, adding superficial and deep hemorrhage to the exudation.

**Photodynamic therapy:* The principle of the procedure is to stimulate photoactivated dye (verteporfin) by infrared laser that destroys the vessels with minimal damage to the retina on the surface, retinal pigment, and choroid underneath by releasing free radicals that cause site-specific vascular occlusion. The amount of laser used is too less to cause damage to the tissue but sufficient to cause the death of endothelial cells, resulting in the obliteration of offending vessels without damaging surrounding tissue.

[†]*Macular star:* The macular star is formed in the outer plexiform layer of the macula due to the deposition of lipids. The macular star does not radiate from a point, as the name may suggest, but the exudates are arranged around a circle like rays of the sun. The common causes of macular stars are neuroretinitis, papilledema, and hypertensive retinopathy. It takes 6–12 months to fade and return to normal with the recovery of vision.

[‡]*Circinate retinopathy:* Circinate retinopathy is a delayed effect of chronic retinopathy. Where exudates are arranged around the edematous macula like a girdle, occasionally, it can be incomplete in the form of a crescent with concavity toward the macula. It has rarely been reported in places other than the circumocular area. Generally, it is bilateral and seen mostly in adults. The common causes are diabetic retinopathy, Coats disease, venous obstruction, Leber disease (multiple miliary aneurysm with retinal degeneration), and senile macular degeneration. Out of these, diabetic retinopathy is the foremost.

Retinal Hemorrhage

To reach its high metabolism, the retina is endowed with a very rich blood supply from two sources, i.e., retinal and chorioretinal. Retinal hemorrhages are a pretty common occurrence in many diseases, both local and systemic; the latter is the more common cause of retinal hemorrhages, less common in children than adults.

Depending upon the system of blood vessels involved, i.e., choroidal/retinal and the caliber of vessels involved, i.e., capillaries and branches, they have been put in the following groups:

- *Intraretinal (capillary):*
  - Superficial
  - Deep
- *Preretinal (branch):*
  - Subhyaloid
  - Vitreous
- *Subretinal (choroidal):*
  - Choroidal hematoma
  - Subretinal neovascularization

Intraretinal hemorrhages are referred to as deep hemorrhages, while hemorrhages in the superficial retinal layers and surface of the retina are called superficial hemorrhages. In long-standing disorders, both may co-exist in the same eye. Both types of hemorrhages are generally bilateral and simultaneous, and they need not be symmetric.

Causes of retinal hemorrhages are given as follows:

- *Traumatic:*
  - Closed or open globe injury.
  - It is common for retinal vessels to be torn in tractional retinal detachment; tears in blood vessels in rhegmatogenous detachment are not uncommon.
- Inflammation is more common in periphlebitis.
- Retinopathy

The most common causes of both types of retinal hemorrhages are given as follows:

1. Retinopathies
2. Blood disorders

The hemorrhages in retinopathies are uncommon in children. Common causes of retinal hemorrhages due to retinopathies in children are sickle cell retinopathy, malignant hypertension, nephritis, and subacute bacterial endocarditis.

Blood disorders that cause retinal hemorrhage are anemia, leukemia, hemophilia, and sickle cell anemia.

- *Miscellaneous:* Papilledema, papillitis periphlebitis, telangiectasis, Coats' disease, Terson's syndrome*, and Purtscher's retinopathy†.

Characteristics of superficial retinal hemorrhages: The hemorrhages are situated in the nerve fiber layer, the source of bleeding being capillaries; they are bright red in color and stand out on the pink retinal background, irregular, flame shaped, lie under the vessels, and fade way within weeks to months even without treatment of the causative factors. They do not leave any trace in the form of pigmentation or fibrosis, only occurring in newer places. There is no method to hasten their clearance or prevent recurrence. The hemorrhages away from the macula may go unnoticed and be discovered on routine fundus examinations for systemic disorders such as hypertension, diabetes or unrelated conditions such as refractive errors. Macular hemorrhages are symptomatic and may cause sudden, profound visual loss.

The common causes of superficial hemorrhages in children are given as follows:

Trauma, direct or indirect, retinitis, papillitis, papilledema, secondary hypertension, and diabetes, a major cause of retinal hemorrhage in adults, are not seen in children, except in the late stages of unmanaged juvenile diabetes. Other causes are leukemia, pernicious anemia, and purpura. They may be in the form of Roth's spot‡.

**Terson's syndrome:* Terson's syndrome is a neurological condition with ocular involvement that may be seen in any age but is more common in adults due to access to subarachnoid blood in the retina via the subarachnoid space. It has been reported in newborns as well.

†*Purtscher's retinopathy (traumatic retinal angiopathy):* This is due to occlusion of the fine capillaries of the retinal vessels following injury away from the eyes. The clinical pictures consist of white exudate-like bodies scattered around the papilla and macula. These white spots are generally accumulations of lipids in the microvasculature.

‡*Roth's spot (Litten's spots/sign):* These are special types of nonspecific, superficial retinal hemorrhage of variable size and number with white centers, mostly seen in children suffering from subacute bacterial endocarditis, anemia, and purpura. They are also associated with hypertension, diabetes, and collagen vascular diseases in adults. The basic pathogenesis is damage to the endothelial cell and plugging of the damaged endothelium with fibrin and platelets. The white center is due to the deposition of fibrin and platelets in the center of the hemorrhage. Like any other superficial hemorrhage, they need no specific treatment and are known to fade away without treatment, leaving no trace. Recurrence in the persistence of the primary cause is common.

Deep hemorrhages: The retinal hemorrhages developing in the deeper layers of the sensory retina are referred to as deep hemorrhages. Due to the compactness of the tissue around them, they cannot spread such as in superficial layers; they are circular, small, and dull red in color; their number and size vary from a microscopic spot to a dot as large as 1 mm. They are most common in the posterior pole, they may be in clusters without coalescing; the clusters are confused as microaneurysms, which can only be differentiated by FFA; the hemorrhages do not stain; they block the dye. The most common cause of deep hemorrhages is diabetes retinopathy, which is not seen in children. The other causes are retinal vein thrombosis, ocular ischemic syndrome, sickle cell retinopathy, and telangiectasia near the macula.

It is common to have both superficial and deep hemorrhages in the same eye. The hemorrhages are bilateral; like all other hemorrhage they do not require any specific treatment and fade away with treatment of the basic cause; they are also known to disappear without treatment.

Both types of retinal hemorrhage have profound diagnostic value in retinopathy of systemic origin and for recording progress, such as in diabetic and hypertensive retinopathy.

The causes of retinal hemorrhages in children are:

- *Retinopathies:* The majority of cases of retinal hemorrhages can be traced to various types of retinopathies. The commonly seen retinal hemorrhages are sickle cell retinopathy, anemia, leukemia, purpura, retinopathy of prematurity, and malignant hypertension.
- *Trauma:* Both closed and open globe injuries cause retinal hemorrhage. It is common for retinal vessels to be torn in rhegmatogenous retinal detachment and tractional retinal detachment.
- *Inflammation:* Periphlebitis is a common cause of retinal hemorrhage in the late second decade or early third decade.
- *Blood disorders:* Anemia, leukemia, purpura, hemophilia, and sickle cell anemia.
- *Miscellaneous:* Retinal telangiectasia, Coats' disease, papilledema, papillitis.
- *Pseudohemorrhages:* Cherry-red spot, macular hole

Subhyaloid (preretinal) hemorrhages: Hemorrhages occurring between the internal limiting membrane and posterior surface of the vitreous without rupture in the vitreous. This is due to its location, which is referred to as subhyaloid or preretinal hemorrhage. The bleeding is from the vessels on the surface or the retina. They are less frequent in children. The most common cause in the late twenties and early third decade is periphlebitis (*Eales' disease**).

Common causes in children are:

Retinopathy of prematurity, primary persistent hyperplastic vitreous, angiomatosis retinae, juvenile retinoschisis, drusen of optic nerve, Coats' disease, untreated juvenile diabetes, Purtscher's retinopathy, and Terson's disease.

Pathologically, it is an occlusive vasculitis of the peripheral retina characterized by periphlebitis, vascular occlusion, hemorrhage, and neovascularization.

Figure 20.20 shows the various phases of Eales' disease.

Vitreous hemorrhage is the predominant cause of sudden loss of vision in Eales' disease. Traditionally, it has been divided into the following stages without clear-cut demarcation between vasculitis, occlusion, and neovascularization. The treatment is to suppress the periphlebitis, preserve loss of vision, and prevent complications with corticosteroids and immunosuppressives. The treatment is very personal, with each patient requiring a different regime. Systemic steroid and anti-immunosuppressive regimes have the advantage of being effective in both eyes at the same time, even looking after the asymptomatic lesion in the contralateral eye.

Clinical features of subhyaloid hemorrhage: The clinical features depend on position, size, time lapsed from onset, and associated ocular and systemic disorders.

**Eales' disease*: Eales' disease is a common cause of sudden, painless unilateral loss of vision in healthy males in their late twenties and early thirties. A spontaneous cure is followed by a period of clear vision with a recurrence that may be as serious as the initial attack or more. The recovery following each is longer than the previous, and the gap between two recurrences is shorter, ultimately leading to a stage of hemophthalmos. Though the disease starts in one eye, the other nonsymptomatic eye may harbor quite advanced disease, making it mandatory to examine the other eye in detail by indirect ophthalmoscope. The exact cause of the disease is not known; in the past, infective processes such as tuberculosis and sepsis in other places of the body were squarely blamed for the disease, and all patients were put on anti-infective drugs for a long time without any satisfactory result. Later on, it was realized that the condition was an autoimmune disease with implications for T-cells and improvements with steroid and immunosuppressive.

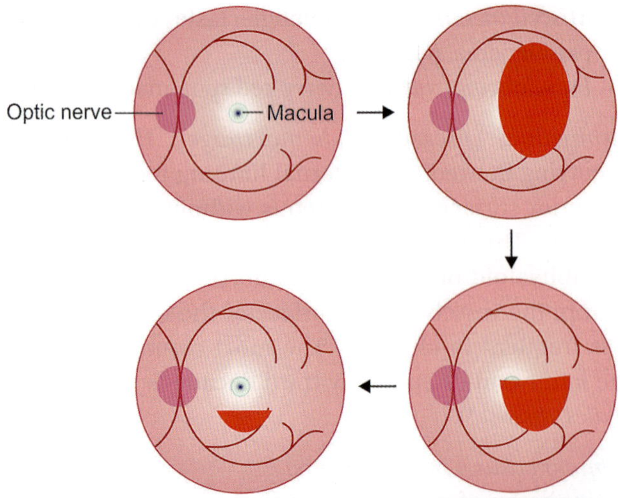

Fig. 20.20: Showing evolution of subhyaloid hemorrhage. (Retinal vessels → vein → periphlebitis → occlusion → hemorrhage → absorption of blood → recurrence → neovascularization → fibrosis → traction detachment)

Symptoms:

- *No symptoms:* Even a large hemorrhage away from the macula, especially in the lower part, may be asymptomatic and go unattended.
- *With symptoms:*
  - A hemorrhage in front of the macula is always associated with sudden unilateral painless loss of vision that worsens within hours to days, from 6/6 to as low as hand movement, retaining accurate projection. Even a large subhyaloid hemorrhage does not result in a loss of perception of light.
  - A patient with a fresh hemorrhage may complain of a red hue (erythropsia), which passes off within a few days; all patients need not complain of erythropsia.
  - The patient may report a slight-to-moderate improvement in vision after a few days, especially if the patient is in an upright position, due to the settling of blood in the lower part of the subhyaloid hemorrhage.
  - Less common is the return to prehemorrhage vision; generally, this happens if the patient has been advised bed rest.
  - A fall of vision may occur in the recumbent position.
  - Rebleeding worsens the improved vision.

Signs:

- Externally, the eye is normal, without congestion, ciliary tenderness, and without anterior chamber reactions. A pupillary reaction is normal, in the long run, the eye may develop an afferent pupillary defect with a gross difference of vision in two eyes.
- The signs are visible on:
  - *Retinoscopy:* There may be a loss of red retinal glow, and small subhyaloid hemorrhage in the visual axis stands out as a large black blotch against the pink retinal glow.
  - *Ophthalmoscopy:* The subhyaloid hemorrhage is best visualized through an indirect ophthalmoscope under full cycloplegia. Examination with a direct ophthalmoscope fails to delineate the borders of the subhyaloid hemorrhage. The advantage of examination by indirect ophthalmoscope lies in the fact that an indirect ophthalmoscope can circumvent even a large hemorrhage with the advantage of stereopsis and a wider field that may harbor the cause of hemorrhage (vasculitis).
  - Subhyaloid hemorrhage is always solitary and does not clot.
  - The appearance of a subhyaloid hemorrhage depends on the duration of hemorrhage.
  - *Appearance of a subhyaloid hemorrhage:* A hemorrhage, if examined within a day or two, looks like a large, bright red, vertically oval, three-dimensional spot larger than the disk in front on the macula between the internal limiting membrane and vitreous. As time passes, the heavy particles of blood settle down at the most dependent part, with a clear or translucent/lighter, noncellular part of blood occupying the upper part with a horizontal line of demarcation in between if the patient is upright. The hemorrhage, though it has an oval, three-dimensional shape, it does not have a formed wall.

Vitreous hemorrhage: In the previous paragraph, we have seen that the vitreous does not have a formed capsule yet; its outer surface keeps the contents contained in itself. Though it has close proximity to the optic nerve and the inter-limiting membrane of the retina, with retinal vessels on its surface sandwiched behind the vitreous, normal vessels do not invade the vitreous body. Moreover, the fully developed vitreous is avascular and semisolid; so long as the outer surface of the vitreous is intact, no vessels invade the vitreous, leaving it transparent. Only when blood vessels disrupt the outer surface does an intravitreal hemorrhage develop. The condition, in short, is referred to as vitreous hemorrhage or, better yet, vitreous hematoma.

The exact cause that disrupts the vitreous is not well understood; it may be a vasoformative factor or a vitreolysis factor.

A small hemorrhage away from the visual axis does not cause symptoms. The symptoms of vitreous hemorrhage do not differ from those of subhyaloid bleeding; the most common cause of intravitreal hemorrhage besides periphlebitis is proliferative retinopathy. Generally, vitreous hemorrhages get absorbed, requiring more time than preretinal hemorrhages, leaving few cells in the vitreous. The vitreous is generally either fluid or gets liquefied, for which there is no established reason. Nonabsorption of vitreous hemorrhage or recurrent bleedings get churned with the fluid vitreous, and a state of hemophthalmos results, obscuring the fundus, which is not visible even by an indirect ophthalmoscope. The liquid vitreous, upon being irritated by blood, releases VEGF that encourages vascular proliferation and rebleeding, which initiates fibrous proliferation in the form of bands. The bands start from the optic nerve head and progress toward the ora. Intravitreal hemorrhages carry a poorer prognosis than preretinal hemorrhages. There is no significant therapeutic benefit to hastening the absorption of blood from the vitreous. The only solution is to do a total vitrectomy followed by a laser.

Subretinal hemorrhage: As the term suggests, these are not true retinal hemorrhages. They are, in fact, choroidal hemorrhages. The hemorrhages occur between the pigment epithelium and the choroid. They are rarely seen in children. The causes of subretinal hemorrhages are trauma, choroidal rupture, high myopia, vascular retinopathy, drusen of the optic nerve head, chorioretinitis, and choroidal neovascularization.

In contrast to the red appearance of retinal and preretinal hemorrhages, the subretinal hemorrhages impart a blackish color to the retina over the hemorrhage, the hemorrhagic area is raised over which the retinal vessels pass. The condition in adults may be mistaken for melanoma of the choroid. The diagnosis is confirmed by USG, FFA, and OCT.

Inflammation of the Retina

Both inflammation and infection of the retina are clubbed under one term of retinitis. Which should logically be reserved for the infection of the retina. Isolated infection of the retina is rare; more common are retinochoroiditis, neuroretinitis, and retinal vasculitis, which is mostly periphlebitis. Retinitis can be divided as follows:

- *Primary:* Infection of the retina only (rare).
- *Secondary:* Infection spreading either from the choroid or, less commonly, from the optic nerve.
- *Associated:* Retinal vasculitis

All microbes that infect adults can infect children. The following paragraphs will comprise a description of an infection caused by organisms that have a propensity for children. The organism can be endogenous or exogenous, rarely unilateral; the latter is common with parasitic infections. Retinitis in children can be acute, subacute, chronic, or recurrent.

Viral retinitis in children: Both RNA and DNA viruses are known to cause retinitis; DNA viruses cause chronic retinitis, while acute retinitis is caused by RNA viruses such as rubella and rubeola. Herpes simplex virus causes predominantly chorioretinitis, while rubella and rubeola cause primarily retinitis. Healthy adults rarely develop viral retinitis but may be seropositive yet asymptomatic for many viruses; viral retinitis is common in neonates due to intrauterine infection. The two common examples are rubella and cytomegaloviruses. Vasculitis is frequent association of retinitis, which is set to be an immune reaction. Retinitis can be generalized or localized, causing pigmentary changes in the retina without attenuation of vessels and diminished night vision. The above two factors differentiated viral retinitis from more serious degeneration, i.e., retinitis pigmentosa. Viral retinitis is often associated with superficial exudates and hemorrhages; gliosis, retinal detachment, secondary glaucoma, and complicated cataracts are long-term effects of viral retinitis. Involvement of the posterior pole predisposes involvement of the optic nerve in various combinations. The common viruses that cause retinitis in children, including neonates, are rubella, herpes, cytomegalovirus, and Epstein–Barr virus.

Rubella retinitis: Rubella retinitis is a part of congenital infection. The end result of this is pigmentary changes in the retina; hence, the condition is also known as embryonic pigmentary retinopathy. This healing is left with pigmentary changes on the periphery with normal vessels and normal dark adaptation, the two cornerstones of the more serious condition of retinal pigmentosa, retinitis pigmentosa.

Rubella retinitis is seen in half of the children born to mothers infected by systemic rubella in the first trimester.

Such children are often likely to develop bilateral cataracts and glaucoma, along with an array of congenital systemic anomalies. It is difficult to diagnose retinitis as rubella retinitis without other signs of generalized rubella in the acute stage.

The macula is spared; hence, central vision remains normal. The fundus shows a paper-salt appearance that should be differentiated from other causes of embryonal retinopathies; this is topped by congenital syphilis, which is differentiated by other systemic involvement and a positive serological test. The other conditions that need differentiation are varicella, cytomegalovirus influenza, and radiation to the mother in the first trimester. The TORCH test is a handy test to screen, but it is not a specific test for rubella. There is no treatment for Rubella retinitis. It is best done by immunizing against rubella well before the mother's planned pregnancy.

Rubeola (measles) retinitis: Rubeola is a common, preventable disorder of childhood. Retinal involvement is rarer than the involvement of the lids, conjunctiva, and cornea. The retina is involved along with the involvement of the central nervous system in subacute necrotizing panencephalitis, a fatal complication of measles, which is a mild, almost universal disease in children. The retinal involvement is bilateral. Involvement of the optic nerve is common, and the end result for a surviving child is chorioretinal scars and optic atrophy. There is no treatment for measles of any kind except immunization, as per the national program of immunization.

Herpes simplex retinitis: Involvement of the retina is always secondary to systemic involvement in neonates in the form of encephalitis; it is also seen in immunosuppressed children in the form of superficial exudates, hemorrhages, occasional sheathing of blood vessels, vitritis, and exudative retinal detachment.

Cytomegalovirus retinitis: With the alarming rise of immunodeficiency in children, the incidence of cytomegalovirus retinitis in children has shown an upward swing. Incidentally, 80% of the general population is seropositive for the cytomegalovirus and goes undetected unless they develop systemic symptoms. When immunity falls beyond a critical level, cytomegalovirus retinitis is diagnosed in two groups of children. They are congenital and acquired. The first is necrotizing retinochoroiditis anywhere on the retina; the macula is the most common site of involvement and may result in consecutive optic atrophy.

The acquired form is seen in children inflicted with HIV, where the virus reaches the retina by hematogenous spread. It starts with unilateral lesions, but soon the other eye gets involved. The condition is vision-threatening in the majority of cases.

Bacterial retinitis: All pyogenic and nonpyogenic bacteria, may they be gram positive or gram negative, are capable of causing retinitis, which is rarely primary. It could be granulomatous or nongranulomatous, congenital, or acquired. The most common congenital retinitis is seen in congenital syphilis in the form of embryopathic pigmentary retinopathy that, on healing, leaves a picture of the pepper-salt fundus without night blindness. Acquired syphilitic retinitis is not seen in children. The treatment consists of treatment for systemic syphilis.

Toxoplasma retinitis: The most common part of the retina involved in toxoplasmosis is the macula. It could be congenital or acquired, and the latter is seen in adults. The first is intrauterine, due to the transmission of infection via the placenta. The third possibility is a stage of reactivation of a healed lesion presenting as a fresh, acquired lesion slightly away from the original macular scar. About 30% of the general population is seropositive and nonsymptomatic. The prevalence is more in developing countries. The systemic involvement in adults is mild or asymptomatic and may go undetected unless the person is immunocompromised. Pregnant women are more likely to pass the infection on to the growing fetus if they acquire toxoplasmosis during pregnancy. 50% of infected mothers are likely to pass the disease to the fetus; the fetus is at danger of getting infected only if the mother acquires the disease during pregnancy. Children born in subsequent pregnancies are safe.

Eighty percent of infants with congenital toxoplasmosis have retinal involvement. The parasites have an affinity for the neural layers of the retina. The condition is bilateral in more than 80% of cases, with predilection for macula. This may be missed unless looked for specifically, or the child has convulsions and hepatosplenomegaly. Convulsion is part of three cardinal features of congenital toxoplasmosis, the other two being chorioretinitis and intracranial calcification. Thus, it is mandatory to get the fundi of every newborn examined if the infant has convulsions or hepatosplenomegaly. The condition, if missed in infancy, is diagnosed only when the child presents with esotropia and is found to harbor a large scar of chorioretinitis in the posterior pole. The typical lesion is larger than the optic disk, with pigmentation on the periphery and a white floor. The conditions should be differentiated from congenital coloboma of the macula. The infective process is no more amenable to treatment at this stage. The child should be observed for reactivation of the disease for many years. The reactivated lesions may be single or multiple, a little away from the original scar. The reactivated condition may be associated with vitritis, vitreous detachment papillitis, and an anterior chamber reaction.

Toxocariasis of the Retina

Toxocara infection of the retina is broadly divided into two types, i.e., macular granuloma and peripheral granuloma. Besides these to there may be larval endophthalmitis.

Macular granuloma: Macular granuloma may begin as submacular lesions that extend to involve the whole macula; as the lesion is limited to the posterior pole, the eye is devoid of anterior chamber reaction. The condition is invariably unilateral, hence going undetected unless the child is brought for squint and found to have uncorrectable diminished vision. Fundus examination reveals a lesion on the macula, which arouses suspicion of retinoblastoma because of its similarity to early retinoblastoma. The macular lesion in toxoplasmosis is an oval, raised mass over which retinal glial tissue develops, that may be large enough to cause a white reflex in the pupillary area.

Peripheral granuloma: This is also a single unilateral lesion with minimal anterior chamber reaction mistaken for more common pars planitis. In appearance, the lesion is raised and oval, from which glial bands develop and grow toward the center, may invade the macula, or may be long enough to reach the disk again, causing a white reflex in the pupillary area.

Larval endophthalmitis: This is the most extensive involvement of the retina and vitreous in toxocariasis. It may be considered an advanced, nonattended form of the above two stages, with a white reflex in the pupillary area. It may terminate in complicated cataracts or secondary glaucoma, ending in blindness.

Retinal Tumors in Children

The retina, being an extension of brain, logically should be home to all brain tumors; fortunately, it is not so, barring astrocytoma of the retina. The most common tumor of the retina is retinoblastoma. The retinal tumors can be benign or malignant; the retina, in spite of its rich blood supply, is an infrequent site of malignant deposits but is not immune to them. The common malignancies that can invade the retina are leukemias and central nervous system lymphomas. The retina can be invaded by growth from the choroid and optic nerve, both of which do not happen in children. The common congenital growths of the retina are mostly vascular; they are hemangiomas—capillary, cavernous, and racemose (Wyburn-Mason); they may be aneurysm and arteriovenous anastomosis. The benign tumors of the retina are generally on the periphery, more common on the temporal side, stationary, or slow progressing. They could be hamartomas or nonhamartomas.

Astrocytoma of the Retina

Basically, they arise from glial tissues. Hamartomas in nature may be isolated or associated with phacomatosis; the most common association is with tuberous sclerosis. Other conditions that may be associated with astrocytomas of the retina are type 1 neurofibromatosis and, surprisingly, retinitis pigmentosa and its variations. The astrocytomas are asymptomatic; they are generally found on routine examination of the fundus in persons with tuberous sclerosis and other phacomatosis.

SUGGESTED READING

1. Abdi F, Aghajani A, Hemmati S, Moosavi D, Gordiz A, Bayatiani ES, et al. Pediatric rhegmatogenous retinal detachment: a meta-analysis of clinical features, surgical success rate, and prognostic factors. Ind J Ophthalmol. 2023;71(3):717-28.
2. Aurora A. Rhegmatogenous retinal detachment and its management. In: Ramamurthy D, Biswas P (Eds). AIOS Ready Reckoner in Ophthalmology, 2nd edition. New Delhi: Jaypee Brothers Medical (P) Pvt. Ltd.; 2017.
3. Bloom MA, Garcia CA. Manual of Retinal and Choroidal Dystrophies. Connecticut: Appleton and Lange; 1981.
4. Elder SD. Layers of the retina in the System of Ophthalmology. London: Henry Kimpton; 1961. pp. 230-1.
5. Galloway NR, Amoaku WMK, Galloway PH, Browing AC. Retinal detachment. In: Galloway NR, Amoaku WMK, Galloway PH, Browing AC (Eds). Common Eye Disease and Management, 5th edition. Switzerland: Springer; 2022. pp. 117-24.
6. Haller J. Coats' disease. In: Rayns SJ (Ed). Retina, 2nd edition. St. Louis: Mosby; 1994. pp. 1443-60.
7. Jay B, Carrot W Albinism. Recent advances. Trans Ophthalmol Soc. 1980;100(4):467-71.

8. Mukherjee PK. Disorder of the retina and vitreous. In: Mukherjee PK (Ed). Children in Pediatric Ophthalmology, 1st edition. Delhi: New Age International; 2005. pp. 393-466.
9. Mukherjee PK. Examination of retina and macula. In: Mukherjee PK (Ed). Clinical Examination in Ophthalmology, 2nd edition. New Delhi: Elsevier; 2016.
10. Natarajan S, Bankeer AS, Nakhwa C. Photodynamic therapy. In: Ramamurthy D, Biswas P (Eds). AIOS Ready Reckoner in Ophthalmology, 2nd edition. New Delhi: Jaypee Brothers Medical (P) Pvt. Ltd.; 2017. pp. 406-9.
11. Nirmalan PK, Krishnaiah S, Nutheti R, Shamanna BR, Rao GN, Thomas R. Consanguinity and eye diseases with a potential genetic etiology. Data from a prevalence study in Andhra Pradesh, India. Ophthalmic Epidemiol. 2006;13(1):7-13.
12. Pandey N. A Descriptive Study of Inherited Retina Dystrophies in a Tertiary Eye Center in Central India.
13. Parameswarappa DC, Jalali S, Khanna RC, Marmamula S, Natarajan R, Mettla AL, et al. Visual impairment and blindness due to retinitis pigmentosa in India: 15-year follow-up of the Andhra Pradesh eye disease study cohort. Ind J Ophthalmol. 2023;71(3):902-8.
14. Parmeggiani F, Sato G, De Nadai K, Romano MR, Binotto A, Costagliola C. Clinical and rehabilitative management of retinitis pigmentosa: Up-to-date. Mol Med Rep. 2011; 12(4):250-9.
15. Reese AB. Telangiectasis of the retina and Coats' disease. Am J Ophthalmol. 1956;42(1):1-8.
16. Seal SK. Blood-retinal barrier. In: Seal SK (Ed). GN Seal's Textbook of Ophthalmology, 5th edition. Kolkata: Current Books International; 2002. p. 293.
17. Sen A, Karkhur S. Vitreous hemorrhage. In: Ramamurthy D, Biswas P (Eds). AIOS Ready Reckoner in Ophthalmology, 2nd edition. New Delhi: Jaypee Brothers Medical (P) Pvt. Ltd.; 2017.
18. Singh I, Visual Pathway in the Textbook of Human Neuroanatomy. 6th ed. New Delhi: Jaypee Brothers Medical (P) Pvt. Ltd.; 2002. pp. 229-31.
19. Vinekar A. Pediatric retinal imaging. In: Ramamurthy D, Biswas P (Eds). AIOS Ready Reckoner in Ophthalmology, 2nd edition. New Delhi: Jaypee Brothers Medical (P) Pvt. Ltd.; 2017. pp. 406-9.
20. Wu L. Coats' disease. In: Fraunfelder FH, Roy HF (Eds). Current Ocular Therapy, 5th edition. Philadelphia: WB Saunders Company; 2000. pp. 607-8.

CHAPTER 21

Disorders of the Optic Nerve in Children

The visual path extends from the retina to the visual cortex, commonly referred to as the retinocalcarine path. It is arbitrarily divided into the retinopapillary complex, optic nerve, chiasma, optic path, lateral geniculate body, and optic radiation. The visual path up to the beginning of chiasma carries ipsilateral visual impulses; thereafter, it carries impulses from both eyes. The lesions in each section have a definite clinical presentation. Out of them, the optic nerve has more clinical features.

APPLIED ANATOMY OF THE OPTIC NERVE

The optic nerve, which is the second cranial nerve, is in fact not a true nerve; it lacks a nucleus and fascicular part. It is a tract of white matter in the brain. It joins ganglion cells of the retina to the brain; it does not have regenerative power; hence, once it is severed, it results in permanent loss of vision. The fibers of the optic nerve can either be afferent or efferent; the former carry visual fibers, while the latter carry pupillary fibers. The optic nerve extends from the optic nerve head to the anterior part of the chiasma in the brain. The length of the optic nerve varies between 3.5 and 5.5 cm, being smaller in children. Topographically, it has been divided into the following parts:

- Intraocular 0.7 mm—the smallest part
- Intraorbital 3.0 cm—the longest part
- Intracanalicular—6.0 mm to 1.00 cm
- Intracranial—1.0 cm

- The smallest intraocular part that is visible on the ophthalmoscope is called the head of the nerve or papilla. The optic nerve is roughly circular, with an average diameter of 1.00 mm in adults and smaller in children. It is nonmyelinated, and its pink color is due to many fine capillaries on the surface. In the absence of a sufficient number of capillaries, the disk loses its pink color, which is replaced by pallor, and the disk of a newborn is paler than that of an adult. A saucer-shaped, eccentrically tilted depression in the middle of the optic nerve head is called the cup of the disk, the floor of which is formed by lamina cribrosa. From the center of the disk, passes the central retinal vessels. The intraocular part itself is divided into two parts, i.e., (1) prelamellar and (2) retrolamellar, with separate sets of blood vessels. The retina stops short at the lateral side of the disk, leaving the choroid to reach up to the border of the disk, forming a choroidal crescent of no clinical significance. The intraocular part passes backward through the scleral canal, which is bridged by the lamina cribrosa.
- The intraorbital traverses in the muscle cone formed by the recti; the nerve in this part is surrounded by orbital fat. The intraorbital part extends from the back of the globe to the beginning of the optic canal. It is covered by the dura, arachnoid, and pia, which are continuous with the meninges of the brain. The dura is outermost, followed by the arachnoid and pia. The former is loosely attached to the optic nerve; the dura is continuous, and with the intracranial dura passing through the optic canal in the orbit, it divides into two parts, namely (1) the outer and (2) the inner. The former becomes the periorbita, and the latter merges with the outer surface of the sclera **(Fig. 21.1)**.

In between the dura and arachnoid is a potential space called subdural space. The space between the arachnoid and pia is called subarachnoid space that ends blindly at the back of the sclera. The space in between is filled with cerebrospinal fluid (CSF). The central retinal vessels pass through the subarachnoid space, entering the space from below. The artery enters

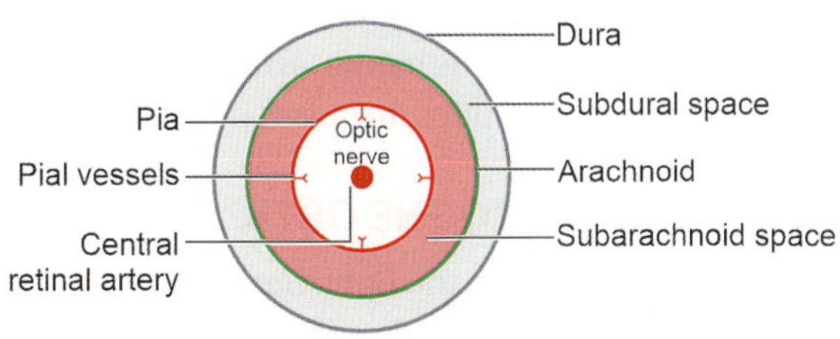

Fig. 21.1: Covering of optic nerve.

the nerve at a right angle, but the vein takes an oblique course, making it vulnerable to raised intracranial tension that impedes the venous flow, resulting in swelling of the disk.

At the apex of the orbit, the nerve is encircled by an annulus of zinc, from which the recti originate. The superior and medial recti at their origin are closely attached to the dural sheath of the optic nerve. Stretching of this attachment causes pain in the lateral and upward movement of the eye in inflammation of the nerve.

Some of the important structures that come in relation to the optic nerve in this course are—lower division of the oculomotor nerve, abducens nerve, nasociliary nerve, sympathetic fibers, and ciliary ganglion, which lie lateral to the nerve in the middle of the cone. The nerve is surrounded by long and short ciliary nerves and posterior ciliary arteries at the back of the sclera. The ophthalmic artery crosses the nerve at the most posterior part.

- The intracanalicular part is most vulnerable to trauma as it is fixed to the bony canal. It is 1.00 cm in length. The nerve in the canal is accompanied by its meninges, ophthalmic artery, and sympathetic fibers.

  The ophthalmic artery is in close proximity with the nerve in various parts of its course. The artery passes under the nerve in the dural sheath; the other structures that come in relation to the nerve are sphenoidal and part of the ethmoidal sinus on the medial side. The wall separating the nerve from the sinuses is paper thin, making the nerve vulnerable to infection from the sinuses.
- The intracranial part of the nerve is about 1.00 cm in length. It is a flattened band that appears as a triangle, with its apex laterally, and lies in the middle cranial fossa. The course of the nerve begins at the posterior end of the optic canal and ends at the anterolateral end of the chiasma. The dura and arachnoid stop at the back of the optic canal, leaving it covered only by pia.

  The nerve initially lies on the diaphragma sellae and then on the anterior cavernous sinus. The internal carotid lies first below the nerve and then takes a lateral position. The ophthalmic artery originates from the internal carotid under the nerve in its middle part.

BLOOD SUPPLY TO THE OPTIC NERVE

The main blood supply to the optic nerve is derived from two sources, i.e., (1) internal carotid and its branches and (2) anterior cerebral artery. The blood supply of the optic nerve varies according to its topographical division, i.e., optic nerve head, intraorbital, intracanalicular, and intracranial. Out of all these, blood supply to the optic nerve head is most important, as it is directly related to many pathological conditions such as glaucoma, papilledema, and ischemic optic neuropathy. The last is not encountered in children. The blood supply of the optic nerve head can be divided into two groups, i.e., (1) retinal and (2) ciliary. The surface of the optic nerve gets its blood supply from the branches of the central retinal artery; the rest of the blood supply to the optic nerve is via short posterior ciliary arteries. However, the retrolamellar area has a dual supply both from retinal and ciliary circulation **(Fig. 21.2)**.

Note:
- The central retinal artery has a short, almost vertical passage in the subdural space. The central retinal vein has a long oblique passage in the subdural space, making it venerable to raising CSF pressure.
- Unlike subdural and subarachnoid space, there is no subpial space around the optic nerve; pia is firmly attached to the optic nerve substance, sending fine capillaries to the nerve.

DEVELOPMENT OF THE OPTIC NERVE

The optic nerve is a conduit between the brain and the retina, which itself is out of pouching of the brain. The optic stalk that joins the forebrain to the optic vesicle is the forerunner of the optic nerve. Incidentally, the embryonic fissure that develops at the lower part of the optic cup also extends into the optic stalk, from the optic cup to the forebrain. The optic stalk grows between the cup and the brain, with a groove underneath. By the end of 6 weeks, axons from the developing retina get into the optic stalk; this is the time when the hyaloid artery also enters the optic nerve, with axons engulfing the hyaloid artery.

By the 3rd month of development, small capillaries develop in the substance; they are the precursors of future pial vessels. The coverings of the optic nerve become obvious by the 7th month. As the axons of the ganglion cells find their way into the optic nerve, some retinal cells get separated from the main body in a small clump of glial tissue to form the optic nerve head.

The optic nerve gets myelinated late in its development; the myelination starts in the lateral geniculate body and spreads toward the sclera. The myelination

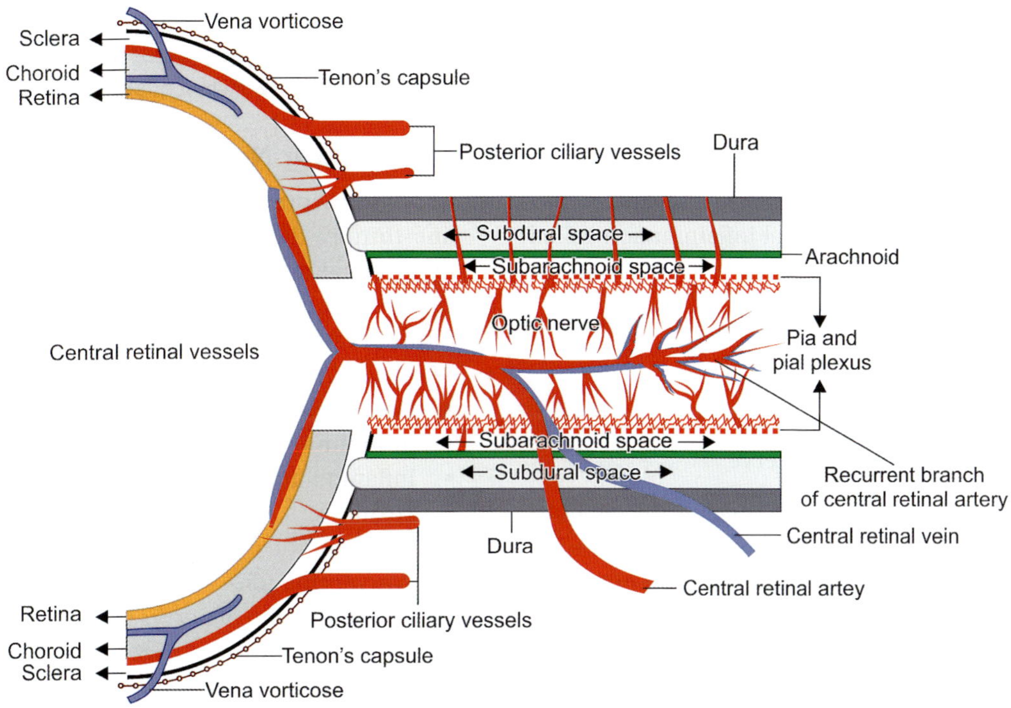

Fig. 21.2: Blood supply of the optic nerve.

is complete and stops short of the lamina. The lamina cribrosa partly develops from the choroid and partly from the sclera.

CONGENITAL ANOMALIES OF OPTIC NERVE

It has been discussed in detail in Chapter 3.

DISORDERS OF THE OPTIC NERVE IN CHILDREN

Disorders of the optic nerve in children are frequent; they are more common than thought to be because some of them may be asymptomatic, especially when uniocular, or they are so subtle that they may go unnoticed. On the other hand, they may be so serious as to cause gross loss of vision alone or be associated with systemic symptoms mostly concerning the central nervous system.

The disorders of the optic nerve are broadly divided into two groups, i.e., (1) congenital and (2) acquired. The latter being more common than the former.

The acquired conditions are given as follows:

- Inflammatory
- Infectious
- Traumatic
- Degenerative
- Dystrophic
- New growths
- Associated with vascular anomalies

Note: Papilledema and optic atrophies are not primary disorders of the optic nerve head; the former is the aftermath of raised intracranial pressure, and the latter is the end result of all infection, inflammation, and degeneration of the nerve.

The common symptoms that bring a child for examination are given as follows:

- Diminished distant vision
- Changes in the field of vision
- Subnormal color vision
- Diminished contrast vision
- Squint
- Amblyopia
- Nystagmus
- Proptosis

The features may be unilateral or bilateral simultaneously; one eye may be affected more than the other, asymmetric or symmetric, stationary or progressive, blinding or nonblinding or they may be confined to the disk only.

OPTIC NEURITIS IN CHILDREN

The term optic neuritis encompasses inflammation/infections of the optic nerve, from disk to chiasma; it may be added to a combination of retinal inflammation called neuroretinitis.

As per the topography of the condition, it can be given as follows:

- Neuroretinitis
- Papillitis—inflammation of the disk
- Neuritis—inflammation of the nerve

Note: Papillitis and neuritis are rarely isolated; the papillitis may spillover the nerve or the other way round.

The other classifications of optic neuritis are axial, paraxial, and transverse.

The nerve may be affected either transversely or longitudinally; the latter can be peripheral or central. The central type involves the macula-papillary fibers, which mostly cause early visual symptoms, including a central or centrocecal scotoma, while the involvement of peripheral fibers causes nerve fiber defects **(Figs. 21.3 and 21.4)**.

There is no clear-cut division between central and peripheral involvement. In severe or long-standing cases, both may merge to cause transverse neuritis. The optic neuritis may occasionally be in patches. The optic nerve inflammation may be localized to the nerve or may be associated with involvement of the central nervous system or spinal cord (myelitis). It can be uniocular or bilateral. The involvement of the other eye is independent of the first; it may or may not be simultaneous, and asymmetry is the rule.

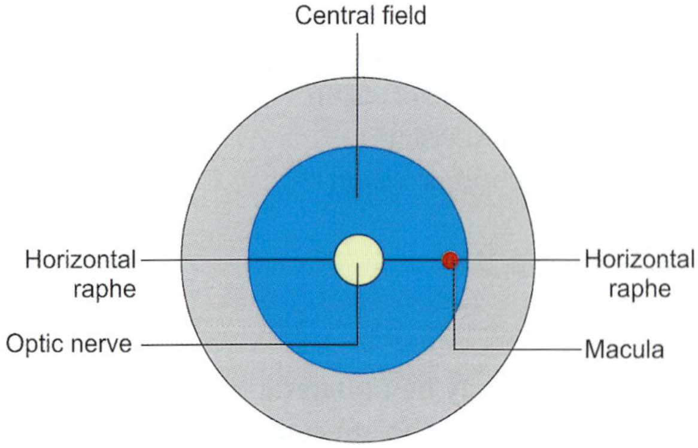

Fig. 21.3: Normal fundus without scotoma.

The triad of symptoms of optic neuritis in all ages is diminished vision, dyschromatopsia, and central field defect; to them, it may be added to the relative afferent pupil.

Causes of Optic Neuritis

- *Idiopathic*—previously, no cause could be found in one-third of the cases. With the availability of better neuroimaging and serological tests, more and more cases can now be assigned to some of the definite forms of causes.
- *The causes are given as follows:*
  - Degeneration
  - Autoimmune disease
  - Inflammation
  - Toxin
  - Genetic
  - Postvaccination
  - Direct invasion of nerves (rare)

Inflammation of the structures that come in close proximity to the nerve, i.e., sphenoidal sinus, ethmoidal sinus, rarely orbital abscess, and panophthalmitis. The infection may travel from the intraocular structure, either by blood vessels or retinal nerve fiber. The latter causing neuroretinitis and the other causing choroiditis near the disk or between the macula and disk, endophthalmitis, and sympathetic ophthalmia, too, may involve the optic nerve.

The orbital causes, besides lid abscess, that cause optic neuritis are posterior orbital cellulitis, orbital apex inflammation, thrombophlebitis, infective granulomas, i.e., tuberculoma, and pseudo-orbital tumors. The noninfective cause is Wegener's granulomatosis, which is a polyangiitis of autoimmune origin. It is a multi-systemic disorder that, if not treated, may last for life with relentless spread. The condition is medically treatable with immunosuppressive drugs. The condition is rare in children.

Systemic Causes

- Infective
- Demyelination
- Toxin
- Hereditary

- *Infective:* The systemic infective causes are tuberculosis; various types of bacterial pneumonia; and viral diseases such as mumps, measles, influenza, and poliomyelitis.

The intracranial infections causing optic neuritis are meningitis, encephalitis, and meningoencephalitis.

- *Demyelination*: In developed countries, demyelination surpasses infection and inflammation as causes of optic neuritis. Multiple sclerosis leads the list of demyelinating disorders; most of them are not seen in children. Other causes are Devic's neuromyelitis optica* and Schilder's disease†.
- *Toxin:* The toxin causing optic neuritis may be considered to be iatrogenic because the chemicals involved are mostly drugs, many of which are antibiotics. Fortunately, they cause optic neuritis only after prolonged use, and their effects are mostly reversible. The list of antibiotics is headed by antitubercular drugs of the first generation; the most often blamed drug is ethambutol, followed by isonex and streptomycin.
- *Hereditary:* Out of many types of hereditary optic neuritis, Leber's optic neuropathy stands out prominently as an inherited optic neuritis seen only in boys. The mothers are the carriers. It starts as a fast deterioration of vision in teens but may inflict it on younger children (see above).

**Devic's neuromyelitis optica (Devic disease)*: Devic's neuromyelitis optica is a disorder of two different parts of the nervous system, i.e., the optic nerve and the spinal cord. It is a disease more prevalent in children and younger adults of both sexes in adults in the third decade and above. The exact cause of the malady is not clear; demyelination is the most commonly blamed factor. It does not follow the traits of multiple sclerosis, which is more common in adults. The other factor that requires explanation is the anatomical distance between two independent lesions sharing a common pathology in the optic nerve and spinal cord. Involvement of the brain is also possible; generally, other cranial nerves are spared.

The following are the modes of presentation of Devic disease:

- Optic neuritis followed by transverse myelitis
- Myelitis preceding optic neuritis
- Simultaneous involvement of the optic nerve and spinal cord.
- Recurrence

Clinically, it has been divided into two types given as follows:

1. Monophasic
2. Relapsing

In the former, the recurrence between two attacks happens over days or weeks, while in the latter, there may be a long gap that may be as long as months or years.

Neuritis may start unilaterally, with the other eye getting involved soon. A child with unilaterally diminished vision may not be aware of it unless the other eye is involved or develops weakness of the lower limbs.

The clinical features of myelitis are variable; they may be weakness in the arms and legs, numbness or frank paralysis, and loss of bladder and bowel control. Children with brain involvement may have stiff necks, headaches, nausea, vomiting, confusion, seizures, or even a coma.

There is no specific investigation to confirm neuromyelitis optica. MRI is not as efficient as in multiple sclerosis, where there is no prophylaxis or definite therapy for neuromyelitis. Steroids are usually given to minimize disability, delay recurrence, and retain vision. Immunosuppressants such as azathioprine and mycophenolate, too, have been used alone or in combination with steroids without uniformly good results.

†*Schilder's disease:* Schilder's disease is a rare condition that starts in childhood, mostly in boys aged between 7 and 12 years. The condition is supposed to be a variant of multiple sclerosis‡ that involves the white matter of the brain. It is an infrequent cause of bilateral optic neuritis. It is a blinding disease of childhood; there are many similarities between it and not only multiple sclerosis but also neuromyelitis optica as well. Basically, it is a demyelinating disease due to leukodystrophy. It is associated with severe neurological deficiency besides profound optic neuritis that ends in postneuritic optic atrophy. Involvement of other cranial nerves is common; there may be cortical blindness§ and nystagmus.

‡*Multiple sclerosis:* Multiple sclerosis is a widely spread neurological disorder due to demyelination. It is an autoimmune disorder. It is the most common cause of optic neuritis in adults, but the involvement of children is less frequent. One-third of cases of multiple sclerosis have optic neuritis; all cases of acute optic neuritis that are considered to be idiopathic ultimately end up in multiple sclerosis; especially in girls, the clinical features wax and wane last for two to three decades; fifteen percent of multiple sclerosis cases present with optic neuritis initially; hence, all cases of optic neuritis should be suspected to be harbinger of multiple sclerosis. Besides the optic nerve, the spinal cord is the next common structure to be involved, and cranial nerves other than the optic nerve are involved less commonly. There may be internuclear involvement; pupillary defects are frequent. Symptoms of optic neuritis in multiple sclerosis share the same clinical features as those in nonmultiple sclerosis. The diagnosis is confirmed by an MRI. Recently, monoclonal antibodies have been recommended as the first line of treatment for multiple sclerosis; otherwise, steroids and immunosuppressants are used to minimize the extent of the disease.

§*Cortical blindness:* Cortical blindness is a severe loss of vision without any detectable cause in the fundus with a normal pupillary reflex caused by bilateral lesions in the visual cortex. It is part of cerebral blindness due to damage to the visual pathways beyond the lateral geniculate body.

The patient generally denies loss of vision; the condition is also known as Anton syndrome.

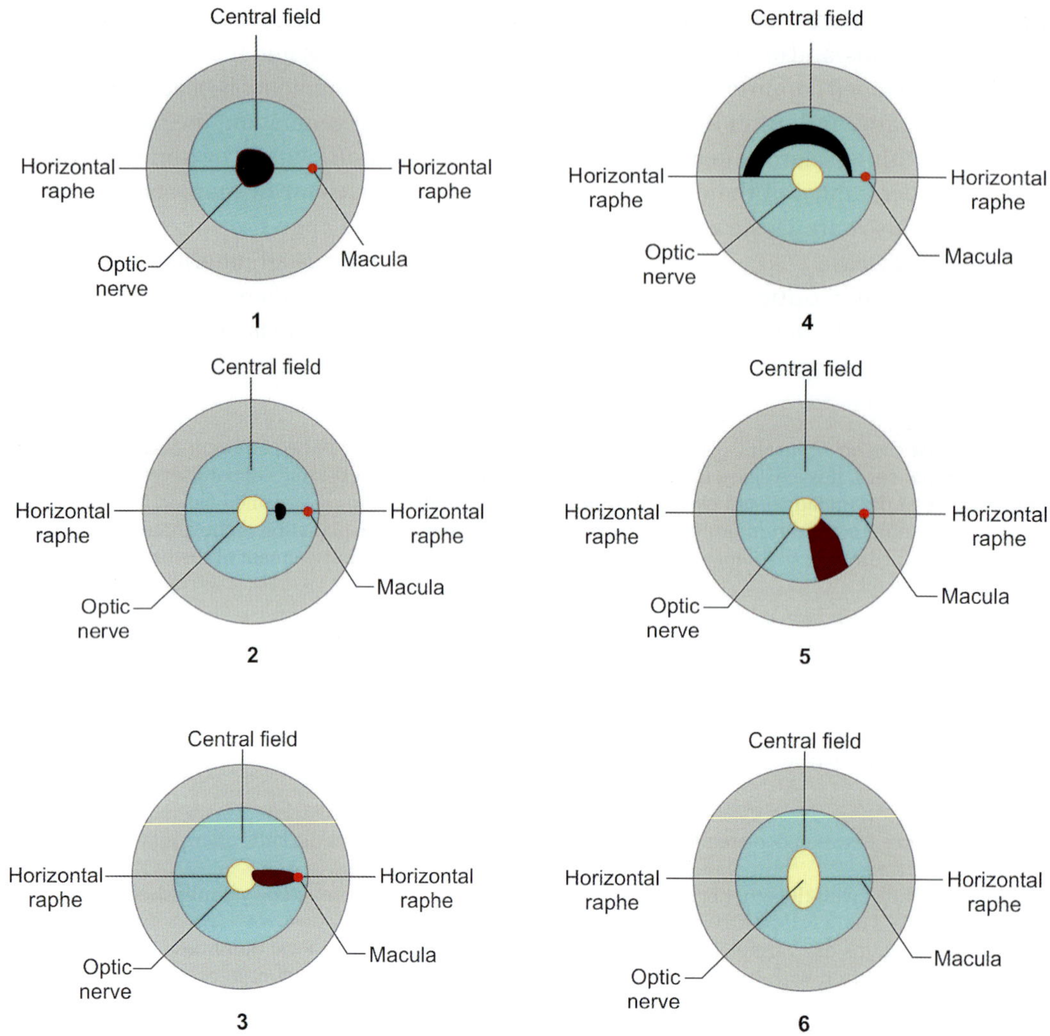

Fig. 21.4: Scotomas of various lesions of the optic nerve: (1) Central scotoma, (2) paracentral scotoma, (3) centrocecal scotoma, (4) arcuate scotoma, (5) sectorial scotoma, and (6) enlargement of blind spots.

General Features of Optic Neuritis

Generally, the condition in children starts as unilateral and acute and then involves the other eye. Optic neuritis in children is more often bilateral, especially under 10 year old; about 70% of optic neuritis in children aged under 10 years have bilateral involvement. There is a reversal in the second decade, where 70% of children have unilateral involvement. Bilaterality follows a definite pattern as per the duration and has been classified given as follows:

- Simultaneous—involvement of the other eye within 2 weeks of the first eye
- Sequential—involvement of the other eye between 2 and 12 weeks
- Recurrent—involvement of the other eye after 12 weeks

Pathogenesis of Optic Neuritis

The pathogenesis is not well elucidated. The most commonly blamed factor is multiple sclerosis, which causes demyelination of the optic nerve with plaques of perivascular cuffing, edema of the nerve sheaths, and breakdown of myelin sheaths.

Symptoms of Optic Neuritis

- Diminished central vision
- Central field defect
- Reduced color sense (red desaturation)
- Poor contrast
- Defective stereopsis

- Neurological deficit (myelitis)
- Pain in movement of the eye

> Unilateral fast disappearing vision in a noncongested eye is a case of acute optic neuritis, or macular in origin, in children.

Diminished Central Vision

The fall of vision is fast; it may fall to 20/200 or even just perception of light within hours to days and may be with pain or without pain on movement of the globe. The child may not be aware of diminished vision in a unilateral case without pain. The vision once reaches the lowest point and remains so for about 2–3 weeks and then starts recovering, even without treatment. The improvement is slower than the decline and may not reach the original level. The third possibility is nonimprovement of vision; this is extremely rare in those under 20 years but more common in adults, which requires neurological evaluation, including neuro-imaging. The diminished vision is generally followed by central scotoma and dyschromatopsia; in a few cases, relative central and centrocecal scotoma may precede the fall of central vision.

Another visual phenomenon with vision loss in optic neuritis is called Uhthoff's phenomenon that causes acceleration of neurological signs and symptoms in demyelinating diseases, especially in multiple sclerosis, when body temperature is raised either by external application of heat to the body such as taking a hot bath or during exercise.

Central Field Defect

Though central and centrocecal field changes are the most common field changes in acute optic neuritis, many other forms of field changes are also encountered. The field changes are more marked for color other than white; the most affected is red. The type of scotoma depends on the position of the retinal nerve fibers involved. **Figures 21.5, 21.6, and 21.7** show the distribution of retinal fibers.

> The field defects do not become evident unless one-fourth of the ganglion cells are lost. The improvement in the field takes longer time than improvement of vision that may take months to years.

Pupillary Changes in Optic Neuritis

Pupillary changes in optic neuritis hold the key to the diagnosis of conduction defects. In unilateral optic neuritis, the most common pupillary change is a relative afferent pupillary defect (RAPD), also known as dynamic anisocoria.

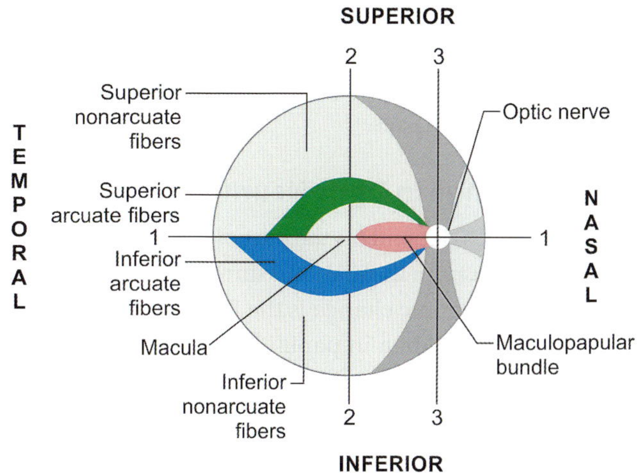

Fig. 21.5: Distribution of retinal fibers in relation to the optic nerve: (1) Horizontal raphe, (2) imaginary line passing through the macula, and (3) imaginary line passing through the optic nerve.

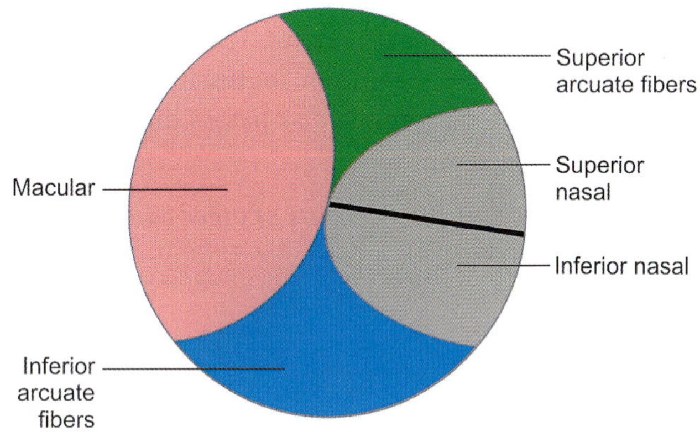

Fig. 21.6: Distribution of retinal fibers at the back of the globe.

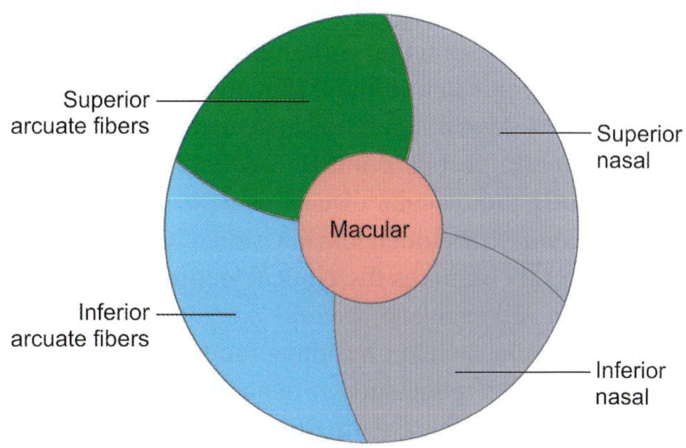

Fig. 21.7: Distribution of retinal fibers at the beginning of chiasma.

In bilateral cases, RAPD does not happen unless there is too much difference between the two eyes. RAPD may be absent if the other eye has preexisting disease, even with equal vision in both eyes.

Fundus Change in Optic Neuritis

Fundus changes depend on the part of the nerve involved and its distance from the disk and surrounding retina. The first ophthalmoscopic change is the filling of the cup; this is rapid and faster than in papilledema. The color of the disk changes from the usual pink to hyperemia, and there may be an increase in the number of capillaries of the disk. The second sign is blurring of the disk margin with edema spreading to the peripapillary retina; the blurring does not have any rule of thumb. In fulminating cases, there may be a few splinter hemorrhages and soft exudates on the disk. This is followed by visible swelling of the disk, which at its maximum is not >+3 D. As the condition passes into the stage of recovery, the edema recedes at a slower speed when compared to its development. The lamina remains obscured even with maximum regression. Sheathing is absent. In the long run, the disk passes into a stage of postneuritis optic atrophy.

The differential diagnosis consists of other causes of disk swelling, which consist of:

- Pseudoneuritis
- Early papilledema
- Hypoplasia of the disk
- Drusen of disk
- Glial tissue on the disk

COMPARISON BETWEEN OPTIC NEURITIS, PAPILLEDEMA, AND PSEUDONEURITIS

Many times, it is difficult to differentiate between early papilledema, optic neuritis, and pseudoneuritis.

Table 21.1 gives differences between the three.

The other important point is to differentiate between optic neuritis and macular disease of acute onset, as both are associated with sudden loss of vision.

Table 21.2 compares the clinical features of an optic nerve lesion and a macular lesion.

Occasionally, a child on routine fundus examinations is found to have a uniocularly swollen disk (it is better not to call uniocular disk swelling papilledema). The child may be asymptomatic. The causes could be ocular or intracranial.

The ocular causes of uniocular disk swelling are given as follows:

- Congenital: Pseudoneuritis, hypoplasia of the disk
- Acquired:
  - Intraocular: Papillitis, neuroretinitis, severe intraocular inflammation, and drusen
  - Intraorbital: Optic nerve glioma, orbital pseudotumor, orbital cellulitis, intraorbital foreign body, and intraorbital parasitic cyst
  - Ocular hypotony
  - Intracranial: Foster Kennedy syndrome, cavernous sinus thrombosis, contralateral eye with unilateral high myopia, and subarachnoid hemorrhage

DIFFERENTIAL DIAGNOSIS OF OPTIC NEURITIS

The disk conditions that require differentiation are given as follows:

- Early papilledema, pseudoneuritis, drusen of the optic nerve, and hypoplasia of the disk
- The condition that produces central or centrocecal scotomas
- Condition that produces dyschromatopsia

DIAGNOSIS OF OPTIC NEURITIS IN CHILDREN

Diagnosis of optic neuritis is not always straightforward; it requires proper history taking and a complete ocular examination that should include:

- *Vision*: Visual acuity, vision with pinhole, refraction under cycloplegia, color vision, contrast and brightness, and central field examination

> Even after improvement of vision to near normal, the color defect and reduced contrast sensitivity may longer for years.

- *Examination of pupil:*
  - Anisocoria: The eye with neuritis generally has a larger pupil.
  - Light reflexes are both direct and indirect. The eye with neuritis has a sluggish pupillary reaction that may dilate further in the presence of light. RAPD is strongly suggestive of neuritis.
- *Examination of fundus:* Examination of fundus by direct ophthalmoscope generally suffices. Disk is hyperemic, lamina is not visible, cup is obliterated, and margins are blurred. The blurring does not follow any rule of thumb; it may spillover the surrounding retina.

TABLE 21.1: Comparison between optic neuritis, papilledema, and pseudoneuritis.

Signs and symptoms	*Optic neuritis (Papillitis)*	*Papilledema*	*Pseudoneuritis*
Age	Any, rare after 50 years	Any rare before the sutures close	Any
Sex	Both	Both	Both
Onset	Acute	Slow	Present from birth
Bilaterality	Generally unilateral	Bilateral	Bilateral, rarely unilateral
Vision	Rapid fall of vision	Good, the fall of vision is late	Normal, may have an error of refraction
Causes of visual loss	Early conduction defect	Involvement of the macula and late conduction defect	Nil
Other visual defects	Defective color sense, stereopsis, and contrast	Transient loss of vision	Nil
Field change	Central or centrocecal, may have a nerve fiber defect	Enlargement of the blind spot was initially normal. Peripheral constriction late	Nil
Pupil	May show an afferent defect	Pupillary reaction is absent if the 3rd nerve is involved or optic atrophy has set in	Nil
Other neurological associations	Generally none	Signs of raised intracranial tension	Nil
Fundus	The variable degree of disk swelling is not >3 D. May be normal initially: blurring of the disk margin, a few flame-shaped hemorrhages, macular star absence, and vitreous haze over the disk	Swollen disks are >3 D. Absence of venous pulsation, edema of the macula, macular star, and may have flame-shaped hemorrhages	Small hyperemic disk, not >3 D. No hemorrhage and no exudate
Fluorescein angiography	Nonspecific, minimal leakage of dye	Vertical pool of dye due to leakage	Normal
CT	No specific change	May show an intracranial lesion	No change
MRI	Shows plaque in the perivascular area, demyelination	Intracranial lesion	Normal

TABLE 21.2: Clinical features of an optic nerve lesion and a macular lesion.

		Lesion	
Macular			***Optic nerve***
1.	Vision	Greatly reduced	Reduced and variable
2.	Metamorphopsia	Is the rule	Negative
3.	Color vision defect	Slight	Gross
4.	Brightness	Not change	Dulled
5.	Photo stress test	Positive	Nil
6.	Pupil	No change	Relative afferent pupillary defect (RAPD)
7.	Amsler grid test	Positive	Negative
8.	Field changes	Central variable	Relative/positive central and centrocecal, rarely nerve fibers defect both types more for the red color

There is no venous congestion. The disk is swollen but not >+3 D; eyes with high myopia and glaucoma may not show swelling of the disk. In severe cases, there may be a few hemorrhages and soft exudates. The rest of the retina, including the macula, is not involved in optic neuritis.

- *Field changes:* Initially, they are relative and soon getting converted to absolute. They are central and centrocecal; rarely causing nerve fiber defects. The field changes are more marked for color (red). The peripheral fields are not affected.
- *Imaging in optic neuritis:*
  - X-ray examination of the skull was the only imaging mode available a few decades ago; it has been replaced by better imaging systems such as MRI and CT. Ultrasonography (USG) has no role in diagnosis.
  - Magnetic resonance imaging: MRI is better than CT in predicting prognosis in optic neuritis due to its ability to pickup demyelination, for which gadolinium-enhanced, fat-suppressed T1- and T2-weighted images are best.

Optical Coherence Tomography

Optical coherence tomography (OCT) was originally developed to find lesions in the retina, especially the macula. Later, due to its utility in the detection of glaucomatous optic nerve changes and changes in retinal fiber layers, it became a routine investigation in glaucoma detection and management. Presently, it is widely used to study the optic nerve head, especially in neuritis; it allows visualization and measurement of the optic nerve head topography and retinal nerve fiber layer thickness.

Visual Evoked Potential

Visual evoked potentials show increased latency with minimal expected amplitude in demyelination of the nerve; it does not show any specific change.

Laboratory Investigation

Batteries for laboratory tests are generally still ordered, though many of them have become obsolete. More reliable tests are antinuclear antibodies, antineutrophil cytoplasmic antibodies, and rheumatoid factors.

MANAGEMENT OF OPTIC NEURITIS

- Treatment of optic neuritis in children does not differ from adult neuritis.
- Many of the cases recover without treatment.
- There is no definitive treatment for its cure.
- The treatment is directed toward ameliorating the symptoms and shortening their duration, minimizing demyelination, and reducing the chances of recurrence.
- Antibiotics have no role in autoimmune and demyelinating diseases; hence, they should be avoided unless a clear-cut infection is present.
- As demyelination is the most common attributable cause, presently the treatment is directed to minimize its effect.
- Treatment is specially indicated for bilateral childhood neuritis and neuritis with recurrence.
- Visual recovery is good in postviral neuritis.
- Steroid responders rarely pass onto multiple sclerosis.

Commonly used therapeutic agents are steroids and immunosuppressive agents. The other drugs used are immunoglobulins and immunomodulators.

Steroids are the only drugs that have been found to be effective; they do not cure optic neuritis, and they only hasten recovery to baseline and reduce the chances of recurrence. It is better to start steroids early in children, especially if there is bilateral involvement. Steroids are better administered under the supervision of a pediatrician, with usual precaution. The most common regimen is intravenous (IV) methylprednisolone for 3 days, followed either by oral methylprednisolone or prednisolone orally tapering, as per the practice of the institute; different schools have different regimens of administration and tapering.

Ancillary Treatment

Children under the age of 10 years who belong to the amblyogenic age group are prone to passing into a state of lifelong amblyopia; hence, all efforts should be taken to minimize it.

SOME SPECIFIC OPTIC NEURITIS IN CHILDREN

The specific types of optic neuritis are given as follows:

- *Infection:* Mostly viral, followed by bacteria
- *Postvaccination:* The vaccinations that cause optic neuritis are Bacillus Calmette-Guérin (BCG), measles, mumps, and rubella (MMR), hepatitis B, rabies, tetanus, and meningitis.
- Neuroretinitis

- Retrobulbar neuritis
- Drug-induced neuritis
- *Demyelination disease:*
    - Multiple sclerosis
    - Devic's neuromyelitis optica
    - Schilder's disease
    - Acute disseminated encephalomyelitis
    - Krabbe disease

Postinfection Neuritis

Both bacterial and viral infections may cause optic neuritis either during the actual infection or following the infection. It may take weeks to months after the actual infection to develop neuritis.

The viruses that cause postinfection optic neuritis are measles, mumps, herpes simplex, and herpes zoster. The herpes zoster ophthalmicus causes both anterior and retrobulbar neuritis simultaneously during or following infection. Bacteria commonly blamed are tuberculosis, syphilis, Lyme disease*, and leptospirosis.

Postvaccination Optic Neuritis

They are more common following immunization against virus infections; the vaccines are MMR, influenza, hepatitis B, and rabies.

The bacterial vaccines that cause optic neuritis are BCG, antitetanus, and antimeningitis. All the vaccines can cause either anterior or retrobulbar optic neuritis, generally a few days to weeks after vaccination. The parents may not have mentioned vaccination in the recent past that has to be found out by specific questions. The clinical presentation of postinfection and postvaccination is similar; both are generally self-limiting and, otherwise, managed as usual with optic neuritis.

Neuroretinitis

Neuroretinitis is relatively rare with variable presentation; hence, it has been called a great mimic. It is an acute, unilateral disorder with disproportionate painless loss of vision. It starts with retinitis spreading to the disk. The infections can either be viral or spirochetal. The viral infections that cause neuroretinitis are herpes simplex, hepatitis B, and acute retinal necrosis syndrome of viral origin. The other causes are syphilis, Lyme disease, and leptospirosis†. The clinical picture consists of painless unilateral loss of vision with the usual features of optic neuritis. The diagnosis lies in a fundus finding of disk swelling and macular edema that may terminate in macular star formation. Treatment is directed toward the primary infection with the usual treatment of neuritis.

Retrobulbar Optic Neuritis in Children

This is an acute, episodic inflammation of the optic nerve behind the globe. It starts in one eye, with no disk change during the initial attack. The condition becomes bilateral within 3 weeks. The presentation in the first attack is accompanied by a loss of central vision with central scotomas. In subsequent attacks, the inflammation spreads anteriorly with disk swelling. Pain in the movement of the eye goes in favor of retrobulbar neuritis. Retrobulbar neuritis is rare in children.

Drug-induced Optic Neuritis in Children

Drug-induced optic neuritis in children does not differ much from adult neuritis. The clinical features depend on the type of drug, its strength, and the duration of use. The neuritis is generally bilateral and slow progressing. The diagnosis is exclusion with a high degree of suspension and a history of drug administration for a long time. Drug-induced neuritis is rarely acute. The common drugs are anti-infective. The most common group of drugs is antitubercular, which is headed by ethambutol. The list of drugs is long; the most frequent drugs that cause neuritis are streptomycin, isonex, chloramphenicol, cimetidine, vincristine, and cyclosporine.

Demyelinating Disorders

The demyelinating disorders that cause optic neuritis are given as follows:

- Multiple sclerosis
- Devic's neuromyelitis optica
- Schilder's disease

**Lyme disease* is an infective condition caused by the bacterium *Borrelia burgdorferi* and *Borrelia mayonii*. The condition is transmitted to humans through the bite of infected black-legged ticks, found mostly in North American states. The typical symptoms are fever, headache, fatigue, and skin rash. The organism is sensitive to broad-spectrum antibiotics such as ceftriaxone.

†*Leptospirosis* is a disease that spreads from animals to humans and is caused by infection with the bacteria *Leptospira*. The most common sources of infection are contact with the urine of infected animals and/or contaminated soil or water. Outbreaks may occur following periods of heavy rain or flooding. Doxycycline is the antibiotic of choice. It has a 90% cure rate.

- Acute disseminated encephalopathy
- Krabbe disease*

Acute Disseminated Encephalopathy

Acute disseminated encephalomyelitis is a demyelinating disorder of the brain and spinal cord, most often following infection and vaccination against bacterial and viral infections. The common vaccinations responsible are MMR in combination or separately, causing optic neuritis as well.

PAPILLEDEMA IN CHILDREN

Papilledema is neither an infection, inflammation, autoimmune disease, nor demyelination. It is a noninflammatory, passive, bilateral edema of the disk, thought to be due to an alteration in the pressure gradient across the lamina.

It is imperative to have raised intracranial pressure to develop papilledema. This is in contrast to pseudopapilledema, which has normal intracranial pressure with local causes such as drusen.

The exact cause of papilledema in any age is not well established except for the fact that if the intracranial pressure is raised enough to be transmitted from the subarachnoid space of the brain to the subarachnoid space around the optic nerve, it will slow down the axoplasmic flow, leading to stasis of fluid and swelling of the disk. There are various theories regarding the etiopathogenesis of papilledema, but none of them are conclusive.

Some of the relevant points in papilledema are given as follows:

> Papilledema is not a disease per se; it is a sign that reflects a serious intracranial disorder causing raised intracranial pressure.

- It is a passive, noninfective, and noninflammatory process.
- Raised intracranial pressure is the harbinger of papilledema.
- Raised intracranial pressure is transmitted around the optic nerve up to the lamina.
- The increased CSF pressure builds up to a level that throttles the nerve fibers in the retrobulbar space.
- The intracanalicular part of the optic nerve is more pressure sensitive.
- Though fluid pressure in the subarachnoid space is increased, it does not affect the nerve transversally.
- There is a collection of axoplasmic fluid in the axons of the nerve.
- The axoplasmic fluid seeps into the extracellular space in front of the lamina.
- The venous flow is slowed or obstructed.
- There is hypoxia/anoxia in the nerve.
- The prelamellar capillaries dilate.
- There is no spontaneous venous pulsation.
- Peripapillary swelling leads to cotton-wool exudates and superficial hemorrhages.
- Vision and color vision are retained until the nerve head goes into a state of atrophy.
- There may be visual obscuration for a few seconds that clears in a few minutes.
- The extent of papilledema is an indication of the pressure gradient between the pre- and retrolamellar spaces.

> Papilledema develops fast and subsides slowly.

Common causes of papilledema in children are given as follows:

> Children will not develop papilledema till the cranial sutures are open.

- *Congenital anomalies:* Various types of craniostenosis/craniosynostosis
- *Trauma:* Traumatic intracranial hemorrhage
  - Intracerebral:
    - Subdural
    - Subarachnoid
- *Infection:*
  - Meningitis/encephalitis
  - Brain abscess
  - Intracranial granuloma
  - Lateral sinus thrombosis
- *Space-occupying lesions:*
  - Tumors:
    - Primary:
      - Benign
      - Malignant
    - Secondary:
  - *Cysts:* Cysticercosis
- *Drugs:*
  - Overdose of fat-soluble vitamins: Vitamins A and D
  - Steroid overdose, sudden withdrawal of steroids
  - Prolonged use of tetracycline
  - Nalidixic acid

**Krabbe disease:* Krabbe disease is a demyelinating disease of infants under 6 months old. The disease involves extensive demyelination of the brain and other parts of the nervous system. It is a fatal disease; the children rarely live >2 years.

- *Miscellaneous:*
  - Pseudotumor cerebri

Subtentorial growths cause more papilledema than supratentorial growths.

Symptoms of Papilledema in Children

To begin with, it may be symptomless. To be followed by symptoms that can be divided into two broad groups: (1) systemic and (2) ocular.

1. *Systemic symptoms*: The systemic symptoms are due to raised intracranial tension.
   They are given as follows:
   a. Pulsatile headache that may be continuous or periodic; the child may get up with a headache.
   b. Nausea and vomiting almost daily may be constant or in bouts. Projectile vomiting in the absence of gastrointestinal (GI) tract involvement goes more in favor of raised intracranial pressure.
   c. Postural blackout.
   d. Diplopia: Mostly horizontal
   e. Pulsatile tinnitus is synchronous with pulses
   f. Fainting attacks
   g. Well-established papilledema may have symptoms of central nervous system involvement.
   h. Fever, neck rigidity with any or many of the above symptoms are indication of infections, i.e., meningitis, encephalitis, or brain abscess.
2. *Ocular symptoms*:
   a. Visual symptoms: Early symptoms consist of blackouts and grayouts, but there is no definite diminished vision or color vision; there are no flashes of light. Reduced vision is a late feature and is due to the onset of atrophic changes in the disk. The other cause of diminished vision is the development of a macular star. Unilaterally diminished vision with altered color vision goes in favor of optic neuritis.
   b. Diplopia: Diplopia is generally horizontal due to the involvement of the 6th nerve; paralysis of the 6th nerve has no localizing importance. The diplopia is present throughout the waking hours without the influence of exercise. Initially, the child may take mild diplopia as blurred vision. Diplopia may diminish with the bilateral involvement of six nerves. Involvement of other cranial nerves and tracts may have localizing importance.
   c. *Fundus changes:* Fundus changes are the most important physical finding in papilledema.
      As per the fundus picture, papilledema is clinically divided into:
      - Early papilledema
      - Established papilledema
      - Chronic papilledema
      - Sequel to papilledema

- *Fundus changes in early papilledema*:
  - The early changes that should alert a clinician are seen at the disk margin as blurring. There is no rule of thumb to predict the spread, i.e., clockwise/anticlockwise. It most commonly starts at the upper pole and gradually spreads on each side downward.
  - There is obscuration of the retinal vessels at the disk margin with peripapillary retinal edema. The development of striation on the retina radiating from the disk, referred to as Paton's folds (line), is due to the lateral extension of disk swelling pushing the retina. There may be one or more such folds without much clinical significance.
  - Hyperemia of the disk is due to an increase in the number of capillaries.
  - The optic cup is maintained in early papilledema; this is explained by the fact that the early changes are peripheral on the disk. The cup remains visible for a long time; early loss of the cup points toward pseudopapilledema.
  - Spontaneous venous pulsation may be absent.
- *Fundus changes in established papilledema:* The fundus changes are an exacerbation of the changes seen in early papilledema given as follows:
  - The blurring of the disk margin engulfs the whole circumference of the disk, and the edema spills into the peripapillary retina.
  - The disk has an intense hyperemic look and may have a few superficial hemorrhages on the surface. It looks like a small pink mushroom.
  - The lamina is no more visible.
  - The swelling of the disk is >+3 D on direct ophthalmoscopy.
  - There may be cotton-wool exudates near the disk, more on the temporal side.
  - Venous pulsation is absent. The presence of venous pulsation goes against papilledema.
  - The retinal vessels seem to dip into the swollen disk.

- *Fundus changes in chronic papilledema:* It takes months to develop changes in the optic nerve head to be called chronic.
    - Glial proliferation takes over vascularization.
    - The disk edema is either maintained or starts receding in spite of the cause remaining unaffected.
    - Hemorrhage starts fading.
    - The color changes from angry red to dirty yellowish white.
    - The exudates take time to fade.
    - The retinal vessels develop sheathing.
    - The cup is permanently lost.
    - The condition is referred to as a champagne cork appearance.
    - The macular changes start subsiding, and the exudates are replaced by scars and light pigmentation.

The general symptoms at this stage persist; the vision is diminished; it may range from 6/60 to no perception; the color sense is maintained, and the field shows peripheral constriction.

Sequels of Papilledema

The sequelae are the effects of prolonged, raised intracranial pressure that may not only affect optic nerve but also the retina and may involve other cranial nerves and neurological tracts, resulting in:

- Postpapilledema optic atrophy*
- Loss of vision
- Loss of field
- Motor in balance
- Squint

Imagining Papilledema

A few decades ago, the X-ray of the skull was the only imaging device available in cases of papilledema. Now, with better imaging devices, it has taken a back seat. Now, it is relevant only in cases of depressed fractures of the skull and retained intracranial foreign bodies, craniostenosis, and hydrocephalus. The two common imaging devices available are given as follows:

1. Magnetic resonance imaging and MRI with contrasts
2. Computed tomography

Magnetic Resonance Imaging and Magnetic Resonance Imaging with Contrasts

Magnetic resonance imaging reflects the position of the dura covering the optic nerve, allowing raised intracranial pressure that is transmitted to the subdural space of the optic nerve. MRI imaging is best done with gadolinium; the other method is MRI venography, which is used for venous thrombosis (rare in children). The MRI depicts changes in the globe, optic nerve, orbit, and optic tract; enlargement of the optic nerve sheath; protruding of the optic nerve head in vitreous; and increased tortuosity of the optic nerve. It also demonstrates changes in raised intracranial pressure before the onset of ophthalmically visible papilledema. The most important change in the globe seen by MRI is the flattening of the posterior sclera.

Computed Tomography in Papilledema

Computed tomography fails to identify early papilledema but can pick up hidden drusen, which is often mistaken for papilledema.

Optical Coherence Tomography

Optical coherence tomography has little role in the diagnosis of papilledema.

Other Investigation Orders for the Diagnosis of Papilledema

Fundus Fluorescein Angiography

Fundus fluorescein angiography is used to differentiate pseudopapilledema such as drusen, pseudoneuritis, high hypermetropia, and glial tissue on the optic nerve from true papilledema. Fluorescein angiography is not always the last word in differentiating between early papilledema and papillitis, both of which show diffuse leaking and staining of the peripapillary retina.

**Postpapilledema optic atrophy*: Postpapilledema optic atrophy is secondary optic atrophy where the diminished edema of the disk that was hyperemic is replaced by a yellow-white color due to gliosis. The gliosis is responsible for the sheathing of the blood vessels as well. Generally, it takes 6 months to 1 year for postpapilledema optic atrophy to develop; it is a permanent feature that does not pass off even following successful lowering of intracranial pressure. The postpapilledema optic atrophic causes peripheral constriction of fields; the enlargement of blind spots that are seen in fully developed papilledema may shrink in size. The condition is generally associated with varying degrees of loss of vision, ranging from the loss of a few lines on Snellen chart to total loss of vision.

Fundus fluorescein angiography shows variable presentation at various stages of papilledema. *They are given as follows*:

- Leak: It may be very little or extensive
- Diffuse: Spread of dye in nerve fiber layers
- Staining of the disk

Field Changes

Field changes are not conclusive in papilledema in contrast to papillitis. The papilledema shows a nonspecific enlargement of the optic disk. This happens only in well-established papilledema due to peripapillary retinal edema. The next field change is constriction of the peripheral field; this is a late feature and denotes the onset of postpapilledema optic atrophy.

Differential Diagnosis of Papilledema

It is not difficult to diagnose fully developed papilledema with systemic features of raised intracranial pressure.

Otherwise, it should be differentiated from the following conditions:

- Papillitis
- Pseudoneuritis
- Drusen of the optic nerve
- Glioma of the optic nerve
- Bergmeister papilla

Causes of Bilateral Disk Edema

The causes of bilateral disk edema can be divided into two broad groups, i.e., those with raised intracranial pressure and those without raised intracranial pressure. The second group consists of a variety of conditions that are put together as pseudopapilledema. The list is headed by the drusen of the optic nerve.

The most important factor is raised intracranial pressure due to any of the following causes:

- *Congenital:* Too small a cranium for an expanding brain (craniostenosis)
- Space-occupying lesions:
    - Intracranial tumors
    - Edema of the brain
    - Retained foreign body
    - Parasitic cysts
- Reduced cerebrospinal fluid (CSF) drainage:
    - Aqueductal stenosis:
        - Congenital
        - Mass pressing over the aqueduct
    - *Damaged arachnoid:* Meningitis, subarachnoid hemorrhage
- Increased CSF production

Causes of Uniocular Disk Swelling in Children that are Confused with Early Papilledema

- Hypoplasia of the disk
- Glial veil
- Opaque nerve fibers
- Tilted disk
- Foster Kennedy syndrome
- Uniocular high hypermetropia
- Hypotony
- Optic neuritis
- Optic nerve tumor
- Unilateral drusen

The disks that are not likely to develop disk edema are given as follows:

- Large coloboma of the disk
- Moderate-to-high myopia
- Already atrophied disk, as in primary or glaucomatous optic atrophy

Management

There is no fixed algorithm that fits all cases of papilledema. It has been pointed out earlier that papilledema is not a disease but an expression of a serious cause. The main pathology is raised intracranial pressure; it is but natural that lowering intracranial pressure will reduce papilledema but not cure unless the cause has been attended to.

The medical treatment is effective only in infective processes, i.e., meningitis, encephalitis, and brain abscess, with specific systemic antimicrobials and judicious use of steroids. Repeated lumber punctures are no more recommended. Surgical treatment is left to a neurosurgeon. The malignant growths are treated by radiation, chemotherapy, and surgery.

OPTIC ATROPHY IN CHILDREN

Optic atrophy per se is not a disease itself; it is after effect of many disorders of the visual path from the retina to optic radiation. A retrogeniculate lesion causes delayed and milder atrophy. Basically, optic atrophy is the death of the axon of the optic nerve secondary to degeneration with obliteration of blood vessels. Lesions nearer to the disk cause more atrophy than those away. It is virtually a scar with a loss of function. The optic nerve may be an isolated feature or may be associated with other neurological deficits.

Optic atrophy in general has been classified in different ways; the following list contains some of them. They can be:

- Congenital/acquired
- Hereditary/nonhereditary
- On the basis of ophthalmoscopic appearance:
    - Primary
    - Secondary
    - Consecutive
- Ascending/descending
- Isolated/with a neurological deficit
- Presynaptic/postsynaptic
- Unclassified:
    - Cavernous optic atrophy
    - Glaucomatous optic atrophy
    - Temporal pallor
    - Bow tie appearance
- The best classification is etiological, supported by biochemical and serological evidence backed by neuroimaging.

They are given as follows:

- Heredofamilial
- Postpapilledematous
- Postneuritic
- Consecutive
- Compressive
- Toxic
- Nutritional
- Metabolic
- Vascular (not seen in children)

Heredofamilial Optic Atrophy

They form a group of congenital optic neuropathies that are generally not apparent at birth but only manifest in childhood.

> Optic atrophies developing beyond the second decade are rarely heredofamilial.

The features that are common to most of the conditions are given as follows:

- Diminished vision: May be sudden, reaching maximum loss within a short period of time or rarely gradual
- Dyschromatopsia
- Central scotomas
- Diminished contrast
- Diminished brightness
- Pupillary changes
- Nystagmus
- May be associated with a neurological deficit
- They may be part of optic abiotrophy
- Associated with chorioretinal abiotrophy
- Storage diseases

The common conditions are given as follows:

- Leber's optic neuropathy
- Kjer's dominant juvenile neuropathy
- Behr's recessive neuropathy
- Optic neuropathy in juvenile diabetes

Heredofamilial optic atrophy (neuropathy) is broadly divided into dominant and recessive forms as depicted in ***Flowchart 21.1***.

Features of congenital dominant forms are given as follows:

- Discovered in the first decade
- Severe vision loss: 6/60 or less
- Achromatopsia
- Nystagmus

Features of infantile form of dominant trait are given as follows:

- Mild-to-moderate vision loss
- Yellow-blue color defect
- Loss of hearing
- Ataxia
- Ophthalmoplegia

Recessive optic atrophies of infancy are always associated with central nervous system involvement with mental retardation, spasticity, and ataxia.

Recessive optic atrophy in childhood is associated with diabetes insipidus, diabetes mellitus, and hearing loss with growth retardation.

Flowchart 21.1: Classification of heredofamilial optic atrophy.

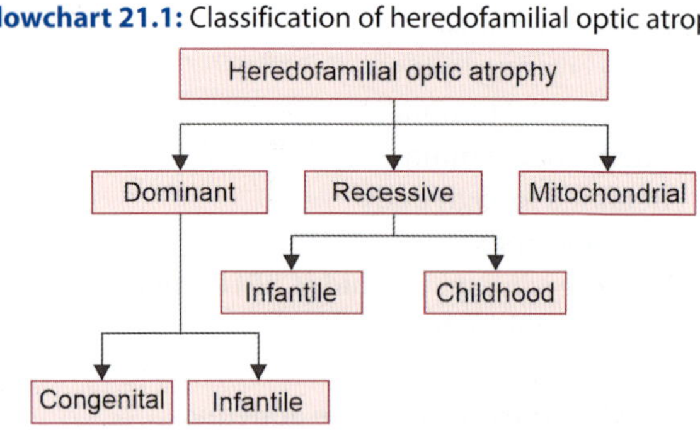

Flowchart 21.2: Features of childhood optic atrophy.

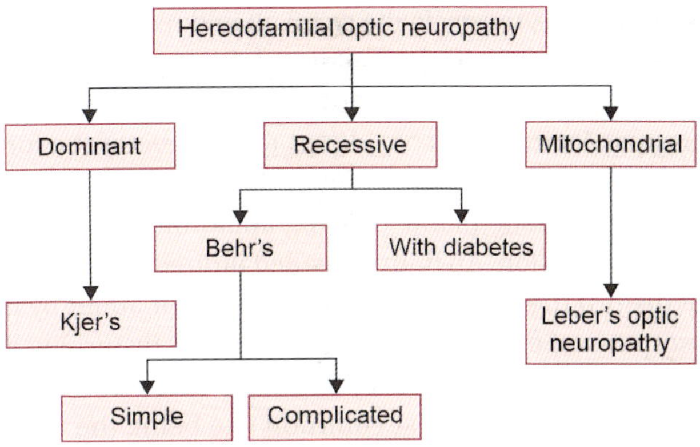

Characteristics of Heredofamilial Optic Atrophy

The conditions are hereditary, occasionally with a positive family history, isolated, or may be associated with central nervous system degeneration.

Flowchart 21.2 shows some of the important features of childhood optic atrophy (neuropathy).

Kjer's Optic Neuropathy

It is an autosomal dominant neuropathy that starts between 4 and 8 years of age and may be delayed up to the end of the first decade. With mild-to-moderate visual loss, the disk shows mild pallor; the child has a blue-yellow color defect, which may be associated with nystagmus with the variable course, and the improvement of vision when present is marginal.

Behr's Recessive Neuropathy

It is a recessive form of juvenile optic neuropathy, which has two forms: (1) simple and (2) complicated. The simple starts in neonates and is often mistaken for congenital; it is diagnosed later when the child is examined for diminished distant vision. Vision is found to be as low as counting fingers near the face; color defects are common. As the condition develops at neonatal age, nystagmus is common. In spite of the great loss of vision, the vision remains stationary, requiring rehabilitation for the child as a visually handicapped person. The condition is more common if there is consanguinity. The complicated form is seen between infancy and the end of the first decade; loss of vision is not as severe as in the former type, which never terminates into legal blindness*; the vision remains between 6/36 and 6/60, and half of the children develop mild-to-moderate nystagmus; the disk is partially pale on the temporal side.

Neuropathy with Juvenile Diabetes

This is a recessive form of optic atrophy, the prominent feature of which is the presence of diabetes mellitus. It is a progressive disorder that becomes apparent in childhood with a severe loss of vision without nystagmus. The disk is markedly pale with a profound color defect; there may be hearing loss, and the condition is progressive.

Leber's Optic Neuropathy

This is a heredofamilial optic neuropathy due to a mitochondrial defect in the mother. This is also known as Leber's disease without causing amaurosis (not to be confused with the less common Leber's congenital blindness, which is a retinal pigmentary dystrophy and not a true neuropathy). The disease starts mostly in puberty; it may be in boys as young as 5 years old, making it difficult to differentiate from other childhood neuropathies; it rarely starts after 30 years. It is a bilateral condition that starts in one eye as a sudden deterioration of painless vision, often confused with acute optic neuritis from childhood. It is mostly seen in boys (90%), and the mother is the carrier who passes the disease onto her children, both boys and girls. The mother may or may not have manifestations of the disease. The girl children become carriers themselves without manifestation. The affected male does not pass it onto his progeny but may have brothers with manifestation. That may be full blown or partial; the maternal uncles, too, may have the disease. The fathers of carriers do not have the disease; this has social importance because it is not the affected male who spread the disorders but his carrier's sister. The defect lies in the mitochondrial DNA of the mother due to mutation.

The clinical picture is typical and begins with rapid deterioration of vision in one eye. The other eye follows soon, and the vision may be 6/60 or less. Then, it progresses slowly to the lowest level and then starts improving, never to reach 6/6. It generally stays at 6/24 or 6/18, which is not correctable.

There is a diminished color sense, stereopsis, and contrast. There is a large, dense central or centrocecal

---

**Legal blindness:* The definition differs from country to country. The most commonly used definition is a person with best-corrected vision <20/200 (6/60) in the better eye with a retained field <20° all-round the fixation.

absolute scotomas, which are surrounded by larger relative scotomas, more for color. The fundus in the initial stage may look normal or may have features of acute neuritis. The common fibers affected are papillomacular. The disk may show microvascular angiopathy in the form of telangiectasia that passes off with time. The rest of the fundus is normal without exudates or hemorrhage.

Management: There is no specific treatment for the conditions; the steroids that are used in the acute stage of optic neuritis have not proved to be effective. The nonspecific drugs are high doses of hydroxocobalamin given intramuscularly initially, to be followed by oral tablets for the next few years. Oral zinc is a common supplement thought to slow the progress and so is oral cysteine. Surgical decompression of the nerve, too, has not shown encouraging results. Children with nonimprovement of vision should not be put in blind schools; they should be encouraged to stay in usual schools with normal children and encouraged to learn professions compatible with low vision.

The summary of clinical features of Leber's optic neuropathies is given as follows:

- The most common symptom is rapid fall in the affected male.
- His male siblings and carrier sisters may be asymptomatic.
- The male siblings may develop partial or fully developed discords.
- Slow improvement in vision. Color vision, contrasts, and stereopsis take a longer time to improve.
- Stage of postneuritic optic atrophy
- Permanent, noncorrectable vision does not culminate in legal blindness.

CONGENITAL OPTIC NEUROPATHY

Congenital neuropathy can either be dominant or recessive; both are often mistaken for heredofamilial optic neuropathy. The heredofamilial optic neuropathy is not present at birth in contrast to congenital neuropathy; the loss of vision later is moderate, in spite of the pale disk. As the condition is congenital, it is very commonly associated with nystagmus. The child may have diminished color vision; there may be a positive history of noncorrectable distant vision in siblings and other members.

TRAUMATIC NEUROPATHY IN CHILDREN

Traumatic optic neuropathy is either missed or the diagnosis is made too late to be managed. It is generally unilateral, followed more commonly by blunt indirect injury to the optic nerve, mostly in the canal, than direct injury to the nerve anywhere in its course. It is defined as neuropathy due to trauma between the globe and the beginning of the chiasma. An injury is considered to be direct if the force that disrupts the optic nerve with loss of vision involves the normal tissue plane, causing anatomical disruption with loss of vision. An injury is called indirect when it does not disturb the tissue plane. This is brought about by the absorption of energy caused by the trauma disturbing the function. The indirect injury is generally sustained away from the nerve; the most common site being the frontal bone, when the shearing force travels backward to the optic nerve or the force is strong enough to move the brain backward, pulling the optic nerve. The trauma may be so trivial as not to attract much attention and is often forgotten until the child notices a unilateral loss of vision on the side of the injury. In cases of craniofacial injuries, the trauma to the optic nerve is generally overshadowed by more visible craniofacial injuries. The mechanism of traumatic neuropathy depends on the site of the injury. In the orbit, the nerve may be avulsed in the retrobulbar space, with or without disrupting its blood supply. The fundus picture is similar to central retinal artery obstruction, i.e., a pale disk without visible blood vessels on the disk surface. There may be some superficial hemorrhage adjacent to the disk margin. The optic canal is the most frequent location to cause damage to the optic nerve in both types of injuries.

The lesion could be any or many of the following:

- Hemorrhage in the nerve
- Edema of the nerve
- The above two, in combination, throttle the blood supply of the nerve
- Bone spicules impinging on the optic nerve
- Retrocanalicular and prechiasmal lesions are due to mechanical disruption of the nerve or its blood supply.

> One of the most common iatrogenic injuries that cause traumatic neuropathy is the retrobulbar injection of an anesthetic agent. This accident has been almost eliminated with the emergence of peribulbar injections.

In the avulsion of the optic nerve, there is a sudden loss of vision amounting to no perception of light, generally associated with mild-to-moderate proptosis and subconjunctival hemorrhage that spreads from the periphery to the center. The condition is generally associated with severe pain that attracts the attention of not only the child but also the clinician, who finds an absence of pupillary reaction and an afferent pupillary defect. The long-term effect of avulsion is the development of primary optic atrophy with its sequelae.

Injury to the nerve behind the entry of the central retinal artery does not produce changes initially. However, after some weeks or months, primary optic atrophy is common.

Bilateral traumatic optic neuropathy is less common; it is mostly seen in close head injuries with the involvement of chiasma. Traumatic optic neuropathy, especially secondary to an indirect injury to the frontal bone or a small laceration on the lateral end of the eyebrow, is more common in boys, but girls are not immune.

> The triad of histories of injury to the frontal bone, unilateral loss of vision, and afferent pupil go in favor of traumatic optic neuropathy.

The condition is confirmed by fundus examination; field examination (when vision is present); and imaging of the cranium, orbit, and paranasal sinuses. X-rays may be helpful in detecting fractures of the cranium; all fractures of the skull need not to be associated with optic neuropathy. The better imaging methods are CT and MRI. CT is better than MRI for outlining fractures. MRI is superior to CT in soft-tissue delineation. MRI is contraindicated in cases suspected of having an intracranial or intraorbital metallic foreign body, which is best visualized by an appropriate X-ray.

Management

Treatment consists of the management of head and oculofacial injuries. This should get priority over its ocular counterpart. Traumatic optic neuropathy is better managed by medical treatment when the child has been stabilized.

The medical management consists of a megadose of IV steroids. The most common drugs used are methylprednisolone (30 mg/kg) as the loading dose, followed by 5 mg/kg for the next 48 hours, or dexamethasone (4 mg/kg) a day. Methylprednisolone is continued for 2–3 days and then replaced by oral prednisolone in a tapering dose as per the protocol of the institute under the supervision of a pediatrician, with usual precaution. If there is deterioration of vision while on an oral steroid, parental methylprednisolone is restarted. If there is no improvement with a steroid, the child may be subjected to surgery by a neurosurgeon. The common procedure is decompressing the optic nerve with or without the removal of the roof of the optic canal. The results are not encouraging.

OPTIC NERVE TUMORS IN CHILDREN

Tumors of the optic nerve are relatively uncommon in all ages; most of them are benign, some carry chances of malignancy, and they can be put into two groups, i.e., in children and adults. They are given as follows:

- Glioma optic nerve
- Neurofibroma type 1
- Meningioma of the optic nerve sheath
- Schwannoma

The last two are seen in adults.

Glioma Optic Nerve

This is also called optic pathway glioma, as it may develop/extend in chiasma. Basically, it is a brain tumor developing round or in the optic nerve. Some authors considered it to be a hamartoma due to its close relations with neurofibroma type 1. It is seen exclusively in children who become symptomatic before 10 years of age, with an average age of 7 years; they may be unilateral or bilateral, which later carries a poor prognosis in both visual and life expectancy. They are known to be stable or even shrink without treatment. The tumors may be isolated or may be associated with neurofibroma type 1. Due to the loss of the *NF1* gene, neurofibroma type 2 has not been reported to be associated with optic nerve glioma. The percentage of association between glioma and neurofibroma ranges between 5 and 50%. This is applicable to optic nerve glioma type 1. Optic nerve glioma with neurofibroma has a better prognosis; both are benign. The counterpart of optic nerve glioma in adults is glioblastoma, which is rarer and potentially malignant. Optic nerve glioma is an important cause of slow-progressing axial proptosis in the pediatric age group. The tumor is an intrinsic pilocytic astrocytoma of the nerve without involving the sheath of the optic nerve.

Topographically, the optic nerve glioma is divided into:

- Orbital
- Intracanalicular
- Intracranial:
  - Prechiasmal
  - Chiasmal
  - Retrochiasmal

Optic nerve glioma per se does not develop in the optic nerve head.

The second and third in the above list are seen in late teens and adults. The tumors of the optic tract may be multicentric. Intracranial tumors developing after the second decade are more likely to be malignant and even fatal.

The orbital glioma of the optic nerve is the second most common cause of unilateral orbital tumors in children, the first being rhabdomyosarcoma.

The optic nerve glioma is benign, showing growing, nonfatal, well-capsulated growth. It most frequently develops in the posterior part of the optic nerve, with a propensity to extend back with marked proptosis in comparison to anteriorly placed growth.

The symptom consists of unilateral diminished distant vision, field loss, and squint. Children brought late may present with visible proptosis; otherwise, proptosis may be minimal and missed unless looked for. The typical proptosis of an optic nerve glioma is axial, nonreducible, nonpulsatile, without bruit, with no change in various positions of the head, and a Valsalva procedure.

The extraocular muscles are not affected; the examiner can insinuate the index finger between the growth and the orbital wall. The tumor cannot be felt by the finger. However, there may be a widening or interpalpebral aperture due to the mechanical effect of the proptosed eyeball. The anterior segment is not involved unless exposure to keratitis secondary to proptosis sets in; the pupillary reaction is conduction defect dependent on vision; lesser is the vision, more is pupillary involvement; ultimately, the afferent pupillary defect is the result.

Posterior segment involvement is limited to optic nerves that range from filling of the cup to full-blown papilledema; postpapilledematous atrophy is the rule. Occasionally, optociliary vessels may be present **(Fig. 21.8)**.

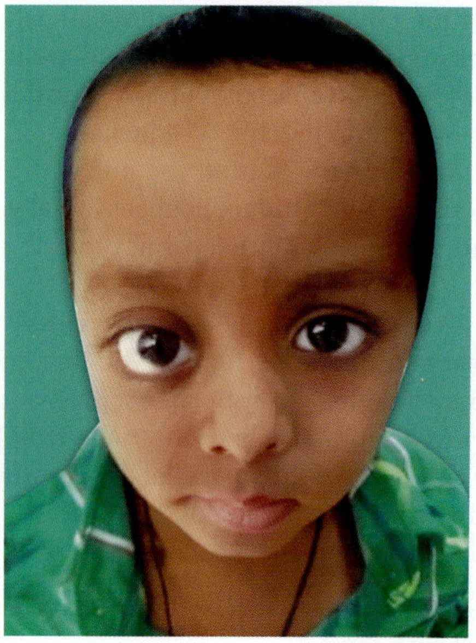

Fig. 21.8: Right-sided moderate optic nerve glioma.

Diagnosis

The diagnosis of optic nerve glioma under 10 years of age is simple. A child with unilateral axial slow-growing proptosis with early loss of vision and an afferent pupillary reaction is most probably suffering from an optic nerve glioma. The presence of a telltale sign of neurofibromatosis anywhere on the body increases the possibility of optic nerve glioma in a child; hence, it is mandatory to look for café-au-lait spots in every case of unilateral proptosis in a child and all cases of neurofibromatosis; the orbit should be examined for covert glioma. The diagnosis is confirmed by an X-ray, CT, and MRI of the orbit.

X-ray of orbit: X-ray findings are divided into X-rays of the orbit and X-rays of the optic foramen, along with the optic canal.

The X-ray of the orbit shows uniform enlargement of the orbit behind the rim; there is no calcification either in the globe or anywhere in the orbit. X-rays show fusiform, diffuse, well-capsulated growth in the orbit.

Both the optic foramen should be examined. A difference of 1.5 mm between the two foramen is suggestive of a glioma on the side of enlargement, with the possibility of intracanalicular extension.

Magnetic resonance imaging of the orbit: MRI is the most useful single imaging method to diagnose optic nerve gliomas. MRI reveals the earliest lesions of the optic nerve; even a subtle lesion becomes obvious in MRI.

Computed tomography: CT is a more important method to detect subtle bony erosion and extension in the optic canal. It is used to find other causes of intraorbital calcification, which is absent in childhood optic nerve glioma but present in optic nerve sheath meningioma, which is not seen in the first two decades.

Differential Diagnosis

Differential diagnosis of all unilateral, slow-progressing proptosis in a child aged under 10 years.

The causes of fast-growing unilateral proptosis should be excluded, especially rhabdomyosarcoma and malignant deposits from other sites, especially sympathetic chains such as neuroblastoma.

Traditionally, for academic interest, the difference between two optic nerve tumors, i.e., optic nerve glioma in children and optic nerve sheath meningiomas in adults, is discussed in **Table 21.3**.

Causes of enlarged optic foramen (in all ages) are given as follows:

- Optic nerve gliomas
- Meningioma of optic nerve sheath
- Neurofibromatosis
- Orbital retinoblastoma
- Rhabdomyosarcoma
- Metastasis
- Aneurysm of the ophthalmic artery

Management

Treatment of optic nerve gliomas is controversial. Only one factor is certain; there is no medical treatment except chemotherapy. The glioma of the intraorbital part of the optic nerve is not as amenable to chemotherapy or radiation as the intracranial growth of the visual path. The intracranial path gliomas are partially sensitive to radiation. The next question comes if surgical intervention is needed and, if needed, what should be the procedure. In the initial stages, the growth may be left undisturbed and observed regularly for an increase in proptosis, a change in field, and a loss of vision. Treatment is not required if the growth is still in the substance of the optic nerve, without proptosis or intracranial extension. The mainstay of surgery is the debulking of the growth, saving the globe and extraocular muscle. The parents should be counseled about the nonrestoration of vision following surgery. The surgery is best performed by a combined team of neurosurgeons and ENT surgeons. Debulking can be achieved via transfrontal, lateral orbitotomy, and transnasal routes. Debulking may reduce the proptosis, resulting in a much desired cosmetic appearance. In cases of unmanageable proptosis with exposure to the cornea, the most common procedure is partial or total tarsorrhaphy. If the cornea is already sloughed, the only option left is enucleation. Chemotherapy and radiotherapy are best left to oncologists and radiotherapists.

GLIOMA OF CHIASMA

Surprisingly, gliomas of chiasma are more common than optic nerve gliomas but are diagnosed less frequently. By the time they are diagnosed, they are quite advanced, without proptosis, with the possibility of intracranial extension. The symptoms of chiasmal gliomas are initially

TABLE 21.3: Difference between optic nerve glioma in children and optic nerve sheath meningiomas in adults.

Features	*Optic nerve gliomas*	*Optic nerve sheath meningioma*
Genetic	Sporadic	Sporadic
Age	Below 10 years	Fourth decade and beyond
Sex	Equal in both sexes	More common in women
Nature	Benign	Benign
Vision loss	Gradual, early loss	Gradual delayed loss
Proptosis	Unilateral	Unilateral
X-ray	Fusiform thickening of the optic nerve, widening of the optic canal, and enlargement of the optic foramen	Doughnut sign that forms a cuff of enhanced tumor mass around the nonenhancing optic nerve that looks like a dot; it also denotes any enlargement of the optic canal, similar to optic nerve glioma; it also reveals hyperostosis of the bone
CT	An intraconal heterogeneous fusiform mass arising from the optic nerve without calcification may show cystic changes	Intraconal homogeneous mass arising from the sheath of the optic nerve with or without calcification and no cystic change
MRI	Fusiform heterogeneous mass arising from the substance of the optic nerve, mixed signal in the T2-weighted image	Fusiform homogeneous mass encasing optic nerve from outside hypolucency signal on T2-weighted image

Note: In short, optic nerve sheath meningioma is seen mostly in women in postmenopausal age with slow and late diminished vision.

the same as those of optic nerve gliomas, i.e., unilaterally diminished vision, central scotomas with or without pupillary change and no proptosis, may have squints, and uncorrectable vision loss. There may be hemianopia on the other side of the center of the chiasma is involved; bitemporal hemianopia indicates extensive involvement. Chiasmal gliomas are more frequently likely to be malignant; they are known to extend in the optic canal, in the pituitary, hypothalamus, and third ventricle that result in internal hydrocephalus, raised intracranial pressure, and other hypothalamic signs, i.e., precocious puberty, obesity, diabetes insipidus, and somnolence. They are known to end in bilateral blindness; the chiasmal lesions do not respond to surgical debulking, and they cannot be removed completely; the chiasma lesions are better treated by radiation and chemotherapy.

TUMORS OF THE OPTIC NERVE HEAD

Primary glioma exclusively of the optic nerve head has not been reported; all the cases are forward extensions of anteriorly placed glioma that may spread into the prelamellar space. The other growths that may be mistaken as gliomas of the optic nerve head are drusen, neurofibromatosis, tuberous sclerosis, and remnants of the hyaloid system. It may be mistaken for growth arising from the disk. An intraocular retinoblastoma may extend into the optic nerve head. Another tumor that invades the optic nerve head is neuroblastoma.

SUGGESTED READING

1. Acheson JF, Burton B, Plant GT. Hereditary optic neuropathy. In: Jackson TL (Ed). Moorfield's Manual of Ophthalmology, 3rd edition. New Delhi: Jaypee Brothers Medical (P) Pvt. Ltd.; 2020. p. 737.
2. Acheson JF, Burton B., Plant GT. Optic nerve tumors. In: Jackson TL (Ed). Moorfield's Manual of Ophthalmology, 3rd edition. New Delhi: Jaypee Brothers Medical (P) Pvt. Ltd.; 2020. p. 740.
3. Badrinath SS. Papilledema. In: Netralaya S (Ed). Clinical Practice and Pattern in Ophthalmology, 1st edition. New Delhi: Jaypee Brothers Medical (P) Pvt. Ltd.; 2004.
4. Chinta S, Wallang BS, Sachdeva V, Gupta A, Patil-Chhablani P, Kekunnaya R. Etiology and clinical profile of childhood optic nerve atrophy at a tertiary eye care center in South India. Indian J Ophthalmol. 2014;62(10):1003-7.
5. Deb AK, Kannan NB, Ramasamy K, Mishra C. Double ring sign in optic nerve head hypoplasia. Indian J Ophthalmol. 2019;67(7):1187.
6. Duke-Elder S. Anomalies of the Optic Disc and Nerve in the System of Ophthalmology. London: Henry Kimpton; 1964.
7. Fraunfelder FT, Fraunfelder FW. Drug-Induced Ocular Side Effects in Clinical Ocular Toxicology, 8th edition. United States: Elsevier; 2020.
8. Karan S. Papilledema. In: Karan S (Ed). Step-by-Step Neuroophthalmology: Clinical Examination and Diagnosis, 1st edition. New Delhi: Jaypee Brothers Medical (P) Pvt. Ltd.; 2006. pp. 295-9.
9. Khadse R, Ravindran M, Pawar N, Maharajan P, Rengappa R. Clinical profile and neuroimaging in pediatric optic neuritis in the Indian population: a case series. Indian J Ophthalmol. 2017;65(3):242-5.
10. Khadse R, Ravindran M, Pawar N, Maharajan P, Rengappa R. Clinical profile and neuroimaging in pediatric optic neuritis in the Indian population: a case series. Indian J Ophthalmol. 2017;65(3):242-5.
11. Kovarik JJ, Doshi PN, Collinge JE, Plager DA. Outcome of pediatric patients referred for papilledema. J AAPOS. 2015;19:344-8.
12. Liu B, Murphy RKJ, Mercer D, Tychsen L, Smyth MD. Pseudopapilledema and association with idiopathic intracranial hypertension. Childs Nerv Syst. 2014;30(7): 1197-200.
13. McCafferty B, McClelland CM, Lee MS. The diagnostic challenge of evaluating papilledema in pediatric patients. Taiwan J Ophthalmol. 2017;7(1):15-21.
14. Mollan SP. Papilloedema. In: Denniston AKO, Murray PI (Eds). Oxford Handbook of Ophthalmology, 4th edition. United Kingdom: Oxford University Press; 2018. p. 758.
15. Mukherjee PK. Congenital pit of the optic nerve. In: Fraunfelder FT, Roy FH (Eds). Current Ocular Therapy, 5th edition. Philadelphia: WB Saunders Company; 1983. p. 558.
16. Mukherjee PK. Disorders of the optic nerve. In: Fraunfelder FT, Roy FH (Eds). Children in Pediatric Ophthalmology, 1st edition. New Delhi: New Age International; 2005.
17. Mukherjee PK. Disorders of the Visual Pathway in Essentials of Neuroophthalmology, 1st edition. New Delhi: Jaypee Brothers Medical (P) Pvt. Ltd.; 2010. pp. 64-141.
18. Samant PM, Samant H, Nabar SN. Optic neuritis. In: Samant PM, Samant H (Eds). Ophthalmology Theory and Practical, 1st edition. Mumbai: Balani Publishing House; 2004. p. 187.
19. Saxena R, Phuljhele S, Menon V, Gadaginamath S, Sinha A, Sharma P. Clinical profile and short-term outcomes of optic neuritis patients in India. Indian J Ophthalmol. 2014;62(3):265-7.
20. Saxena R, Singh D. Optic neuritis. In: Ramamurthy D, Biswas P (Eds). AIOS Ready Reckoner in Ophthalmology. New Delhi: Jaypee Brothers Medical (P) Pvt. Ltd.; 2017. pp. 543-4.
21. Yen EA, Graves JS, Bensen LA, Wassmer E, Waldman A. Pediatric optic neuritis. Neurology. 2016;87(9 Suppl 2): S53-8.

CHAPTER 22

Childhood Glaucoma

Glaucoma is not a single disease. It is an enigmatic syndrome complex that causes irreversible diminished vision in all ages, ranging from newborns to ripe old ages if not managed in time. About 2% of the general population over the past four decades has been infected by glaucoma of some type or another. Incidence rises with age.

The three cornerstones of the syndrome are: (1) A rise in intraocular pressure (IOP), (2) a loss of peripheral field, and (3) changes in and around the disk with ancillary changes in the ocular coat. In the past, the rise of IOP was squarely blamed for all the maladies that were seen concurrently with changes in the optic nerve and field. There is no doubt that field changes are not independent of changes in the optic nerve. This started another debate, i.e., are the optic nerve changes independent of IOP? Are they primary or tension related?

Childhood glaucoma differs greatly from glaucoma in adults. The childhood glaucoma is far less frequent than adult glaucoma. Statistically, all childhood glaucoma, when put together, does not exceed one in 10,000 live births. Adulthood glaucoma does not have prominent clinical features that have to be suspected and confirmed. Childhood glaucoma, especially in children under 3 years of age, has prominent clinical features that are so obvious that caregivers, neonatologists, or even a general physician can find something amiss in a child suffering from congenital glaucoma, more so when it is unilateral or grossly asymmetric in two eyes. **Flowchart 22.1** shows a rough classification of childhood glaucoma.

To better understand childhood glaucoma, it is imperative to recapitulate knowledge of the following:

- The applied anatomy of the anterior segment is related to:
  - Production of aqueous (drawing)
  - Drainage of aqueous (drawing)
  - Surgical anatomy (drawing)
- Development of angle anterior chamber (AC) and anterior segment
- Clinical methods of examination of a child's eye with reference to glaucoma
- Genetic involvement in the production of childhood glaucoma
- A universally accepted classification of childhood glaucoma
- Standardization of management

Flowchart 22.1: Classification of childhood glaucoma.

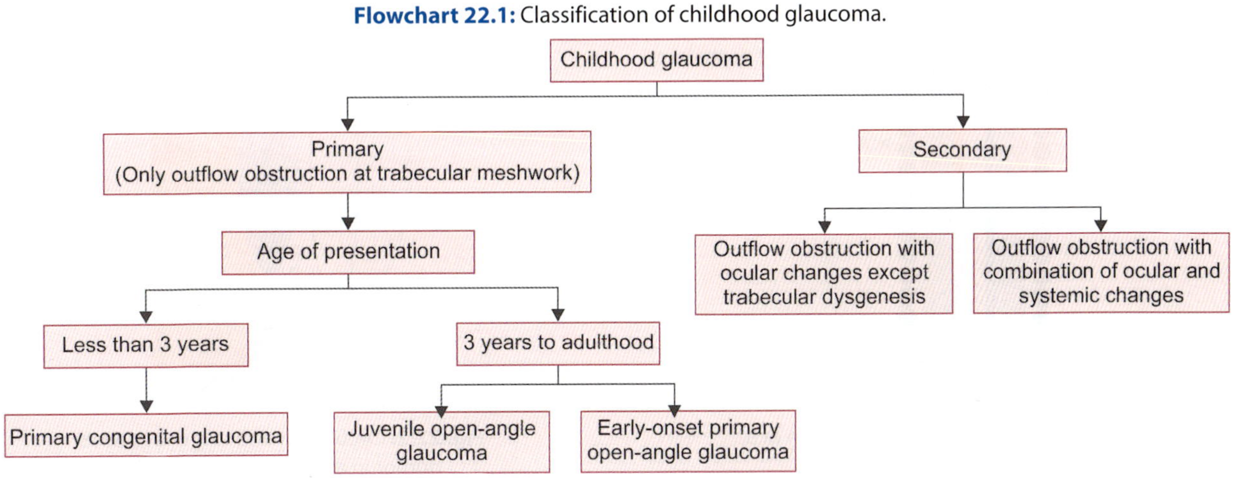

Applied anatomy of the anterior segment related to childhood glaucoma is concerned with the:

- Production of aqueous humor
- Drainage of aqueous humor
- Surgical anatomy of glaucoma

The only structure related to the production of aqueous is the ciliary body; to be more specific, it is the ciliary process complex that plays the most dominant part in the production of aqueous. The ciliary muscle has no role in the production of aqueous, and it is indirectly related to its drainage. There are about 70–80 ciliary processes that start in the ciliary body and project centrally, such as fingers. Each ciliary process consists of blood vessels in the stroma, covered by epithelium **(Flowchart 22.2)**.

The epitheliums of the ciliary process are forward extensions of the retinal epithelium, hence neuro-ectodermal in origin. According to the presence of pigment, they are divided into two types, i.e., (1) pigmented and (2) nonpigmented, each composed of a single layer of cuboidal cells **(Fig. 22.1)**.

The pigmented epithelium is superficial to the non-pigmented epithelium and corresponds to the pigmented epithelium of the retina. The two layers are firmly adherent to each other without a potential space in between; hence, they are not liable to be separated such as the retina. A tuft of blood vessels traverses each ciliary process longitudinally. The arteries and their corresponding terminals unite in capillary formation. Structurally, they resemble choroidal vessels minus choriocapillaris; the vessels are lined by fenestrated endothelium. The space between the blood vessels and the epithelium is filled by a delicate stroma; the ciliary process does not contain any muscle. It comprises of collagen and mucopolysaccharides.

STRUCTURES RELATED TO DRAINAGE OF AQUEOUS HUMOR

Aqueous humor is a vital fluid that supplies nutrition to the lens, and corneal endothelium acts as an optical medium, removes metabolic byproducts, and maintains intraocular pressure.

The aqueous humor is formed in the posterior chamber from the ciliary processes. To be effective, the aqueous humor needs to circulate in the AC. The production of aqueous humor is a continuous process, as its circulation and exit from the AC **(Fig. 22.2)**.

Aqueous humor from the posterior chamber passes into the AC through the pupil, and after circulating in the AC, it exits through the angle. Obstruction, either at the level of the pupil or angle, or both, impedes the exit of the aqueous humor, resulting in a rise in IOP, followed by a chain of events that constitute glaucoma.

Flowchart 22.2: Various parts of the ciliary process.

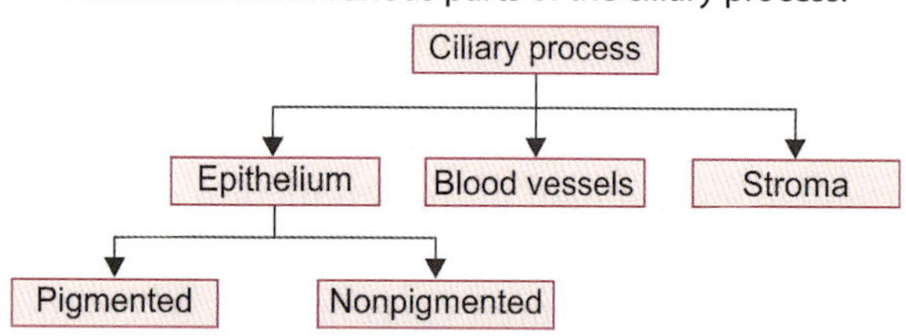

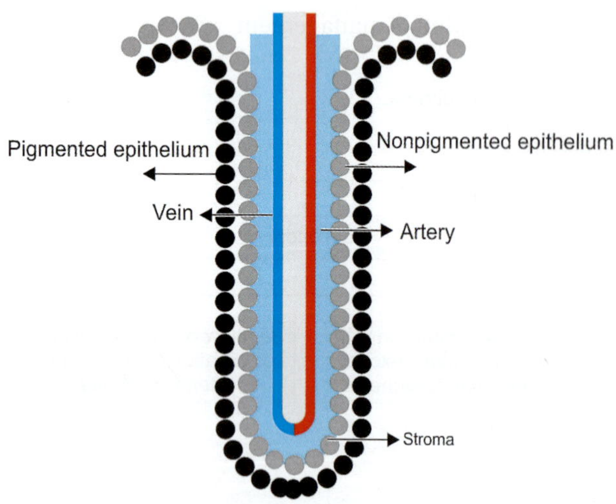

Fig. 22.1: Diagrammatic representation of a section of a ciliary process.

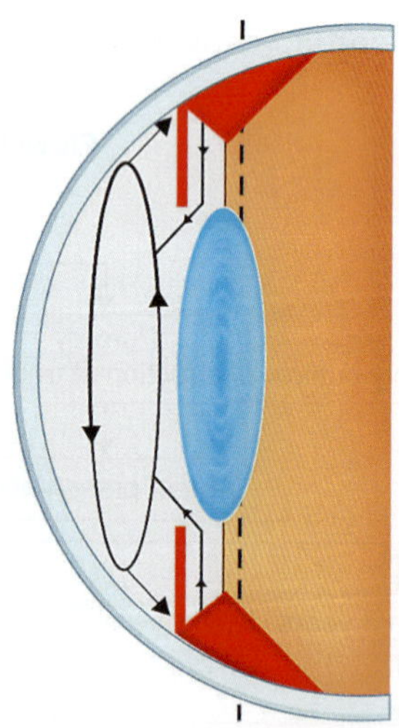

Fig. 22.2: Circulation and exit of aqueous humor in anterior chamber (AC).

ANATOMY OF ANTERIOR CHAMBER

A diaphragm formed by the ciliary body, zonules, and lens/after cataract/intraocular lens (IOL) divides the interior of the eye into two unequal chambers given as follows **(Fig. 22.3)**:

1. A large vitreous chamber is occupied by the vitreous and lined by the retina.
2. A smaller aqueous chamber filled with aqueous humor.

In the absence of the lens, the line demarcating the two chambers is lost. The vitreous per se does not have any role in the production of glaucoma, except in aqueous misdirection syndrome **(Fig. 22.4)**.

The aqueous chamber is divided into two unequal spaces, i.e.:

1. Small posterior chamber
2. Larger AC

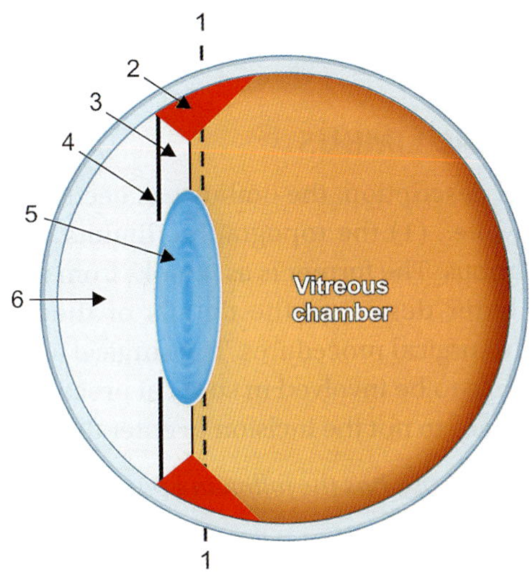

Fig. 22.3: The chambers of the eye are: (1) an imaginary line showing two chambers of the eye, (2) ciliary body, (3) posterior chamber, (4) iris, (5) lens, and (6) anterior chamber.

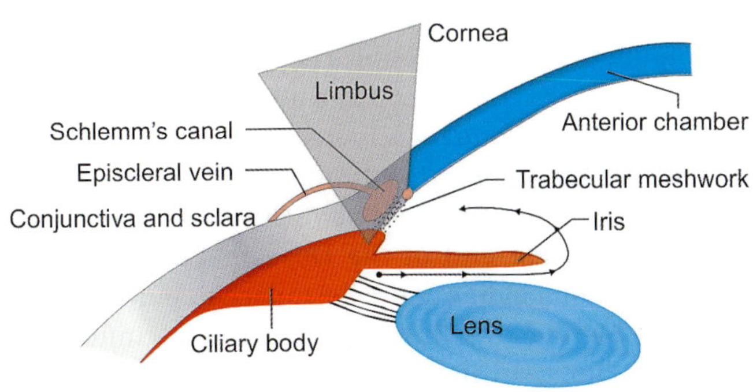

Fig. 22.4: Surgical anatomy of the limbus anterior chamber and aqueous flow.

The *posterior chamber* is bounded on the anterior surface by the posterior surface of the iris all around, the lens, the anterior surface of the zonules, and the ciliary process forming the posterior surface. The ciliary processes arising from the ciliary body projecting in this space are dipped in aqueous humor that fills the posterior chamber.

> The anterior chamber may be called the center of the stage, where most of the activities related to glaucoma take place.

The *AC* is a planoconvex space with a posterior flat surface formed by the anterior surface of the lens, IOL in the bag, or after cataract. The posterior surface has a deficiency in the center in the form of a pupil that acts as a conduit between the posterior and anterior chambers for the aqueous to flow freely between the posterior chamber and AC. The flow of aqueous humor is one-way from behind forward; a small chunk of the ciliary body constitutes the periphery of the posterior plane.

> The dome of the anterior chamber is formed by the posterior surface of the cornea, lined by endothelium that also lines the anterior surface of the iris, except for the crypts. The angle of the anterior chamber is the most important part related to glaucoma. It has been called the cockpit of glaucoma.

The junction of the two surfaces of the planoconvex space is the angle of the AC. The space being planoconvex has maximum depth in front of the pupil, gradually getting reduced to zero as the two surfaces merge.

> The depth of the anterior chamber is genetically determined.

The depth of the AC of a full-term baby is slightly less than that of an adult. It takes 2 years for the AC to attain adult depth.

The angle formed by the confluence of two surfaces is roughly 45°. It is visualized by gonioscope, ultrasound biomicroscopy (UBM), and optical coherence tomography (OCT). Under physiological conditions, the angle is not blocked by maximum mydriasis.

Parts of the angle visible on gonioscopy are given as follows:

- The scleral spur is a sharp posterior lip of the scleral sulcus to which the ciliary body is anchored all around. The scleral spur is the most important and constant landmark for gonioscopy.
- The scleral sulcus is a shallow groove that runs concentric with the pupil on the inner side of the AC under the limbus.

- Trabecular meshwork is a sieve-like structure that runs across the scleral sulcus between the periphery of the cornea and the scleral spur. The trabecular meshwork has three sources of origin, i.e., (1) cornea, (2) sclera, and (3) uvea. The meshwork is triangular in section, with its apex toward Schwalbe's line, and the base is attached to the scleral spur.
- Schwalbe's line denotes the line to which the meshwork is attached on the inner side of the cornea. Schwalbe's line denotes the thickened peripheral end of the Descemet's membrane.
- Schlemm's canal is a channel of irregular caliber, running all around the angle of the AC. The canal is formed by converting the scleral sulcus into a channel by the trabecular meshwork. It is akin to a venous channel with an endothelial lining. The canal is not only irregular in diameter but also in its course. At places, the canal breaks into tributaries only to join the main circle again. The outer side of the canal drains into the episcleral vessels, which ultimately open into subconjunctival vessels. The episcleral veins open into the anterior ciliary veins. One side of the triangle faces the AC, and the other side faces the lumen of Schlemm's canal.

The structure related to the surgical anatomy of glaucoma is the limbus ***(Fig. 22.5)***.

The limbus is a nonspecific area on the outer surface of the globe. It represents the junction of the cornea on one side and the sclera and conjunctiva on the other side. It is neither connected with the production nor drainage of aqueous but is of utmost surgical importance. In surgical processes, such as antiglaucoma surgeries, the anterior part consists of all structures between the end of Bowman's membrane and the termination of Descemet's membrane. The limbus is a circular, ill-defined area, roughly 1.00 mm wide, all around the cornea. It partially encroaches on the periphery of the cornea. As the cornea and scleral curvature are not equal, their junction is not smooth but steep on the corneal end. For ease of identification, the limbus is divided into two circles and two zones.

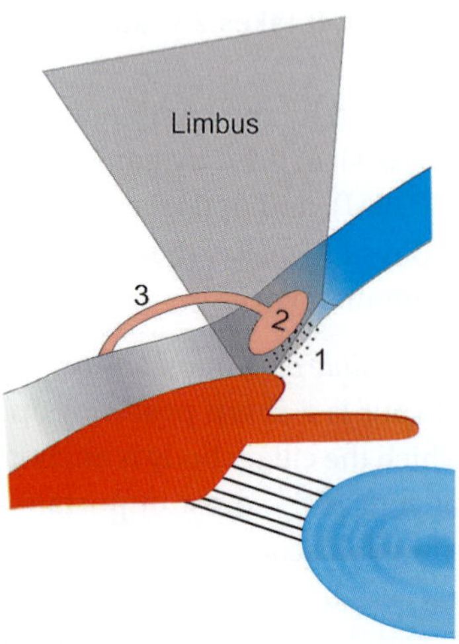

Fig. 22.5: An enlarged view of the limbus.

The circles are formed by insertion of conjunctiva and Tenon's capsule. This overlies the termination of Bowman's membrane, which is 1 mm shorter than the stroma and Descemet's membrane. This portion of the limbus lies over the scleral spur. Over Schwalbe's line lies an imaginary line in between the two limbal borders, called the midlimbal line, representing the two parts of the limbus with two colors, one bluish, representing cornea and the other gray, denoting the sclera. The limbus topographically is not a perfect circle; its position around the cornea is variable, and the width is irregular. The limbus is rich in vasculature and is a source of stem cells.

SURGICAL LIMBUS

For ease of description, the limbus has been divided into two forms, i.e., (1) the topographic limbus and (2) the surgical limbus. The former is as it looks from the surface, and the latter describes the details of the structures involved in surgical procedures. The surgical limbus is the specific place to be involved in surgical procedures. It is a specified place to put the incision to enter the AC.

The surgical limbus has the following parts:

- Anterior border
- Posterior border
- Mid-limbal line

- *The anterior border* is a place where the conjunctiva is anchored to the corneal periphery. It overlies the end of the Bowman's membrane. On removing the conjunctiva and the Tenon's capsule, a bluish hue is seen in an area that is 1.00 mm all around.
- *The posterior border* is situated over the scleral spur. It is 1.00 mm posterior to the mid-limbal line.
- *The mid-limbal line* lies over Schwalbe's line, which represents the end of the Descemet's membrane. The mid-limbal line is the best place to enter the AC. Entry behind this line is most likely to injure the ciliary body; an incision more forward may injure the meshwork and predispose to iris injury and iris prolapse.

Development of Limbus

The limbus is a complex structure consisting of both embryonic, ectodermal, and mesodermal tissues. The surface ectoderm is responsible for the corneal epithelium. The rest of the cornea is mesodermal in origin. The limbus is a conglomeration of the conjunctiva, Tenon's capsule, cornea, sclera, and uvea. To understand the embryogenesis of the limbus, it is essential to recapitulate the development of the above tissues in general and the angle in particular.

DEVELOPMENT OF ANTERIOR CHAMBER

The study of the development of the AC requires a more detailed description because most of the changes causing childhood glaucoma depend on its developmental anomalies.

The AC is a space containing aqueous humor. Logically, its development should be simple and secondary to the development of its boundaries. However, it is not so simple—paradoxically, the AC, which should be a space filled with aqueous, is in fact a solid structure until its formation is complete. Statistically, the number of congenital anomalies in the eyes due to maldevelopment of the AC is far more than expected. The maldevelopment of the AC is responsible for many syndromes and childhood glaucoma.

The development of the AC can be broadly divided into two parts given as follows:

1. Development of the AC proper
2. Development of angles and drainage channels

Development of the Anterior Chamber Proper

The presence of the AC becomes evident at the 20.00 mm stage and keeps developing till birth. At birth, the AC is fully developed but narrower than in adults. It is filled with circulating aqueous humor. The AC develops following the separation of the lens from the surface ectoderm. The surface ectoderm is left behind, giving rise to the corneal epithelium. At this stage, waves of mesoderm originating from the optic cup creep between the corneal epithelium and the lens to be converted into the corneal stroma and its endothelium. It also gives rise to the iris stroma. The space between the mesodermal iris and corneal stroma is the future AC. The mesoderm gets atrophied to accommodate the developing AC. Till the 5th month, the cavity remains very narrow, developing fast thereafter, parallel with the development of the rest of the anterior segment.

Development of the Angle of the Anterior Chamber

The development of the angle of the AC is influenced by the embryogenesis of the cornea, sclera, and uvea. The tissues at the angle become obvious at an early stage of gestation. It develops slowly. It is fully developed just before birth. The Schlemm's canal develops 2 months earlier than the angle.

Development of Trabecular Meshwork

The trabecular meshwork develops from the mesenchyme that originates from the optic cup.

Development of Schlemm's Canal

The Schlemm's canal develops as a vascular channel at the gap in the angle at the posterior plane, only to shift gradually anteriorly in relation to the iris. The canal is lined by endothelium. During the development of the angle of the AC, the Schlemm's canal and trabecular meshwork are the structures that differentiate least and last.

> The overall development of the anterior chamber and its angle is genetically determined. Genes that regulate development are divided into three broad groups, each with a specific purpose. They are structural genes, regulatory genes, and cell-specific genes.

Summary of the Development of the Anterior Chamber and its Angle

- Development involves both the ectoderm and the mesoderm (mesenchyme).
- The presence of an AC becomes evident at an early stage of gestation as a chink in mesoderm.
- The mesoderm surrounding the optic cup grows centrally between the cornea and the iris.
- The growth of mesoderm is intermittent in waves. The first wave gives rise to all the corneal structures but the epithelium.
- The corneal epithelium is the ectoderm.
- The second wave forms the pupillary membrane, which will disappear at birth.
- The keratocytes of the cornea are products of the third wave.

- The AC expansion is accompanied by the absorption of mesoderm.
- By the 3rd month, the iridocorneal recess (angle) develops.
- By the 7th week, the trabecular meshwork develops from the neural crest mesenchymal cells, and at the same time, the Schlemm's canal develops as venous channels.
- By the 15th week, the corneal endothelium and the iris epithelium meet at an angle.
- The angle is well formed at birth but continues to develop to adult size till 1st year.
- Schlemm's canal and the trabecular meshwork are the structures that differentiate last.
- The AC and its angle are genetically mediated.
- The genes that control development are structural genes, regulatory genes, and cell-specific genes.
- All the structures involved in the formation of the AC are mesenchymal. The mesenchymal cells develop from the neural crest.
- The anomalies caused by the defect in migration and differentiation of neural crest cells are collectively called neurocristopathies, which were previously called mesodermal dysgenesis/AC cleavage syndrome.

Primary congenital glaucoma is due to a defect in the normal maturation of the chamber angle.

Congenital Anomalies of the Anterior Chamber and its Angle

We have seen that:

- The angle of the AC develops, replacing the mesodermal tissue between the corneal stroma and lens complex.
- The anomalies in the angle of the anterior are few.
- When present, some are major causes of glaucoma in infants and children.
- Most of them are genetically determined.
- Some are present at birth or may manifest in adolescence. Occasionally, they are sporadic.
- All of them are not associated with glaucoma.

It is difficult to classify them under a single classification. The anomalies may involve single or multiple structures. On the basis of the tissue involved, they may be: as shown as in **Table 22.1**.

Table 22.1 shows congenital anomalies of the AC on the basis of the tissue involved.

TABLE 22.1: Congenital anomalies of the anterior chamber.

Tissues involved	*Clinical manifestations*
Cornea	• Axenfeld anomaly • Axenfeld syndrome • Posterior keratoconus
Iridocorneal	• Rieger anomaly • Peters anomaly
Trabeculum	• Trabecular dysgenesis
Iridocorneal endothelial	• Chandler's syndrome • Cogan–Reese syndrome
Iris	• Progressive iris atrophy • Aniridia • Persistent pupillary membrane • Essential iris atrophy • *Anomalous pupil:* – Corectopia – Polycoria – Coloboma of iris

SPECIFIC IRIDOCORNEAL SYNDROME

Axenfeld Anomaly (Posterior Embryotoxon)

This is the mildest and most asymptomatic form of dysgenesis of the AC. Unlike other congenital anomalies, it is devoid of subnormal vision and does not cause glaucoma unless a peripheral iris is attached to it. Posterior embryotoxon is seen in 30% of individuals as a wide ring 1.00 mm inside the limbus on slit-lamp examination. It may be a complete or fragmented ring. The cause of the condition is not well understood. The most common hypothesis is the thickening of the end of Descemet's membrane and the central shift of Schwalbe's line. If the iris is adherent to Schwalbe's line, the condition is called Axenfeld syndrome, which is invariably associated with congenital glaucoma.

The Axenfeld anomaly does not require treatment. In the case of Axenfeld syndrome, glaucoma needs to be kept under control. Axenfeld syndrome may be associated with hypertelorism.

Rieger Anomaly and Rieger Syndrome

This anomaly is the further exacerbation of mesodermal dysgenesis in the AC without systemic features. Systemic features, when associated with Rieger anomaly, are called Rieger syndrome. Both are associated with variable glaucomatous changes.

Rieger anomaly consists of:

- Prominent Schwalbe's line
- Iris strand attached to prominent Schwalbe's line
- Hypoplasia of the iris; patches of iris atrophy leading to corectopia, polycoria, and pseudocornea
- Glaucoma

Rieger syndrome consists of Rieger anomaly with congenital anomalies of the teeth, cranium, and face.

Peters Anomaly

Peters anomaly is the most advanced form of mesodermal dysgenesis and the rarest of all AC malformations that may involve the lens. The features are a combination of ocular and systemic changes. The features are present at birth and are bilateral.

They are given as follows:

- Central corneal leukoma
- Localized defect in Descemet's membrane and endothelium in the area of leukoma
- Iris is attached to the leukoma without atrophy
- Anterior polar cataract
- Keratolenticular adhesion
- Shallow slit like an irregular AC
- Pupillary deformity
- Glaucoma
- Other features are given as follows:
    - Persistent hyperplastic primary vitreous
    - Retinal dysplasia
    - Microphthalmos
- The etiopathogenesis of the above features is not well understood. There are three grades of anomalies given as follows:
    1. Axenfeld and Rieger syndrome with central corneal opacity at the level of Descemet's membrane, absent endothelium under the corneal opacity, and an iris attached to the periphery of the opacity.
    2. Central defect in Descemet's membrane and endothelium without Axenfeld or Rieger changes.
    3. Corneal changes are similar to those in grade II with lenticuloirido changes in addition.
- Systemic involvement consists of various degrees of craniofacial and skeletal abnormalities. There may be mental retardation.
- The disease is nonprogressive, and management is directed toward the glaucoma, cataracts, and corneal opacity.
- Overall visual results are poor.

Cogan–Reese (Iris Nevus) Syndrome and Chandler's Syndrome

In the past, they were considered to be different entities. Presently, they are thought to be a single malady with variable presentation. They are sporadic, uniocular, and potentially blind without systemic involvement. It is more common in females and is not present in childhood. It may become evident in the late teens. The main symptoms are diminished vision and glaucoma. The causes of diminished vision and glaucoma are the proliferation of corneal endothelium all over, spreading over the iris, causing defects in the iris, and corneal edema caused by epitheliopathy. Defective vision is a cause that brings the patient for consultation. The morphological defect in the iris attracts early attention, bringing the child for consultation. Cogan–Reese syndrome with multiple flat-dark nodules on the iris is called iris nevus syndrome.

Chandler's syndrome consists of:

- Hammered silver discoloration of the corneal endothelium, best seen on specular microscope
- Mild-to-moderate glaucoma
- No iris incarceration in the cornea
- Deformity of the pupil
- The specific endothelial cells visible on specular microscopy are called iridocorneal epithelial cells (ICE).
- Corneal edema is independent of glaucoma.
- Rarely, the anterior lens capsule may be invaded.
- The condition is differentiated from posterior polymorphic dystrophy and Fuchs' endothelial dystrophy, which is seen in the fourth to seventh decade and is bilateral.

Essential Iris Atrophy

This consists of atrophic changes in the irises that are uniocular and not manifesting at birth. Though listed as a disorder of the iris, it is in fact a disorder of the corneal endothelium. The endothelial changes are associated with the proliferation of Descemet's membrane that invades the angle of the AC, associated with changes in the iris stroma, and the formation of peripheral iridocorneal adhesion with a secondary rise of IOP.

The earliest iris changes are thinning of the stroma, discovered on routine examinations on suspicion of raised IOP.

Things are first discovered under high power as areas of transillumination in the thin area, which is replaced by a full-thickness hole in the iris. By the time, the holes are progressing in the mid-periphery, and the peripheral anterior synechiae start developing. Generally, the peripheral anterior synechiae first develop 180° away from the hole. The reverse may also happen, i.e., the synechiae precede the holes. The number of holes varies. The holes lead to a distorted pupil. The condition becomes apparent in late teens as iris atrophy. Glaucoma develops in adulthood. Glaucoma is difficult to manage. Essential iris atrophy is considered a variant of Chandler's syndrome by some authors.

Trabeculodysgenesis and Primary Congenital Glaucoma

From the discussions in the previous pages, it is obvious that congenital anomalies of the AC involve three tissues in combination or in isolation to cause glaucoma.

The tissues are given as follows:

1. Cornea
2. Iris
3. Trabeculum

The congenital anomalies of these tissues are collectively called neurocristopathy.* Isolated involvement of the trabeculum is the cause of primary congenital glaucoma, often erroneously referred to as buphthalmos.

> All large eyes are not glaucomatous. All eyes with trabeculodysgenesis will have glaucoma. All infantile eyes with raised tension will lead to buphthalmos.

A buphthalmic eye is an eye enlarged in all directions, including the cornea. The causes of such enlargement can be primary or secondary.

PRIMARY CONGENITAL GLAUCOMA

Primary congenital glaucoma is a rare disorder compared to adult primary glaucoma but a more devastating cause of rapidly developing blindness in children. Younger the child, greater the chance of losing vision. Adult glaucoma is one of the five major causes of blindness in the world. About 2% of the population above 40 years of age suffers from some kind of glaucoma. The exact percentage of children who suffer from glaucoma is not known. The available statistics is relevant only for primary congenital glaucoma, which is one in 10,000 live births. The adult primary glaucoma that causes blindness is slow, progressive, and almost symptomless. However, awareness of adult glaucoma is quite high in the general population and among practicing healthcare workers due to the relentless spread of information regarding adult glaucoma.

In contrast to this, childhood glaucoma under 3 years is always symptomatic unless it is mild. Loss of vision is fast. A nonverbal child does not complain of diminished vision but cannot ignore or hide watering, photophobia, or blepharospasm, which makes parents realize that all is not well with the child's eyes. Surprisingly, a child with primary glaucoma is otherwise healthy.

Classification of Primary Congenital Glaucoma

It is difficult to have a universally accepted classification of childhood glaucoma.

**Neurocristopathy:* Neurocristopathies are a group of congenital anomalies of the body due to pathological changes in the cells of the neural crest. Neurocristopathies may affect any structures arising from the neural crest. The cells give rise to both ectodermal and mesodermal cells; hence, in neurocristopathies, both types of cells are involved. The cells arising from neurocristopathies are pluripotent, i.e., they develop into an array of diverse cells during embryogenesis. In the eye, they are responsible for the maldevelopment of tissues involved with the development of the angle of the AC.

The maldevelopments are given as follows:

- Cornea—stroma and endothelium
- Trabecular meshwork
- Ciliary body
- Sclera

The following ocular structures do not develop from the neural crest:

- Fibers of extraocular muscles
- Endothelium of all the ocular and orbital structures

Examples of oculoneurocristopathy are given as follows:

- Posterior embryotoxon
- Axenfeld anomaly and syndrome
- Rieger anomaly and syndrome
- Peters anomaly
- Albinism
- Sturge-Weber syndrome
- All primary congenital glaucomas are neurocristopathies.

Note: Aniridia is not a neurocristopathy.

The various divisions and their subdivisions are given as follows:

- Genetics
- Age wise
- As per the tissue involved:
  - Single tissue involved
  - Multiple tissues involved
  - Involvement of nonocular tissue
- Etiology
- Width of the angle

Genetics

- *Hereditary:* Only 10% of cases are inherited as autosomal recessive.
- *Sporadic:* 90% of cases are sporadic.
- *Familial (second):* A sibling has a 5% chance of getting the disorder. This rises to 25% in the third sibling.
- *Consanguinity:* Incidence—rises many folds if parents are consanguineous.

Age of the First Presentation

- *Neonatal:* These are detected in infants <1 month. These are the cases that have raised IOP in utero.
- *Infantile (seen under):* 2 years
- *Late onset:* Developing at about 2 years
- *Juvenile:* Develops between 2 years to puberty

Tissues Involved

- Only ocular
  - Single tissue involved, i.e., trabecular dysgenesis
  - More than one tissue is involved:
    - Iridotrabecular dysgenesis
    - Iridodysgenesis
    - Iridocorneal dysgenesis
    - Corneal dysgenesis
- Associated with nonocular tissues—nonocular tissues commonly involved are dental and facial, which are not responsible for raising tension.

As Per Etiology

- *Primary:* Trabeculodysgenesis, wide angle
- *Secondary:* Multiple causes

As Per the Width and Angle of the Anterior Chamber

- Wide angle
- Narrow angle

Note: It is common for an eye with congenital glaucoma to have overlapping of above findings.

The most widely accepted classification was proposed by Duke Elder in 1964, which still seems to be the most practical.

He divided congenital glaucoma given as follows ***(Flowchart 22.3)****:*

- Neonatal
- Infantile
- Juvenile
- Early development of adult primary glaucoma

Following are various types of congenital glaucoma:

- *Congenital open angle:*
  - Neonatal
  - Infantile
  - Juvenile
- *Anterior segment dysgenesis:*
  - Axenfeld syndrome
  - Reiger anomaly
  - Reiger syndrome
  - Peters anomaly
  - Sclerocornea
  - Posterior polymorphous dystrophy
  - Chandler-Reese syndrome
- *Associated with systemic anomalies:*
  - Trauma
  - Uveitis
  - Iatrogenic (steroid)
- Secondary causes of congenital glaucoma

Besides these, there are common causes of secondary childhood glaucoma, such as:

- *Trauma:*
  - Accidental closed globe
  - Accidental open globe
  - *Surgical:*
    - Aphakia
    - Pseudophakia
    - Malignant glaucoma

Flowchart 22.3: Classification of congenital glaucoma.

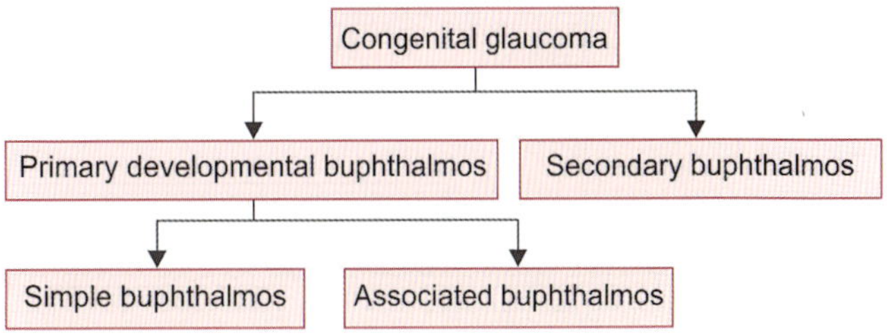

- *Uveitis:*
  - Congenital (rare)
  - Acquired
- Steroid induced
- Lens induced
- Aphakia and pseudophakia
- Intraocular malignancy

Another classification used presently is mentioned in **Flowchart 22.4**.

> - There is no condition where there is overproduction of aqueous.
> - Secondary glaucoma results due to ocular defects rather than without ocular defects.
> - Primary and secondary glaucoma may coexist, worsening each other.
> - All eyes under 3 years with raised intraocular pressure will develop buphthalmos and optic nerve changes. Eyes developing raised intraocular pressure after 3 years will not develop buphthalmos but will have optic nerve changes.

Clinical Features of Primary Congenital Glaucoma

General Information

The condition is rarer than adult glaucoma. However, it is a major cause of diminished vision in children that may be as severe as to be put in the category of legal blindness. This may even happen under constant supervision and an accurate diagnosis.

Like glaucoma in all ages, vision once lost is not retrieved, except for the part that has been lost by anterior segment changes. It is seen in one in 10,000 to one in 20,000 live births. It is more frequent in children with consanguineous parents. It is slightly more common among boys.

It is bilateral in about 70% of cases; when unilateral, the other eye may follow suit. Hence, in all uniocular cases, the other eye should be examined and followed regularly. In bilateral cases, both eyes may have symmetric involvement. Unilateral cases attract attention earlier than symmetric bilateral cases **(Figs. 22.6 and 22.7)**.

Seventy-five percent of cases seek consultation in the first year; twenty-five percent are present at birth or within a month of birth and may be misdiagnosed as nonglaucomatous epiphora. Primary congenital glaucoma is not associated with systemic disorders that may be correlated to glaucoma.

About 80% of cases are sporadic. The rest are autosomal recessives. In sporadic cases, 5% of siblings have a chance of developing the disease. This increases to 25% for subsequent siblings.

> An enlarged globe is not a sure sign of glaucoma.

Symptoms

The triad of symptoms that should point toward primary congenital glaucoma are given as follows:

- Watering
- Photophobia
- Blepharospasm

All the above symptoms should be explored individually before declaring the child to be glaucomatous **(Fig. 22.8)**.

***Flowchart 22.5** depicts the genesis of the triad of symptoms.*

Flowchart 22.4: Another classification of childhood glaucoma used currently.

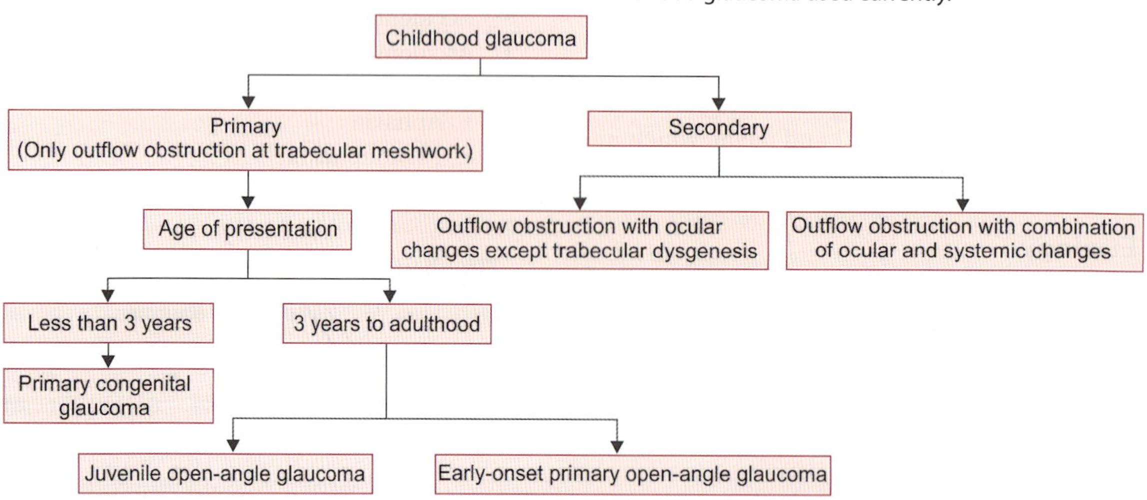

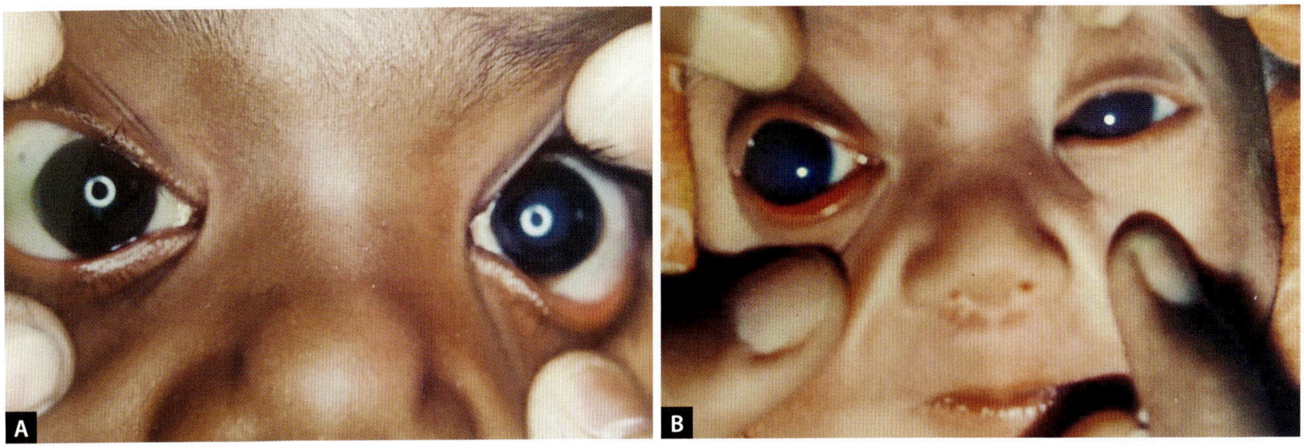

Figs. 22.6A and B: (A) Moderate bilateral congenital glaucoma; (B) Severe bilateral congenital glaucoma.
Courtesy: Dr Somen Misra.

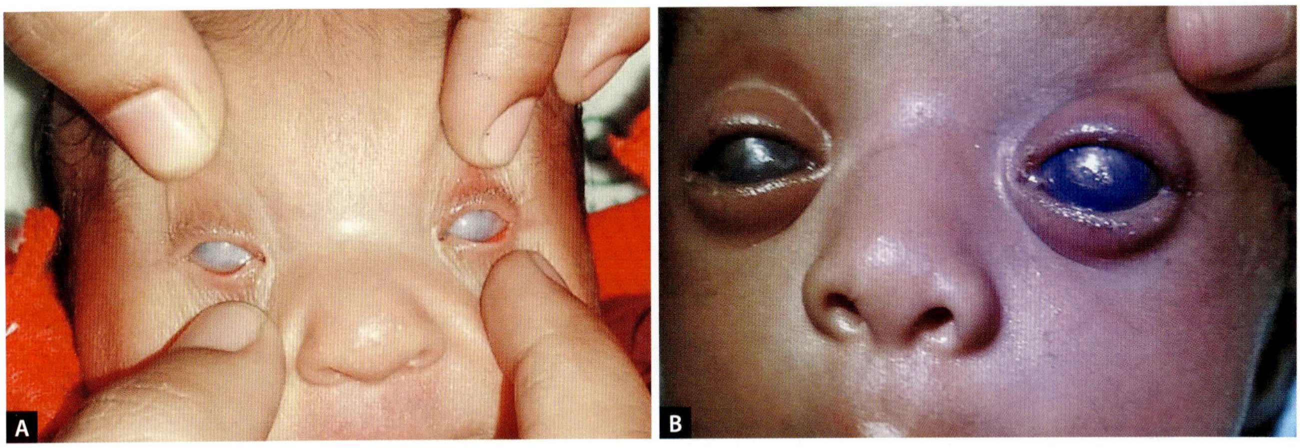

Figs. 22.7A and B: (A) Bilateral congenital glaucoma in a newborn; (B) Bilateral congenital glaucoma in an infant.
Courtesy: Professor ML Garg.

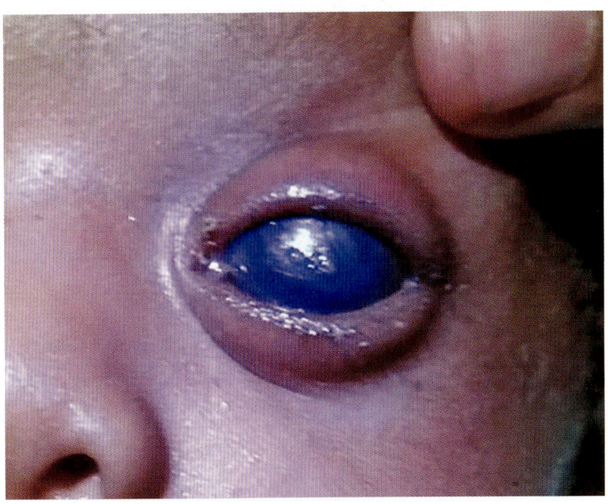

Fig. 22.8: Epithelial edema in congenital glaucoma.
Courtesy: Professor ML Garg.

Genesis of a Triad of Symptoms

The salient features of primary congenital glaucoma are given as follows:

- *Rise of intraocular tension:*
  - A child with primary congenital glaucoma may have raised IOP at birth.
  - The normal parameters of intraocular tension at various ages in children are given as follows:
    - *At birth:* 10 mm Hg
    - *At 3 years:* 12.5 mm Hg
    - *At 9 years:* 14.0 mm Hg
  - A difference of >5.00 mm Hg between two eyes is a red flag.
  - In cases of established primary congenital glaucoma, the tension may be as high as 80.00 mm Hg.

Flowchart 22.5: Genesis of the triad of symptoms.

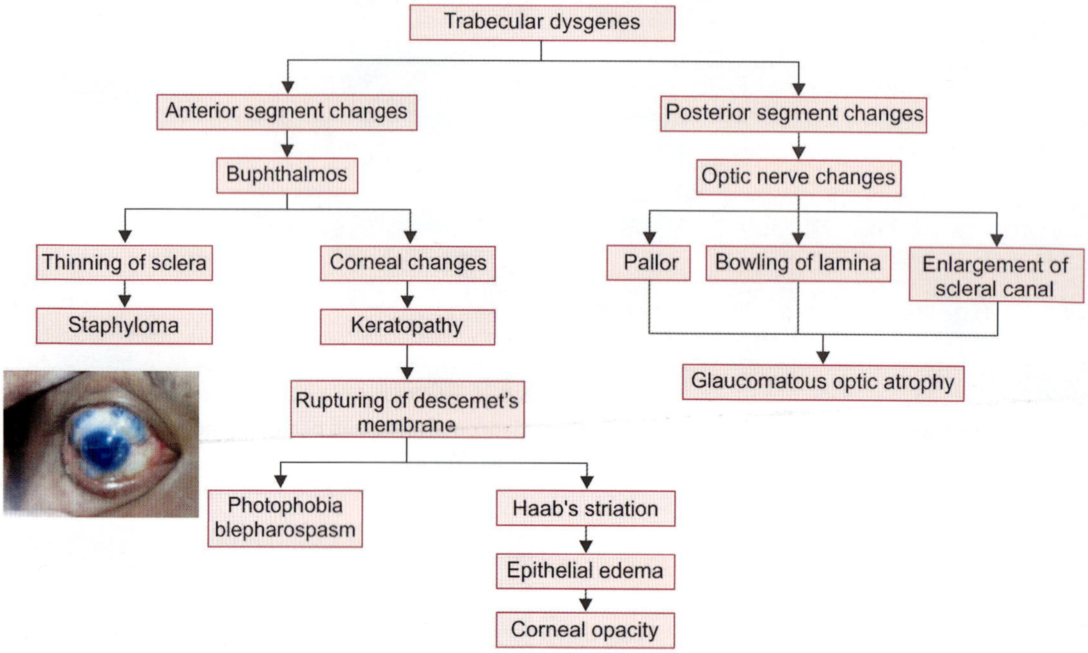

- The rise in tension is fast. The child may present with acute symptoms of lacrimation, photophobia, and blepharospasm due to decompensation following a rupture in Descemet's membrane.

- *Globe in primary congenital glaucoma:* Most of the changes visible on oblique illumination are in the anterior segment.
    - *Corneal changes:* The most spectacular and symptomatic changes are seen in the cornea, which comprises of:
        - *Diameter:* The corneal diameter of a full-term normal child is 9.5–10.5 mm. It increases by 0.5–1.0 mm in first 12 months to reach 12.0 mm and remains so for the rest of the life. Corneal diameter of >12.0 mm in the first year requires investigation to exclude glaucoma.
        - *Maximum enlargement:* It occurs at the corneoscleral junction
        - The other ominous sign is an asymmetry in diameter in two eyes.

Corneal diameter >13 mm at any age goes in favor of glaucoma.

- Unilaterally large corneas noted by parents are more likely to be due to raised intraocular tension.
- Corneal diameters >13 mm are not likely to change following successful surgery.

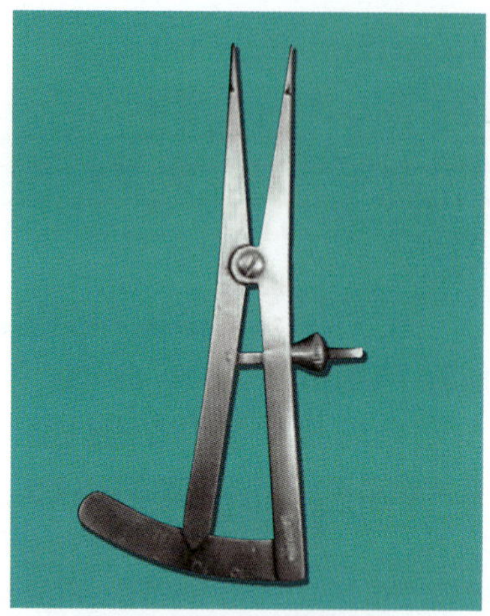

Fig. 22.9: Corneal caliper.

- In advanced cases, the diameter may be as high as 13–18 mm.
- Filtering surgeries always produce some degree of astigmatism.
- The best way to measure corneal diameter is to measure it with a corneal caliper under local anesthesia **(Fig. 22.9)**. The cornea should be measured both in horizontal and vertical meridians.
- The cause of the enlargement of the corneal diameter is its enhanced stretching in all

directions. The stretching is more in the pre-equatorial region. It is maximum in the anteroposterior axis, followed by horizontal, and least in the vertical meridian.
- Irregular stretching of cornea/sclera is a contributing factor in producing irregular myopic astigmatism.
- The cornea stops enlarging after 3 years, but the sclera keeps enlarging even thereafter.

The common manifestations of corneal stretching other than increased diameter are given as follows:

- Flattening of the central cornea causes a relative decrease in curvature myopia.
- *Rupture in Descemet's membrane:* As the cornea stretches, Descemet's membrane gives way, resulting in striated opacities of various shapes and sizes. The ruptures in the center of the cornea are horizontal and linear. Those on the periphery are curved and concentric with the pupil. The ruptures in Descemet's membrane in primary congenital glaucoma are referred to as Haab's striations.
- Rupture causes imbibement of the fluid in the corneal stroma, making it hazy and reducing vision.
- As the Descemet's membrane is less elastic than the stroma, it ruptures before the stroma.
- Persistent IOP is the cause of the stromal scar, which is one of the causes of irregular astigmatism and failure to regain age-matched vision following successful surgery.
    - *Scleral changes*: The scleral changes run concurrent with corneal changes. They are given as follows:
        - Irregular stretching of the sclera all round.
        - Stretching is more in the pre-equatorial region, with a maximum in the anteroposterior axis.
        - Irregular stretching is one of the causes of irregular astigmatism that is supplementary to corneal changes.
        - Due to more stretching on the anteroposterior axis, the globe has:
            - An appearance of pseudoproptosis.
            - The eyeball assumes the appearance of an eggshell.
            - The corneal scleral sulcus is obliterated, imparting a significant change in the surgical limbus and position of the ciliary body that may cause accidental placement of a sclerotomy during surgery.
            - Sclera becomes so thin that the uvea underneath gives a bluish discoloration, replacing the white color of the sclera. The discoloration may be all around or in patches. This is followed by the development of ciliary and equatorial staphylomas. The size and extent of staphylomas depend on the level of IOP and the duration of raised tension. If the tension remains very high and persists, it results in annular staphyloma. The staphylomas may regress completely or partially following successful filtering surgery.
            - Stretching of the sclera also influences the configuration of whole of the anterior segment; they are peripheral shifts of the scleral spur to which the ciliary body is attached, hence the shift of the ciliary body.
            - *Stretching of zonules:* This leads to snapping of the zonules, resulting in subluxation of the lens and ultimate dislocation.
            - *Flattening of lens:* This contributes to the deepening of AC, tremulousness of the iris, and a reduction in curvature myopia.

Flowchart 22.6 *summarizes the effect of stretching the globe.*

Anterior Chamber Changes in Primary Congenital Glaucoma

The depth of the AC depends on the time of onset, duration of raised IOP, and level of IOP. The AC is uniformly deep but less than aphakic unless the lens has been dislocated.

Causes of the deep AC in primary congenital glaucoma are given as follows:

- *Corneal:*
    - Increased curvature
    - Thinning of the cornea
- *Iris:*
    - Stretching of the iris leads to overall thinning of the iris substance
    - *Tremulousness of iris:* So long as the zonules are intact, the iris is nontremulous. The mildest tremulousness should be investigated for subtle subluxation. Mild tremulousness should first be seen under high magnification without dilatation and then with full mydriasis to examine the zonules.
    - Iris in primary congenital glaucoma is light-colored.

Flowchart 22.6: Effect of stretching of the globe.

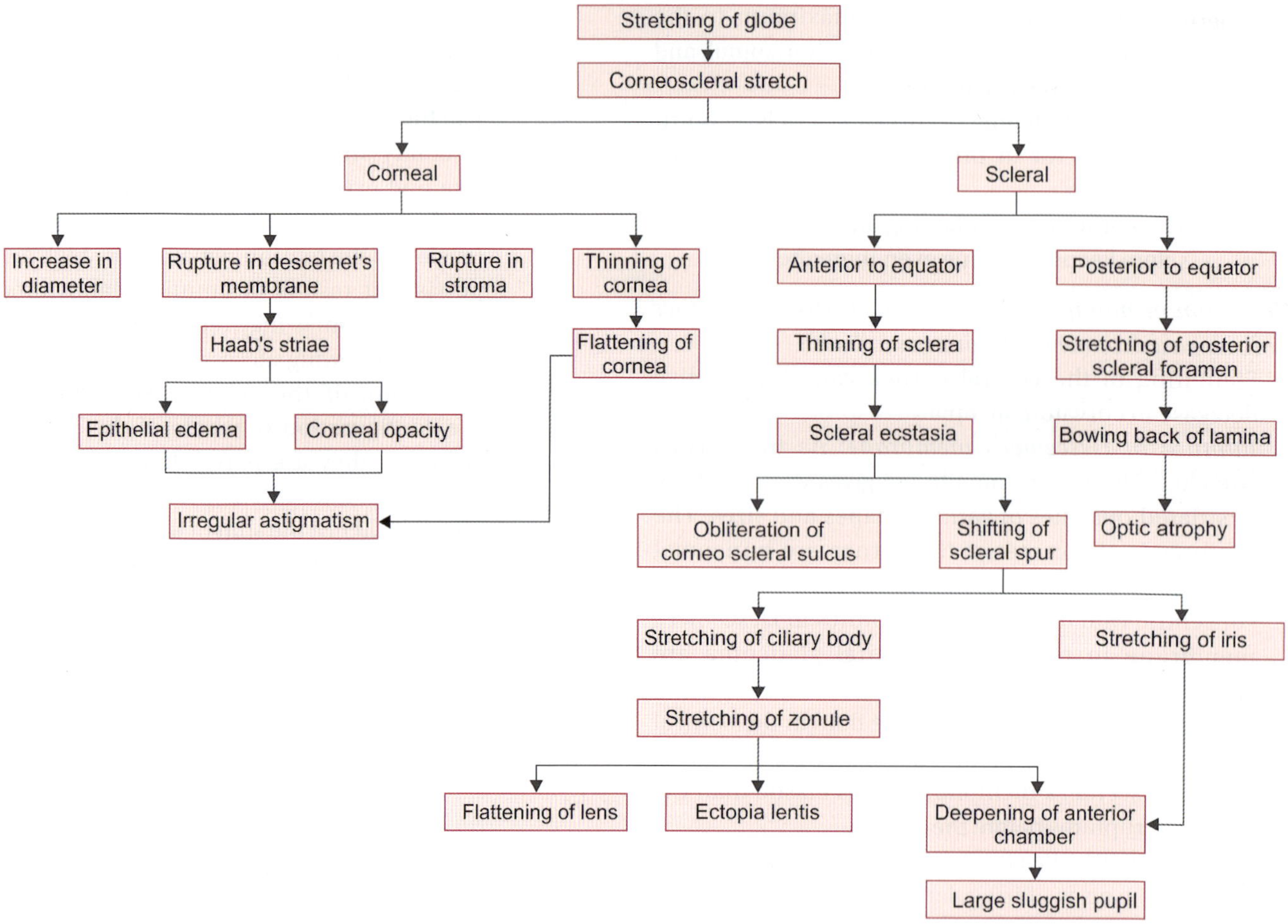

- *Lens:*
  - Stretching of zonules leads to flattening of lenses.
  - Disruption of zonules leads to subluxation that may end up in dislocation.
  - Once the lens is dislocated, the eye assumes the appearance of clinical aphakia
- *Angle of the AC:*
  - The angle is wide.
  - Presence of abnormal tissue points toward the possibility of secondary congenital glaucoma.
  - Barkan's membrane may be present
- Choroid, retina, and vitreous do not show any changes that can be correlated to congenital glaucoma except neural rim changes around the optic disk.
- *Optic disk:*
  - Neural rim changes—visible on OCT
  - Bowing back of lamina
  - Pallor of the disk
  - Glaucomatous cupping

The optic disk changes are reversible until 3 years of age. Thereafter, they become permanent and progressive.

Fundus Examination in Primary Congenital Glaucoma

Fundus can be examined by:

- Direct ophthalmoscope
- Direct ophthalmoscope on Koeppe goniolens
- Indirect ophthalmoscope with +30 D
- Slit lamp with +14 D
- Optical coherence tomography

The fundus changes in primary congenital glaucoma are given as follows:

- Confined to the optic disk and its neuroretinal rim.
- To appreciate the disk changes, it is better to recapitulate the appearance of an infantile disk without glaucoma.

Normal disk in children is given as follows:

- The disk does not show much difference from the adult disk.

- It looks smaller than an adult disk due to infantile hypermetropia and a small eyeball.
- The disk may be as pink as an adult disk or may be slightly pale. A white disk is a suspicious disk.
- Fundus changes are mostly pressure dependent and, hence, reversible.
- The cup does not regress after 3 years of age.
- Once the pressure is reduced to normal, the cupping stops. This is true until 3 years of age.
- The disk changes develop faster in children compared to adults with matching IOP.
- The disk can be seen fairly well, even without mydriasis.
- The disk is best seen with a direct ophthalmoscope over Koeppe goniolens.
- Cup–disk ratio of 0.5 and asymmetry between the two eyes are always suspicious.
- Disk in children tolerates raised IOP better than adults.
- The other examinations, such as corneal diameter, gonioscopy, and fundus examination, should be done in the same sitting.
- The loss of neural tissue in the vertical pole is an ominous sign.
- The scleral canal in children increases more horizontally.
- Cupping starts early in children but reverses if tension is brought low.
- The field changes do not regress.
- Asymmetry in the disk is a bad sign.

Tonometry in Primary Congenital Glaucoma

Intraocular tension can be easily recorded in a newborn under local anesthesia as an office procedure. Care should be taken not to exert pressure on the globe while separating the lids. Speculum is better avoided in recording intraocular tension. The tension is best recorded by noncontact handheld tonometers such as the tonopen, Perkin's handheld, and Goldmann tonometers.

In the absence of these, the tension can safely be recorded by a Schiotz tonometer. The most accurate measurement is recorded under general anesthesia, keeping in mind that the general anesthetic drugs modulate IOP in either way. Some are known to cause a rise in IOP; others lower it. A rough guideline is that depolarizing agents such as succinylcholine raise IOP while nonpolarizing agents lower it.

The list of drugs that cause a rise in intraocular pressure is given as follows:
- Succinylcholine: First 4–6 minutes
- Ketamine
- Nitrous oxide

Out of them, ketamine is the best. It leaves the child awake and cooperative. The only drawback is that it is a mild hallucinogen.

The list of drugs that lower intraocular pressure are all inhalants such as halothane and sevoflurane.

No attempt should be made to record IOP in a struggling child. **Table 22.2** shows normal intraocular tension as per age.

A child presenting with established primary congenital glaucoma generally has an IOP of 40 ± 5 mm Hg. In advanced cases, it may be as high as 80 mm Hg.

Three years of age is the cutoff age between primary congenital glaucoma and juvenile open-angle glaucoma. The diagnosis of juvenile primary glaucoma is often based on cupping.

Flowchart 22.7 shows the topographical basis of trabecular anomalies.

Ocular Examination Under Anesthesia in Primary Congenital Glaucoma

If it is found that the child does not cooperate or stand by the examination procedure in the outpatient department, a detailed examination under general anesthesia is ordered. An examination under general anesthesia should be done in the operating room. Anesthesia should be administered only by a competent anesthetist trained in pediatric anesthesia. Though most of the procedures do not require elaborate preanesthetic workups, it is still better that the child can be examined by a neonatologist or pediatrician the day before. Generally, an antibiotic drop is taken four times a day, a day before. The anesthetist should discuss the procedure and its utility with the parents and obtain informed consent as per the practice of the institute. It takes 10–30 minutes to finish the complete examination of the eye.

TABLE 22.2: Normal intraocular pressure (IOP) as per age.

Age	*IOP (mm Hg)*
Birth	9.6
1 year	10.6
2 years	12.0
12–16 years	15.5

Flowchart 22.7: Topographical basis of trabecular anomalies.

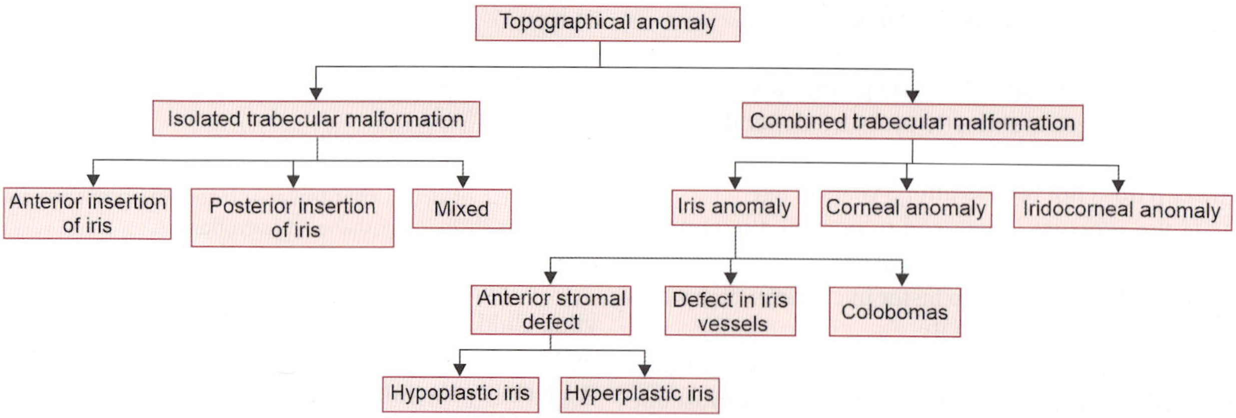

All the examinations should be preceded by an examination of vision with appropriate age-matched methods.

The examination can be divided into two parts, i.e.:

1. Examination of the anterior segment
2. Examination of the posterior segment

1. *The examination of the anterior segment includes*:
   a. Examination of the cornea by handheld slit lamp
   b. Measurement of corneal diameter by corneal calipers
   c. Recording of intraocular tension
   d. Ultrasonography
   e. Optical coherence tomography
   f. Ultrasonic biometry
   g. Refraction by streak retinoscope
   h. Gonioscopy
   i. Keratometry
2. *Examination of the posterior chamber includes*:
   a. Optic nerve
   b. Neuroretinal rim
   c. The whole periphery should be examined for any hidden malignancy, i.e., retinoblastoma.

Fundus can be examined by:

- Direct ophthalmoscope alone
- Direct ophthalmoscope over Koeppe's lens
- Indirect ophthalmoscope
- Fundus photography

> Direct gonioscopes are devices of choice because both eyes can be examined at the same time with one gonioscope over each eye.

Gonioscopy in Primary Congenital Glaucoma

Normal Neonatal Angle

It differs from the adults' angle in many ways:

- The angle of a neonate is narrower or absent.
- The trabecular structure is translucent and smooth.
- The iris is scalloped.
- There may be fine capillaries over the iris.

Gonioscopic Findings in Primary Congenital Glaucoma

- High insertion of the iris in the scleral spur
- Prominent trabecular tissue
- Hypoplasia of the iris stroma
- Barkan's membrane (the presence of Barkan's membrane has been under scrutiny since the beginning, so much so that it has been labeled as a theoretical tissue supposed to run across the trabecular meshwork obstructing the outflow).
- Lister's morning mist (fluffy tissue in peripheral iris)
- Loch monster sign (vascular loop in the angle)
- Iris may be inserted into the trabecular meshwork
- Iris insertion may be flat or concave
- Thickened trabecular beam
- In Sturge–Weber and rubella syndrome, the angle may be normal even with a raised IOP.

Ultrasonography (The Immersion Method of Ultrasonography is the Preferred Mode)

The normal axial length is 17.5–20.00 mm at birth. It should be 22.00 mm in 1 year. Following successful surgery, it should reduce by 1 mm, denoting the success of the surgery. Axial length is increased in congenital myopia.

Ultrasound Biometry

Ultrasound biometry is a noninvasive imaging procedure to examine the anterior segment in primary congenital glaucoma. It gives magnification similar to that of a clinical light microscope. It delineates corneal edema, iridocorneal changes in the depth of the AC, and the position of the lens.

Optical Coherence Tomography

Optical coherence tomography is yet another noninvasive method of examining optic nerve and nerve fiber layer thickness. The nerve fiber layer is the first to be affected in congenital glaucoma; it also shows changes in the angle of the AC.

Optical coherence tomography shows:

- Configuration of angle of AC
- Thickness of:
  - Retinal nerve fiber layer
  - Ganglion cell complex
- Optic cupping

Etiopathogenesis of Primary Congenital Glaucoma

The exact mechanism is debatable. The probable contributing factors given below play an important role, alone or in combination:

- The angle is premature.
- The angle and anterior uvea of a full-term child with primary congenital glaucoma are developmentally similar to that of a 7–8-month-old fetus.
- There is an abnormality in the cleavage of the angle.
- Failure of the iris and ciliary body to separate from the trabecular meshwork.
- The ciliary body is attached more anteriorly than normal.
- Presence of the so-called Barkan's membrane, the Loch monster sign, and Lister's morning mist.
- The condition is an isolated trabecular dysgenesis without involving the cornea or iris.
- The iris and ciliary body should recede in the case of the normal eye.
- Its failure to recede results in primary congenital glaucoma.
- Involvement of the cornea and iris will cause secondary congenital glaucoma.

Differential Diagnosis of Primary Congenital Glaucoma

This is divided into two parts, i.e.:

1. The child already has established glaucoma.
2. If the condition is glaucoma, it is primary congenital or it is due to other congenital anomalies of the anterior segment, i.e., posterior embryotoxon, Axenfeld anomaly, Rieger anomaly, Rieger syndrome, Reese syndrome, and Peters anomaly.

This differentiation is important because, on the basis of the type of congenital glaucoma, management depends on it to a large extent.

The symptoms that may be confused with primary congenital glaucoma or vice versa are given as follows:

- Watering
- Blepharospasm
- Large cornea
- Cloudy cornea

- *Watering:* The most common cause is congenital nasolacrimal duct obstruction. The other causes are given as follows:
  - Ophthalmia neonatorum
  - Corneal abrasion
  - Herpetic keratitis
  - Rubella keratitis
  - Uveitis
- *Blepharospasm:* The most common cause is a large traumatic epithelial defect.
- *Large cornea:* Normal corneas with congenital ptosis may be mistaken for corneas larger than normal, which can easily be excluded by comparing with the contralateral eye or measuring with corneal calipers.

One of the common causes of large corneas is megalocornea:

- A cornea >12.00 mm at birth is called megalocornea. Clinically, large corneas are put into two groups, i.e., (1) simple megalocornea and (2) anterior megalophthalmos. The former is nonprogressive, nonblinding, and polygenic, with only clinical findings of a cornea larger than normal, i.e., bright with normal AC depth and intraocular tension. The eyes are generally myopic.
- An eye with a large cornea other than the megalocornea is called an anterior megalophthalmos. The features are given as follows:
  - X-linked recessive
  - Bilateral
  - Progressive
  - The cornea is larger than normal.
  - Iris anomaly
  - Widened ciliary rim
- *Cloudy cornea:* The cornea of a full-term normal child should be clear and bright. In some neonates, the cornea may have some haze at birth that passes off in a few days.

  The other causes of cloudy cornea besides primary congenital glaucoma are given as follows:
  - *Trauma:* Mostly in forceps delivery.

- *Infection:* Rubella and herpes simplex.
- Sclerocornea*
- Trisomy 13†
- *Congenital corneal dystrophies:*
  - Congenital endothelial dystrophy
  - Posterior polymorphous dystrophy
  - Congenital stromal dystrophy
  - Errors of metabolism.

Following is a summary of the common anterior segment dysgenesis that is associated with congenital glaucoma.

- *Posterior embryotoxon:* It consists of anterior displacement of Schwalbe's line visible on bright oblique illumination of a slit lamp with an iris attached to it as a ridge protruding in AC; the attached iris may be thin as a thread or wide; the condition is without glaucoma.
- *Axenfeld syndrome:* Above findings with raised intraocular tension without any systemic features.
- *Rieger anomaly:* Above defects with congenital anomalies of the iris: pseudopolycoria, corectopia, without glaucoma.
- *Rieger syndrome:* Above findings in children with anomalies of the face and teeth, mental retardation, and glaucoma.
- *Peters anomaly:* Central corneal opacity, iris attached to the opacity, lens touching corneal opacity. The cause of opacity is the absence of Descemet's membrane glaucoma.

Systemic syndromes with congenital raised intraocular tension are given in ***Table 22.3****.*

TABLE 22.3: Systemic syndromes with congenital raised intraocular tension.

Syndrome	*Clinical features*
Sturge–Weber syndrome	• Skin hemangioma overdistribution of the trigeminal nerve • Intracranial hemangioma resulting in convulsions and intracranial calcification • Conjunctival and episcleral hemangioma • Choroidal hemangioma • Anomalies of the angle
Lowe syndrome	• Oculocerebral renal syndrome • X-linked recessive • Male preponderance • Cataract • Aminoaciduria • Mental retardation • Glaucoma
Neurofibromatosis	• Plexiform neurofibroma of the skin • Café-au-lait spots • Lisch nodules on the iris • Angle anomaly • Glaucoma
Trisomy 13	Patau syndrome

SECONDARY GLAUCOMAS IN CHILDREN

The following conditions may be associated with raised intraocular tension in children:

- Aphakia
- Pseudophakia
- *Trauma:*
  - Angle recession
  - Traumatic hyphema
  - *Juvenile xanthogranuloma:* It is a benign rare histiocytosis seen mostly in infants and children with ocular, cutaneous, and systemic involvement by yellow nonmalignant growth. Ocular involvement is seen in <1% cases as spontaneous hyphema, which terminates in secondary glaucoma. The skin and ocular lesions have a tendency to resolve without treatment. It is frequently associated with raised intraocular tension. The exact cause is not known.
- *Anterior uveitis:*
  - Juvenile rheumatoid arthritis
  - Rubella

**Sclerocornea* is a rare congenital anomaly of the anterior part of the eyeball, i.e., the cornea and sclera, where there is no differentiation between the transparency of the cornea and sclera. The cornea becomes as opaque as the sclera. The corneoscleral sulcus is either obliterated or very shallow. It can be peripheral, leaving a central cornea, or it may be totalis, i.e., the whole of the cornea is scleralized. It is polygenic and may be associated with other systemic syndromes.

†*Trisomy 13*—Patau syndrome is a rare condition where the newborn has a very short lifespan. Most of them die within the first month. They are generally associated with multiple ocular disorders.

- Steroid induced
- *Pupillary block:* Ectopia lentis, spherophakia, microphakia, and microspherophakia
- Retinopathy of prematurity
- *Intraocular malignancy:* Retinoblastoma

MANAGEMENT OF CHILDHOOD GLAUCOMA

The management of childhood glaucoma is difficult and frustrating. It is palliative.

The aim of management is given as follows:

- Give relief from lacrimation and photophobia
- Reduce IOP soon enough to:
  - Salvage maximum vision
  - Prevent damage to the optic nerve
- Keep the child under observation for changes in refractive error and manage amblyopia:
  - The first part of management consists of early diagnosis.
  - The second part is to counsel the parents regarding:
    - Poor results of treatment
    - Limited role of medication
    - Informing them that surgery is the definitive treatment Single surgery may not be enough - Repeat surgeries may be required The child in spite of successful surgery may remain visually challenged.

The management can be divided into the following:

- *Definitive:*
  - Surgery
  - Laser
  - Combination
- *Palliative:* Medical
- Ancillary

MEDICAL TREATMENT

Medical treatment has a limited role in the present day management of raised intraocular tension in children.

- They are given to keep the tension low until surgery.
- Miotics have no role to play (pilocarpine is used to constrict the pupil to do goniotomy, trabeculotomy, or trabeculectomy).
- The most widely used drug in the short term is a carbonic anhydrase inhibitor (CAI), either orally (Diamox) or topically (dorzolamide). Oral Diamox lowers IOP faster than topical dorzolamide. Diamox is given orally at 10 mg/kg of body weight in three divided doses. Oral Diamox should be prescribed to children with all precautions needed in administering sulfa drugs in consultation with neonatologist/pediatrician. Local drops are safer.
- *Beta-blockers:* The most widely used beta-blocker is timolol maleate 0.5% two times a day. Beta-blockers administered even as local drops have their own systemic side effects.
- Other antiglaucoma drugs used in adult glaucoma are either not effective or contraindicated in children.

SURGICAL TREATMENT

Surgery is the best treatment available. Surgical treatments available are given as follows:

- *Paracentesis:* No more used
- *Goniotomy:*
  - Direct goniotomy in a cloudy cornea
  - Goniotomy with an operating gonioscope with clear cornea
- Goniopuncture
- Trabeculotomy*
- Trabeculectomy*
- Trabeculotomy with trabeculectomy*
- Glaucoma implants
- *Laser:* The types of laser procedures available are given as follows:
  - Laser trabeculoplasty
  - Cyclophotocoagulation:
- Transscleral by neodymium-doped yttrium aluminum garnet (Nd:YAG)
- Endoscopic by diode and krypton
- Cyclocryodestruction.

Flowchart 22.8 is a summary of the various types of surgical procedures available for congenital glaucoma.

Goniopuncture

Goniopuncture is an almost blind procedure for making a single puncture in the trabecular meshwork without operating a gonioscope with a specially devised goniotome. It consists of entering the AC through a clear cornea. The knife passes across the constricted pupil to reach the opposite angle, only to emerge at the limbus without puncturing the conjunctiva **(Fig. 22.10)**.

*With or without antifibrotic substances.

Flowchart 22.8: Types of surgical procedures available for congenital glaucoma.

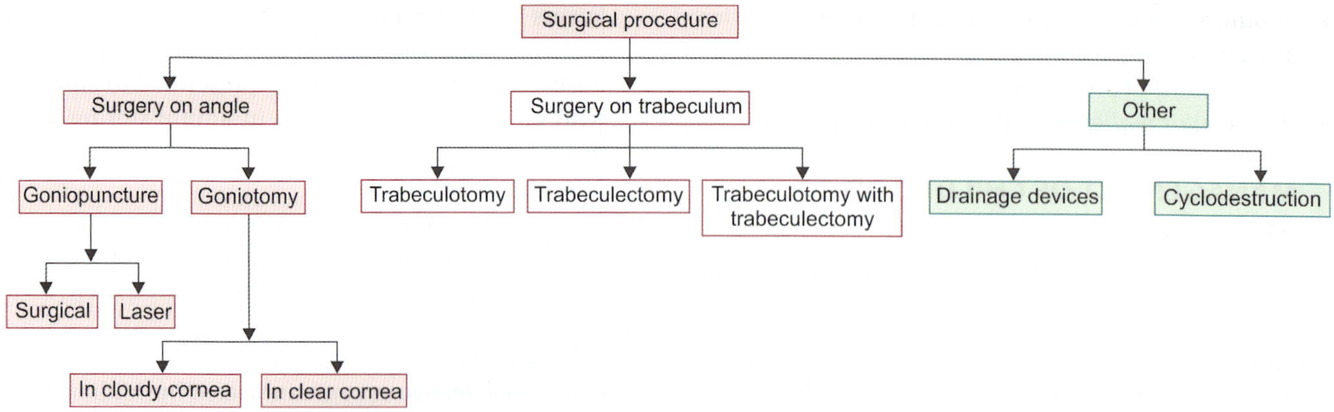

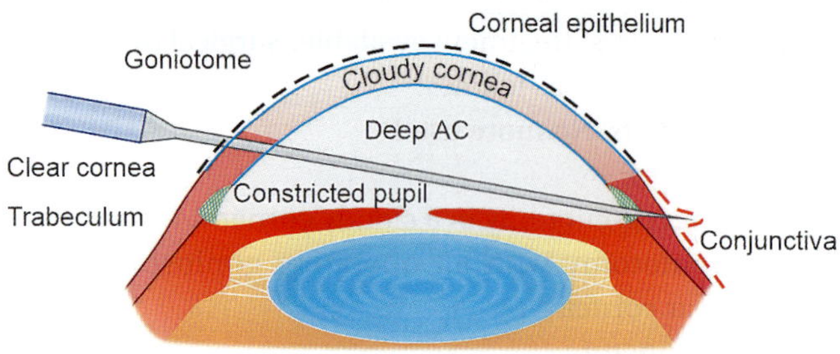

Fig. 22.10: Outline of goniopuncture. (AC: anterior chamber)

The various modifications of goniopuncture are given as follows:

- After deep sclerotomy
- After canaloplasty

The former creates a pool called Descemet's window to allow the escape of aqueous humor from AC. This may later form a filtering bleb.

Trabeculotomy ab externo is also called nonpenetrating trabeculotomy, in which Schlemm's canal is exposed and stripped off under a large scaffold.

Goniotomy

It is to incise the trabecular face with a goniotome under a goniotomy lens and microscope under general anesthesia in an eye with a clear cornea.

Trabeculotomy

External Trabeculotomy

The conjunctiva is incised and undermined to expose the sclera. A vertical incision is given at the limbus to expose Schlemm's canal. Schlemm's canal is cut. The two cut ends are identified, and a specially designed trabeculotome is passed in one cut-end until the whole of the trabeculotome passes concentric with the limbus. The arm of the trabeculotome is swept toward the pupil like a wiper to split the canal. The trabeculotome is withdrawn. The procedure is repeated in the other end. The conjunctival is replaced, and the eye is bandaged.

Internal Trabeculotomy

Internal trabeculotomy, also called TRAB360, is a newer glaucoma procedure belonging to a group of glaucoma surgical procedures known as microinvasive glaucoma surgery (MIGS). This procedure is similar to the *trabectome* and another procedure called gonioscopy-assisted transluminal trabeculotomy (GATT). Unlike trabeculectomy or tube shunt surgery, which bypass the internal drainage system to filter fluid outside the globe, these procedures are designed to improve eye pressure by enhancing drainage through the natural internal drainage pathway. Specifically, this procedure involves stripping the trabecular meshwork to expose the internal drainage canal called the Schlemm's canal, which then has access to the remainder of the drainage system known as the collector channels. In effect, stripping the trabecular meshwork removes much of the resistance to the flow of internal eye fluid, allowing the internal eye fluid to drain faster and more efficiently, resulting in lower eye pressure. However, in those patients who have poor outflow through the collector channels, this procedure may only have limited effectiveness. Determining the status of the collector channels cannot be made prior to surgery but can be assessed indirectly during surgery. Scarring at the site where the tissue is removed may cause a block in the flow of internal eye fluid and limit the success of surgery.

A small incision is made in the clear part of the cornea, and using a specialized viewing lens, a device is inserted into the eye, and the trabecular meshwork is pierced. Then, the canal is threaded with a special stent for its entire length around the eye (thats why it is called a 360 trabeculotomy) and then pulled to strip the meshwork. This maneuver will result in considerable reflux bleeding, which sometimes requires an injection of gel-like material to control the bleeding. Most of the time, the blood clears, and the eye pressure decreases significantly.

Trabeculectomy

It is a modified subsclerotomy filtering surgery that establishes communication between the AC and the subsclerotomy space/subconjunctival space.

The steps, in short, are given as follows:

- Anesthesia
- Traction suture
- Conjunctival incision
- Injection of antifibrotic agents, such as fluorouracil (5FU) and mitomycin C
- Cautery/bipolar cautery
- Scleral flap shaping
- Scleral flap dissection
- Paracentesis
- Sclerostomy
- Peripheral iridectomy
- Suturing the scleral flap
- Conjunctival sutures
- Subconjunctival antibiotic injection

Trabeculectomy with Trabeculotomy

It is a combined procedure of usual trabeculectomy with trabeculotomy added to it, performed with the help of a special Harms trabeculotome.

Cyclodestructive Surgeries

Cyclodestructive surgeries are used to reduce the function of the ciliary body, thus preventing the formation of aqueous. These methods are kept reserved for cases where multiple surgeries have failed. The results can be achieved by:

- Diathermy (no more used)
- Cryo (rarely used)
- Cycloablation by ultrasound
- Laser (commonly used)

The laser procedures can be done with or without an endoscope.

The common procedures are given as follows:

- Cyclophotocoagulation
- Micropulse diode

Glaucoma Implants

Glaucoma drainage devices (GDDs) work by regulating the flow of aqueous from the AC to the subconjunctival space through a small device, one end of which is placed in the AC and the other end connected to this device in the subconjunctival space away from the limbus between the two adjacent recti. The principle is to regulate the flow from AC out without allowing the AC to collapse.

CHILDHOOD SECONDARY GLAUCOMAS

The list of disorders that cause glaucoma under 15 years of age is long. Some of them are genetically determined, may be congenital or acquired, may be associated with only ocular disorders or with systemic disorders, may be post-traumatic, postuveitic, associated with malignancy, or iatrogenic (steroid induced).

The ocular anomalies that are associated with raised IOP are given as follows:

- Anterior chamber cleavage syndrome: Iridocorneal dysgenesis
- Iridotrabecular dysgenesis
- Posterior polymorphous corneal dystrophy
- Sclerocornea
- Aniridia

Systemic syndromes associated with raised IOP are given as follows:

- Sturge–Weber syndrome
- Neurofibromatosis
- Marfan syndrome
- Marchesani syndrome
- Lowe syndrome
- Reiger syndrome
- Peters anomaly
- Mucopolysaccharidosis

Secondary causes of raised IOP in the eyes other than ocular dysgenesis are given as follows:

- *Trauma:*
    - *Acute:*
        - Hyphema
        - Trauma to the angle
    - *Chronic:* Sequel to angle recession
- Steroid induced

- Uveitis
- Retinoblastoma
- Lens related
- *Postoperative:*
  - Aphakia
  - Pseudophakia
- Retinopathy of prematurity

TRAUMATIC GLAUCOMA IN CHILDREN

Traumatic glaucoma in children is more common than primary congenital glaucoma, glaucoma associated with AC dysgenesis, and systemic congenital anomalies put together. Trauma of both types, i.e., closed globe and open globe injuries, is capable of causing raised intraocular tension. The factors could be mechanical or nonmechanical. The former is more likely to cause glaucoma. The nonmechanical causes are headed by chemical injuries. Alkalis cause more glaucoma than acids of the same strength and identical exposure time. The cause of glaucoma in chemical injuries lies in the fact that they cause initial shrinkage of the coat of the eye, followed by a series of changes in the anterior segment.

The immediate effect of an open-angle injury on ocular tension is a precipitous fall in IOP that may or may not be accompanied by an extrusion of intraocular structures, ranging from minimal (i.e., a small iris prolapse) to as massive as the extrusion of all the intraocular contents. Such a calamity is beyond the retrieval of the function of the eye.

Following a small penetrating injury, the eyeball becomes soft without recordable intraocular tension. Larger open globe injuries, if not repaired, keep on leaking with nonrecordable tension. In a few cases, the wound heals, and tension builds up that may overshoot the physiological level mostly due to the post-traumatic deformity of the angle.

The rise of intraocular tension may be acute and short-lived, may be persistent, and may develop months later. All post-traumatic glaucomas do not have a similar presentation, and their management depends on the nature of the injury.

One of the common divisions of traumatic glaucoma is given as follows:

- *Following a closed globe injury:*
  - *Mechanical:*
    - Contusion
    - Concussion
  - Chemical
- *Following a penetrating injury:*
  - Surgical
  - Accidental:
    - With a retained foreign body
    - Without retained foreign body

CHILDHOOD GLAUCOMA DUE TO CLOSED GLOBE INJURY

These are generally unilateral unless there is a sudden increase in ambient atmospheric pressure, as happens in the explosion of a big cracker in a closed room. There is generally a fall in IOP, following a blunt injury due to a short-lived ciliary shutdown. In a few hours, the tension starts rising and may reach age-matched IOP and remain so unless the following factors intervene:

- *Blood in the AC:*
  - Whole blood
  - Blood constituents
- *Lens:*
  - *Increased in size:* Sudden or delayed swelling.
  - *Position:*
    - Subluxation
    - Entrapment in the pupil
    - Dislocation in the AC
    - Rupture of the capsule:
      - Phacolytic
      - Phacotoxic
    - Aphakia
- *Vitreous:* Vitreous in the AC
- Angle:
  - Debris in angle
  - Recession of the angle (delayed)

The hemogenic glaucomas can be:

- Total hyphema (red cell glaucoma)
- Hemolysis of blood
- Ghost cell glaucoma

GLAUCOMA DUE TO TOTAL HYPHEMA

Glaucoma following closed globe injuries depends on the amount of blood in the AC and its duration. Following a blunt injury, the globe is compressed anteroposteriorly, almost obliterating the AC. This forces the aqueous toward the angle. The force may tear the iris from its root, resulting in iridodialysis. It may be severe enough to cause laceration of the ciliary body facing the pupil. It may cause cyclodialysis or result in a recession of the angle of the AC. The normal iris does not bleed even when it is cut during surgical iridectomy or sphincterotomy, unless the iris is inflamed or vascularized. However, due to an unexplained mechanism, the iris bleeds when torn from its root, in contrast to the ciliary body, which is prone to bleed even following mild trauma.

Bleeding may start immediately or be delayed for hours or days. The amount of blood varies from specks of blood to as much as to fill the whole of the AC. The former is visible on a slit lamp, while the latter is obvious on oblique illumination, even with parents noticing it.

The effect of total hyphema is twofold, i.e., injury causing traumatic miosis and obliteration of meshwork. The small pupil may be blocked by blood in the AC, which is less frequent than blood-obliterating meshwork.

The RBCs, being heavier, settle down at the most dependent part, i.e., the lower part of the AC, if the child is upright. Initially, the hyphema moves with the position of the head. A small hyphema may disappear in a few days, even without treatment. Blood filling the whole of the AC behaves differently. The most common effect of large hyphema is the fast rise of IOP, which adds extra pain to an already painful eye. The vision is reduced to the perception of light or, at the most, hand movement close to the face. The conjunctiva is congested with circumciliary congestion. If the child is made to sit erect for a few hours, the heavy RBCs settle down at the bottom of the AC, allowing aqueous to drain again from the opened-up trabecular meshwork at the upper part. This reduces pain and improves vision. Initially, the blood is bright red in color with a horizontal border toward the pupil. With time, blood starts clotting, which is seen as a change of color, i.e., from bright red to brown and ultimately black. Due to some ill-understood mechanism, the clot assumes a spherical appearance that is referred to as a black ball. By the time blood clots, the aqueous in front of the pupil starts clearing up from total opacity to translucency and ultimately clears. Though the aqueous may look clear, in fact, some RBCs remain suspended in the aqueous, visible only with high power and good illumination, which may be mistaken for an aqueous flare.

Glaucoma due to total hyphema can be divided into the following groups:

- *Acute glaucoma:* Hemogenic glaucoma
- *Delayed:* Hemolytic and ghost cell glaucoma
- Angle-recession glaucoma

In hemogenic glaucoma, the macrophages engulf the particulate materials in the aqueous, such as hemoglobin, inflammatory cells, lens particles, and residual viscoelastic substances that are large enough to obstruct the trabecular meshwork, resulting in the rise of intraocular tensions.

The macrophages themselves assume a red tinge and are seen circulating in the aqueous. The trabecular meshwork, too, becomes red-tinged. These changes, along with raised intraocular tension, constitute hemolytic glaucoma, which is a self-limiting secondary open-angle glaucoma. The tension may take a few weeks to months within physiological limits. This time lapse may be long enough to cause changes in the optic nerve and field. In contrast to this, the other variety, which is also secondary glaucoma, is caused not by macrophages but by RBCs themselves. These cells are called ghost cells, which are deformed RBCs from which hemoglobin has been lost. Normal RBCs are malleable enough to squeeze through the meshwork, but the ghost cells do not pass through the already swollen trabeculum and cause a rise in IOP.

Management

Management consists of anticipating the possible development of hemogenic glaucoma following a closed-angle injury through frequent follow-up, i.e., vision, best-corrected vision, and measurement of IOP. If glaucoma is detected, it must be treated with standard antiglaucoma drugs.

> Epinephrine derivatives, prostaglandin analogues, and miotics are contraindicated in hemorrhagic glaucoma.

If antiglaucoma drugs fail, the best option is surgery, which may be as minor as paracentesis to as extensive as a filtering operation.

Management of Hyphema-induced Rise of Intraocular Pressure in Children

- Bed rest for a few days. It helps clear blood from the AC. If the hyphema does not subside after 48 hours, an attempt must be taken to reduce the IOP by medical means, which include the following:
  - Oral CAI in a dose of 10 mg/kg/day with potassium supplement and all the precautions required while administering CAI.
  - Oral glycerin in doses of 1 cc/kg/day in two divided doses.
  - Intravenous mannitol.
- Prevent rebleeding by administrating aminocaproic acid at a dose of 50 mg/kg/day. The efficacy of this drug has not been well established.

All the above drugs should be administered in consultation with a pediatrician and an anesthetist.

If tension does not come down in 48 hours of medical treatment, a simple guarded paracentesis of AC is indicated. The AC may have to be flushed with a balanced salt solution. If this fails to remove the clotted blood, stabbed valve incisions are made 1.00 mm inside the limbus, one on the temporal side and the other on the nasal side. Through one, viscoelastic is introduced to force the clot out. Pressing the lower lip of the wound helps it drain. The viscoelastic should be washed with balanced salt solution (BSS), followed by introducing a bubble of sterile air. The eye is bandaged with antibiotics and homatropine.

The eye is watched for rebleeding for a week, and the IOP is monitored.

ANGLE-RECESSION GLAUCOMA

This is delayed-acquired uniocular wide-angle glaucoma, more common in boys following a closed globe injury. The glaucoma may develop in eyes that had hyphema in the past or even without hyphema. It generally develops months to years after a blunt injury. However, it may develop earlier than 12 months. This makes it mandatory for exploring the possibility of blunt injury in the past in all cases of uniocular wide-angle glaucoma in adolescence and young adults. Simple angle recession happens in 20–90% of eyes with blunt injuries. Only 10% of them may develop angle-recession glaucoma. Angle recession following a blunt injury may be as small as 10° to >270°. However, a 360° recession has not been reported. Recession <180° is not likely to develop glaucoma or may develop years later. The most common extent of recession to end up in glaucoma is between 180° and 270°. Glaucoma developing in eyes <20°–30° is most likely due to preexisting primary open-angle glaucoma that may be obvious by other signs of glaucoma, most probably of genetic origin.

The recession of the angle per se is not the cause of glaucoma. To understand the pathogenesis, the following factors must be kept in mind:

- *Effect of a blunt injury to the ciliary body:*
  - There is a tear between the circular and longitudinal fibers of the ciliary body.
  - The anterior ciliary arteries may be involved, causing bleeding.
  - A tear in the ciliary body may be associated with irido- and cyclodialysis.
- *Changes in the trabecular meshwork:* As it has been pointed out, the causes of the rise of IOP cannot be explained on the basis of the recession of angle alone. It may be accompanied by changes in trabecular meshwork as well, which are given as follows:
  - Degenerative process involving trabecular meshwork following the original hyphema or rebleeding.
  - Scarring in the trabecular meshwork, obliterating the pores.
  - Development of a membrane that is hyaline in nature extends from the end of Descemet's membrane—over the meshwork—over the anterior iris surface.
  - In rare instances, the membrane may shrink and cause secondary angle closure.

The angle recession may be associated with rupture of the pupillary margin, trauma to the sphincter, mydriasis, split in the iris stroma, pseudopolycoria, iridodonesis, phacodonesis, zonulolysis, and ectopia lentis.

The other eye may have open-angle glaucoma unrelated to trauma following an applicable genetic trait.

Investigations

- High degree of suspicion in all cases of unilateral secondary open-angle glaucoma, with special reference to a history of blunt injury in the eye under examination.
- Repeated recording of the IOP, fundus examination, and field examination.
- *Gonioscopy:* Gonioscopy is the gold standard of all investigations. The initial gonioscopy should be done with Koeppe's direct gonioscope. Both eyes should be examined simultaneously to compare the two eyes.

Gonioscopic changes in angle-recession glaucoma are given as follows:

- Widening of the ciliary band—that may not be uniform all over
- Paleness of the scleral spur
- Whitening of meshwork
- Sprinkling of meshwork with pigment
- Widening of the angle

Other less commonly used investigations are given as follows:

- Ultrasound biomicroscopy
- Optical coherence tomography of the anterior segment

Management

Management of the condition is similar to that of wide-angle glaucoma in that, most of the time, in response to local medical treatment that consists of aqueous suppressants such as CAIs, beta-blockers, and alpha-agonists; prostaglandin analogues are not preferred because of their tendency to cause inflammatory reactions. In cases of medical treatment failure, surgical intervention is required, which could be laser trabeculoplasty or routine filtering operations.

STEROID-INDUCED GLAUCOMA

This is acquired secondary open-angle glaucoma seen under 20 years of age, more often in males. It is avoidable iatrogenic reversible glaucoma due to the use of steroids in steroid responders. It takes at least 3 weeks of constant use of steroids to develop the disease. The only exception is the intravitreal injection of triamcinolone acetonide, where the rise may be fast, if not abrupt. Fortunately, such an incidence is rarer in children.

Steroid use in all its forms can cause steroid-induced glaucoma. The list is headed by ocular drops, both clear solution or suspension. Steroid-containing ointments also cause the malady. The other routes are subconjunctival injection, periocular injection of clear solution, or depot. The depot steroids available for ocular use are triamcinolone acetonide and methylprednisolone acetate.

Nonocular routes of administration that cause glaucoma are oral tablets, subcutaneous depot, skin ointment, nasal inhalants, nasal sprays, nasal drops, and intra-articular injection.

All children receiving steroids do not develop glaucoma. Only children who are steroid responders are likely to develop glaucoma. The incidence of steroid-induced glaucoma is rare in nonresponders. A history of primary open-angle glaucoma, myopia, and diabetes in parents makes children more vulnerable to steroid-induced glaucoma. All steroids are not equally responsible for steroid-induced glaucoma. Glucocorticosteroids are more likely to cause glaucoma in a shorter period of time than nonglucocorticosteroids.

The steroids that cause glaucoma the most are:

Prednisolone, prednisone, dexamethasone, betamethasone, triamcinolone, and rimexolone are less potent than others. Fluorometholone causes the least rise in the presser.

Frequency, strength, and duration of use of steroids also influence the duration of the onset and range of IOP. In the uniocular use of steroids, the other eye may also have a marginal rise. The common conditions that contribute to the development of steroid-induced glaucoma are spring catarrh, uveitis in children, recurrent bilateral phlycten, aphakia, pseudophakia, sympathetic ophthalmia, keratoplasty, and interstitial keratitis. The steroid is responsible for the rise of IOP, independent of the primary pathology that may be a contributory factor. Out of the above list, spring catarrh is the most common cause because:

- It may start even at <3 years of age
- It requires frequent use of strong steroids to achieve quick results
- Requires prolonged use of steroids

The next in the list is pseudophakia in children, which requires a low dose of steroids for months to years in low concentrations but less frequently. The exact mechanism of the steroid-induced rise of IOP is not well understood; the condition is basically an impediment to outflow that can be brought about by a combination of predisposing factors, i.e., structural and biochemical changes in the trabecular meshwork. The important predisposing factors are response to the steroid, family history of open-angle glaucoma, and prolonged use of the steroid for systemic pathology.

The trabecular changes in steroid-induced glaucoma are given as follows:

- Accumulation of polymerized glycosaminoglycans in trabecular meshwork
- Accumulation of debris in trabecular meshwork
- Reduced phagocytosis in the trabecular meshwork
- Inhibition of prostaglandin
- The above factors work in various combinations

Though most of the steroid-induced glaucoma is secondary open angle, preexisting secondary angle closures such as following uveitis and trauma may worsen the pressure-raising effect of the steroid.

Clinical Presentation

Clinical presentation is similar to primary open-angle glaucoma in adults, i.e., almost symptomless, without congestion.

Various methods of presentation include:

- Discovered on routine fundus examinations for conditions other than glaucoma.

- *Diminished distant vision:* The child is brought to be prescribed glasses as the child does not see writing on the board in the class or views television from a short distance.
- Squint
- Amblyopia
- *Buphthalmos:* Children under 3 years who have been put on a strong steroid for >3 weeks, more than three times following an IOL implant, may present with buphthalmos and be mistaken for having primary congenital glaucoma.

Examination

The following features are found:

- Noncorrectable visual loss
- Raised IOP that falls to normal on withdrawal of the steroid
- Open angle
- May have steroid-induced cataracts that may stop progressing. Steroid-induced cataracts may be enhanced in presenile age.
- Glaucomatous optic atrophy
- Nerve fiber layer defect on OCT
- *Field changes:* Matching disk changes that are irreversible
- Noncongested eye
- *Large sluggish pupil:* The size of the pupil depends on the duration of the IOP and the height of the persistently raised pressure.

Differential Diagnosis

- Milder form of primary congenital glaucoma of delayed onset.
- Juvenile glaucoma.
- Early onset of primary open-angle glaucoma.
- *Low-tension glaucoma:* An adult presenting for the first consultation fails to confirm that he has been on steroids since childhood. It may be mistaken for low-tension glaucoma.

Management

Management consists of the following steps:

- *Prevention*:
    - Steroid-induced glaucoma should be anticipated in all children receiving steroids in any form in general and local eye drops in particular.
    - All children under steroids should have their vision and intraocular tension recorded every 3–6 months.
    - If tension is found to show an upward swing, the strength and frequency of the steroid should be reduced.
    - If pressure remains still high, the glucocorticosteroids should be replaced by nonglucocorticosteroids.
    - If the IOP still remains high, antiglaucoma medicines should be added.
- *Medical treatment:* It is better to start with a single antiglaucoma drug. If that fails, a second drug may be required.
- *Surgical treatment:* If lowering of the dose of a steroid along with antiglaucoma treatment fails, then only surgery is considered. Any modern filtering surgery may be undertaken.

INFLAMMATORY GLAUCOMA (GLAUCOMA ASSOCIATED WITH UVEITIS)

Inflammatory glaucoma is a common complication of anterior uveitis; posterior uveitis does not cause glaucoma except when systemic steroids are used to combat it. The entity is often overshadowed by the overwhelming features of anterior uveitis and hence missed. It is a secondary glaucoma that, unlike steroid-induced glaucoma, can have both a wide angle or a narrow angle.

It can be divided into the following groups:

- *Open angle:*
    - Acute
    - Chronic
- *Angle closure*:
    - Synechial closure
    - Occludable angle
    - Preexisting narrow angle
    - With seclusion pupillae
- *Steroid induced:* Initially, there is ocular hypotension due to ciliary shutdown that is followed by a rise to normal to stay at a normal level or an overshoot to be glaucomatous.
- *Acute inflammatory open-angle glaucoma:* This is caused due to spread of inflammation to the trabeculum, resulting in edema and obliterating the pores of the trabeculum, which is worsened by thick aqueous and inflammatory debris.
- *Chronic inflammatory open-angle glaucoma:* This develops within a few days to a few months of the onset of acute anterior uveitis and is secondary to scarring

of the trabecular meshwork, impeding outflow. Trabeculitis may linger for many weeks and then develop a scar.

Secondary Angle Closure Inflammatory Glaucoma

- *Synechial angle obstruction:* This is more common in granulomatous anterior uveitis, where extensive peripheral anterior synechiae all around may close the angle in a zip manner. It is more common if the angle is relatively narrow and occludable, which is inevitable due to the use of strong mydriatic and cycloplegic. Prolonged use of strong steroids worsens the condition. A paradoxical situation may occur in prolonged chronic granulomatous uveitis when the ciliary body goes into a stage of hyposecretion, narrowing the angle, and a second wave of posterior synechiae forms, resulting in a pseudoangle that blocks the outflow and causes the IOP to rise.
- *Occludable angle:* This happens in narrow angles with a swollen iris and the use of atropine.
- *Preexisting* narrow angle predisposing and worsening above two situations.
- *With seclusion pupil:* Generally the pupil is small with annular synechiae that prevent aqueous to flow from the posterior to the anterior chamber, causing iris bombe and glaucoma.

Clinical Features

Clinical features are variable. They differ in acute and chronic anterior uveitis.

The *acute stage* is overshadowed by features of acute anterior uveitis, i.e., circumciliary congestion, ciliary tenderness, keratic precipitates (KPs), aqueous flare/hypopyon, edematous iris, and constricted irregular pupil with normal AC depth.

An unexplained pain at this stage points toward the possibility of inflammatory glaucoma, which should be confirmed by tonometry, UBM, and OCT of AC.

The vision is variable. It is mandatory that, in all cases of anterior uveitis, the visual acuity and IOP can be monitored regularly.

The *chronic stage* does not show active signs and symptoms but has telltale evidence of previous anterior uveitis, i.e., old KPs and irregular small pupil/occlusion/seclusion pupil. The angle is generally open; it may be occludable or may have a pseudoangle. The IOP has been raised.

The conditions that are prone to developing inflammatory glaucoma are given as follows:

- Juvenile rheumatoid arthritis
- Herpes zoster
- Herpes simplex
- Post-traumatic status

Note: Sarcoid, Fuchs' heterochromic iridocyclitis, and Posner–Schlossman syndrome are causes of postinflammatory glaucoma in adults, not met with in children.

Management

Management may be divided into two parts given as follows:

1. Management of anterior uveitis
2. Management raised the IOP

In the acute stage, anterior uveitis must be treated vigorously in the initial days of hypotony using atropine. After a few days, weak parasympatholytic drugs such as homatropine, tropicamide, and cyclopentolate should replace atropine; only mydriatics such as phenylephrine have hardly any therapeutic role in acute anterior uveitis.

Steroids are added in adequate dose, strength, and frequency.

If the patient is steroid sensitive, weaker steroids or nonglucocorticosteroid drugs in higher doses and frequencies may be used.

Nonsteroidal anti-inflammatory drugs are poor substitutes for steroids. If necessary, immunosuppressant drugs may replace steroids or be added to steroids.

Immunosuppressant drugs take a long time to be effective; hence, they are not initially suitable for acute uveitis. In such cases, they should be supplemented with steroids and steroid tapered as per the practice of the institution.

Raised IOP is kept under control by standard antiglaucoma drugs.

Pilocarpine and the latanoprost group of drugs are contra-indicative in acute anterior uveitis.

If medical treatment fails, the alternative left is any of the surgical procedures.

GLAUCOMA FOLLOWING OPEN GLOBE INJURY

Open globe injuries that cause glaucoma are given as follows:

- Surgical
- Accidental

Surgical Causes of Traumatic Glaucoma

Many of the surgical procedures, both intra- or extraocular procedures (retinal surgery), can lead to a rise in IOP that may be immediate or delayed. The common intraocular surgeries that cause glaucoma are given as follows:

- Needling
- Aspiration
- Lensectomy
- Aphakia
- Pseudophakia
- Repair of corneal/corneoscleral wound
- Penetrating keratoplasty
- Vitrectomy
- Encircling bands for retinal detachment

LENS-RELATED GLAUCOMA

Lens-related glaucomas are more frequent causes of raised IOP than many others. They can happen at all ages, but they are more common and severe in children. The lens-induced glaucomas are multifactorial.

They are given as follows:

- Prolonged, shallow, or absent AC
- Distortion of angle
- Viscoelastic is left at an angle
- Lens particle in angle
- Anterior chamber IOL
- Combination of uveitis, glaucoma, and hyphema
- Pupillary block by vitreous, residual lens matter
- Inflammatory glaucoma
- Steroid-induced glaucoma
- Genetically narrow angle
- Nanophthalmos
- Congenital anomalies of the AC
- Decentered IOL
- Malignant glaucoma

The mechanism consists of the following:

- Initially, there is a fall in IOP following lens surgery, with or without IOL, for 1–2 days.
- By that time, the IOP builds up, reaches the physiological level, and remains so.
- If the rise of IOP overshoots the physiological limit, glaucoma sets in, which may be acute if large lenticular debris/lots of viscoelastic is left or if vitreous obstructs the pupil. Otherwise, the rise of IOP is gradual.
- A child following lens surgery should be comfortable and pain free without watering.
- An irritable child with congested, watering eyes has either acute inflammatory glaucoma or postoperative glaucoma that should require prompt attention.

Management

In acute cases, the tension should be brought down by oral acetazolamide, beta-blockers, and local CAIs. If there is too much lens matter or viscoelastic, they may be drained by standard procedure.

An iridectomy at the time of lens surgery prevents pupillary block and the rise of IOP.

Steroids should not be withheld for the apprehension of steroid-induced glaucoma in acute postsurgical glaucoma.

Atropine per se is not contraindicated in the acute stage. However, it may be replaced by short-acting cycloplegics.

The chronic rise of postoperative IOP should be anticipated and, when present, treated by local anti-glaucoma drugs, minus pilocarpine and latanoprost.

MALIGNANT GLAUCOMA

Malignant glaucoma is also known as aqueous misdirection glaucoma, ciliary block, and ciliary lenticular block glaucoma. This is an unfortunate postsurgical, rarely post-traumatic, situation that is less common in children but worth keeping in mind. This follows any surgery where the AC is entered. It is more common following filtering surgeries. However, even minor procedures such as needling or peripheral iridectomy for acute congestive glaucoma in adults have been reported to cause the disorder. A raised IOP prior to a surgical procedure is more likely to precipitate it. It has even been reported following a laser iridotomy and the use of a strong miotic in the presence of iridotomy/iridectomy done earlier.

There are many theories regarding the mechanism of the rise of tension in malignant glaucoma.

Some common observations are given as follows:

- It is no doubt a secondary glaucoma of sudden onset in phakic/pseudophakic or aphakic eyes.
- It can happen in the eyes even with normal tension.
- More common following filtering surgery
- More common in smaller eyes, i.e., high hypermetropia
- Nanophthalmic eye (not to be mistaken for choroidal effusion syndrome in nanophthalmos)
- Difficult to treat medically
- Miotics worsen the condition.
- Systemic ocular hypotensive drugs such as acetazolamide give better results.
- Strong mydriatics bring relief.

The most widely accepted theory is that there is an intense pupillary block that causes the pooling of aqueous in the posterior chamber. The aqueous not finding its way to the AC causes a noninflammatory pupillary block and peripheral anterior synechiae, which force the unimpeded formation of aqueous behind the vitreous, pushing the vitreous forward, shifting the zonule lens, iris diaphragm forward, pulling the vitreous centrally, or associated with cyclospasm.

Diagnosis

A correct diagnosis is a matter of exclusion. The conditions that should be excluded are given as follows:
- Ciliochoroidal detachment, which causes hypotony
- Choroidal effusion syndrome is seen in nanophthalmos.
- Intraocular pressure decentering
- Suprachoroidal hemorrhage

The disorder manifests within a day or two following surgery with unexplained pain, watering, and a fast deterioration of vision. On slit-lamp examination, there is corneal edema. The AC is shallow or absent and may be unequal in depth. Surprisingly, the iridectomy is invariably patent. The AC is without lens material or viscoelastic substance. The tension is very high.

Ultrasound biomicroscopy and anterior segment OCT are helpful in confirming the diagnosis. UBM shows swelling of the ciliary body, forward shifting of the ciliary body, anterior shift of the iris-lens complex, anterior shift of the lens, pupillary block, relaxation of the zonule, narrowing of the angle, and closure of the angle.

By anterior segment OCT, the changes are similar to UBM but of lower resolution. The added advantage of OCT is that it gives an objective and quantitative estimate of the condition. The OCT is a noncontact procedure and, hence, does not require coupling. The only disadvantage of OCT is that it is not being effective beyond the iris.

Management

Management of malignant glaucoma is difficult and frustrating. It consists of two parts given as follows:
1. Medical
2. Surgical

The first part (medical) consists of:
- Fast reduction of IOP by:
  - Intravenous mannitol
  - Oral acetazolamide
  - Oral glycerin
- *Relief of ciliary block:*
  - Strong mydriatic cum cycloplegic such as atropine 1% drop two times a day. In children, atropine should be used with the usual precaution.
  - Frequent strong steroid drops.

The second part (surgical) consists of:
- Laser iridotomy to relieve pupillary block
- Surgical iridectomy
- Formation of the AC once the tension has been brought down therapeutically, supplemented by paracentesis and iridectomy
- Incision of the anterior vitreous face with anterior vitrectomy
- Laser lysis of the anterior vitreous face
- Total vitrectomy

LENS-INDUCED (PHACOGENIC) GLAUCOMA IN CHILDREN

Lens-related glaucomas were pretty common following needling and aspiration in the past. The incidence has come down following better management of congenital and traumatic glaucoma in children.

The lens can cause glaucoma in the following ways:
- Congenital
- Acquired

Both can be with an intact lens capsule or without an intact lens capsule.

The congenital lenticular changes causing glaucoma may be:
- *Phacotopic (position of lens):* Ectopic lentis:
  - Subluxated
  - Dislocated
    - In the AC
    - In the posterior chamber (rarely cause glaucoma)
  - Lens entrapped in the pupil
- Phacomorphic* (shape of lens)
  - Spherophakia
  - Microphakia
  - Microspherophakia

**Phacomorphic* glaucoma is caused due to a relatively congenital small and spherical lens that blocks the pupil as a ball in the socket, causing a rise of tension due to the pupillary block to which the factor of angle closure is added, worsening the matter. The pupillary block is relieved by mydriasis, hence called glaucoma inversus or paradoxical glaucoma. Repeated attacks are prevented by peripheral surgical iridectomy or laser iridotomy.

The other causes of phacogenic glaucoma are given as follows:

- Intumescence
- Leak of lens material (phacolytic glaucoma):
  - Leak of lens protein with an intact capsule
  - Liberation of cortical matter following injury:
    - Accidental—closed or open globe
    - Surgical

Intumescence of the lens is generally seen among adults with age-related cataracts but can happen in children with unattended congenital cataracts or traumatic cataracts with an intact capsule. Basically, it should also be thought to be a phacomorphic glaucoma where a swollen lens obstructs the pupil and causes a secondary angle block, which may be acute or chronic. The management is phacoemulsification with posterior chamber intraocular lens (PCIOL) and constant watch on IOP in view of impending or existing secondary glaucoma.

PHACOLYTIC GLAUCOMA

This occurs when the lens protein seeps through the intact lens capsule of a soft cataract. The cause of the leak is not known. The most accepted theory is that heavy protein particles clog the pores of the trabecular meshwork, obstructing the flow of aqueous. Some of the macrophages present in aqueous engulf the protein particles, resulting in an increase in the size of macrophages that become too big to pass through the meshwork, resulting in the accumulation of aqueous in AC and ultimately the rise of IOP. It is generally seen in age-related cataracts and rarely seen in children, with neglected complete congenital cataracts or cataracts following blunt injury. This happens mostly in underdeveloped countries.

The only symptoms are mild pain in the eyes and headaches. Generally, vision is very low due to dense cataracts. If tension builds up fast, colored halos may be seen. The signs consist of circumciliary congestion, corneal edema, large fat KPs, AC flare, soft cataracts, and raised IOP.

Management

Management consists of reducing IOP medically and removing cataracts by standard microsurgical procedure with PCIOL.

The other conditions that should be differentiated are glaucoma secondary to anterior uveitis, acute narrow angle glaucoma (not seen in children), and lens particle glaucoma.

LENS PARTICLE GLAUCOMA

This is common in unattended traumatic glaucoma following a penetrating injury to the lens capsule, liberating cortical matter in AC. The cortical matter cannot be drained by natural processes. So, they not only obstruct the meshwork, but they may be large enough to fill the whole of the AC, resulting in the rise of IOP even when the angle is wide. The same can happen following lens surgery if cortical matter is not fully removed during lensectomy, worsened by residual viscoelastic in AC. The clinical features are similar to phacolytic glaucoma, and management is removal of cortical matter, fully, with or without PCIOL.

PHACOANAPHYLACTIC GLAUCOMA (PHACOANTIGENIC)

This is less frequent than the above two. It is a delayed inflammatory process, a cell-mediated condition where lens protein acts as an antigen. It is more common in persons who have been sensitized to lens protein previously by lensectomy in the contralateral eye. The clinical features are akin to the conditions mentioned above.

The management is given as follows:

- Reduction of IOP medically
- Cycloplegia
- Intense use of strong steroids
- Removal of lens matter if left behind, followed by primary or secondary PCIOL

JUVENILE GLAUCOMA

Juvenile glaucoma comprises an array of raised IOPs, both secondary and primary. The former is more frequent and easy to diagnose than the latter. Latter's are better treated than formers. Thus, juvenile glaucoma per se is divided into two groups:

1. Secondary juvenile glaucoma:
   i. Wide angle
   ii. Narrow angle
2. Primary developmental juvenile glaucoma.

Primary Developmental Juvenile Glaucoma

It is considered to be a subset of primary open-angle glaucoma, manifesting before the third decade, i.e., between 3 and 30 years. The average age of presentation is 18 years. It is equally common in both sexes, bilateral, with a strong family history of primary open-angle glaucoma and myopia. The person may develop type 2 diabetes later. The patients themselves have a higher tendency of axial myopia with its sequelae. It is autosomal dominant in nature, with mutations in chromosomes 1-1q21-q23. There is debate regarding the exact cause of the disorder.

The two most contested theories are given as follows:

1. Late onset of primary congenital glaucoma where trabeculodysgenesis is so less and so localized that it does not completely shut outflow of aqueous but enough to impede outflow over years to cause glaucoma. There may be a spurt in the rise of IOP during puberty. The partial trabeculodysgenesis has not been demonstrated on gonioscopy.
2. Early onset of primary open-angle glaucoma because there are no visible angle anomalies on gonioscopy, i.e., history of trauma, uveitis, prolonged steroid use, absence of stigma of primary congenital glaucoma, i.e., enlarged cloudy cornea, lacrimation, and photophobia. Field and fundus changes are similar to primary open-angle glaucoma in adults.

Symptoms

- Being primary open-angle glaucoma, most of the time it is symptomless.
- The patient may present with diminished distant vision that comes out to be axial myopia.
- On fundus examination, the disk shows change similar to those seen in chronic glaucoma.
- Optical coherence tomography shows neuroretinal changes.
- Typical field changes.
- Raised IOP that may be in the range of 30–40 mm Hg.
- If there is a rapid rise in IOP, the patient may complain of colored halos.
- On inquiry, the patient may admit increased dark adaptation.
- Unattended advanced cases may be aware of peripheral field loss.

Signs

- The eye may be noncongested.
- The cornea may be marginally large but not >13 mm.
- There may be some epithelial edema.
- The AC does not show flare or pigmentation.
- The pupil is large and sluggish, without signs of inflammation or trauma.
- Tension is high with diurnal variation and a positive provocative test for primary open-angle glaucoma.
- Fundus shows various changes in raised IOP depending on duration and range of IOP.
- The cases are generally bilateral but may occasionally be unilateral, making it mandatory for regular checkups of the IOP, fundus, and field in the supposed to be normal eye.

Management

The first thing to do is to correct myopia to avoid amblyopia and improve your lifestyle. The second step is to bring down IOP by:

- Beta-blockers
- Local CAIs
- Systemic CAI is rarely required.
- Prostaglandin analogue
- Miotics are no more in vogue, though they are known to reduce tension with thrice a day instillation of 2% drops.

If medical treatment fails to give the desired result, the choice left is surgery. The most common surgery is trabeculotomy with trabeculectomy, with or without an antifibrotic agent. Laser procedures do not give the desired result. If the tension does not come down with surgery, local drops may be added to achieve the desired effect. Glaucoma implants are rarely required.

SUMMARY OF DRUGS USED TO LOWER INTRAOCULAR PRESSURE IN GLAUCOMATOUS EYES IN CHILDREN

It has been noted earlier that the aqueous is formed by ciliary processes in the posterior chamber at a constant rate. From the posterior chamber, it finds its way to the AC through the pupil and leaves the AC through the angle of the AC at a constant rate. A delicate balance between production and drainage is of utmost importance to maintain the physiological firmness of the globe for the optical integrity of the eye.

There are no conditions where there is overproduction or overdrainage of aqueous in a normal eye. The only condition to produce glaucoma is an obstruction of outflow, resulting in raised IOP to a pathological level that damages the optic nerve and nerve fiber layer.

Hence, the drugs that can lower the tension therapeutically available are given as follows:

- That reduces production.

- Increases drainage through trabecular meshwork/uveoscleral drainage. The latter is responsible for only 10% of drainage.

The drugs can be used as local drops or systemic medicine, either orally or intravenously, either alone or in combination. It is common practice to use an oral hypotensive agent with local drops. The drops can also be used as monotherapy or polytherapy. When used in combination, they enhance the efficacy of each. Intravenous administration is meant for a fast reduction of IOP for a short time.

The other division consists of:

- Those that decrease aqueous formation
- Those that increase trabecular outflow
- Those that decrease production along with an increase in trabecular/uveoscleral outflow
- Those that increase uveoscleral outflow
- Those that reduce vitreous volume without interfering with the production or drainage of aqueous
- Physical method of bulbar compression. This most probably extracts fluid from the vitreous and forces the fluid out of the trabecular. This has a transient IOP-lowering effect.

Table 22.4 shows the ocular hypotensives used in children according to their mode of action:

- Drugs that decrease the production of aqueous
- Drugs that increase outflow are cholinergic drugs that can be direct acting or indirect acting. None of them are used in children nowadays.

TABLE 22.4: Drugs for ocular hypotensives used in children.

Nature	*Name of the drug*	*Dosage*
Alpha-2 selective adrenergic agonist	• Apraclonidine (0.5–1%) • Brimonidine (0.2%)	• Two times a day • Two times a day
• *Beta-blockers:* – Nonselective – Selective	• Timolol maleate (0.25–0.5%) • Betaxolol (0.25–0.5%)	• Two times a day • Once or twice a day
• *Carbonic anhydrase inhibitor:* – Oral – Local	• Acetazolamide (5–10 mg/kg daily) • Dorzolamide (2%) • Brinzolamide (1%)	• Three divided doses • Three times a day • Three times a day

- *Drugs that increase uveoscleral outflow are:*
  - *Prostaglandin analogues:*
    - Latanoprost 0.005% (once a day)
    - Travoprost 0.004% (once a day)
    - Bimatoprost 0.03% (once a day)
  - *Alpha-2 agonist:* Brimonidine 0.2% (twice a day)
- *Hyperosmotic agent:*
  - *Intravenous:* Mannitol—1.5–2 g/kg intravenously (IV) infused over 30–60 minutes.
  - *Oral:* Glycerol—1–1.5 g/kg per day in divided doses.
- *Miscellaneous:* These do not have pressure-reducing effect. They are supplementary to the above drugs.
  - *Steroids:* To reduce associated postoperative inflammation
  - *Cycloplegics:* They reduce pupillary block

SUMMARY OF SURGICAL PROCEDURES IN CHILDHOOD GLAUCOMA

Surgery is the second option, except in primary congenital glaucoma, where surgery is the management of choice. Surgical procedures can be classified according to the location of its position.

They are given as follows:

- *Iris procedure:*
  - Iridectomy
  - Iridotomy
- *Angle procedure:*
  - Nonfiltering:
    - Goniotomy
    - Goniopuncture
    - Trabeculotomy
  - *Filtering:*
    - Trabeculectomy
    - Trabeculectomy with trabeculotomy
- *Others:*
  - Paracentesis (only for short-term IOP lowering)
  - Glaucoma devices
  - Cyclodestructive

SUMMARY OF LASER PROCEDURES IN CHILDHOOD GLAUCOMA

The common laser procedures used in childhood glaucoma are given as follows:

- *Peripheral iridotomy:* Nd:YAG laser
- *Laser trabeculoplasty:* Nd:YAG laser
- Laser iridoplasty
- Cyclodestruction with a diode laser

ALGORITHM OF MANAGEMENT OF CHILDHOOD GLAUCOMA

Medical treatment gets precedence over surgery and laser in all glaucomas except primary congenital glaucoma, where surgery is the method of choice; medicine is given to keep IOP low until the infant is able to stand general anesthesia. Lasers are ineffective in primary congenital glaucoma.

In other glaucomas, medicines are administered to keep the tension low. Medicines do not remove the cause; they only modulate production, outflow, or both. Once the drugs are withdrawn, the eye returns to a state of high tension. Polytherapy has to replace monotherapy many times when monotherapy is ineffective.

Surgery can be a primary procedure, generally done if polytherapy fails. Surgery is also not meant to undo the pathology but to create an extra passage for the aqueous to drain. It is no way interferes with aqueous production. Surgery may have to be supplemented with medicine if the surgical result is suboptimal. Repeat surgeries may be required.

Laser surgery is rarely a primary procedure. Glaucoma valves are used in recalcitrant cases in the second decade.

SUGGESTED READING

1. Agarwal HC, Sood NN, Kalra BR. Clinical presentation of congenital glaucoma. Indian J Ophthalmol. 1983;31: 619-22.
2. Allingham RR, Damji KF, Freedman S, Moron SE, Rhee DS. Embryology of the eye. In: Allingham RR, Damji KF, Freedman S (Eds). Shields's Textbook of Glaucoma, 6th edition. Gurgaon: Wolters Kluwer; 2020. p. 610.
3. Aziz A, Fakhoury O, Matonti F, Pieri E, Denis D. Épidémiologie et caractéristiques cliniques du glaucome congénital primitif [Epidemiology and clinical characteristics of primary congenital glaucoma]. J Fr Ophtalmol. 2015;38(10):960-6.
4. Brian F, Lin SC, Cuong V. Glaucoma. In: Chern KC, Zogam ME (Eds). Ophthalmology Review Manual. Philadelphia: Lippincott Williams & Wilkins; 2000.
5. Brian F, Lin SC, Cuong V. Glaucoma. In: Shera KC, Zegans MF (Eds). Ophthalmology Review. Philadelphia: Lippincott Williams & Wilkins; 2000. pp. 283-344.
6. Chan JY, Choy BN, Ng AL, Shum JW. Review on the management of primary congenital glaucoma. J Curr Glaucoma Pract. 2015;9(3):92-9.
7. Cibis GB. Congenital corneal clouding. In: Cibis GB (Ed). Decision Making in Pediatric Ophthalmology. St. Louis: Mosby; 1993. pp. 120-1.
8. Cibis GB. Neurocristopathy. In: Cibis GB (Ed). Decision Making in Pediatric Ophthalmology. St. Louis: Mosby; 1993. pp. 140-1.
9. Cibis GM. Neurocristopathy. In: Cibis GM (Ed). Decision Making in Pediatric Ophthalmology. St. Louis: Mosby; 1996.
10. Dada T, Sidhu T, Midha N, Gupta S. Diagnosis and management of primary open-angle glaucoma. New Delhi: AIOS; 2020. p. 29.
11. Dada T, Sidhu T, Verma S, Tomar A, Shakrawal J. Diagnosis and management of primary angle closure disease. New Delhi: AIOS; 2018.
12. Elder SD, Cook C. The Limbus in the System of Ophthalmology, 1st edition. London: Henry Kimpton; 1963. pp. 170-8.
13. Elder SD. Buphthalmos. In: Elder SD (Ed). System of Ophthalmology, 1st edition. London: Henry Kimpton; 1964. pp. 548-85.
14. Hoskins HD, Shaffer RN, Hetherington J. Anatomical classification of the developmental glaucomas. Arch Ophthalmol. 1984;102(9):1331-6.
15. Idrees F, Vaideanu D, Fraser SG, Sowden JC, Khaw PT. A review of anterior segment dysgeneses. Surv Ophthalmol. 2006;51(3):213-31.
16. Kaushik S, Mishra D. Embryology of the anterior chamber. In: Mishra D, Bhushan P, Singh M (Eds). Essentials in Ophthalmology. New Delhi: Elsevier; 2019.
17. Madgula IM, Anand N. Long-term follow-up of zonulo-hyaloido-vitrectomy for pseudophakic malignant glaucoma. Indian J Ophthalmol. 2014;62(12):1115-20.
18. Mandal A, Netland P. The Pediatric Glaucomas, 1st edition. London: Elsevier; 2006.
19. Mandal AK, Bhatia PG, Gothwal VK, Reddy VM, Sriramulu P, Prasad MS, et al. Safety and efficacy of simultaneous bilateral primary combined trabeculotomy-trabeculectomy for developmental glaucoma in India. Indian J Ophthalmol. 2002;50:13-19.
20. Mandal AK, Chakrabarti D. Update on congenital glaucoma. Indian J Ophthalmol. 2011;59 Suppl(Suppl 1):S148-57.
21. Mandal AK, Gothwal V, Bagga H, Nutheti R, Mansoori T. Outcome of surgery on infants younger than 1 month with congenital glaucoma. Ophthalmology. 2003;110:1909-15.
22. Mandal AK, Matalia JH, Nutheti R., Krishnaiah S. Combined trabeculotomy and trabeculectomy in advanced primary developmental glaucoma with a corneal diameter of 14 mm or more. Eye (Lond). 2006;20:135-43.
23. Mandal AK.Current concept of management of primary congenital glaucoma. Indian J Ophthalmol. 1993;41:51-70.
24. Mandal AK. Long-term surgical and visual outcomes in Indian children with developmental glaucoma operated on within 6 months of birth. Ophthalmology. 2004;111: 283-90.
25. Murdoch I. How I approach trabeculectomy surgery. Commun Eye Health. 2006;19(59):42-3.

26. Nema HV, Singh VP, Nema N. Development of the Eye and its Adnexa, 2nd edition. New Delhi: Jaypee Brothers Medical (P) Pvt. Ltd.; 1997. pp. 130-40.
27. Samant PM, Samant HP, Nahar SM. Glaucoma. In: Samant HP, Nahar SM (Ed). Ophthalmic Theory and Practical, 1st edition. Mumbai: Balani Publishing House; 2004. pp. 60-1.
28. Sinha S, Krishnadas R. Primary congenital glaucoma. In: Ramamurthy D, Biswas P (Eds). AIOS Ready Reckoner in Ophthalmology, 2nd edition. New Delhi: Jaypee Brothers Medical (P) Pvt. Ltd.; 2017.
29. Tripathi BJ, Tripathi RC. Neural crest origin of human trabecular meshwork and its implications for the pathogenesis of glaucoma. Am J Ophthalmol. 1989;107(6): 583-90.
30. Wagner RS. Glaucoma in children. Pediatr Clin North Am. 1993;40(4):855-67.
31. Walton DS. Glaucoma. In: Harley RD (Ed). Pediatric Ophthalmology, 2nd edition. Philadelphia: WB Saunders; 1983. pp. 585-98.
32. Walton DS. Infantile glaucoma. In: Fraunfelder F, Ray FH (Eds). Current Ocular Therapy, 5th edition. Philadelphia: WB Saunders; 2000. p. 483.
33. Waring GO, Rodrigues MM, Laibson PR. Anterior chamber cleavage syndrome. A stepladder classification. Surv Ophthalmol. 1975;20(1):3-27.

CHAPTER

23 Disorders and Errors of Refraction in Children

The study of refraction in children is more complex than in adults. It is more dynamic and subject to frequent changes until a particular age.

Neither the child's eye nor the refraction is compressed form of the adult eye, though it is 66% of the adult size.

The study of refraction denotes the dioptric status of an eye in relation to the photosensitive layer of the retina.

Table 23.1 *gives a comparison of the eyes of a newborn and an adult in relation to refraction.*

The eyes of newborns increase in length by 0.1 mm every year until they are 14 years old.

The vision of a newborn as per estimation by an optokinetic drum is given in **Table 23.2**.

Following are the methods employed to estimate the type and extent of the error of refraction in children:

- Retinoscopy under cycloplegia (most effective)
- Autorefraction
- Subjective (better avoided)

The factors responsible for poor vision in newborns are given as follows:

- Immature visual connection between eyes and brain
- Foveal immaturity
- Partial development of the macula
- Absent myelination of the optic nerve
- *Prematurity:* A preterm baby is invariably myopic
- Opacity in media
- Any or many of the above

For normal development of vision, a child should have:

- Equal retinal stimulation
- Equally clear retinal image in two eyes
- Proper alignment

TABLE 23.1: Comparison between the eyes of a newborn and an adult in relation to refraction.

Features	***Newborn***	***Adult***
Vision	20/200	20/20
Axial length (mm)	17–18	24
Shape	More spherical	Slightly elongated
Corneal diameters (mm)	9.5–10.5	12
Corneal curvature (mm)	6.6–7.4	7.4–8.4
Keratometry (D)	52.00	42–44
Astigmatism	Universal	Selective
Lens	Almost spherical	Ellipsoid
Accommodation	15 D	Age related
Refraction	Mild hypermetropia (+3 D)	Emmetropia

TABLE 23.2: Expected vision at various ages.

Age	***Vision***
Birth to 2 weeks	20/200
6 months	20/100
3 years	20/50
3–5 years	20/20

To understand the various refractive statuses of a child, it is essential to understand a few fundamentals of optics.

For the purpose of calculating the dioptric value of the eye, following factors are taken into consideration:

- The eye is imagined as a reduced eye.*
- The rays of light are taken to traverse from left to right.

**Reduced eye (Donders'):* The living eye has so many curvatures, refractive indices, and diopters that are difficult to calculate any one factor in isolation. To overcome this problem, many ophthalmologists and physicists have devised many optical models called reduced and schematic eyes, with minor differences in each.

The Donders' model of reduced eye is one of them and is most widely used due to its clarity **(Fig. 23.1)**.

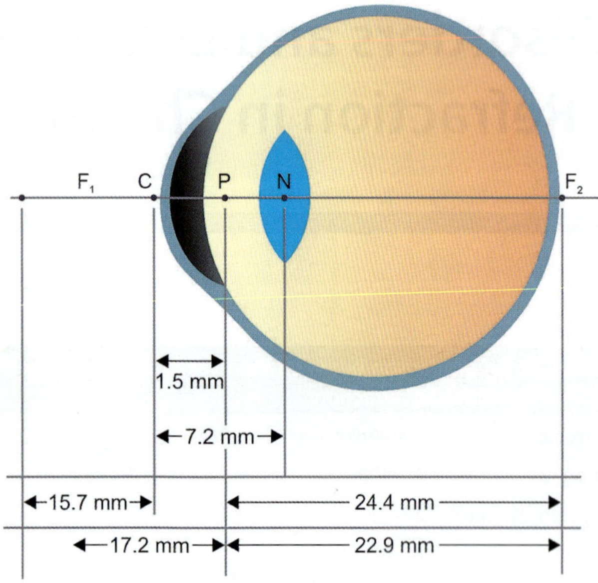

Fig. 23.1: Outline of reduced eye.

- All rays are considered paraxial.
- All elements are aligned on the visual axis.
- The total dioptric value of the eye is taken as +60 D.
- The refractive index of the eye is considered to be 1.367.
- The converging power of the cornea is +43 D.
- The refractive index of the lens is 1.4.
- The dioptric power of the lens is +17 D.
- Accommodation is maximum at birth, i.e., 15 D, which is reduced with age; an adult has accommodation of +3 D.

It is an imaginary model meant to calculate various components of the optical system of the eye with little clinical use.

The features of Donders' reduced eye are given as follows:

- It is a single unit of curved surface.
- The eye is considered to be a perfect transparent sphere.
- The sphere has a refractive index of 1.336.
- The refractive index of air is taken as 1.00.
- The refractive index of aqueous is 1.3.
- The diopter of the reduced eye is taken as +60 D.
- The converging power of the cornea is +43 D.
- The refractive index of the lens is 1.41.
- Dioptric power of the lens is +17 D.
- Accommodation is maximum (+15 D) at birth and diminishes with age.

TYPES OF ERRORS OF REFRACTION IN CHILDREN

Children share the same errors of refraction as adults. The eyes of newborns have mild hypermetropia and astigmatism, i.e., +3 Dsph and 2.5 D CYL, respectively, both of which pass off by 2–3 years. If this does not happen, the child is said to have an error of refraction and will probably need correction either optically or surgically.

An eye without error of refraction is called emmetropic, and an eye with error of refraction is called ametropic.

Emmetropia is defined as the refractive state of an eye where parallel rays are brought to pinpoint focus on the photosensitive layer of the retina in all meridians with accommodation at rest. In contrast to this, if the parallel rays are not brought to pinpoint focus on the photosensitive layer of the retina with accommodation at rest, the condition is called ametropia. In ametropia, the parallel rays form a circle of diffusion (blur) rather than a pinpoint image. The circle of diffusion may be circular or oblong; the size of the circle of diffusion depends on refractive error. Higher the error, larger the circle of diffusion; spherical errors produce circular blur, and astigmatism produces elliptical blur.

The emmetropic eye is a physiologically ideal eye; hence, like all physiological parameters, it is an exception.

TYPES OF AMETROPIA

Ametropia can be of the following types, irrespective of age:

- Myopia
- Hypermetropia
- Astigmatism

Anisometropia

Anisometropia is a state of refraction when there is a difference in the error of refraction between two eyes. Theoretically, any difference in power between two eyes should be considered anisometropia. In clinical practice, a difference of 2 D is considered to be anisometropia. Anisometropia can be of the same sign but of different diopters, i.e., anisomyopia. Both eyes have myopic refraction, one more than the other. Similarly, both eyes can be hypermetropic of different diopters, called anisohypermetropia.

Less common combinations are given as follows:

- One eye is emmetropic, and the other eye is myopic/hypermetropia.

- One eye is hypermetropic; the other is myopic.
- The least common combination is the difference in cylindrical value both in diopter and axes in two eyes.

Following are the factors that lead to ametropia:

- Axial length of the eyeball
- Refractive index of optical components
- Curvature of an optical component
- Position of the lens

Accommodation per se does not cause an error of refraction but affects it, i.e., improves or worsens it.

- *Axial length:* Axial length in a newborn is 17 mm; it increases to 24 mm by 5 years, and any change in the ultimate length will result in ametropia. One millimeter of deviation in length will cause 3 D of ametropia either way. Twenty-three millimeters of axial length will result in +3 D hypermetropia, and an eye with 25 mm of axial length will have –3 D myopia **(Figs. 23.2 and 23.3)**.
- *Refractive index:* The refractive indices that influence the dioptric value of the eye are cornea, lens, aqueous, and vitreous. Out of the four, the last two are negligible

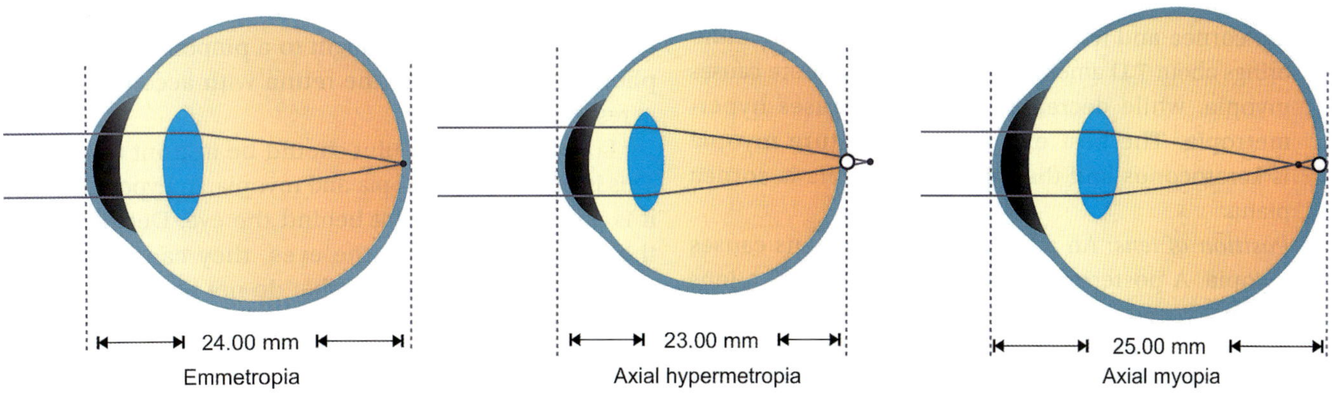

Fig. 23.2: Various types of axial ametropia.

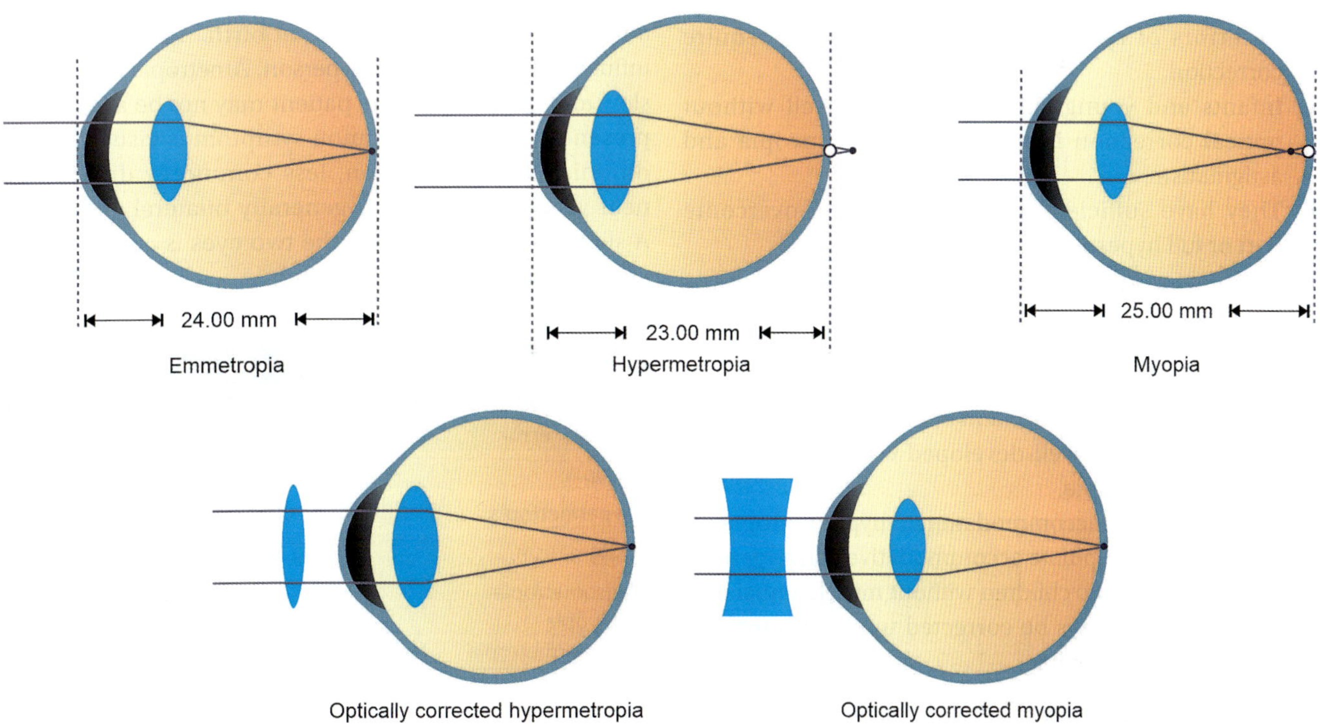

Fig. 23.3: Various types of axial ametropia and the principles of their optical correction.

in causing ametropia. The most common part of the optical system that causes ametropia is the lens. The normal refractive index of a lens is 1.39; an increase in the refractive index of the lens causes myopia, and a decrease causes hypermetropia. There is no fixed formula to predict the change in refraction due to alteration.

The two common examples of index ametropia are hyperglycemia and central nuclear sclerosis, both of which cause index myopia. Hypoglycemia causes index hypermetropia.

- *Curvature of the optical component:* The two curved components in the refractive system of the eye are the cornea and lens. A change of 1 mm in curvature brings about 7 D ametropia. Increased curvature causes myopia, while decreased curvature causes hypermetropia. The best example of curvature myopia is keratoconus and that of hypermetropia is cornea plana.
- *Position of lens:* An anterior shift of the lens causes myopia. A posterior shift and the absence of a lens cause hypermetropia. Aphakia is the single most important cause of high hypermetropia, i.e., +10 D.

Principles of Correction of Ametropia (Error of Refraction) in Children

- All errors of refraction in children do not require correction.
- Infants and young children do quite well without optical correction in low to moderate myopia and astigmatism.
- They have sufficient accommodation to overcome part or full hypermetropia as well.
- The main purposes of optical correction are given as follows:
    - Improve vision both for the distant and the near.
    - Give equal vision to two eyes.
    - Assist in the development of the visual system.
    - An intact and well-developed visual system mitigates amblyopia.
    - To replenish accommodation in hypermetropia.
    - To help manipulate accommodative convergence.
    - Hypermetropic children without muscle imbalance need not always be corrected unless it interferes with their schooling.
    - All aphakic children should be corrected either by suitable glasses or, better yet, by contact lenses.
    - Refractive power in childhood aphakia is known to reduce over a period, requiring frequent adjustment.
    - Childhood myopia increases with age up to 18 years and stabilizes after that.
    - Children under 8 years with *amblyogenic refractive factor** should be given optical correction.

AMETROPIA

Ametropia is a group of refractive conditions where parallel rays, i.e., those arising from the far point of the eye under consideration, are not brought to a pinpoint focus on the photosensitive layer of the retina with accommodation at rest.

Logically, the far point should be in front of the eye. This is true for emmetropia and myopia. In hypermetropia, it is a hypothetical point behind the eye. Depending on the refractive status of the eyes, they can be divided into two groups: those eyes that do not have any error of refraction are called emmetropic eyes, and those eyes that have error of refraction are called ametropic eyes. About 70–80% of the population are emmetropic, i.e., without error of refraction. Some races are more prone to be ametropic than others. Ametropia mostly develops after birth; rarely, it is present at birth. Ametropia is not influenced by the sex of the person. Ametropia is generally slow and progressive. The patient may not be aware of its presence. The most common symptom is visual, mostly diminished distant vision, less commonly diminished near vision. Ametropia is generally bilateral and equal. A slight variation between the two eyes is common, not amounting to clinical anisometropia.

TABLE 23.3: The effect of error of refraction on the amblyogenic range.

Types of error	*Amblyogenic range*
Myopia	−2.00 D to −3.00 D
Hypermetropia	+4.00 D to +5.00 D
Astigmatism	1–2 Dcyl
Anisometropia • Myopia • Hypermetropia	 −2.00 D to −3.00 D +1.00 D to +1.5 D

Amblyogenic refractive factors* in children are given in **Table 23.3.

As per refractive status, ametropia is divided into three groups, each with its own subgroups.

The various types of ametropic conditions are given as follows:

1. Myopia
2. Hypermetropia
3. Astigmatism

Myopia

Myopia is defined as the refractive status of an eye where parallel rays are brought to focus in front of the photosensitive layer of the retina with accommodation at rest.

Accommodation moves the image farther away from the retina, worsening myopia **(Fig. 23.4)**.

- The term nearsightedness for myopia is relevant.
- The term farsightedness for hypermetropia is irrelevant.

Though the term nearsightedness is relevant, it is no more used in clinical practice. Myopia is also referred to as nearsightedness, correlating it to its main symptom of diminished distant vision and good near vision.

A low degree of myopia is the most common type of refraction error in children. It is the most prevalent cause of diminished distant vision that is gradual and painless. It may be so insidious that the child may not know its existence and may even consider it to be natural. Myopia is not common in infants, except for congenital myopia. However, premature children are more likely to have myopia that disappears by 1 year, except in those who develop retinopathy of prematurity (ROP). Low myopia is equally distributed among boys and girls. However, a higher degree of myopia above –5 D is more common in girls.

No race is immune to myopia. Some races have a higher prevalence than others.

Myopia has a strong hereditary predisposition. It can be autosomal dominant when one parent is myopic or autosomal recessive when both parents are myopic. If both parents are myopic, 50% of children are likely to be myopic; this percentage is reduced to 25% if only one parent is myopic. About 25% of myopic children do not have any genetic predisposition but are capable of passing the gene on to the next generation. It is common to have myopia in a few or all siblings. Myopia can be traced among grandparents as well as first cousins. The incidence of myopia is more among urban children when compared to rural children. The incidence is more in children of developed countries; the overall incidence is showing an upward swing; it is estimated that in 2000, it was 20% in children, which is likely to be as high as 52% in 2050, the cause of which remains a riddle. Increased near-work and environmental factors are the two most common factors blamed.

The optics of myopia is less complicated than those of hypermetropia. We have seen that in myopia, the parallel rays from the far point, real or apparent (myopic far point), are focused in front of the photosensitive layer of the retina with accommodation at rest. In myopia, the parallel rays meet to form a pinpoint, and the sharp image is away from the retina, nearer to the nodal point. After forming the pinpoint image, the rays continue until they reach the retina, where instead of a pinpoint image, the rays form a circular blurred image. The distance between the pinpoint image and retina denotes the converging power of the optical system. Longer the distance, higher the myopia. The size of the circle of blur is also proportionate to the myopic power; larger the circle, greater the power.

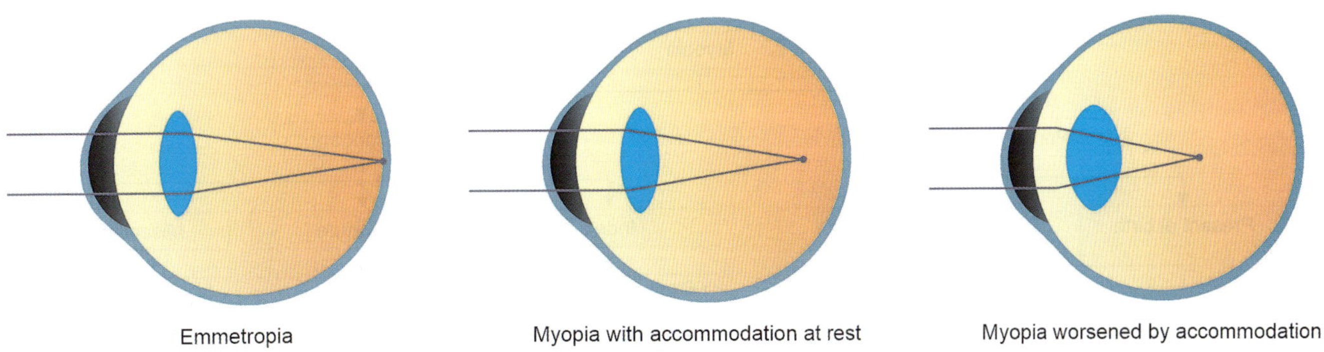

Fig. 23.4: The effect of accommodation on myopia.

There are three mechanisms by which the rays can converge in front of the retina given as follows:

1. Without increasing the converging power of the optical system, as in axial myopia.
2. Increasing the converging power of the system:
   i. *Curvature:* Keratoconus, lenticonus, and spherophakia
   ii. *Refractive index:* Central nuclear sclerosis and hyperglycemia
3. Shifting of the lens

Ninety percent of children have bilateral myopia; the power in two eyes is seldom equal (isometric). However, the difference in power is generally so small that it cannot be called clinical anisometropia. Rarely, the child has unilateral myopia, which is generally congenital, high in power, but stationary. Though their dioptric power does not increase, they are equally prone to the same complications seen in progressive and pathological myopia.

Mechanism of Production of Axial Myopia

The average axial length of a full-term normal baby is 17 mm, against an adult axial length of 24 mm. One millimeter of shortness of the axis makes the eye +3 D hypermetropia. As per this formula, the eye of a newborn should be $7 \times 3 = 21$ D hypermetropia; in reality, the newborn child's eye is only +3 D hypermetropia. This riddle is solved by the fact that the cornea and lens of a newborn are far more curved than adults, and a 1.00-mm change in curvature leads to 7 D ametropia. Thus, the inherent curvature of the cornea and lens negates the effect of increased axial length; the above argument is just one part of the solution. The second part consists of a gradual increase in the axial length of the eye from 17 to 24 mm. We have seen that 1 mm of increase in axial length imparts 3 D of convergence. Both facts acting in unison make the eye emmetropic by 5–6 years.

By 5–6 years, the increment in length should stop to remain emmetropia. If the length continues to grow, the eye becomes myopic by 3 D for every millimeter increment.

Conversely, if the eye fails to increase in length to become 24 mm by 5 years, it remains hypermetropic (axial).

> In childhood myopia, the refractive power of the eye is too strong for the axial length.

If the eye at birth has a length of >17 mm, the child will be born with congenital myopia; similarly, if the length overshoots 24 mm at 5–6 years and continues to grow, the child will become a case of progressive/pathological myopia.

Classification

The crudest classification is to divide childhood myopia into congenital and acquired types. The former is far less frequent than the latter.

The other classification is to divide childhood myopia into two groups, i.e., (1) primary and (2) secondary. **Flowchart 23.1** shows various types of childhood myopia as per this classification.

Other ill-defined terms used in clinical practices are school myopia, college/high school myopia, pathological myopia, degenerative myopia, malignant myopia, and pseudophakic myopia.

Syndromes associated with childhood myopia are given as follows:

- Marfan syndrome
- Homocystinuria

Flowchart 23.1: Classification of myopia in children.

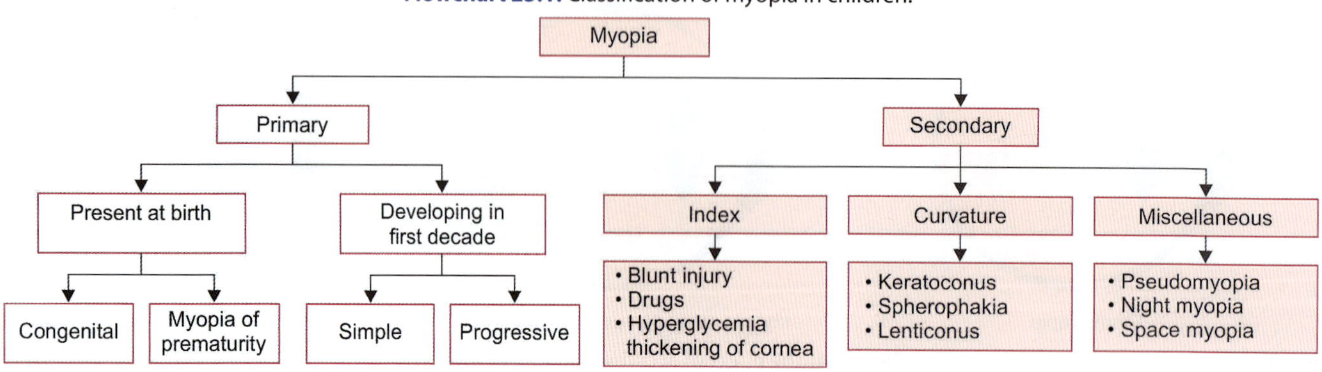

- Rubella syndrome
- Down syndrome
- Albinism
- Retinopathy of prematurity

The better classification of childhood myopia is based on the anatomical configuration of the eye.

- *Axial:* This is the most frequent type and can be simple (minimally progressive) or progressive; to this may be added pathological myopia.
- *Curvature:* It is caused following—keratoconus, lenticonus, and spherophakia. The first being more common than the latter two.
- *Index:* Rare in children but can be seen in adolescents suffering from uncontrolled type 1 diabetes, blunt injury, thickened cornea, and myopia of pseudophakia.
- *Displacement of the lens:* Anterior subluxation.

The abovementioned conditions are acronymed as ACID.

Clinical Presentation of Childhood Myopia

Clinical presentation depends on the following:

- The extent of myopia, i.e., low, moderate, and high.
- The extent of progression, i.e., nonprogressing and progressing.
- *Laterality:* Binocular/uniocular

A child with uniocular myopia may not be aware of diminished vision in the affected eye.

The most common complaint is diminished distant vision with good near vision. A child with low binocular myopia may not complain; moderate myopia is generally detected in schools where the child cannot see the letters on the blackboard. A child with high myopia, i.e., >–5 D, has an obvious diminished distant vision that is noticed by parents as well.

To overcome diminished distant vision, the child squeezes the lids to produce a pinhole effect to improve vision.

The child's good near vision in the presence of diminished distant vision is explained on the following facts:

- The myopic far point is a finite point.
- The myopic far point is situated in front of the eye.
- Rays arising from the myopic far points behave like parallel rays.
- They are focused on the retina without accommodation.
- If the myopic far point is within a near point, the child can see small prints without glasses.
- The myopic eye is conditioned not to accommodate.
- Keeping a small object near the eye slightly enlarges the image.

Reciprocal of the far point is the power of the spectacle at the anterior focal point, i.e., the far point of 25 cm will require –4 D for distant correction.

The external appearance of the eyes does not reveal the presence of mild-to-moderate myopia.

Children with high myopia have large eyes that may be phoric or tropic, and the cornea is larger than the emmetropic eye; the anterior chamber (AC) is slightly deeper than emmetropia, and the pupil is larger but central and circular, reacting briskly to direct and indirect light. The presence of relative afferent pupillary defect (RAPD) is a bad sign; it may indicate extensive retinal degeneration and retinal detachment, causing unequal and severe loss. Age-related cataracts are common at any age but not in childhood. A myopic child may suffer from glare due to a large pupil; children with high myopia may have diminished night vision. Myopia (>6 D) is a potential danger to vision.

Specific Types of Myopia in Children

Simple myopia (developmental myopia): Ten percent of children under the age of 15 years suffer from some error of refraction or other. Ninety percent of them suffer from myopia. Simple myopia is the most common form of myopia in children. The exact cause is not known. It has a strong hereditary predisposition and may run in generations in the family, with siblings and first cousins affected.

The type, extent, and progress of myopia in all the members follow a similar pattern. It is generally bilateral and isometric, and the association of mild astigmatism is common. The spherical value has a tendency to increase. The increment stops in the teens. The value of the cylinder rarely changes, though the axis may change within 10° on either side.

Simple myopia is a slow-progressing error of refraction; it is so insidious that the child does not complain, and parents do not realize it unless the child starts going to school and complains that he cannot read the letters written on the blackboard. At home, the child prefers to sit nearer the TV than others. The child keeps the book too close to his face while reading. The belief that the condition is precipitated by near work has not been clinically substantiated.

The sudden surge in power at puberty, the role of diet in containing power, and general health have not been substantiated.

The increase in power is gradual and not related to the use of myopic correction. Only 15% show a moderately fast increment requiring a yearly change of power. Unless the child has developed amblyopia, vision in both eyes can be improved to 6/6 with correction.

Generally, the first glasses prescribed range between –1.00 and –2.00 D may be with or without mild astigmatic correction.

In spite of the glasses, the power grows for 9–10 years and becomes stationary, not exceeding –5.00 to –8.00 D. There is yet another type of simple myopia with slow progression and fully correctable vision that starts at about 15 years. It also starts with –1.00 to –1.50 D but rarely increases to –2.00 or –2.50 D over the years. The difference between initial and final power in this group does not exceed >1 D. This is called high school or college myopia.

Another feature of simple myopia is muscle imbalance. The far point (punctum remotum) is at a finite distance in front of the eye. Higher the power, shorter the punctum remotum. As punctum remotum is within or nearer than the nearest point, the child does not need to accommodate. If the child accommodates, the image moves away from the retina, making it more blurred. The child learns not to accommodate.

Convergence remains within the normal range or may exceed the range. This results in dissociation between accommodation and convergence, resulting in exophoria that may lead to intermittent exotropia and frank exotropia. Occasionally, excess convergence may lead to exophoria/exotropia.

The child suffers from glare and may have asthenopia. Anisometric eyes may squint and be amblyopic.

Signs: There may be no signs that may point toward the presence of myopia of a low grade or a simple type. The child may be accused of squinting deliberately. In fact, the child does not squint. What he does is to produce a pinhole effect by narrowing the interpalpebral aperture to improve vision.

A child with moderate myopia may keep his chin up.

Negative angle kappa is common that leads to pseudo-convergent squints. Myopic eyeballs are larger than emmetropic and hypermetropic eyes, giving an impression of pseudoprotosis. Cornea is larger, AC is deeper, and pupil is bigger than emmetropia, but pathological fundus changes are few most of the time. The fundus picture is within normal limits.

The vitreous may show a few floaters that too when the myopia is in excess of –5.00 D; other changes consist of the temporal crescent and lattice degeneration, which are innocuous. The latter puts the child at risk of developing peripheral holes that may result in retinal detachment in adulthood.

Myopia per se does not cause color deficiency; the presence of color defect with myopia is a coincidence.

Diagnosis: The diagnosis of simple myopia is not difficult. A school-going child with a history of bilateral poor distant vision, good near vision, short reading distance, positive family history of visual acuity not <6/60 with good projection of light, and improved vision by three to four lines with pinholes is most probably a myopic child.

The error should conform under complete cycloplegia. It is better to perform retinoscopy under atropine in children <5 years old to avoid pseudomyopia. In non-cooperative children, retinoscopy should be better verified on an autorefractometer, especially if there is associated astigmatism.

Management: While managing myopia in a child, the parent should be counseled. They must be told:

- There is no medical treatment for any error of refraction.
- Enriched diets have no effect on the error of refraction.
- There are no exercises to improve vision.
- The power of the glasses will increase in spite of the regular use of glasses.
- Regular use of glasses will not reduce the power of glasses.
- Regular use of glasses diminishes the chance of amblyopia.

Purpose of treatment: The purpose of treatment is to bring the rays arising from the myopic far point to a pinpoint focus on the retina. Properly corrected myopia helps develop accommodation and convergence, preventing squints. Well-corrected myopia prevents amblyopia. The two methods available for the above purposes are given as follows:

1. Optical
2. Surgical

Optical: Optical methods are a spectacle and a contact lens.

Surgical: The surgical methods are contraindicated in children.

The practice is to give minimum power with maximum and comfortable vision.

The principle involved in determining power is based on the following factors:

The reciprocal of the myopic far point is the power of the glass in spectacle, placed at the anterior focal plane.

This can be achieved by the following ways:

- Subjective
- *Objective:*
    - Retinoscopy
    - Autorefraction

Subjective method: The subjective method of determining the power of an eye is a rough and crude method of asserting power in children. Myopic children, when tested subjectively, may get overcorrected. Pseudomyopia is more likely to be introduced by the subjective method; it fails to determine the correct axis of astigmatism. It may be used in children who already have glasses prescribed following retinoscopy under cycloplegia in the past.

Objective method:

- *Retinoscopy:* Retinoscopy in children should be done under complete cycloplegia. It is better to avoid retinoscopy under simple mydriatic without cycloplegia, i.e., phenylephrine.
- *Autorefraction:* This is not as accurate as retinoscopy under cycloplegia. It is useful in nonverbal children and mentally underprivileged children. It is good for large-scale school screening.

How to prescribe glasses to myopic children?

The practice is to prescribe minimum power with maximum comfort, keeping a balance between accommodation and convergence to give comfortable near vision.

Astigmatism should be corrected fully and on the correct axis. The power of the axis does not change with age in simple myopia.

The disadvantage of myopic spectacle corrections is that they minify the image. A child who was accustomed to a blurred but large image finds a minified, bright image uncomfortable. This happens more if the child is overcorrected. A spectacle may not be acceptable to a first-time user teen due to its cosmetic blemish. Prescribing glasses to children is not as simple as in adults; they cannot appreciate the difference between two low spheres, and similarly, they are not able to differentiate between two adjacent axes in astigmatism. Infants under 3 years with <–4.00 D can do without glasses unless they reach school, at which point they should be given full correction. The purpose of prescribing myopic glasses under 3 years is to stimulate the macula to avoid amblyopia.

All these are negated by contact lenses that give a larger image and a larger field without cosmetic drawbacks. Children under 15 years may not be able to manage contact lenses. Hence, they are better prescribed after 15 years of age.

Progressive myopia: This type of myopia is less common than simple myopia. Other terms used to denote progressive myopia are pathological myopia, degenerative myopia, and even malignant myopia without a clear line of demarcation. The clinical features common among the conditions are a relentless increase in myopic power by 4–5 D yearly. The progress stops in the third decade. In the most cases, the vision rarely improves to 6/6. The condition is always associated with degeneration of the vitreous and macula. Involvement of the macula is common and causes nonimprovement with the best correction. The condition starts as simple myopia at 4–5 years old. Initially, the vision can be improved to 6/6 with glasses. Then, the power starts increasing relentlessly by 3–4 D annually without improving to 6/6 in the next 5–6 years; the power stabilizing at this stage at –10 to –15 D; in a few eyes, the power keeps on increasing till the third decade and gets established at –20 to –30 D.

The condition has a strong racial and hereditary predisposition. It is more common in girls.

Symptoms: As expected, the most common symptom is diminished distant vision with good near vision.

The next symptom is the appearance of black spots in the space. If the spots develop under 5 years, the child may not complain. Spots developing later may make the child aware of them. The opacities are in the vitreous and move with the movement of the eyes. They are called muscae volitantes. These spots, per se, do not require any treatment. A sudden spurt in number, size, and density, along with flashes of light, is red flags that may herald retinal detachment. The muscae are generally bilateral.

Children with pathological myopia have poor dark adaptation and are mistakenly diagnosed as night blind and treated with vitamin A.

The cause of diminished scotopic vision does not lie in the dioptric system of the eye but in the presence of extensive peripheral retinal degeneration. Various types of tropias are common in children with pathological myopia; the most common among them is esotropia due to excess convergence and underaction of the lateral rectus.

Sudden loss of vision, loss of field, and flashes of light point toward the presence of rhegmatogenous retinal detachment. A large vitreous hemorrhage causes a sudden, painless loss of vision. A tiny hemorrhage on the macula may cause a profound loss of central vision.

Signs: Signs of pathological myopia do not differ much from simple myopia except for large eyes, a wide palpebral aperture, and reduced vision to count figures with good near vision. The child may keep the book as close as a few inches from their face to read.

Elongated eyeballs may produce pseudoproptosis; the cornea is large, with a diameter not exceeding 13 mm. A cornea >13 mm should be examined to exclude congenital glaucoma. Retinoscopy under complete cycloplegia shows a dull retinal glow that moves slowly against the movement of the mirror. As minus lenses are added, the glow becomes brighter and moves faster until the point of reverse is reached. A concave mirror retinoscope gives better results. The retinoscope may reveal –15 to –20 D of myopia. Once the retinal glow becomes bright, large vitreous floaters may become visible. A large choroidal pattern may stand out as white lines in a pink glow. The other cause of white reflex is a retinal detachment; the absence of fundal glow without lenticular opacity denotes vitreous hemorrhage.

A fundus examination is best done with an indirect ophthalmoscope. A +30 D plano-convex lens is better than +15 or +20 D; though it has lesser magnification, it has a larger peripheral field.

The fundus findings can be divided into two categories given as follows:

1. Peripheral lesions
2. Central (posterior polar) lesions

It is not uncommon to have a combined picture. The peripheral changes are less vision-threatening. They are due to the enlargement of the eyeball laterally. The peripheral lesions are various forms of degeneration, i.e., lattice, snail track, and cystoids. The above three are harmless until holes develop in them, enhancing the chances of rhegmatogenous detachment and making myopia a common cause of retinal detachment. A blunt injury to an eye with pathological myopia increases the chances of retinal detachment by many folds. Central changes are more numerous than peripheral; they involve many structures in various combinations, i.e., the optic disk, macula, choroid, vitreous, and even the sclera.

Optic nerve changes in progressive myopia: They can be divided into two phases: (1) early and (2) late. The early changes start in the second decade. The changes in the optic nerve are not in isolation; they are concurrent with changes in the choroid and macula.

A crescent develops at the temporal side of the optic nerve; it is widest toward the macula, with concavity toward the center of the disk extending from the upper pole to the lower pole.

The width of the crescent is directly proportionate to myopia; higher the myopia, wider is the crescent. Occasionally, the crescent may develop on the nasal side; still rarely, the changes may be all around the disk. The probable cause of the myopic crescent is the failure of retinal pigment to reach the border of the disk along with retraction of the choroid. The retinal vessels are seen to traverse the crescent. The sclera shines through it; the edges may have clumps of uveal pigment; there is no vision in the area of the crescent; hence, it is a cause of horizontal enlargement of the blind spot.

The overall color of the disk is lighter than that of emmetropia and hypermetropia. The optic disk itself looks larger; the enlargement of the disk is optical rather than anatomical. The cup is proportionately large with a normal cup–disk ratio.

Retinal changes: As the eyeball enlarges axially, it drags the retina and choroid along with it. The retina becomes thin, pale, and more transparent, making the underlying choroidal vessels visible. The picture may begin as a tessellated (tigroid) fundus, which is a physiological condition. The retina may develop atrophic patches. Sometimes, there may be patches of retinal hemorrhage.

The exact cause of chorioretinal changes is not well elucidated. There are two theories. The first is mechanical stretching, mostly in the retroequatorial sclera. The second is hereditary, which is presumed to be an abiotrophy mechanism independent of scleral stretching.

Choroidal changes: Choroidal changes are concurrent with retinal changes; they are noninflammatory and degenerative. Stretching of the choroid may be a contributing factor in the onset of progressive myopia.

The choroidal vessels become visible through the pale retina. Due to some ill-understood mechanism, the choriocapillaris and retinal pigment epithelium get atrophied. Only large choroidal vessels stand out, only to disappear in the years to follow, leaving bare areas of the sclera visible through the retina. The patches of choroidal atrophy resemble postinflammatory patches of choroiditis. The patches of choroidal atrophy do not cross the equator.

Changes in Bruch's membrane: They are less frequent than chorioretinal degenerative changes and are supposed to be the effect of overall stretching of the choroid, leading to rupture of Bruch's membrane. They have an appearance similar to angioid streaks, which are not related to progressive myopia. The ruptures present as fine yellow irregular lines with branching. They develop more frequently in younger myopes. The brakes are called lacquer cracks, and the presence of lacquer cracks is an ominous sign. They herald subretinal and choroidal neovascularization (CNV) that may result in choroidal hemorrhage.

Changes in macula: Of all the retinal changes that cause loss of central vision, macular lesions top the list. There are two types of changes, i.e., (1) retinal and (2) vascular. The retinal changes consist of thinning of the ganglion cell layers, accompanied by cystic degeneration, followed by atrophy that may terminate in macular hole formation. The vascular changes are essentially uveal in origin. First, there is thrombosis of choroidal vessels that are either accompanied or followed by hemorrhage, which spreads to the macula. The macular change is characterized by a bright circular patch of hemorrhage surrounded by a pale ring. The change is called Förster–Fuchs' spot or Fuchs' fleck. Förster–Fuchs' spot has been reported in nonmyopic eyes as well. The incidence of Fuchs' spots increases with the duration of myopia; they are generally bilateral and predispose to hole formation.

Changes in sclera: In pathological myopia, the main fault lies in the dimension of the globe. The globe enlarges in all directions, i.e., anterior, posterior/lateral. The anterior–posterior elongation has more optical influence, while lateral expansion is responsible for fundus changes.

The changes in the sclera consist of not only thing of fibers but also in size of the fibers. The sclera is said to be poor in both quality and quantity of fibers. This leads to the enlargement of the retroequatorial sclera to 15 sq cm from the 9 sq cm of a normal sclera. The stretching is more marked at the posterior pole that involves the macula, disk, and papillomacular bundle. Higher the power, more are the chances of thinning. The stretching may spill outside this area as well. The myopic power needs not always be above 10 D; it may be as low as 6–8 D. Higher the power, more are the changes.

The most important myopic change in pathological myopia in the sclera is posterior scleral staphyloma, also known as scarpa staphyloma. It is a hallmark of pathological myopia. Clinically, posterior staphylomas have been divided into two groups, i.e., (1) primary (simple) and (2) secondary (compound). Eyes with myopic posterior staphylomas are more likely to go blind in the fifth decade when compounded by other chorioretinal changes.

The posterior scleral staphyloma has a variable size, from one disk to several disk diameters. The myopic staphyloma is best visualized by an indirect ophthalmoscope. A direct ophthalmoscope requires adding extra minus lenses to focus. Retinoscopes too require different powers to focus on the edge and bottom of the staphyloma. For example, they require –6 D to reach the end point at the nonstaphylomatous area; they may require –8 or –9 D to see the bottom of the staphyloma. The opening of the staphyloma on the retinal surface is circular, and the retina along with its vessels dips into the staphyloma.

The other methods to visualize posterior staphyloma are ultrasonography (USG) (both A and B scans), optical coherence tomography (OCT), and computed tomography (CT).

Changes in vitreous: Vitreous changes are very common in pathological myopia. The changes are liquefaction of the vitreous, vitreous floaters, and posterior vitreous detachment. The vitreous changes are heredodegenerative, not proportionate to the extent of refraction.

Other changes: Other changes are diminished scotopic vision not amounting to real night blindness, poor dark adaptation, restricted peripheral field, glare, photopsia, weak zonules, and the early onset of age-related lenticular opacity.

Pathological myopia is the most common cause of CNV in young. The two common causes of CNV in progressive myopia (not seen under 15 years) are (1) lacquer cracks and (2) myopic choroidal patches. Primary glaucoma has been observed more in myopic patients at an early age (not exactly in childhood).

Management of progressive myopia in children: The principles involved in the management of progressive myopia in children are the same as in adults. Adult progressive axial myopia gets stabilized by the third decade unless it is superseded with central nuclear opacity.

They have the following options:

1. Spectacles
2. Contact lens
3. Spectacle glass over the contact lens
4. Refractive surgery
5. Clear lens extraction with or without intraocular lens (IOL)
6. Phakic IOL

Only the first three options are suitable for children. It is not always possible to predict if a child with simple myopia will pass into a state of progressive myopia or if his refraction will be stabilized at –5 to –6 D.

A positive family history of progressive myopia in parents is forewarning.

Most of the time, the best-corrected vision with pathological myopia is not better than 6/18 to 6/12.

The cause of the nonimprovement of vision is not optical but pathological changes in the posterior pole. It is better to undercorrect pathological myopia by –1.00 to –2.00 D for comfortable, distant, and hearing vision. With an increase in power, the image gets minified. The second cause is bilateral amblyopia.

The other problem is the yearly increment in power by –3 to –4 D to reach as high as –18 to –20 D. This is in contrast to simple myopia, where the increase is seldom >–1 to –1.5 D annually, stabilizing at puberty.

With the increased dimension of the globe, the pupil also gets enlarged, causing glare. This can be minimized by giving tinted glasses. The pupil retains pupillary reactions unless there are pathological changes in the posterior pole. RAPD is common in unilateral high myopia.

Increased power is associated with an increased weight of the spectacle that causes the heavy glasses to slide down the nose; this in turn reduces the clarity of the image, and the child develops the habit of pushing the glass up frequently.

To overcome this, it is better to give plano-concave glasses with a flat surface toward the cornea or a myodisk that has power only in the central 15.00 mm.

While prescribing the glasses, the parents should be counseled on the following points:

- The glasses are being given to improve distant vision and retain binocular good vision; otherwise, the child will develop bilateral amblyopia.
- The glasses are neither meant to stop progression nor reduce, increment, or cure myopia.
- The glasses are not specific for reading; they are meant to be worn throughout the waking hours.
- A child can read small prints without correction. The glasses maintain a near-physiological balance between accommodation and convergence. Hence, the child should be discouraged from reading without distance correction glasses.
- There is no medicine or exercise that reduces power or helps get rid of glasses. There are no food supplements that are not effective against myopia.

Recently, a new concept has been tried to retard the progress of myopia by using atropine sulfate at a subtherapeutic strength of 0.01% once a day for the rest of the life. The results so far are not encouraging. The other drug that is being tried is pirenzepine, an antimuscarinic substance commonly used to treat peptic ulcers.

The alternatives to spectacle are contact lenses, which can be prescribed by the end of the first decade. One of the advantages of a contact lens is that it reduces minification, hence giving better vision; moreover, it is devoid of peripheral distortion. The child does not need to move the head to increase the field that is achieved by moving the eye. The greatest advantage of contact lenses is that contact lenses are more acceptable cosmetically.

Hypermetropia (Hyperopia)

Considering the refractive status of the eye at birth that is moderately hypermetropic, with accommodation of 15 D, it is expected that hypermetropia should be the most common error of refraction, which is far from the truth; only 10–15% of children between 5 and 6 years in ametropia clinics are hypermetropic. In contrast to orthoptic clinics, where more children with squints are hypermetropic.

The eye that has hypermetropia of +2.5 to +2.00 D at birth should get neutralized by 10 years and become emmetropic, yet 35% of eyes remain hypermetropic up to 16 years; most of them are asymptomatic. They do not complain and do not require correction, in contrast to myopia, which is always symptomatic and requires correction.

The term farsightedness that is commonly used for hypermetropia is not relevant because a child may have diminished distant as well as near vision [absolute hypermetropia (AH), nanophthalmos, and aphakia].

Hypermetropia is a state of refraction in the eye where parallel rays are brought to focus behind the photosensitive layer of the retina when accommodation is at rest. In emmetropic eyes, parallel rays form a pinpoint sharp image on the retina, while in hypermetropia, the parallel rays form a circular image on the retina. The circular image is blurred; the size of the blurred circle depends on the amount of hypermetropia; higher the hypermetropia, larger the circle of blur.

Hypermetropia may be thought to be an underdeveloped eye with variable accommodation. The hypermetropic eye is shorter than not only the myopic but even the emmetropic eye. Generally, the axial shortening is not >2 mm that makes an eye +6.00 D hypermetropic; this is true for simple hypermetropia that amounts to 95% of all hypermetropic eyes. Eyes with more hypermetropia are always pathological; examples are nanophthalmos and aphakia.

Hypermetropia is universal and generally bilateral, symmetric, and isometric. High anisometropic eyes are generally amblyopic and resistant to usual antiamblyopic treatment. It is equally seen in children of both sexes, has a strong hereditary predisposition, and may run in families. Hypermetropia is a common cause of deprivation, amblyopia, and esotropia.

Hypermetropia can be:

- Congenital:
  - Nanophthalmos
  - Microphthalmos
- Developmental (most common types)
- Acquired:
  - Aphakia
  - Pseudophakia
  - Growth is pushing the globe from behind.
  - Central serous retinopathy
  - Internal ophthalmoplegia

The better classification based on the anatomical configuration of the eyeball is given as follows:

- Axial
- Curvature
- Index
- Displacement of the lens

Axial Hypermetropia

Axial hypermetropia is the most common type of hypermetropia. Shorter the anterior–posterior length, higher the hypermetropia; one millimeter of shortening causes 3 D of hypermetropia. Shortening >2.00 mm is rare.

- A longer eye can be emmetropic if the optical components are weak.
- A shorter eye can be emmetropic if dioptric power is >+58.7 D (60 mm roughly).

Primary shortening of axial length is hereditary and developmental; it is brought about by the failure of the eye to be emmetropic by 5–6 years. Secondary shortening is not real shortening; it is always pathological, brought about by forward shifting of the retina, as in central serous retinopathy, posterior scleritis, shallow central retinal detachment, and mass pushing the sclera forward. Nanophthalmos and microphthalmos are two congenial causes of axial hypermetropia.

Curvature Hypermetropia

Curvature hypermetropia is less common than axial hypermetropia and is always pathological. Physiologically, the cornea acts as a strong converging device. At birth, it is +55.3 D, which gets reduced to +43 D by 3 years. One millimeter of flattening of the cornea results in +6 D hypermetropia. The lens at birth is almost spherical but gets flattened as the child grows. If the lens overshoots this limit, the eye will suffer from lens-induced curvature hypermetropia. Lens-induced curvature hypermetropia is far less common than cornea-induced. The only cause of lens flattening is buphthalmos. The causes of corneal flattening are corneal plana, microcornea, microphthalmos, leaking wounds, and overcorrection by refractory surgery.

Index Hypermetropia

Index hypermetropia is the least common type of hypermetropia in children. It is occasionally seen in dehydrated children and type 1 diabetes under insulin for the first time.

Other causes of hypermetropia are posterior shift of the lens, overcorrection of myopia by refractive surgery, wrong calculation of IOL power, overcorrection of myopia by phakic IOL, and overcorrection of myopia by contact lenses.

Highest amount of index hypermetropia is seen in aphakia.

Accommodation and Hypermetropia

Points to remember:

- The parallel rays are focused behind the photosensitive layer of the retina.
- Rays arising from the retina are divergent and seem to meet behind the globe.
- Hypermetropic image is smaller than emmetropic and myopic eye because the retina of the hypermetropic eye is away from the nodal point.
- Accommodation plays an important role in correcting hypermetropia, either totally or partially.

- Myopia is always worsened by accommodation.
- Excess accommodation for distance converts the emmetropic eye of a child to pseudomyopia.
- Accommodation is completely abolished by strong cycloplegia.
- Simple mydriatics such as epinephrine and phenylephrine have no influence on accommodation.
- Other causes of total loss of accommodation are aphakia and internal ophthalmoplegia.
- As per available accommodation, hypermetropia can be latent or manifest.

Latent Hypermetropia

Latent hypermetropia (LH) is hypermetropia that is corrected by the inherent tone of the ciliary muscle; this is physiological. It ranges between 0.5 and 1.00 D. This is measured as the difference between total and manifest hypermetropia (MH) after accommodation has been abolished completely by a strong cycloplegic.

Manifest Hypermetropia

Manifest hypermetropia is divided into two types, i.e., (1) facultative hypermetropia (FH) and (2) AH **(Flowchart 23.2)**.

Flowchart 23.3 shows one of the popular classifications of hypermetropia.

Another classification in vogue as per clinical features of hypermetropia is given in ***Flowchart 23.4****.*

Facultative Hypermetropia

Facultative hypermetropia is hypermetropia that is corrected by accommodation. This is over and above the LH, and the child remains 6/6 and N5 without glasses. The condition is clinically revealed by putting plus lenses in front of the eye in a gradual increment until it remains 6/6. Most of the children have FH that gets converted to absolute with age and by the sixth decade. When whole hypermetropia is converted to AH, it requires optical correction.

Absolute Hypermetropia

Absolute hypermetropia is hypermetropia that is not corrected by accommodation. It is rare in children; when present, the vision is between 6/12 and 6/24, and it requires plus lenses to improve vision.

Following examples show an algorithm for various components of hypermetropia:

- Total hypermetropia is arrived by retinoscopy under atropine and shows +5 D of hypermetropia.
- Out of this 0.5 D, there is LH.
- A child's MH is +5.0 D – 0.5 D = +4.5 D.
- Out of this +1.5 D, there is FH.
- The child has AH +4.5 D – 1.5 D = +3.0 D.

Flowchart 23.2: Division of hypermetropia as per accommodation.

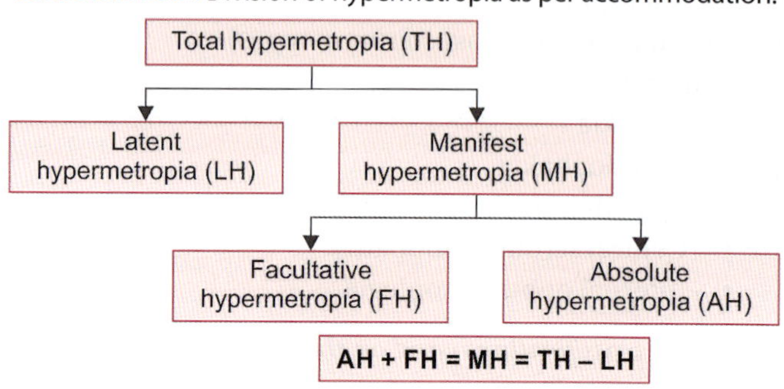

Flowchart 23.3: Alternate classification of hypermetropia.

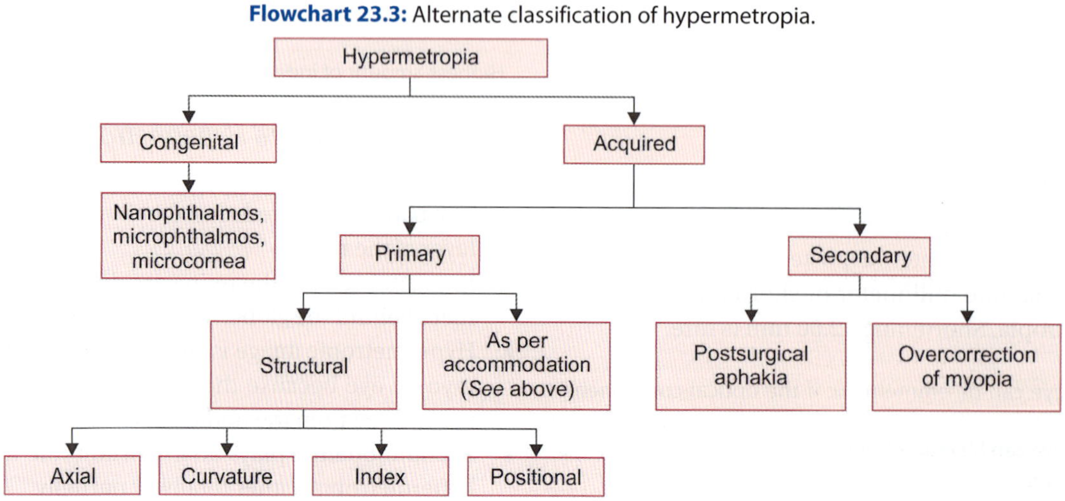

Flowchart 23.4: Clinical classification of hypermetropia.

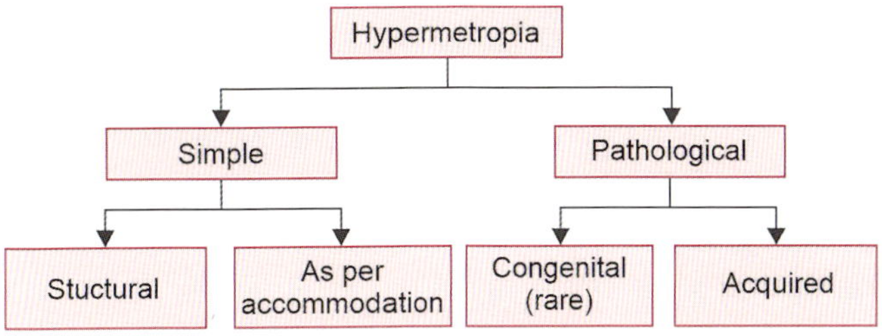

A newborn child cannot have AH because a newborn with +2.5 to +3.00 D hypermetropia has accommodation of +15 D.

Symptoms of Hypermetropia

The symptoms depend more on physiological factors, i.e., accommodation, than on anatomical factors such as axial length, curvature, and index of the refracting component.

A child with low hypermetropia may be asymptomatic. Hypermetropia is discovered during routine fundus examinations under cycloplegia.

Other symptoms that bring the child for the examination can be both with normal vision and subnormal vision.

They are given as follows:

- *Asthenopia (eye strain and ocular fatigue):* Asthenopia can be without visual loss or with visual loss.
  - *Asthenopia without visual loss:* This is seen in moderate FH, where a large part of accommodation is used for clear, distant vision. To have good vision during the waking hours, the child has to keep the eye constantly accommodated. It becomes worse for near work. This constant exertion leads to asthenopia symptoms of tiredness of the eye, the child rubs the eyes even when not itching, mild intolerance to light, watering, and frontal headache. The child is more likely to complain of the above symptoms on returning from school but not on holidays. However, persistent headaches in children should be investigated for other causes of headaches that may themselves reveal hypermetropia.
  - *Asthenopia with diminished vision:* This happens when FH is no more neutralized by accommodation, and the eye is on the verge of passing into a state of AH. The child has fleeting episodes of diminished distant vision that, in the next few months, pass into a state of persistent diminished vision. This may be precipitated by ill health. Generally, diminished distant vision is preceded by difficulty in reading letters and blurring of lines.
- *Diminished distant vision:* Once a stage of AH has been reached, the distant vision remains diminished. This stage may be mistaken as simple myopia, and an inexperienced optician may supply a pair of minus glasses, resulting in pseudomyopia.

  Pseudomyopia: The child may overaccommodate to achieve good distant vision; this overaccommodation results in overshooting emmetropia, bringing the rays in front of the retina, resulting in myopia. A similar situation arises when a hypermetropic child is prescribed a minus lens without refraction under cycloplegia. To overcome spectacle-induced pseudomyopia, the best is to advise the child not to use glasses for 3 days, followed by retinoscopy under atropine. Simple mydriatic that is good for examination of the fundus has no role in suspected errors of refraction.
- *Squint:* A child turns up with esotropia and is found to have hypermetropia.
- *Other symptoms:*
  - The child keeps the book too close to read. A child with high hypermetropia is expected to keep the book away for clear near vision, but this particular child keeps the book too near. The answer to this paradox is that letters kept near the eyes give moderate magnification sufficient for good near vision.
  - Recurrent styes, chalazia, and blepharitis in children with the above symptoms should be refracted under cycloplegia and if necessary given glasses for constant use.

Signs of Hypermetropia

- On a cursory look, the eye with low-grade hypermetropia does not show any peculiarities to differentiate it from emmetropia or low-degree myopia.
- An eye with high hypermetropia is smaller than emmetropia with emmetropia, a small cornea, shallow AC, and a small pupil.
- A flat, small cornea with a coloboma of the iris points toward pathological hypermetropia.
- On close look, the child has an asymmetry of face. Hypermetropia is more on the side of asymmetry and is invariably astigmatic.

- Pseudodivergent squint is due to the large positive angle kappa.
- *A positive Brückner test** may be present in uniocular hypermetropia, denoting amblyopia.
- Esophoria may be present.
- Esotropia may be the cause of bringing the child of examination and found to have high hypermetropia, i.e., +4 to +6 D. The esotropia is mostly accommodative.
- Refraction under cycloplegia shows a bright retinal glow that moves with the movement of the retinoscope. Higher the power, brighter and smaller the glow that moves faster than in emmetropia.
- Fundus is best examined with a direct ophthalmoscope, in contrast to myopia, which is better visualized by an indirect ophthalmoscope.
    - The overall size of the visible fundus is smaller than emmetropia.
    - The retina has shot silk appearance.
    - The disk is small and may be mistaken for papillitis. This appearance is called pseudoneuritis.
    - The blood vessels reflect more light, similar to those seen in arteriosclerosis.
    - The foveal reflex is bright but situated a little away from the disk than emmetropia.
    - No peripheral degeneration is seen.
    - The fundus is nontessellated.

Management of Hypermetropia in Children

The aim of treatment is to bring the image on the retina at the same time keeping the relation between accommodation and convergence within the physiological limit with good near vision.

Theoretically, this can happen by increasing axial length, curvature of the cornea, refractive index of the eye, and increasing the accommodation. Out of all the above, only accommodation is liable to modification. However, the curvature can be changed by refractive surgery, which is contraindicated in children.

The only practical way left is to prescribe plus lenses. While prescribing plus lenses, the following points must be kept in mind:

- Age of the child
- Amount of refraction
- Visual requirement
- Associated muscle imbalance

Thus, two methods of management of hypermetropia are given as follows:

1. Optical
2. Surgical

Optical methods are given as follows:

- Spectacle
- Contact lens
- Combination

Surgical methods are not indicated in children.

Optical correction:

The mere presence of hypermetropia is no indication of the need to prescribe glasses.

The protocol for prescribing glasses should be planned keeping in mind given as follows:

- All hypermetropes, irrespective of age, need not be treated, in contrast to myopia, where myopia is better treated.
- Teens may tolerate hypermetropia up to +3 D without glasses.
- Hypermetropes under 10 years of age should be refracted under atropine.
- Manifest hypermetropia up to +1 D may not be treated unless it is causing symptoms.
- The initial lens should be sufficient enough to give up to 6/6 vision. The power is increased over months until the MH has been reached.
- The donor's recommendation is to add one-fourth of the latent power to the manifest to keep the ciliary body relaxed.
- Accommodative squints should be fully corrected.
- Unilateral hypermetropia is invariably associated with amblyopia; this should be treated vigorously by standard treatment for amblyopia.

**Brückner test:* The Brückner test, also known as the "transillumination" test, is a simple outdoor procedure that can be performed even on infants. It does not require mydriasis. All that is required is a moderately bright beam of light from a direct ophthalmoscope. The procedure is to throw light from the ophthalmoscope from a distance of about 1 m; the light should fall on both pupils at the same time. An eye without opacity in the media will give a pink circular glow in the pupil in a normal eye. The brightness of the glow in two eyes should be equal. An unequal glow in one eye is suggestive of an abnormality. In squinting, the fixing eye has a bright reflex. The amblyopic eye has a dull reflex; a white reflex is suggestive of leukocoria.

- Bilateral high hypermetropia, i.e., +6 to +8 D, causes bilateral amblyopia even when the powers in two eyes are isometric. They should be given a full correction.
- All the hypermetropic children who have been prescribed optical devices should be examined twice a year; at least the axial length has increased as a part of normal growth, and the eye is left overcorrected.
- Astigmatism, when present, should be fully corrected. It is common for the spherical power to change, but the cylindrical power is generally constant.
- The dioptric power of the contact lens and the spectacle lens is not the same. The power of the contact lens is more than that of a spectacle lens.
- It is better to prescribe contact lenses after the hypermetropia has stabilized. However, contact lenses are strongly recommended in cases of uniocular hypermetropia and high anisometropia.
- Children with diminished vision and accommodative squints should be corrected. If the hypermetropia exceeds +3 D, the child should be encouraged to use glasses constantly. If the hypermetropia is <+3 D, the child may use the spectacles for near work only.
- In children above 6 years, full correction is advocated, in contrast to children under 6 years old.
- The power should be less by 1.5 to 2.00 D than postcycloplegic power.

Pathological Hypermetropia

The two common causes of pathological hypermetropia are nanophthalmos and aphakia. The former has been discussed earlier.

Aphakia: Total or partial absence of a lens from the pupil is called aphakia. Optically, aphakia is a total and significant cause of index hypermetropia. The most common cause of aphakia is the surgical removal of the lens. Spontaneous absorption of the lens or trauma also causes aphakia, which is indistinguishable from surgical aphakia, i.e., extracapsular lens extraction.

Other causes of aphakia are dislocation of the lens, mostly in vitreous chamber and rarely in the AC. Still rare is its extrusion outside the globe following a blunt injury. The common causes of dislocation of the lens are given as follows:

- Syndromes:
  - Marfan syndrome
  - Marchesani syndrome
  - Homocystinuria

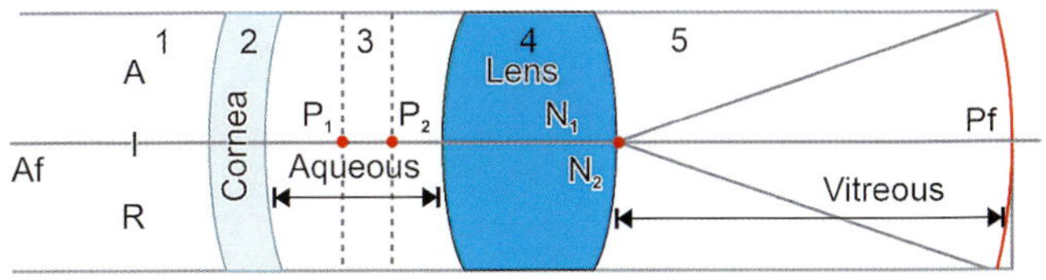

Fig. 23.5: Cardinal points of the phakic eye.

- Trauma
- Miscellaneous:
  - Long-standing anterior uveitis
  - Buphthalmos
  - Congenital (extremely rare)

Optics of aphakia: To understand the optics of aphakia, it is better to recapitulate the basics of the refraction of an eye.

Figure 23.5 depicts cardinal points as per Donders' reduced eyes and the optics of the aphakic eye.

Numbers from 1 to 5 show the refractive indices of various optical components given as follows:

1. Air: 1 μ
2. Cornea: 1.337 μ
3. Aqueous: 1.377 μ
4. Lens: 1.42 μ
5. Vitreous: 1.335 μ

Af is the anterior principal focus, 15.7 mm in front of the cornea; Pf is the posterior principal focus, 24.4 mm behind the cornea; N_1 and N_2 are the two nodal points in the posterior part of the lens; and P_1 and P_2 are the two principal points in the AC **(Figs. 23.6 and 23.7)**.

To understand the salient features of the refractive status of an aphakic eye, the following should be kept in mind.

Phakic eye:

- Normal phakic emmetropic eye has a dioptric power of plus 60 D.
- Out of this, +43 D is corneal.
- The rest of the power is contributed by a crystalline lens.

Aphakic eye:

- The absence of a lens leaves the eye less converging, i.e., +43 D.
- The aphakic eye is nearer to Donders' reduced eye.
- In a reduced eye, the anterior focal plane is 17.2 mm in front of the cornea, and the posterior focal plane is 24.4 mm from the cornea.

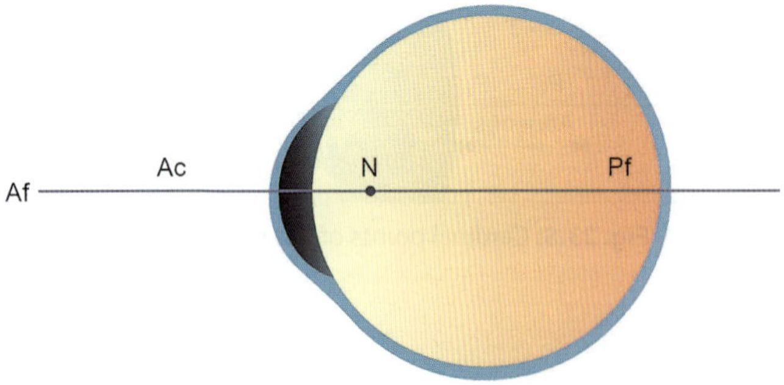

Fig. 23.6: Dimension of Donders' reduced eye (Ac – N = 7.2 mm, Af – Ac = 15.7 mm, and Ac – Pf = 24.4 mm). (Af: anterior focal plane; Ac: anterior corneal plane; N: nodal point; Pf: posterior focal plane)

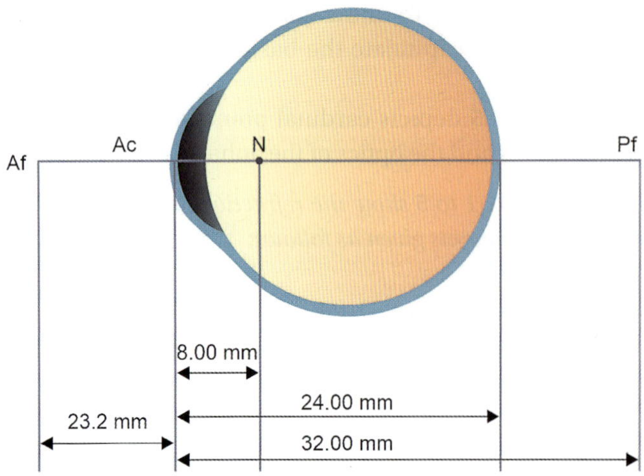

Fig. 23.7: Dimension of the aphakic eye (that was emmetropic when phakic).

- The two principle points are taken to be on the cornea.
- The two nodal points are taken to be as one and situated 8.00 mm from the anterior corneal surface.
- The changes brought about by the absence of the lens are given as follows:
  - It shifts the anterior focal plane to 23.3 mm in front of the anterior corneal surface.
  - The posterior focal plane is shifted to 31.00 mm from the anterior corneal plane.
  - This can be corrected by a +10 D lens put in the anterior focal plane, a +20 D lens in the posterior chamber, or a contact lens.
  - A spectacle lens put in the anterior focal plane is as an effective as a plus 17 D in situ.
  - If the eye was emmetropic before it became aphakic, it will require a plus 10 D to correct the refraction; a hypermetropic eye in the same situation will require >+10 D, and a myopic eye will require less.
  - The most frequently used formula to find out postsurgical power is A = +10 D +1/2a, where A stands for postoperative power and a stands for preoperative spectacle power.

For example:

- A preoperative myopia of –5 D will require a lens of +10 D + (5/2) = +10 – 2.5 = +5 D sphere.
- In the case of –20 D, the correction required will be +10 D + (20/2) = 10 – 10 = 0 D.
- A –10 D will not be neutralized but will require a spectacle correction of +5 D.
- A +5 D preoperative hypermetropia will require a +5 D and not +15 D.
- Theoretically, an eye that is 31 mm long should be –21 D. This depends on the formula 31 – 24 = 7 mm × 3 = 21 D and should not require any aphakic correction. This is not possible due to the fact that eye 21 D myopia has so many pathological changes in the posterior pole that it does not permit the vision to improve.

> The refraction in aphakia is static refraction because the eye has no accommodation; hence, there is no need for cycloplegia. The retinoscopy can be done under simple mydriatic, irrespective of age.

Loss of accommodation in aphakia is corrected by adding a plus 3 D sphere in spectacle; this near correction is a state of fixed focus. Hence, a patient requires two separate sets of glasses, one for near work and another for intermediate distance for writing and eating, etc. All aphakic lenses do not tolerate bifocal, trifocal, or progressive lenses.

- Magnification following spectacle is the most unwanted feature of aphakia. It may be as high as 25–33%. The cause of magnification lies in the combined optics of the aphakic eye and lens placed at the anterior focal plane. The spectacle-corrected aphakic eye behaves like a Galilean telescope, where the lens in the spectacle acts as objective and a hypothetical minus lens inside the eye acts as the eyepiece. A magnification of 33% will mean that a 1.00 m object will look 1.33 m high. Magnification leads to uncomfortable diplopia.
- The magnification is better tolerated if:
  - Both eyes are aphakic.
  - Both eyes have almost equal power.

- The other eye has very poor vision due to advanced cataracts, corneal opacity, deep amblyopia, fundus changes, and a high degree of squinting.
- Diplopia is most troublesome in uniocular aphakia when the other eye has good vision and no magnification.
- Diplopia is caused due to high ametropia and aniseikonia, which are accentuated in uniocular corrected aphakia.
- Diplopia in uniocular aphakia can be reduced by:
    - No power is given to the operated eye.
    - Occlude the normal eye. The child is most likely to reject this situation due to the inherent magnification of spectacle correction in the operated eye.
    - The diplopia can be avoided or reduced if the magnification is brought to 5–7%, which is the borderline of accepted magnification.
    - The methods to reach this situation are contact lenses, IOL, and refractive surgery (not indicated in children).

- Another inherent defect of postoperative aphakia is a high degree of astigmatism, against the rule.
- The next difficulty with aphakia is loss of near vision, which is corrected by adding a plus sphere to the distant correction as per retinoscopy and the requirements of the child.
- The usual distant correction in uncomplicated aphakia ranges between +9 and +11 D spheres as per retinoscopy. A high myopia will require <+9 D spheres, while a high hypermetropia will require >+11 D spheres for distant correction.
- To this is added a plus cylinder at 180°, ranging between +1 and +5 Dcyl.
- The disadvantages of spectacle correction in aphakia that makes it unpopular among other methods of aphakia correction are given as follows:
    - Anisometropia
    - Aniseikonia
    - Magnification
    - A spectacle-corrected vision of 6/6 is in fact equal to 6/9 or 6/12 in an emmetropia eye.
    - Spherical and prismatic aberration
    - Ring scotomas
    - Addition for a near defect
    - Cosmetic blemish

Contact lens correction in aphakia:

- Contact lenses are prescribed either as per keratometry or retinoscopy findings.
- The power of the contact lens is more than spectacle correction.
- Contact lenses fail to correct astigmatism completely, which may require spectacle correction over the contact lens. Toric contact lenses are not suitable for aphakic eyes.
- The associated loss of accommodation is not corrected by the contact lens unless the contact lens is multifocal, which itself is not generally tolerated by children.
- Features of contact lens correction in aphakia are given as follows:
    - A contact lens is put on the cornea nearer the nodal point.
    - The power of a contact lens is more than the power of a spectacle.
    - Magnification by contact lens is far less than in spectacle correction (33%); the magnification given by contact lens varies between 8 and 10%, which is nearer to the tolerable limit of 5% magnification. A child may tolerate up to 8% magnification.
    - Contact lenses abolish peripheral aberration and peripheral distortion.

The advantages of contact lenses over spectacle corrections are given as follows:

- Reduced anisometropia, aniseikonia, and magnification
- A better visual outcome
- Better acceptance
- Reduced chances of diplopia
- Enlarged field
- The child needs not turn the head or raise the chin to have better vision
- No ring scotomas
- The disadvantages of contact lenses are given as follows:
    - They cannot be used on infants or children under 5 years.
    - Children may not be able to maintain proper hygiene with their contact lenses. They are difficult to fit.
    - Costly

Intraocular lens correction for aphakia in children: Intraocular lens correction has become the most effective method of aphakia correction, and it is considered to be the gold standard. It can be primary or secondary; the first is more preferred than the latter. Theoretically, it can be AC, pupillary chamber, or posterior chamber. The first two are no more in vogue; the posterior chamber IOL can be put either in the sulcus or in the bag; the latter is more preferred. The power of the IOL is more than the power in spectacles or contact lenses; it can be roughly calculated by multiplying the aphakic correction following refraction by factor 1.8. The best method of choosing the power of IOL is the biometer. The other advantage of IOL is the absence of astigmatism. IOL does not correct defective near vision that requires spectacle correction. Other methods of reducing near power are to make the eye mildly myopic, leaving a child with distant vision from 6/12 to 6/9. This gives fairly good near vision without additional correction; children as young as 3 months old are known to tolerate contact lenses.

Astigmatism

Statistically, astigmatism is the most common error of refraction if all ametropia are put together from birth to ripe old age.

The eyes of all newborns are astigmatic to various degrees; they may be as high as two cylinders. Ninety percent of astigmatism at birth gets neutralized by 6 months. The amount of astigmatism that does not pass off by the first year persists as clinical astigmatism. Preterm children are more prone to higher astigmatism.

Paradoxically, the large astigmatism of premature births may get reduced or completely neutralized in infancy, in contrast to the astigmatism of full term that may persist for the rest of life. The exact cause of the above two phenomena is not known.

Astigmatism is defined as a state of ametropia where all parallel rays do not come to focus with or without accommodation on the photosensitive layer or retina; they are focused either in front of or behind the retina in various combinations. The condition becomes worse when the child is accommodated, even in hypermetropia.

> The eyes in which the rays are brought to focus to pinpoints are called stigmatic eyes.

In astigmatic eyes, the rays are focused in the planes. These planes are called focal planes in contrast to the focal points of the stigmatic eye. The astigmatic eyes behave like torus as opposed to spheres of stigmatic eye. The rays of the astigmatic eye are focused as in Sturm's conoid **(Fig. 23.8)**.

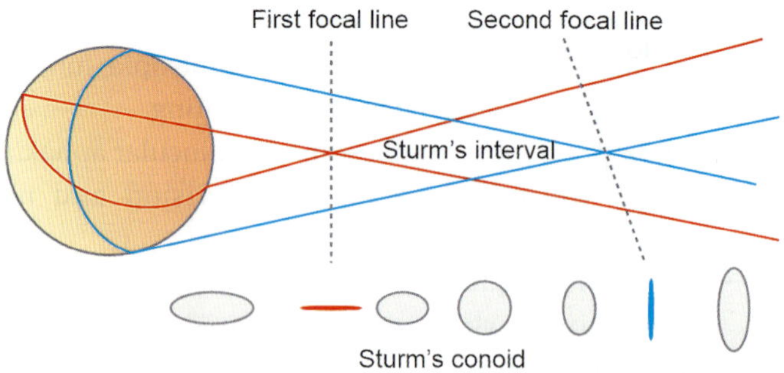

Fig. 23.8: Optic of Strum's conoid. Blue line represents less curved surfaces and their rays, and red line represents more curved surfaces and their rays.

The distance between two planes is called the focal interval or Sturm's interval that represents the value of the cylinder that will merge the two planes in one. Farther they are from each other, larger will be the cylindrical value. The circle of least confusion in Sturm's conoid represents the spherical value. In simple astigmatism, there is no spherical component. In other types of astigmatism, a definite spherical value is required.

Role of Accommodation in Astigmatism

In previous paragraphs, we have seen that myopia is worsened by accommodation, and hypermetropia is reduced or corrected by accommodation. In contrast to this, accommodation even in hypermetropic astigmatism worsens the condition.

The value of the cylinder that abolishes the focal interval does not change with accommodation. The axis of the cylinder is not affected by accommodation.

Classification of Astigmatism

> A pure stigmatic eye is a rarity.

Astigmatism has been classified variously; it can be congenital or acquired. Congenital astigmatism can be divided into three types according to their progression **(Flowchart 23.5)**.

- Most of the eyes in preterm babies are astigmatic, which regresses only to be neutralized in infancy.
- The astigmatism of a full-term baby usually persists for the rest of life.
- Persistent astigmatism of the full term is better called developmental.
- Astigmatism above 3 Dcyl is considered to be high astigmatism.
- Astigmatism of more than six cylinders has not been reported in primary astigmatism.

Flowchart 23.5: Classification of astigmatism.

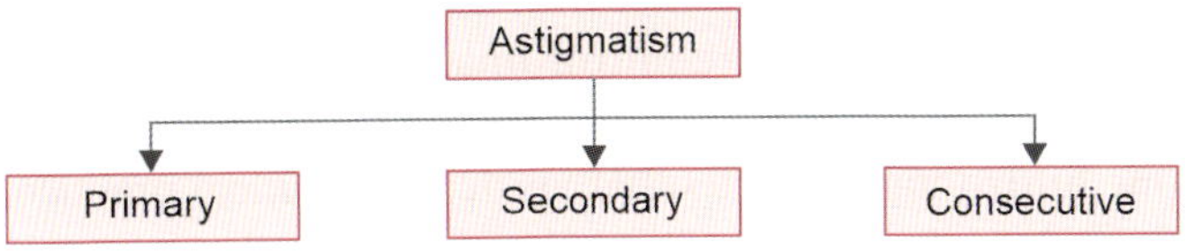

When no cause can be attributed to astigmatism, it is called primary. Ninety percent of astigmatism in children is primary; when some cause can be found for astigmatism, it is called secondary. The incidence of secondary astigmatism increases with age.

The causes of secondary astigmatism are (in all ages) given as follows:

- Trauma:
  - Accidental
  - Surgical
    - Classical lens extraction
    - Small incision cataract extraction
    - Intraocular lens (phaco procedure—least astigmatism)
    - Postglaucoma surgery
    - Postdetachment surgery
    - Postkeratoplasty
    - Postlaser-assisted in situ keratomileusis (LASIK)
- Degeneration
- Dystrophy

Primary Astigmatism

This is the most common type of astigmatism that is present at birth and lingers for a whole life without change in diopter. Ninety percent of astigmatism is due to the cornea; the remaining parts are the lens and still less retina; in fact, retinal astigmatism is better put in the category of secondary astigmatism.

Extracorneal astigmatism is called residual astigmatism that cannot be measured separately from total astigmatism. In fact, corneal astigmatism is mostly at the air corneal junction and can be measured by a keratometer. The other methods of measuring total astigmatism are the mirror retinoscope, streak retinoscope, and autorefraction.

The subjective method is not suitable for children under the age of 10 years and is best avoided in all ages. The total primary astigmatism is said to be proportionate to spherical power. In children with nonpathological myopia, spherical and cylindrical components develop simultaneously.

- *Corneal astigmatism can either be regular or irregular:* The characteristics of regular astigmatism are given as follows:
  - It is the most common type of primary astigmatism.
  - It has two meridians.
  - Refraction in each meridian is uniform throughout the axis.
  - Refraction changes smoothly from one meridian to the other.
  - The main axes are vertical or horizontal and at right angles to each other.
  - In a few cases, the axes are not at the right angle, i.e., one is at 20° and the other is at 120° and are called bioblique astigmatism. The sum of angles of a cylinder in bioblique is never 180°, which is the hallmark of the sum of angles at the right angle.
- *Regular corneal astigmatism can either be with the rule or against the rule:* The division is based on the steepness of the vertical meridian.

  Astigmatism with the rule:
  - In all emmetropic eyes, the vertical meridian is steeper by 0.25 D; hence, the vertical meridian is more myopic by –0.25 D cylinder in comparison to the horizontal meridian, which is emmetropic. This is physiological; hence, it is considered to be the rule and needs not be corrected. The explanation for this is supposed the pressure exerted by the lids over the globe.
  - The astigmatism with the rule is that astigmatism requires a minus cylinder at 180° with a variation of 20° on each side or a plus cylinder at 90° ± 20°.
  - Children are more often likely to have astigmatism with the rule that there is a minus cylinder at the horizontal axis and a plus cylinder at the vertical axis.

Astigmatism against the rule: It is a regular astigmatism where the horizontal meridian is more curved. This is less common than astigmatism with rules. It is corrected by a plus cylinder at 180° or a minus cylinder at 90°. The cause of astigmatism where the horizontal meridian is more curved is not well understood. People in the fifth decade and above are more often astigmatism against the rule.

Oblique Astigmatism

It is that type of regular astigmatism where the two meridians are at right angles to each other but not at 180°

or 90°; they are generally at 45° and 135°, i.e., one axis in the right eye is at 45°, its corresponding axis in the left eye will be at 135°, and vice versa. In oblique astigmatism, the sum of two axes is 180°.

Classification of astigmatism as per errors of refraction is given in ***Flowchart 23.6****.*

Simple Myopic Astigmatism

In this type of astigmatism, one of the meridians is emmetropic and the other is myopic. If the child accommodates the myopic points, they move away from the retina, making it more myopic, and the emmetropic point also moves forward by the same power, converting the meridian myopic, thus changing the eye from simple myopic astigmatism into compound myopic astigmatism, worsening the far vision **(Fig. 23.9)**. The child gives up accommodation in favor of less blurred vision. The condition is corrected by a single minus cylinder at an angle as per retinoscopy. The value of the cylinder is generally the same in two eyes, and the axis is identical. The most common axis met with is horizontal. Otherwise, at such angles, they are mirror images of each other, i.e., 45° in one eye and 135° in the other; it is very rare to have one horizontal and the other vertical. In clinical practice, the value of a cylinder is rarely more than that of a 3 D cylinder.

Compound Myopic Astigmatism

In this type of refraction, all the meridians are ametropic and myopic, one more than the other. They come to focus in two different focal planes in front of the retina. If the child accommodates both, the myopic planes move forward, making them more myopic and worsening the vision. The condition is corrected by a myopic sphere and a myopic cylinder at an appropriate angle, elicited by a retinoscope. The value of the cylinder is the difference between the meridians, and the value of the sphere is the lower power, i.e.,

Flowchart 23.6: Various possibilities of astigmatism.

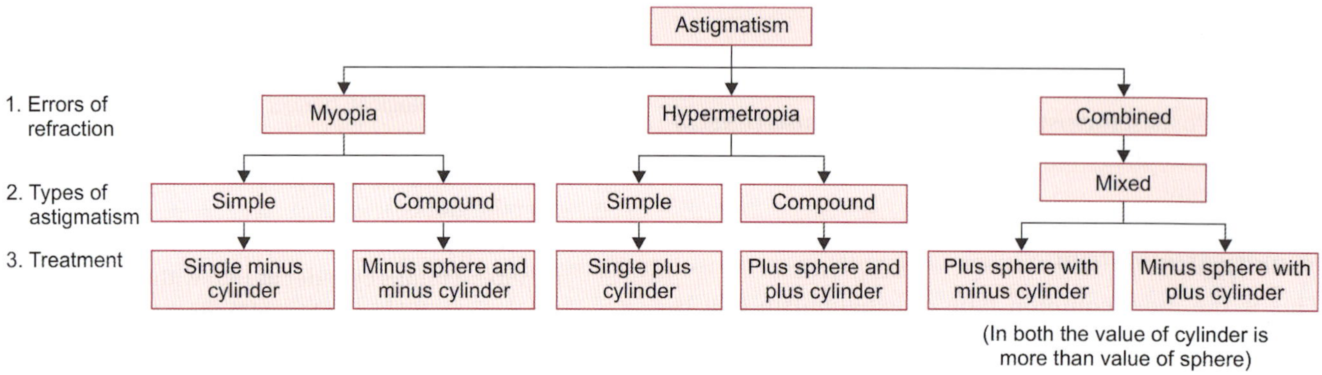

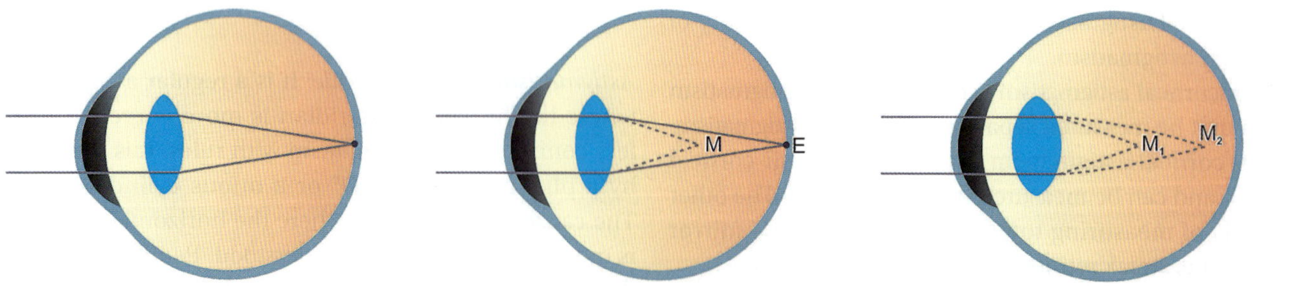

1 Emmetropia

2 Simple myopic astigmatism with accommodation at rest

3 Effect of accommodation in simple myopic astigmatism point M in figure 2 moves to point M_1 and point E shift 2 point M_2. Distance between M and E in figure 2 is equal to distance between M_1 and M_2 in figure 3

Fig. 23.9: The effect of accommodation on myopia.

–4 –5.5
–3 ┼ –3 Adding –1.5 to this makes it –4.5 ┼ –4.5
–4 –5.5

Refractive power at two meridians in compound myopic astigmatism.

The difference between the two meridians is 1.0 D. This is the value of the cylinder that will be required to correct the astigmatism. Here, the lower value is 4.5 D, which the child will require as a spherical value. The power of the glass will be –4.5 D sphere with –1.00 Dcyl at 180°.

The condition is corrected by prescribing a minus spherocylinder as per retinoscopy.

Simple Hypermetropic Astigmatism

In this error of refraction, one meridian is emmetropic and the other is hypermetropic. If the child accommodates to bring the hypermetropic meridian in the retina, the emmetropic meridian moves forward, and they behave with simple myopic astigmatism. If the child continues to accommodate, both the meridians move away from the retina, and the eye becomes compound myopic astigmatism, which is worse than the original simple hypermetropic astigmatism. This forces the child to give up accommodation **(Fig. 23.10)**.

Simple hypermetropic astigmatism is corrected by a single plus cylinder, as per retinoscopy under cycloplegia.

Compound Hypermetropic Astigmatism

Here, both the meridians are hypermetropic. The effect of accommodation will be given as follows:

- If the hypermetropia is so high that accommodation does not bring either of the planes on the retina, the eye remains hypermetropic astigmatic with reduced spherical value. The child may prefer vision with accommodation and keep accommodating.
- Accommodation brings one meridian to the retina, and the other moves forward without reaching the retina. The eye is converted to simple hypermetropic astigmatism with accommodation.
- Both planes move in front of the retina, and the eye is converted into compound myopic astigmatism.
- In cases of very high hypermetropic astigmatism, one meridian moves in front of the retina, becoming

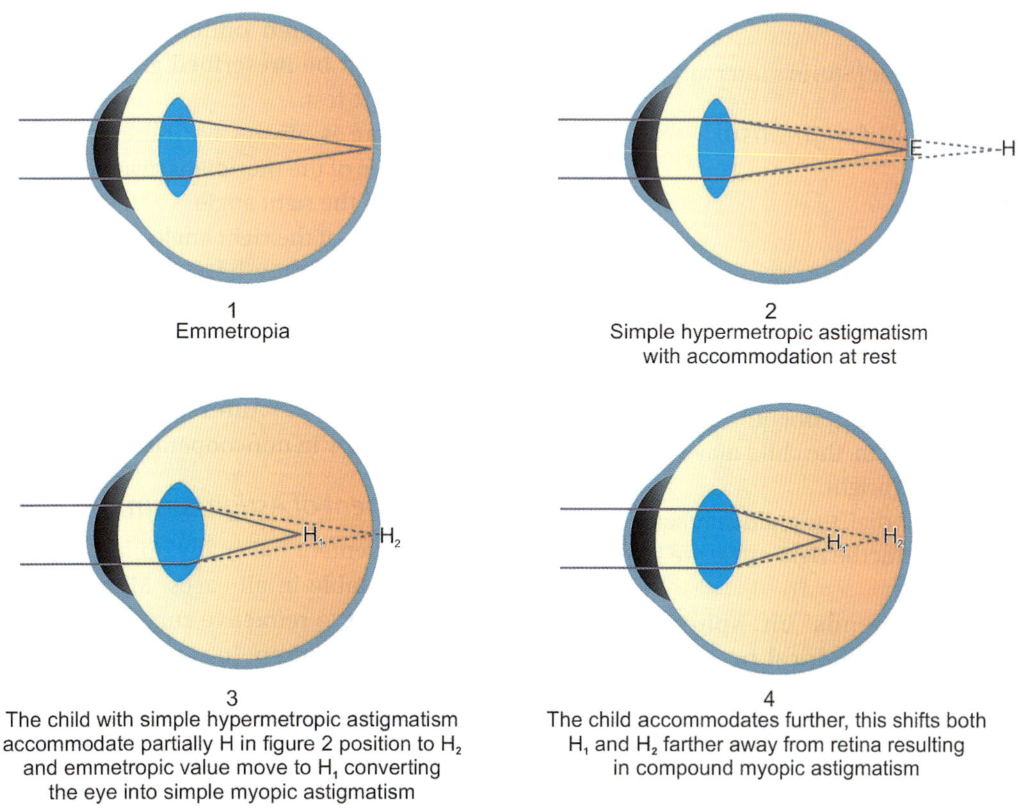

Fig. 23.10: Effects of accommodation on hypermetropic astigmatism.

myopic, and the other, in spite of accommodation, fails to reach the retina, so the eye is converted into mixed astigmatism.

The best method to manage compound hypermetropic astigmatism is to refract the eye under complete cycloplegia and prescribe plus spherocylinder as per retinoscopy.

Mixed Astigmatism

This is that error of refraction where one plane is in front of the retina (myopic), and the other plane is hypermetropic. Accommodation worsens the condition as accommodation converts the eye into compound myopic astigmatism. The eye without accommodation surprisingly has unexpectedly good vision, so the child opts not to accommodate. The condition is corrected by sphere and cylinder of opposite signs, i.e., a plus sphere with a minus cylinder or a minus sphere with a plus cylinder. The value of the cylinder is always more than the value of the sphere. The condition is best corrected by a contact lens.

Regular Astigmatism

Features of regular astigmatism are given as follows:

- Regular astigmatism is always congenital.
- The anterior corneal surface is responsible for regular astigmatism.
- The power of a cylinder (Sturm's interval) is constant.

Signs and Symptoms of Astigmatism

Signs:

- *External appearance:*
  - There may be no sign.
  - Some children tilt their heads to compensate for the axis of astigmatism.
  - The child may narrow the interpalpebral fissure to neutralize some of the spherical components but not the cylindrical component.
  - On the astigmatic fan, the child may see some lines that are clear and bright.
  - On the astigmatic dial, the child may see some lines clearly, but those at the right angle are blurred.
- *Vision:*
  - Vision loss depends on spherical power compounded by cylindrical power; a child with –3 sphere and one cylinder will have vision between 6/36 and 6/60 out of that major part will be due to spherical error. Only –3 D sphere will improve its vision to 6/12. To improve vision to 6/6, the child will require –1 cylinder at the appropriate axis.
  - A low astigmatic may not complain of diminished vision, especially in simple astigmatism.
  - Loss of vision due to simple astigmatism is not >6/12 to 6/18.
  - Vision with pinhole may not improve as much as in pure spherical error; for example, an eye with 6/18 vision will improve to 6/6 or better in the case of spherical error, but an astigmatic with the same vision will improve to 6/12 or 6/9 but will improve with the required cylinder in the correct axis to 6/6 or better.
  - The power of the cylinder in regular astigmatism may be unexpectedly high, i.e., a child with spherical error will improve to 6/6 or better from 6/12 to 6/18 by ±0.5 Dsph, but to reach the same clarity, the child will require ±1.25 to ±1.75 cylinders.
  - An astigmatic child may not be able to tell the direction of the arms of E in vision drum equally in both horizontal and vertical directions, i.e., he is able to indicate the vertical lines correctly but not the horizontal or other way round.
- *Retinoscopy:*
  - The extent of the error of refraction should always be evaluated under cycloplegia, and the child should be prescribed glasses after the postcycloplegic test.
  - There is always a difference in the retinoscopy value of the meridians given as follows:
    - At the right angle
    - Not at the right angle
    - There may be scissor movement in oblique astigmatism.
- *Keratometry:* Keratometry may be employed if parents do not agree to refraction under cycloplegia.
- *Autorefraction:* Autorefraction is an alternative to retinoscopy in noncooperative children.

Management of Astigmatism

The management has many options, not all of which are equally suitable in all cases. Management ranges from no treatment to refractive surgery. The latter are contraindicated in children. In some instances, more than one method gives the best result; the most common example is spectacle correction over contact lenses.

- If there is no eye strain, asthenopia, amblyopia, or muscle imbalance and the child is comfortable with his vision, no treatment is required. However, this child should have a yearly visual assessment to exclude amblyopia, and they should be refracted under cycloplegia to detect spherical errors that may creep with age.

- Optical

  Optical corrections consist of:
  - Spectacles
  - Contact lens
  - Combination
  - Refractive surgery (not indicated in children)

Spectacles: Spectacles are the most commonly used optical devices in treating all errors of refraction and presbyopia, astigmatism being no exception. The advantages of spectacles are that they are economical, give a good visual result, do not require eye–hand coordination, and hardly need any maintenance. They are available in various sizes, shapes, and colors; they are generally unifocal, but some children may require bifocals.

- Simple astigmatism is corrected by a single cylindrical lens of the required power at the required axis.
- Compound astigmatism is corrected by a sphere and cylinder of the same sign.
- Mixed astigmatism is corrected by a sphere and a cylinder of opposite signs. The dioptric power of the cylinder is always more than spherical.

> - While prescribing the cylinder, its power and axis should be as per retinoscopy.
> - There is no scope for overcorrection or undercorrection in the cylinder.

- In mixed astigmatism, the combination that is most comfortable should be prescribed. For instance, it is to be decided if the child should be given a plus sphere with a minus cylinder at 180° or a minus sphere with a plus cylinder at 90°.
- Children are more comfortable with the minus cylinder at 180° and the plus cylinder at 90° because they are more physiological.

There are various methods of verifying the power and axis of a cylinder.

They are given as follows:

- Retinoscopy by streak retinoscope
- Autorefraction
- Keratometry
- Jackson cross-cylinder
- Astigmatic fan
- Astigmatic dial
- Fogging

Theoretically, Jackson cross-cylinder is the best out of all. The greatest disadvantage is a lack of child's attention and cooperation. Only children above 10 years are suitable for this method.

In the case of spectacles prescribed for astigmatism, the fitting of the spectacle should be good and stable. An ill-fitting spectacle invariably results in the shifting of the axis on either side of the desired axis, making it ineffective. Rectangular frames are better than circular ones.

Contact lenses: Contact lenses are a good alternative to spectacles for astigmatism. They should be prescribed only when the child can manage the contact lens without parental help.

Parents should see that the contact lenses are clean and maintained as per the instructions of the manufacturer. Contact lenses mostly correct spherical requirements in moderate to high compound astigmatism.

Moderate astigmatic errors can be fully corrected by contact lenses. Rigid gas-permeable contact lenses are better than soft lenses. High astigmatism is best corrected by toric contact lenses, which are otherwise not very comfortable for children.

Refractive surgery: Refractive surgery in astigmatism does not give as satisfactory a result as in stigmatic ametropia.

Moreover, they are indicated only after 20 years of age.

Irregular Astigmatism

Irregular astigmatism is astigmatism where:

- Power varies on the same axis.
- There may be more than two axes.
- Power from one meridian to the outer changes abruptly.
- The defect causing irregular astigmatism lies mostly in the cornea.
- There is no change in axial length in any meridian.
- The corneal curvature itself may be variable.
- Irregular astigmatism is mostly acquired.
- When congenital, they are missed at birth.
- Irregular astigmatism can be unilateral.
- Common causes of irregular astigmatism in children are given as follows:
  - Limbal dermoid
  - Keratoconus
  - Corneal scar:
    - Postinflammatory
    - Post-traumatic status

 - Pseudopterygium
 - Keratectasia
 - Corneal foreign body
- Most of the time, the principal meridians are separated by an angle other than 90°.

Symptoms of irregular astigmatism: The symptoms vary according to the extent of astigmatism. The common symptoms are given as follows:

- Diminished vision
- Scattering of light
- Glare

The vision may improve with single or multiple pinholes and stenopic slits but not with spectacle glasses.

Various types of contact lenses are prescribed with variable results; the best results are achieved by keratoplasty.

Anisometropia

Anisometropia is the refractive state of eyes that have different refractions in two eyes. In contrast to isometropia, which has equal refraction in both eyes, isometropia is an ideal physiological condition; hence, like all physiological statuses, it is a rarity. Logically, any difference in refraction between two eyes is anisometropia. Clinically, eyes are said to be anisometropic when the difference in refraction between two eyes is >2.5 D.

Before the clinical significance of anisometropia is discussed, it is essential to pay attention to the magnification produced by lenses that are employed to correct anisometropia.

- One diopter of the lens in a spectacle causes a 2% change in image.
- Hypermetropics cause magnification.
- Myopia causes minification.
- The difference in the size of images between two eyes is called aniseikonia*.
- A difference of 2 D will produce a change of 4% between two images, which is well within the tolerable limit; a difference of 5% and above of aniseikonia will result in diplopia, suppression, and amblyopia. The first symptom after spectacle correction of anisometropia is diplopia, in which the child may give up spectacles. The most common example is unilateral aphakia corrected by spectacle when the other eye has a normal or near-normal vision.
- Though 2 D of anisometropia is generally well tolerated, yet some children may not be comfortable with such a small difference. In contrast to this, some children may tolerate as much as 4 D of difference.
- Antimetropia is an anisometropia where refraction in two eyes is of a different type, i.e., one eye is myopic and the other eye is hypermetropic. The child uses a hypermetropic eye for distance and a myopic eye for near, retaining binocular vision; they do not develop amblyopia and squint. The children prefer to be without glasses than with glasses.
- The term monovision is used to denote the following:
 - The child is habituated to use one eye; the other eye is either suppressed or amblyopic; the amblyopic eye is invariably a squinting eye.
 - One eye is used for distance and the other for near.
- One degree of aniseikonia corrected introduces 1° of change is size that is roughly 1%.
- To have good binocular vision, the retinal images should be iseikonic. However, the two eyes are able to fuse up to 2% of aniseikonia physiologically.
- Children with hypermetropic anisometropia are more prone to develop muscle imbalances that may initially be latent to become manifest with the passage of time.
- Eye with more power is prone to be amblyopic and squint.

Etiology of Anisometropia

About 5% of persons with errors of refraction are clinically anisometropic. Undetected or untreated anisometropia is an important cause of amblyopia. Seventy-five percent of children with esotropia are anisometropic.

Anisometropia can be congenital or acquired. Most children are mildly anisometropic at birth. The defect passes away in a few months. The part of anisometropia that is not corrected by this time lasts for the rest of life. No cause is found in congenital anisometropia; congenital anisometropia is generally nonpathological. Most of the congenital anisometropia are genetic and follow the genetics of the type of error of refraction, i.e., myopia/hypermetropia, they suffer from.

**Aniseikonia:* Aniseikonia is the difference in size or shape of an object between two eyes. Besides anisometropia, it can even be physiological. Other causes of aniseikonia are neurological and retinal; the last two are less frequent than optical.

Flowchart 23.7: Classification of various possibilities of anisometropia.

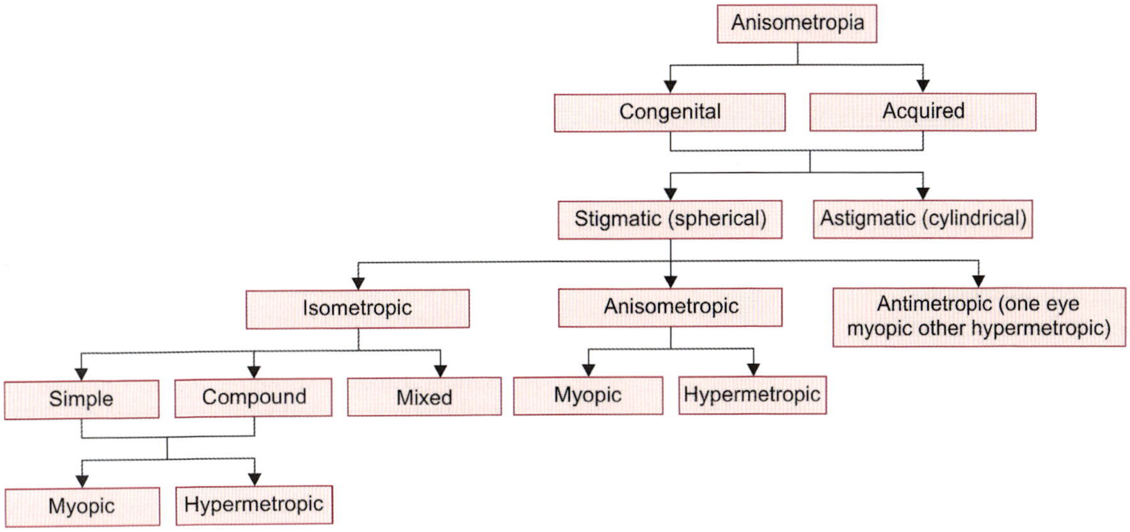

The most common cause of acquired anisometropia is unilateral aphakia; other causes are wrong calculation of the power of the IOL, keratoconus, and postkeratoplasty status.

Flowchart 23.7 shows various types of anisometropia.

Symptoms of Anisometropia in Children

- Asymptomatic
- Uniocular diminished distant vision in the eye with higher error.
- Diminished vision in both eyes, one eye more than the other.
- Diminished distant vision in both eyes due to antimetropia; this child uses a myopic eye for near and hypermetropic eye for distance.
- The child is brought with squints and is found to be anisometropic.
- Asthenopia
- If one eye is ametropic and the other is emmetropic, the child keeps the ametropic eye closed.

Management of Anisometropia

Management of anisometropia is not as easy as isometropia, especially in children; if it is not treated before the age of 8 years, it passes into a state of permanent suppression and squinting. Loss of binocularity is proportionate to the degree of anisometropia. In anisometropia, <2.5 D binocular vision may be present.

Anisometropia should be detected and treated as early as possible to avoid troublesome amblyopia.

Eyes with high errors do not improve as much as eyes with low errors, and this should be a clue to the presence of anisometropia. Anisometropia is best diagnosed by refraction under cycloplegia. It may be detected by the Brückner test as well, where the eye with the higher error has a duller red reflex.

The aim of treatment is not only to correct ametropia but also to reduce aniseikonia.

This is achieved optically.

The first choice is to treat anisometropia optically as early as possible to avoid amblyopia.

The various optical methods available to treat anisometropia are given as follows:

- An effort should be made to correct anisometropia above 1 D when detected in children under 8 years.
- This can be fairly achieved in anisometropia up to 3 D.
- When the difference between two eyes is 3 D or more, the eye with higher power should be undercorrected.
- It is better to give equal power to both eyes.
- Spectacles are no answer to high anisometropia, such as uniocular aphakia. They are better treated by contact lenses.
- To avoid unilateral aphakia in children, the best alternative is a planned phaco with posterior chamber intraocular lens (PCIOL). This will negate the difference in magnification in the affected eye.

- If the eye is already unilateral aphakic, the options are given as follows:
  - Contact lens to the aphakic eye
  - Secondary IOL
  - Refractive surgeries (this is not indicated in children)
- In contrast to high hypermetropia anisometropic, high myopic anisometropia is treated by:
  - Contact lens
  - Clear lens extraction
  - Clear lens extraction with IOL
  - Intraocular lens over clear lens

SUGGESTED READING

1. Agrawal LP. Principles of Optics and Refraction, 2nd edition. New Delhi: CBS Publishers and Distributors; 1979.
2. Curtin BJ. The posterior staphyloma of pathological myopia. Trans Am Ophthalmol Soc. 1977;75:67-86.
3. Elder SD. Astigmatism in Duke Elder's Practice of Refraction, 9th edition. New Delhi: BI Churchill, Livingston; 1989.
4. Elder SD. Congenital Aphakia in System of Ophthalmology. London, UK: Henry Kimpton; 1964.
5. Elder SD. Ophthalmic Optics and Refraction. In: Elder SD (Ed). System of Ophthalmology. St. Louis, Missouri, USA: Mosby; 1970.
6. Elder SD. The Foundation in Ophthalmology. London, UK: Henry Kimpton; 1962.
7. Khurana AK. Theories and Practice of Optics and Refraction, 1st edition. New Delhi: BI Churchill Livingstone; 2001.
8. Mukherjee PK. Clinical Examination in Ophthalmology, 2nd edition. New Delhi: Elsevier; 2016.
9. Mukherjee PK. Manual of Optics and Refraction, 1st edition. New Delhi: Jaypee Brothers Medical (P) Pvt. Ltd.; 2015.
10. Mukherjee PK. Ophthalmic Assistant, 1st edition. New Delhi: Jaypee Brothers Medical (P) Pvt. Ltd.; 2013.
11. Safir A. Charlse M. Refraction in Children in Pediatric Ophthalmology, 2nd edition. Philadelphia, PA, USA: WB Saunders; 1983. pp. 277-92.
12. Singhal NC. Principles and Practice of Refraction and Optics, 1st edition. New Delhi: Jaypee Brothers Medical (P) Pvt. Ltd.; 1996.
13. Tongue AC, Grin TR. Refractive errors and glasses for children. In: Tongue AC, Grin TR (Eds). Decision making in pediatric ophthalmology. St. Louis, MO, USA: Mosby; -1993. pp. 186-7.
14. Venkatesh P, Verma Tewari HK. Macular and Allergic Diseases in Clinical Practice in Ophthalmology, 1st edition. New Delhi: Jaypee Brothers Medical (P) Pvt. Ltd.; 2003.

CHAPTER

24 Muscle Imbalance in Children

To understand muscle imbalance, it is imperative to discuss about the anatomy and physiology of the extraocular muscles, which are as follows.

In order to move the eyes, there are six extraocular muscles attached to the globe, each with a different action that requires specialized nerve supply by cranial nerves. The eyes move either voluntarily or reflexively. All the extraocular muscles are striated and supplied by cranial nerves third, fourth, and sixth for motor functions. The sensory supply to the extraocular muscles is through the fifth nerve. The extraocular muscles are not supplied with an autonomic nervous system.

The extraocular muscles act around three imaginary axes X, Y, and Z **(Figs. 24.1A and B)**, called the axes of Fick. The X axis passes horizontally from one end of the globe to the other, through the point of rotation round which the globe revolves; the Z axis passes vertically through the center of rotation; and the Y axis passes anteriorly and posteriorly through the center of rotation. The center of rotation lies 12–13 mm posterior to the cornea in the horizontal plane.

Table 24.1 shows action of extraocular muscles in various positions.

The extraocular muscles are put into two groups, i.e., those essentially concerned with horizontal movements of the globe and those meant for cyclovertical movements. The former group consists of two muscles, namely (1) the medial rectus (MR) and (2) the lateral rectus, with the main functions of horizontal movement; their muscle planes coincide with the visual axis of the eye. The cyclovertical muscles are the superior rectus (SR) and inferior rectus (IR) and the superior and inferior obliques. The four recti originate from the apex of the orbit and are inserted in front of the equator. They are also involved in the retraction of the globe; their paralysis results in the protraction of the globe. The two obliques have an effective origin at the rim of orbit and are inserted behind the equator of globe. The obliques give a retracting influence on the globe.

CYCLOVERTICAL MUSCLES

Due to their complex actions, they require a detailed description.

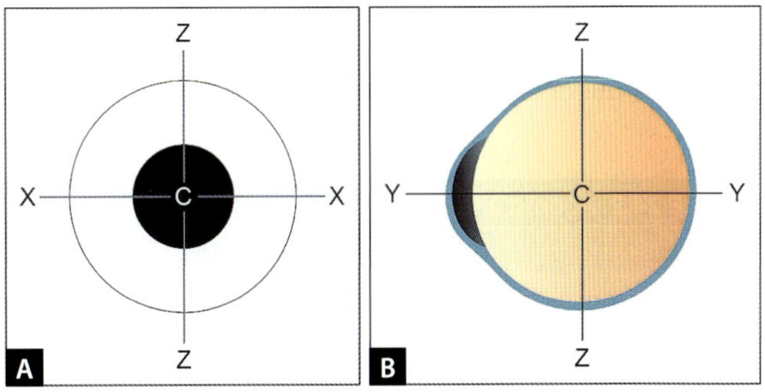

Figs. 24.1A and B: Axes of Fick. (A) Axis Z and X; (B) Axis Y and Z. (C: center of rotation; XCX: horizontal axis; YCY: anteroposterior; ZCZ: vertical axis)

TABLE 24.1: Action of extraocular muscles.

Muscle	*Primary action*	*Best position of action*	
Medial rectus	Adduction	Primary	
Lateral rectus	Abduction	Primary	
Superior rectus	Elevation (intorsion and adduction)	Elevation (only at 23° abduction)	Intorsion (only in 67° adduction)
Inferior rectus	Depression (extorsion and adduction)	Depression (only at 23° abduction)	Extorsion (only at 67° adduction)
Superior oblique	Intorsion (depression and abduction)	Intorsion (only at 39° abduction)	Depression (only at 51° adduction)
Inferior oblique	Extorsion (elevation and abduction)	Extorsion (only at 39° abduction)	Elevation (only at 51° adduction)

- The four cyclovertical muscles are superior and inferior recti and superior and inferior obliques.
- The superior and inferior recti are supplied by a single cranial nerve, i.e., the oculomotor.
- The superior oblique (SO) gets its motor supply from the fourth cranial nerve, which does not supply any other extraocular muscle.
- The inferior oblique (IO) shares its motor supply with the IR from the inferior division of the third nerve.
- The muscle plane of the cyclovertical does not coincide with the visual axis in primary position.
- The recti form an angle of 23° with the visual axis, while the obliques form an angle of 51°.

Some terms used in clinical practice about the action of extraocular muscles are given as follows.

Agonist and Antagonist Muscles

These are terms used to denote the action of more than one muscle at a particular movement.

- *Agonist*: The agonists are prime movers in the required direction.

No muscle acts alone.

- *Antagonist*: The antagonist in the same eye acts directly against the agonist.

Note: In abduction of the right eye, the right lateral rectus muscle is the agonist; the right superior and IO muscles are the synergists. The right medial, superior, and inferior recti are the antagonists.

***Table 24.2** shows agonist and antagonist muscles of the eye.*

Synergist Muscle

A synergist is a muscle that increases the action of a specific muscle in a particular gaze. They contract at the time of action; they work with the agonist in the same eye to produce the desired movement. The example is that superior rectus is synergist to inferior oblique in elevation; it is also synergist to superior oblique in intorsion.

Antagonist: The muscles that are inhibited (relaxed) are called antagonists.

Yoke Muscle

They are also known as contralateral synergists. They are pairs of agonist muscles with the same primary action, one from each eye that works together in binocular movement in one direction (version). Yoke muscles are the primary muscles in each eye that accomplish a given version (e.g., for right gaze, the right lateral rectus, and left medial rectus muscles) **(Table 24.3 and Fig. 24.2)**.

Duction

Duction is the movement of one eye, i.e., abduction stands for lateral movement, and adduction means

TABLE 24.2: Agonist and antagonist muscles and their actions as per the muscle involved.

Actions	*Agonist (synergist)*	*Antagonists*
Dextroversion	Right lateral rectus + Left medial rectus	Right medial rectus + Left lateral rectus
Dextroelevation	Right superior rectus + Left inferior oblique	Right inferior rectus + Left superior oblique
Dextrodepression	Right inferior rectus + Left superior oblique	Right superior rectus + Left inferior oblique
Sursumversion	Right superior rectus + Left superior rectus and *Right inferior oblique + Left inferior oblique*	Right inferior rectus + Left inferior rectus and *Right superior oblique + Left superior oblique*
Deorsumversion	Right inferior rectus + Left inferior rectus and *Right superior oblique + Left superior oblique*	Right superior rectus + Left superior rectus and *Right inferior oblique + Left inferior oblique*
Levoversion	Right medial rectus + Left lateral rectus	Right lateral rectus + Left medial rectus
Levoelevation	Right inferior oblique + Left superior rectus	Right superior oblique + Left inferior rectus
Levodepression	Right superior oblique + Left inferior rectus	Right inferior oblique + Left superior rectus

(dextro: right; deorsumversion: downgaze; duction: movement of both eyes at a given time; levo: left; sursum: upward; version: movement of one eye)

The vertical recti are the chief elevator; they are supplemented by obliques to a lesser extent.

TABLE 24.3: Action of yoke muscles in various cardinal gazes.

Direction of gaze	*Muscles involved*
Up and right	RSR and LIO
Up and left	LSR and RIO
Right	RLR and LMR
Left	LLR and RMR
Down and right	RIR and LSO
Down and left	LIR and RSO

(LIO: left inferior oblique; LIR: left inferior rectus; LLR: left lateral rectus; LMR: left medial rectus; LSO: left superior oblique; LSR: left superior rectus; RIO: right inferior oblique; RIR: right inferior rectus; RLR: right lateral rectus; RMR: right medial rectus; RSO: right superior oblique; RSR: right superior rectus)

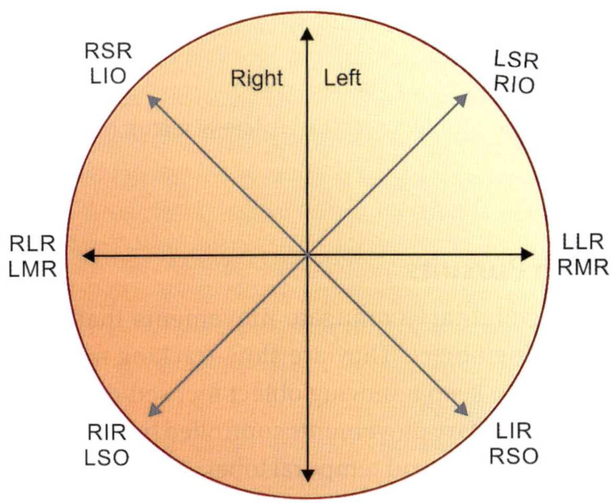

Fig. 24.2: Yoke muscle in various gazed. (LIO: left inferior oblique; LIR: left inferior rectus; LLR: left lateral rectus; LMR: left medial rectus; LSO: left superior oblique; LSR: left superior rectus; RIO: right inferior oblique; RIR: right inferior rectus; RLR: right lateral rectus; RMR: right medial rectus; RSO: right superior oblique; RSR: right superior rectus)

medial movement. The elevation of one eye is called sursumduction, the depression of one eye is called deorsumduction, and the term "cycloduction" is used to denote rotation either medially or laterally. Incycloduction means movement of the 12 o'clock position medially, while excycloduction stands for dipping of the 12 o'clock position laterally **(Fig. 24.3)**.

Versions

These are binocular movements in the same direction, i.e., conjugate movements. The versions are examined in the following diagnostic directions: Dextroversion means right-sided binocular movements, while levoversion means left binocular movements. Dextroelevation stands for bilateral right-up movement, dextrodepression represents left-down movement, and sursumversion means moving both eyes up. Deorsumversion is moving both eyes down **(Figs. 24.4 and 24.5)**.

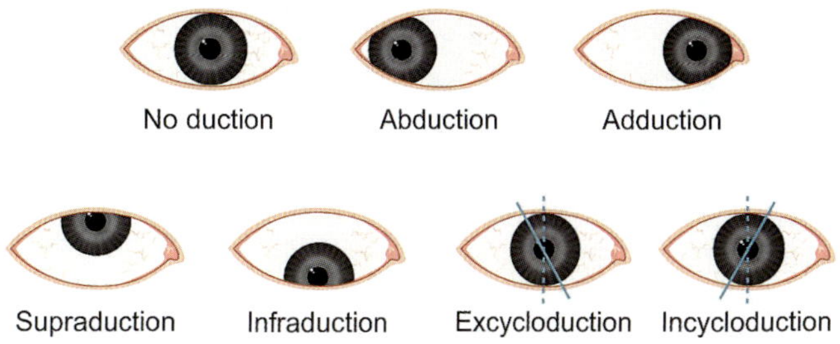

Fig. 24.3: Duction of the right eye.

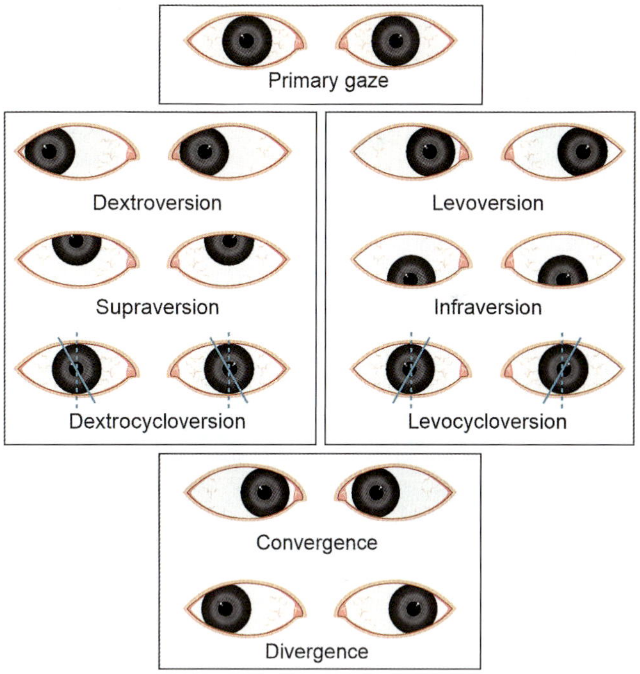

Fig. 24.4: Types of versions of eyes.

The importance of the testing version lies in the fact that a paralysis of extraocular muscles missed on examination of duction becomes obvious on the testing version.

Vergence

Disconjugate eye movements are called vergence. They are referred to as disjunctive, nonconjugate; they are slow movements of both eyes meant to find and fix objects at different distances. The objects need not to be stationary.

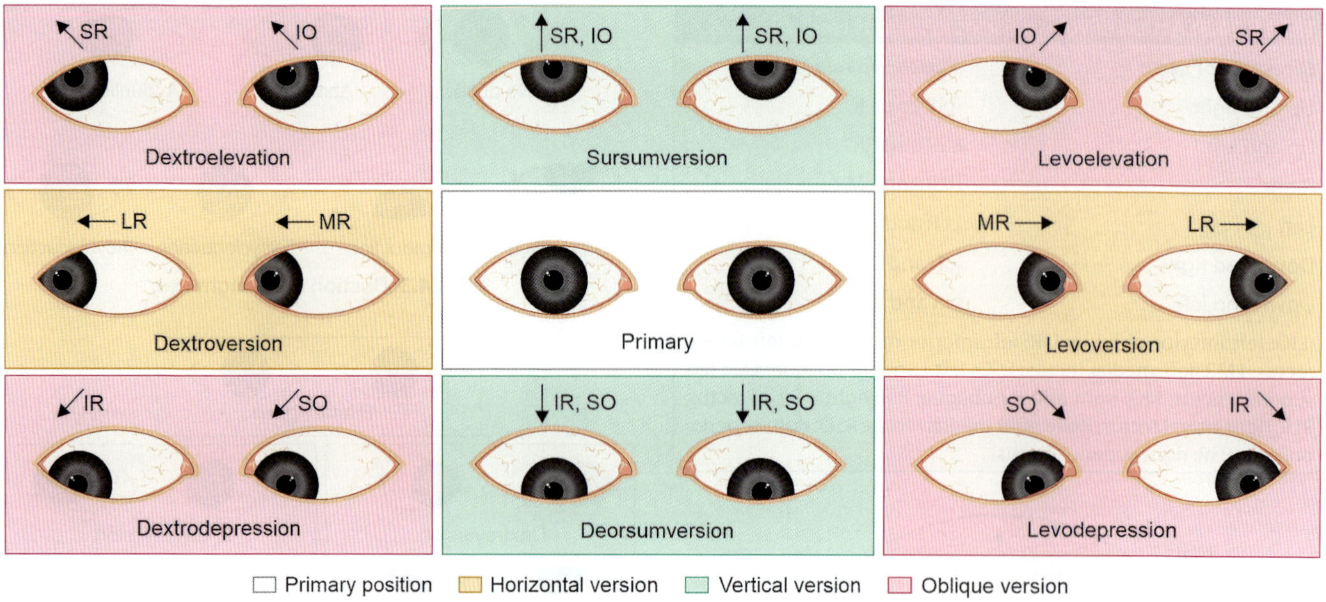

Fig. 24.5: Muscles involved in version (binocular movement). (IO: inferior oblique; IR: inferior rectus; LR: lateral rectus; MR: medial rectus; SO: superior oblique; SR: superior rectus)

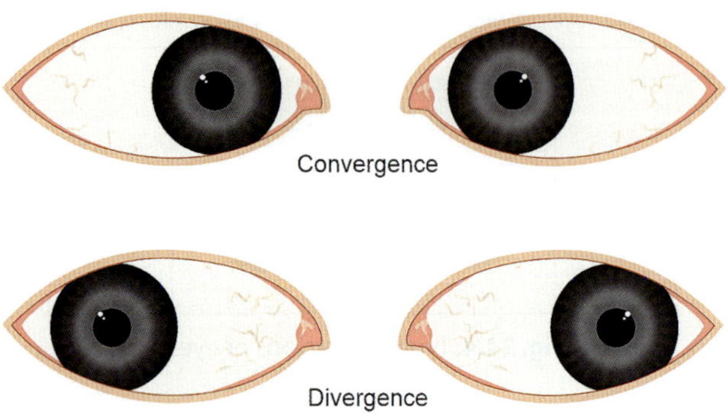

Fig. 24.6: Vergence of eyes.

The eyes move in opposite directions to allow both foveae to maintain fixation at the same time, even when the object moves near or away. The former is called convergence, and the latter is called divergence **(Fig. 24.6)**. The advantages of vergence are bifoveal fixation, binocular single vision (BSV), and stereopsis.

Saccades

Saccades are rapid conjugate movements that can be voluntary or involuntary. Due to a quick burst of activity, the eyes quickly change fixation from one fixation to another object of regard. They are present from birth. They can be in any of the following directions, i.e., horizontal, vertical, or oblique.

Smooth Pursuits

They are voluntary conjugate movements that follow a slow-moving object. They are slow-tracking movements of the eyes to keep a moving object focused on the fovea. They are voluntary movements controlled by the ipsilateral parietal, occipital, and temporal lobes.

Vestibulo-ocular Movements

They are meant to maintain ocular position in altered head and body positions.

Cardinal Positions of Gaze

The cardinal positions are six, brought about by a single muscle and its yoke muscle. They are right up, right, right down, left up, left, and left down.

Besides these, there are three gazes, i.e., (1) straight up, (2) straight down, and (3) convergence.

Flowchart 24.1 shows cardinal gazes and the muscles involved.

Gaze

Gaze is the ability to look at an object of interest steadily for a long time. In clinical practice, they are primary, secondary, and tertiary.

Flowchart 24.1: Cardinal direction of gaze.

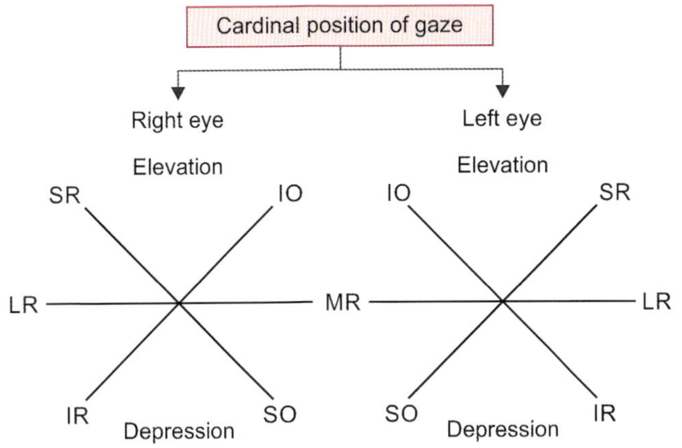

(IO: inferior oblique; IR: inferior rectus; LR: lateral rectus; MR: medial rectus; SO: superior oblique; SR: superior rectus)

Note:
- The superior rectus and inferior obliques are elevators.
- The inferior rectus and superior obliques are depressors.

Primary Gaze

Primary gaze can fix an object beyond 20 feet (far point) with the head straight and accommodation at rest. Secondary positions can be right, left, up, and down gazes. The tertiary positions are oblique positions of the eyes.

Conjugate Movements

Conjugate movements are meant for bilateral fixation of an object. It is a coordinated movement of two eyes at the same direction. It is also called yoked movement; it can be in any direction and may have saccadic or smooth pursuit.

Overaction and Underaction of Extraocular Muscles

An extraocular muscle is said to be overacting when it moves excessively into the field of action in version. The reverse of this is referred to as underaction **(Fig. 24.7)**.

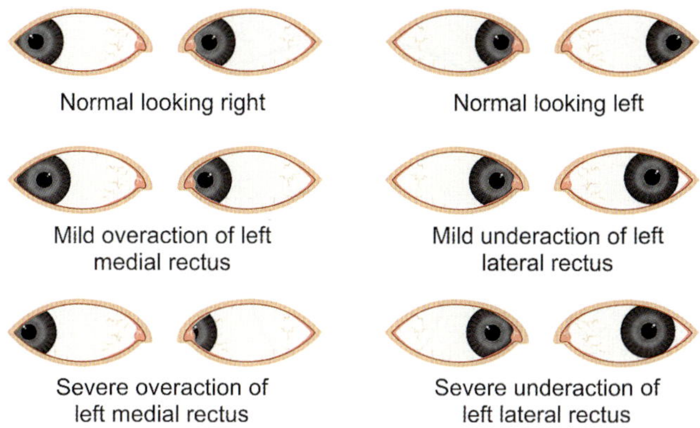

Fig. 24.7: The overaction and underaction of horizontal muscles.

LAWS GOVERNING THE ACTION OF EXTRAOCULAR MUSCLE MOVEMENT

There are two laws, i.e., Hering's and Sherrington's. The former is also called the "law of equal innervations," while the second is called the "law of reciprocal innervations." Hering's law states that synergists of one eye get equal and simultaneous innervations for its movement, i.e., the number of innervations to the right MR is exactly the same as that of the left lateral rectus and inhibits the right lateral rectus exactly the same as the left MR.

TABLE 24.4: Action of various muscles in different positions.

Muscles	*Primary*	*Secondary*	*Tertiary*
Medial rectus	Adduction	Nil	Nil
Lateral rectus	Abduction	Nil	Nil
Superior rectus	Elevation	Intorsion	Adduction
Inferior rectus	Depression	Extorsion	Adduction
Superior oblique	Intorsion	Depression	Abduction
Inferior oblique	Extorsion	Elevation	Abduction

Sherrington's law states that increased action of an extraocular muscle is associated with reduced contraction of its antagonist. For example, during convergence, there is increased contraction of both medial recti with diminished contraction of both lateral recti.

APPLIED ANATOMY OF EXTRAOCULAR MUSCLES

Each extraocular muscle is meant for a specific purpose. The movements can be primary, secondary, or tertiary.

Table 24.4 shows muscles involved in primary, secondary, and tertiary positions.

It has been noted that the four recti take their origin from the annulus of Zinn and pass forward to be inserted in front of the equator. The length of the recti varies; the inferior rectus being shortest, and all the recti are not inserted in the globe at the same distance from the limbus. The medial rectus is inserted nearest to the limbus, i.e., 5.5 mm, and the superior rectus is farthest, i.e., 7.7 mm. From the limbus, the inferior rectus is inserted at 6.5 mm and the lateral rectus at 6.9 mm. The points of insertion are depicted in the "spiral of Tillaux" **(Fig. 24.8)**.

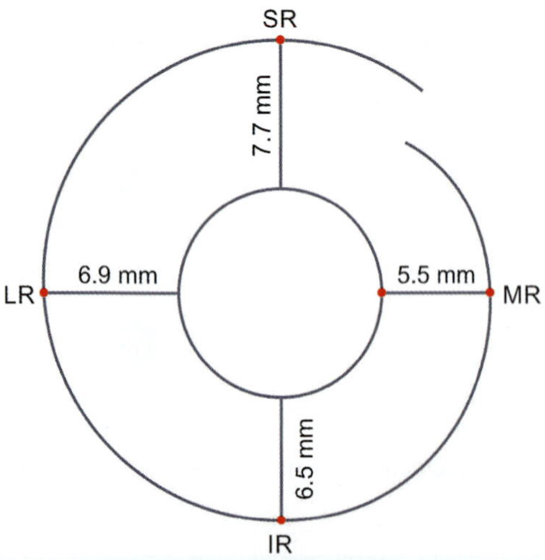

Fig. 24.8: Spiral of Tillaux. (IR: inferior rectus; LR: lateral rectus; MR: medial rectus; SR: superior rectus)

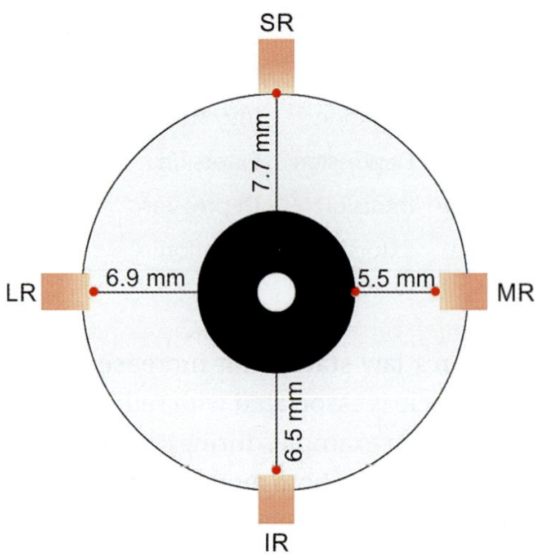

Fig. 24.9: The distance of the recti from the limbus. (IR: inferior rectus; LR: lateral rectus; MR: medial rectus; SR: superior rectus)

TABLE 24.5: Dimension of tendons of the recti.

Muscle	*Length of tendon (mm)*	*Width of tendon (mm)*	*Type of insertion*
Superior rectus	10.5	10.00	Obliquely linear
Inferior rectus	5.5	10.00	Convex, apex toward the cornea
Medial rectus	3.7	10.00	Straight, linear
Lateral rectus	8.8	10.00	Linear, vertical

The recti are inserted by tendons of different lengths **(Fig. 24.9)**.

Table 24.5 shows dimensions of recti muscles.

The following is the summary of the insertion and nerve supply of the obliques:

- The obliques are inserted behind the equator. The superior oblique is inserted obliquely, the anterior end of the insertion is 13.5 mm from the limbus, and the posterior end is 18.5 mm away from the limbus.
- The inferior oblique is inserted behind the equator by an oblique insertion with convexity upward. The posterior end of the insertion lies 1.5 mm from the macula. The anterior end of the insertion lies just under the insertion of the lateral rectus.
- The obliques either do not have tendons at their insertion or have very short tendons. They are attached to the sclera in a curved manner **(Figs. 24.10A and B)**.
- All the recti get their blood supply from the scleral surface.
- The insertion of the recti is almost straight; the insertion of the obliques is curved.
- Out of six extraocular muscles, four, i.e., MR, SR, IR, and IO, get their nerve supply from the third nerve. The lateral rectus gets its nerve supply from the sixth nerve and the superior oblique from the fourth nerve.
- The obliques are inferior to the corresponding recti, i.e., the SO lies under the SR above the sclera, and the IO lies under the inferior rectus between the IR and orbital wall **(Fig. 24.11)**.

The actions of cyclovertical muscles in primary and secondary gaze are given in **Table 24.6**.

The action of synergist muscles and their position of gaze are given in **Table 24.7**.

The summary of cyclovertical action is given as follows:

- *Elevation:* Superior rectus and inferior oblique
- *Depression:* Inferior rectus and superior oblique
- *Intorsion:* Superior rectus and superior oblique
- *Extorsion:* Inferior rectus and inferior oblique

The sequels of extraocular muscle underaction are given as follows:

- Secondary underaction of the contralateral antagonist
- Contraction of the direct antagonist
- Overaction of contralateral synergist

ANATOMY OF EXTRAOCULAR MUSCLES (IN BRIEF)

The muscles can be horizontally acting or cyclovertically acting.

- *Horizontally acting:* Medial and lateral muscles

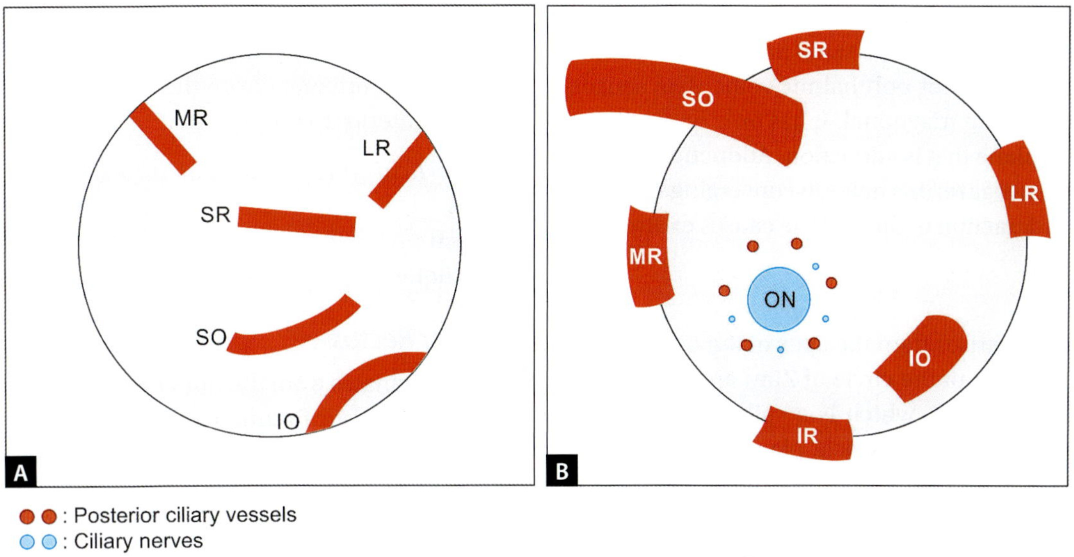

Figs. 24.10A and B: (A) Relation of recti and obliques as seen from above; (B) Insertion of the oblique and recti from behind. (IO: inferior oblique; IR: inferior rectus; LR: lateral rectus; MR: medial rectus; ON: optic nerve; SO: superior oblique; SR: superior rectus)

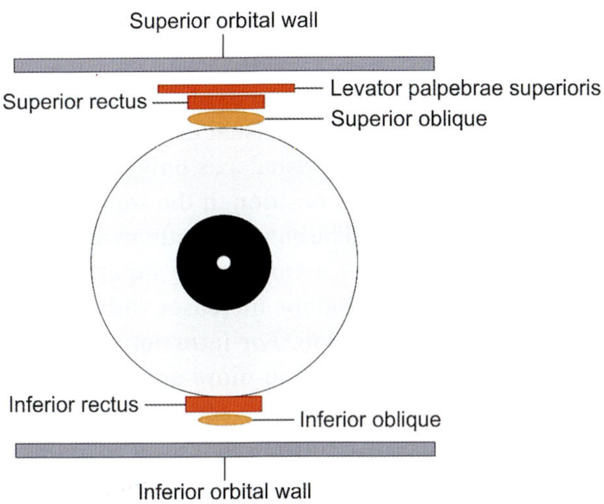

Fig. 24.11: The position of obliques in relation to the recti and orbital wall.

TABLE 24.6: Primary and secondary actions of cyclovertical muscles.

Cyclovertical muscles	*Primary action*	*Secondary action*
• *Recti:* – Superior rectus – Inferior rectus	• Elevation • Depression	• Adduction and intorsion • Adduction and extorsion
• *Obliques:* – Superior oblique – Inferior oblique	• Intorsion • Extorsion	• Depression and abduction • Elevation and abduction

TABLE 24.7: Direction of action synergist muscles.

Synergist muscles	*Direction*
Right superior rectus and left inferior oblique	Up and right
Left superior rectus and right inferior oblique	Up and left
Right lateral rectus and left medial rectus	Right
Left lateral rectus and right medial rectus	Left
Right inferior rectus and left superior oblique	Down and right
Left inferior rectus and right superior oblique	Down and left

- *Cyclovertically acting:* Superior and inferior rectus and superior and inferior obliques

Horizontally Acting Recti

Medial Rectus

This is a straight muscle. The plane of the muscle coincides with the visual axis of the eye. It originates at the apex of the orbit from the medial side of the circle of Zinn. It is 41.0 mm (actually 40.8 mm) in length. It passes forward between the medial wall of the orbit and the globe in the horizontal meridian of the eyeball. The anterior 3.7–4.5 mm (mean 4.0 mm) is its tendon, which is 10.3 mm wide that inserts in the sclera in a vertical linear fashion 5.5 mm away from the limbus. Its insertion is nearest to the limbus when compared to other extraocular muscle insertions (see "spiral of Tillaux"). It is innervated by the lower division of the third cranial nerve, which pierces the muscle from its ocular surface. It gets its blood supply by two twigs of the anterior ciliary artery. The venous drainage is through the corresponding veins of the same name that drain into the superior and inferior ophthalmic veins. The sensory supply is through the trigeminal. It has only one action in the horizontal plane that is adduction. Adduction is better in slightly lowered gaze; this helps in converging the eye to near work. Underaction of this muscle causes exotropia.

Lateral Rectus

The lateral rectus arises from the apex of the orbit, mostly from the lateral part of the circle of Zinn and partly from the spina lateralis recti, which is a spike in the greater wing of the sphenoid. Its muscle plane coincides with the visual axis; it has only one horizontal action, i.e., abduction. Its average length is 41 mm. It passes between the lateral orbital wall and the globe. Its tendon is about 9.0 mm in length and 9.2 mm wide. It gets inserted in front of the equator, 7.0 mm from the limbus, in a vertical line. It is innervated by the abducens nerve, which pierces the muscle from the inner surface.

> It gets its blood supply from a single anterior ciliary artery; all other recti get their blood supply by two anterior ciliary arteries.

Its venous drainage is via the veins of same name that drain in the ophthalmic vein. Its sensory supply is through the trigeminal. The action of the lateral rectus is best for distant fixation in a slight-up gaze.

The upper border of the lateral rectus almost reaches the lower border of the lacrimal gland, along with the lacrimal artery in the anterior part of the orbit. The tendon of the inferior oblique lies between the lateral rectus and the globe at its insertion.

Cyclovertical Muscles

There are two recti—the superior and inferior recti—and two obliques—the superior and the inferior obliques. The actions of the cycloverticals are more in number and more complex in nature when compared to horizontally acting muscles. They have all three actions, i.e., primary, secondary, and tertiary, in different gazes. Their long axes do not coincide with the visual axis in primary position. The two cyclovertical recti are adductors, while the two obliques are abductors. The superior cycloverticals, the SR and SO, are intorters. The two inferior cycloverticals are extorters.

> The primary action of all the cyclovertical is best in abduction.

The obliques have an effective origin in front of the globe and insertion behind the equator; in contrast to this, the recti originate from the apex of the orbit and are inserted anterior to the equator.

Cyclovertical muscles are put into two groups given as follows:

1. Recti
2. Obliques

Superior Rectus

The SR originates from the upper part of the circle of Zinn. Lateral to the optic foramen and sheath of the optic nerve, it travels forward under the roof of the orbit. Its average length is 42 mm. Its tendon is 5.5 mm in length and 10.5 mm wide at the insertion, which is 7.7–7.8 mm away from the limbus. The tendon does not insert in a straight line but has a mild convexity forward. The superior rectus lies under the levator and above the superior oblique. Its insertion is farthest from the insertion of any other recti (spiral of Tillaux).

In primary position, the long axis of the superior rectus forms an angle of 23° with the visual axis. The axis of the muscle coincides with the visual axis only when the eye is abducted at 23°. At this position, if the superior rectus contracts, the eyeball will be elevated without any torsion. Elevation is the primary action of the superior rectus. The ability to elevate the globe increases with abduction and decreases in adduction. For intorsion, the eyeball rotates to 67° medially; it is no more an elevator but is an intortor, which is a secondary action of the superior rectus. Adduction is the tertiary action of the superior rectus. Thus, the superior rectus is an elevator, intortor, and adductor of the globe. It is supplied by the upper division of the third nerve. It gets its blood supply by two anterior ciliary arteries. It has its corresponding venous drainage. Its sensory supply is through the trigeminal. One of its protective reflex actions is Bell's phenomenon. The superior rectus and inferior rectus work together as adductors but oppose each other as cyclovertical muscles.

Inferior Rectus

The IR takes its origin from the circle of Zinn traveling anteriorly and slightly downward under the globe and is inserted in the sclera 6.0 mm from the limbus in a slightly curved manner with convexity toward the limbus. The length of the muscle is 40.0 mm with a tendon of

5.0 mm length, and the width of the tendon is 10.0 mm at its insertion. The IO passes under it near the globe. The IR and IO have an intimate relation with the nonstriated muscle of the lower lid. The IR is joined to the ligament of Lockwood to give mechanical support to the globe from below. This prevents the globe from sinking down if there is a loss of bony support at the floor of the orbit. It follows the direction of the SR; its long axis is at an angle of 23° with the visual axis in primary position.

When the eyeball is abducted at 23°, the axis of the muscle and the visual axis coincide. It is a depressor of the globe that increases with abduction and is reduced in adduction. The primary action of the IR is depression. Its secondary action is extorsion, which is best at 67°; the tertiary action is being adduction.

Thus, the IR is a depressor, extortor, and adductor.

Cyclovertical Obliques

The two oblique muscles with cyclovertical action are superior and inferior obliques.

Superior Oblique

The SO differs from other extraocular muscles due to its length; it has the longest muscle belly and tendon. The muscle is divided into a long and a short part; the shorter part is the effective part of the muscle. The other point that differentiates it from other cyclovertical muscles is that it is supplied by a single cranial nerve, i.e., the trochlear nerve. The other cyclovertical muscles are supplied by the 3rd cranial nerve. This property of the SO being supplied by a single cranial nerve is shared by the lateral rectus that is supplied by a single cranial nerve, i.e., abducens. Due to peculiar position, the SO muscle is most liable to injury. Congenital anomalies of extraocular muscles are maximum in the SO **(Fig. 24.12)**.

It takes its origin at the apex of the orbit outside the circle of Zinn; its actual origin is from the periosteum of the body of the sphenoid, slightly above and medial to the optic foramen.

The muscular part of the muscle is 40.0 mm that runs forward, medially, and upward up to the trochlea, situated at the superomedial angle of the rim of the orbit. At this position, it passes over the pulley, after which it is converted wholly as a 20.0-mm long tendon. The tendon changes its direction backward, downward, and laterally under the SR to be inserted at the sclera in a wide area behind the equator in the posterolateral quadrant.

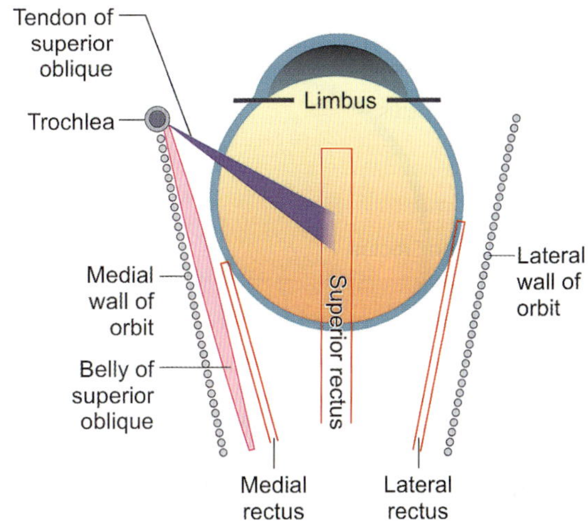

Fig. 24.12: The relation of the superior oblique to the superior and lateral rectus.

The muscular part of the muscle is called the direct part, and the tendon is referred to as the reflected part. The passage of the muscle over the trochlea is the effective origin of the muscle. The temporal side of the insertion is nearer to the limbus compared to the medial part. The temporal end is inserted 14.0 mm from the limbus, and the medial end is inserted 19.0 mm from the limbus. The insertion of the muscle is rounded with convexity away from the limbus. The posterior end of the insertion is near the vortex vein.

The plane of the muscle forms an angle of 54° with the visual axis, in which it is most effective. The muscle contracting at 54° is the best position for the globe to intort, which is the primary action of the superior oblique. The secondary function of the muscle is depression, while the tertiary action is abduction. The muscle is supplied by a fourth cranial nerve that enters the orbit outside the circle of Zinn, supplying the muscle belly from the orbital surface.

The muscles get its blood supply from the superior muscular branch of the ophthalmic artery. The muscle lies outside the muscle cone of the recti, and its motor nerve enters the orbit outside the circle of Zinn. As the motor supply is from outside the muscle cone, it is least affected by retrobulbar anesthesia but is well anesthetized by peribulbar injection.

Inferior Oblique

The inferior oblique too has some peculiar properties that differentiate it from other cyclovertical muscles, specially the two recti.

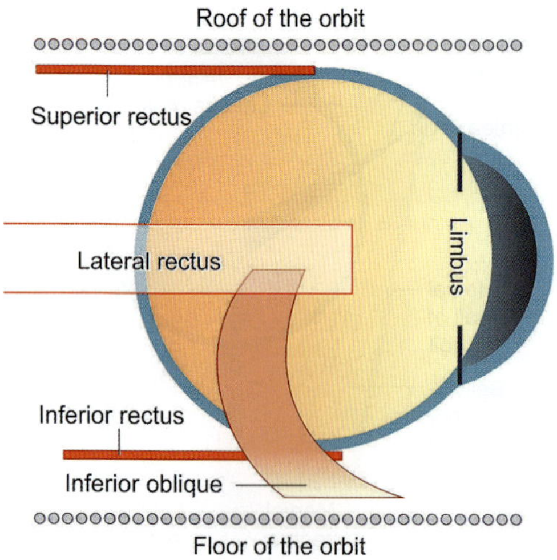

Fig. 24.13: Relation of inferior oblique to lateral rectus and inferior rectus.

The differences are given as follows:

- It is the shortest and bulkiest extraocular muscle, with a length of 37.0 mm, in contrast to the average of 40.0 mm of other extraocular muscles.
- The tendon is very short or may be absent; in such eventuality, the muscle is directly inserted to the sclera.
- It is the only extraocular muscle that has a true anterior origin from the inferomedial part of the rim of the orbit.
- Its insertion is very near the fovea.

After origin, the muscle passes posteriorly and laterally between the floor of the orbit and the inferior rectus within Lockwood's ligament. It is inserted 17.0 mm away from the limbus, 1.0 mm anterior, and below the fovea. The anterior end of the insertion lies in the same plane as the lower end of the insertion of the lateral rectus. The insertion of the muscle is under the lateral rectus **(Fig. 24.13)**.

The action of the IO is complex. Its primary action is extortion, best in abduction. The secondary action is elevation, and the tertiary action is abduction.

The motor supply is through the inferior division of the third cranial nerve. It gets its blood supply from the inferior orbital artery and the medial muscular branch of the ophthalmic artery.

The muscle is most likely to be injured in a fracture of the floor of the orbit. The action of cyclovertical muscle is depicted in the following mnemonic:

SINRAD
S – IN – R – AD

where, S: two superior muscles, i.e., the superior rectus and the superior oblique; IN: intorsion; R: cyclovertical recti; AD: adduction.

TABLE 24.8: Action of extraocular muscles.

Muscle	*Functions*
Superior rectus	• Elevation increasing in abduction becomes nil when adducted • Intorsion increases as the eye is adducted • Adduction
Medial rectus	Adduction
Inferior rectus	• Depression increasing in abduction becomes nil in adduction • Extrusion increasing in adduction • Adduction
Lateral rectus	Abduction
Superior oblique	• Intorsion increasing in abduction • Depression increasing in adduction • Abduction
Inferior oblique	• Extorsion increasing in abduction • Elevation increasing in adduction becomes nil in abduction • Abduction

The above abbreviations are explained given as follows:

- The superior's, i.e., SR and SO, will intort.
- The inferior's, i.e., IR and IO, will extort.
- The two recti will adduct.
- The obliques will abduct.

The mnemonic is applicable only to cyclovertical muscles.

Table 24.8 shows summary of the action of extraocular muscles.

APPLIED ANATOMY OF CRANIAL NERVES IN RELATION TO EXTRAOCULAR MUSCLES AND THEIR DISORDERS

The cranial nerves involved in ocular movement are given as follows.

Oculomotors (two branches): Trochlear and abducens. The oculomotor nerve serves the superior, inferior, medial recti, and inferior oblique. The trochlear and abducens supply single muscle each; the former supplies the superior oblique, while the latter supplies the lateral rectus.

Disorders of cranial nerves without involving central neural paths will produce only ocular signs and symptoms. The neural paths involved in disorders of extraocular muscle, directly or indirectly, are given as follows:

- Frontomesencephalic path
- Parieto-occipital temporal mesencephalic path
- Occipitomesencephalic path

Flowchart 24.2: Effects of single and multiple cranial nerve palsies.

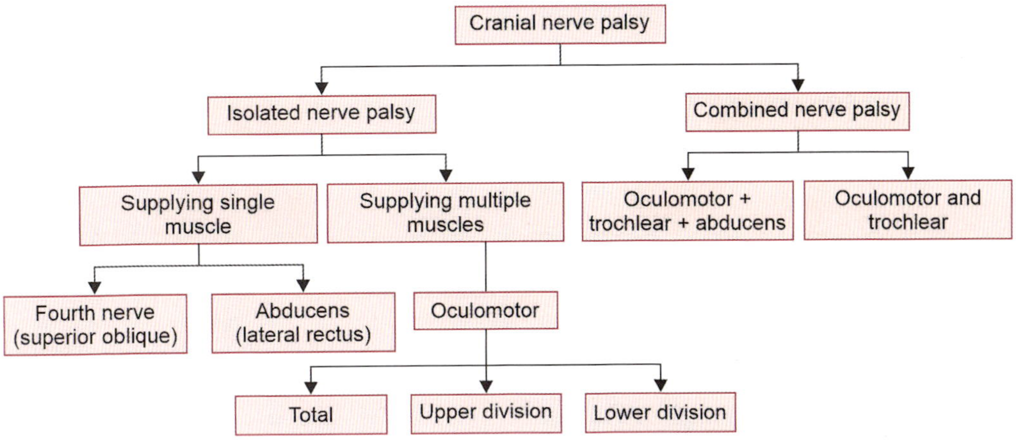

- Paramedian pontine reticular formation
- Labyrinthine pontine path

Examples of cranial nerves without involving neural tracts can be divided as follows:

- Single cranial nerve supplying only one extraocular muscle, i.e., isolated fourth or sixth nerve palsy
- A single nerve supplies multiple extraocular muscles:
  - Total third nerve palsy
  - Partial third nerve palsy
- Multiple cranial nerve palsy:
  - Third, fourth, and sixth
  - Third and fourth

***Flowchart 24.2** summarizes cranial nerve involvement in ocular disorders.*

Table 24.9 shows lesions of the third cranial nerve and neural tracts in relation to the eyes.

BRIEF DESCRIPTION OF THE CRANIAL NERVES INVOLVED IN OCULAR PALSIES

Oculomotor Nerve

This is the third cranial nerve that supplies more than one extraocular muscle; it also supplies the intraocular muscles of the iris and ciliary body through the parasympathetic chain. It has its nucleus in the midbrain that is the largest among all the nuclei serving the extraocular muscles; its nucleus is divided in two groups, i.e., paired and unpaired nuclei **(Fig. 24.14)**.

The paired nuclei are arranged in three subgroups to supply the ipsilateral MR, IR, and IO. The unpaired nucleus supplies the SR. The caudal central nucleus is called the Perlia's nucleus; it supplies the levator.

TABLE 24.9: Various syndromes and their clinical features.

Syndrome	***Neurological involvement***
Weber	Ipsilateral third nerve palsy with contralateral hemiplegia
Claude	Ipsilateral third nerve palsy with contralateral ataxia
Benedikt	Ipsilateral third nerve palsy and contralateral hemiplegia with contralateral ataxia
Nothnagel	Cerebellar ataxia with a third nerve palsy on the same side
Raymond	Ipsilateral sixth nerve palsy, contralateral hemiplegia, and facial paralysis
Fisher syndrome (modified Guillain–Barré syndrome)	Bilateral oculomotor palsy, ataxia, and areflexia
Jacob	Total third, fourth, and sixth nerve palsy; trigeminal neuralgia; and amaurosis

The parasympathetic fibers that control accommodation and light reflexes originate in the Edinger–Westphal nucleus. The SR and SO muscles have their motor nuclei on the contralateral side.

The nucleus of the fourth nerve is below and near the nucleus of the IR. The third nerve nucleus complex is well connected with the neural tracts that lie in its path.

*The function of paired nuclei is given in **Table 24.10**.*

The characteristic nuclear third nerve palsy is given as follows.

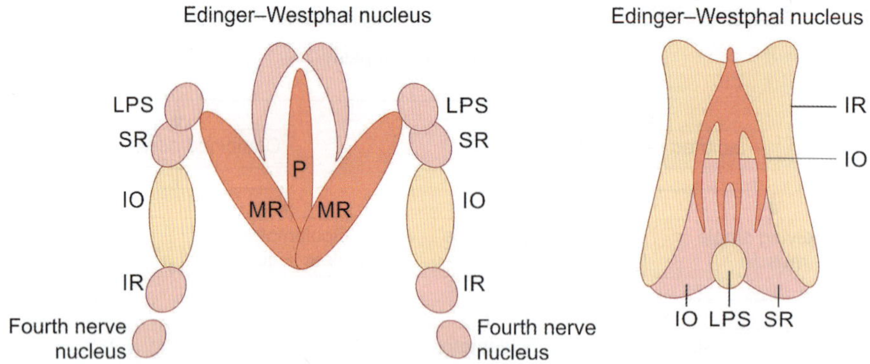

Fig. 24.14: Distribution of subnuclei of 3rd nerve 'P' in Perlia's nucleus. (IO: inferior oblique; IR: inferior rectus; LPS: levator palpebrae superioris; MR: medial rectus; SR: superior rectus)

TABLE 24.10: Lesions of paired nuclei and their clinical features.

Nucleus involved	***Muscle affected***
Dorsolateral nucleus	Ipsilateral inferior rectus
Intermediate nucleus	Ipsilateral inferior oblique
Ventromedial nucleus	Ipsilateral medial rectus
Nucleus mass of the superior rectus	Contralateral superior rectus

Nuclear

Nuclear lesions are rarer. The features of a nuclear lesion comprise of:

- Bilateral ptosis
- Bilateral superior rectus palsy with bilateral ptosis
- Superior rectus and levator palsy with contralateral third nerve palsy
- Bilateral third nerve palsy
- Bilateral external ophthalmoplegia
- Bilateral internal ophthalmoplegia

The nuclear lesions of the third nerve are governed by Daroff's rules, which divides them into three groups. They are given as follows:

1. *Conditions that are obligatory for nuclear involvement*:
   a. Bilateral third nerve palsy without ptosis
   b. Unilateral third nerve palsy with contralateral SR paresis
   c. Bilateral ptosis
2. *Conditions that exclude a third nerve nuclear lesion*:
   a. Unilateral ptosis
   b. Unilateral internal ophthalmoplegia
   c. Unilateral external ophthalmoplegia is associated with normal contralateral superior rectus.
3. *Conditions that may or may not be nuclear*:
   a. Bilateral third nerve palsy
   b. Bilateral ptosis
   c. Bilateral internal ophthalmoplegia
   d. Bilateral medial rectus palsy

The explanations for such selective manifestations are given as follows:

- Each superior rectus is supplied by its nucleus on the other side.
- The nuclei of the two elevators are single and central.
- A large lesion may involve all the nuclei, causing bilateral total third nerve palsy.
  The nuclei are supplied by the posterior cerebral artery.

Like all cranial nerves, the oculomotor nerve is divided into the following parts:

- Nuclear
- Fascicular
- Basilar
- Intercavernous
- Intraorbital

Fascicular Part

The fascicular part passes through the red nucleus medial to the cerebral peduncle **(Fig. 24.15)**. A lesion of the fascicular part at this level produces a symmetric lesion of the muscle supplied by individual nuclei and tract lesions, i.e., Weber, Benedikt, Claude, and Nothnagel syndromes.

Basilar Part

The nerve passes through the subarachnoid space under the posterior cerebral artery and above the superior cerebellar artery, lateral to the basilar artery. The nerve passes parallel to the posterior communication artery. The fourth nerve also passes between the posterior cerebral and superior cerebellar arteries on the lateral side of the third nerve; in this space, the nerve does not

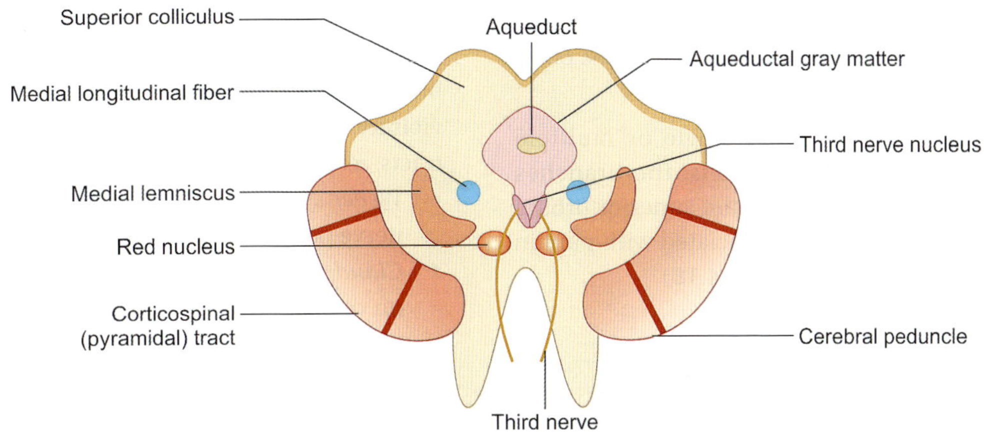

Fig. 24.15: Section through the fascicular of the third nerve showing its relation to the red nucleus and other neural tracts.

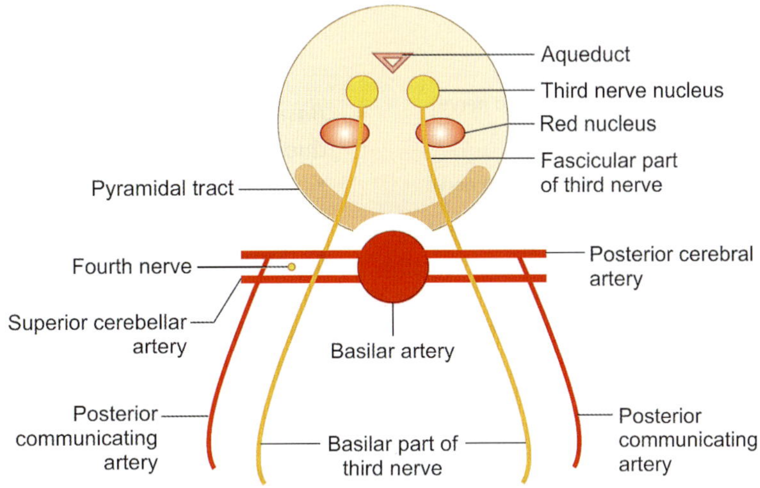

Fig. 24.16: The position of the third nerve in the fascicular and basilar parts.

come in relation with any nerve tract or cranial nerve; hence, lesions in this area do not have any neurological deficits, barring extraocular muscles. This is the most frequent site to involve the third nerve **(Fig. 24.16)**.

Intercavernous Part

In this space, the third nerve comes in proximity to many anatomical structures of ocular importance. The nerve passes between the posterior clinoid process and the free edge of the tentorium, piercing the dura. In the posterior part of the cavernous sinus, it lies near the roof of the cavernous sinus and then passes laterally to reach the lateral wall of the cavernous sinus. During its remaining course in the cavernous sinus, it remains embedded in the lateral wall of the cavernous sinus above the fourth nerve, ophthalmic, and maxillary nerves. The fourth nerve crosses the third nerve to be above and medial to the oculomotor nerve until it leaves the sinus. The third nerve divides into superior and inferior divisions at the anterior end of the cavernous sinus **(Fig. 24.17)**.

The superior division is smaller and supplies the SR and the levator, while the larger inferior division supplies the medial and IR along with the IO. The inferior branch also carries the fibers of the parasympathetic nerve to the ciliary ganglion.

Intraorbital Part

The two divisions leave the cranium to enter the orbit through the superior orbital fissure. The superior division passes over the optic nerve to supply the SR from its ocular surface. Some fibers pierce the SR to reach the levator above. The inferior division reaches the IR, MR, and IO from their orbital surfaces. The branch to the IO also gives a branch to the ciliary ganglion.

> The cranial nerves in the orbit do not come in the proximity of any neural tract; hence, lesions of the cranial nerve in the orbit do not have any systemic neural deficit.

The lesions may involve either single or multiple cranial nerves in various combinations; the branches of the fifth nerve also travel through the superior orbital fissure; hence, the conditions are associated with pain in the distribution of the fifth nerve **(Fig. 24.18)**.

Clinical Features of Third Nerve Involvement

- *Nuclear:* Nuclear lesions are rarer in all ages; they are rarer in children (see above).

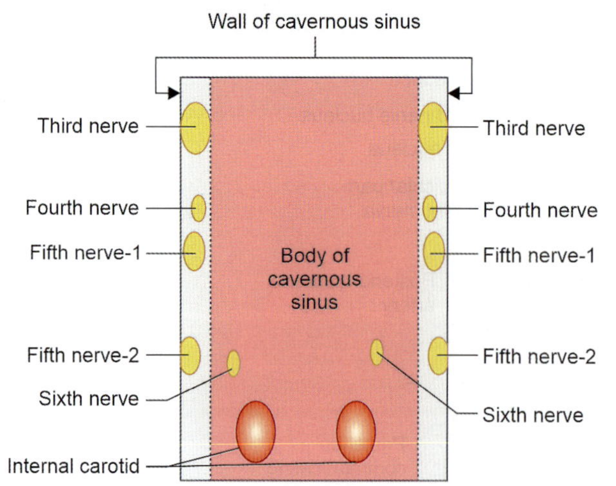

Fig. 24.17: Cavernous sinus and its relation with internal carotid and cranial nerves in the wall.

- *Fascicular:* The fascicular part of the third nerve is small, but its involvement causes multiple syndromes because the nerve passes either through or in the vicinity of other nuclei (the red nucleus) or neural tracts, resulting in the following syndromes:
  - *Weber syndrome:* This consists of ipsilateral third nerve palsy with contralateral hemiplegia.
  - *Claude syndrome:* This consists of third nerve palsy on one side with ataxia/tremor on the other side due to involvement of the red nucleus.
  - *Benedikt syndrome:* The clinical features are more seen in Claude syndrome due to the involvement of the corticospinal tract besides the red nucleus.
  - *Nothnagel syndrome:* This is caused due to involvement of the superior cerebellar peduncle, causing ipsilateral third nerve palsy and cerebellar ataxia.
- *Basilar:* The basilar part of the third nerve is important due to its close relation to the following arteries:
  - Basilar
  - Posterior cerebral
  - Superior cerebellar
  - Posterior communicating artery

The lesions do not involve any other cranial nerve or neural tract; they are generally painful and involve the pupil. The common cause of their involvement is vascular, which is less common in children. The other cause of involvement of the third nerve is uncal herniation* due to extradural hematoma that presses the nerve trunk over the

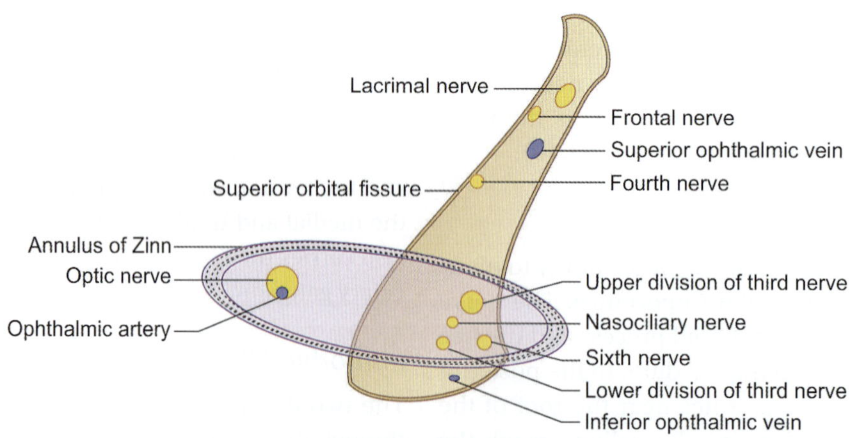

Fig. 24.18: Various structures passing through the superior orbital fissure and circle of Zinn.

**Uncal herniation* is caused due to rise of intracranial pressure that forces the brain to herniate from one intracranial compartment to another. It may press the third nerve that results in parasympathetic underaction on the side of affected nerve, resulting in dilatation of the pupil not reacting to light.

tentorial edge, causing total third nerve palsy with a fixed dilated pupil.

- *Trauma:* The most common traumatic lesion of the cranial nerve is involvement of the fourth nerve, followed by the third nerve. Both are seen in closed head injuries, with involvement at two different levels. The common site for involvement of the oculomotor nerve in a closed head injury is between its exits from the pontomedullary junction to its entry in cavernous sinus. Rarely, the nerve may be avulsed near the brainstem, causing total 3rd nerve palsy. The nerve may be forced down over the tentorial edge. The other possibilities of traumatic involvement of the third nerve are given as follows:
  - Hemorrhage in the nerve
  - Contusion of the nerve during its passage in the interpeduncular space

Such lesions are associated with fractures of the base of the skull, loss of consciousness, and Hutchinson's pupil*.

- *Cavernous sinus:* The third nerve lies in the wall of the cavernous sinus, along with the fourth nerve and two branches of the fifth nerve. The fourth nerve enters the sinus inferior to the third nerve only to change its course to be superior to the third nerve. The other nerve, which comes in relation to the third nerve, little medial to it, is the sixth nerve. The sixth nerve differs from the third, fourth, and fifth nerves in not being embedded in the wall of the sinus but in the substance of the sinus **(Fig. 24.17)**.

  Due to their location in the cavernous sinus, the nerves are not involved in isolation. They produce paralysis/paresis of various extraocular muscles. The sympathetic chain is also involved. The involvement of the fifth nerve is the cause of pain and loss of sensation along its distribution. Generally, the pupil remains undilated. The explanation of the phenomenon is that there are two diagonally opposite processes acting simultaneously. Logically, paralysis of the third nerve should dilate the pupil, which is counteracted by associated miosis due to the involvement of the parasympathetic, resulting in a state similar to incomplete Horner's syndrome†. Aberrant regeneration‡) of the third nerve is common.
- *Orbital*: The oculomotor nerve divides into two branches:
  1. A small twig is meant for the superior rectus and levator.
  2. A large twig is meant for the MR, IR, and IO.

The lower twig also carries the parasympathetic nerve. The orbital lesions are rarely isolated and complete. They are associated with multiple cranial nerves traversing the orbit. The sixth nerve involvement is more common than

---

Hutchinson's pupil* is an important bedside clinical sign of great diagnostic and prognostic value in cases of intracranial fast-growing mass of any nature. It consists of mydriasis due to compression of the oculomotor nerve on the side of the lesion. Initially, the pupil on the side of the lesion is constricted, and then it starts to dilate to its maximum. In the last stage, both the pupils dilate completely **(Fig. 24.19).

†*Horner's syndrome (oculosympathetic syndrome)*: The condition is rare in children, but when present, it is congenital in 5% of cases. It is generally unilateral and consists of mild ptosis, miosis, and anhidrosis. It is caused due to involvement of the cervical sympathetic chain in various levels. It is not vision threatening.

‡*Aberrant regeneration*: Out of all cranial nerves, two cranial nerves, i.e., the third and seventh nerves, are known to regenerate following trauma or inflammation. The regeneration of the seventh nerve causes crocodile tear§ on movement of the jaw. The causes of regeneration of the third nerve are trauma, neoplasm, and rarely vascular. The condition is associated with the sprouting of axons from the affected nerve. The newly sprouted axons do not follow the usual course of the third nerve; they are misdirected to muscles to which they are not meant for. The condition appears 3–4 months following the onset of the third nerve, which could be partial or total. It is mostly unilateral.

§*Crocodile tears syndrome (Bogorad syndrome)* is a gustatory lacrimation seen following regeneration of the seventh nerve months to years after facial palsy. It is a unilateral phenomenon of shedding tears while eating or drinking.

The two forms of aberrant regeneration of the third nerve are given as follows:
1. Without involvement of the third nerve in the past
2. Following acute oculomotor palsy during recovery

The condition is unilateral, always associated with paradoxical movement of extraocular muscle, mostly the levator. The paradoxical movements are divided into three following groups:
1. *Pseudo-Graefe's sign*: Elevation of the lid on attempted movement of the inferior and medial rectus
2. *Inverse Duane syndrome*: Adduction or retraction of the globe on an attempted vertical gaze
3. *Pseudo-Argyll Robertson pupil*: Light near dissociation on attempted convergence

The exact cause of the condition is not known. There is no specific treatment for the condition; the treatment is directed toward the primary cause of third nerve palsy. The surgical management comprises various surgical processes directed toward ptosis and squinting by combination of various surgical processes.

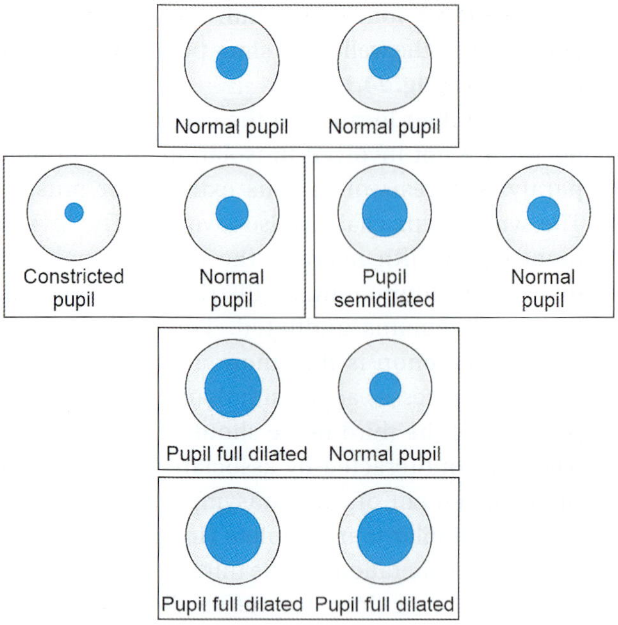

Fig. 24.19: Various stages of Hutchinson's pupil due to a right-sided brain lesion.

fourth nerve. The condition is commonly accompanied by mild proptosis. Pupillary involvement is common in the involvement of lower divisions. Involvement of the fifth nerve is associated with pain radiating on the distribution of the fifth nerve, resulting in painful ophthalmoplegia*.

Other less common paralysis of the oculomotor nerve are given as follows:

- *Cyclic oculomotor palsy:* This rare condition is thought to be congenital in origin or traumatic. It is a unilateral condition. The acquired form becomes obvious in early childhood. The condition has two phases. The first is the paralytic phase. In the second spastic phase, the former consists of partial involvement of the third nerve, resulting in ptosis, paresis of muscles supplied by it, including cycloplegia. The child presents with mild-to-moderate ptosis; the eye is abducted and moved downward. The second phase starts with twitching of the lids, retraction of the lids, miosis, and spasm of accommodation. The eye then goes into an

---

**Painful ophthalmoplegia:* Ophthalmoplegia with pain is more common in multiple cranial nerve palsies due to the passage of the nerves through the superior orbital fissure. Isolated involvement of the third nerve can also result in painful ophthalmoplegia to a lesser extent. Painful ophthalmoplegia is less common under 20 years; when present, it is generally associated with ophthalmoplegic migraine. The other causes which are seen in adults are aneurysms of the following arteries, i.e., basilar artery, posterior communicating artery, and intracavernous aneurysm. The most common cause of painful ophthalmoplegia in adults is diabetic neuropathy. Followed by a posterior communicating artery aneurysm. The causes of painful ophthalmoplegia in children besides ophthalmoplegic migraine† are cavernous sinus thrombosis, Gradenigo syndrome, parasellar growth, and sinusitis.

†*Ophthalmoplegic migraine:* It is a commonly missed diagnosis because of its varied clinical features. It sets in before 10 years of age; it has been reported in infants as well. Generally, there is a family history of migraine; it lacks the usual aura of migraine; it starts acutely with pain in and around the eyeball with hemicrania on the side of the involved eye; it may be associated with nausea or vomiting. The eye is not congested; there is no tenderness in the eyeball. Diplopia is the cornerstone of the syndrome due to the involvement of extraocular muscles. The most common muscles are those supplied by the third nerve; less common are muscles supplied by the fourth and sixth nerves. Involvement of more than one cranial nerve is not uncommon; there are no neurological deficits. The paralysis is transient, subsiding within a month without sequel or with residual paresis. Recurrence is common, and spontaneous recovery has been reported. The optic nerve is not involved. The exact cause is not clear; some authors do not consider it to be a form of migraine, in spite of the fact that the child with ophthalmoplegic migraine may develop classical migraine in adulthood. The other theory is that edema and dilatation of the internal carotid in the cavernous sinus impinging the third nerve. Keeping in mind spontaneous recovery without sequelae, the condition is treated with systemic analgesics. A severe condition requires neurological workup with usual neuroimaging.

‡*Tolosa-Hunt syndrome:* This is a nonspecific chronic granuloma of the anterior cavernous sinus and/or superior orbital fissure, singularly or in combination, sparing the apex of the orbit.

The condition is also called as superior orbital fissure syndrome; if the condition extends in the orbital apex, it is called orbital apex syndrome. The former does not involve the optic nerve. The Tolosa-Hunt syndrome may start acutely with unilateral pain in the distribution of the fifth nerve, diplopia, and mild proptosis. Spontaneous recovery is common; otherwise, it becomes chronic. There is no rule of thumb regarding the involvement of cranial nerves; it may begin as the involvement of a single nerve and remain so. More common is the involvement of multiple cranial nerves; the ocular palsies are generally partial, and involvement of the pupil is not uniform. Pupil may be normal, miotic, or mydriatic, depending on the involvement of the division third nerve and the involvement of the sympathetic chain. Involvement of the fifth nerve is common and is the cause of hemicrania. The condition was supposed to be due to chronic infections such as tuberculosis and syphilis and was treated as such without much relief until it was realized that the condition was the result of a localized autoimmune disorder responding to a systemic steroid. In children, it is often bilateral. The diagnosis is by exclusion of neoplasms and vasculopathy. The common investigations ordered are total blood count, including an erythrocyte sedimentation rate (ESR), X-ray, computed tomography (CT), magnetic resonance imaging (MRI), ultrasonography (USG), and fine-needle biopsy. The steroid administered in proper dose and frequency provides immediate relief from pain, associated with an improvement in vision. The paresis of muscles takes a longer time to be cured. The differential diagnosis consists of ophthalmoplegic migraine in children, especially when it is periodic.

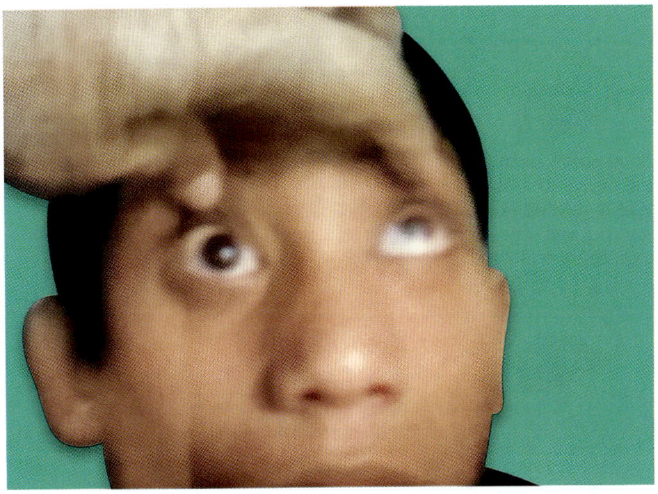

Fig. 24.20: Photograph of a boy with right double elevator palsy.

abducted position. The phases last for a few minutes. The exact cause is not known.
- *Double elevator palsy*: This is an uncommon unilateral, congenital condition with subnormal elevation in the horizontal gaze. The most probable cause is hypoplasia of the nucleus serving the levator, resulting in pseudo- or true ptosis that may be mild to moderate. The eye in primary gaze is hypotropic with retained Bell's phenomenon. The chin is elevated. Elevated chin with hypotropia assures absence of amblyopia **(Fig. 24.20)**.

The three different types of double elevator palsy are given as follows:
1. Prominent IR and normal SR function
2. Weakness of elevation, negative forced duction test, and diminished SR function
3. Combination of the above two

Differential diagnosis consists of:
- Brown syndrome
- Congenital fibrosis of the IR
- General fibrosis syndrome
- Anomalous superior and IR insertion
- A blow-out fracture of the orbit is a prominent cause of acquired double elevator palsy

Management

There is no medical treatment; associated errors of refraction and amblyopia must be treated by an appropriate method before surgical intervention is contemplated. Surgical treatment is the definitive treatment, especially with vertical deviation and abnormal head posture.

Double Depressor Palsy

Double depressor palsy is less common than double elevator palsy. It is most probably due to the congenital ipsilateral underaction of the depressors, i.e., IR and SO that the affected eye is hypertropic.

Involvement of the Trunk of the Third Nerve

It can be partial or total.

Partial Involvement

It is caused due to involvement of the upper division of the third nerve, mostly in the cavernous sinus; it causes simultaneous paralysis of the superior rectus and levator on the same side, resulting in mild-to-moderate ptosis, diminished Bell's phenomenon, and hypotropia. The pupil is spared.

Total Nerve Palsy

This is due to the involvement of both branches of the third nerve, causing paralysis of all the muscles supplied by the third nerve. Involvement of fourth, fifth, and sixth nerves is common with total third nerve palsy. The pupil is spared in basilar involvement that should, otherwise, cause paralysis of the internal muscles of the eye. However, involvement of the nerve in the cavernous sinus results in involvement of the sympathetic chain, which should cause miosis; thus, involvement of the nerve in the orbit leaves the pupil with two opposing factors, which results in a normal pupil. Isolated total third nerve involvement results in complete ptosis; on lifting the lid, the eye is found in a down-and-out position **(Figs. 24.21A to D)**.

Initially, the symptoms are mild ptosis with crossed diplopia (false image being higher, upper end tilted toward the paralyzed side) as depicted in **Figure 24.22**.

As the condition worsens, the ptosis increases to become complete, covering the pupil. Pupillary obscuration causes the disappearance of diplopia, which again becomes obvious on lifting the lid. The eye cannot be adducted or elevated, and it is intorted.

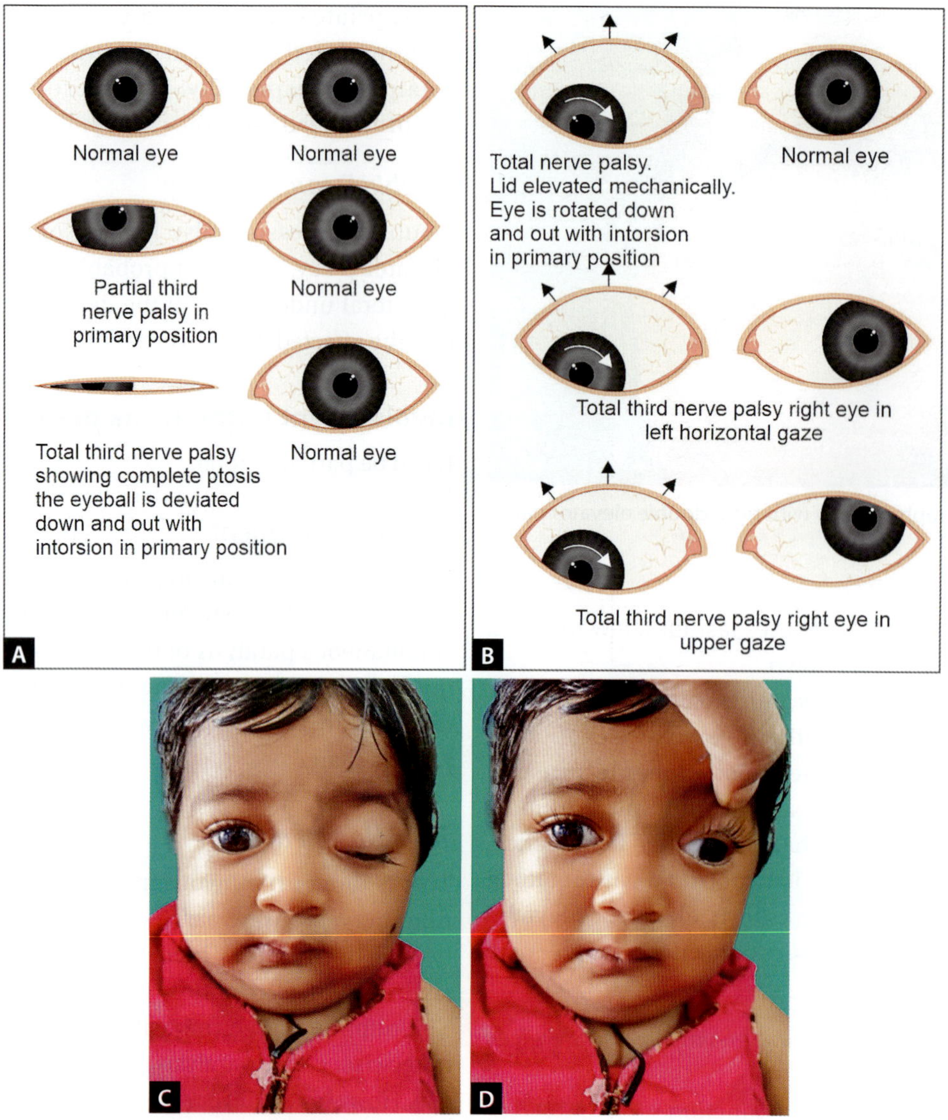

Figs. 24.21A to D: Total third nerve palsy in a child.
Courtesy: Dr Anand Deshpande.

Clinical Features of Paralysis of Individual Muscles Supplied by the Third Nerve

Paralysis of individual muscles is rare; when it presents, it is generally due to a congenital anomaly of either the muscle or its nerve supply. Selective involvement of individual muscles is generally traumatic.

Superior Rectus

Isolated paralysis of the SR is rare; most of the time, it is associated with the levator under action. In the primary position, the eye is slightly depressed with absent Bell's phenomenon. When the paretic eye fixes, the sound eye becomes hypertropic due to overaction or IO of the sound eye. The chin is raised, and the head is tilted toward the sound eye.

Medial Rectus

Individual paralysis of the MR is rarer. The most common cause of MR underaction is its incarceration in the medial orbital wall following a fracture of the medial wall; in this situation, the eye is tethered to the fracture, causing esotropia, in contrast to the nontraumatic case, which is generally congenital, causing exotropia due to overaction of the lateral rectus. There is no abnormal head posture.

Inferior Rectus

A congenital anomaly of the muscle or its nerve supply causes underaction of the muscle. A more common cause is trauma entrapping the muscle in the fractured floor of the orbit. The depression of the involved eye is restricted; this is accompanied by an underaction of the SO of the contralateral eye along with an overaction of the ipsilateral SR. The chin is depressed, with the face turned to the side of the involved eye.

Inferior Oblique

The most common cause of IO palsy is trauma, either to the muscle itself or its incarceration in the fractured floor of the orbit. The congenital anomaly is it, as in double depressor palsy. The eye in primary position is hypotropic. In fixing the sound eye, the affected eye becomes hypertropic; during vertical movement, there is restriction of conjugate movement.

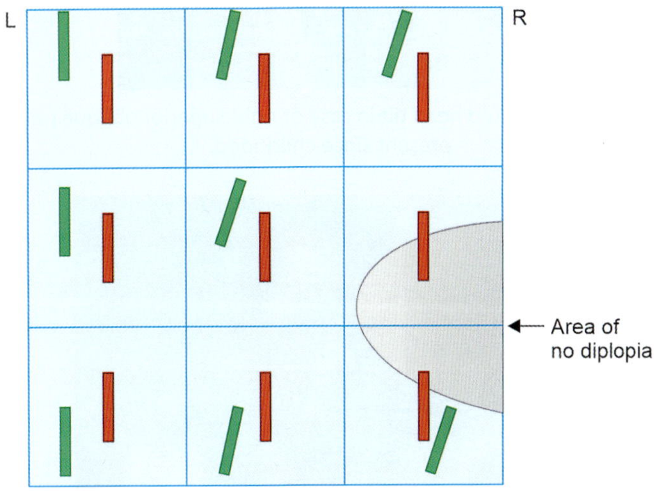

Fig. 24.22: Diplopia charting in third nerve palsy.

Trochlear Nerve

This is the fourth cranial nerve, with the following features:

- It has the longest intracranial course.
- It is the thinnest cranial nerve.
- It is only the cranial nerve that decussates completely.
- The nerve decussates dorsally.
- It is only the cranial nerve that emerges from the brain posteriorly.
- It has the smallest fascicular course.
- Its fascicular and nuclear parts are so near to each other that lesions of them cannot be separated individually.
- It innervates the contralateral single extraocular muscle, i.e., the SO.
- It enters the orbit through the superior orbital fissure outside the annulus of Zinn.
- It is not affected by retrobulbar anesthesia.
- It is paralyzed by peribulbar anesthesia.
- No neural tract comes in close proximity to the nerve throughout its course, barring the sympathetic chain and medial longitudinal fasciculus **(Fig. 24.23)**.

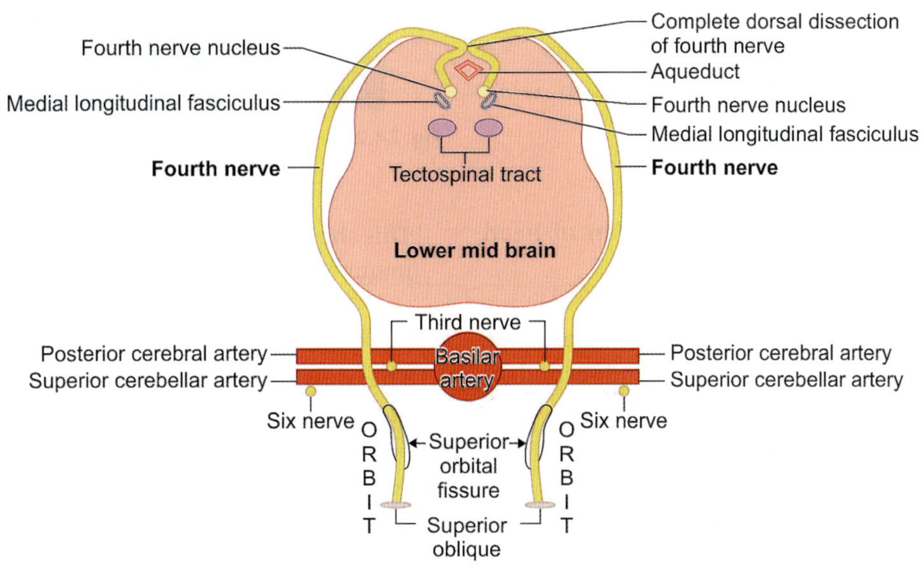

Fig. 24.23: Origin, dissection, and course of the fourth nerve.

CHARACTERISTICS OF TROCHLEAR NERVE PALSY

The common features of fourth nerve palsy are vertical squint, vertical diplopia, and compensatory head posture. Out of the three nerves that cause paralysis of extraocular muscles, it is less frequent than the third and sixth nerves in children. The two frequent causes of fourth nerve palsy are congenital and trauma; infection and neoplasm too have their share. Vasculopathy such as diabetes, arteriosclerosis, and hypertension, which are common causes of fourth nerve palsy in adults, is not seen in children. The palsy can be unilateral or bilateral; the congenital palsy may be present at birth but missed; it is common for it to be asymptomatic until it gets decompensated in the fourth to fifth decades.

Congenital Fourth Nerve Palsy

About one-third of all vertical squints are caused by congenital anomalies of the superior oblique and/or its nerve supply. The congenital palsy of the SO can be put into two distinct groups, i.e., childhood and adult.

The clinical features of congenital SO palsy are given as follows:

- There is a strong family history, and many of the members in different generations may have the anomaly that can be seen in old family photographs.
- The affected members may have manifested squints without binocular fusion.
- The affected eye is hypertropic in its primary position.
- Marked head tilt **(Figs. 24.24 and 24.25)**
- Diplopia is absent in compensatory head posture.
- The child may read with one eye closed to avoid troublesome vertical diplopia.
- Facial asymmetry is common.
- AV syndrome is common.
- Diplopia becomes obvious on correction of head posture.
- The antagonist may show contracture.
- The eye may develop comitance, causing an absence or reduced difference between primary and secondary deviations.
- Suppression in the affected eye causes the disappearance of diplopia.
- The adults may develop diplopia at as late as the fourth to fifth decade, for which no apparent cause can be detected except old family group photographs.

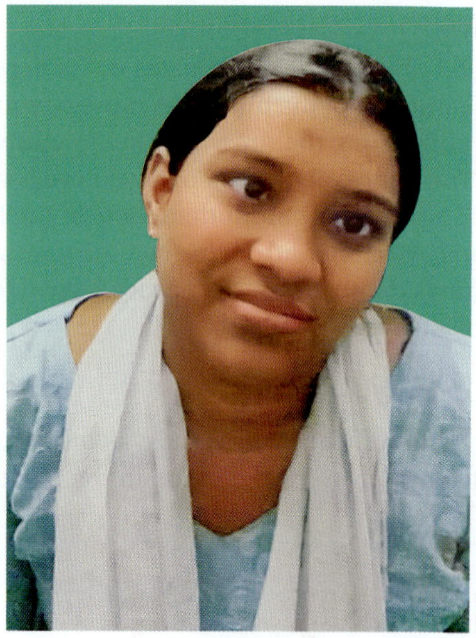

Fig. 24.24: Marked head tilt in case of right superior oblique palsy present since childhood.

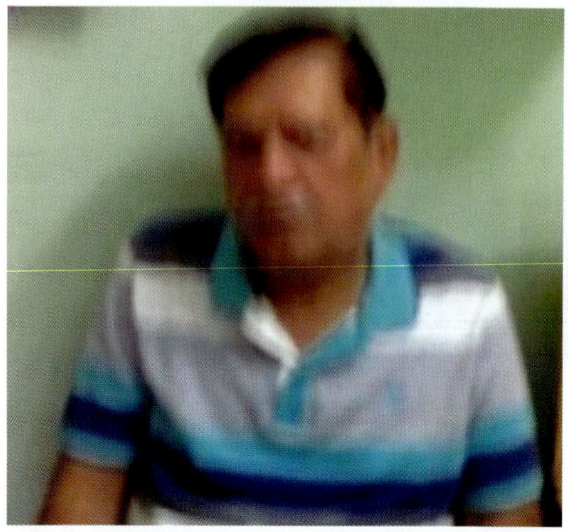

Fig. 24.25: Head tilt and face turn in recent left superior oblique palsy in adults.

This shows abnormal head postures in more than one member of different ages.

Effect of Congenital Superior Oblique Palsy

- The palsy may be present at birth and remain unchanged throughout life.
- The squint may be so small that the child is able to fuse two images even without compensatory head posture.
- The child may have binocular vision in particular gaze.
- The squint may be latent, intermittent, or becoming constant.

Unilateral Fourth Nerve Palsy

Involvement of one eye in the fourth nerve palsy is more frequent than both eyes. It could be congenital or acquired. The feature of recent unilateral fourth nerve palsy differs from that of long-standing palsy.

The features of recent palsy are given as follows:

- Ipsilateral, hypertropia in primary position
- Hypertropia increases on moving the eye medially.
- Hypertropia increases if the head is tilted on the same size.
- The child may complain of vertical diplopia.
- The hypertropia and head tilt may be noticed by the parents.
- Hypertropia has a tendency to become concomitant.
- Diplopia is minimized due to suppression.
- The deviation is best measured by a double Maddox rod test.
- It can be detected on synoptophores with specific torsion slides.
- The excyclotropia is generally about 7°.
- The child tolerates excyclotropia up to 4° only after which it becomes symptomatic.
- If the child fixes with paralyzed eye, the sound eye shows hypotropia.

Summary of Action of the Superior Oblique

The main functions of the muscles consist of:

- Depression of the eye in adduction
- Intorsion in abduction

> Fourth nerve paralysis produces ipsilateral hypertropia, diminished depression, and worsening in adduction. Extorsion worsening on abduction with compensatory contralateral head tilt and depression of the chin.

Bilateral Fourth Nerve Palsy

- Bilateral fourth nerve palsy is more difficult to diagnose.
- The most common cause is trauma (a closed head injury).
- The next cause is a congenital anomaly.
- Asymmetries are frequent.
- There is no head tilt except chin down.
- In symmetrical palsy, there is no vertical deviation in the primary position.
- Orthophoria is more common than eso- or exodeviation.
- There is left hypertropia on the right gaze and right hypertropia on the left gaze.
- Diplopia is present in all gazes, except the upgaze.
- Excyclotropia may be as high as 20°.
- Excyclotropia increases in downgaze.
- Bielschowsky head tilt test is positive on both sides.
- Measure the vertical deviation in the upright position and then in the supine position; a 50% decrease in the supine position is positive.
- Both contralateral synergists, i.e., both inferior recti, show overaction.
- Children with asymmetry may develop ocular torticollis*.
- The V pattern is common.

Summary of Bilateral Fourth Nerve Palsy

- Chin down without/with a tilt
- Bilateral inability to adduct in downgaze
- Reversing hyperdeviation
- Excyclotorsion >10°
- Prominent V pattern

Topical Diagnosis of Fourth Nerve Palsy

- It can be unilateral or bilateral.
- The nerve may be involved in isolation or in various combinations with the underaction of the third and sixth nerves.
- The sympathetic chain is involved in a nucleofascicular lesion.
- No neural tract is involved in isolated fourth nerve palsy.

Table 24.11 *shows differences between unilateral and bilateral SO palsy.*

> *Head posture in superior oblique palsy*
> Chin down → Bilateral palsy → Contralateral head tilt → Unilateral palsy

Figure 24.26 shows the three steps of the Bielschowsky three-step test.

PRINCIPLES OF THE BIELSCHOWSKY TEST

> Oblique abductors are best tested in adduction.
> The head turns where the eyes do not.

**Ocular torticollis:* It is a form of abnormal head posture that may consist of any of the following, alone or in combination, i.e., head tilt, face turn, elevation, or depression of the chin. Superior oblique palsy is the most common cause of ocular torticollis.

TABLE 24.11: Differences between unilateral and bilateral superior oblique palsy.

Features	***Unilateral***	***Bilateral***
Head posture*	Depressed chin, face turned toward sound side, head tilted toward sound side	Only chin depression
Cover test in primary position	Hyperdeviation	Slight or no hyperdeviation
Extortion	Mild	Moderate
Lateral version	No reversal of diplopia in the lateral version	Reversal of diplopia in the lateral version
Bielschowsky test	Positive when head tilted toward affected side	Positive when head tilted toward any side
Diplopia	Vertical, torsional	Diplopia only when decompensated

**Head posture in superior oblique palsy:* Tilting the head to the side opposite the affected eye, sometimes accompanied by a chin-down position, to reduce vertical diplopia and improve binocular vision.

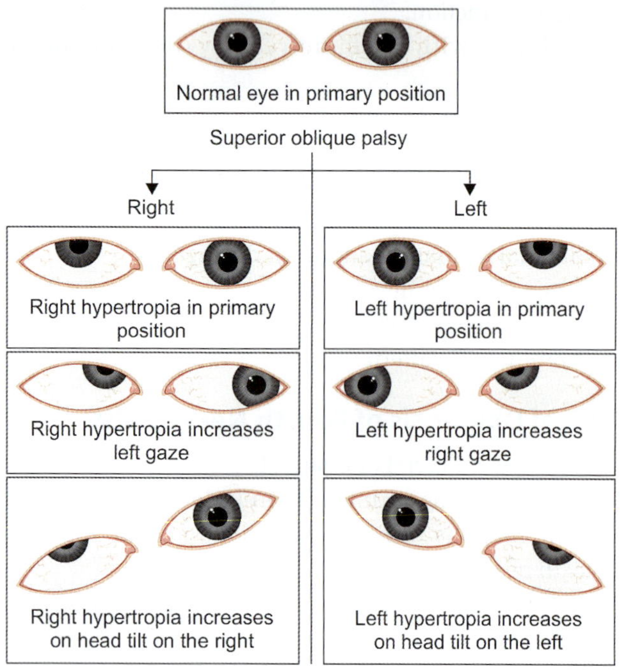

Fig. 24.26: Three steps of the Bielschowsky test in the right and left eyes separately.

Interpretation of the Bielschowsky Three-step Test

- Cyclovertical squint may be caused by the involvement of eight cyclovertical muscles.
- To pinpoint the single-offending muscle, three steps are required.
- First step:
  - Find out if the right or left eye is hypertropic.
  - In the case of right hypertropia, the offending muscles can be four, i.e.,
    - Two underacting and depressors of the right eye, i.e., the right SO and the right IR.
    - Two underacting elevators belonging to the left eye, i.e., the left SR and the left IO.
- Moving the eyes horizontally—observe if hypertropia increases on the right or left.
  - If hypertropia increases on the right gaze, the number of offending muscles is reduced to two but not in the same eye. They may either be the right IR or the left IO.
- Head tilt: The head is tilted alternately to the right and left.
  - If hypertropia increases in right head tilt, the paralyzed muscles are right SO.
- Characteristics of the right SO are given as follows:
  - Right hypertropia in the primary position
  - Right hypertropia increases in the left gaze.
  - Right hypertropia increases with right head tilt.

Causes of Right Hypertropia

- Right SO palsy
- Left IO palsy
- Right IR palsy
- Left SR palsy

Causes of Left Hypertropia

- Left SO palsy
- Right IO palsy
- Left IR palsy
- Right SR palsy

Diplopia in the Fourth Nerve Palsy (Fig. 24.27)

- Diplopia is uncrossed.
- The diplopia is worse on looking down.
- The false image is lower than the true image.
- The upper end of the false image is tilted toward the true image.
- The distance between the two images increases on looking down and toward the sound side.
- The inclination increases when looking down toward the paralyzed side.

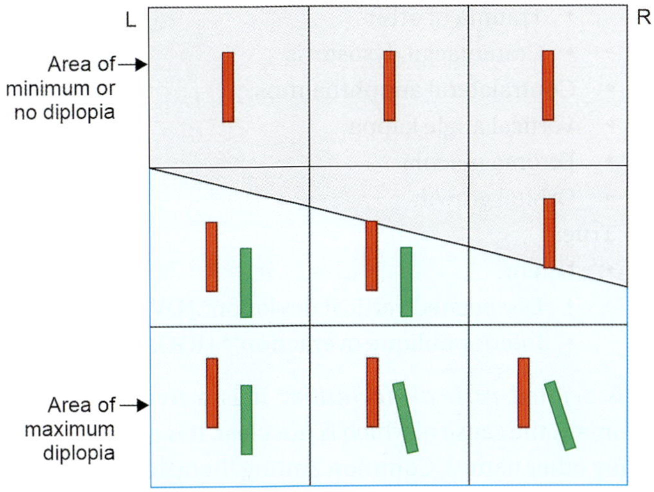

Fig. 24.27: Diplopia chart of right superior oblique palsy.

Acronym for head tilts of oblique muscles

> **IS - SO**
> Which means:
> - Underaction of **I**nferior oblique will cause head tilt on the **S**ame side.
> - Underaction of **S**uperior oblique will cause head tilt on the **O**pposite side.

NEUROLOGICAL CHARACTERISTICS OF FOURTH NERVE PALSY

The neurological characteristics of the third and sixth nerves are discussed under following levels: nuclear, fascicular, basilar, cavernous, and orbital part. The fourth nerve is an exception.

> The nucleus and fascicles of the fourth nerve are so close to each other that makes it impossible to differentiate between a nuclear and a fascicular lesion.

There are no neural tracts or vessels in its proximity of fourth nerve nucleus, presence of these pinpoint level of lesion of the third and sixth nerves. The only structure that passes near the fourth nerve in the fascicles is ocular sympathetic. Hence, it is logical to call them as nuclear fascicular lesions.

Nuclear Fascicular Lesion

The lesion at this level produces contralateral SO palsy that may be associated with Horner's syndrome.

TABLE 24.12: Clinical features of fourth nerve palsy at different levels.

Level	*Clinical features*
Sympathetic path	Horner's syndrome—same side with superior oblique palsy—other side
Medial longitudinal fascicle	Internuclear ophthalmoplegia—same side Superior oblique palsy—other side
Superior cerebellar peduncle	Superior oblique palsy—other side Ataxia and intention tremor

A lesion at the anterior medullary velum causes bilateral SO palsy.

Infrequent causes are given as follows:
- Involvement of medial longitudinal fascicle resulting in ipsilateral internuclear ophthalmoplegia* and contralateral superior oblique underaction.
- Involvement of superior cerebellar peduncle causes ipsilateral ataxia, tremors, and contralateral SO palsy.

A summary of nuclear fascicular fourth nerve palsy is given in **Table 24.12**.

Basilar

The fourth nerve, after its exit from the midbrain winds, found the brainstem and passed between the posterior cerebral and superior cerebellar arteries, lateral to the third nerve (see Figure above), to enter the cavernous sinus. At this location, the nerve is likely to be impinged against the tentorium following a head injury that causes paralysis of the SO on the same side without any other localizing sign.

Cavernous Sinus

The fourth nerve, due to its close proximity to other cranial nerves at this level, is never isolated; it is involved in multiple cranial nerve palsies that include the third, fifth, sixth, and oculosympathetic.

Orbital

The orbital lesions can either be:
- *Traumatic* causing injury either to the muscle itself or the trochlear over which it passes, happens following injury to the superomedial aspect of the orbital rim.
- *Neural* due to involvement of the third and sixth nerves.

**Internuclear ophthalmoplegia*: It is caused by a lesion in the medial longitudinal fasciculus, which is responsible for the coordination of various ocular movements. It consists of the inability to perform conjugate lateral gaze, along with ophthalmoplegia. The common cause is damage to interneurons between two cranial nerve nuclei. The common nuclei involved are the third and sixth nerves. Damage to the fourth nerve is uncommon in this condition.

Causes of Fourth Nerve Palsy in Children

- In one-third of cases, the cause cannot be pinpointed.
- It is mostly congenital and traumatic. Infection is less common than the former two.
- Vasculopathy, which is a major nontraumatic cause of fourth nerve palsy, does not seem to cause fourth nerve palsy in children.
- Other causes of vertical squints are given as follows:
  - Pseudovertical squint
  - True vertical squint

The causes of pseudovertical squints are given as follows:

- Craniofacial dysostosis
- Orbital asymmetry
- Orbital growth
- Ectopia of macula
- Microcornea **(Fig. 24.28)**

  The last two are less frequent than the former three.

A true vertical squint that can be:

- Latent/manifest
- Concomitant/paralytic
- The spread of comitance is common in paralytic vertical squints

  Causes of vertical squint are given in **Flowchart 24.3**.
- Pseudo[#]:
  - Contralateral lid retraction
  - Ipsilateral mild ptosis
  - Asymmetry of orbit:
    - Trauma of orbit
    - Craniofacial dysostosis
  - Contralateral anophthalmos
  - Vertical angle kappa
  - Ectopia macula
  - Orbital growth
- True:
  - Latent:
    - Dissociated vertical deviation* (DVD)
    - Inferior oblique overaction** (IOOA)

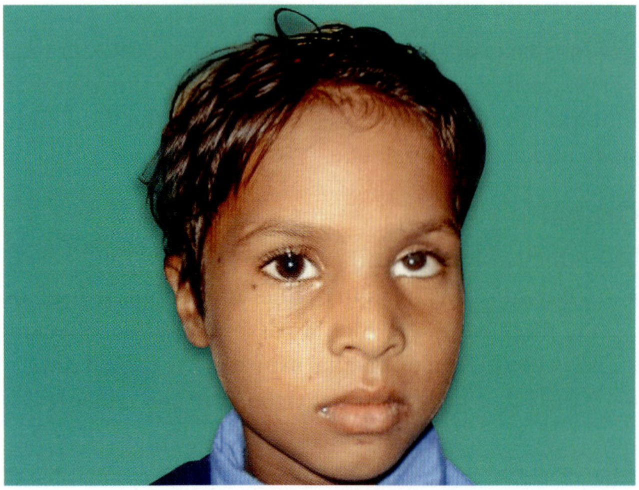

Fig. 24.28: Microcornea left eye presenting as pseudohypertropia.

Dissociated vertical deviation:* It is a neuromuscular anomaly, the cause of which is not clear. It is also known by many other names. Common among them are dissociated hyperdeviation, alternate sursumduction, and alternate hyperphoria **(Fig. 24.29).

As the last term indicates, it is basically a latent squint that manifests undercover; however, in some instances, when the child is tired or daydreaming, one of the eyes may deviate upward.

It is a binocular disorder with variable asymmetry in two eyes. The difference may be so much that one eye seems to divert all the time and the other looks normal.

It can be intermittent or constant; it may be associated with any type of squint. The most common deviation associated with the condition is infantile esotropia. The age of first detection is after 18 months of age. It can also be an isolated feature without a squint. Its association with squints is more frequent than without.

It is rare, after 18 months, to acquire a squint. If a squint is acquired after 18 months, in the case of an infantile squint, it takes about 2 years for the dissociated vertical deviation (DVD) to set in. Half the children with infantile esotropia are at risk of developing DVD. It is not only seen as a primary condition but may develop following successful surgery of infantile esotropia, which develops about 2 years following surgery. This makes it imperative to inform the parents about its possibility that they may require another surgery later.

The cover test is a handy test to unmask latent DVD.

- The eye is occluded by a Spielmann translucent occluder, through which the movement of the eye can be appreciated.
- The child fixes it with the other eye.
- The affected eye undercover deviates slowly up.

Flowchart 24.3: Different types of vertical squint.

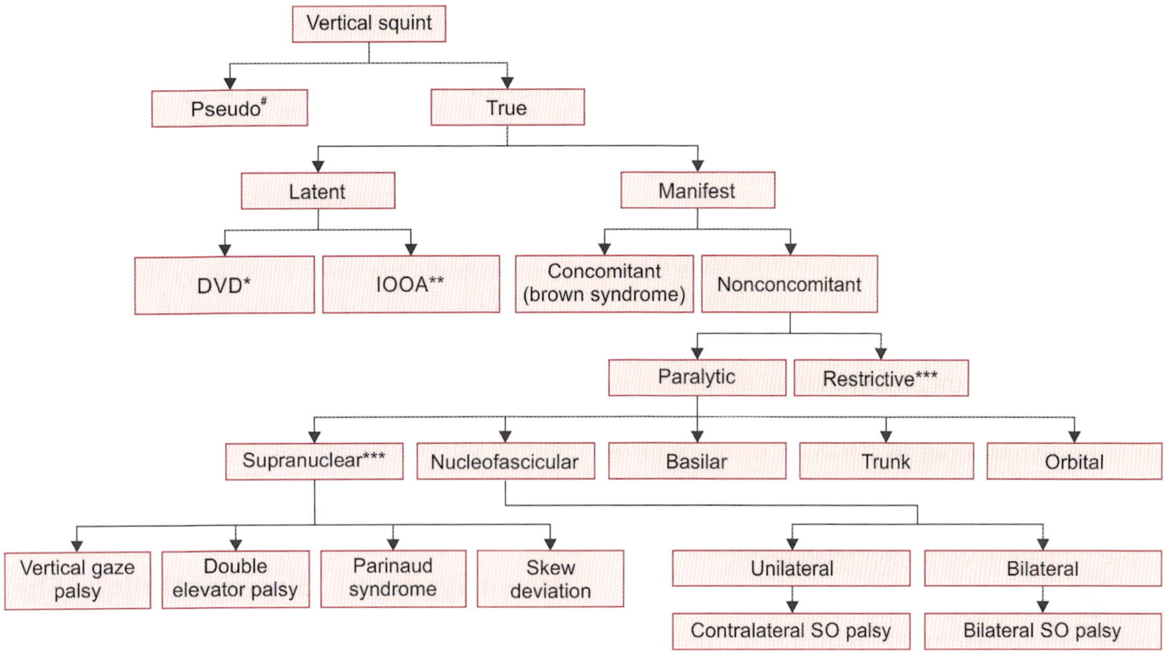

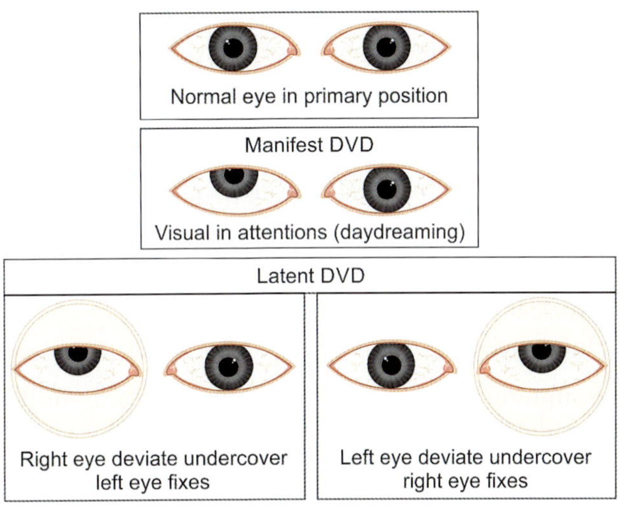

Fig. 24.29: Upward displacement of eyes under translucent Spielmann occluder* separately. When the right eye deviates undercover, the left eye takes fixation and vice versa. (DVD: dissociated vertical deviation)

Note: **Spielmann occluder* is a mildly frosted scratch-proof lens that is used as a translucent occluder. The occluder provides total form; occlusion yet allows the examiner to note the position of the eye behind the occluder with inducing suppuration.

- The drift is more marked if the cover is maintained for a long time.
- The deviation is more for distance.
- On removing the cover, the eye gradually comes down to primary position or may become hypotropic.
- The deviation is measured by a base-down prism in front of the deviating eye.
- The next step is to shift the occluder to the other eye, which starts deviating.

The other common features of DVD are given as follows:

- Manifest/latent nystagmus
- Extorsion of the deviated eye
- The eye in torts in downgaze
- Binocular single vision is possible in DVD.
- It may be associated with the AV pattern.
- It may be associated with oblique muscle overaction.
- The other test employed to differentiate the other conditions where the eye undercover deviate up is alternation in hyperphoria. The two conditions are differentiated by the dark wedge test. In the test, a *Sbisa bar** is placed

**Sbisa bar (Bagolini filter)*: This instrument consists of a series of red filters of varying densities (a photometric neutral density filter). The lightest red color is at one end, and the darkest red color is at the other end. The instrument is generally used to measure the depth of suppression in amblyopia, for which the test is done at one-third of a meter, in contrast to the Bielschowsky phenomenon, where the test is done at 6 m. The bar is placed before the fixing eye in increasing density until diplopia develops. The strength of the density gives the depth of the suppression.

before the fixing eye with provision to increase the density of the filter. The eye under the translucent occluder is found to drift down and even dip below the horizontal line if DVD is present. The next step consists of reducing the density of the filter and observing the eye undercover, which starts upward drift again. The phenomenon is absent in alternating hypertropia.

- There may be associated oblique muscle overaction that can be inferior oblique overaction (IOOA) or, rarely, SO overaction.

***Inferior oblique overaction:* It is as common as DVD following successful treatment of infantile esotropia; its occurrence is less common in exotropia **(Fig. 24.30)**.

There is no hypertropia in IOOA in primary gaze, which is best seen in adduction. Secondary hypertropia is seen with the underaction of the antagonist SO. The other feature is pseudoparesis of the contralateral SR.

V phenomenon: Latent nystagmus is common. The negative Bielschowsky phenomenon differentiates it from DVD. The cause of the condition is not clear; both mechanical and surgical procedures have been implemented to be the cause.

Superior Oblique Overaction

This is less common than IOOA; it can be primary/secondary, unilateral, or bilateral. When bilateral asymmetry is frequent enough to take it as unilateral, unless proved otherwise, all bilateral cases are primary; vertical deviation in the primary position is common in unilateral cases. The side of overaction of the SO results in hypotropia; association of the A pattern is common.

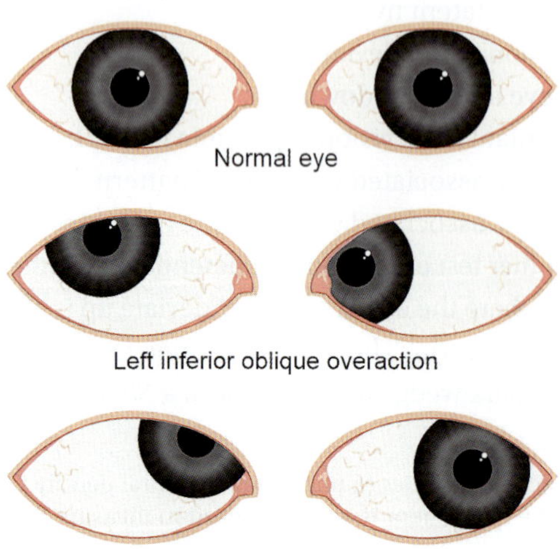

Fig. 24.30: Inferior oblique overaction in the left and right eyes.

Inferior Rectus Muscle Palsy

The other cause of vertical deviation is IR palsy. The causes could be congenital maldevelopment of the muscle belly or its defective insertion. Out of all the acquired causes of trauma, this is the most frequent. Fracture of the floor of the orbit is the most common cause, with or without incarceration of the IO. The eye in primary position is hypertropic in cases of nonincarceration of the muscle, in contrast to hypotropia when the muscle is entrapped. Abnormal head posture consists of turning the face to the paretic side, chin depressed, and head tilted to the same side. It is not seen in infantile esotropia, either before or after surgery.

Brown Syndrome (Superior Oblique Sheath Syndrome)

Causes of Nonconcomitant Vertical Squint

These are due to the involvement of cyclovertical muscles. Involvement of muscles may be restricted to one muscle in one eye or involve multiple muscles in one or both eyes in various combinations. The nonconcomitant vertical squint can be neurological or restrictive.

The neurological causes may be given as follows:

- Supranuclear
- Nuclear
- Infranuclear

The supranuclear lesions can produce not only vertical deviation but also horizontal deviation. The vertical deviations due to supranuclear lesions are given as follows:

- Vertical gaze palsy (VGP)
- Skew deviation
- Double elevator palsy
- Parinaud syndrome

Vertical Gaze Palsy

Vertical gaze palsy is a conjugate, bilateral limitation of the eye movements in upgaze and/or downgaze. This is under the bilateral cerebral and brainstem centers.

The following are the types of VGP:

- Inability to look up
- Inability to look both up and down

- Inability to look down (rarest)
- Transient vertical down deviation is seen in neonates without any neurological significance and does not require any treatment or further investigation.
- Vertical gaze palsy in infantile hydrocephalus, i.e., associated with retraction of the upper lid, gives a setting sun appearance to the eye. This is in contrast to the condition mentioned above. This requires investigation and treatment; the treatment falls under neurosurgical intervention. The causes are hydrocephalus, tumors, injury, and arteriovenous malformation.

Skew Deviation

Skew deviation is a supranuclear defect; there is divergence of the eyes in the vertical plane, which is large. It may vary in different positions of gaze. The deviation is more in uniocular lesions. There is no restriction on the forced duction test. No single muscle can be pinpointed as the cause of skew deviation on the Parks–Bielschowsky three-step procedure. The condition may be associated with internuclear ophthalmoplegia. The most common cause is a posterior fossa lesion that is confirmed by CT and MRI. Other causes are vestibular or cerebellar. It may develop in congenital esotropia, for which no cause is detectable. The pathology is generally ipsilateral to the involved eye.

Parinaud Syndrome

This is an acquired lesion. It is bilateral; there is paresis of upgaze. In an attempt to look up, the eyes converge. The pupils are semidilated, there is light near dissociation, and there may be lid retraction on downgaze. This is seen more commonly in children with the setting sun sign of hydrocephalus. Other common cause is a tumor of a pineal body.

The nuclear and infranuclear lesions have been discussed in lesions of the third, fourth, and sixth nerves.

The other lesions are (as already discussed above) given as follows:

- Dissociated vertical deviation
- Brown syndrome
- Inferior oblique overaction
- Superior oblique overaction
- Inferior rectus muscle paresis
- Superior oblique myokymia (not seen in children)

The restrictive causes of vertical squint are given as follows:

- Fracture floor of the orbit
- Myasthenia gravis
- Dysthyroid ophthalmopathy
- General fibrosis syndrome
- Progressive external ophthalmoplegia

CHARACTERISTICS OF ABDUCENS (ABDUCENT) NERVE PALSY

The characteristics of the third, fourth, and sixth nerves have been discussed in detail above. The following is a consolidation of the same, where the features of the nerves have been compared to each other. It has been noted earlier that the abducens is the sixth cranial nerve, which has a long intracranial course, second only to the fourth nerve. There are some similarities between the two; both innervate single extraocular muscles. However, there are some dissimilarities between the two; the sixth nerve does not decussate anywhere in its course, while the fourth nerve decussates completely in the dorsal part of the midbrain to form the nerve trunk that supplies the contralateral SO. While the sixth nerve supplies the ipsilateral lateral rectus, the third nerve partially decussates; the fourth nerve does not come in relation with nuclei of other cranial nerves or neural tracts except oculosympathetic. The sixth and third nerves differ from the fourth nerve in this respect due to their vicinity to other neural paths. The fourth and sixth nerves do not develop aberrant regeneration, which is seen in the third and seventh cranial nerves. In spite of its long intracranial course, isolated sixth nerve palsy does not have any localizing value. The sixth nerve nucleus lies near the medial longitudinal fiber that joins the contralateral MR nucleus in the third nerve complex. The sixth nerve fasciculus passes through the pyramidal tracts. The sixth nerve may be involved at any age, between newborn to old age. The fascicular part of the sixth nerve may be associated with involvement of the oculosympathetic. Diagnosis of an isolated sixth nerve is many times difficult due to masquerading pathologies. *They are given as follows*:

- Duane syndrome
- Moebius syndrome
- Infantile esotropia
- Spasm of the near reflex
- Myasthenia
- Thyroid eye disease
- Entrapment of the medial rectus in a fractured medial wall of the orbit

Like all cranial nerves serving extraocular muscle, the sixth nerve lesions can also be the following:

- Supranuclear
- Nuclear
- Infranuclear:
    - Fascicular
    - Basilar
    - Intracavernous
    - Intraorbital

Supranuclear

The supranuclear lesions are difficult to diagnose and are mostly seen in old age; however, children are not exempt from all of them. The supranuclear lesions are not due to an isolated lesion of the sixth nerve. The lesions are associated with lesions of the paramedian pontine reticular formation (PPRF).

They are given as follows:

- Horizontal gaze palsy
- Loss of pursuits (slow)
- Loss of saccades (quick)
- Internuclear ophthalmoplegia
- One-and-a half syndrome
- Tonic gaze deviation
- Locked-in syndrome

Nuclear

Nuclear lesions are infrequent when compared to infranuclear lesions.

> An isolated sixth nerve palsy is never nuclear. It is either associated with lesions in the nuclei for horizontal gaze or the seventh nerve nucleus.

The nuclear lesions of the sixth nerve produce the following conditions:

- Ipsilateral abduction failure
- Ipsilateral seventh nerve palsy
- Ipsilateral horizontal gaze palsy
- Ipsilateral Horner's syndrome

Infranuclear

Fascicular

The fascicular lesions are caused due to lesions in the brainstem or anterior inferior cerebellar artery syndrome. *They are of the following types*:

- Dorsal pones lesion (Millard–Gubler syndrome): Ipsilateral sixth nerve palsy and contralateral hemiparesis due to involvement of the pyramidal tract.
- Dorsolateral pons (Foville syndrome): Horizontal conjugate gaze palsy due to involvement of PPRF. Ipsilateral fifth, seventh, and eighth nerve palsy and Horner's syndrome.
- Combination of the two (Raynaud's syndrome): Ipsilateral sixth nerve palsy and contralateral hemiparesis **(Fig. 24.31)**.

Basilar

The common causes of sixth nerve palsy in children in its basilar course are given as follows:

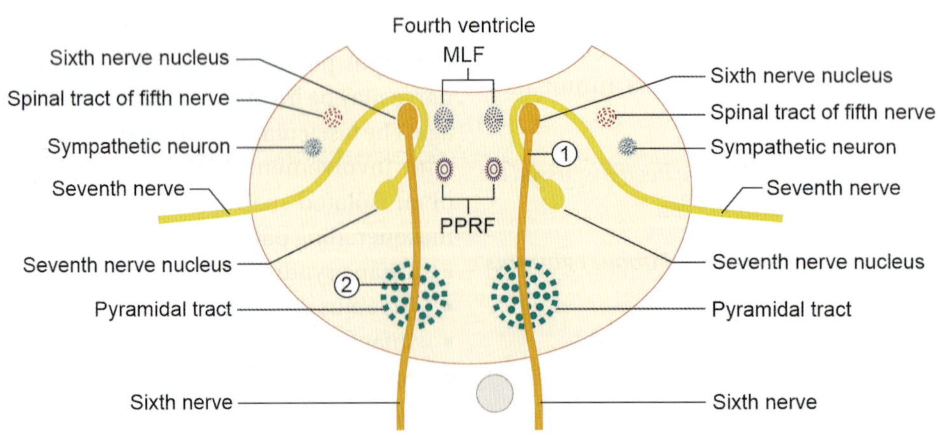

Fig. 24.31: Section through the lower pons showing the relation of the sixth nerve to other structures. (1) Lesion at this level will produce Foville syndrome; (2) Lesion at this level will produce Millard–Gubler syndrome; A combined lesion is called Raymond's syndrome. (MLF: medial longitudinal fasciculus; PPRF: paramedian pontine reticular formation)

- Raised intracranial pressure
- Gradenigo syndrome
- Trauma

Note: Acoustic neuromas and nasopharyngeal tumors, which are causes of sixth nerve palsy in adults, are not seen in children.

Raised intracranial pressure: The brainstem is pushed down due to raised intracranial pressure, pulling the sixth nerve along with on both sides, stretching the sixth nerve on the apex of the petrous bone. This causes bilateral sixth nerve palsy without any localizing signs. The causes of raised intracranial pressure are posterior cranial fossa tumors and pseudotumor cerebri. It can happen following an uncontrolled lumber puncture in severely raised intracranial tension.

Gradenigo syndrome: This used to be a major cause of unilateral sixth nerve palsy in children the World over before the advent of chemotherapy; it is still prevalent in underdeveloped countries. Where earache is a prominent and early symptom, it is not considered to be of any importance in children, which may be a harbinger of serious conditions such as otitis media that end in infection of the petrous bone and subdural abscess formation. Due to the close proximity of the sixth nerve to the petrous bone, the nerve is frequently involved in otitis media. The syndrome consists of unilateral sixth nerve palsy without involvement of any other neural tract, infranuclear facial palsy, facial pain due to involvement of the first division of the fifth nerve, and diminished hearing. This is explained in **Figure 24.32**.

Trauma: A direct injury to the petrous bone causes sixth nerve palsy due to its proximity to the sixth nerve, which may cause unilateral isolated sixth nerve palsy in all ages. The other form of bilateral sixth nerve palsy is a closed head injury where the skull is compressed horizontally, causing a transverse fracture of the temporal bone or base of the skull. A combination of bilateral sixth and seventh nerve palsy, bleeding and leak of cerebrospinal fluid (CSF) through the external ear, ecchymosis over the mastoid that presents as a crescent-shaped bruise over the mastoid, and ecchymosis of the lids (Raccoon sign*) is called Battle's sign†. It is a serious surgical condition that is best managed by a neurosurgeon.

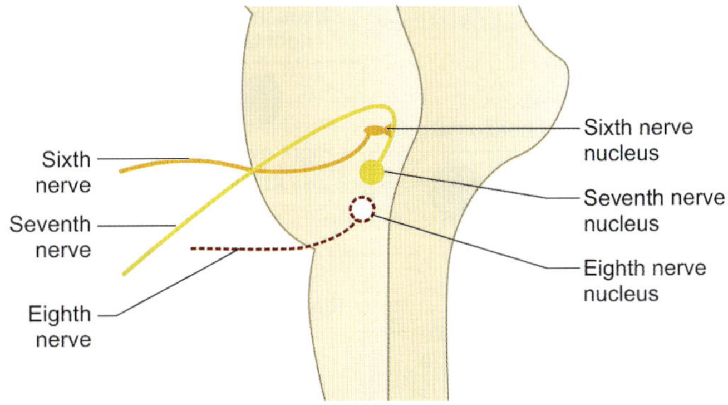

Fig. 24.32: The relative positions of the sixth, seventh, and eighth nerves causing Gradenigo syndrome.

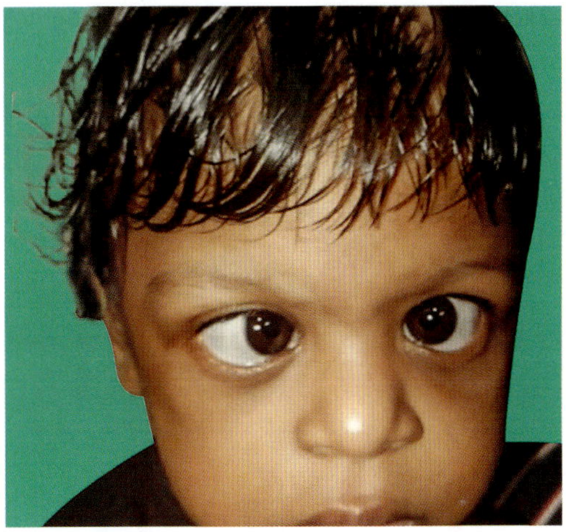

Fig. 24.33: Lateral rectus palsy in a child.

CHARACTERISTICS OF SIXTH NERVE PALSY

The sixth nerve supplies the ipsilateral lateral rectus that has only one function, i.e., abduction. The involvement of the sixth nerve can be put into two brought categories:

1. Isolated sixth nerve palsy
2. Sixth nerve palsy with other neurological signs

Characteristics of an Isolated Sixth Nerve Palsy

Isolated sixth nerve palsy has no localizing value.

- Convergent squint **(Fig. 24.33)**.
- Head turned toward the affected muscles without change in position of chin or tilting of head.

*The *Raccoon sign* comprises unilateral or bilateral progressive periorbital ecchymosis associated with edema. It is also referred to as the "raccoon eyes" and the "panda sign," due to the similarity between the clinical picture and the raccoon eye/panda sign. This is a red flag denoting fractures of the base of the skull involving the anterior cranial fossa.

†*Battle's sign* is due to bruising over the mastoid process due to the result of a head injury, mostly the base of the skull.

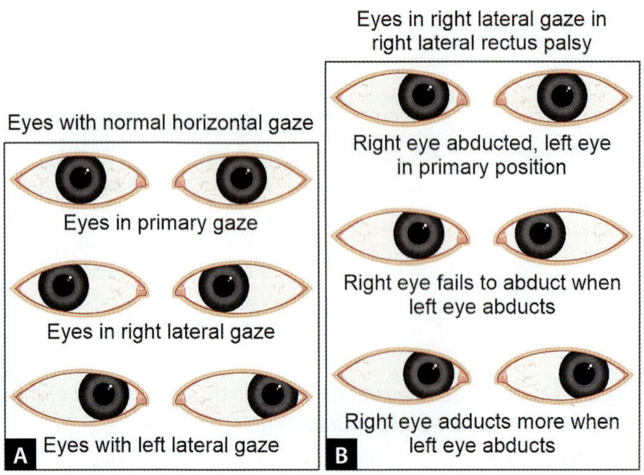

Figs. 24.34A and B: An abduction defect in the right lateral rectus palsy.

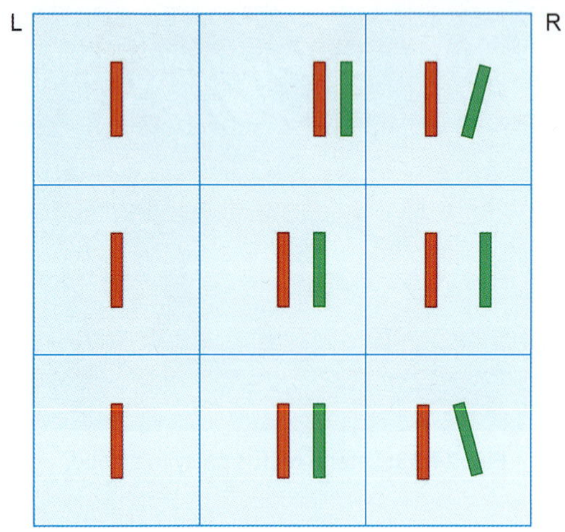

Fig. 24.35: Diagram showing diplopia chart of isolated right lateral rectus palsy.

- Restricted abduction **(Figs. 24.34A and B)**.
- Homonymous horizontal diplopia.
- Diplopia worsens on looking toward the involved sign **(Fig. 24.35)**.
- Bilateral paralysis of the sixth nerve produces diplopia in all gazes.
- Paralysis of the unilateral sixth nerve is far more frequent than bilateral.

Sixth Nerve Palsy with Other Neurological Signs

It has been discussed above.

Common causes of sixth nerve palsy in children are given as follows:

- Congenital
- Trauma
- Infection
- Inflammation
- Demyelination
- Neoplasm

Congenital

Most of the congenital cases are bilateral. *They are given as follows*:

- Developmental anomaly of the lateral rectus
- Birth trauma
- Maternal infection
- Hereditary

The developmental anomalies that are present with the underaction of the sixth nerve are given as follows:

- Moebius syndrome
- Duane syndrome
- Strabismus fixus
- General fibrosis syndrome

Differential Diagnosis of Sixth Nerve Palsy in All Ages

The differential diagnosis of sixth nerve palsy consists of many unrelated nonneurological conditions that produce mechanical restrictions of the lateral rectus. The conditions can be congenial or acquired. *They are given as follows*:

- Infantile esotropia
- Moebius syndrome
- Duane retraction syndrome
- Fractured medial wall of the orbit
- Strabismus fixus
- General fibrosis syndrome
- Alternate-day esotropia
- Conjunctival shortening syndrome
- Spasm of the near reflex
- Break in fusion of congenial esophoria
- Infantile esotropia
- Nystagmus blockage syndrome

Besides these, myasthenia and thyroid myopathy are two systemic conditions that may masquerade any motor palsy.

The diagnosis of recent lateral palsy is not difficult. However, occasionally, the child with nonparalytic esotropia may fail to abduct the involved eye, i.e., infantile esotropia. In such a situation of simulated sixth nerve palsy, it is essential to find out if the lateral rectus in question is really paralytic. The best way to demonstrate the action of the lateral rectus in such conditions is to patch the straight eye for a few hours. This will move the eye laterally in cases of pseudoparalysis of the lateral rectus but not in paralyzed lateral rectus. The only exception is entrapment of the MR in a fracture of the medial wall of the orbit, which is confirmed by a forced duction test. The child with lateral rectus palsy has his face turned toward paralyzed muscle to avoid diplopia. The other advantage of face turning is the increased temporal field on the side of the paralyzed lateral rectus. The child with prolonged lateral rectus palsy may cross-fix with the paralyzed eye, such as in infantile esotropia. Doll's eye reflex* is negative in the lateral rectus.

Long-term Effects of Extraocular Muscle Palsy

- Presentation of acute ocular palsy greatly differs from chronic palsies
- Some cases may present with palsy of one particular muscle only to involve other muscles later. This happens frequently in thyroid, eye disease, and myasthenia gravis.
- Following are the changes that are seen in other muscle/muscles when one muscle is involved:
  - Overaction of the ipsilateral antagonist
  - On long term, the ipsilateral antagonist may end up in contracture.
  - Secondary inhibition of the contralateral antagonist (underaction)
  - By the time secondary changes (sequels) take place, the other muscles get primarily involved.
  - Compensatory head posture: The child may overcome diplopia by keeping the head in an abnormal position.
  - Suppression and amblyopia are common in children with manifest squints.

Benign Abducens (Abducent) Palsy

Transient lateral rectus palsy due to viral infection is occasionally seen in children; it has been called by various terms, the most popular being benign sixth nerve palsy. This happens after a nonspecific upper respiratory tract infection 2–3 weeks after the viral infection, as painless paralysis with a mild-to-moderate sixth nerve underaction. It has a benign course lasting for a month or two, clearing over 3 months without leaving any trace. Sixth nerve palsy in children and adolescence is common following bacterial infection that also clears with treatment of bacterial infection; on rare occasions, it may develop following various vaccinations. The condition is not a harbinger of any serious neurological disorder.

CONCOMITANT SQUINT

General Consideration

Squint has been defined variously; the overall essence of all of them is a loss of parallelism between the visual axes of the two eyes, except in convergences. In a squint, one of the visual axes are directed toward the object of interest (fixation), and the other visual axis drifts away from the point of fixation (squinting eye).

Normally, the visual axes of the two eyes are parallel to each other in all gazes except convergence, where they meet at a point on the point of convergence; in contrast to this, when the eyes look at a point beyond a far point, they diverge slightly, which, when projected back, meets at an imaginary point behind the eye. Physiological convergence is more pronounced than divergence.

Epidemiology of Squint

Five percent of children suffer from some types of malalignment of the eyes. About 20% of the population belongs to the pediatric age group. This makes the number of children suffering from squint, a staggering figure. The incidence of squint is evenly distributed among all races, affecting boys and girls equally. It can be present at birth or acquired later. It has a strong hereditary predisposition; it is not uncommon to see siblings to have same type of squint, and it is also common among other members of the same family. Squint is a multifactorial, multigenic disorder. The most common condition that brings a child for consultation is frank squint; the other form of presentation is seen in children who have been brought for complaints other than squint, which is generally diminished vision, and are found to have squint that may be overt or covert.

> It is a misconception that the child will outgrow squint.

In the following conditions, the squint seems to be cured:

- A first-time parent may be scared at bizarre eye movements of a neonate and seek ophthalmic consultation to exclude squints. All that has to be done

---

**Doll's eye reflex* is a positive oculocephalic reflex based on vestibulo-ocular reflex; it is used in the examination of third, sixth, and eighth nerve palsies. In this test, the child moves the head opposite to the rotation of the head.

by a medical person is to counsel the parents, assuring them that the bizarre movement will disappear by few months, and the eyes will be straight. If the child does not have straight eyes and normal movements by 3 months, the child should be investigated for squints or nystagmus.

- The child has a pseudoconvergent squint due to the broad nose bridge and epicanthic fold. The nose bridge will become narrow, and the epicanthic fold will disappear, abolishing the suspected squint.
- The child has developed and abnormal head postures to avoid diplopia, which masks mild squints as seen in Brown syndrome.

What Keeps the Eyes in Alignment?

There are many factors that keep the eyes aligned (straight). The most important among them is BSV.

Binocular single vision is an asset. A lack of it is a liability.

Points to remember regarding BSV are given as follows:

- Binocular single vision is a conditioned reflex acquired at infancy.
- At birth, the eyes lack coordinated movement in the absence of a central mechanism; by 6 weeks, fixation starts developing; by 6 months, it is fully developed; BSV is well developed at 6 years.
- The mechanisms of BSV are given as follows:
    - Each eye receives a single image of object of interest.
    - Images in two eyes are independent of each other.
    - A centrally acting mechanism fuses them in a single image.
    - If they are not fused, there will be no BSV, and the child will see two images, i.e., diplopia.
    - The ability to fuse two separate images is called BSV or haplopia.
    - Fusion requires:
        - Equally clear image in two eyes
        - Correct alignment of two images
    - Binocular single vision will permit normal retinal correspondence
    - A child with congenital squint lacks central BSV but is capable of developing peripheral bilateral single vision.
    - The BSV is a property of the fovea that permits alignment of each eye at the same time in all gazes.
    - Fusion and stereopsis are not possible in the absence of BSV.
    - Anomalies of BSV are given as follows:
        - Abnormal retinal correspondence (ARC)*
        - Confusion leading to diplopia†
        - Suppression‡
        - Amblyopia

**Abnormal retinal correspondence*: Normal retinal correspondence stimulates anatomically corresponding points of each retina and corresponding points in the visual cortex to result in a single image. It is a central faculty; absence of normal BSV leads initially to confusion, followed by diplopia; some degree of BSV is possible in tropia. The abnormal BSV can be partially corrected by suppression, ARC, and abnormal head postures.

†*Confusion*: It is the result of corresponding retinal points being stimulated by two different objects. It is the state of seeing different objects in the same location. It is a major factor to cause amblyopia. The mechanism is as follows: In heterotropia, the fovea of the fixing eye sees the object of interest clearly, while at the same time, the deviation eye sees something other than what is seen by the fixing eye. This makes the brain to superimpose the two images formed at different places. This creates states of confusion, which is result of two corresponding retinal points being excited by two different objects. The patient is unaware of this phenomenon.

‡*Suppression*: It is a binocular temporary phenomenon of central origin seen in squinting eyes; the child is not aware of it. It is an attempt to avoid binocular vision disability, and it is a protective mechanism initiated by the onset of squints; hence, it is not seen in fixing eyes. Initially, all children with recent squints learn to suppress; it disappears if the nonsquinting eye is covered, and the squinting eye is made to fix. Suppression eliminates confusion and diplopia. It can be facultative or obligatory, central, or peripheral. In central inhibition, the image of the squinting eye is neglected; the fovea of the nonsquinting eye takes over dominance. It is mostly seen in uniocular esotropia. If there is a large area over which the suppression is spread, the area is called as area of the suppression scotoma. They are present in both types of horizontal squints. The esotropic suppression scotoma is seen nasally, while the exotropia produces a temporal suppression scotoma. There are two types of suppression scotomas, i.e., facultative and obligatory. The former develops in the eye in deviation, and as soon as the eye takes off fixation, the suppression scotomas disappear. The condition is seen in alternating squints. The latter is present even when the squinting eye takes up fixation, mostly in uniocular esotropia. In such a situation, the suppression is initially facultative that turns obligatory with the passage of time. It is tested by Worth's four dot test§, four-dimensional (4D) base-out prism, red glass test, and synoptophore.

§*Worth's four dot test*: This is a simple outdoor procedure that uses the principle of binocular dissociation by presenting images of the same shape and size in two different colors. It can be done at 6 or 1 m; the panel of the former is generally incorporated in the distant vision drum, which consists of a panel of dark color with four circles of equal size arranged in a diamond fashion. The colors of the circle are two green, one red, and one white; the same can be used on the glass of a large torch for examination at 1 m **(Figs. 24.36 and 24.37)**.

The test is usually done in an illuminated room, and the child should have fairly good vision. The test is generally not done under 10 years of age because the child may not appreciate the procedures and their interpretation. The child wears a red-green glass, red in front of the right. First, the child is asked to close the left eye and sees the spots with the right eye. He will see one red spot, the green spots will not be appreciated, and the white spot will look lighter than the red. The next step is to repeat the same with the right eye closed. The child will see three green spots. When an orthophoric child looks with both eyes open, he sees one red, two green, and one white **(Fig. 24.37A)**. The white may have a shade between red and green. In the case of left suppression, the patient will see two red **(Fig. 24.37B)** and one pink (white) spot with right suppression, patient will see three green spots **(Fig. 24.37C)**. If the patient sees five lights, the patient has diplopia **(Fig. 24.37D)** and normal correspondence. If the patient sees four spots in the presence of ocular deviation, the patient has anomalous retinal correspondence (ARC). The test can be used to diagnose in unilateral loss of vision in malingering; it cannot be used to test color vision.

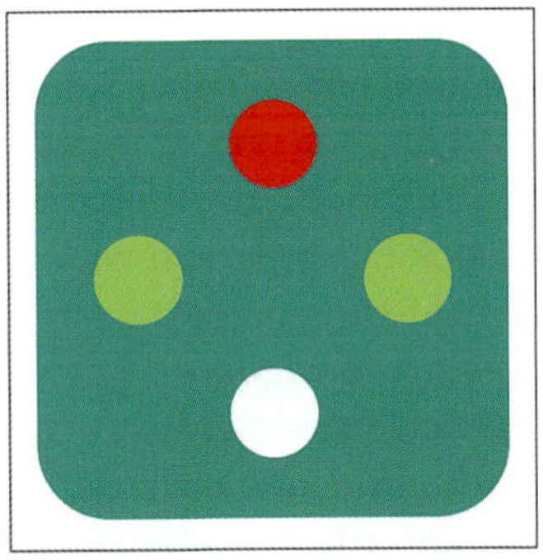

Fig. 24.36: Panel of Worth's four dot test.

Eccentric Fixation

Eccentric fixation is seen in unilateral squints where the object is fixed by a retinal point other than the usual fovea without change in the principle of visual direction. It is most commonly seen in esotropia and microtropia of longstanding. According to location, these points can be parafoveal, paramacular, paracentral, centrocecal, and erratic. The condition is diagnosed by a specially modified ophthalmoscope called visuoscope*.

Diplopia

Diplopia, in short, means seeing two images of a single object of interest with both eyes open. It happens when one object stimulates two noncorresponding retinal points, i.e., the fovea of the fixing eye and the extrafoveal point in the squinting eye. It can be binocular or uniocular; the former disappears with closing any of the eyes, and most of the time points toward a serious pathological condition such as paralysis of one or more extraocular muscles. The uniocular diplopia disappears only on closing the affected eye. The causes of uniocular are milder than binocular, and the child tolerates them better.

The causes are given as follows:

- Subluxated lens
- Iridodialysis
- Displaced intraocular lens (IOL)
- Recent corneal opacity

The binocular diplopia can be crossed (heteronymous) or uncrossed (homonymous) **(Figs. 24.38A and B)**.

The second image in binocular diplopia may be in the same plane, shifted vertically, or tilted. The second image is generally fainter than the primary image. It can

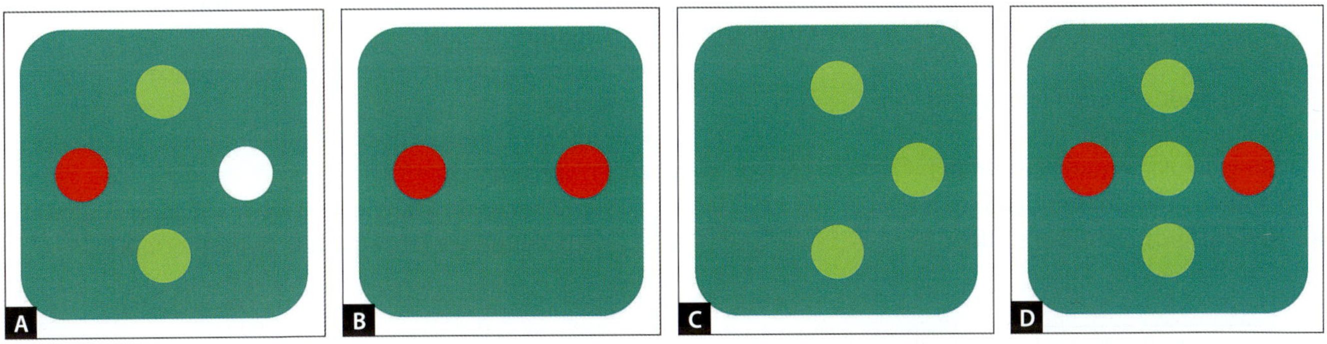

Figs. 24.37A to D: Result of Worth's four dot test. (A) Normal. (B) Left suppression. (C) Right suppression. (D) Diplopia.

*The visuoscope is a specialized direct ophthalmoscope to detect and evaluate eccentric fixation. A cross-hair target is added to the direct ophthalmoscope, which is projected on the macula of the unoccluded eye.

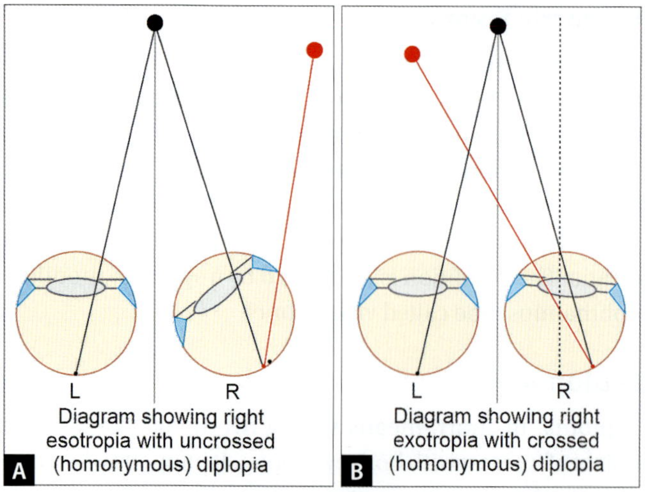

Figs. 24.38A and B: (A) Homonymous and (B) Heteronymous diplopia.

be horizontal or vertical; esotropia causes uncrossed diplopia, while exotropia produces crossed diplopia **(Figs. 24.38A and B)**. The direction of diplopia depends on the involvement of affected muscle/muscles, i.e., lateral rectus palsy causes horizontal diplopia that increases in lateral gaze; the second image is not tilted or vertically shifted. Diplopia is felt more in acute paralytic squints. In spite of deviation, concomitant squint does not result in diplopia because of ARC*, suppuration, and amblyopia.

The objective angle of a squint is the actual measurement of deviation as seen best on a synoptophore; the angle denoted in the synoptophore is called the objective angle of the squint.

> The difference between objective and subjective angles is the angle of anomaly; in normal retinal correspondence, the two angles are equal.

The situations where ARC is most likely to develop are given as follows:

- Small angle of concomitant esotropia
- Infantile esotropia
- Congenital alternating esotropia
- Esotropia develops under 3 years of age
- Residual postoperative squint

The situations where ARC is not likely to develop are given as follows:

- Concomitant divergent squint
- Concomitant convergent squint in adults
- Convergent concomitant large angel squint

In contrast to this, ARC is an adaptation to avoid diplopia in the squint; the adaptation takes this at the level of the cortex. The ARC may lead to an area that may be called pseudomacula; ARC may be associated with some degree of suppression of amblyopia.

SQUINT

Squint is a misalignment of visual axis in relation to each other. The visual axis is an imaginary line joining the point of interest in the space and the fovea. In a normal person, the two visual axes are parallel to each other in primary gaze and in all directions, the only two exceptions being convergences and divergences. In spite of there not being parallel, the angle of convergence or divergence is equal in two eyes. In the position of rest in normal persons, the two visuals are actually slightly divergent, which is of no consequence. This ideal condition is called orthophoria.

Orthophoria is an ideal physiological state; hence, like any physiological position, it is rare. It is present even when fusion is broken artificially (cover test). A person may be orthophoric but look like a person with a squint. This is due to anatomic configuration of the face, lids, and orbit. These conditions are designated pseudosquints. The causes of which are given as follows:

- *Prominent epicanthic fold:* Gives an appearance of a convergent squint, which is abolished by obliterating the epicanthus. It also disappears with age.
- *Hypertelorism:* Gives an appearance of a divergent squint.
- *Facial asymmetry:* Gives an appearance of a vertical squint.
- *Unilateral ptosis:* Gives an appearance of hypertropia.
- *Error of refraction:*
    - Large positive angle kappa gives an appearance of a pseudodivergent squint in hypermetropia.

**Anomalous retinal correspondence:* Normal retinal correspondence is the preferred physiological status where the image of the fovea in one eye corresponds with the image on the contralateral fovea. It is fully developed in adulthood; once established, it cannot be erased; hence, ARC is seen only in childhood. Younger the child, smaller the degree, and longer the duration of squint, more is ARC. It is frequent in infantile esotropia and less common in exotropia and vertical squint. Clinically, it has been put in two groups, i.e., harmonious and unharmonious. In the former, the angle of anomaly is equal to the angle of squint; in the lateral, the subjective angle of squint is less than the objective angle.

- Negative angle kappa, in myopia, gives an appearance of a pseudoconvergent of squint.

If the eye deviates on breaking the fusion, it is called heterophoria (latent squint). All orthophoric eyes do not need to have good vision. Nonorthophoric eyes generally have poor vision; however, reverse vision is also possible. Orthophoria eyes have a central corneal reflex, and none of the eyes move undercover. The pseudosquints, too, are orthophoric.

> An apparent convergent squint worsens a true convergent squint and neutralizes a divergent squint. Similarly, an apparent divergent squint worsens divergence.

Properties of Pseudosquints

- The corneal reflex is always central.
- The eyes do not move undercover.
- The pseudoconvergent squint gradually disappears due to the fading of epicanthus as the child grows.
- The pseudosquint in hypertelorism is a permanent feature, independent of age.
- Pseudosquints due to errors of refraction generally disappear with correction.

Effect of Fusion in Keeping the Eyes Orthophoric

- A high degree of fusion is a predisposing factor in keeping the eyes in a state of orthophoria.
- The breakdown of fusion results in the onset of latent squint, and the condition is called heterophoria.
- In already broken-down fusion, the eye passes into a state of visible squint called heterotropia.
- In between latent and true squint lies a state of intermittent heterotropia.

Classification of Squints

Squints have been classified variously given as follows:

- As per age:
  - Congenital
  - Acquired

The former is less common than the latter.

- The acquired squint can be:
  - True squint or pseudosquint (see above):
    - Tropia
    - Phoria
- As per side:
  - Unilateral
  - Alternate
  - Bilateral

The last is far less common than the former two.

- Concomitant or nonconcomitant: Nonconcomitant can either be paralytic or restrictive.
- Constant or intermittent

***Flowchart 24.4** gives a summary of the classification of squints.*

Flowchart 24.4: Classification of squints.

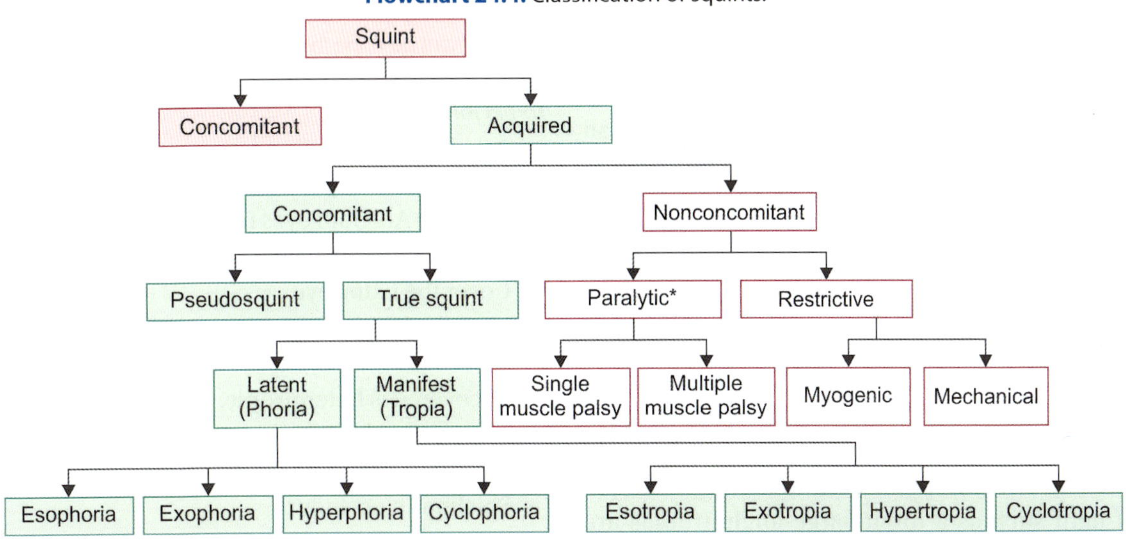

**Paralytic squint:* Paralytic squints can either be primary or may simulate it; it develops due to secondary changes seen in nonparalytic squints of longstanding following decompensation. The cause of which could be general debility, acute illness, inadequate fusional reserve, prolonged near work, or long hours on the computer. The recovery in such conditions may be fast or slow; the later heralds decompensation.

Causes of congenital squint are mostly myogenic; they are given as follows:

- Duane retraction syndrome
- Brown syndrome
- Moebius syndrome
- Strabismus fixus
- Double elevator palsy
- Congenital fibrosis of extraocular muscles
- Congenital extraocular myopathy

Phorias

Phorias are a latent state of malequilibrium of the visual axes. They are not visible when the eyes are fixed with good fusion. Hence, the patients and observers are not aware of their presence. Once the latency breaks down by abolishing fusion by covering any of the eyes, the eye undercover deviates, only to come back to original position when the cover is removed.

The causes of decompensation are given as follows: The phorias are equal in both eyes. In some conditions, such as excessive near work, fatigue, or illness, it may not be possible to maintain fusion; in such cases, they deviate even without cover. This is called decompensation of phoria, and the eyes develop tropias of the same direction, i.e., esophoria getting converted into esotropia and exophoria is converted to esotropia. The recovery on removal of the cover may be fast or slow; slow recovery heralds decompensation (for details, see below).

Tropias

The tropias are manifest squints that are visible to the observer; the child may or may not be aware of small deviations. A large deviation, besides having poor vision, is a cause of embarrassment to the child. Hence, a child with tropia avoids looking straight into the eyes of observer. The tropias are so obvious that they do not require a cover test to diagnose; however, a cover test is required to differentiate between paralytic and nonparalytic squints and to find out if the condition is unilateral or alternate. The angle or deviation may be constant or variable.

Tropias, both concomitant and nonconcomitant, do not require any test; except for examination by a simple source of light such as a torch, large-angle tropias are obvious even on ambient room illumination. Difficulty arises in the diagnosis of small angle deviations, which requires extra methods. The most common test performed to distinguish between phoria and tropia and various causes and types of tropia are the cover test.

Cover Test

A cover test is a qualitative test that does not require elaborate equipment. The prerequisites are given as follows:

- Sufficient vision in each eye to fixate
- Both eyes have a central fixation.
- The eyes are freely mobile.

The test is divided into two steps:

1. Cover test
2. Cover–uncover test

The test requires:

- A proper fixating target
- For distance optotypes at 6 m
- For a near-near vision chart
- A torch light is not a good fixation target for distance as it stimulates accommodation.
- *Occluder:* The occluder should be an object that covers the eye from brow to chin; it can be an opaque or translucent (Spielmann occluder). They could be handheld or spectacle mounted; the examiner's palm is the most handy occluder.

The procedure comprises of two parts.

The first part confirms heterotropia. The steps are given in ***Figure 24.39***.

The test can be done in ambient light.

To perform the test:

- Ask the patient to fix a target at 6 m for distance and 33 cm for near
- *Observe:* Are both eyes fixing or does one seem to fixate and the other deviates (squints).
- Cover the fixing eye
- Note the behavior of the squinting eye
- If the squinting eye takes up fixation, it means the eye uncovered is heterotropic.
- The eye undercover deviates by the same degree in the same direction; this is best observed through a Spielmann occluder.

The second part:

It confirms heterophoria:

- Ask the patient to fix the target, as in the first part.

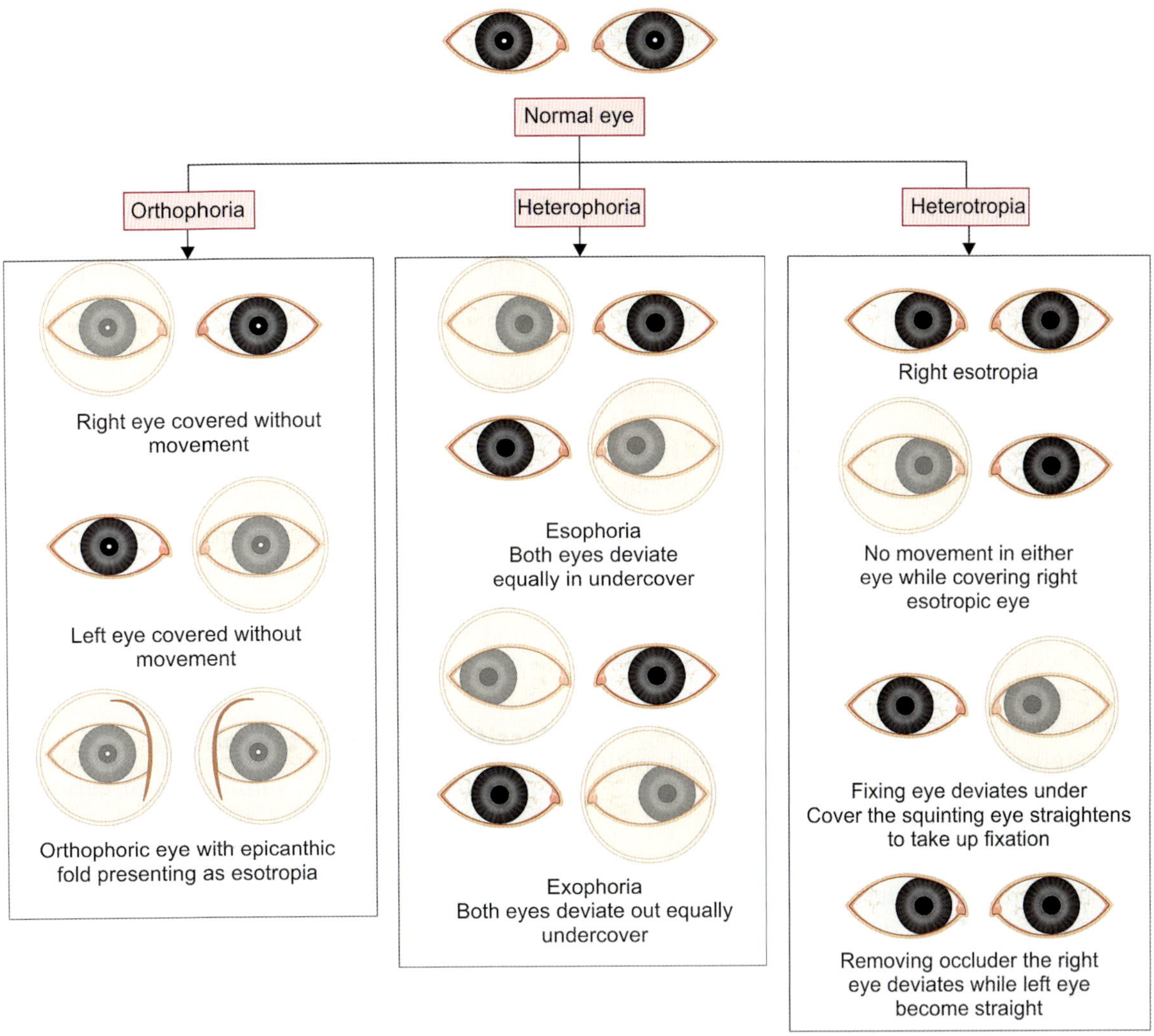

Fig. 24.39: Cover test showing the difference between pseudosquint, phoria, and tropia.

- Observe if:
  - Both eyes fix when not occluded.
  - If one eye fixes the other, the other eye is heterotropic.
  - If there is no movement in any eye when covered and uncovered, the two possibilities are given as follows:
    - There is no phoria.
    - There is microtropia that requires additional confirmation.
- Any eye may be covered to break fusion; if there is phoria, the eye undercover will deviate.

On removal of the occluder, the eye moves to take up fixation.

Interpretation of the cover-uncover test:

- It is a qualitative test to be confirmed by a prism and cover test.
- It confirms the presence of malalignment (latent/manifest squint).
- It denotes the direction of deviation (i.e., eso/exo/vertical).
- It shows visual dominance.
- It can predict the presence of amblyopia.

***Table 24.13** shows a summary of interpretation of cover test.*

The other tests employed to break the fusion are given as follows:

- Dissimilar images falling on two foveae—the Maddox rod test

TABLE 24.13: Interpretation of cover test.

Result	***Squint***
No shift to alternate cover testing	Orthophoria
No shift on the cover–uncover test, with a shift on the alternate cover test	Phoria
Shift on both cover–uncover and alternate cover test tropia	Tropia
Small shift on cover–uncover testing with a larger shift on alternate cover testing	Monofixation syndrome is to be confirmed by specific tests

- Two images have different colors (red glass test).
- Separate images are being projected on two foveae—the Maddox wing.

Etiology of Heterophoria

The etiology is not well understood. It is multifactorial; it has a strong genetic background. The factors given below act alone or in combination:

- Uncorrected error of refraction:
    - Hypermetropia is frequently associated with esophoria.
    - Myopia is more associated with exophoria.
    - Emmetropes are not immune.
- Children are more likely to develop esophoria.
- Muscular anomalies:
    - Faulty origin
    - Faulty insertion
    - Poorly developed muscle
    - Defective innervations: Muscles in each eye getting different tonic innervations.
- Other causes include debilitating disease, fatigue, psychosomatic disorder, drugs, and toxins.

Types of Heterophoria

As heterophoria is not apparent, it has to be elicited to be diagnosed. The child or onlookers are not aware, so long as the fusion is intact. Its presence is elicited by a simple cover test and its modification. As per the direction of the eye undercover, the heterophoria can be:

- *Esophoria:* The eye deviates nasally undercover and moves temporally on removal of the cover.
- *Exophoria:* The eye deviates out undercover and takes up fixation on removal of the cover.
- *Hyperphoria/hypophoria:* One eye moves up in relation to the other eye undercover and returns to the original position on removal of the cover. Presently, the term hypophoria is not used in clinical practice.

The phoria is not designated as right or left; they are marked as plus and minus, i.e., esophoria is marked by the plus sign and exophoria by the minus sign.

- In phoria, the degree of deviation is the same in each eye undercover for a given distance. They are different for far and near.
- *Cyclophoria:* These are the least common. In this condition, there is a tendency for one eye to rotate either inward or outward in relation to the other undercover. There is no condition where the two eyes rotate in opposite directions.

Classification of Heterophoria

Flowchart 24.5 shows summaries of various types of phorias.

Diagnosis of Heterophoria

The diagnosis of heterophoria is more tricky than heterotropia. The parents may wonder why the child is being made to go under so many tests when there is no squint in either eye.

The diagnosis starts with:

- *Symptoms:* The child may be symptom free. Most of the children are not aware of its presence, in contrast to heterotropia, which is so obvious.
- The symptoms, when present, are the aftermath of decompensation*.
- The children who are found to have phoria can be grouped in following two groups:
    1. Those seeking help for visual causes
    2. Those with symptoms of decompensation

**Decompensation of heterophoria:* The exact causes of decompensation are not well understood. Decompensation depends on the available reserve of neuromuscular faculty; better the neuromuscular reserve, lesser the chances of decompensation. In decompensation, the eyes that were straight without cover tend to develop visible deviation undercover; this is preceded by slow recovery when the cover is removed. The symptoms of decompensation are mild, recurring, and irritating; they are headache, vague eye pain in a noncongested eye, recurrent styes, chalazia, chronic conjunctivitis, glare, and the running of letters during prolonged reading and working on a computer. The other complaint is difficulty in changing focus from distant to near and vice versa. The most sure evidence of decompensation is the appearance of a visible squint (tropia).

Flowchart 24.5: Classification of phoria.

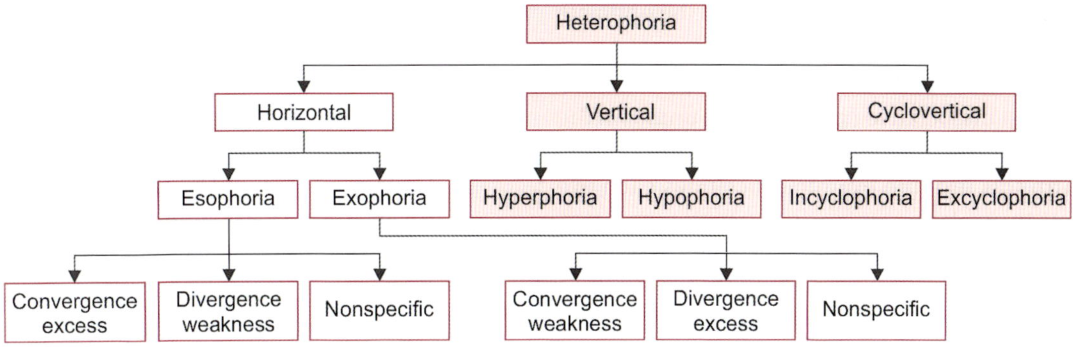

Examination of Cases of Latent Squint

- The first and foremost examination is a complete history of the disorder, including the presence of the disorder in the family, i.e., parents and other blood relations.
- *Visual acuity:* The most important part of the examination is the recording of age-matched vision. The parents may object because they feel that the child has normal vision, and the test is a waste of time, not realizing that the child may have occult hypermetropia, to which the symptoms are directly related.
- *Retinoscopy:* Retinoscopes should be performed under complete cycloplegia with appropriate cycloplegic. Simple mydriatics are not sufficient to unmask and underline hypermetropia.
- Look for facial asymmetry
- Exclude causes of pseudosquints
- The most important examination is the cover test. In fact, all children presenting for consultation for any symptom should be tested for visual acuity and undergo a cover test.
- Prism and cover test
- Maddox rod and Maddox tangent test
- Maddox wing test for near
- Synoptophore examination
- Measurement of accommodation
- Measurement of convergence
- Complete ocular examination.

Cover Test

This is a very handy test that can be done in the office without any special instrument, even in ambient illumination most of the time. *The steps consist of:*

- The child is explained that this is a painless, simple procedure that will not hurt him.
- The child is made to look at a distant object. This will relax accommodations.
- One of the eyes is covered, and the other eye fixes the distant object.

Note: A child with diminished vision in one eye will resent covering the eye with better vision.

- After a few seconds, the cover is removed, and movement of the eye is noted. In cases where a translucent lens (Spielmann occluder) has been used, the movement of the eye can be observed without removing the cover.
- Movement in any direction denotes heterophoria; if the eye moves out to take up fixation, the eye has esophoria moved undercover, in a convergent position. The reverse means exophoria; in hyperphoria, the eye moves down.
- The test is repeated for near.
- The test should be performed both with and without glasses.
- If the child is known to have an error of refraction with phoria, the best correction that eliminates phoria should be noted.
- If full correction does not improve phoria, other methods to treat it should be contemplated.

Types of Cover Test

- *Cover test*: This is an objective method for finding out the presence, type, and magnitude of strabismus, both phoria and tropia. It reveals the presence and extent of phoria and the direction of deviation.
- *Cover–uncover test*: This test not only identifies a tropia but also differentiates it from a phoria. The test is done by using an opaque occluder.
- *Unilateral cover test*: This is done by covering the fixating eye in tropia and observes its movements. If

the eye was exotropic, covering the fixating eye will cause an inward movement; in esotropia, the opposite will happen.

- *Alternate cover test (cross-cover test)*: The alternate cover test is the best dissociative cover test that unmasks the total deviation that includes both tropia and phoria. To perform this test, the examiner occludes each eye alternately in quick succession.
- *Prism and alternate cover tests*: The first part is to perform an alternate cover test and then introduce a prism over one eye to measure the deviation. The power of the prism is increased until the eye stops moving.
- *Other tests:*
  - *Maddox rod test*: The child sits in a semidarkened room 6 m away in front of the Maddox tangent. The Maddox rod is traditionally put in front of the right eye **(Fig. 24.40)**. The child sees a red streak that can be rotated by 180°. The child is asked to locate the streak on the Maddox tangent, and the position of the red streak is noted first on a horizontal scale and then on a vertical scale. In orthophoria, the streak passes through the central light of the scale; otherwise, it passes away from the central light. The streak may be on either side of the light depending on the type of squint; the distance of the streak from the central light is directly read from the scale inscribed on the Maddox tangent. The test fails to differentiate between phoria and tropia.

    Maddox rods (grooves) placed horizontally; Maddox rods (grooves) placed vertically.
  - *Red glass test*: This is similar to the Maddox rod test. In this test, instead of a Maddox rod, a red glass is used. The procedure is the same as in the Maddox rod test. If the vision is unequal, the glass is put in front of the better eye to prevent suppression of the poorer eye. The red glass should be dark enough, so that the patient sees only the central light of the Maddox scale. This test fails to differentiate between phoria and tropia.
  - *Synoptophore test*: The instrument is a haploscope that presents two different images in two eyes through two separate tubes and presents them as one if the eye is orthophoric. The instrument is also called an amblyoscope. The large table-mounted amblyoscope is called a major amblyoscope, and the handheld version is called a minor or portable amblyoscope. This is a multipurpose instrument used in the office; its functions are both diagnostic and therapeutic. *The uses of the instrument are given as follows*:
    - Measurement degree of deviation
    - Used for cover tests and alternate cover tests
    - Measure the range of fusion
    - Detect suppression
    - Detect retinal correspondence
    - It measures subjective and objective angles of deviation, which are used to determine the angle of the anomaly. What is the difference between the objective and subjective angles of squint*? If both are equal, it is concluded that the patient has simultaneous perception and normal correspondence.
  - Last but not least, it is used in the treatment of both tropia and phoria.

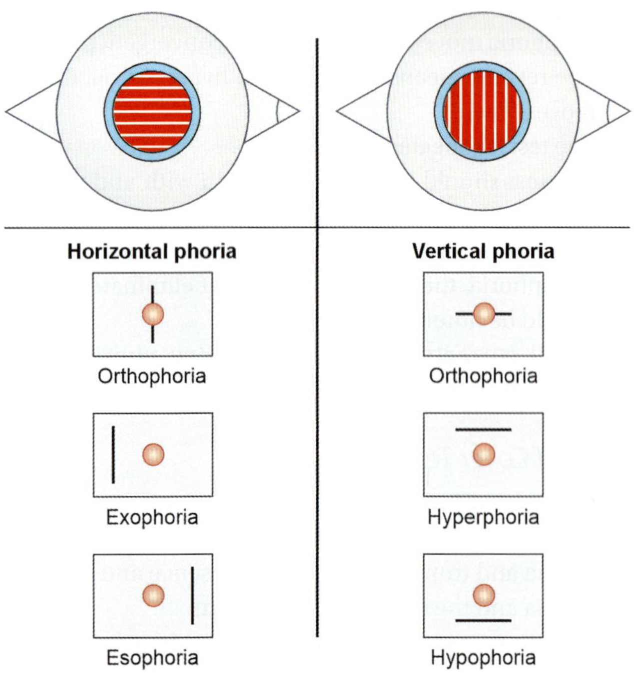

Fig. 24.40: Result of Maddox rod test.

Measurement of Phoria for Near

Phorias for the near are most easily measured by the prism and cover test. The most accurate measurement is

**Objective and subjective angles of squint*: The objective angle is the motor deviation or the angle of deviation of the eye that is seen. The subjective angle is the sensory deviation or how far off the extrafoveal retinal point is from the actual fovea.

given by the Maddox wing test that not only measures the horizontal squint and its degree but also gives the degree and angulation of the cyclophoria.

Detection and Measurement of Cyclophoria

Though simple cover test gives and approximate information regarding cyclophoria, cyclophoria itself requires minute observation during the cover test; the measurements are more accurate when done by following instruments:

- Maddox wing
- Double Maddox rod, one usual red and the other white
- Maddox double prism

Double Maddox Rod Test

The devices required for the tests are one red and one white Maddox rod, a 6 D prism, and a white fixation light. The red Maddox rod is put in front of the eye supposed to have cyclodeviation, while the white rod is put in front of the other eye. Both rods are kept parallel to each other at the 90° mark of the trail frame, producing two parallel vertical streaks, one red and the other white. The prism is put behind the white rod to separate two images vertically. The prism needs not to be used in cases of already present vertical deviation. If both the streaks are parallel, the eye is orthophoric. In cases of cyclodeviation, the red streak will be inclined to the white line. The next step is to rotate the red streak until both lines become parallel, denoting the magnitude and direction of cyclodeviation without differentiating between phoria and tropia **(Fig. 24.41)**.

Maddox Double Prism Test

Maddox double prisms consist of two prisms, each of 4 prism diopters (PD) in strength, mounted on a lens ring with bases against each other. The double prism is put in the trial frame in front of one eye; the other eye is left uncovered without any lens or prism. The patient is given a white sheet of paper that has a line drawn in the middle. The patient keeps the paper at its usual reading distance in such a way that the black line is horizontal **(Fig. 24.42)**.

The two prisms in the trial lens separate the line away from each eye. Thus, a patient without cyclophoria will see three parallel lines. The central line is the line seen by the eye without prism. The other two lines, one above and one below the central line, are formed by the two prisms. If the central line is oblique to the two parallel lines, the patient has cyclophoria or cyclotropia.

DETAILS OF VARIOUS TYPES OF HETEROPHORIA

Esophoria

Here, the eyes move inward following dissociation, common in children; adults are not exempted; hypermetropic children are more prone than myopic and emmetropic. The condition is divided into the following types:

- *Converges excess:* Esophoria is more for near than distance.
- *Divergence weakness:* Exophoria is more for distance than near.

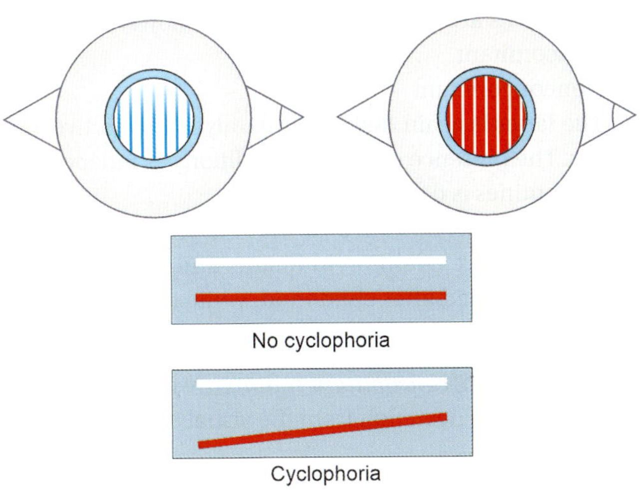

Fig. 24.41: Result of a double Maddox rod with a red rod in front of the right eye.

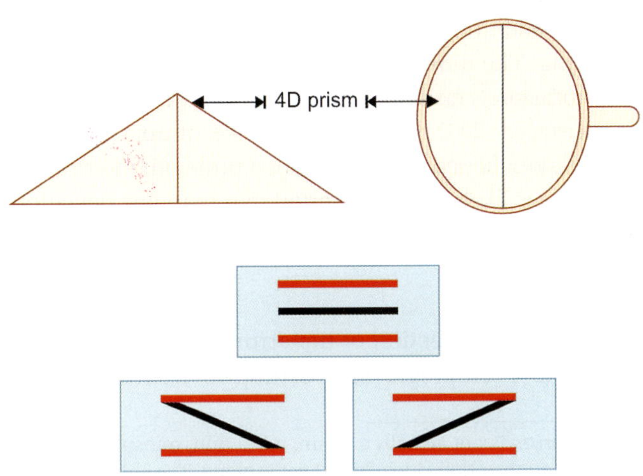

Fig. 24.42: Interpretation of Maddox double prism test.

- *Combination:* There is not much change in the near or distant deviation.

The following is an outline of the management of esophoria:

- Correction of any error of refraction seen under complete cycloplegia. The glasses are meant for constant use.
- *Orthoptic treatment:* We have seen that fusion is the factor that keeps the eyes in alignment in heterophoria. When the eye becomes decompensated, efforts should be made to improve fusion. The methods used are divergence exercises of synoptophore (synoptophore exercises in no way strengthen the extraocular muscles).
- Home stereogram exercise
- Bar reading in the case of convergence excess
- *Prism:* It may sometimes relive symptoms; children using glasses accept prism better than those who do not use glasses.
- *Fresnel prism*:* It may be pasted over the spectacle glasses.
- Surgery is rarely required.

Exophoria

In exophoria, the eyes diverge when dissociated. They are of three types. They are given as follows:

1. *Divergence excess:* The angle of the exodeviation is more at a distance by ≥10 PD. This should be differentiated from pseudodivergence excess, where divergence is ≥10 PD at a distance, which is reduced after 1 hour of monocular occlusion.
2. *Convergence weakness:* Here, exophoria is greater for near than distance.
3. *In between the two*, there is not much difference between near and distance deviation.

The condition should be differentiated from intermittent exotropia. The difference lies in the amount of deviation; exophoria rarely exceeds 20 D prism, while intermittent exotropia exceeds 20 D prism. Intermittent exotropia is prone to suppression; hence, diplopia is not a problem. Intermittent exotropia is likely to be converted into manifest deviation, which does not happen in exophoria.

Management

It consists of correction of the error of refraction under complete cycloplegia and orthoptic treatment. The treatment is required only if there is a possibility of exophoria being converted into exotropia.

Hyperphoria

Hyperphoria is less common than horizontal phorias; generally, the deviation is less in hyperphoria. When compared to the deviation of a horizontal squint, a small deviation such as 2–3 D is sufficient to be symptomatic. In vertical squint, fusional amplitude is also less, and asthenopic symptoms are more marked. The management consists of the correction of the error of refraction and the prescription of a prism, based down in hyperdeviation and base up in hypodeviation. The power of the prism is equally divided between two eyes, it is better to correct one-third to one-half of the deviation by the prism.

Cyclophoria

This is the rarest of all phorias, with a maximum symptom even with a minimum deviation. It is most of the time missed unless specifically looked for; the eyes are examined with the Maddox wing, Maddox double rod, and Maddox double prism. Excyclophoria is more common than incyclophoria. The condition is mostly associated with vertical phoria. The management is better directed toward vertical deviation.

Heterotropia (Manifest Squint)

Heterotropias consist of a group of ocular deviations that are obvious to the onlooker. The child may not be aware of it unless he grows up to realize the cosmetic blemish. The condition becomes very obvious in photographs. Heterotropias are of two types given as follows:

1. Concomitant
2. Nonconcomitant

The latter is again divided as paralytic, restrictive, and kinetic. The presence of the last conditions as independent clinical entities is questionable.

Concomitant squint outnumbers nonconcomitant squint. It is more common in infants and young children that get plateaued after childhood, while the incidence of incomitant squint increases with age.

Characteristics of concomitant squints are given as follows:

- It is a visible deviation from the visual axis of any eye.

**Fresnel prism* is not actually a prism. It is a thin, transparent sheet of plastic that has angular grooves to give a prismatic effect on one side of the sheet; the other side of the sheet is plane. The sheet is pasted on the spectacle glass by the plane adhesive surface as per the requirements of the patients.

- The deviation in the two eyes is constant with regard to time and degree, i.e., the deviation is visible all the time throughout waking hours; the angle of deviation does not change with gaze.
- The object of interest is fixed by one eye at a time, and the other eye drifts.
- The eye looking at the object of interest is called the fixing eye, and the other is squinting eye.
- The eyes move freely in all directions of gaze, as against paralytic squints, where there may be restriction of movement in some gazes.
- There is no limitation of ocular movement, which is a hallmark of paralytic squint*.
- The squint is called intermittent if there is a period of straight eye in between the deviations.
- The squint is called uniocular if it is present in the same eye all the time.
- If squint manifests in each eye at different times, it is called alternate squint.
- Manifest squint can be convergent, divergent, or vertical**.
- A combination of horizontal and vertical deviations is also possible.
- Deviation may differ for distant and near.

Table 24.14 depicts the difference between nonparalytic and paralytic squints.

TABLE 24.14: Difference between paralytic and nonparalytic squints.

Features	***Nonparalytic (concomitant)***	***Paralytic (incomitant)***
Heredity	May have a hereditary predisposition	Nonhereditary; the systemic cause involved may be hereditary
Age of first presentation	Children are more prone to present with concomitant squint	Any
Onset	Usually gradual	Sudden in case of paralytic squint, gradual in restrictive squint, except entrapment of muscle
Diplopia	Generally, there is no diplopia	• Major complains • The extent of diplopia is variable with head position • Diplopia is most marked in recent cases and may pass off with time, over months
Head posture	Normal	Abnormal head posture is the rule
False projection	Not a problem	Common in initial days
Cross fixation	May be present	No cross-fixation
Visual acuity	Squinting eyes generally have poor vision	Diminished vision cannot be attributed to cause squint
Ocular movement	Normal	Restricted in the direction of action of the involved muscle
Angle of squint	Same in all directions of gaze	The angle of the squint varies with various gazes
Primary and secondary deviations	Equal	Secondary is more than primary
Neural path: • Afferent • Efferent	 • Faulty • Normal	 • Intact • Faulty
Abnormal retinal correspondence	Possible	Generally, it does not develop
Amblyopia	Common	May or may not develop
AV syndrome	Common	Absent
Cyclovertical deviation	Less common	More frequent
Systemic disorder	Not present	Common
Doll's head phenomenon	May have to be elicited	No role
Secondary changes in muscle	None	Frequent
Spontaneous recovery	Nil	May be
Change to concomitancy	Already concomitant	Possible
Forced duction test	No role	Useful in restrictive squint

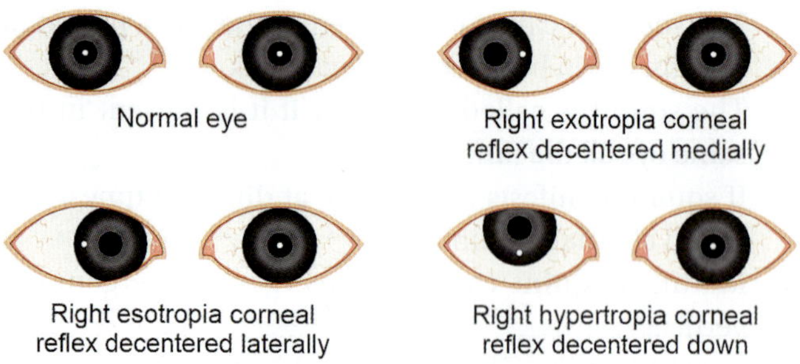

Fig. 24.43: Types of tropias.

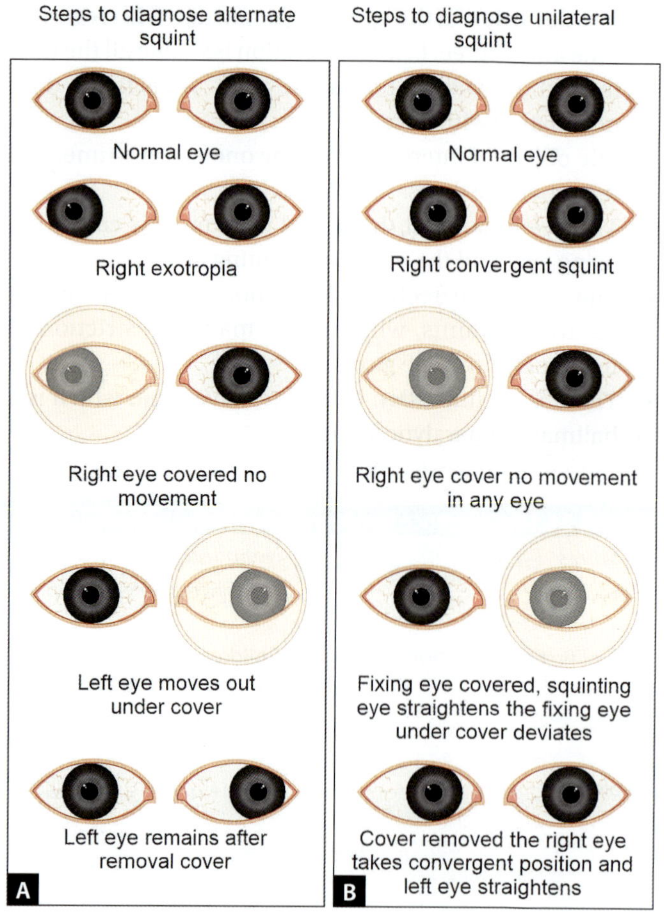

Figs. 24.44A and B: (A) Alternate and (B) Uniocular squints.

Types of tropias are shown in **Figure 24.43**.

Besides the direction of heterotropia, they can also be divided into the following groups as per laterality.

They are unilateral (monocular) and alternate (binocular). Unilateral heterotropia is more frequent now than later.

Figures 24.44A and B show steps to diagnose alternate and uniocular squints.

A squint is said to be unilateral when one of the eyes squints constantly and the other eye fixes. Covering the fixing eye, the squinting eye takes up the fixation, and the fixing eye deviates undercover. The deviation in two eyes is the same; as soon as the cover is removed, the previously covered eye takes up fixation and the other eye deviates.

In an alternate squint, if the fixing eye is covered, it deviates undercover; the angle of deviation is the same as that of the squinting eye, removal of the cover, the eye remains deviated.

Primary and secondary deviations:

- *Primary deviation* is the deviation of the "squinting eye" when the "normal eye" fixes (i.e., X°).
- *Secondary deviation* is the deviation of the "fixing" eye when the "squinting" eye is made to fix. The secondary deviation is always greater than the primary deviation (i.e., $X^{\circ++}$). This is due to Hering's law of equal innervations **(Figs. 24.45A and B)**.

Etiology of Concomitant Squint

Like phorias, the causes of concomitant squints are also not well established. The causes are multifactorial, where more than one facture may be operative.

The two theories put forward by Duane are based on the fact that the medial recti are responsible for nearness and convergence, while the lateral recti are responsible for distance and divergence.

The types are given as follows:

- Medial rectus dysfunction, also known as near dysfunction
- Lateral rectus dysfunction, also known as distance dysfunction

The concomitant squint may present as follows:

- *Primary dysfunction:* The disorder starts without being latent.
- Starting a as latent squint and getting decompensated so much that the eye fails to revert to orthophoria. The common sequence is → Phoria → Intermittent tropia → Constant tropia.
- Spread of comitance in case of congenital dysfunction.
- Other contributory factors are given as follows:
    - *Hereditary:* A 10–15% of concomitant squints show genetic traits.
    - *Idiopathic:* The following conditions are difficult to put under a definite cause:

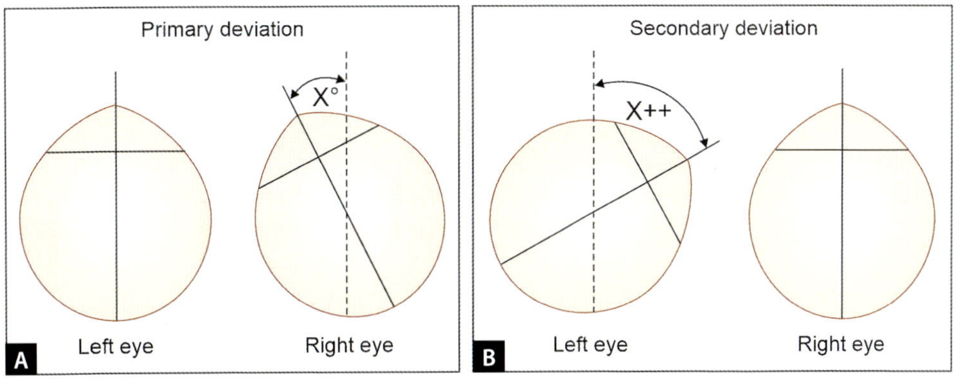

Figs. 24.45A and B: Difference between primary and secondary deviations. (A) Left eye is the fixing eye. The right eye is a squinting eye. The angle of deviation of the right eye is X°. This is the primary deviation; (B) The right eye is made to be fixed; it straightens. The fixing eye deviates in the same direction with an angle of deviation more than X°, i.e., X^{o++}. This is a secondary deviation.

    - Congenital development of extraocular muscle (i.e., mostly abnormal insertion).
    - Squeal of congenital paralysis of extraocular muscles. A child with congenital paralysis may recover, leaving its direct antagonist in a state of contracture, resulting in its underaction.
- Vision:
    - It is not unusual for some squinting eyes to have normal or near-normal vision; this is generally found in alternators and those who cross-fixate.
    - Diminished vision in one eye: The eye with less vision generally squints.
    - Diminished in both eyes; an eye with poor vision is more likely to develop squints.
    - Absence of vision in one eye
    - Amblyopia

Dissociation between accommodation and convergence: This is one of the most common causes of squinting in children. In hypermetropia of a moderate degree, the child accommodates more to see clearly. This stimulates convergence, producing a convergent squint. In contrast to this, myopic eye does not require accommodation to see clearly; hence, there is diminished convergence, resulting in external deviation. A child with congenital myopia has a very short far point and can see only near objects. To see near things, he has to converge more than an emmetropia, and this results in a convergent squint.

Evaluation of Squint in Children

Basically, evaluation procedures are the same in all ages, with little modification in children. Children are more likely to present with concomitant squints. The incidence of nonconcomitant squints is more in adults; this does not mean that adults are immune to the development of concomitant squints. Children are far more predisposed to amblyopia, which requires precise diagnosis and treatment in childhood, i.e., under 8 years. Amblyopia can be the cause or effect of squint. Parents are more worried about cosmetic blemishes than amblyopia; it should be emphasized upon them that a child with amblyopia is left without treatment. The child will remain with subnormal, uncorrectable vision that may be detrimental to many jobs later in life.

Evaluation of squint is divided into following heads:

- History
- Complete ocular examination
- Specific examinations related to squint

History

History is an important part of the evaluation of a squint; many a time, it gives clues to the probable cause, type, and investigation that will be required. The first information sought should be at the time of first detection, which may be by parents or caregivers.

- Noticed at birth:
    - Congenital esotropia
    - Congenital exotropia (rare)
    - Congenital lateral rectus palsy
    - Restrictive squint
    - Infantile esotropia
    - Secondary esotropia:
        - Retinoblastoma
        - Congenital toxoplasma scar

- Between 6 months and 3 years:
  - Concomitant squint
  - Paralytic squint
- Above 3 years:
  - Concomitant squint
  - Paralytic squint

Time of onset:
- Acute:
  - Viral infection
  - Paralytic squint
  - Phoria breaking into tropia
- Cyclic (rare)

Summary of history taking:
- *Time of onset:* Acute/gradual
- Constant or intermittent
- Unilateral/bilateral
- Diurnal variation
- *Diplopia:* Sudden, gradual, progressive, resolution, and pain
- *Types of diplopia:* Horizontal, vertical, and torsional
- Abnormal head posture
- Associated systemic features
- Family history
- Birth history
- Past history of treatment
- Use of glasses and its effects
- History of trauma

Laterality:
- Uniocular
- Alternate
- Bilateral (rare; they are never concomitant)

Movement of the eye: Do both eyes move equally in all direction?

Diplopia (Figs. 24.46 to 24.48)

Diplopia is a subjective feeling of seeing a single object as two with both eyes open; it disappears with the closing of any of the eyes, in contrast to the disappearance of the second image on the closure of the eye with pathology. This is called uniocular diplopia, which in fact is polyopia, where instead of two images, multiple images are seen. The condition is rarer than binocular diplopia. Binocular diplopia happens following malalignment of the visual axes in the squint. The most common cause being paralytic squint. In diplopia, the object of interest stimulates the fovea of one eye, and the image is called

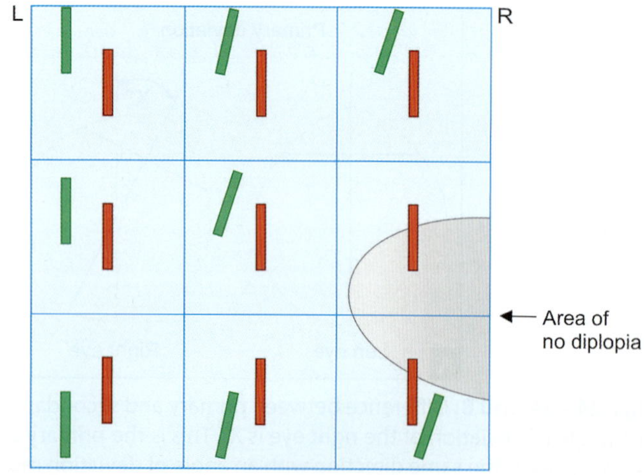

Fig. 24.46: Diplopia charting in multiple muscle involvement (third nerve palsy).

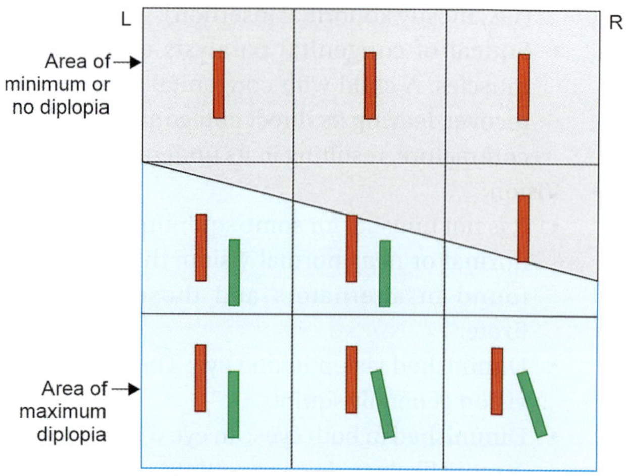

Fig. 24.47: Diplopia charting in single muscle involvement (fourth nerve palsy)

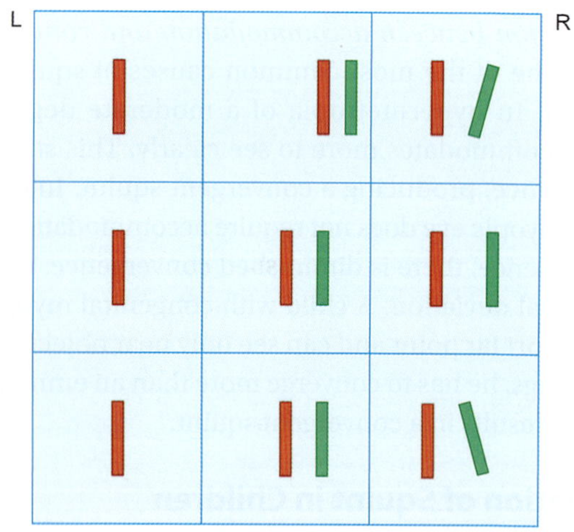

Fig. 24.48: Diplopia charting in single muscle involvement (sixth nerve palsy)

the true image; the image in the other eye is formed on an extra foveal place. This image is called a false image, which is fainter than the true image. It is generally displaced, horizontally or vertically. Horizontal displacement is seen in the involvement of the lateral rectus and medial rectus. Vertical displacement is seen in the underaction of cyclovertical muscles.

The vertical false image may be straight or inclined toward the true image. The false image is projected in a direction opposite to the deviation of the eye. If the eye is deviated nasally, the false image is projected outward, as in convergent strabismus, this diplopia is called uncrossed or homonymous; in the case of divergent squint, the diplopia is crossed or heteronymous. The crossed diplopia is seen in the underaction of the adductor, i.e., the medial rectus and inferior rectus. Uncrossed diplopia is seen in the underaction of the abductor, i.e., the lateral rectus, superior and inferior obliques.

If the eye is deviated upward, its image is projected downward. In nonconcomitant squint, the diplopia varies in different gazes; the diplopia becomes worse in the fields of action of the involved muscle. The worsening is reflected as increase in distance between the two images. Multiple muscle palsies produce both horizontal and vertical. While paralysis of a single muscle shows either horizontal or vertical deviation, as seen in lateral rectus palsy, Paralysis of the superior oblique produces the separation of two images with tilting.

Diplopia is a diagnostic feature of paralytic squint; it not only pinpoints the muscle/muscles but also their grade of involvement; more is the underaction, more will be deviation and diplopia. The diplopia is generally constant throughout the waking hours; however, in restrictive squints, it may vary during the same day, the most common example being myasthenia gravis, where the diplopia increases after physical exertion. The diplopia chart has a prognostic value. The diplopia is measured by the distance between two images in all positions of gaze, utilizing a red-green goggle, a single-red lens, a Maddox prism, and a Hess screen. In paralytic squint, the diplopia is most marked in the acute stage. The other causes of diplopia are convergence spasm, paralysis of convergence, or paralysis of divergence.

Abnormal head posture is seen in all paralytic squints. It is best observed in: Superior oblique palsy and lateral rectus palsy.

- Restrictive squint
- AV pattern (older children)
- Nystagmus blocking esotropia

NYSTAGMUS

Children with paralytic squints may keep one eye closed to avoid diplopia. This is more common in exodeviation.

Family History

In about 10% of cases, there may be a family history of some type of squint or other, the type of squint is generally the same, i.e., horizontal or vertical. It is common to have a positive family history among parents or siblings.

Relevant Ocular Examination in Children with Squint

The relevant examinations are given as follows:

- Recording of vision
- Refraction
- Fundus examination
- Brückner test

Recording of Vision

Recording vision is difficult in children under 5 years. Children above 5 years are generally tested for vision by methods employed for adults with necessary modifications.

Recording of vision depends on the age of the child; it is difficult in infants and preverbal children, requiring much attention and perseverance.

The vision should be taken in:

- To give confidence to the child, both eyes together should be tested first. The child is more comfortable with both eyes open. Vision in both eyes together is better than in a single eye, i.e., a child with 6/18 in the right eye and 6/24 in the left will have 6/9 or better when both eyes are tested together, unless the other eye has very poor or no vision.
- Both eyes separately, the child resents the closing of the eye with better vision.
- *Vision with pinhole:* A child with tropia may not be able to locate the pinhole.
- *Vision with glasses:*
    - Each eye separately
    - Both eyes are together
- Find out the power of the glasses.

- If the vision is not fully corrected by the glasses the child is using, try to find out which glasses that give the best correction and may require refraction under cycloplegia.
- Do the glasses have near additions?
- History of frequent changes of glasses (myopia)

Refraction

All eyes, irrespective of vision, in the presence of a squint should be refracted under age-matched cycloplegia to unmask hypermetropia, overcorrection of myopia, the power of the cylinder, and its precise angle. If the result of previous refraction under cycloplegia is available, the child may be examined on autorefractor in subsequent visits.

Fundus Examination

The advantage of using cycloplegia is that it leaves a widely dilated pupil suitable for ophthalmoscopy of both types.

> All cases of esotropia should be examined for the presence of occult retinoblastoma.

Brückner Test

Brückner test is a simple, objective, and handy office procedure that does not require much of a child's attention. It is an objective test. It can be done in infants also; it is as simple as Hirschberg test. This is performed by a pen torch. Brückner test is done in a manner similar to that of a distant direct ophthalmoscope by a direct ophthalmoscope, not requiring dilatation of the pupil in normal children. It reveals the presence of ametropia and amblyopia. A child with a low grade of ametropia will have an equally bright retinal glow when seen through a direct ophthalmoscope from half a meter of distance without putting any lens in the peep hole. The first step is to locate Hirschberg reflex; this will reveal a squint. The second step is to compare the brightness of the retinal glow in two eyes. The test is said to be positive if the brightness is asymmetric in two eyes. The eye with a higher refractive error will give brighter reflex.

Diagnosis of Heterotropia

- The diagnosis of large-angle tropias is not difficult. The parents are always aware of it; even children in their teens may be aware of it and be embarrassed by it.
- The first step is to find out if the squint is a true or pseudosquint.
- Once the pseudosquint has been excluded, the next step is to find out if the true squint is paralytic or nonparalytic.
- This confirms the presence of a concomitant squint.
- *Cover test:* This is the most important office procedure that is mostly neglected.
  - It reveals the presence of phoria in the straight eye.
  - It differentiates between:
    - Pseudo and true squint
    - Uniocular and alternate squints
    - Paralytic and nonparalytic squint

  The test should be performed for far and near.

MEASUREMENT OF THE ANGLE OF THE SQUINT

Hirschberg Test

This is yet another easy and handy office procedure that requires nothing but a pinpoint light from a torch **(Fig. 24.49)**.

To perform the test:

- The child keeps both eyes open and fixes an object at 6 m with his head straight.
- A bright pinpoint light is directed on the eye from 33 cm; this gives a bright shining spot on the anterior surface of the cornea.
- In the absence of tropias, the bright spot will be centered on the pupillary area.
- Any decentering of the light denotes the presence of tropia.

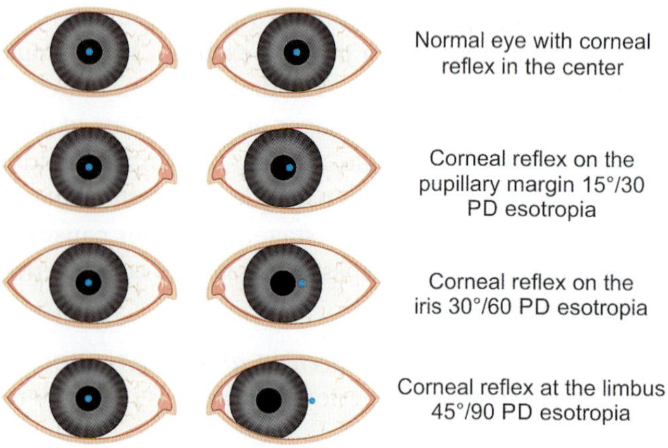

Fig. 24.49: Steps of Hirschberg test.

- The light is decentered to the opposite side of the deviation of the eye, i.e., if the eye deviates out, the spot will be shifted nasally and vice versa.
- Each millimeter of decentering denotes 7° or 14 PD of squint.

Other causes of decentering of the corneal reflex are given as follows:
- A positive angle, Kappa, may look like an exodeviation.
- A negative angle, Kappa, may look like an esodeviation.
- In cases of eccentric fixation in an amblyopic eye, the light reflex remains decentered on covering the contralateral eye.
- Ectopia macula.

Krimsky Test (Prism Reflex Test)

This is a subjective test that is more accurate than the Hirschberg test, which is the first part of the Krimsky test. To perform the test, the corneal light reflex is noted, followed by placing a prism of increasing strength in front of the eye with a decentered corneal reflex. For esodeviation, the prism is put base out, and in exodeviation, base in. The prism shifts the corneal reflex toward the center; the power of the prism that brings the corneal reflex to the center gives the amount of squint. The prerequisite of the test is that the child should fix the light with the dominant eye, the cornea should be transparent and bright, and the observer should place himself exactly in front of the child to avoid parallax from the prism. The test is not influenced by eccentric fixation; a large angle of Kappa may create confusion. The test is suitable even in eyes with poor vision in one eye.

Perimeter Test

This is another office procedure suitable for grown-up children.

The steps are given as follows:
1. The child with both eyes uncovered sits on the Lister perimeter with chin on the chin rest and fixes the central white dot. One of the eyes deviates.
2. A pinpoint light is moved on the arc of the perimeter from periphery to center until the reflex is centered in the deviating eye. The position of the light is read on the arc of the perimeter; this gives a rough idea of the angle of the squint.

Examination on Synoptophore

This is the gold standard for detecting and treating squints in all ages. It is a multipurpose optical haploscope that brings different images from two eyes into a single frame. It is the most accurate method for measuring the squint both far and near in all gazes; it measures the squint, binocular vision, and detects suppression and amblyopia. It is also used to treat suppression and amblyopia.

Besides measuring the angle of squint, it also measures the objective and subjective angle of squint* and angle of anomaly†, presence of ARC‡ and its type, the grades of vision§, range of fusion, after image testing, and AC/C.

Simultaneous macular perception is absent in manifest squint. There may be a suppression scotoma with variable size and location as per the type of squint. In esotropia, the scotoma is relatively small and placed on the nasal side of the disc. In exotropia, the scotoma is large and seen on the temporal retina, which may include the fovea. In uniocular squint, the scotoma does not change its position; it may predispose to strabismic amblyopia. Stereopsis binocular fusion may be absent in concomitant squint.

Stereopsis Test

The stereopsis is tested by the following methods:
- Two-pencil stereopsis test
- Titmus fly test

**Objective and subjective angle of squint*: The objective angle is motor deviation, i.e., visible; in contrast to this, subjective angle is sensory deviation that represents the distance between extrafovea and fovea. The difference between the two is the angle of the anomaly.

†*Angle of anomaly:* The angle of anomaly is the difference of objective angle minus subjective angle. It is equal in normal retinal correspondence. In unharmonious, the angle is not equal.

‡*Types of ARC:* The types of ARC are harmonious, unharmonious, and paradoxical. In a harmonious ARC, the subjective and objective angles of the squint are equal. In an unharmonious ARC, the objective angle is more than the subjective angle.

§*The grades of vision are given as follows:*
- Simultaneous macular perception (most primitive)
- Superimposition
- Sensory fusion
- Motor fusion
- Stereopsis (most advanced)

- TNO test
- Random-dot stereo test
- Frisby stereo test
- Lang stereo test
- Holmes stereoscope
- Keystone stereoscope
- Asher law stereoscope

The therapeutic uses of synoptophore are given as follows:
- Treatment of amblyopia
- Management of suppression
- Treatment for ARC
- Fusional exercises

Suppression is tested by:
- Worth's four dot test
- Synoptophore
- Four-diopter prism test*
- Bagolini striated glass test†
- Red glass test

Interpretation

- The patient sees only one slanting streak, showing that the other eye is suppressed.
- If the patient sees two streaks forming a perfect cross, the eye is orthophoric with central fixation and normal retinal correspondence.
- If there is a perfect cross and the spot of light is deviated from the center, the patient has ARC.
- If the spot of light is in one of the streaks and the other streak breaks in two parts at 45° away from the spot of light, the eye is straight with foveal suppression and normal retinal correspondence.
- If the eye squints under the same condition, it has ARC **(Figs. 24.50A to D)**.

The concomitant squint, in order of frequency, can be:
- Horizontal:
  - Pure horizontal:
    - Esotropia
    - Exotropia
  - Associated with the vertical component:
    - Dissociated vertical deviation
    - Inferior oblique overaction
    - Superior rectus underaction
    - AV pattern

Note: The first three are seen in esotropia. The AV pattern is seen in both eso- and exotropia.
- *Vertical:* Hypertropia (the term "hypotropia" is no more in use.)
- *Torsional:*
  - Incyclotropia
  - Excyclotropia

ESOTROPIA

Concomitant esotropia is the most common esodeviation seen in children. It can be unilateral or alternate; it may be congenital or acquired. The deviation may vary with distance; it may be associated with a vertical component. Amblyopia is common.

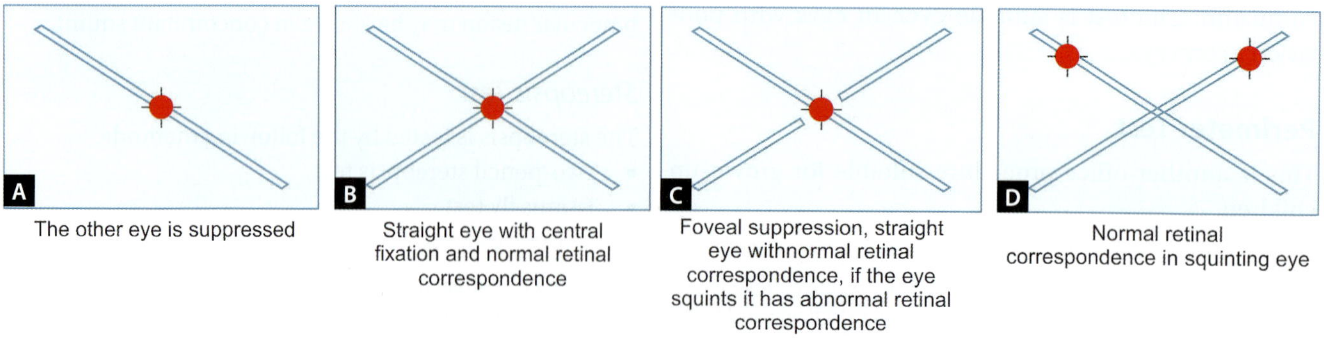

Figs. 24.50A to D: Result of Bagolini striated glass test.

**Four-diopter prism test:* 4 D prism tests are an objective, nondissociative test to assess binocular visual function in microtropia, or central suppression. To perform the test, the child is made to sit in front of a distant target with both eyes open. The examiner puts a 4 D prism base out in front of any eye and observes the fellow eye. The test is repeated in both eyes.

†*Bagolini striated glass test:* This is a subjective test performed in a squint clinic. The test is used to find out about microtropia, diplopia, and suppression. The device consists of two translucent glasses mounted in a ring in a fashion similar to any glass in a trail set that can be put in the trail frame. The Bagolini glass consists of lenses without power with imperceptible parallel scratches. When the lenses are put in the trail frame, the child sees the spot of light at 6 m as a streak. Bagolini glasses are put one in front of each eye, irrespective of its visual axis. The striations are so adjusted that one is aligned at 35° and the other at 145°, thus the two streaks form a cross with the spot in the center.

Flowchart 24.6: Types of esodeviation.

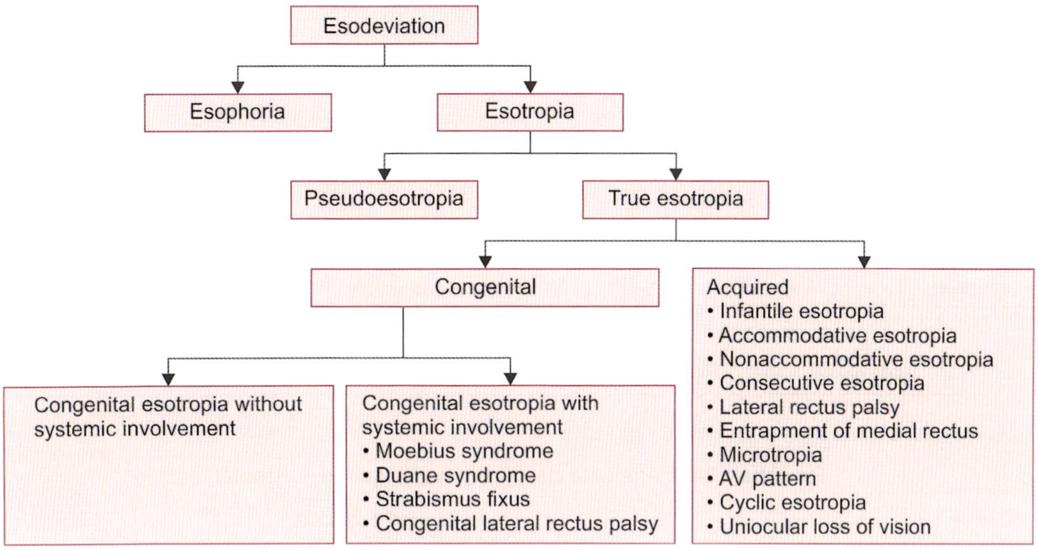

Flowchart 24.7: Acquired esotropia.

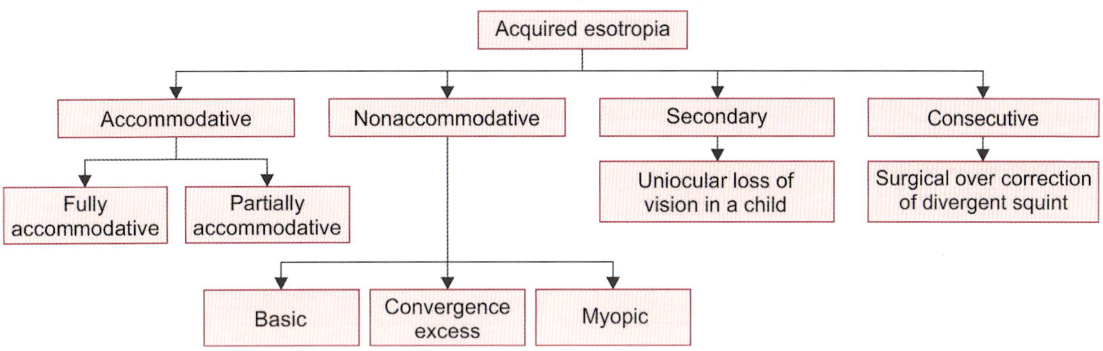

The causes of esodeviation in children are given in **Flowchart 24.6**.

Esotropia in Children

Clinically, esotropia has been put in two broad groups: (1) congenital and (2) acquired. Noorden (1990) divided acquired esotropia as shown in **Flowchart 24.7**.

*The other classification is based on accommodation, which is given in **Flowchart 24.8**.*

*The other more extensive classification is given in **Flowchart 24.9**.*

Yet another classification in vogue is given as follows:

- Age wise:
  - Early onset
  - Late onset
- Period wise:
  - Intermittent
  - Constant
  - Cyclic
- Distance wise:
  - Near point
  - Far point
- According to accommodation:
  - Fully accommodative
  - Partially accommodative
- Miscellaneous:
  - Convergence excess
  - Consecutive*
  - Secondary†

**Consecutive:* Esotropia generally follows surgery that has left the eye overcorrected. It may be constant or intermittent.

†*Secondary:* This is constant esotropia secondary to visual loss. Seen in children under 2 years.

Flowchart 24.8: Classification of esotropia.

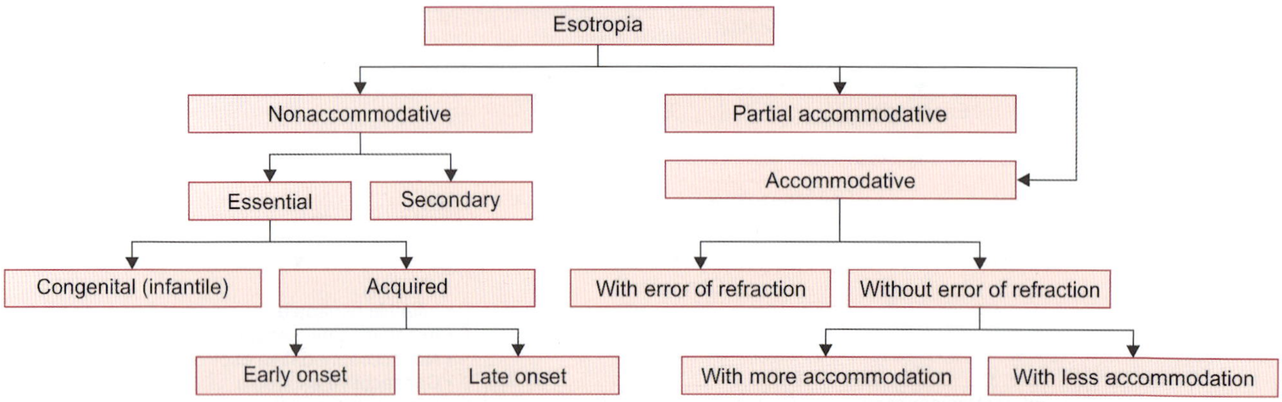

Flowchart 24.9: Alternate classification of acquired esotropia.

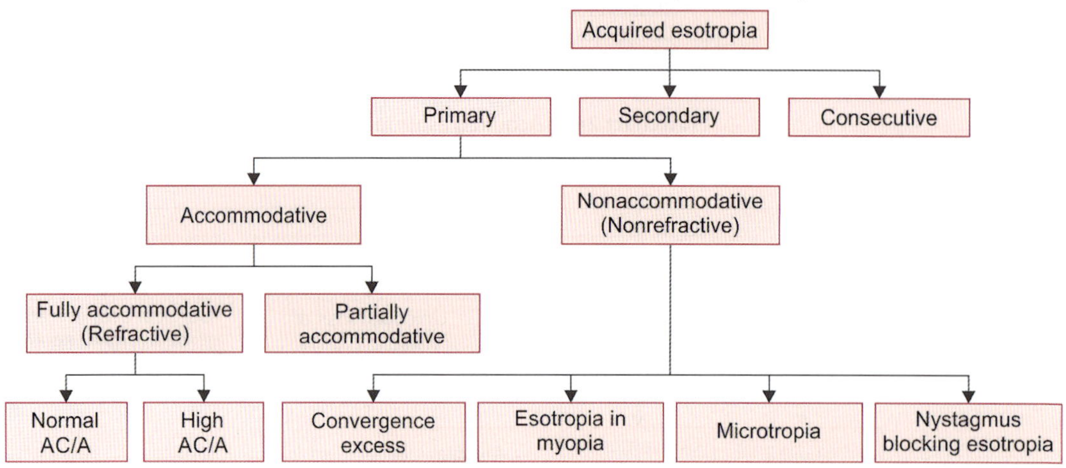

Congenital (Infantile) Concomitant Esotropia

It is better to refer to it as infantile esotropia because it is rarely present at birth, becoming obvious only after 2–3 months and surely before 6 months. An esotropia present at birth is most probably due to congenital sixth nerve palsy or one of the congenital restrictive squints. Infantile esotropia, seen in 1% of all live births, may have a genetic predisposition. Some of the siblings may show abduction restrictions. It is equally seen among boys and girls. Premature infants are more prone to develop infantile esotropia. All children with esotropia by 6 months of age should be examined by an ophthalmologist. Because it may be a harbinger of a permanent loss of binocular vision. The other factor that must be kept in mind in a child with infantile is that esotropia has more chance of retinoblastoma than in straight eye. That, if missed, may be fatal.

Characteristics of Infantile Esotropia

- It is rarely present at birth.
- If present at birth, it is most probably not concomitant.
- The common age to present is between 2 and 6 months.
- It is seen in about 1% of all deliveries.
- Its occurrence cannot be predicted.
- It has a high genetic predisposition.
- It is unilateral.
- Vision is generally good; diminished vision when present is independent of squint.
- Amblyopia is common, which may not develop if the child alternates.
- The error of refraction when present is low and mostly hypermetropia.
- Alternate fixation is common.
- It is a large, angled squint, i.e., between 30 and 40 PD.
- Deviation is equal for far and near.

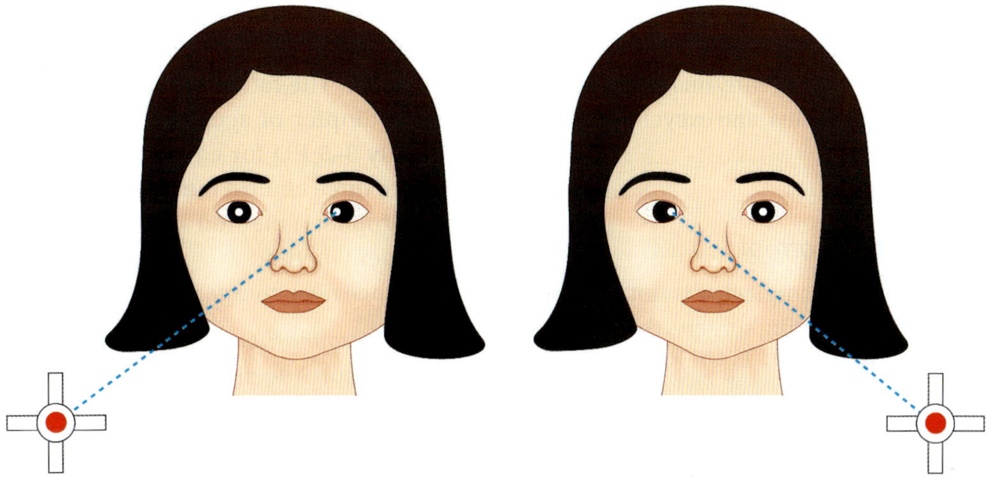

Fig. 24.51: Cross-fixation in a child.

- The child has a tendency to cross-fixate, i.e., the child fixes the right field with the left eye and vice versa **(Fig. 24.51)**.

Note:
- This may be mistaken as bilateral involvement.
- Abduction is poorer than adduction.

The presence of abduction in such a case can be demonstrated by the following methods.

The first method is given as follows:
- Cover the fixing eye and observe the squinting eye.
- An object that may interest the child, such as a feeding bottle, is brought in the field of vision.
- The object of interest is moved from side to side.
- If the squinting eye follows the object of interest, the child has normal abduction, ruling out lateral rectus palsy.

The second method is given as follows:
- Keep both the eyes of the child open.
- The object of interest is put in front of the child.
- The child is allowed the fix.
- The child will fix with the nonsquinting eye.
- The child's head is rotated horizontally.
- This will invariably reveal the presence of abduction in the squinting eye.

The third method is: If the above two methods fail to demonstrate abduction, the fixing eye is patched for a few hours; generally, this forces the squinting eye to fix and move laterally, exposing the presence of abduction. Sometimes, it may take 2–3 days for the test to show the result.

The fourth method is: The examiner holds the child in two extended arms, face to face. The examiner whirls himself by 360° with the child in the same position. The child will have conjugate deviation; the test is repeated in reverse direction. A positive result comprises of a demonstration of abduction and adduction in both eyes. The mechanism involved is stimulation of the oculovestibular reflex.
- Hence, it may be mistaken as congenital sixth nerve palsy.
- *Dissociated vertical deviation*: There are two situations where DVD may be present:
  - Developing by 2 years
  - Developing after a few years following a successful initial surgery, requiring reoperation
- *Inferior oblique overaction*: The condition of diminished convergence in upgaze presenting as a V pattern. IOOA is absent in DVD; generally, this may also develop following primary successful surgery, requiring reoperation.
- *Unilateral superior oblique paresis*: The condition is less frequent than DVD and IOOA.
- *Nystagmus*: Nystagmus is common; it can be latent or manifest.
- There is no neurological defect.

Differential Diagnosis of Infantile Esotropia

It consists of:
- Variant of esotropia in infants. They are: Congenital esotropia syndrome, consisting of infantile esotropia with superior oblique overaction, DVD, and V syndrome.

- Ciancia syndrome—consists of infantile esotropia with a bilateral abduction defect.
- Lang syndrome—consists of the early onset of esotropia with torticollis, DVD, nystagmus, and excyclodeviation.
- Abnormal head posture
- Manifest latent nystagmus

Management of Infantile Esotropia

The management is essentially surgical; it is not corrected by skepticism. Before contemplating surgery, the following factors should be given attention.

Error of refraction: All children with infantile esotropia should be refracted under complete cycloplegia, and when found to have an error of refraction, it should be corrected.

- The most common type of error of refraction met with is low hypermetropia.
- If the error of refraction is found to be >+3 D, an accommodative factor should be considered and dealt with the standard method.
- Instead of mild hypermetropia, the child may be mildly myopic. The child should be slightly undercorrected, which gives a better result.

Management of amblyopia: Management of amblyopia should get priority over surgery. It should be vigorously treated by standard methods.

Surgery: Surgery is the gold standard treatment for infantile esotropia; early surgical intervention gives the best result. Before surgery is planned, the child should be given the best correction; an alteration is the cornerstone of success. The chances of postoperative DVD and IOOA should be kept in mind; it is better to counsel parents about a second surgery years later. That may require 2–3 years following the first successful operation. The two types of surgeries that are done in infantile esotropia are:

- Bilateral equal recession of the medial rectus
- Recession of the medial rectus with appropriate resection of the lateral rectus in the same eye

Accommodative Esotropia

It is better to discuss the role of accommodation in a squint before proceeding further.

Role of Accommodation in a Squint

The eyes have an inherent tendency to converge with accommodation. Accommodation is measured in diopters, while convergence is measured in PD. The ratio between accommodations associated with convergence is called AC/A. The ratio denotes the convergence required for each diopter of accommodation. The normal AC/A is roughly 3–5 PD for each diopter of accommodation. There are three clinical methods to assess them:

1. Heterophoria method
2. Gradient method
3. Distance near comparison

1. *The heterophoria method is given as follows:*
   a. Measure the distant deviation with a prism diopter (D) at 6 m
   b. Measure the near deviation in the prism diopter (N) at 1/3 m
   c. Measure the interpupillary distance in centimeters (PD)
   d. Calculate AC/A by following formula:

$$AC/A = PD + \frac{(N - D)}{\text{Near measurement in diopter}}$$

2. *Gradient method:* The method is as follows:
   a. Correct the error of refraction fully
   b. Measure the deviation through the glasses
   c. Measure the deviation without the glasses
   d. Calculate by the following formula:

$$AC/A = \frac{\text{Difference between far and near deviation}}{\text{Diopter of glasses}}$$

3. *Distance near comparison:* This is a less effective method than the former two; it gives a rough estimate of AC/A when the ratio is high. It is useful only in esotropia. It is a comparison between distant and near deviations. If the near deviation is >10 PD, the child has an abnormally high AC/A ratio. Nonrefractory accommodative esotropia is associated with a high AC/A ratio. The hypermetropia in these children is age-matched.

Fully Accommodative Esotropia

It is the most common esotropia in the pediatric age group with a simple diagnosis and effective nonsurgical treatment, i.e., optical, in contrast to infantile esotropia, where surgery is the treatment of choice, except for children presenting late, who will have a better result following surgery. However, antiamblyopia treatment gets precedence over all treatments.

TABLE 24.15: Clinical features of accommodative esotropia.

Features	*Clinical presentation*
Age of onset	Seen between 6 months and 6 years, the average being 2.5 years
Heredity	Strongly hereditary
Deviation	Uniocular, variable for near and distant, may be intermittent. That becomes constant; the angle of deviation is not very large, ranging between 20 and 45 PD, in contrast to infantile esotropia, where the deviation is >45 PD
Amblyopia	Is common but not deep, amenable to antiamblyopia treatment
Error of refraction	Ranging between +4 and +7 D; the squinting eye has more hypermetropia
AC/A	Normal between 3 and 5 D
Near-distant relation	Normal, when present, is not >10 PD
Correction	Fully corrected by plus glasses
Paradox	It is expected that children with high hypermetropia will have more accommodating squints, which is not true; children with hypermetropia >+8 D do not develop accommodative squints because they have bilateral amblyopia that forces them to give up accommodation, reducing esotropia. These children do not improve with glasses
Spontaneous recovery	There may be a reduction in hypermetropia as the child grows. The conditions may pass into partially accommodative squints or nonaccommodative squints
Surgery	Not needed until the eye is straight with glasses
Binocular single vision	Is it possible to see far and near when hypermetropia is fully corrected
Retinal correspondence	Anomalous retinal correspondence
Associated ocular features	DVD and IOOA

(DVD: dissociated vertical deviation; IOOA: inferior oblique overaction)

Characteristics of fully accommodative esotropia: **Table 24.15** gives the characteristics of fully accommodative esotropia.

Etiology of Accommodative Esotropia

There are two factors that work in tandem. They are given as follows:

1. Uncorrected hypermetropia
2. Abnormally high AC/A ratio

An emmetropic child needs not to accommodate to see clearly at far point, a myopic eye becomes worse with accommodation. The condition that benefits from accommodation is hypermetropia.

Uncorrected hypermetropia: Children with accommodative esotropia, generally have uncorrected hypermetropia of low grade. If the child uses accommodation in excess to correct this small amount, it becomes esotropic. The above fact does not unravel the complete mechanism involved in accommodative esotropia. The second part is the insufficiency of functional fusion; as long as fusional divergence is sufficient, the child does not develop a manifest squint. Occasionally, the child may develop esophoria that may become intermittent and result in esotropia as the divergence breaks down.

Abnormally high AC/A ratio: So long as AC/A is within 3–5 D, the child does not develop squint; it happens only when AC/C is high.

Management

Optical: The cornerstone of the management of accommodative esotropia is spectacle correction following refraction under complete cycloplegia with utmost attention to astigmatism both in power and axis. Logically, a child should be prescribed full cycloplegic correction. Most of the time, the child does not accept full spherical cycloplegic correction. It is better to give the correction that gives the best vision and is tolerable. The power of the glasses may be required to be diminished with an increase in age; hence, it is mandatory that the child is examined yearly and the required adjustment made.

Full hypermetropic correction for distance, most of the time, keeps the eyes straight both for far and near. In some children, this may not correct the squint fully. They may require addition for near in the form of bifocal.

Orthoptic: Orthoptic treatment is a nonoptical or surgical treatment. It requires cooperation of the child and caregivers; it is suitable for children above 10 years with hypermetropia <+3 D.

Surgery: Surgery is not required so long the squint is purely horizontal. Development of DVD and IOOA may require surgery.

Accommodative Esotropia with High AC/A

In case of fully accommodative esotropia AC/A is within normal limits. Children with high AC/A have more esodeviation for near than distance. Some children may even be orthophoric for distance. They may have various errors of refraction varying between low hypermetropia to mild myopia; even emmetropia has been found frequently. Chances of high AC/A is more in low hypermetropia, low myopia, and emmetropia. High hypermetropia is associated with more or less normal AC/A; they are not fully corrected by glasses, some esotropia is rule.

Management

Management consists of correction of error of refraction for distant vision and adding plus lenses for near deviation. *Comparison between infantile and accommodative esotropia is shown in* ***Table 24.16***.

TABLE 24.16: Comparison between two common esotropias in children.

Features	***Infantile esotropia***	***Accommodative esotropia***
Age of onset	Before 6 months	Average 30 months
Angle of deviation	34–50 PD	Average 20 PD
Laterality	Uniocular	Uniocular
Alteration	Very common	Nil
Cross fixation	Common	Nil
Refraction	Moderate hypermetropia does not exceed +2 D	+4 to +7 D is common
Restriction of abduction	Common but no underaction of the lateral rectus	No restriction of abduction
Intermittency	Absent	May be present as intermittent esotropia
Deviation	Equal for far and near	Esotropia slightly more for near
Vertical deviation	DVD and inferior oblique overaction common	DVD and IO over action may be present
Nystagmus	Very common	Absent
Amblyopia	Common, alternators do not develop	May be present but not deep
Management	Surgery is the treatment of choice	Glasses will correct esotropia for far and near

(DVD: dissociated vertical deviation; IOOA: inferior oblique overaction; IO: inferior oblique)

Partially Accommodative Esotropia

This is a condition between accommodative and nonaccommodative esotropia. In this condition, some esodeviation is left after full spectacle hypermetropic correction, even with bifocal. The two explanations for the phenomenon are:

- The child was an infantile esotropic that has acquired an accommodative element, increasing hypermetropia; the final hypermetropia may be far more than the initial hypermetropia.
- The child had accommodative esotropia, to which nonaccommodative elements has been added following decompensation. Generally, in such cases, the additional finding is hypertrophy of the medial rectus. The amount of residual esotropia is constant, the same for far and near; amblyopia is the rule.

Management

Management consists of surgery along with the continuation of glasses that give the best corrected vision for near and distant, even after surgery.

Nonaccommodative Acquired Esotropias

Nonaccommodative acquired esotropia may be any of the following:

- Basic
- Convergence excess
- Esotropia in myopia

Basic

The characteristics of basic, nonaccommodative acquired esotropia are given as follows:

- Generally, it becomes obvious after 6 months of age that it does not develop after 10 years.
- Unilateral with diminished vision in a deviated eye without any error of refraction error of refraction when present is mild to moderate.
- Accommodation is within the normal limit.
- There is only a slight difference between far and near.
- Initially, the deviation is small, with a tendency to increase with age.
- The squinting eye is amblyopic.
- The deviation is not corrected by glasses.
- Surgical treatment is a definitive treatment.
- The surgical procedure commonly used is bimedial recession with conjunctival recession.

Convergence Excess Esotropia

The characteristics of the conditions are given as follows:

- It develops between 2 and 3 years.
- Distant deviation is low.
- Near deviation is between 20° and 40°.
- The child may be emmetropic and may have mild hypermetropia.
- Accommodation is normal.

Management: The management consists of surgery, depending on the extent of esotropia.

Other Types of Esotropia

There are a few types of less common esotropia seen in children. They are given as follows:

- Microtropia
- Esotropia in myopia
- Cyclic esotropia
- Nystagmus blocking esotropia
- Consecutive esotropia
- Secondary esotropia
- Esotropia on DVD and IOOA
- Acute esotropia

Microtropia (Monofixation Esotropia)

Microtropia is often missed unless looked at specifically. It is a unilateral condition with a small degree of deviation. In spite of its small deviation, it is always associated with mild-to-moderate amblyopia.

The characteristics of the conditions are given as follows:

- It does not improve with age, requiring proper management.
- It may be seen following either infantile esotropia or a sequel to surgery for infantile esotropia.
- The angle of deviation is not marked that ranges between 8 and 10 PD or less.
- Central fusion
- There is facultative macular scotoma best demonstrated on the Worth's four dot test and the Bagolini test.
- Cover and cover-uncover test may fail to demonstrate its presence.
- The best method to demonstrate the presence of the condition is a 4 PD base-out.
- The condition is more common in anisometropic amblyopia.
- Parafoveal fixation and peripheral fusion are present with harmonious ARC and normal stereopsis.
- There are three grades of microtropia; they are given as follows:
  1. Primary constant
  2. Primary decompensation
  3. Consecutive microtropia

Management: Microtropia is treated is variously by orthoptics, surgery, and prisms.

Esotropia in Myopia

Esodeviation is common in myopia. Myopic children have good near vision with diminished distant vision that may progress so slowly that the child may not notice its presence. The child may consider it to be a normal phenomenon unless found on regular checkup.

Children with moderate, uncorrected myopia have good near vision. Accommodation worsens far vision. The child is left with the option of converging to have good near vision. The child may give up accommodation altogether, thus developing a convergent squint.

Treatment consists of correction of myopia and surgical undoing of remaining esodeviation.

Cyclic Esotropia

This is a rare esotropia, the cause of which is not well understood. It is seen in children between 3 and 4 years, often mistaken as intermittent esotropia, which itself does not follow a fixed cycle of occurrence, which is the rule in cyclic esotropia that alternates with a straight eye. The gap between orthophoria and heterotropia may vary between 24 and 96 hours. The typical cycle consists to a large angle esotropia for a day or two, followed by a straight eye gap of the same duration. Such cyclic occurrences are not permanent. They last for a few months to years, followed by constant esotropia. Amblyopia develops only when the eye develops a permanent squint.

Nystagmus Blocking Esotropia

Children with congenital or infantile esotropia often have nystagmus that may be manifest nystagmus or manifest-latent, independent of deviation. Some children who have nystagmus without a squint are known to get rid of nystagmus by converging. This phenomenon is called nystagmus blocking esotropia. This is often mistaken for infantile esotropia with nystagmus.

Treatment is difficult. Recession of both medial recti with myopexy behind the equator is the most commonly used surgical procedure.

Consecutive Esotropia

This is a sequel of surgery for exodeviation. This is transient and associated with diplopia; if esotropia persists after a few weeks, the condition should be reviewed and treated. The possibility of amblyopia should always be kept in mind, as in other types of esotropia in children.

EXOTROPIA

Exotropia is the manifest deviation of any of the eyes outward.

Exotropia in children is as common as esotropia. The normal position of the eye at rest is slightly divergent, which is physiological; it is very small to the extent of imperceptibility; hence, the eyes are considered to be orthophoric.

Cause of Exodeviation

Flowchart 24.10 depicts various types of exodeviation.

General Features

- It can be congenital or acquired.
- There may be a hereditary predisposition.
- Exotropia is more common among girls.
- Can be uniocular or alternate.
- They generally begin as exophoria, pass into intermittent exotropia, and finally end as constant exotropia.
- An exotropic eye may not need to go through stages of exophoria.
- It can be:
  - Equal for far and near
  - Greater for distant
  - Greater for near
- The angle may increase with time.
- The angles of deviation in exotropia are generally large.
- Errors of refraction when present are generally small without any predilection for a specific type.
- Suppression is common.
- Amblyopia is less frequent when compared to esotropia.
- Exotropic eyes generally have poor adduction.
- Adduction defect may be mistaken as medial rectus under action.

Flowchart 24.10: Causes of exotropia in children.

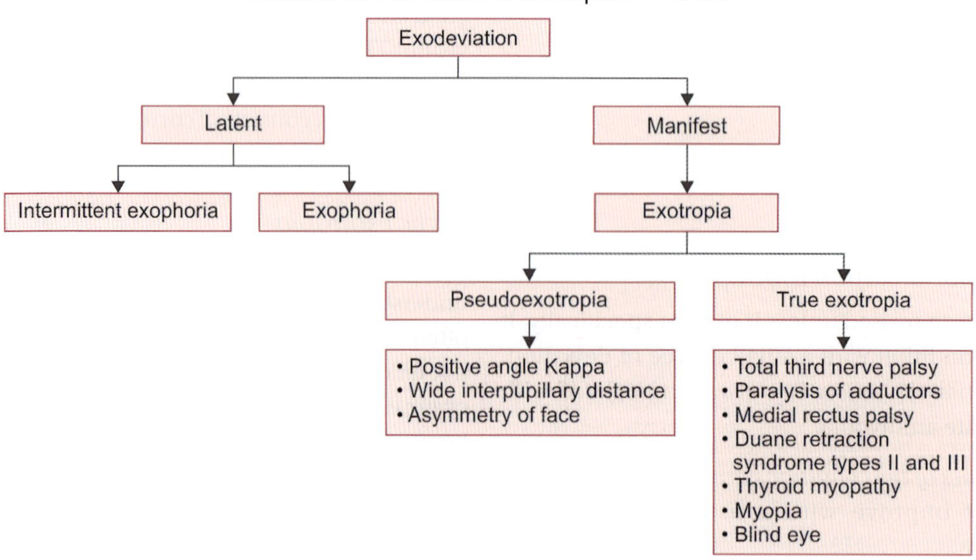

Various Modes of Development of Exotropia

- Orthophoria → Intermittent exophoria → Intermittent exotropia → Constant exotropia → Increase in exotropia
- An eye with esotropia converts to straight eye and then passes in state of exotropia (this is less common than the first.)
- Consecutive exotropia following over correction of esotropia
- Secondary exotropia developing in eyes that have long-standing poor vision with amblyopia, due to:
  - Anisometropia
  - Uncorrected unilateral aphakia
  - Unilateral:
    - Cataract
    - Corneal opacity
    - Macular scar
    - Optic atrophy

Note:

- Unilateral loss of vision under 5 years of age may result in either eso- or exotropia. Out of the two, esotropia is more common.
- There is a reversal after 5 years when exotropia is more common than esotropia.

Classification of Exotropia

Flowchart 24.11 shows the classification of exotropia.

The other common classification used is shown in **Flowchart 24.12**.

Specific Types of Exotropia

- Essential exotropia
- Intermittent exotropia
- Exotropia for distance/near
- Convergence paralysis
- Divergence excess
- Congenital exotropia

An *essential exotropia* is a primary concomitant exotropia without binocularity, neurological defect, anatomical defect, or detectable cause.

Intermittent exotropia is the most common exotropia and most common type out of all squints seen in children. The most common age is between 4 and 5 years, but not before 2 years, which is common in esotropia in children.

The intermittency becomes obvious when the child is tired, ill, or daydreaming. The parents may bring the child up, complaining that the child often squints, on examination, no squint latent or manifest is found. Depending on the information of the parents, it becomes imperative that the child may be examined many times in the same sitting. This unravels hidden deviations. It is well recorded that intermittent exotropia may disappear spontaneously in about three-fourths of cases. However, deviation may increase over the years in remaining children. The deviation does not change with time. The child may have normal distant vision, or there may be a loss of one to two lines on Snellen's charts. In such cases, the error of refraction is mild. The child has binocularity in the primary position. Stereopsis is good when the eyes

Flowchart 24.11: Types of exotropia.

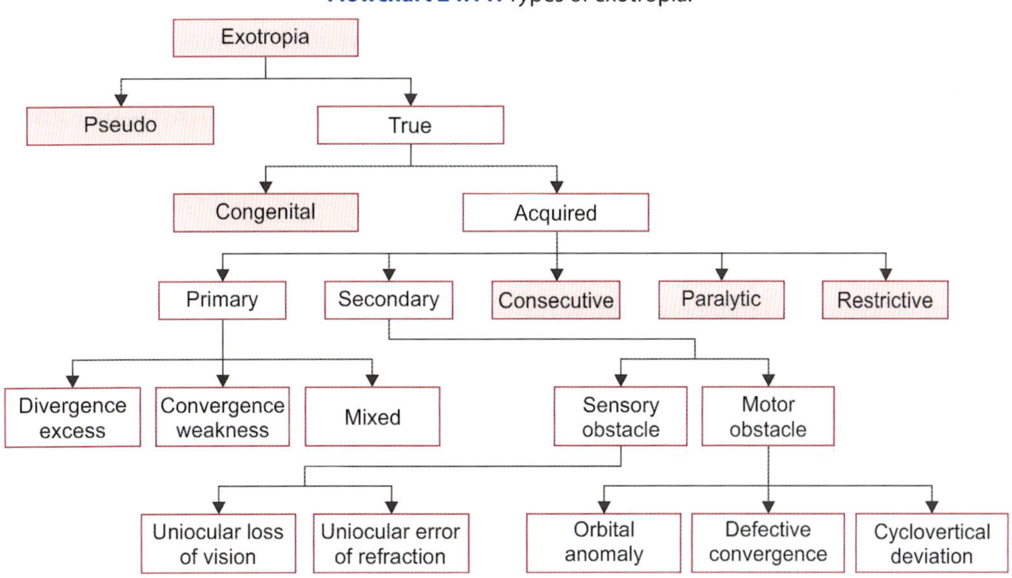

Flowchart 24.12: Alternate classification of exotropia.

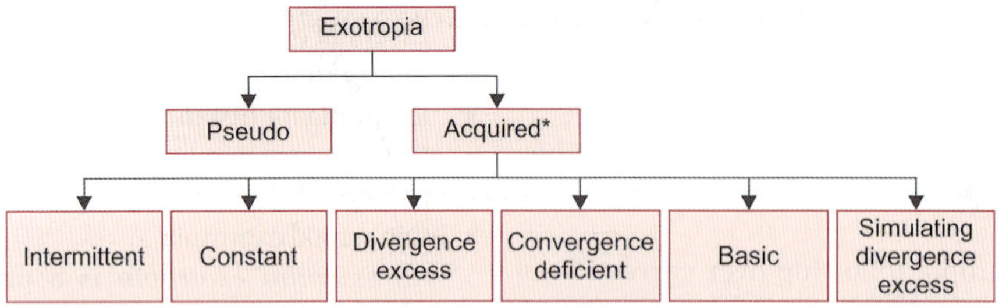

Acquired:* Acquired exotropia begins in infancy, is a high degree of squint ranging between 40° and 80° PD, the deviation is constant, and shows alternation. The child has homonymous fixation; the error of refraction when present is low generally myopic, correctable by glasses; amblyopia is less frequent and when present, it is mild. There is no optical treatment; the definitive treatment is surgical, which consists of recession of both lateral rectus and resection of both medial recti.

are straight and bifoveal fusion without suppression. Suppression develops only when there is exotropia. The child may not be aware of the squint, but when the child looks in a mirror, the image is formed very near the eyes that abolishes deviation. The onlookers are the first to notice the deviation, which the child may deny that is obvious in photographs; few children complain of diminished vision and asthenopia. The child with exotropia closes the deviating eye in bright light. Both types of alphabetic deviation have been noticed, with the V pattern being more common; DVD is less common than in the esotropia of childhood and so is nystagmus.

The condition can be divided into:

- Divergence excess
- Convergence deficient
- Basic
- Pseudodivergence

Divergence Excess

Exotropia is more for the distant; it is better to measure far vision beyond the usual 6 m. The difference between the far and near deviations is >15 PD. The near deviation may just be exophoria, occasionally. On relaxing accommodation by putting a +3 D in front of each eye, the near and far deviations are examined again, and there is generally no difference between the two.

Convergence Deficient

The difference between the near and distant deviations is found to be >15 PD with full correction. It may be present with diminished accommodation, as is common in myopes who do not require accommodation, hypermetropes >6 D who give up accommodation for comfort with low AC/A may have convergence-deficient exotropia.

Basic

Most of the time, there is no difference in deviation for far and near; when present, it is not >15 PD. The condition may be taken as a combination of the above two.

Pseudodivergence

This is also called simulated divergence excess when examined for the first time; the distance deviation is >15 PD than the near deviation. The difference decreases to 10 PD if the eye is patched for half an hour. The eye is again examined immediately after removing the patch, which prevents the development of fusion. The other diagnostic test is to put a +3 D lens in front of both eyes. The near deviation becomes equal to the far deviation.

Management of Intermittent Exotropia

- No treatment is required if intermittency is not converted to constant exotropia.
- The mode of management depends on the age and severity of the condition.
  It consists of the following:

Optical

- *Glasses* are prescribed in children with significant errors of refraction. Myopia is fully corrected, while hypermetropia is undercorrected. The best practice could be the correction that gives the best vision with comfort for the near and distant.

- *Prisms* are not used as frequently as glasses; they are more suitable for small deviations with negligible effect on a large degree of exotropia.

Orthoptics

The orthoptics treatment requires the cooperation of the child and the caregivers because the results are not immediately appreciable; it takes a few weeks to months to be effective. The purpose of the treatment is to strengthen convergence and eradicate suppression.

Surgery

Surgery is the definitive treatment better performed at about 4 years because chances of suppression increase after 4 years, which hampers the result of surgery. A small degree of exotropia is left without any treatment, or when treatment is contemplated, orthoptic treatment should get preference in divergence excess exotropia. The surgery consists of the recession of both lateral recti. This null exodeviation may leave the child with mild esotropia.

In basic exotropia, recession of the lateral rectus with resection of the medial rectus is the surgery of choice; recurrence should be corrected by a base in the prism; myopia is overcorrected; and hypermetropia is undercorrected by 1 D.

Exotropia for Distance/Near

Exotropia can be for distant and near, with a difference in clinical presentation. *They are shown in **Table 24.17**.*

Convergence Paralysis

This is a rare systemic condition of near exotropia where convergence is reduced with intact accommodation and miosis. The paralysis is of acute onset with diplopia for near, due to a lesion in the corpora quadrigemina of the third cranial nucleus. The treatment is directed toward the primary cause.

TABLE 24.17: Difference between near and distant exotropia.

Distance	***Near***	***Symptoms***
Exotropia	Orthophoria	Nil
Intermittent exotropia	Orthophoria or exophoria for near	Symptoms for distance
Exotropia	Exotropia	Suppression scotoma for distant
Exotropia	Intermittent exotropia	Binocular vision only for near
Exotropia	Exotropia	Loss of binocular vision

Congenital Exotropia

Congenital exotropia is less common when compared to congenital esotropia. When present, it becomes evident by 2 months of age; then, features are a large angle deviation (40–80° PD), equal for far and near; without cross fixation, the fixation is homonymous. Alternation is common; this prevents the development of amblyopia error of refraction when present is low. It is managed by surgery when the infant is grown up enough to withstand general anesthesia but not later than 2 years; the aim of the surgery is to reduce the deviation within 10 PD. The surgery should be preceded by a correction of the error of refraction.

Consecutive and secondary exotropias:

Consecutive exotropia: It is an iatrogenic status following the correction of esotropia. This is more common in esotropic eyes with high hypermetropia. The time lapse between initial surgery and the development of exotropia may be as long as 2 years but may develop soon after the surgery.

Secondary exotropia: This is generally seen in unilateral, longstanding visual loss. The causes attributed are amblyopia, anisometropia, uniocular aphakia, uniocular corneal opacity, and optic neuritis. If the child develops diminished vision after 5 years, exotropia is the rule, in contrast to developing diminished vision before 5 years, which can result in both eso- and exotropia. The other causes are nonoptical; they are scarring of the medial rectus following trauma that may be accidental or surgical; paresis of the medial rectus may present as exotropia.

Alphabetic Pattern of Squint

"An abnormal variation in the amount of horizontal deviation as the eyes move from the straight up to straight downgaze."

These constitute a group of horizontal ocular squints either missed or misdiagnosed because of a failure to anticipate their presence and perform a simple cover test in primary, up-and-down gaze. Alphabetic syndrome is defined as:

To understand this phenomenon, it should be remembered that the eyes diverge slightly when looking straight. The deviation increases little on vertical gaze. This is taken as physiological. In some cases of horizontal squint, the divergence increases in both up and down more than this physiological limit. The combination of horizontal deviation with enhanced deviation in vertical gazes has been designated as A, V, X, and lambda due to their imaginary resemblance to these letters. Out of the four conditions, A and V patterns are more common; some authors doubt the presence of the last two.

The exact cause of the phenomena is not well elucidated; there are three schools of thought. They are given as follows:

1. Horizontal muscle theory
2. Vertical muscle theory
3. Oblique muscle theory

Horizontal Muscle Theory

The horizontal muscle involvement is based on the presumption that lateral recti act better in upgaze; the reverse is true for medial recti; thus, the V exo pattern is attributed to overaction of the lateral rectus, and eso, A to underaction of the medial rectus.

***Table 24.18** is a summary of horizontal muscle theory.*

Vertical Muscle Theory

The vertical muscle involvement is based on the assumption that the vertical recti are adductors; hence, a weak superior rectus would result in abduction in the upgaze. **Table 24.19** summarizes the vertical muscle theory.

TABLE 24.18: Clinical features of action of rectus muscle in AV syndrome.

Muscle action	*Deviation*
Overaction of lateral rectus	V exotropia
Underaction of lateral rectus	A exotropia
Overaction of medial rectus	V esotropia
Underaction of medial rectus	A esotropia

Note:
- Medial rectus is involved in esotropia.
- Lateral rectus is involved in exotropia.

TABLE 24.19: Oblique muscle involvement in AV syndrome.

Deviation	*Muscle action*	
Pattern	*Overaction*	*Underaction*
A eso/exo	Superior rectus	Inferior rectus
A eso/exo	Superior oblique	Inferior oblique
V eso/exo	Inferior rectus	Superior rectus
V eso/exo	Inferior oblique	Superior oblique

The gist of the above theories is given as follows:

- The horizontal muscle theory is based on the assumption that the fault lies in horizontally acting muscles only.
- The vertical muscle theory is built on the presumption that the A and V patterns are due to the symmetrical underaction of vertically active muscles.
- The third group believes that both the horizontally and vertically acting muscles are at fault.
- Because there is no single opinion on the cause of the condition, the mode of treatment also varies greatly.

A pattern is defined as laser divergence in upgaze than downgaze. It can be A esotropia or A exotropia.

The V pattern is defined as more divergence in the upgaze than in the downgaze. It can be V esotropia or V exotropia.

Figures 24.52A and B explain the outline of AV syndrome.

Figures 24.53A and B explain horizontal muscle theories in AV syndrome.

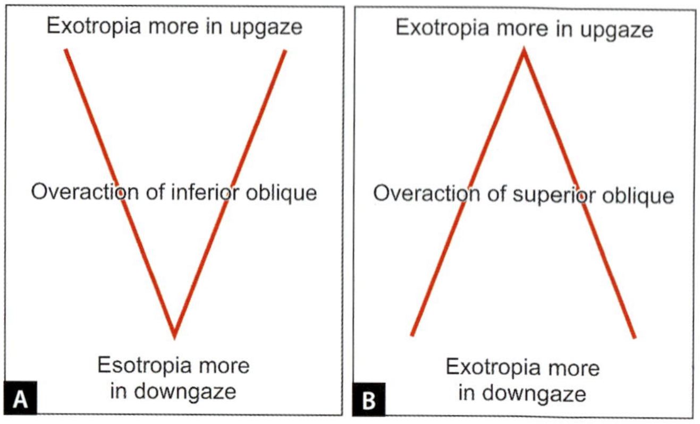

Figs. 24.52A and B: Outline of AV syndrome.

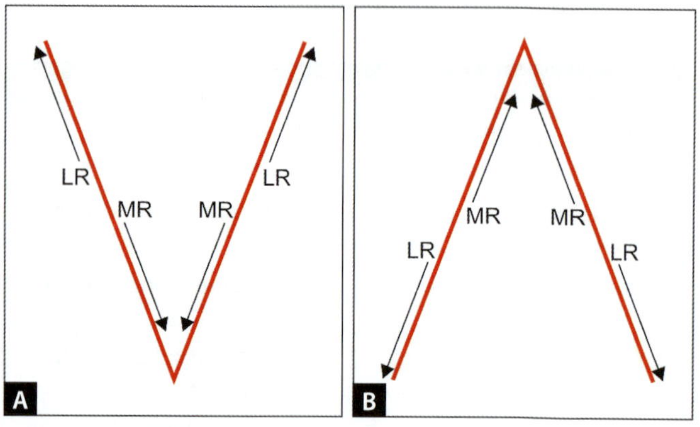

Figs. 24.53A and B: Diagrammatic explanation of AV syndrome.

Characteristics of the AV Pattern

See **Table 24.20**.

Summary of Muscle Action in AV Syndrome

See **Table 24.21**.

Diagnosis

Diagnosis is simple if the vertical deviation is kept in mind while doing the cover test. To achieve this:

- Make the child fix an object at 6 m, keeping both eyes open
- Measure the type and degree of squint in the primary position
- Ask the child to look up by 30° and measure the deviation
- Ask the child to look down by 30° and measure the deviation

Figures 24.54A and B show various patterns in up- and downgazes.

TABLE 24.20: Clinical features of AV pattern.

Deviation	*Clinical features*
A esotropia	Chin-up, mongoloid palpebral fissure, overaction of the superior oblique, underaction of the inferior oblique, and underaction of the lateral rectus were measured by the alternate cover test and prism
A exotropia	Chin down; normal palpebral fissure with overaction of the superior oblique, inferior oblique, and medial rectus; and high insertion of the lateral rectus
V esotropia	Antimongoloid palpebral fissure, superior oblique underaction, lateral rectus overaction, inferior oblique overaction, and high insertion of the medial rectus
V exotropia	Antimongoloid features include inferior oblique overaction, medial rectus overaction, superior rectus underaction, and low insertion of the lateral rectus

TABLE 24.21: Effects of over- and underaction of muscles in AV syndrome.

Syndrome	*Muscle action*	*Involved muscle*
A	Overaction	IO, SR, LR, SO
V	Underaction	SO, IO, IR, LR

(IO: inferior oblique; IR: inferior rectus; LR: lateral rectus; SO: superior oblique; SR: superior rectus)

Figures 24.55A to D show AV syndrome in the presence of a horizontal deviation.

Treatment

The treatment of the condition is essentially surgical. A small degree of deviation needs not to be corrected, except for the management of errors of refraction and amblyopia. Surgery is required only when the condition is symptomatic or has become a cosmetic embarrassment to the child.

There are many surgical procedures available; the most common is transposition of horizontal muscles, as shown in **Table 24.22**.

Note:

- The procedures are effective only when there is no dysfunction of the extraocular muscle.
- The mnemonic for the procedures is *MALB*, where *M* stands for medial rectus, *L* for lateral rectus, *A* for apex, and *B* for below.
- Transposition is accompanied by recession/resection of horizontal muscles as required.

Figures 24.56A and B represent the basis of the procedures.

Paralytic Squint

Paralytic squint is less frequent than concomitant squint in children. The clinical picture of paralytic squint in children and adults is similar. A childhood paralytic squint may present as a concomitant in adult life. The paralytic squint can be congenital or acquired in children.

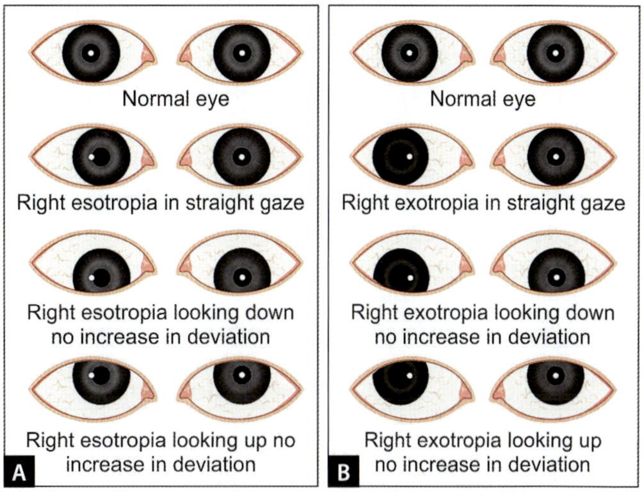

Figs. 24.54A and B: (A) Esotropia in up- and downgaze; (B) Exotropia in up- and downgaze.

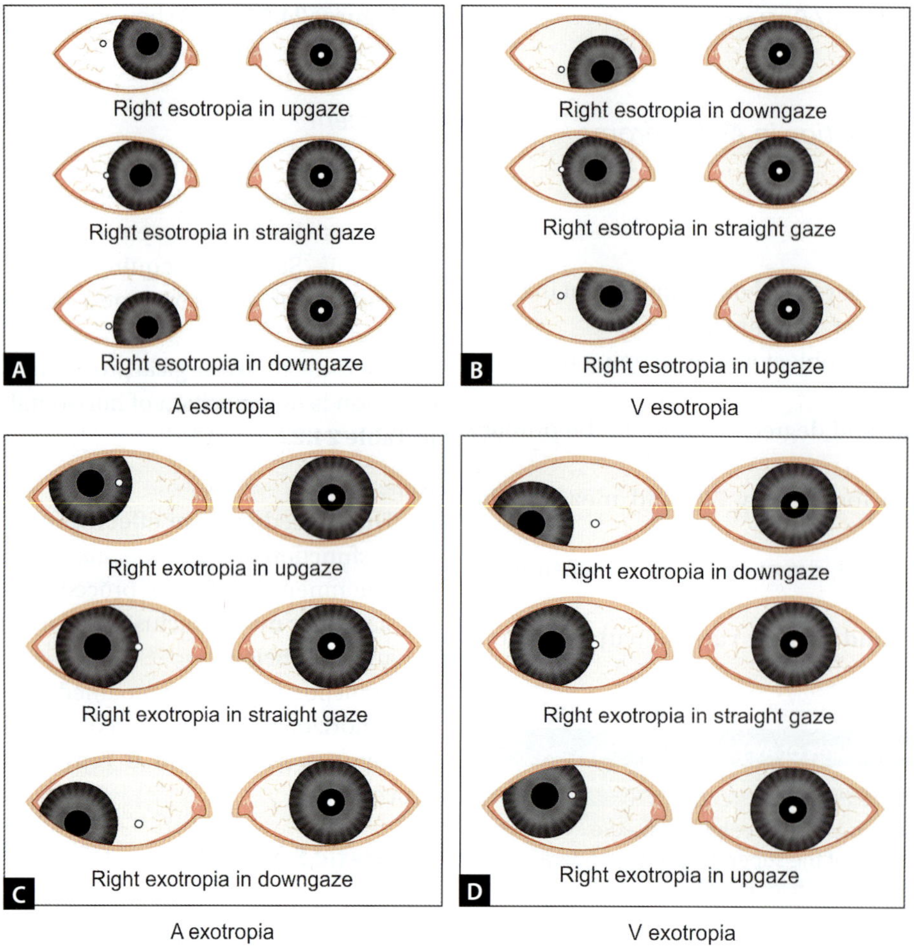

Figs. 24.55A to D: Effects of AV pattern on horizontal squint.

TABLE 24.22: Outline of surgery for AV pattern.

Features of pattern A	***Surgical procedure***
Overaction of the superior rectus and inferior oblique	Weakening of the muscles
Underaction of medial rectus, lateral rectus, and inferior oblique	Strengthening muscles, i.e., move medial rectus up and lateral rectus down
Features of pattern V	***Surgical procedure***
Overaction of the medial rectus, lateral rectus, inferior rectus, and inferior oblique	Weakening of the muscles
Underaction of superior rectus and superior oblique	Strengthening muscles, i.e., move the medial rectus down and the lateral rectus up

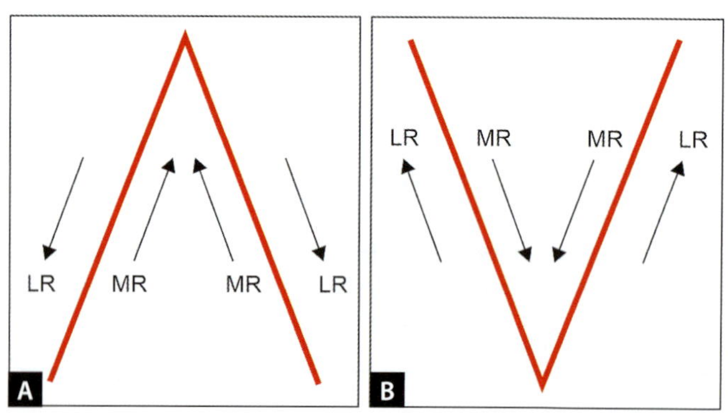

Figs. 24.56A and B: The direction of transposition of horizontal muscles in the (A) A and (B) V syndrome. (LR: lateral rectus; MR: medial rectus)

Absence of action by an extraocular muscle is called paralysis, while weakness is referred to as paresis. The term "palsy" is a nonspecific term used to denote any of the above. Paralytic squints are generally acute on onset, may linger for a long time, develop pathological sequelae that change the clinical presentation in the long run, and may behave like nonparalytics.

The sequelae are given as follows:

- Contracture of the ipsilateral antagonist
- Overaction of the contralateral synergist
- Inhibition of contralateral antagonists

Following are examples of the sequelae of paralysis of the left lateral rectus:

- Contracture of the left medial rectus
- Overaction of the right medial rectus
- Inhibition of the right lateral rectus
  Paralytic sequelae in children are generally unilateral.

Symptoms of Paralytic Squint

- The most common symptom is diplopia. An infant who does not complain of diplopia but may have abnormal head posture may learn to avoid diplopia by closing one eye, which attracts the mother's attention. The person who discovers the second symptom, the deviation, or diplopia, may be pronounced in a particular direction or may be equal in many gazes. In the initial stages, the child may be disturbed with nausea, vomiting, and giddiness. The verbal child may complain of headaches along with the above symptoms, but a preverbal child may just be irritable.
- The second symptom that brings the child for consultation is an abnormal position of the eye.
- Observant parents may notice limited or absent movement of the eye in one or more than one direction involvement of the third nerve may be accompanied by ptosis.
- Abnormal head posture may yet be another sign noted by parents.

Signs of a Paralytic Squint

- Generally, paralytic squint is a uniocular phenomenon. The exception being bilateral involvement of the fourth nerve in a closed head injury and bilateral paralysis of the sixth nerve.
- Abnormal head posture
- Deviation
- Limited movement:
  - Less marked in vertical muscle movement
  - Most marked in involvement of recti
  - Least involvement of obliques
- False projection:
- Diplopia

Abnormal head posture: The most common sign that leads to the diagnosis of paralytic squint is abnormal head posture. On questioning, it turns out to be of recent origin.

In paralysis of horizontal muscle, the face is turned toward the paralyzed muscle, i.e., paralysis of the lateral rectus causes a more pronounced head turn than the medial rectus. The horizontal muscle palsy does not cause tilting or changes in the position of the chin, which are marked in the oblique muscle palsy.

A head turned toward the right is seen in:

- Right lateral rectus palsy
- Left MR palsy
- Duane retraction syndrome, types 1 and 3
- Right MR contractures

A head turned toward the left is seen in:

- Left lateral rectus palsy
- Right MR palsy
- Duane retraction syndrome, types 2 and 3
- Contractures of the left medial rectus
  Turing of the head is not only seen in paralytic squints but also in restrictive squints. This happens less commonly than the former.

They are given as follows:

- Duane retraction syndrome types 2 and 3
- Third nerve palsy
- Medial rectus underaction
- Lateral rectus contracture
  Other causes of head turn are infantile esotropia with nystagmus and, rarely, DVD. The other sign that leads to a diagnosis of paralytic squint is ptosis of recent origin in third nerve palsy. However, unilateral hypertropia due to cyclovertical muscle palsy produces minimal pseudoptosis. Frequent closure of one eye is yet another clue to paralytic squinting. The face is turned to the right in paralysis of the right lateral rectus and left MR. Isolated medial rectus is far less common than lateral rectus. The face is turned left in paralysis of the left lateral rectus or right MR palsy.

Position of the chin:

- Paralysis of elevators, i.e., SR and IO, causes chin up positions.
- Paralysis of the depressor, i.e., IR and SO, causes depression of the chin.

The causes of the abnormal position of the chin are given as follows:

- *Elevation of chin:*
  - Inferior oblique palsy
  - Superior rectus palsy

- Double elevator palsy
- Brown syndrome
- Thyroid myopathy
- Fracture floor of orbit
- A esotropia
- V exotropia

  Elevation of the chin is common in all types of ptosis, i.e., congenital or acquired, unilateral/ bilateral, with normal SR/with SR underaction.

▪ *Depression of the chin:*
- Superior oblique palsy
- Inferior rectus palsy
- Superior oblique palsy
- Inferior rectus palsy
- Thyroid myopathy
- V esotropia
- A exotropia

Head Tilt

Paralysis of the right superior oblique causes tilting of the head to the right, while paralysis of the left superior causes tilting of the head to the left.

> In cases of SO palsy, the head is both turned and tilted to the opposite side.

Ocular Deviation

It is generally the parents who first notice ocular deviation in one eye, which changes with a change of gaze. It is at its maximum when the child tries to move the eye in the direction of the normal action of the paralyzed muscle. The deviation may be abolished if the eye is moved to the opposite; the deviation is most pronounced in paralysis of the lateral rectus. The deviation is mild enough not to be noticed by parents in cyclovertical involvement.

There are two types of deviation, i.e., primary deviation and secondary deviation. The former is the deviation of the paralyzed eye when the normal eye fixes. The secondary deviation is the deviation of the sound eye when the fixing eye is covered and the squinting eye takes up fixation **(Figs. 24.57A and B)**.

> Secondary deviation is always more than primary deviation in paralytic squints.

Limitation of Movement

The movement of the eye is restricted in the direction of normal action of the paralyzed muscle, i.e., paralysis of the right lateral rectus will result in underaction of the right lateral rectus. The limitation should be examined in both induction and version in all gazes.

False Projection

This is demonstrated by occluding the nonsquinting eye and forcing the paralyzed eye to take upfixation. In this process, the paralyzed muscle gets an increased impulse, and the image is formed away from its normal position. To elicit this good eye, it is covered, and the child is asked to

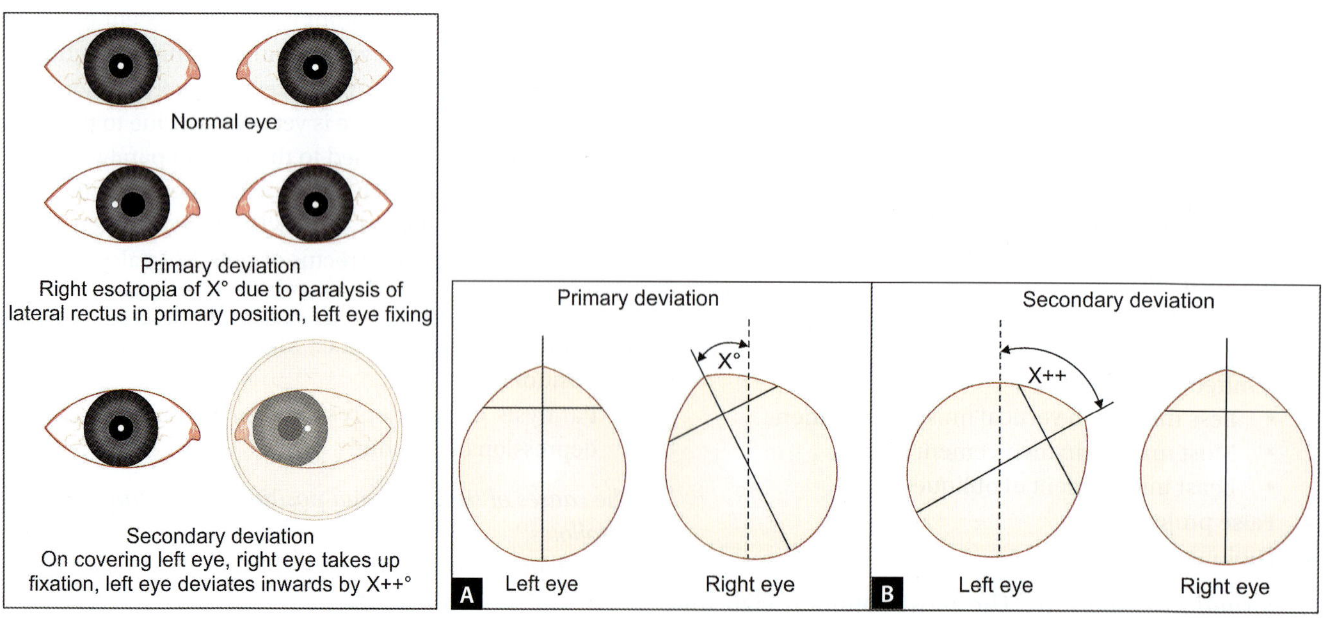

Figs. 24.57A and B: (A) Primary and (B) Secondary deviations in paralytic squint.

touch the finger of the examiner in front of him. The child will fumble and try to grasp the image.

Diplopia

The evaluation of diplopia begins the movement. The child enters the consultant's chamber. To avoid diplopia, he may have:

- An abnormal head posture
- Keep one eye closed
- Frequently blink to refocus the image
    - The first part of the evaluation is to ascertain if the complaint is really diplopia or polyopia. Polyopia is unlikely in children.
    - If it is confirmed to be diplopia, the next step is to find out if it is uniocular or binocular. Uniocular diplopia is again rare in children.
    - Binocular single vision is called haplopia when both eyes are open. This is physiological and the aim of all squint management.
    - Sometimes the patients may complain of foggy vision instead of diplopia, especially when the angle of the squint is small and the second image partly overlaps the original image.
    - Intermittent diplopia is more common in restrictive squints than paralytic squints.
    - The causes of intermittent diplopia may be ocular or systemic. The systemic causes are myasthenia, thyroid ocular disease, and multiple sclerosis. The ocular causes are decompensation of phoria, spasm of the near reflex, and nystagmus blocking syndrome.
    - Enquire if diplopia is:
        - *Horizontal:* Pure horizontal diplopia happens in lesions of the horizontal recti.
        - Vertical
        - Mixed
    - If there is a separation of images, find out the distance between them; separation is maximum in the field of action of paralyzed muscle. Vertical separation is characteristic of lesion of vertically acting recti (isolated paralysis of vertically acting recti is few).
    - *Tilting of image:* Tilting of image is seen as paralysis of obliques.
    - Involvement of cyclovertical muscles gives a mixed type of separation.
    - A child may have a frank paralytic squint without diplopia.

This happens in:

- The pupil is covered by a lid (third nerve palsy).
- One of the eyes has very poor vision.
- Over a period, the child has developed:
    - Suppression and amblyopia
    - Assumed head posture that neutralizes diplopia

The next part is the actual evaluation. This is done by dissociating the two images by changing the color of each image by red-green diplopia glasses. This qualifies and quantifies the position of images; the subjective deviation quantifies nine positions. The following observations are noted:

- Direction of maximum separation
- Distance between two images
- Level of two images
    - Same
    - One higher than the other
    - One of the images is tilted.
- To which eye does the outer image belong? The outer image represents the position of the image formed by the affected muscle. To find out the side of the eye to which the image belongs, the following steps are required: Put the red-green glass in front of the eye; traditionally, the red glass is put in front of the right eye. The red glass produces a red image, while the green glass produces a green image.
- The diplopia is homonymous (uncrossed) or heteronymous (crossed). The former is caused due to underaction of abductors, i.e., the lateral rectus, superior and inferior obliques. The latter is caused due to underaction of adductors, i.e., MR, superior and IR.
- Identify the overacting and underacting muscles
- Hold a white streak of light about a meter away
- The streak would look red when seen by the right eye and green by left. In the case of paralytic squint, the two images will be separated by some distance; one will be toward the midline and the other away from the midline. In the absence of paralytic squints, the images will overlap. Ask the patients to close any eye and enquire; which image has disappeared. This will identify the image formed by each eye and denote if the image is central or peripheral. The far image belongs to the affected eye; this is made clear by the following explanation:

    In the case of left lateral rectus palsy, the outer image belongs to the left eye, maximum separation happens in levoversion. In the case of right medial rectus palsy, the peripheral image belongs to the right eye **(Figs. 24.58 to 24.60)**.

Figures 24.58 to 24.60 show diplopia in third, fourth, and sixth nerve palsy, respectively.

In the case of right medial rectus palsy, the peripheral image belongs to the right eye.

The diplopia can be evaluated by the following methods:
(Children under 10 years old may not cooperate)

The first test is simple, not requiring any elaborate instruments. All that is required is:

- A pair of red-green goggles, the colors of which are complementary to each other, thus mutually excluding the field of action of each muscle.
- A bright and sharp linear white light
- In the absence of this, a lighted candle will suffice.
- The child is counsel that the test is noninvasive, painless but requires the child's cooperation as it is important for treatment and follow-up.
- The child puts on the red-green glasses, red in front of the right eye, and looks at the white streak kept at 1-m distance.

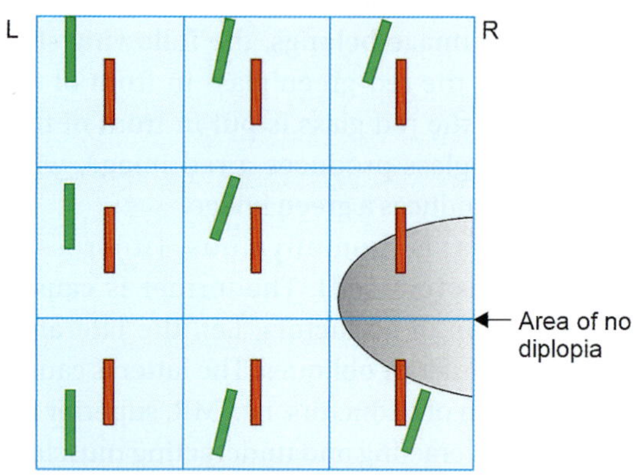

Fig. 24.58: Diplopia charting in third nerve palsy.

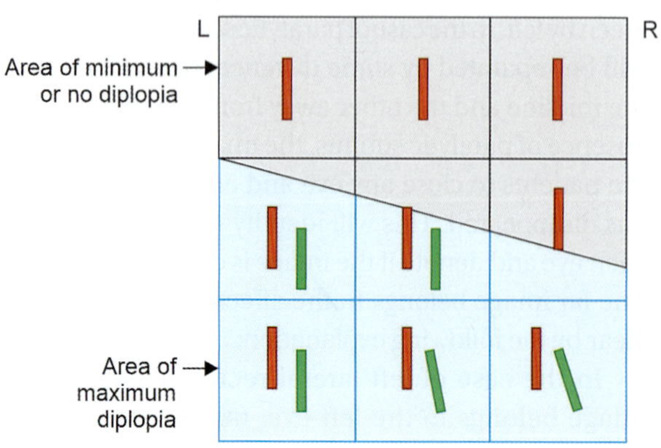

Fig. 24.59: Diplopia chart of right superior oblique palsy.

- The child is asked to close the left eye; as the child looks through the red glass, the light looks red, then the child closes the right eye and sees the streak as green (putting red glass in front of the right is conventional).
- As the child opens both eyes, he develops diplopia and sees one red and one green streak.
- Then, the child opens both eyes to fix the light with the head straight and moves the eyes only, keeping the streak fixed, and the streak is moved in the ninth quadrant of the gaze.
- If there is no paralysis of any extraocular muscle, the two images will be superimposed; otherwise, they will be separated either horizontally or vertically. The images will not only be separated in all directions but tilted in the case of a cyclovertical squint. Paralysis of horizontal muscles does not cause tilting, and the images are at the same height in all positions.

Hess Screen Test

The next test for diplopia is the Hess screen. The principle involved is the same as in diplopia charting, i.e., both are based on Hering's law of equal innervations.

- Both are subjective tests.
- Both are dissociative tests.
- Both exclude the field of action by red and green glasses. The glasses should be dense enough to make the red and green spots visible on the Hess screen*.
- Both indicate the eye and the muscle involved.
- The Hess screen has the advantage of differentiating between paralytic and restrictive squints. It also differentiates between underacting and overacting muscle/muscles.

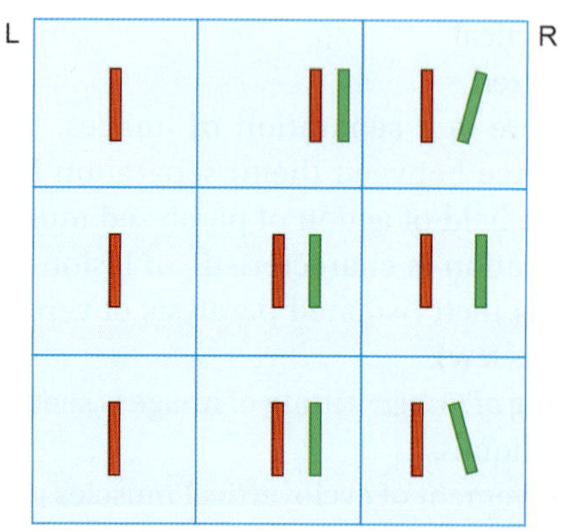

Fig. 24.60: Diplopia chart of isolated right lateral rectus palsy

Hess screen*: The Hess screen test is done either on Hess's board or screen **(Fig. 24.61).

- It also differentiates between primary and secondary deviations.

The board consists of a flat gray or black surface kept vertically in front of the patients. The pattern of the chart is the same for the board and the screen. The board is 3 × 3 feet and is mounted on the wall. The chart is not really square but concave on all four sides, with concavity in the wards. The surface of the board is divided into nine diagnostic squares; they are made up of 144 small squares by two sets of lines: vertical and horizontal. This divides the board into two parts: a smaller central part and a larger outer square; the smaller forms an angle of 15°, while the outer forms an angle of 30°. These two squares have specific diagnostic values. The lines themselves substantiate an angle of 5° on the eye at 0.5 m. The junction of the vertical and horizontal lines can either be marked from outside or illuminated from behind by electrically operated red bulbs (**Figs. 24.62A to C**).

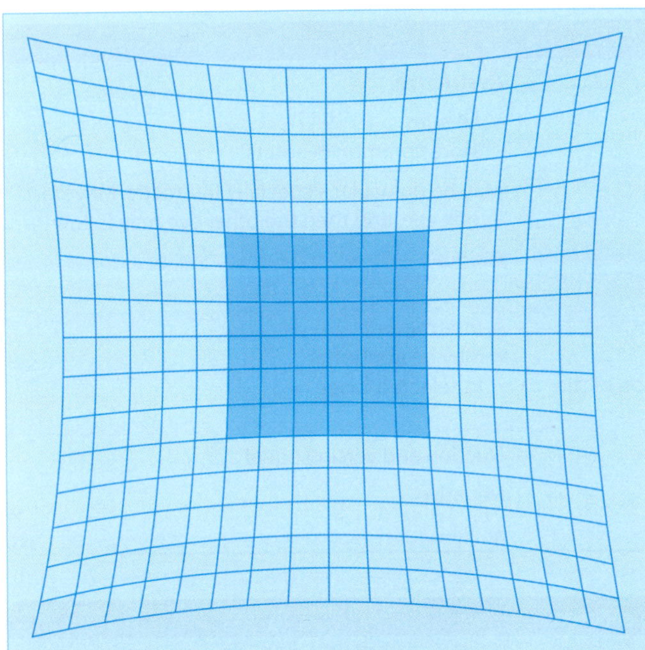

Fig. 24.61: Hess screen.

The spots are illuminated individually by a controlling panel by the examiner; otherwise, the examiner puts a red laser spot on the required junction and asks the patient to put a green spot on it, superimposing the red spot. Of course, putting red-green glasses—red—in front of the right eye. The red glass represents the point of fixation. The patient uses a green streak of light from a suitable source.

In the absence of diplopia, the patient will correctly superimpose the red spot on the green streak. In diplopia, the green spot will be away from the red spot. The first part of the test consists of charting the central small square, which gives the primary deviation. The outer square is tested, and then the outer-deviation indicates secondary deviation, under/overaction muscles, and sequelae of paralysis. The smaller chart gives the extent of maximum restriction in the main action of the paralyzed muscle; the larger chart represents expansion in the main action of the yoke muscle.

In the next part of the test, the glasses are interchanged, putting red in front of the left eye and green in front of the right. The test is repeated in the same manner as in the first part. The results are plotted on two separate papers or fed into a programmed computer. The prerequisites for the Hess test are given as follows:

- Counseling the child
- Making the child aware of the red spot and its relation to the green streak
- The child is instructed to keep the head straight and stationary, and the child is demonstrated how to move the eyes in all quadrants with the stationary head.

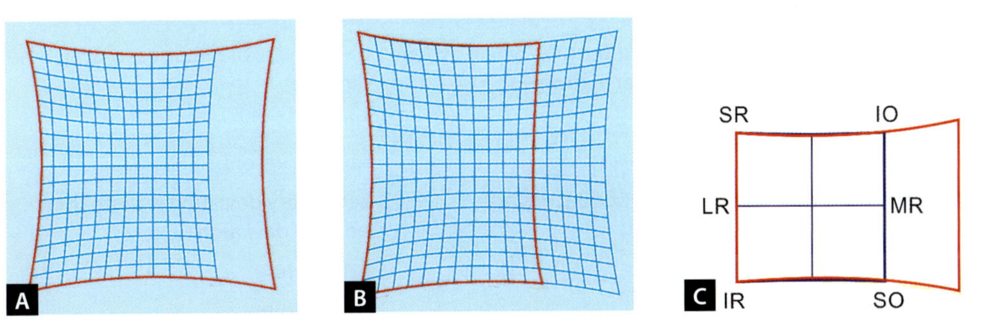

Figs. 24.62A to C: Hess chart of right lateral rectus palsy. The smaller chart represents the right lateral rectus; the larger chart shows overacting medial rectus, left eye. (IO: inferior oblique; IR: inferior rectus; LR: lateral rectus; MR: medial rectus; SO: superior oblique; SR: superior rectus)

- The child should put on the best correction glasses.
- The two eyes should have almost equal vision.
- Exclude amblyopia
- The child should have foveal fixation with normal retinal correspondence.

Forced Duction Test

There are two types of forced duction tests, i.e., active and passive. The purpose of the test is to differentiate between paralytic and restrictive squints in children. It is done under short-acting general anesthesia without succinylcholine. Once the child is anesthetized, the eyeball is grasped at the limbus by a toothed forceps. The eyeball is rotated in the direction of the muscle that is underacting; if it moves freely, the agonist is paralyzed; if no movement occurs, the eye has a mechanical restriction, either entrapment or fibrosis. The restriction can be graded between 1 and 3. The first is the absolute restriction seen in superior oblique sheath syndrome and thyroid ocular disease. The second is the uniform restriction seen in muscle contracture. The third, also known as the leash phenomenon, is where normal resistance is followed by a sudden increase, as seen in long-standing extraocular muscle palsy with restriction of the antagonist.

*Comparison between paralytic and restrictive squints is given in **Table 24.23**.*

*Comparison between clinical features of congenital and acquired paralytic squints in children is shown in **Table 24.24**.*

TABLE 24.23: Difference between paralytic and restrictive squints.

Features	*Paralytic*	*Restrictive*
Age	• All ages • More common in adults	• All ages • More common in adults
Side	Generally uniocular	May be uniocular, especially traumatic. May start in one eye, and then the other eye may follow
Onset	Sudden	Gradual
Complaints: • Diplopia • Head posture • Restriction of movement	 • Constant • Abnormal • In the direction of the main action of the muscle involved	 • Intermittent • May be abnormal • In selected cases
Duction versus version	Duction more than version	Duction and version equal
Muscle changes	Positive	Negative
Globe retraction	Negative	±

TABLE 24.24: Difference between congenital and acquired squints in children.

Features	*Congenital*	*Acquired*
Age	May be present at birth or noticed in the neonatal period	Any age
Onset	Intermittent	Acute
Head posture	The child is unaware of the changed head posture, which, when pointed at, does not correlate to an ocular feature	Child aware of it utilizes to overcome diplopia
Changes in vertebrae	Scoliosis±	Nil
Diplopia	Intermittent or in a certain gaze	Always present
Concomitance	Usually concomitant with equal primary and secondary deviation	Secondary deviation is more than primary deviation
Suppression	Almost always present	Late feature
Amblyopia	Almost always present	Late feature
ARC	Usual	Late

(ARC: abnormal retinal correspondence)

MANAGEMENT OF PARALYTIC SQUINT

A paralytic squint is not an ocular feature. It is not corrected by glasses; local drops have no role to play. The management is divided into two parts: (1) immediate and (2) late. The former consists of patching any of the eyes with a prism with the base away from the normal muscle.

Instead of a prism mounted on the trial set, a Fresnel prism that can be pasted on the glass in the trial frame is used.

The next management step consists of injecting Botox under supervision into the overacting muscle. The surgical treatment should be deferred for at least 6 months from the onset. The principle is to strengthen the weak muscle and weaken the overactive muscle by the standard method.

Systemic conditions such as myasthenia gravis and thyroid myopathy should be treated to the best level by a physician. Most of the time, medical treatment will correct the squint. The unresolved squint should be managed surgically, 6 months after the maximum benefit of medical treatment has been achieved.

SUGGESTED READING

1. Anstice NS, Thompson B. The measurement of visual acuity in children: an evidence-based update. Clin Exp Optom. 2014;97(1):3-11.
2. Bajandas, FJ, Kline LB. Supranuclear and internuclear gaze pathways. In: Bajandas, FJ, Kline LB (Eds). Neuro-Ophthalmology Review Manual, 3rd edition. New Delhi: Jaypee Brothers Medical (P) Pvt. Ltd.; 1989. pp. 43-65.
3. Banks MS, Salapatek P. Acuity and contrast sensitivity in 1-, 2-, and 3-month-old human infants. Invest Ophthalmol Vis Sci. 1978;17(4):361-5.
4. Bhate M, Adewara B, Bothra N. Strabismus in pediatric orbital wall fractures. Indian J Ophthalmol. 2023;71(3):973-6.
5. Dadeya S, Kaur S. Basic Examination of Strabismus. New Delhi: Delhi Ophthalmological Society; 2022.
6. Datta H. Anatomy of extraocular muscles and their fascia. In: Datta H (Ed). Strabismus, 1st edition. New Delhi: Jaypee Brothers Medical (P) Pvt. Ltd.; 2004. p. 10.
7. Denniston AKO, Murray PI. Oxford Handbook of Ophthalmology, 4th edition. Oxford: Oxford University Press; 2018.
8. Elder SD, Wybar KC. Extrinsic Muscles of the Eye in System, 1st edition. London: Henry Kimpton; 1961. pp. 414-63.
9. Glasser S. Eye movement characteristics and recording techniques. In: Glasser S (Ed). Neuro-Ophthalmology. London: Harper and Row; 1978. pp. 187-98.
10. Jackson TL. Moorfield's Manual of Ophthalmology, 3rd edition, New Delhi: Jaypee Brothers Medical (P) Pvt. Ltd.; 2020.
11. Jethani J, Dave P. The subjectivity of objective evaluation of torsion on fundus photographs by practicing strabismologists. Indian J Ophthalmol. 2018;66(9):1301-3.
12. Karlsson VC. Extraocular muscle anatomy and function. In: Karlsson V (Ed). Ocular Motility, 1st edition. New Delhi: Jaypee Brothers Medical (P) Pvt. Ltd.; 1989. pp. 1-11.
13. Karna S. Step by Step Neuro-Ophthalmology Clinical Examination and Diagnosis, 1st edition. New Delhi: Jaypee Brothers Medical (P) Pvt. Ltd.; 2006.
14. Lyle KT, Wybar KC. The extrinsic ocular muscles and related fascia. In: Lyle KT, Wybar KC (Eds). Lyle and Jackson's Practical Orthoptics in Treatment of Squint, 1st edition. New Delhi: Jaypee Brothers Medical (P) Pvt. Ltd.; 1994. pp. 8-14.
15. Lyle TK, Wybar KC. Paralytic strabismus. In: Lyle TK, Wybar KC (Eds). Lyle and Jackson's Practical Orthoptics, 1st edition. New Delhi: Jaypee Brothers Medical (P) Pvt. Ltd.; 1994. pp. 528-75.
16. Manley DR. Cyclic esotropia. In: Nelson LB, Harley RD, Olitsky SE (Eds). Harley Pediatric Ophthalmology, 2nd edition. Philadelphia: WB Saunders Company; 1983. pp. 233-40.
17. Mukherjee PK. Clinical Examination in Ophthalmology, 2nd edition. New Delhi: Elsevier; 2016.
18. Mukherjee PK. Essentials of Neuro-Ophthalmology, 1st edition. New Delhi: Jaypee Brothers Medical (P) Pvt. Ltd.; 2010.
19. Mukherjee PK. Manual of Optics and Refraction, 2nd edition. New Delhi: Jaypee Brothers Medical (P) Pvt. Ltd.; 2022.
20. Mukherjee PK. Pediatric Ophthalmology, 1st edition. New Delhi: New Age International; 2005.
21. Natchair G. Syndrome of Neuro-Ophthalmic Significance in Neuro-Ophthalmology: a Manual for Postgraduate Students. Madurai: Aravind Eye Hospital; pp. 27.1-27.
22. Nema HV. Extraocular Muscles in Anatomy of the Eye and its Adnexa, 2nd edition. New Delhi: Jaypee Brothers Medical (P) Pvt. Ltd.; 1991. pp. 77-84.
23. Noorden GK. Binocular Vision and Ocular Motility, 4th edition, St. Louis: Mosby; 1990.
24. Prager TC, Zou YL, Jensen CL, Fraley JK, Anderson RE, Heird WC. Evaluation of methods for assessing visual function of infants. J AAPOS. 1999;3(5):275-82.
25. Prasad VN. Prospect of Goswami's theory for false projections and diplopia screens. J All India Ophthalmol Soc. 1970;18(4):183-4.
26. Rohatgi JN. Acquired paralytic squint. In: Rohatgi JN (Ed). Squint Basic and Clinical Aspects, 1st edition. New Delhi: CBS Publishers; 2003. pp. 197-201.
27. Rosenberg MA. Ocular motor system. In: Peyrnan GA, Sander DR, Goldberg MF (Eds). Principle and Practice of Ophthalmology, 1st edition, New Delhi: Jaypee Brothers Medical (P) Pvt. Ltd.; 1987. pp. 1951-4.

28. Rowe F. Extraocular muscle anomaly and innervation. In: Rowe F (Ed). Clinical Orthoptics, 1st edition. London: Blackwell Science; 1997. pp. 3-12.
29. Rowe F. Method of Measurements of Ac/A Ratio in Clinical Orthoptics, 1st edition. Oxford: Black Science; 1997. p. 58.
30. Salmon JF. Kanski's Clinical Ophthalmology: A Systemic Approach, 9th edition. New Delhi: Elsevier; 2020.
31. Saxena R, Sharma P; Pediatric Ophthalmology Expert Group. National consensus statement regarding pediatric eye examination, refraction, and amblyopia management. Indian J Ophthalmol. 2020;68(2):325-32.
32. Sharma P. An overview of strabismology. In: Sharma P (Ed). Strabismus Simplified, 1st edition. New Delhi: Modern Publishers; 1989. pp. 1-8.
33. Suttle CM. Visual acuity assessment in infants and young children. Clin Exp Optom. 2001;84(6):337-45.
34. Thomas R, Braganza A, George T. Practical approach to diagnosis of strabismus. Indian J Ophthalmol. 1996; 44(2):103-12.

CHAPTER

25 Nystagmus

Nystagmus is not a disease but is a manifestation of many diseases that could be not only vision-threatening but may be crippling or even life-threatening as well may involve the central nervous system. Nystagmus does not lead to blindness; the reverse may be true.

There are about a dozen definitions of nystagmus used in clinical practice; the central point round which they are built is a disturbance of ocular posture.

In normal fixation for distance, the eyes are motionless and move smoothly in a coordinated fashion in various desired directions of gaze without oscillation.

Normal fixation requires afferent and efferent paths with an intact intracerebral connection. A fault in any of them leads to an uncoordinated oscillation of the eyes, generally in both eyes.

The most widely used definition of nystagmus is "involuntary, periodic, repetitive oscillations of the eye that are rhythmic." The patient may not be aware of it. The condition should be differentiated from oscillopsia, which is the movement of a visual image due to a defect in the oculovestibular path.

In addition, it may be:

- Binocular/uniocular, the former is more common. It is thought that the conditions presenting as uniocular are really an asymmetric variation of binocular nystagmus, where the intensity of oscillation is more marked in one eye. The other possibility is that the eyes without oscillation will ultimately pass into full-blown bilateral nystagmus.
- It may be congenital or acquired.
- It may be present in a particular gaze or all gazes.
- It can be physiological or pathological. The physiological nystagmus becomes apparent only under certain conditions. Examples of physiological nystagmus are given as follows:
    - Fatigue (Rare)
    - End point nystagmus—seen in extreme lateral gaze, is very mild, and disappears as the eyes come to the primary position. It is seen in all individuals without any clinical importance.
    - Optokinetic nystagmus

OPTOKINETIC NYSTAGMUS

Optokinetic nystagmus is an artificial method of precipitating oscillations in the normal eye. It requires a specially constructed cylinder that can be rotated around a central axis. The outer surface of the drum has alternate strips of black and white lines. The rotation of the drum presents black and white lines alternatingly to the eyes, producing nystagmus **(Fig. 25.1)**.

Faster the rotations, quicker the oscillations; the movement stops with the stopping of rotation. The reflex is not developed before 6 months of age. The optokinetic drum is used to detect the following conditions besides the precipitation of nystagmus:

- *Is there vision in the eye?:* This is used to ensure the presence of vision in preverbal children and infants and also in Malinger, who claims not to have a perception of light.

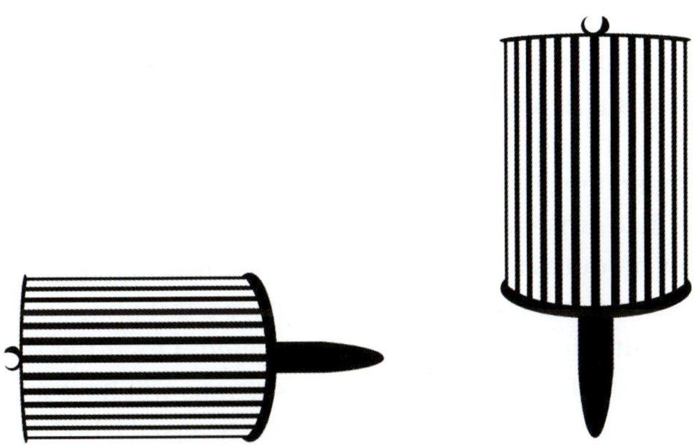

Fig. 25.1: Optokinetic drums.

- *Detection of vision:* By changing the width of the strips, a rough estimate of vision can be assessed.
- *Detect the integrity of:*
  - Frontomesencephalic tract
  - Occipitomesencephalic tract

Other physiological nystagmus are given as follows:
- Rail road nystagmus
- Miners' nystagmus
- Vestibular-evoked nystagmus

RAIL ROAD NYSTAGMUS

This is a modified form of nystagmus based akin to principle of the optokinetic drum; it is seen in passengers looking out of windows in a moving train. The passenger looking outside the window is not aware of the oscillations of his eyes. The person looking in the eyes of the person can see the oscillation faster the speed, more frequent are the oscillations.

That stops as the train halts.

MINERS' NYSTAGMUS

This is seen in persons who work for hours in reduced illumination, commonly in underground coal mines. The nystagmus is pronounced in up-horizontal gaze mostly. The person has difficulty fixing the point he wants to. It is not seen in children. It consists of nystagmus, diminished vision, photophobia, and diminished scotopic vision.

VESTIBULAR-EVOKED NYSTAGMUSWW

The vestibular apparatus plays an important role in maintaining ocular posture without involuntary movement; hence, the interruption of its function produces nystagmus. The two commonly used procedures to produce nystagmus are (1) caloric stimulation and (2) acceleration (deacceleration of the body). This procedure is used in diagnosing vestibular nystagmus.

It is a neurological test to evaluate vestibulo-ocular reflex. In caloric nystagmus test, fluid, irrespective of its temperature, is used to irrigate the external auditory canal; the fluid evokes convention current in the semilunar canal. This produces temperature-dependent nystagmus. If cold water is used, the nystagmus will have a fast phase in the opposite direction of the side irrigated, i.e., if the right canal is irrigated, the resulting nystagmus will have a fast phase toward the left side. This will be reversed if hot water is used. Each side is evaluated separately. It is depicted in mnemonic COWS that is Cold Opposite and Warm on the Same side.

PATHOLOGICAL NYSTAGMUS

Nystagmus can either be congenital or acquired. Congenital nystagmus is always pathological.

The pathological causes are put into two categories given as follows:
1. With ocular pathology
2. Extraocular pathology

1. *Ocular causes*: *The list is long; it comprises of* bilateral congenital cataract, bilateral macular scar due to congenital toxoplasmosis, optic nerve hypoplasia, macular hypoplasia, Leber's congenital amaurosis, achromatopsia, congenital stationary night blindness, albinism, aniridia, cone dystrophy, bilateral corneal opacity, and retinopathy of prematurity (ROP).
2. *The extraocular causes* of nystagmus are neurological, in origin, they may involve the vestibular system, brainstem, posterior fossa, cerebellum, or spinal cord.

Rule of 2-4-6

Nystagmus of ocular origin roughly follows the rule of 2-4-6 in relation to the age of onset. It is summarized given as follows:
- If the child has very poor vision before 2 years of age, there are 100% chances of nystagmus in the child.
- If the child has poor central vision at 4 years, there are 50% chances of developing nystagmus.
- No nystagmus will develop if the child acquires poor central vision by 6 years of age.

CLASSIFICATION OF NYSTAGMUS

Nystagmus is classified variously; the common division is given as follows:
- Morphology
- Plane
- Amplitude
- Frequency
- Degree

Some terms used to specify nystagmus are given as follows:
- Congenital/acquired
- True/pseudonystagmus (nystagmoid)
- *Latency:*
  - Manifest

- Latent
- Manifest latent
- *Laterality:*
    - Unilateral
    - Bilateral (this is the rule)
- *Morphology:*
    - Jerk
    - Pendular
    - Mixed
- *Plane:*
    - Horizontal
    - Vertical
    - Rotatory
    - Mixed
- *Phase:*
    - Slow—initiating (pursuit)
    - Fast—correcting (saccade involuntary fast movement of the eyes as they change from one point of gaze to another)
- A null zone is a plane in which the nystagmus is least, may be left, right, or in convergence. The child learns to locate this null zone and keeps his head turned to it to have the best vision. Abnormal head posture is a clue to field loss.
- Direction—this indicates the direction of the fast phase.
    - Horizontal
    - Vertical
    - Oblique
    - Seesaw—one eye moves up and the other down, the rising eye in torts and the other extorts
- *Amplitude:*
    - Small
    - Large
    - The amplitude is best seen on a slit lamp
- Frequency—this is the number of oscillations/second; it is measured as cycles/second or in Megahertz. A rough estimate is rapid or slow; the former is >5 Hz, while the latter is 1–2 Hz.
- Intensity—this is arrived by multiplying amplitude by frequency
- *Conjugacy:*
    - Conjugate
    - Dissociated
- Sensory deficit nystagmus
- Motor deficit—congenital idiopathic

Flowchart 25.1 depicts various classifications in vogue.

Congenital motor nystagmus following occlusion of one eye behaves differently and is grouped in the following types:

- Latent
- Manifest
- Manifest latent

- *Latent nystagmus:* It is defined as a motor nystagmus that is bilateral and horizontally developing when any preferably fixing eye is covered, and the eye beats toward the other eye. It is a conjugate jerk nystagmus developing mostly in congenital esotropia. The child may not have any symptoms, hence being unaware of its presence.
- *Manifest nystagmus:* It is the nystagmus that is obvious even when both eyes are fixed; the parents are aware of it and bring the child for examination; the child may be embraced and prefers to look downward, avoiding looking into the eyes of the person he is talking to. It is bilateral, horizontal, and conjugate; it may be jerk or pendular, reduced in convergence. The child may assume an abnormal head posture.
- *Manifest latent nystagmus:* This is a manifest nystagmus that becomes obvious when the dominant eye is covered.

The terms manifest latent seem to be confusing; **Table 25.1** differentiates manifest nystagmus.

Flowchart 25.2 shows the classification of nystagmoid movements.

Alternate classification of nystagmus on the basis of onset is depicted in **Flowchart 25.3**.

Some specific terms are used that may be confused with true nystagmus given as follows:

- *Ocular dysmetria:* This is overshooting of the gaze on changing the gaze. It is caused by a disorder of the cerebellum. Overshooting of both eyes results when the gaze is shifted from the left to the primary position in a lesion of the left cerebellum. A right cerebellar lesion will result in its opposite form of overshoot.

  Overshoots are followed by to-and-fro oscillation. It is due to a lesion such as encephalitis. It is generally accompanied by myoclonus and ataxia. It may be due to neuroblastoma.
- *Ocular flutter:* This is a pendular nystagmus that is horizontal and spontaneous during fixation or after fixation. It has a small amplitude. It is caused due to lesion in the paramedian pontine reticular formation.

Flowchart 25.1: Classification of nystagmus.

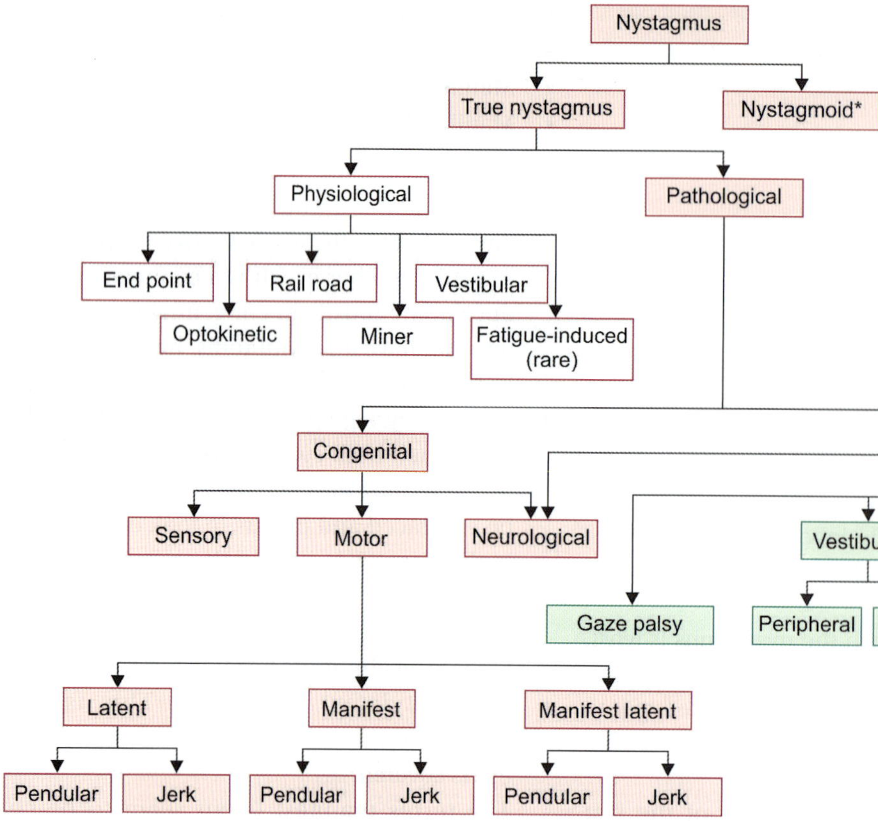

**Nystagmoid:* Nystagmoids are involuntary eye movements. Differing from true nystagmus, i.e., without much clinical importance, not fitting in accepted definitions. They are square wave jerks, ocular flutter, opsoclonus, superior oblique myokymia, and voluntary nystagmus.

***Vestibular:* Vestibular dysfunction can be in the end organ, nerve, or nucleus. The prominent symptom is vertigo. The causes are labyrinthitis, Ménière's syndrome, vascular trauma to the brainstem, and neoplasms.

****Miscellaneous:* The examples are spasmus nutans, nystagmus blockage syndrome, seesaw nystagmus, and upbeat and downbeat nystagmus.

TABLE 25.1: Difference between manifest and manifest latent nystagmus.

Features	*Manifest*	*Manifest latent*
Covering the fixing eye	No change	Nystagmus becomes more marked
Type	Pendular	Jerk
Vision	Equal in both eyes	Binocular vision is better
Effects of abduction	No change	Increases
Esotropia	When present, infantile but less common	Always associated with infantile esotropia

Flowchart 25.2: Classification of nystagmoid movements.

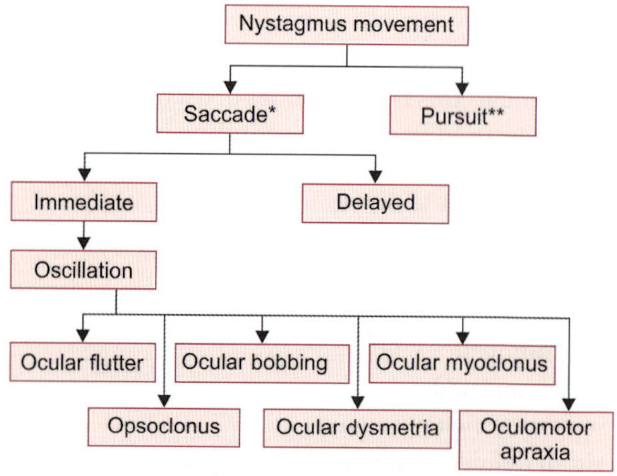

*Saccades are primarily directed toward stationary targets.

**Pursuits are used to track small moving objects; they require an intact fovea.

Flowchart 25.3: Alternate classification of nystagmus on the basis of onset.

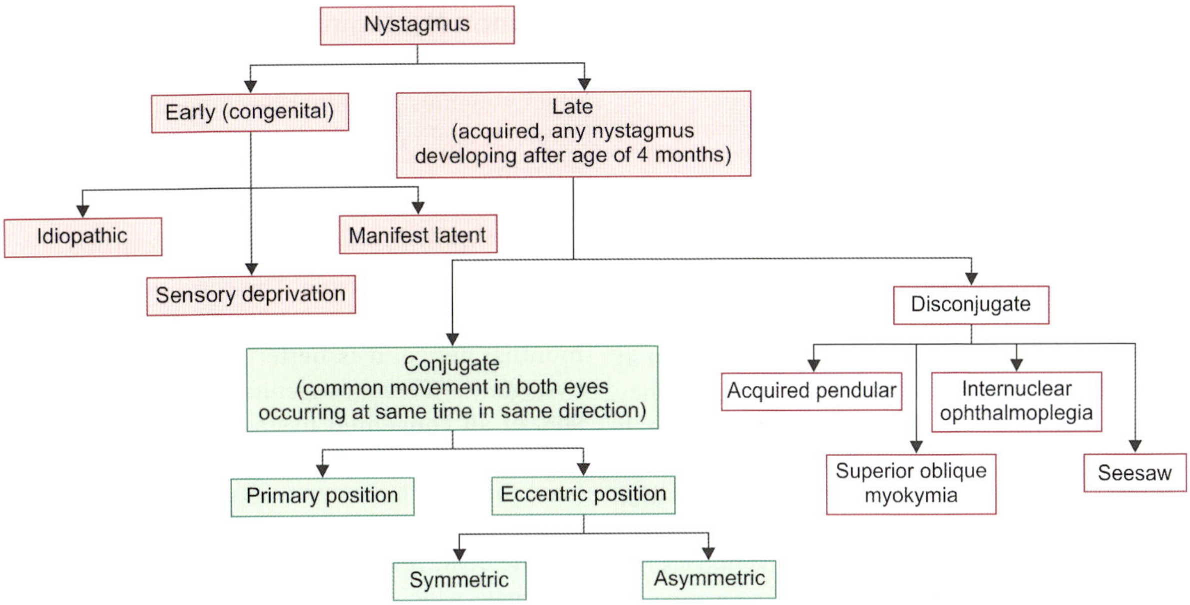

- *Opsoclonus*: This is a rare oscillation. It comprises repetitive, irregular, multidirectional conjugate movement.
- *Ocular myoclonus:* This is to-and-fro; it continues pendular oscillation of cerebellar origin. The oscillations are multidirectional. Its amplitude varies in various directions. It is generally associated with the myoclonic movement of the lids and palate.
- *Oculomotor apraxia:* It is a congenital condition of failure of saccade. The infant cannot look around till the head movements develop; even with the development of head movements, the saccades are absent. Once the eyes fixate, the head comes back to its central position.
- *Ocular bobbing:* This occurs due to a brainstem lesion. It consists of repeated downward movements of the eyes. The eyes remain in a downward gaze for a few seconds, only to go back to their central position. The movement in two eyes may be disconjugate. It must be differentiated from downbeat nystagmus.
- *Spasmus nutans:* It is an acquired episodic form of ocular oscillation that starts by 1 year and disappears by 3 years; it is associated with movement of the head. If it persists after 3 years, the child should be examined and investigated for sensory–visual disorders or intracranial lesions. The oscillations are asymmetric, have a small amplitude, and have a high frequency. They may rarely be unilateral, but when bilateral, they are asymmetric, giving the false impression of being monocular. No neurological or ocular defects are found.

Characteristics of Congenital and Infantile Nystagmus

- Nystagmus present at birth or noticed before 2 months is labeled as congenital nystagmus. No definite cause can be attributed to it.
- Nystagmus developing between 2 and 3 months is a sensory deficit; there are cone dystrophy, rod monochromatopsia, rod cone dystrophy, and albinism.
- More common causes of sensory deficit nystagmus are given as follows:
  - *Anterior segment:* Bilateral congenital cataract, buphthalmos, aniridia, Peters anomaly, and albinism.
  - *Posterior segment:* Foveal hypoplasia, foveal toxoplasmosis, ROP, persistent hyperplastic primary vitreous, familial exudative retinopathy, retinal detachment, achromatopsia, congenital optic atrophy, hypoplasia of the disk, and coloboma of the disk.

Congenital nystagmus is always pathological.

Characteristics of Various Types of Morphological Nystagmus

Morphological nystagmus is divided into two forms given as follows:

1. Pendular
2. Jerk

1. *Pendular nystagmus:* The eyes move like a pendulum in the horizontal plane with equal speed and amplitudes, less commonly seen in the vertical plane; the cause is sensory deprivation (see above). It is a slow and smooth nystagmus. It is present at birth or acquired by 2 months of age. The frequency and amplitudes are reduced during convergence. It persists in dim light but stops following the closure of the eyes; it could be hereditary that becomes obvious during infancy and lasts for the rest of the life. It is seen in many members of the family with good vision. The other common causes of pendular nystagmus are miners' nystagmus, lesions of the brainstem, drug toxicity, and spasmus nutans. Acquired pendular nystagmus develops in one-eyed persons with brainstem lesions and drugs.
2. *Jerk nystagmus*: In this nystagmus, the first phase is slow, and the second phase is faster and saccadic. It is customarily identified with the rapid phase. The slow phase is fundamental and pursuit. The rapid phase is compensatory. Jerk nystagmus can either be congenital or acquired. It is broadly divided into gaze paretic and vestibular; the former is seen in upper brainstem disorders. It is characterized by slow movement toward the lesion and a fast jerk to the opposite side. The vestibular nystagmus is a horizontal or rotational jerk nystagmus in primary gaze generally associated with vertigo. It can be due either to a central or peripheral lesion of the 8th nerve and its connection; the peripheral type of nystagmus is reduced in central fixation.

The other causes are end point, optokinetic, gaze paretic, congenital jerk nystagmus, and vestibular latent nystagmus.

Mixed Nystagmus

It is a rare form when there is a pendular nystagmus in the primary gaze and a jerk nystagmus on misaligned eyes.

Clinical Presentation of Some Common Nystagmus

In the clinical classification of nystagmus, we have noted that nystagmus can either be congenital or acquired. The former is again separated into groups that are afferent and efferent.

Congenital/Infantile Afferent Nystagmus

The terms are debatable. The condition is rarely present at birth, generally developing in the first few weeks to months; hence, it is better to label them as infantile nystagmus. Afferent congenital infantile nystagmus forms 90% of all congenital nystagmus. They are secondary to ocular motor disorders. The list of causes is many (see above). The other nonocular cause is a cortical defect acquired within a few days of birth.

The features of infantile nystagmus are bilateral conjugate, which is reduced in convergence and increased in fixation. One of its characteristics is that it is abolished during sleep. The near vision improves with convergence.

Congenital/Infantile Efferent Nystagmus

The condition is far less common than its afferent counterpart. This was formerly referred to as congenital motor nystagmus and is currently termed as idiopathic infantile nystagmus. The condition has detectable abnormal head posture and has null point* in eccentric gaze.

Acquired Nystagmus

The list of acquired nystagmus is pretty long.

They are given as follows:

- Gaze paretic
- Gaze evoked
- Vestibular
- Seesaw
- Upbeat
- Downbeat
- Periodic upbeat
- Nystagmus blockage syndrome

- *Gaze paretic nystagmus:* This is acquired following gaze palsy either due to intraocular ophthalmoplegia, failure of saccade pursuit, or vestibular underaction.

**Null point:* The null point is the distance where the eyes stop moving during the movement of the nystagmus.

It is a nystagmus of slow frequency horizontal, slow gaze paresis with eyes rotated toward side of lesions, followed by a fast jerk nystagmus with eye away from the side of session.

- *Gaze-evoked nystagmus:* It occurs only in various gazes and is absent in the primary position with fast components in the direction of gaze. It can be drug-induced; posterior fossa lesions such as trauma, tumors, ischemia, demyelination, and even myasthenia and thyroid eye diseases have been blamed.
- *Vestibular nystagmus:* It is a jerk nystagmus that is invariably horizontal and less commonly rotatory, accompanied by symptoms of vestibular disorder that can either be central or peripheral. The central type is due to brainstem disorders such as stroke, tumor, trauma, and demyelination. The causes of peripheral vestibular nystagmus consist of neuritis, ischemia, and trauma.
- *Seesaw nystagmus:* It is mostly acquired. Rarely, it can be congenital. It is a pendular nystagmus where one eye elevates and the other depresses at the same time; the upgoing eye intorts and the downgoing eye extorts. It is caused by trauma, vertebrobasilar insufficiency, and tumors.
- *Upbeat nystagmus:* It is always seen in the primary position. It has a fast upbeat and is caused by brainstem and cerebellar disorders. It can be congenital.
- *Downbeat nystagmus:* It is associated with a fast downward component. Pressure at the foramen magnum is one of the major causes. It is associated with a posterior fossa disorder.
- *Periodic upbeat nystagmus:* This is an infrequent type of nystagmus that is generally acquired; it is caused by other neurological and ocular causes. It may improve if the ocular causes are treated.
- *Nystagmus blockage syndrome:* It is an acquired condition seen in infantile esotropia. The characteristic features are the nystagmus of either eye. It is a compensatory method to improve vision in the horizontal nystagmus that increases in abduction and decreases in adduction. The oscillations are dampened in convergence, and the child likes to put the eye in adduction. They turn the head in the direction of fixing the eye; this is generally associated with amblyopia and should not be confused with cross-fixation.

LOCALIZATION OF THE CAUSE OF NYSTAGMUS

- History will reveal if it is congenital or acquired
- Family history may be present in nonvision-threatening and nonfatal nystagmus
- Comprehensive ocular checkup to exclude ocular causes
- Probable neurological location of the lesion in a specific nystagmus

Table 25.2 shows the types of nystagmus in relation to the position of the lesion.

INVESTIGATION IN NYSTAGMUS

The investigations start with a history of the present illness and family history, followed by a comprehensive ocular examination. As more than half of children with infantile nystagmus have retinal involvement, it is mandatory to examine the fundus by indirect ophthalmoscope. Examination of the macula by +90 D lens is a difficult task due to the rapid to-and-fro movement of the eye. X-rays have limited use except in suspected trauma. CT is less useful than MRI. MRI is the gold standard of imaging.

The conditions that require imaging are given as follows:

- Associated with neurological signs
- Unilateral nystagmus
- Asymmetric nystagmus
- Cyclovertical nystagmus
- Disconjugate nystagmus
- Presence of neurological signs
- All oscillations other than horizontal

The following additional tests are recommended for children in the second decade:

- ENT evaluation includes a caloric test and a postural test.
- Complete neurological workup

TABLE 25.2: Types of nystagmus on the basis of anatomic location.

Nystagmus	*Location*
Upbeat	Posterior fossa
Downbeat	Cervicomedullary
Seesaw	Chiasma
Convergence retraction	Dorsal midbrain
Gaze evoked	Posterior fossa
Gaze paretic	Cortex

MANAGEMENT

Management of nystagmus in children is difficult and frustrating, except in systemic causes such as trauma, tumors, and infection. Responses to specific treatments are generally given by specialists in specific fields such as neurosurgery, neurology, oncology, and pediatrics. The ophthalmologist's role in such a situation is limited.

The ophthalmologist is concerned with improving vision and cosmetic appearance by reducing nystagmus, managing squint amblyopia, and correcting head posture.

The above can be done by given as follows:

- Medically
- Optically
- Surgically

The medical treatment consists of an array of many drugs of diverse action, either singularly or in combination. They are gamma-aminobutyric acid (GABA) agonists, sedatives, tranquilizers, and anticonvulsants. The latest to enter this list are local carbonic anhydrase inhibitor drugs.

The commonly used systemic drugs are gabapentin, baclofen, clonazepam, valproate, and carbamazepine. They should be administered in consultation with a pediatrician. Many of the drugs cause drowsiness and, hence, may interfere with a child's routine, especially in schooling. The most commonly used carbonic anhydrase inhibitor is brinzolamide, given one drop in each eye three times a day. It takes about 7–10 days to be effective; the mode of action of the drug in alleviating nystagmus is not well understood.

Retrobulbar botulinum toxin type A has been tried without an unequivocal result.

The aim of optical correction is to salvage maximum vision, retain vision, and prevent amblyopia; all of them are better said than done. They are spectacles, contact lenses, and prisms.

The squint is corrected by surgery and a prism. The purpose is to reduce the null zone, weaken the strong muscle, and put the eye in a position with the least nystagmus.

SUGGESTED READING

1. Aygit ED, Ocak OB, İnal A, Fazıl K, Akar S, Gokyigit B. The effects of topical carbonic anhydrase inhibitors in the treatment of nystagmus. Int Ophthalmol. 2018;38(1):265-9.
2. Dell'osso LF, Hertle RW, Leigh RJ, Jacobs JB, King S, Yaniglos S. Effects of topical brinzolamide on infantile nystagmus syndrome waveforms: eye drops for nystagmus. J Neuroophthalmol. 2011;31(3):228-33.
3. Karan S. Nystagmus evaluation. In: Karan S (Ed). Step-by-Step Neuro-ophthalmology Clinical Examination and Diagnosis, 1st edition. New Delhi: Jaypee Brothers Medical (P) Pvt. Ltd.; 2006.
4. Kothari M. Clinical management of nystagmus. In: Lal H, Verma L, Biswas P (Eds). Ready Reckoner in Ophthalmology, 2nd edition. New Delhi: Jaypee Brothers Medical (P) Pvt. Ltd.; 2017. pp. 699-708.
5. Mollan SP. Nystagmus. In: Denniston AKO, Murray PI (Eds). Oxford Handbook of Ophthalmology, 4th edition. United Kingdom: Oxford University Press; 2018. pp. 802-6.
6. Mukherjee PK. Examination of an Eye with Nystagmus in Clinical Examination in Ophthalmology, 2nd edition. New Delhi: Elsevier; 2016. pp. 387-92.
7. Mukherjee PK. Nystagmus in Essentials of Neuro-ophthalmology, 1st edition. New Delhi: Jaypee Brothers Medical (P) Pvt. Ltd.; 2010. pp. 337-53.
8. Mukherjee PK. Nystagmus in Pediatric Ophthalmology, 1st edition. New Delhi: New Age International; 2005. pp. 628-35.
9. Sarvananthan N, Surendran M, Roberts EO, Jain S, Thomas S, Shah N, et al. The prevalence of nystagmus: the Leicestershire nystagmus survey. Invest Ophthalmol Vis Sci. 2009;50(11):5201-6.
10. Tilikete C, Jasse L, Pelisson D, Vukusic S, Durand-Dubief F, Urquizar C, et al. Acquired pendular nystagmus in multiple sclerosis and oculopalatal tremor. Neurology. 2011;76:1650-7.

CHAPTER 26

Amblyopia

Amblyopia is a common, chronically acquired disorder of form sense (vision). About 2–5% of children are affected by this malady. It is one of the most missed and misdiagnosed disorders of nonimproved vision. It can be unilateral or bilateral; the former is more common and graver than the other. It is commonly associated with squints. The vision loss is about 2–3 lines, i.e., 6/12–6/18 on the Snellen chart. The condition does not fulfill the criteria to qualify as blindness; it leaves the child handicapped professionally and socially, with a financial drawback in adult life. A person with unilateral amblyopia may not be employed for jobs that require 6/6 vision in each eye. No race is immune, involving both sexes equally, without a fixed hereditary pattern; however, various disorders commonly associated with amblyopia, like strabismus, errors of refraction, cataracts, and ptosis, follow their distinct hereditary pattern not related to amblyopia. It is a disorder of the first decade of life, may begin in infancy, and progresses until the child is 6–8 years old; thereafter, it stops progressing. Coincidentally, from infancy to 8 years of age is the most suitable period for successful treatment. An initial good response in treatment does not eliminate the possibility of recurrence. Recurrences are difficult to treat.

There is no universally accepted definition of amblyopia. The most widely followed definition is "Symptomatic disturbance of form, sense (vision), and/or binocular interaction in the critical period, i.e., birth to 6 months of age without any detectable reason."

The mechanism is most probably central in origin; vision cannot be improved with optical devices. An amblyopic eye is anatomically within normal limits with reduced function.

The pathophysiology of amblyopia is as elusive as its definition and classification. The most accepted hypothesis is abnormal binocular interaction. To have a good binocular interaction, it is essential to have a well-developed visual pathway. The second contributory factor is the nonformation of a sharp image on the macula, either due to strabismus, an error of refraction, or obstructions like cataracts and ptosis.

In the previous chapters, we have seen that the macula starts developing early in utero; the development is not complete at birth. The development continues up to 6–7 years after birth. Any obstruction in the formation of a sharp image on the macula during this period causes amblyopia.

CLASSIFICATION OF AMBLYOPIA

Amblyopia has been classified in various ways:

- An amblyopia that fits strictly in its definition of diminished vision and for which no cause is detected is sometimes called as true amblyopia.
- If any cause is detected, like congenital cataract ptosis, etc. It is called deprivation amblyopia.
- Amblyopia from poor vision resulting due to deviation of the visual axis from the fovea centralis to a point elsewhere on the retina where vision is less acute is called amblyopia ex-anopsia, commonly seen as strabismus.
- Both terms have become obsolete.
- The other two terms of the past are functional and organic amblyopia. The former is amenable to treatment, and the other irreversible. The organic causes are, most of the time, congenital.

Relations with squints and amblyopia are as elusive as hens and eggs. The perpetual question remains: which came first? It has not yet been settled if squint causes amblyopia or vice versa. The problem becomes more confusing when amblyopia is present without a squint. It is not rare for squinting eyes not to be amblyopic under 6 years.

NOMENCLATURE IN AMBLYOPIA

Amblyopia, as a clinical entity, has been known for more than three centuries. Yet it has not received much attention because it does not lead to blindness, is never acute or painful. There are many terms which may be interchangeable or may have altogether different meanings.

Some of the nomenclatures used in relation to amblyopia are:

- Strabismic amblyopia
- Ametropic amblyopia
- Congenital amblyopia
- Amblyopia of arrest
- Amblyopia of extinction
- Amblyopia ex-anopsia
- Stimulus deprivation amblyopia
- Organic amblyopia
- Functional amblyopia

Out of the list given above, only the first and second are clinically relevant at present. Confusing terms which are not amblyopia are:

- Toxic amblyopia and nutritional amblyopia, which are entirely different from the amblyopia under discussion they do not fit into the definition of amblyopia.
- Amaurosis is a complete loss of vision that has no detectable pathological lesion. It could be congenital or acquired, mostly due to lesions of the optic nerve, brain, or even spinal cord (rare).

Amaurosis fugax is a sudden, unilateral loss of vision due to intraocular vascular causes. Nowadays, it has been proved that it can be binocular as well in rare instances. The condition is not seen in children and is not related to amblyopia.

CLINICAL FEATURES OF AMBLYOPIA

- Amblyopia is an acquired anomaly of cortical origin.
- It is never acute and painful.
- It may start at birth and progress up to 6–7 years. Thereafter, it becomes stationary.
- The development of strabismic and ametropic amblyopia after 7–8 years is rare.
- Acute loss of vision without any ophthalmoscopic cause is most probably a toxic amblyopia.
- Amblyopia is uniocular in 90% of cases.
- The most common cause of bilateral amblyopia is uncorrected or partially corrected myopia.
- Amblyopia is sometimes confused with suppression.
- Amblyopia, if not treated before 8 years, becomes permanent.
- An amblyopic eye is not a blind eye.
- Vision loss due to amblyopia is only two to three lines on the Snellen chart, i.e., 6/12–6/18.
- Parents may not have knowledge of amblyopia in a straight eye.
- Strabismic amblyopic children report earlier due to obvious cosmetic blemishes.
- The difference of two lines in the Snellen chart or three log MAR, or two octaves is diagnostic. The eye with less vision is amblyopic.
- Amblyopic eyes can be picked up by a simple Bruckner's test (Bruckner).

Bruckner's Test

This is a simple procedure to master that should be used more often than at present. It may be called a modified distant direct ophthalmoscopy. It is used as a screening method in the office to detect strabismus and amblyopia in nonverbal infants and toddlers who do not cooperate for other methods of examination.

The only instrument required is a direct ophthalmoscope with medium illumination. There is no need to dilate the pupil. The infant should be awake because a pupil in sleep is smaller than an undilated normal pupil. The aperture of the ophthalmoscope is put at maximum without any lens in the peep hole.

The light of the ophthalmoscope is put on and held about a meter from the face of the child. The spot of light should be large enough to cover both pupils simultaneously. It is better to focus the iris in each eye.

The corneal reflex is located in relation to the limbus, as in the Hirschberg test. A decentered corneal reflex denotes a manifest squint.

Then attention is moved to the pink reflex in the pupil. Asymmetry in the brightness means a positive test. The squinting eye has a brighter reflex. The test can detect microtropia as well.

The eye with a brighter reflex may have amblyopia. It is not a very effective test in straight-eye amblyopia. As the light entering the pupil is parallel, it can pick up ametropia and white reflex in the pupillary is:

- *Crowding phenomenon:* To test the crowding phenomenon, vision is recorded in both eyes separately. Obviously, the amblyopic eye has less vision than the best-corrected vision in the other eye. It will be observed that the child is more comfortable when single optotypes are pointed in isolation to the amblyopic eye but are unable to recognize the letter of the same size from the same distance when asked to read the letters in a line.

- *Vision with a neutral density filter:* When a neutral density filter is put in front of a nonamblyopic eye with the best correction, the vision drops by one to two lines. In the case of amblyopic eyes, the vision remains unchanged or may improve by one to two lines. This happens because an amblyopic eye has better scotopic (peripheral) vision than a nonamblyopic eye.
- An amblyopic eye may have eccentric vision.
- An amblyopic strabismic eye may have subnormal movement.
- Color vision in amblyopia is normal.
- The dark adaptation is well developed.
- Contrast sensitivity is poor.
- There may be a relative afferent pupillary defect.
- Nystagmus, when present, is latent.
- Ametropic amblyopia may have poor near vision.
- Strabismic amblyopia may be accompanied by ametropia.

Examination of Suppression by a Worth-Four-Dot Test

The patient sits at a distance of 6 meters from the worth-four-dot panel. The panel has four circular, translucent colored discs against a dark background. The panel can be illuminated from behind. One of them is white, two are green, and the remaining one is red **(Fig. 26.1)**.

Some panels have two reds and one green. The patient is tested with best corrected vision. Both eyes are kept open during the examination. The patient wears red green goggles with red in front of the right eye and looks at the illuminated panel. He is asked to tell the numbers and color of the spots seen.

- If the patient sees all four spots, he has normal fusion and no suppression.
- Sees two reds; he has suppression of the left eye.

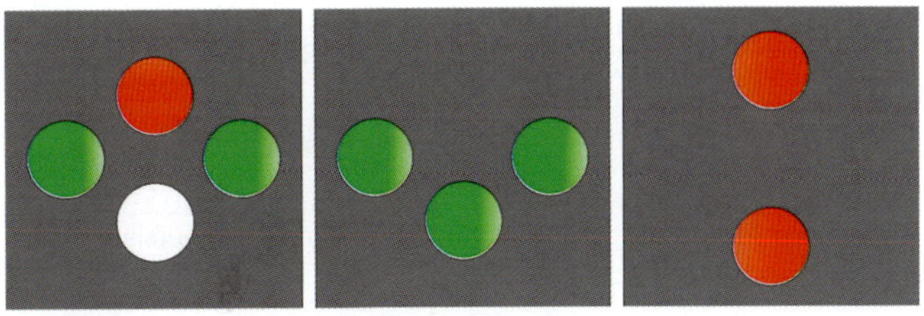

Fig. 26.1: Test for suppression on the worth-four-dot test.

- If he sees three green discs, he has suppression in right eye.
- If the patient sees that the red and green lights alternate, he has alternate suppression.

Clinical Features of Strabismic Amblyopia

- The child has an obvious squint, or microtropia.
- The child habitually fixes it with one eye.
- Children with alternate fixations do not develop amblyopia.
- Children with esotropia develop amblyopia early and deep.
- Congenital esotropia have cross-fixation, so they generally do not develop amblyopia.
- Vertical deviations are less prone to develop amblyopia because of their compensatory head posture.

Crossfixators and hypertropes are almost immune to amblyopia.

- Children with microtropia, in spite of small deviations, have more amblyopia than large-angle squints.
- The incidence of amblyopia is more in strabismic patients than in pure ametropic.
- There is no direct relation between the degree of squint and amblyopia.
- The depth of amblyopia is more duration-oriented than the age of onset.
- Earlier the squint develops deeper is the amblyopia.
- Deeps amblyopias are accompanied by more subnormal vision and are difficult to treat.

Suppression in all cases of amblyopia is at the level of the cortex.

Clinical Features of Ametropic (Straight-eyed) Amblyopia

- It is less common than strabismic amblyopia.
- Parents may not be aware of it, hence the late diagnosis.
- If both eyes have a high error of refraction, they may have difficulty in school due to amblyopia.
- *It is seen in various types of errors:*
  - No significant error
  - Both eyes have an equal but high error of refraction (isometropia).
  - One eye has an error of refraction; the other in normal.
  - One eye has more error than the other (anisometropia).

   - Both eyes have errors of refraction of different types (one myopic, the other hypermetropic).
   - Anisohypermetropia produces more amblyopia than anisomyopia.
   - One to two diopters of hypermetropic anisometropia is sufficient to cause amblyopia in contrast to anisomyopia of 3–4 D.
   - Uncorrected high errors of refraction cause bilateral amblyopia.
- The eyes have fairly good binocular function.
- Stereopsis is good.
- There is no known relation between the degree of anisometropia and the depth of amblyopia.
- Unilateral, uncorrected hypermetropia is likely to end as strabismic amblyopia.

DIAGNOSIS

Diagnosis of amblyopia is not difficult in strabismic amblyopia. In fact, in all cases of squint, amblyopia should be looked for and, when present, should be treated before the management of the squint is planned.

To diagnose amblyopia, the following steps are taken:
- Test the vision in both eyes separately
- *Note:* Best corrected vision
- *Test for:*
   - Vision with a neutral density filter
   - Crowding phenomenon
   - Bruckner's test
   - Refraction under cycloplegia
   - Test for suppression
   - Fundus examination

TREATMENT

Management of amblyopia is encouraging if:
- If diagnosed early
- Treatment is started early.
- Treatment is continued for sufficient time under supervision.
- Treatment is continued until the vision in both eyes is equal.
- Regular follow-up until the child is 7 years old.

This protocol should be preceded by counseling the parents.

The parents cannot comprehend the far-reaching effect of amblyopia in a straight amblyopic eye. All they are interested in is the improvement of vision in ametropia.

Parents of children with strabismic amblyopia are more interested in cosmetic correction than amblyopia.

It should be emphasized to them that the success of treatment depends on their cooperation.

The first step in the management of amblyopia is to remove obstructions like ptosis and cataracts.

All cases of amblyopia should be refracted under cycloplegia, and the child is prescribed the best possible correction as per retinoscopy, with special attention to astigmatism.

Small children may not cooperate in finding the exact amount and degree of astigmatism. Astigmatism correction in such children may be checked on autorefraction.

This should be followed by occlusion.

> Occlusion should proceed with squint correction and be followed if necessary.

Occlusion is the gold standard of treatment for amblyopia.

Unilateral, prolonged occlusion alone is no more practiced.

There are many methods and modifications of occlusion in vogue. The best results have been reported with complete and constant occlusion, the duration of which depends on the age of the child.

Flowchart 26.1 shows outline of management of amblyopia.

Table 26.1 gives the common question asked about occlusion.

Flowchart 26.1: Management of amblyopia.

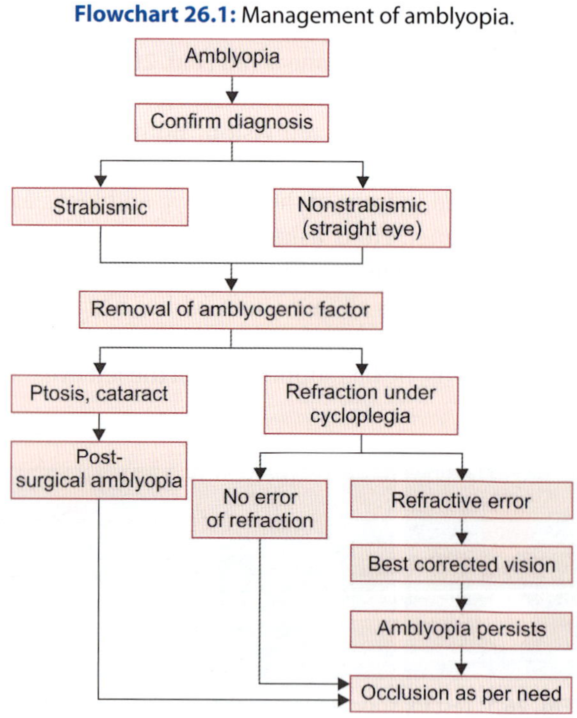

TABLE 26.1: Common questions about occlusion.

Problem	*Suggestion*
1. When to start occlusion	As soon as amblyopia is confirmed
2. How long should the occlusion be continued?	Till vision, both eyes have been equalized
3. When should occlusion be given up?	After 3–4 months, if there is no improvement in vision
4. What type of occluder should be used?	Complete and constant, the best occluders are patches fixed to the skin 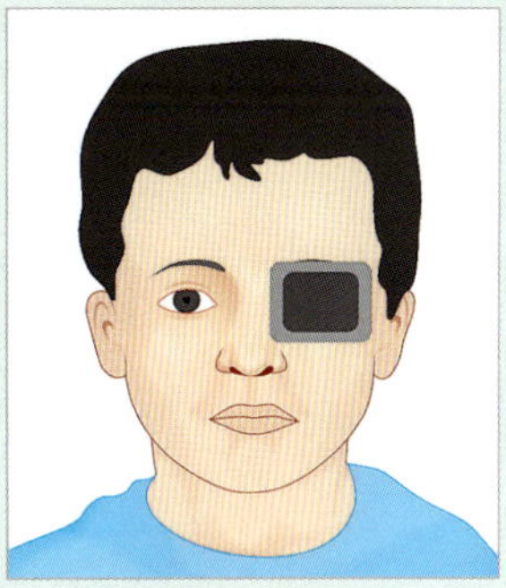 Patch occluder
5. What other occluders are available?	i. Spectacle mounted: • Doyens occluder 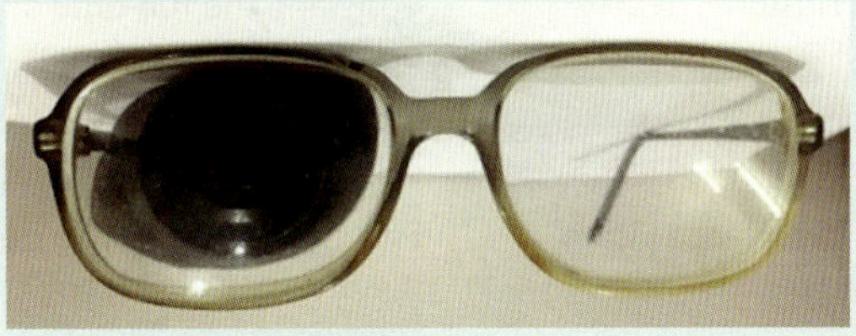 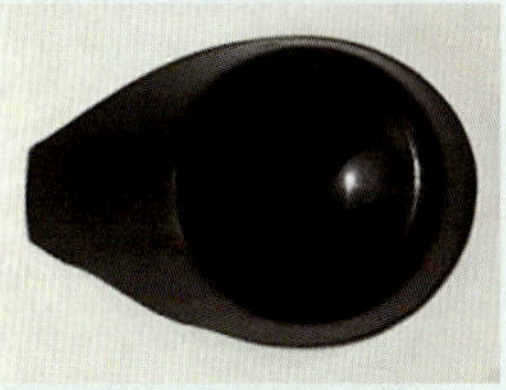 • Ground-glass occluder 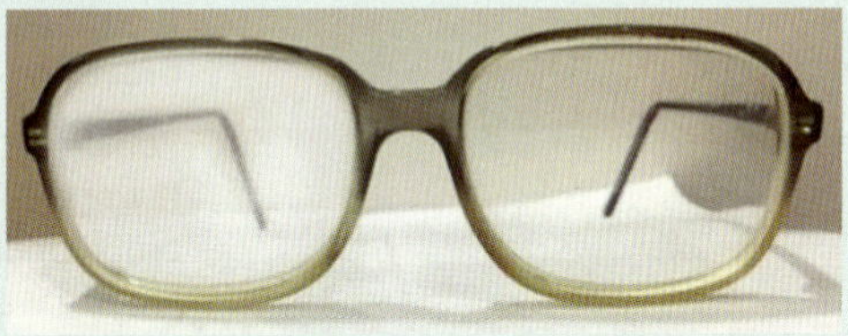 • Opaque occluder 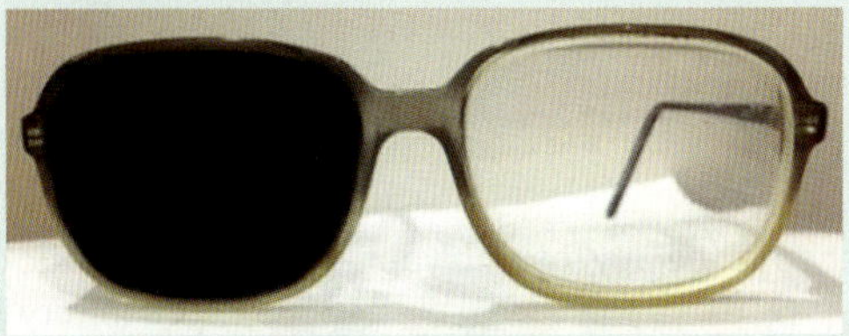 The disadvantage of spectacle-mounted occluders is that the child may peek over the occluder, negating the effect of occlusion ii. Opaque contact lens
6. What should be the gap between visits after occlusion has been started?	It depends on the age of the child; a child under 1 year should be examined every week, while a child over 4 years old may be examined every month

Contd...

Contd…

Problem	***Suggestion***
7. Is there any rule of thumb for the duration of occlusion?	The duration of occlusion is very personalized, but the rule generally followed is 1 week for each year of age
8. What should be looked for during visits?	Vision should be noted in both eyes under the same condition, i.e., the same Snellen chart at the same distance with the same illumination, if possible, by the same person. It is better to note vision on an E or C chart because a child aged 4–5 years may memorize the letters. The other trick is to ask the child to read from right to left instead of usual left to right
9. Are there any chances of vision sliding down to the preocclusion level?	This is possible up to the age of 8–9 years
10. What is occlusion amblyopia?	• It is an uncommon paradoxical state of diminished vision developing in an occluded eye • This generally develops in strabismic amblyopia of early onset, generally following complete prolonged occlusion; however, it can occur even in the early days of complete occlusion. The best method to prevent it is constant monitoring of vision in both eyes during visits. The other suggested method is to occlude the normal eye for a few hours each day; this is supposed to be effective up to 6 years of age. The best treatment is an early diagnosis
11. What are the methods to improve retained vision through occlusion?	This can be done by part-time occlusion of the better eye for up to 8–9 years
12. What is conventional occlusion?	Constant and full-time occlusion of the better eye is called conventional occlusion
13. What is inverse occlusion?	Intermittent occlusion of the nonamblyopic eye in-between conventional occlusions of the amblyopic eye
14. Are there any methods to enhance vision in amblyopic eyes during patching of nonamblyopic eyes?	Encouraging a child to do extra work near worklike. Threading beads, tracing pictures, plying jigsaw puzzles, and playing video games. They have been claimed to be effective
15. Are there methods other than occlusion in the treatment of amblyopia?	They consist of penalization, CAM vision stimulators, pleoptics, a red filter, and the therapeutic use of levodopa. Except for penalization, the rest have not proved to be effective
16. What is penalization?	Penalization is a nonoptical method of reducing vision in the better eye. It works best in hypermetropic eyes in children with mild to moderate amblyopia. In this process, 1% atropine ointment is put in the better eye twice a week. The advantage of the method is that it is cosmetically better accepted than occlusion. The disadvantage is glare and diminished near vision; the child may be allergic to atropine; and some children may develop toxic reactions
17. What is inverse occlusion?	Inverse occlusion is occluding the amblyopic eye in contrast to usual practice of occluding the better eye. This based on presumption that it improved binocular vision
18. What is dichoptic therapy for amblyopia? 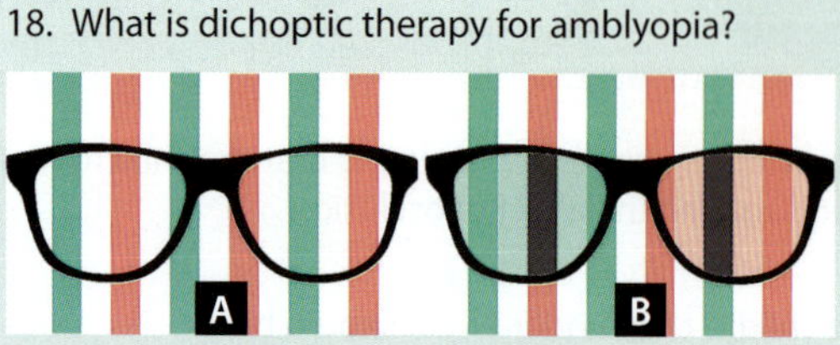 A: Strip seen through white glasses B: Strip seen through dichoptic glasses	Dichoptic treatment of amblyopia improves binocular vision by reducing inhibitory interactions at the level of the visual cortex. In this, the stimulus presented in two eyes is different. The test consists of—the child puts on a spectacle with one red and other green plane glass and looks at a chart with alternate red and green stripes of the same width with a white stripe in between the two colors. The procedure is based on the principle of diplopia glasses, where the red stripe is seen through the red glass and the green stripe through the green glass

SUGGESTED READING

1. Adams GGW, Timms C. Amblyopia. In: Jackson TL (Ed). Moorfields Manual of Ophthalmology, 3rd edition. New Delhi: Jaypee Brothers Medical Publisher; 2020. pp. 659-60.
2. All India Ophthalmological Society. (2017). All India Ophthalmological Society Guidelines, National, Expert-Based Consensus Statement Regarding Paediatric Eye Examination, Refraction, and Amblyopia Management, AIOS Focus Group Meeting, 22nd October, 2017. [online] Available from https://boamumbai.com/wp-content/uploads/2023/12/Paedamblopia.pdf. [Last accessed March, 2025]
3. Anstice NS, Thompson B. The measurement of visual acuity in children: an evidence-based update. Clin Exp Optom. 2014;97:3-11.
4. Dadeya S, Kaur S. (2021). Basic Examination of Strabismus, Delhi Ophthalmic Society (D.O.S.). [online] Available from https://www.researchgate.net/publication/349348910_Basic_Examination_of_Strabismus. [Last accessed March, 2025]
5. Dadeya S, Khurana C. (2009). Diagnosis and Treatment of Childhood Amblyopia, AIOS CME Series 18. [online] Available from https://www.aios.org/cme/cmeseries18.pdf. [Last accessed March, 2025]
6. Ghauri AJ, Abbott J, Lucilla B. Amblyopia. In: Denniston AKO, Murray PI (Eds). Oxford Handbook of Ophthalmology, 4th edition. London: Oxford University Press; 2018. pp. 868-9.
7. Mukherjee PK. Clinical Examination in Ophthalmology, 2nd edition. New Delhi: Elsevier; 2016.
8. Mukherjee PK. Manual of Optics and Refraction. New Delhi: Jaypee Brothers Medical Publisher; 2015.
9. Mukherjee PK. Ophthalmic Assistant, 1st edition. New Delhi: Jaypee Brothers Medical Publisher; 2013.
10. Mukherjee PK. Paediatric Ophthalmology, 1st edition. New Delhi: New Age International; 2005.
11. Pavan-Langston D, Azar N. Treatment of Amblyopia. In: Pavan-Langston D (Ed). Manual of Ocular Diagnosis and Therapy, 6th edition. Philadelphia: Wolters Kluwer; 2008.
12. Pediatric Eye Disease Investigator Group; Repka MX, Kraker RT, Dean TW, Beck RW, Siatkowski RM, et al. A randomized trial of levodopa as treatment for residual amblyopia in older children. Ophthalmology. 2015; 122(5):874-81.
13. Prager TC, Zou YL, Jensen CL, Fraley JK, Anderson RE, Heird WC. Evaluation of methods for assessing visual function of infants. J AAPOS. 1999;3:275-82.
14. Saxena R, Sharma P; Paediatric Ophthalmology Expert Group. National consensus statement regarding paediatric eye examination, refraction, and amblyopia management. Indian J Ophthalmol. 2020;68:325-32.
15. Sharma P. Strabismus Simplified, 1st edition. New Delhi: Modern Publisher; 1999.
16. Suttle CM. Visual acuity assessment in infants and young children. Clin Exp Optom. 2001;84:337-45.
17. Vijayalakshmi P. Strabismus (Squint) and Amblyopia. Paediatric Ophthalmology: A Practitioners' Guide. Madurai: Aravind Eye Hospitals and Postgraduate Institute of Ophthalmology;
18. Vimla M. Guideline for treatment of amblyopia and various modalities available for the same. In: Ramamurthy D (Ed). Ready Reckoner in Ophthalmology, under the aegis of AIOS. New Delhi: Jaypee Brothers Medical Publisher; 2010.

CHAPTER 27

Anesthesia in Pediatric Ophthalmology

Jaya Lalwani

> The secret to success in anesthesia in all ages lies in paying utmost attention to details.

Most ocular surgeries in adults are done under topical or infiltration anesthesia or a combination of both, unless the patient desires or requires otherwise.

Short-term surgical procedures can be done under topical anesthesia in children in the second decade with little persuasion and counseling. Some of them may cooperate with infiltration anesthesia as well.

It should be kept in mind that a child is not a compressed adult. Their therapeutic requirements are different from adults. The anatomy and physiology in children are different from adults, so are drug doses and tolerance. This is true for all branches of medicine; anesthesia being not an exception. The management of childhood anesthesia depends on consideration of pediatric anatomy, physiology, altered pharmacology and psychology of the child. The role of parents cannot be underestimated. Ocular anesthesia in children can be broadly divided into the following categories:

- Topical
- Infiltration
- Combination of the above two
- General

> Ophthalmologists should refrain from administrating general anesthesia in any form in all ages.

Pediatric ocular anesthesia should preferably be administered by an anesthetist well versed with pediatric variables. The children require specially designed laryngoscopes and tubes as per size and not age of the child. The high risk of complications and mortality should be kept in mind. Complications are more common in underweights and prematures.

Preterms obey no laws of physics. Abnormalities are more in gestation between 25 and 30 weeks. The candidates for pediatric ophthalmic anesthesia can be broadly divided into two groups as per priority:

- Planned surgeries
- Emergency surgeries

Both types of surgeries can be divided into two groups anticipating the time required to complete the surgical procedure.

They are:

- Short-term procedures
- Long-term procedures

The procedures belong to the first group are:

- Syringing of lacrimal passage
- Probing of lacrimal passage
- Measurement of corneal diameter
- Recording of the IOP
- Detailed examination of the cornea by hand-held slit lamp
- Removal of foreign bodies
- Refraction by streak retinoscopy
- Removal of sutures
- Adjusting sutures
- Gonioscopy
- Ultrasonography
- Keratometry for the calculation of intraocular lens (IOL) power
- Detailed examination of the fundus by indirect ophthalmoscopy
- Laser capsulotomy for posterior capsule opacification (PCO)
- Biopsy of conjunctiva
- CT and MRI
- Intra-arterial chemotherapy

To the second group belong following surgical procedures:

- All oculoplasty surgeries
- Keratoplasty
- All surgeries on the lens, with or without IOL
- All glaucoma surgeries
- Squint surgeries
- Retinal detachment surgeries
- Vitrectomy
- Enucleation and evisceration

Before starting anesthesia, the operating surgeon should:

- Identify the child
- Mark the eye to be operated
- Recheck the above two
- Confirm the surgery to be performed

The surgeon should inform the anesthetist before:

- Injecting fluid in nasolacrimal duct
- Using diathermy and cautery

The anesthetic procedure starts with:

- Preanesthetic check by anesthetist backed by neonatologist/pediatrician and some pathological tests, especially urine examination for reducing substance, amino acid, and level of hemoglobin
- This is followed by counseling the parents regarding the procedure, the duration of anesthesia, and talking to the child above 5 about surgery. This calms the child.
- Anesthetists should enquire about:
    - Gestation period of the child at the time of birth; premature children even years after birth remain at poor-anesthetic risk.
    - History of congenital infections, especially rubella, should be noted and required precautions taken.
    - History of allergy
    - History of recent upper respiratory infections should be taken. Children with upper respiratory infections are better off not being exposed to planned surgery.
    - History of recent and prolonged medication, especially steroids, should be noted.
    - History of asthma should get appropriate treatment.
    - History of bleeding disorder should be managed well in advance.
    - Past history of complications during and following surgery under general anesthesia in the child, parents, and siblings noted.
- An informed consent as per practice should be obtained, both for anesthesia and surgery.

The real procedure is divided into:

Preanesthetic fasting: The risk of swallowing regurgitated material is present in one in ten thousand children undergoing general anesthesia, both long and short. This is partially eliminated by keeping the child starved before induction. Each institution has its own protocol. The general outline defers for fluids and solids. The outlines consist of clear fluids like tea, fruit juice, and sugary drinks can be allowed up to 2 hours before anesthesia.

Breast milk and top milk is restricted until 4 hours before anesthesia. Semisolid is restricted 8 hours before.

Administration of preoperative and intraoperative antibiotics is managed by the operating surgeon. Many surgeries require good mydriasis that should be obtained by parasympatholytic drugs like atropine, home atropine, cyclopentolate, and tropicamide, alone or in combination. The strength of a sympathomimetic drug like phenylephrine should not exceed 2.5%.

Preanesthetic sedation:

The best preanesthetic medicine is:

- Proper counseling
- The aim of preanesthetic medication is:
    - To calm the child
    - To let the child allow smooth induction
    - Child awakens after surgery in a short time.
    - Has less bucking, coughing, and vomiting in the postoperative period
- In the past, many drugs have been used, some simple hypnotics, others antihistamines or anxiolytics, singly or in combination, orally or intramuscular. Infants do not require preanesthetic medications. Older children and adolescents may be nervous or even jittery. The common drugs used as preanesthetic sedations are:
    - Midazolam
    - Alprazolam
    - Diazepam
    - Dexmedetomidine
    - Ketamine
    - Clonidine

Out of the above, the most frequently used drug is midazolam. It is considered to be the best that can be used even in neonates. It is used in children before a procedure without anesthesia or as a preanesthetic medication, causes drowsiness, reduces anxiety the child does not remember the details of the procedure. It is administered orally in doses of 0.5–0.75 mg/kg. It has a rapid onset that reaches its peak in 30 minutes. It does not interfere with cardiorespiratory function.

Ketamine: This is an anesthetic agent designated as dissociative anesthesia used at the beginning of general anesthesia and to maintain it. It actually does not cause hypnosis but a state of trance unless administered intravenous. It is an analgesic as well as an antidepressant. The greatest disadvantage of the drug is that it is a hallucinogen. It can be used as an adjunct to other anesthetic agents or singly for short-term anesthesia and analgesia.

Ketamine is the only agent when used intravenous, acts as a strong hypnotic and analgesic. It is a mild bronchodilator and preserves the airway reflex. As a preanesthetic agent, ketamine can be given orally as well as injection in a dose of 1–2 mg/kg intravenous (4–8 mg/kg intramuscular) for children between 1 and 6 years. A combination of oral midazolam and ketamine in a 1:1 ratio is better than each used singly. Midazolam, when used in combination with ketamine, reduces the chances of hallucinations and nightmares and helps the child to forget the surgical processor. It is contraindicated in patients with increased intraocular pressure and open globe injuries.

Etomidate: It is a new drug for short-acting IV anesthesia to induce general anesthesia and sedation for short procedures like tracheal intubation, paracentesis of AC, removal of foreign body, and sutures.

Clonidine: It is basically a centrally acting alpha-agonist with multiple diverse therapeutic uses, including hypertension in adults and attention-deficient hyperactivity in children.

As preanesthetic sedative, it is used in dose of 4 µg/kg. It reduces dose of main anesthetic agent. It has a slower onset as compared to midazolam. It reduces intraoperative bleeding and postoperative pain. It is an anxiolytic as well. It takes about an hour to be effective.

Dexmedetomidine: It is also a centrally acting alpha-agonist. It is anxiolytic, sedative, and analgesic without respiratory depression. It increases anesthetic effect of all anesthetic agents, irrespective of the route of administration.

The anesthetic sedatives can be used via various routes, i.e., oral, intramuscular, and intravenous; they can even be used intranasal, sublingual, or rectal.

Preanesthetic secreto-suppressants: They are anticholinergic drugs. The drugs are bronchodilators, reduce saliva and secretion, and modulate heart rate. The two commonly used drugs are atropine and glycopyrrolate. Both can be used intramuscular or intravenous. These drugs have no anesthetic potential. They are neither sedatives nor analgesics. The main purpose of their use is to decrease secretion and facilitate intubation. Glycopyrrolate is 5–6 times more potent than atropine as an antisialogogues, which exhibits a selective, prolonged effect on salivary secretion in the sweat gland. Glycopyrrolate per se has minimal cardiovascular, central nervous system (CNS), and ocular side effects.

The dose of preanesthetic sedatives and cholinergic drugs should be decided by anesthetist.

The actual induction of anesthetic agents can be:
- Inhalation
- Intubation

The two commonly used drugs prior to intubation are:
1. Pentothal
2. Propofol

1. *Pentothal* can itself be used as a short-term anesthetic or to facilitate endotracheal intubation.
2. *Propofol* is a sedative-hypnotic agent used as a general anesthetic drug and to maintain general anesthesia. Propofol induces sleep before actual induction and maintains the level of general anesthesia; it can be used in infants as old as 2 months.

The anesthesia can be administered in two ways, i.e.:
1. Inhalation
2. Intravenous
3. Intramuscular

The most commonly used drugs for inhalation are:
- *Halothane (fluothane):* Used to start and maintain anesthesia
- Sevoflurane
- Isoflurane
- Desflurane
- Nitrous oxide

The commonly used drugs for endotracheal intubation are: Etomidate, ketamine, and propofol. Commonly used neuromuscular blocking agents for the same purpose are succinylcholine and rocuronium.

Paradigm of anesthetic procedures in children for ophthalmic surgery: Different institutions have their own protocols of administering anesthesia.

The following passage gives steps of anesthesia in children. Preanesthetic checkups—counseling parents—informed consent of parents—speaking to the child above 10 years—dilatation of pupil—preoperative antibiotic drops—preanesthetic sedation—injection of secreto-suppressant (atropine/glycopyrrolate)—IV pentothal/propofol—IV succinylcholine (succinylcholine is the best muscle relaxant. However, it should be better avoided in strabismus and ptosis surgery)—inhalation/intubation—monitoring during surgery—extubation—postanesthetic recovery

Endotracheal versus laryngeal mask airway: Although endotracheal anesthesia is more suitable for children at risk of aspiration, the laryngeal mask airway has been developed and accepted as a means to secure the airway without risk of aspiration. Laryngeal mask airway is safe and effective in such condition; it causes less rise of intraocular pressure that is common with endotracheal anesthesia during intubation and extubation. Other advantages of a laryngeal mask airway are: It is less invasive, causes minimal injury to the airway, and causes less laryngospasm and bronchospasm. The laryngeal mask airway is an advanced airway alternative to endotracheal intubation, with all the functions of the endotracheal tube retained. The laryngeal mask airway is put in the pharynx to provide ventilation, oxygenation, and the administration of anesthetic gases. Causes less bucking and coughing during recovery.

Some of the advantages attributed to endotracheal intubation are:

- It maintains the airway
- Ventilation is controlled
- No gastric bloating
- No gastric aspiration
- Works on a lighter depth of anesthesia
- Offers ease of removable of secretion

Anesthesia can be induced by the following methods:

- Inhalation induction
- Intravenous induction

- *Inhalation induction:* It is suitable for children of all ages following premedication. In the process, the concentration of inhaled anesthetic can be controlled to produce a smooth transition from awakeness to anesthesia. Once the child loses consciousness, ventilation is maintained manually. The drugs used are listed above.
- *Intravenous induction: It* is a fast technique of induction. If the child is still jittery, 50–70% nitrous oxide can be used to facilitate setting the intravenous line. The mode of action of nitrous oxide as an anesthetic agent is not well understood; it is the oldest and most frequently used gas in anesthesia, and it is generally supplemented by thiopental, halothanes, and diazepam. At the end of nitrous oxide anesthesia, oxygen is mandatory to flush out retained nitrous oxide, besides being an anesthetic agent. It is an analgesic as well, most probably acting at the level of the pain center in the brain.

Propofol is a short-action barbiturate used in the induction maintenance of anesthesia and sedation in children during anesthesia, administered intravenously. It decreases conciseness and memory. The next drug used in intravenous induction is sodium thiopental, which is an ultra-short barbiturate marketed as pentothal.

Some of the uncommon but serious complications of general anesthesia in children are—oculocardiac reflex, hypothermia, malignant hyperthermia, unexpected dehydration, and subglottis edema.

RECOVERY FROM ANESTHESIA

The surgeon should inform the anesthetist a few minutes before completion of the surgery for a smooth recovery from anesthesia. The surgeon should keep the cornea of the other eye wet and lubricated by putting an antibiotic ointment in the nonoperated eye during the surgery and after. Once the anesthesia is over, the head of the child should be turned to one side; this prevents aspiration. The child is kept under observation in the recovery room until he is out of anesthesia. The child may be drowsy for some time after he recovers from anesthesia. The child is generally kept in the ward for the next 24 hours; during this time, he is encouraged to drink liquid and semi-solid food. Generally, there is no need to restrict his movement. Postanesthetic vomiting is managed as per the protocol of the hospital.

SUGGESTED READING

1. Cibis GW. Evaluation under anaesthesia. Decision Making in Paediatric Ophthalmology. St. Louis, Missouri: Mosby; 1993.
2. Danas MH. Anaesthesia for paediatric patient for surgery of eye. In: Harley RD (Ed). Paediatric Ophthalmology, Volume 2, 2nd edition. Philadelphia: WB Saunders Company; 1983.
3. Mestad PH. Anaesthesia in Decision Making. In: Cibis GW, Tongue AC, Stass-Isrn ML (Eds). Paediatric Ophthalmology. St. Louis, Missouri: Mosby; 1993.
4. Vohra SB, Mathewson P, Denniston AKO, Murray PI. Surgery: Anaesthetics and perioperative care. In: Denniston AKO, Murray PI (Eds). Oxford Handbook of Ophthalmology, 4th edition. London: Oxford University Press; 2018. pp. 1040-7.

CHAPTER

28 Basic Genetics in Ophthalmology

With the ever-increasing scope of genetic engineering and gene therapy, the study of genetics has become more routine teaching in ophthalmology; hence, it is imperative for all ophthalmologists that they must have basic knowledge of the genetics of ocular diseases. Genetics is commonly discussed in every disease, with the exception of infection and trauma. It is needed for a clinician to be competent to have knowledge of some disorders that run in families. The genetic disorders of the eye can involve the eyes only or may be associated with systemic disorders.

> Systemic genetic disorders associated with the ocular component are generally severe, serious, and even fatal.

Genetic disorders of the eye can be:

- *Congenital anomalies:*
  - Ocular
  - Ocular with systemic involvement
- *Dystrophies:* They themselves are congenital. May not be apparent at birth.
- Malignancies retinoblastoma

Trauma and infectious diseases cannot be correlated to genetic anomalies.

Much study of human genetics has been done in ophthalmology because the eye is an ideal model to study genetics and the disorders are apparent on routine examination. However, some conditions may require specific tests to confirm their existence.

Due to some unexplained factors, the eyes are more prone to suffer from genetic disorders than other organs. By and large, the ophthalmologist should be able to predict the risk of many genetic disorders, which may be common or rare, not only to reach a precise diagnosis but also to predict:

- Prognosis
- Fatality
- Possibility of passing in the following generation

The rare diseases are generally severe (blinding/fatal). To be able to have basic knowledge of ophthalmic genetics, the clinician should be:

- Well versed with standard terminology
- Understand symbols
- Draw pedigree chart
- Able to decipher the pedigree chart

To reach a definite genetic pattern, the following steps should be taken:

- *History:* Was the anomaly present at birth or manifested latter?
- *Family history:* Is there a history of the same disease among:
  - Parents
  - One of the parents
  - Sex of the affected parent
  - Grandparents (paternal/maternal)
  - Siblings
  - First cousins
- Consanguinity

> In the absence of family history, the condition is called sporadic.

> Genetic disorders are transmitted by spouses but not shared among themselves.

Terms commonly used in genetics:

- *Heredity:* Passing on physical and mental characteristics from one generation to another
- *Generation:* A group of living organisms from ancestors during the same period. The average period of time between the births of parents to birth of offspring is considered for calculating a generation. Generally, a mother's lifespan is given weightage.
- *Gene:* It is a basic unit, both physical and functional. It is made up of a self-replication sequence of DNA (deoxyribonucleic acid) nucleotides.
- *Genealogy:* It is the study of a family, tracing their history and lineage.

- *DNA and RNA*:
  - *DNA* is a strand of deoxyribonucleic acid. It is a code. It determines the characteristics of living organisms. It is a molecule of two chains made up of nucleotides wrapped around each other that forms a double helix carrying genetic instructions. Each nucleotide has the following substances: sugar, phosphate, and nitrogen. The DNA in the cell nucleus is called nuclear DNA. DNA in mitochondria is called mitochondrial DNA.
  - *RNA* is a single-stranded molecule. As against DNA, which is a double-stranded nucleus, DNA is self-replicating, while RNA cannot replicate on its own. RNA is found in the nucleus and cytoplasm. RNA is synthesized from DNA. *All living* organisms have both DNA and RNA. A virus has either DNA or RNΛ, but not both.
- *Mitochondria:* These are visible under a light microscope. They can replicate themselves, and they contain DNA, RNA, and enzymes. They can synthesize their own protein. The mitochondria are located in the cytoplasm of the cell and are responsible for the energy of the cell and its metabolism.
- *Chromosome:* A chromosome is a strand of DNA. The DNA in chromosomes contains genetic properties. The number of chromosomes is constant for each species. Cells with a pair of homologous chromosomes are called diploid, in contrast to haploid that have only one set. For human species, the diploid number is 46, or 23 pairs. The gametes contain 23 chromosomes out of which 1 is the sex chromosome and the rest are called autosomes.
- *Gamete:* It is a mature haploid (male or female germ cell) that can join another of the opposite sex. The united product is zygote.
- *Zygote (joined/yoked):* It is a byproduct cell following fertilization between two gametes.
- *Genome:* The genome of a zygote is a combination of DNA in each gamete, containing all the genetic information in a new individual in the form of eukaryotic cells.
- *Eukaryotic:* It means a true nucleus. They contain a specialized structure called organelles.
- *Organelles:* They are membrane-bound structures called Golgi bodies and mitochondria.
- *Golgi bodies:* The Golgi bodies are a cluster of flattened vesicles associated with the endoplasmic reticulum. The Golgi bodies produce lysozyme.
- *Autosome:* The chromosomes other than sex chromosomes are called autosomes.
- *Sex chromosomes:* Either the X or Y chromosome. At fertilization, the chromosome from the sperm and ovum meet to result a zygote, that latter develops in an embryo. The sex chromosome of ovum is always X but male sex chromosome can be either by X or Y.

During fertilization, the male chromosome may contribute either X or Y to the female sex chromosome; thus, the embryo may have either XY or XX chromosomes but never YY.

The embryo with XX will produce a female, and XY will result in male offspring **(Fig. 28.1)**.

X chromosomes carry more genetic material than *Y*.

All chromosomes are:

- *Not of the same size and shape*
- *All chromosomes exist in pairs.*
- *Chromosomes are two strands joined together.*
- *The junction is known as centromere.*
- *The centromere divides the chromosome into two parts, one longer than the other. The long part is labeled "q" while the other "p"* **(Fig. 28.2)**.

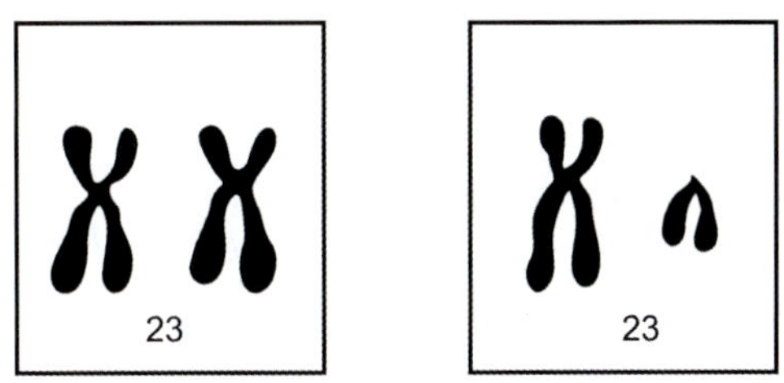

Female Male

Fig. 28.1: Male and female chromosomes.

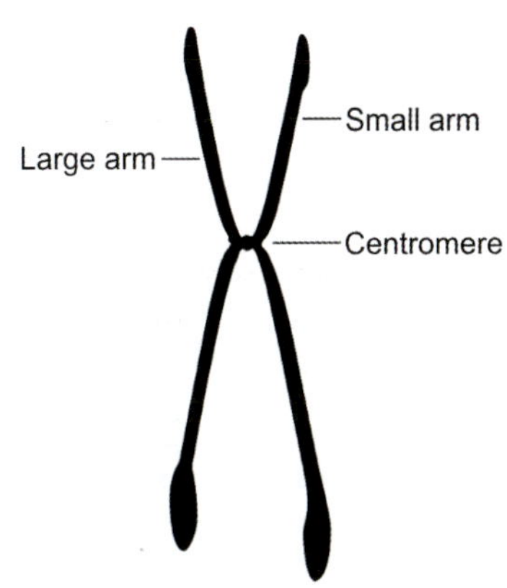

Fig. 28.2: Position of centromere in a typical chromosome.

- *Staining technique of chromosomes is called banding. Chromosomes are stained deeply with basic dyes. They are better visualized during mitosis.*
- *Chromosome pairs are numbered according to size from 1 to 22. The largest pair is designated 1* **(Fig. 28.3)**.
- *X and Y are not numbered* **(Fig. 28.3)**.
  They are also put in several groups (A-G) **(Fig. 28.3)**.
- *Grouping depends upon the size and position of centromere* **(Fig. 28.2)**.
- *Homologous chromosomes are a pair of chromosomes, one from each parent that have same gene length, gene position and centromere location, i.e., same traits, one from mother and other from father.*
- *Heterologous chromosomes are chromosomes present on different loci which cannot undergo genetic recombination.*
- *Alleles:* They are alternative forms of individual genes that occupy a particular locus on a chromosome. An organism with two different alleles is called heterozygous.
- *Dominant and recessive:* It is defined as relation between alleles of one gene where the phenotype of one allele masks the role of the other, situated in the same locus. The first allele is termed dominant, and the second is recessive.

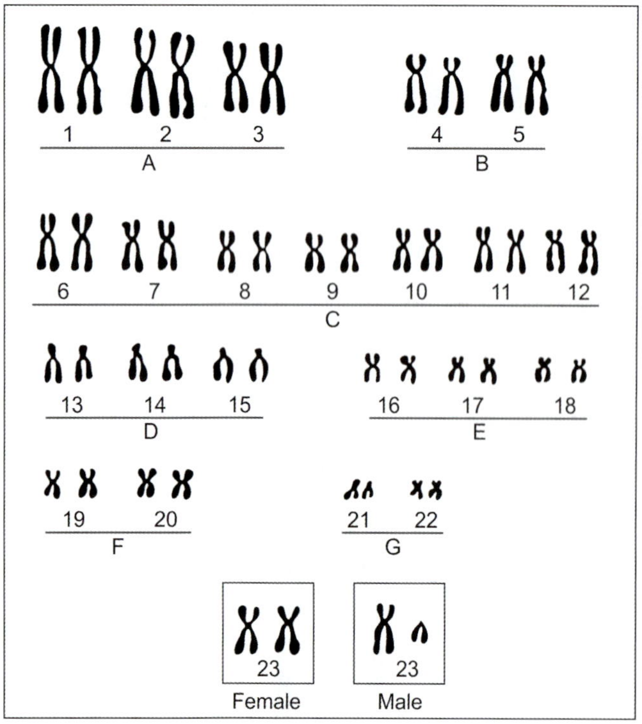

Fig. 28.3: Human chromosomes (male and female).

- *Heterozygous:* Heterozygous are two members with a particular heredity that are not the same; neither of the two allelic pairs are the same in a given gene.
- *Homozygous:* Both the genes of an allele pair are the same.
- *Genetic counseling:* It is the application of knowledge about human genetics to prospective parents about the possibility of hereditary diseases. In some straightforward cases, the ophthalmologist is able to give advice. Single-gene disorders are most accurately predicted regarding their recurrence.
- *Genetic engineering:* It is an ever-expanding specialization in the genetics of living organisms. It is the synthesis, change, repair, and replacement of genetic material by artificial means.
- *Gene therapy:* Human gene transfer is mostly in the trial stage with great therapeutic potential. In simple terms, it is the transfer of beneficial nucleic acids into the offending cell for therapeutic purposes. Some of the ocular diseases that may benefit from gene therapy are—retinitis pigmentosa, Stargardt disease, age-related macular degeneration, few uveitis, and some glaucomas.
- *Forme fruste:* An inherited disorder that is so mild that it is difficult to distinguish it from normal variation.

General information:

- The eye is an ideal model for studying *genetics.*
- Genetics is the study of *heredity* and its variation in living organisms.
- *A gene* is the basic unit of genetics.
- *Genealogy* is the continuous tracing of ancestors.
- A gene is made up of *DNA* that codes for specific proteins in nature.
- DNA is found in the cell *membrane and mitochondria.*
- Each gene has a fixed position on *the chromosome.*
- Genes are self-replicating sequences of DNA nucleotides.
- Hereditary peculiarities are controlled by a pair of genes.
- The gene pair that controls the trait is called *the allele.*
- Alleles in the gene can either be *dominant* or *recessive.*
- If both genes are the same, they are called *homozygous*; otherwise, they are called *heterozygous.*
- Offspring inheriting the same gene from both parents are homozygous. They have two identical genes inheriting.
- Inheriting one of the gene pairs is called *hemizygous.*
- The first allele is dominant, and the second allele is recessive.

- A recessive gene does not express itself, and a dominant gene expresses a *trait*.
- The gene position in a chromosome is called *the locus*.
- A gene is called *holandric* if it is located in Y chromosome. They can only be passed by *males to sons*. These are Y-linked features.
- A *hologynic* gene is passed from *mother to daughter*.
- An individual's genetic profile is called *a genotype*.
- A trait is a distinguishing feature. It is inherited when transmitted through *germ cells*.
- A *recessive trait* manifests only in *the phenotype* when both alleles are recessive.
- Genes present either *in the X or Y chromosomes* that determine sex are called *sex-linked genes*.
- The females have *homologous* genes, i.e., X-X. In males, they are *heterologous* X-Y.

Some extra terms used in genetics:

- *Penetrance:* It denotes how often hereditary features manifest. It is the proportion of individuals carrying the allele of a gene.
- *Expressibility:* It measures the extent to which a given genotype is expressed at the phenotype level.
- *Phenotype:* The phenotype shows actual physical characteristics, i.e., height of an individual, color of eye, etc. The characteristics may be directly visible or may become obvious by some specific tests, as in the blood group.
- *Genotype:* Genotype is the complete information regarding hereditary. It represents the pair of genes responsible for a particular characteristic. It is a genetic make-up, inherited from parents.

Mutation: Mutation is a random structural change in the sequence of DNA nucleotides and means the transformation to one characteristic from other due to a change in a gene capable of transmitting to offspring. It is brought about by:

- Changes in genes
- Permanent variation in genetic structure

It may be a change from parents or may be through gradual variation over generations. Mutation without clinical manifestation is called nonpenetrant. This trait is present in the genome but does not manifest itself. A trait that manifests itself is called penetrant trait. Mutation is generally with/without an obvious cause. The gene, due to mutation, occupies the same locus as in original gene. The new gene is allelic to the gene from which it has developed.

Pleiotropism: It is the multiple effects of a single mutation, as in Rieger syndrome.

Heterogeneity: Multiple genes cause a single syndrome, i.e., Marfan's syndrome.

Inheritance: The overall effect of all the traits inherited is called inheritance. This is brought about by DNA in germ cells. If a trait is inherited from one parent only, it is called alternative inheritance.

Inheritance is the process of producing new classes. The classes from which new classes originate are called base classes. The new classes are called derived classes, which have all the potential of the base class. The derived class can refine the characteristics of the base class.

Autosomal dominant disorder: Autosomal dominant disorders are caused by mutations in non-sex chromosomes carrying the autosomal gene. The person with autosomal dominant disorder has only a copy of the gene inherited from either parent with a disorder containing mutation. If one parent has the mutation and the phenotype, 50% of the offspring are likely to be affected.

Autosomal recessive disorder: A person with autosomal disorder recessive disorder should have two copies of an abnormal gene. The gene is located on one of the autosomes. Both males and females are equally affected. A person with only one recessive gene is a carrier without any clinical features and is not even aware of his/her career status unless they have an offspring with the particular disease. The chances of developing the same disease in subsequent pregnancies are one in four (25%). Males cannot be carriers because they only have one X chromosome.

Sex-linked disorders: These characteristics are controlled by genes on the sex chromosome; hence, they depend on the sex of the carrier. The disorder can be dominant or recessive. The different types of carriers are:

- *Mother carrying mutation:* The son has a 50% chance of inheriting the gene. The son will have a phenotype. The daughter has a 50% chance of inheriting the gene and will become a carrier.
- *Father carrying mutation:* The daughter has cent percent chance of getting the gene and becoming a carrier. The son will not inherit the gene.

Points to note about sex-linked disorders are:

- When the gene is located either on the X or Y chromosome (sex chromosome or allosome), the condition is called an X-linked disorder.
- X-linked inheritance can either be dominant or recessive.
- The common sex-linked recessive disorder is red-green blindness **(Flowchart 28.1)**, hemophilia A and B, ocular albinism, and some retinitis pigmentosa **(Flowchart 28.1)**.
- The disorder is more common in males.
- The mother of the affected male is the carrier.
- Half of the male offspring of the carrier mother will be affected.
- All the males sired by the affected male will be normal.
- The mother carries the mutation in sex-linked mitochondrial inheritance.

Some more terms commonly used in genetics:

- Karyo means nucleus.
- Karyocyte stands for nucleated cell.
- Eukaryotic cells have a nucleus that is surrounded by a membrane that harbors genetic material.
- Karyotype means a human chromosome lined up in pairs. This is the number and appearance of chromosomes in the nucleus of an eukaryotic cell.
- The isochromosome is a chromosome that differs from ordinary chromosomes in—form, size, or behavior. It is an abnormal metacentric chromosome. It is formed by the duplication of one arm of a normal chromosome with the other arm missing. However, both arms of the metacentric chromosome are identical. They are produced by transverse splitting of the centromere. Both arms belong to the same side. They are of the same length with similar genes, being mirror images of each other.
- Abiotrophic disease is a disease that is present at birth but does not manifest itself at birth, only to manifest later, e.g., retinitis pigmentosa.
- *Familial:* This concerns traits that run in many members of a family. The number of persons involved in more than expected in general population.
- A carrier is a person who has a hereditary characteristic that is not manifest, but the person can transmit it to the offspring.
- *Polysomy:* The organism has at least one extra chromosome, i.e., 47 instead of 46.
- *Trisomy:* It is presence of three chromosomes of the same nature instead of a normal pair. It is an example of polysomy. It could result in trisomy (8, 9, 16, and 22). The person has 47 instead of the usual 46 chromosomes.
- Monosomy is a condition of having a diploid chromosome complement in which one chromosome lacks its homologous partner.
- *Translocation:* It is exchange of DNA among chromosomes at the time of meiosis.

Flowchart 28.1: Autosomal sex-linked inheritance.

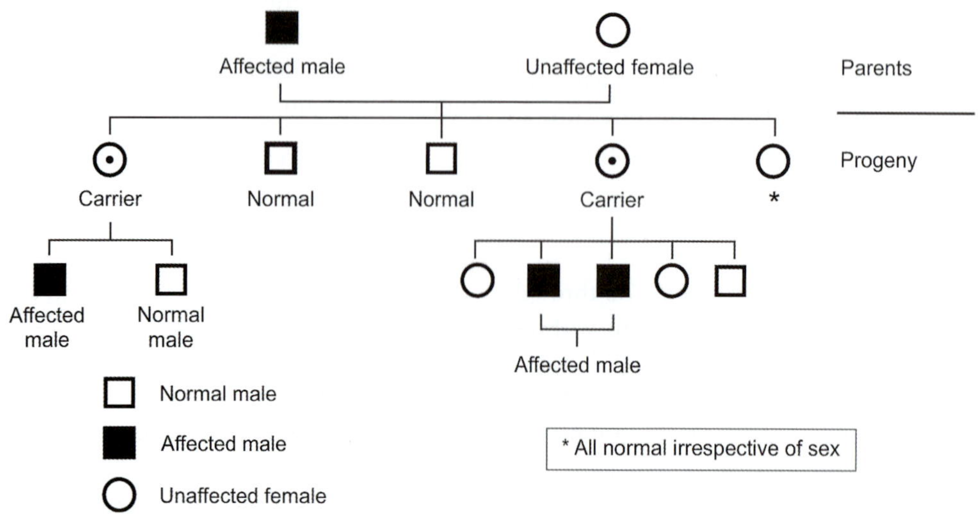

Flowchart 28.2: Common inherited disorders.

Inheritance

- **Autosomal**
  - **Dominant**
    - Aniridia
    - Anterior embryo toxon
    - Correctopia
    - Rieger's anomaly
    - Cataract (some)
    - Ectopia lentis*
    - Corneal dystrophy
    - Horizontal tropia
    - Jaw winking
    - Glaucoma (some)
    - Some retinitis pigmentosa
    - Uveal coloboma
    - Retinoblastoma (some)
    - Craniofacial anomalies
    - Alport's syndrome
    - Wardenberg's syndrome
    - Marfan's syndrome
    - Juvenille glaucoma
    - Phacomatosis
    - Congenital stationary night blindness
    - Keratoconus
  - **Recessive**
    - Aniridia
    - Anterior embryo toxon
    - Ectopia lentis*
    - Horizontal squint
    - Congenital glaucoma
    - Albinism
    - Homocystinuria
    - Alport's syndrome
- **Sex-linked**
  - **Dominant**
    - Nystagmus
    - Xero derma pigmentosa
    - Alport's syndrome
  - **Intermediate**
    - Ocular albinism
    - Retinitis pigmentosa (some)
  - **Recessive**
    - Leber's optic atrophy
    - Megalocornea
    - Esotropic nystagmus

Ectopia Lentis* - Example of ploygenecity of ectopia lentis
1. Simple ectopia lentis
2. Other ocular symptoms associated with ectopia lentis-
   - Aniridia
   - Uveal coloboma
   - Ectopia lentis et pupillae
   - Retinitis pigmentosa
   - P. H. P. Vitreous
3. Systemic disorders associated with ectopia lentis
   - Marfan's syndrome
   - Homocystinuria
   - Weill-Marchesani syndrome
   - Ehlers-danlos syndrome
   - Rieger's syndrome

- Meiosis is a special type of cell division that reduces the chromosome number by half, creating four haploid cells, each genetically distinct from the parent cell that gave rise to them.
- *Mitosis:* It is type of cell division where the daughter nuclei get a similar number of chromosomes as per a specific species.

Genetic disorders may develop from any of the following in isolation or in combination:

- Abnormal number of chromosomes
- Deviation from the normal number of chromosomes
- Abnormal mitochondrial DNA
- Environmental interaction of genes
- Variation in the amount of material
- Autosomal disorders follow the Mendelian law of segmentation and assortment.
- The manifestation of a genetic disorder is not always predictable.

Flowchart 28.2 shows common inherited disorders. They may be present at birth or may manifest later. Some of the disorders have dual or triple inheritance (polygenicity).

Symbols used to trace pedigree ***(Fig. 28.4)****:* This may differ in different countries.

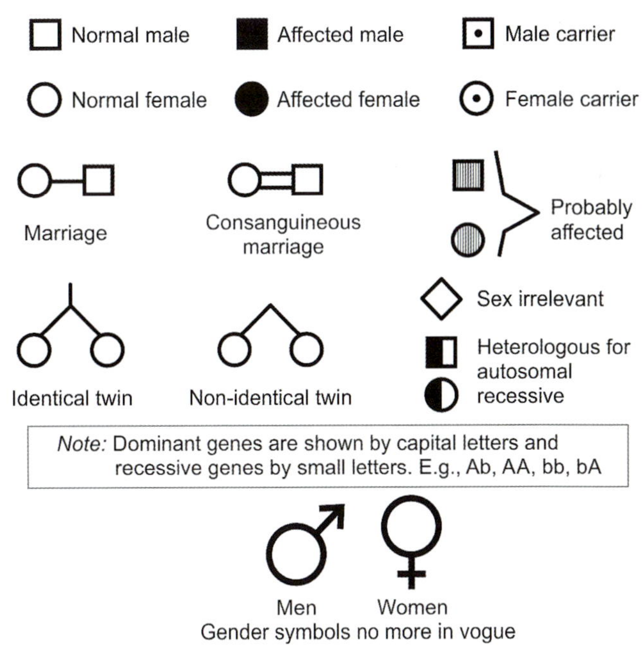

Fig. 28.4: Various symbols used in tracing the pedigree.

Flowchart 28.3 shows various types of inheritance patterns.

Flowchart 28.4 shows autosomal recessive inheritance.

Characteristics of autosomal recessive inheritance:

- Males and females inherit autosomal recessive traits equally from their parents.
- All children of affected parents are carriers.
- Traits are usually passed by two carriers.
- They have one recessive and one dominant gene.

Flowchart 28.5 shows the effect if both parents are carriers.

*Summary of characteristics between autosomal recessive **(Flowchart 28.6)** and autosomal dominant **(Flowchart 28.7)***: To understand the difference between the two. It is imperative to be remembered.

- Any chromosome other than the sex chromosome is autosomal.
- The first allele is dominant, and the other is recessive.

Flowchart 28.3: Various types of inheritance patterns.

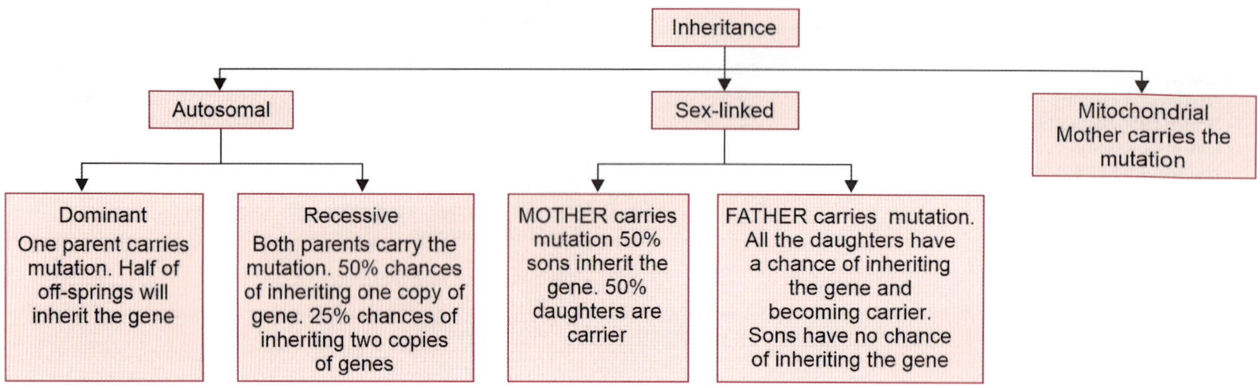

Note: The dominant autosomal gene may have the following rare exceptions:

1. The trait is seen in every generation.
2. It is equally distributed among sons and daughters.
3. Affected person always have affected parents.
4. On an average, 50% of the progeny of affected persons will be affected.

Flowchart 28.4: Autosomal recessive inheritance.

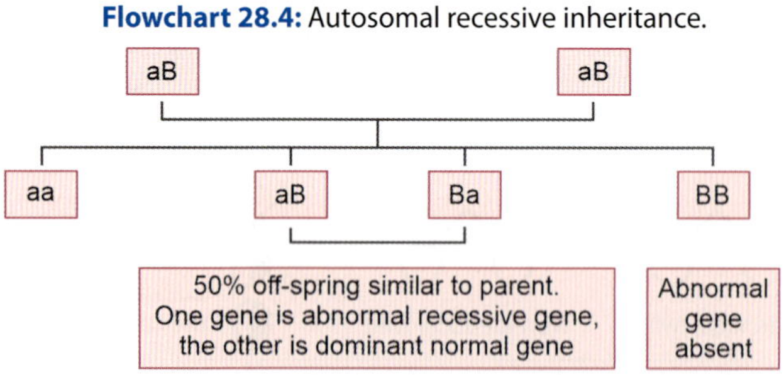

(a: abnormal gene; B: dominant normal gene)

Flowchart 28.5: Effect on progeny if both parents are carriers.

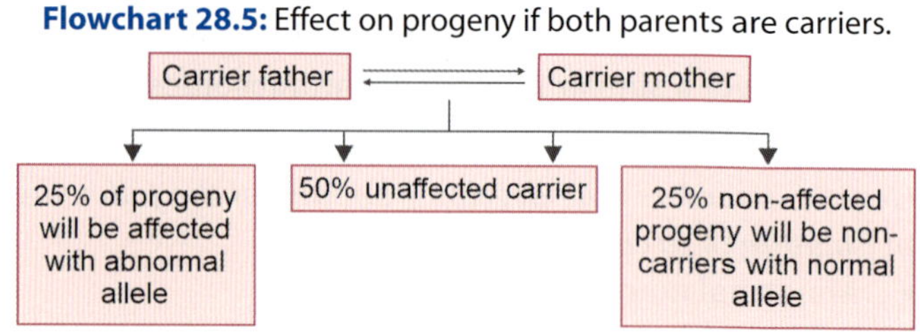

Flowchart 28.6: Sex-linked recessive.

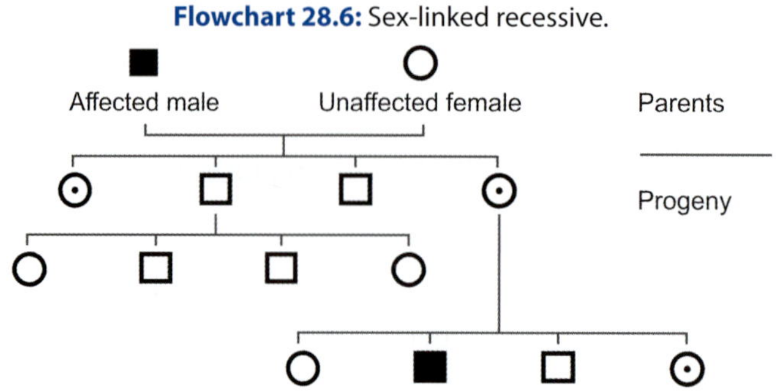

Flowchart 28.7: Sex-linked dominant.

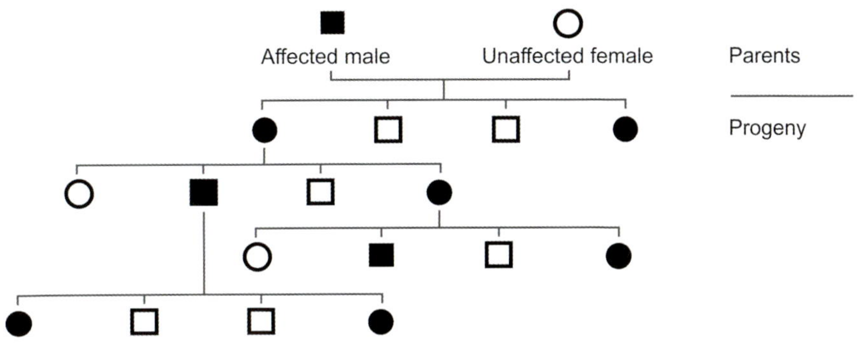

- *Autosomal recessive:*
  - Manifest in a single generation (horizontal configuration)
  - Both sexes are equally affected.
  - 25% of the offspring of heterozygous are affected.
  - 50% of the offspring of heterozygous parents are heterozygous.
  - Consanguinity is common.
  - 50% of offspring are carriers.
- *Autosomal dominant:*
  - Affected persons are vertically distributed.
  - Both sexes are equally affected.
  - Both sexes may produce affected children.
  - 50% of the offspring of affected parents show similar abnormalities.
  - Traits appear in every generation.
  - The gene is located in one of the 22 pairs of autosomes.

SUGGESTED READING

1. Bogger WP, Peterson RA. Basic Genetic Principles: Pediatric Ophthalmology. In: Pavan-Langston D (Ed). The Manual of Ocular Diagnosis and Therapy, 3rd edition. Boston: Little Brown; 1991.
2. Clarke CA. Genetics in General Medicine. In: Perkins E, Hill DW (Eds). Scientific Foundation of Ophthalmology. London: William Henimun Medical Book; 1977.
3. Cross HE. Principle and Practice of Ophthalmology, Volume III, 1st Indian edition. New Delhi: Jaypee Brothers Medical Publisher; 1987.
4. Denniston AKO, Murray PT. Genetics: Pediatric Ophthalmology. Oxford Handbook of Ophthalmology, 1st edition. New Delhi: Oxford University Press; 2006.
5. Duke Elder S. Heredity in Symptoms of Ophthalmology, Volume VIII. London: Henry Kimpton 1962.
6. Nirmalan PK, Krishnaiah S, Nutheti R, Shamanna BR, Rao GN, Thomas R. Consanguinity and eye diseases with a potential genetic etiology. Data from a prevalence study in Andhra Pradesh, India. Ophthalmic Epidemiol. 2006;13(1):7-13.
7. Park K. Genetics and Health. In: Park K (Ed). Text Book of Preventive & Social Medicine, 25th edition. Jabalpur: Banarasidas Bhanot Publishers; 2019. pp. 889-91.
8. Riordan-Eva P. Genetic Aspects of Ocular Disorders. In: Vaughan D, Asbury T, Riordan-Eva P (Eds). General Ophthalmology, 15th edition. New York: Appleton & Lange; 1999.
9. Schaffer DB. Genetics and Ophthalmology. Text Book of Ophthalmology, 9th edition. Philadelphia: WB Saunder; 1979.
10. Shastry BS. Pharmacogenomics in Ophthalmology. Discov Med. 2011;12(63):159-67.
11. Singh AD, Damato BE. Clinical Ophthalmic Oncology Basic Principles (Cancer Genetics), 3rd edition. New York: Springer; 2019. pp. 79-86.
12. Singh JR. Genetics in Ophthalmology. In: Dutta LC (Ed). Modern Ophthalmology, Volume II, 2nd edition. New Delhi: Jaypee Brothers Medical Publisher; 2000.
13. Singh M, Tyagi SC. Genes & Genetics in Eye Diseases: A Genomic Medicine Approach for Investigating Hereditary and Inflammatory Ocular Disorders. Int J Ophthalmol. 2018;11(1):117-34.
14. Verma B. Genomics in Community Ophthalmology. Indian J Comm Ophthalmol. 2021;1(2):17-32.
15. Wadhwani M, Vashisht P, Saxena R. Prevalence & Causes of Childhood Blindness in India. Indian J Ophthal. 2020; 68(2):311-5.

CHAPTER 29

Disturbance of Vision other than Visual Acuity in Children

Visual acuity (VA) is a measure of the ability of the eye to distinguish shapes and the details of objects at a given distance.

Clinically, visual acuity comprises distant vision, near vision, color vision, and field of vision.

The causes of the above factors are ocular except for some field defects, which are considered peripheral. Besides this, there are many causes that may be associated with the above symptoms and have a systemic background; they are called central. Most of them involve neuro-visual paths. They are also known as symptomatic disturbances. Many of them are followed by the term "blindness," i.e., night blindness, color blindness, or day blindness, without meeting the laid-down criteria of blindness. The terms are mostly used in clinical practice, more as habits than academic accuracy. They are:

- Nyctalopia (night blindness)
- Day blindness
- Color blindness
- Chromatopsia
- Metamorphopsia
- Amaurosis
- Amblyopia
- Scotoma
- Visual aphasia
- Agnosia*
- Dyslexia
- Defective contrasts

Out of the aforementioned long list of symptoms, the most important is night blindness because it is a mostly acquired condition that is fully preventable and treatable. The incidence of the condition has been mostly eliminated in all countries due to the administration of vitamin A as part of the national immunization program in all developing and underdeveloped countries.

"Visual Agnosia": Visual Agnosia is a rare neurological disorder where person finds it difficult to process the visual impression.

NIGHT BLINDNESS (NYCTALOPIA)

Night blindness is a state of diminished vision in reduced light (scotopic vision) accompanied by prolonged dark adaptation and abnormal electroretinogram (ERG).

Night blindness is mostly acquired. It is said to be developmental when associated with pathology in the retina resulting in constricted fields, vascular attenuation of vessel pigmentation, and consecutive optic atrophy. As seen in retinitis pigmentosa and its allied conditions, the condition may be confined to the eye only or may be associated with a systemic condition.

Acquired Night Blindness

Acquired night blindness is the most common form of night blindness in children, followed by developmental and congenital causes, respectively. The most frequent cause of acquired night blindness in children is vitamin A deficiency, which is brought about by suboptimal supply, as in malnutrition, increased requirement, as seen in measles, and increased elimination, as seen in recurrent diarrhea. The factors rarely act alone; a combination of two or more makes the situation worse.

The daily requirement of dietary vitamin A in retinol activity equivalents (RAE) is given in the following **Table 1**.

Formally, vitamin A was measured in international retinol units, which have been replaced by RAE, which make 1 IU of retinol equivalent to 0.3 μg of RAE and 1 IU of supplemental β-carotene equivalent to 0.3 μg of RAE.

**Agnosia* is inability to interpret sensations and hence, recognize things, typically as a result of brain damage. It can be visual or nonvisual.

TABLE 29.1: The daily requirement of dietary vitamin A in retinol activity equivalents (RAE).

Age	*Recommended amount*
Birth–6 months	400 µg RAE
Infants 7–12 months	500 µg RAE
Children 1–3 years	300 µg RAE
Children 4–8 years	400 µg RAE
Children 9–13 years	600 µg RAE

Night blindness associated with vitamin A deficiency is generally associated with xerophthalmia (see disorder of the conjunctiva); however, it may precede, accompany, or follow xerophthalmia.

The World Health Organization (WHO) recommends the following regime for prevention and treatment of xerophthalmia that will eliminate night blindness as well.

Under this strategy, every infant 6–11 months and every child 1–5 years are to be administered vitamin A every 6 months. The recommended schedule is as follows: 6 months to 5 years: one doze of 100,000–200,000 IU/ every 6 months. A child must receive a total of nine oral doses of vitamin A by its fifth birthday.

However, different countries have modified this regime to suit their local requirements.

Under this strategy, vitamin A is supplied in two forms: Oral and intramuscular. The former is used mostly as a preventive method and less frequently in cases of clinically apparent vitamin A deficiency. For oral use, vitamin A is supplied in colored capsules, i.e., red and blue. The red capsule contains 200,000 IU of vitamin A, while the blue capsule contains 100,000 IU.

Night blindness due to vitamin A deficiency develops over weeks or months, depending on the supply of vitamin A and its requirements. It is enhanced in the presence of protein-caloric malnutrition; generally, it begins gradually, and the child complains of the dimness of ambient light in the room in the evening, which terminates fast into total night blindness. The child finds it difficult even in familiar surroundings; at the end, he even cannot locate his food kept in front. The condition returns to normal in daylight. Vitamin A deficiency by itself does not cause diminished vision or loss of field. There are no vascular changes.

The condition is reversible by administration of vitamin A, as per clinical pictures. The other acquired causes of night blindness in children are less frequent; they are slower in onset and associated with corresponding field defects. The conditions are high myopia with associated extensive retinochoroidal degeneration and juvenile glaucoma.

It is not difficult to diagnose the cause of diminished night blindness due to vitamin A deficiency in malnourished children. The difficulty arises in children in the last years of the first decade when the child presents with only night blindness; at this stage, the first condition that should be kept in mind is retinitis pigmentosa. That can be differentiated by a simple therapeutic test, which consists of the administration of intramuscular vitamin A. In the case of night blindness due to avitaminosis A, the child will show dramatic improvement in 14 hours, while it will have no effect on retinitis pigmentosa.

DAY BLINDNESS

This is far less common than night blindness and is not known to cause blindness. The condition comprises a constriction of the pupil that results in marginally reduced distant vision. The other causes are in the cornea or in the lens; a corneal opacity in front of the pupil in bright light brings down the vision greatly; similarly, opacities in the posterior pole also reduce vision disproportionately, which is compounded by a constricted pupil. A less common cause is a large macular lesion.

The condition is often confused with glare and photophobia. The former is intolerance to light without loss of vision, commonly seen in coloboma of the iris (congenital or surgical), aniridia, albinism, myopia, and mydriasis (therapeutic or neurological).

In photophobia, the child involuntarily closes the lids in the presence of light. The child may turn his face away from the light or bury his face under a pillow. The cause lies in irritation of the trigeminal nerve. The cause could be ocular, i.e., interstitial keratitis, phlyctenular keratitis, fascicular ulcer, corneal abrasion, corneal ulcer, buphthalmos, hydrops of the cornea, or acute iridocyclitis. The systemic causes are meningitis, encephalitis, and congenital achromatopsia.

Other symptomatic disturbances of vision in children are:

Related to Light

Photopsia

This represents seeing flashes of light. This is due to irritation of the visual elements of the retina. This is a serious symptom that is almost always a warning of the development of retinal detachment, especially in myopic children and eyes that have sustained injury.

Cases of photopsia should not be dismissed casually. All children complaining of flashes of light should undergo a complete ocular examination. Which should include indirect ophthalmoscopy with scleral indentation?

Rarely, cerebral irritation may also cause flashes of light.

Related to Color

Chromatopsia

In this condition, a person gets a colored hue on a light colored object, i.e., a white-washed wall, white cloth, etc. This is mostly due to faulty absorption of a particular color due to changes in the lens, or it may be drug-induced. They are:

Erythropsia (Seeing Red): This is common following lens extraction in the first few days. Occasionally, a child with a fresh, thin blood film in front of the pupil or a fresh vitreous hemorrhage can complain of red colored vision. It also occurs in snow blindness.

Cyanopsia (Seeing Blue): This is also a common complaint after a lens extraction.

Xanthopsia (Seeing Yellow): The most common cause is jaundice. There is a big list of drugs that cause xanthopsia.

Related to Shape

Metamorphopsia

Metamorphopsia comprises distorted shapes. As best demonstrated on the Amsler grid, each eye should be examined separately. The most common cause is an acute macular lesion. The other cause is recent retinal detachment extending into the posterior pole.

Related to Size

Micropsia

When the things took smaller than their actual size. This is due to the crowding of cones. In contrast to this, minification is smaller image formation on the retina by minus glasses, as is seen in myopic correction without involving the macula.

Macropsia: When things look larger than their actual size due to the separation of cones.

Magnification: Magnification is an optical phenomenon where the size of the object is optically enlarged, as in high hypermetropic correction, aphakic correction by glasses and magnifiers.

Minification: Like magnification, this is also an optical phenomenon where the image of the object looks smaller than it actually is. This is brought about by myopic correction and examination by the Hruby lens.

COLOR BLINDNESS

Color blindness per se does not cause diminished vision; hence, it is in appropriate to put it under the category of legal blindness, though some of the pathological conditions may be associated with the defect. It should better be called failed color perception. Human eyes have highly developed color sense; the color sense depends on the wave length of the light, and human eyes can differentiate 200 shades of color between 380 and 760 nm. The visible spectrum is commonly referred to as white light, which is a mixture of all the colors. The white color is produced when all the visible wavelengths falling on the object are reflected back. An object looks black because it has absorbed all the visible wavelengths. Objects look colored when only a particular wavelength is reflected back.

Ultraviolet light has the shortest wavelengths, i.e., below 400 nm, while infrared light ranges between 800 and 1.00 mm. It is, in fact, electromagnetic radiation that produces heat.

> The cones are endowed with color sense; the rods are not involved in color sense.

The colors generated in the cones are transmitted to the optic pathway like white light. Hence, disorders of the optic nerve produce diminished acquired colored sense, which is reversible, while a true color defect is permanent, not amenable to treatment. There are three types of cones that are responsible for red, green, and blue color sense. The cones contain three different types of pigment, one each for red, green, and blue. The distributions of pigment containing cones do not have a uniform distribution. The central part is devoid of blue-pigment-sensitive cones. Red, green, and blue are the primary colors, their mixers, in various proportions, produce different colors. The condition of absence of color sensation is suffixed by the term anopia; thus, red, green, and blue color defects are called protanopia, deuteranopia, and tritanopia, respectively.

This property of cones to produce different colors have been utilized to create pseudo-chromatic plates to diagnose color defects. The color defects are brought about by the following factors:

- Absence of all pigments in cones produces total absence of color. The condition is called achromatopsia which is an extremely rare congenital hereditary condition. A child with achromatopsia sees everything as black and white or in shades of gray.
- One out of the three pigments is abnormal—this is called anomalous trichromacy, the condition is further divided in three groups depending on absence of pigment. They are:
    - Abnormal red sensitive cone—called protanomalous color defect.
    - Abnormal green-sensitive cone—called deuteranomalous color defect.
    - Abnormal blue-sensitive cone—called tritanomalous color defect.

  The last is rare.

Defects of the optic nerve and faulty absorption of light by the lens are two causes of the acquired color defect.

Sensitivity to color depends on brightness, hue, and saturation. Hue denotes the ability to perceive color. While saturation refers to the dominant wave length, saturation depends on the presence of white in the combination; the lesser the white, the purer the combination.

Classification of Color Blindness

All types of color blindness are congenital; however, only achromatopsia is present at birth; rest are detected after 5 years and remain stationary without remission or exacerbation; hence, they are preferentially referred to as developmental **(Flowchart 29.1)**.

Flowchart 29.1: Classification of color blindness.

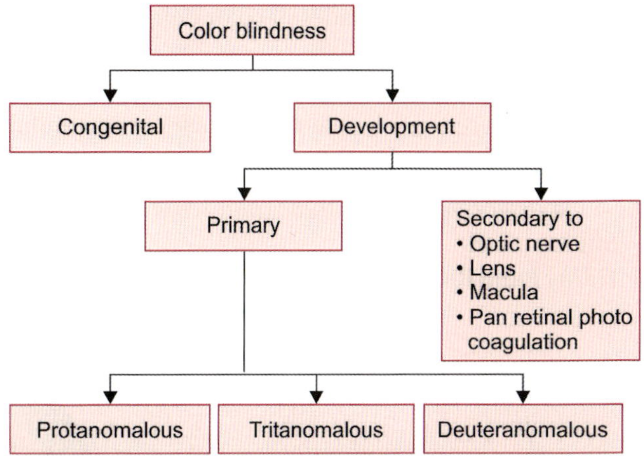

Color blindness is universal, with some races showing a preponderance. It is exclusively seen in boys; 8–10% of boys suffer from some type of color defect or other. Color blindness among girls is a clinical curiosity; girls and boys suffer from secondary color defects equally. Women are carriers but do not suffer from color blindness due to X-linked in heritance. The condition is bilateral and of the same type. The preponderance of the defect in boys makes it mandatory for boys to be examined for color defect when they enter the school, or at least when they can understand the procedure. It is surprising that most of the colors blind do not find it difficult to negotiate traffic signals; most probably due to the brightness of the signal, a boy learns to call a leaf green and a rose red by experience. The faculty of color sense is hampered in misty weather; thus, candidates for loco drivers are specially examined on the Edridge green lamp.

The following **Figure 29.1** shows Edridge Green Lantern.

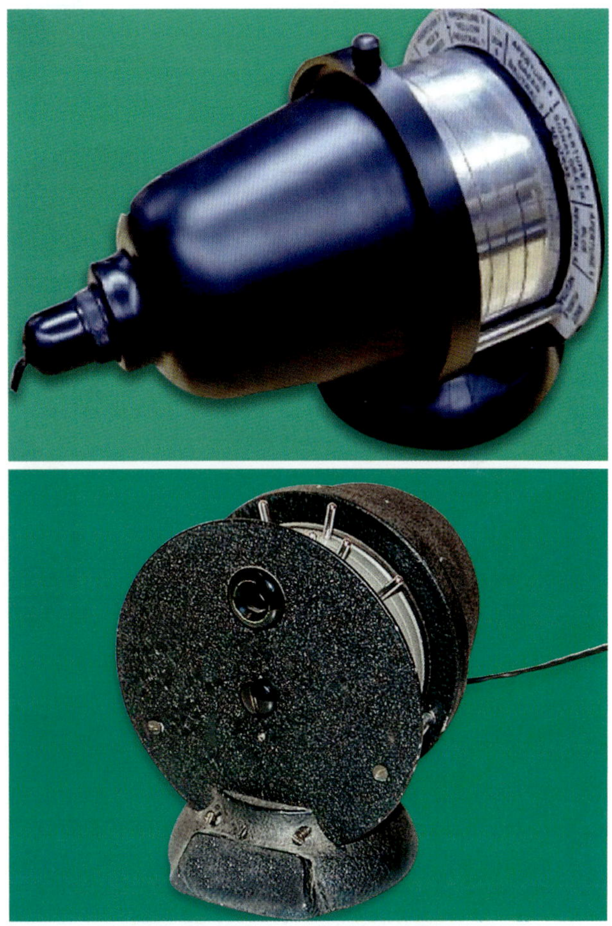

Fig. 29.1: Edridge Green Lantern.

The pseudo-Ishihara plates use fifteen hues to differentiate between various grades of color defects. It is good for red, green defects only.

The following **Figure 29.2** shows Abridged Ishihara plates to detect red-green defects and their corresponding index.

The other devices used to examine color sense are:

- Stilling plates
- Hardy Rand Rittler (blue defect)
- *Farnsworth hue discrimination test:* Farnsworth D-15 test.
- Farnsworth Munsell 100 hue test.
- Nagel's anomaloscope (not suitable for blue defects).
- Sloan achromatopsia test (for total color defect).
- Holmgren's wool test (a complicated and time-consuming test).
- Intersociety color council aptitude test (too many negative tests).

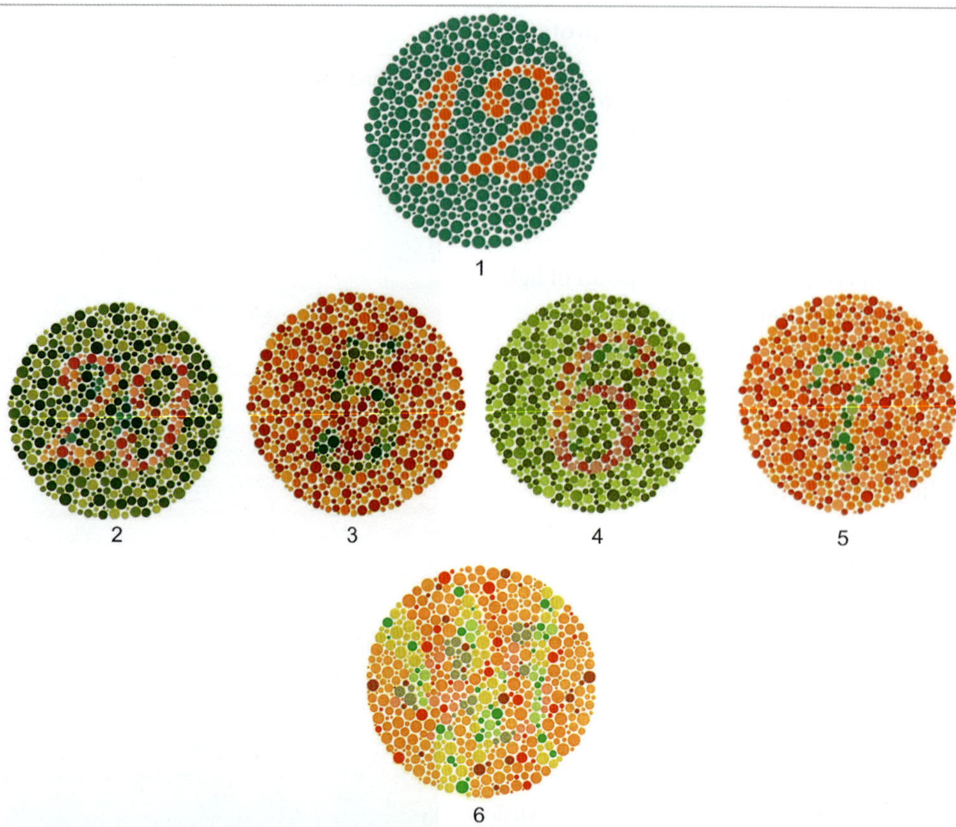

Figure	Normal person	Person with Red-Green deficiency	Person with total color blindness
1	12	12	12
2	29	70	X
3	5	2	X
4	6	X	X
5	7	X	X
6	X	5	X

Fig. 29.2: Abridged Ishihara plates and its index.

Other devices, other than pseudo-Ishihara plates and Edridge green lamps, are not commonly used in clinical practice. The others are available in higher centers for specific examinations.

SCOTOMAS

Any defect in the field of vision produces a scotoma. Scotoma is defined as diminished or absent vision in a particular part of the field, which may be central or peripheral; scotomas exclusively within 30° are called central scotomas. The remaining are peripheral; it is not possible to have both types in the same eye; the peripheral field may encroach upon the central field in extensive peripheral defects. The vice versa has not been reported; there are some scotomas that are better demonstrated on colored isopters than with white. Isopters are the points that represent visual thresholds in the fields.

A scotoma is called absolute if the size and density of the scotoma does not change with the size, color, or illumination of the isopters. The scotomas are referred to as relative if the size and density of the scotomas change with illumination. A scotoma is called positive that makes a person aware of, it is generally acute. If the patient is not aware of a scotoma, it is called a negative. The best example of a negative scotoma is a blind spot. A steep scotoma represents a defect where the margin of the scotoma does not change with size; in contrast to this, if the borders of a scotoma change with the size of the target, the scotoma is called sloping. The scotoma can be uniocular or binocular, congruous or noncongruous.

A scotoma is called congruous when it is similar to its counterpart in the other eye, both in size and shape. They can be homonymous or heteronymous, as shown in the following **Flowchart 29.2**.

Flowchart 29.2: Bilateral field defect.

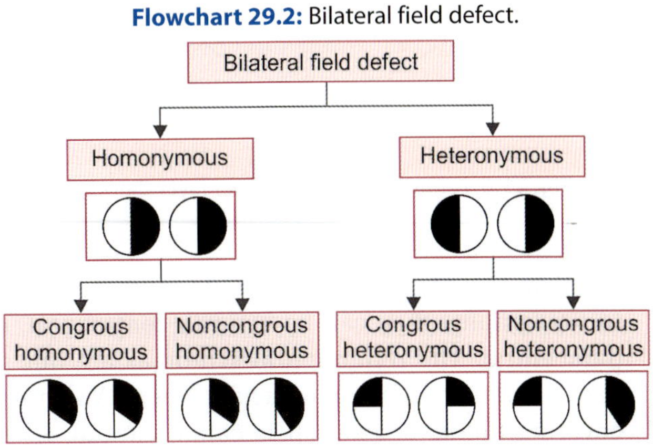

Figures 29.3 and 29.4 show the various levels of lesion that produce scotomas (field defect) unilateral/bilateral and unilateral field defect.

Scotomas have been classified according to their location. *They can be:*

- Chorioretinal **(Fig. 29.5)**
- Neuroretinal **(Fig. 29.6)**
- Neural
  - Optic disc
  - Optic nerve
  - Chiasma
  - Optic tract
  - Geniculate
  - Retrogeniculate
    - *Optic radiation:* Temporal/parietal
    - Cortical

Scotomas due to lesions from the disc to the visual cortex are given in **Figure 29.7**.

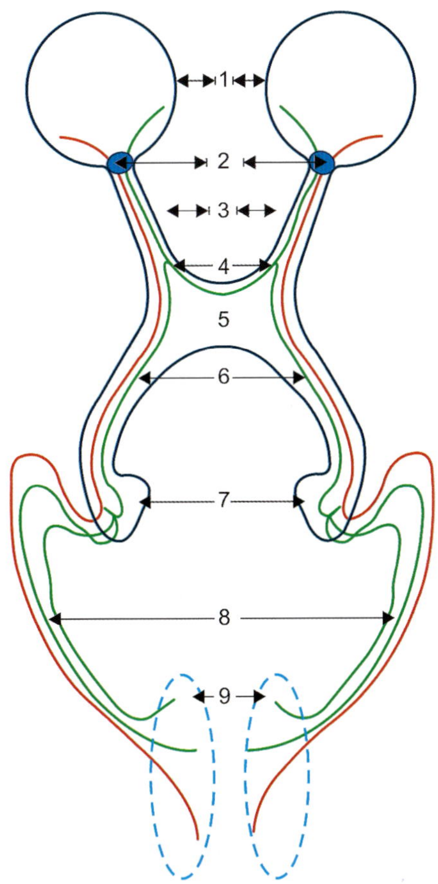

Fig. 29.3: Levels of lesion that produce scotomas (Field defect) unilateral/bilateral. (1. Neuroretina; 2. Papilla; 3. Optic nerve; 4. Anterior chiasma; 5. Chiasma; 6. Optic tract; 7. Lateral geniculate body; 8. Optic radiation; 9. Visual cortex).

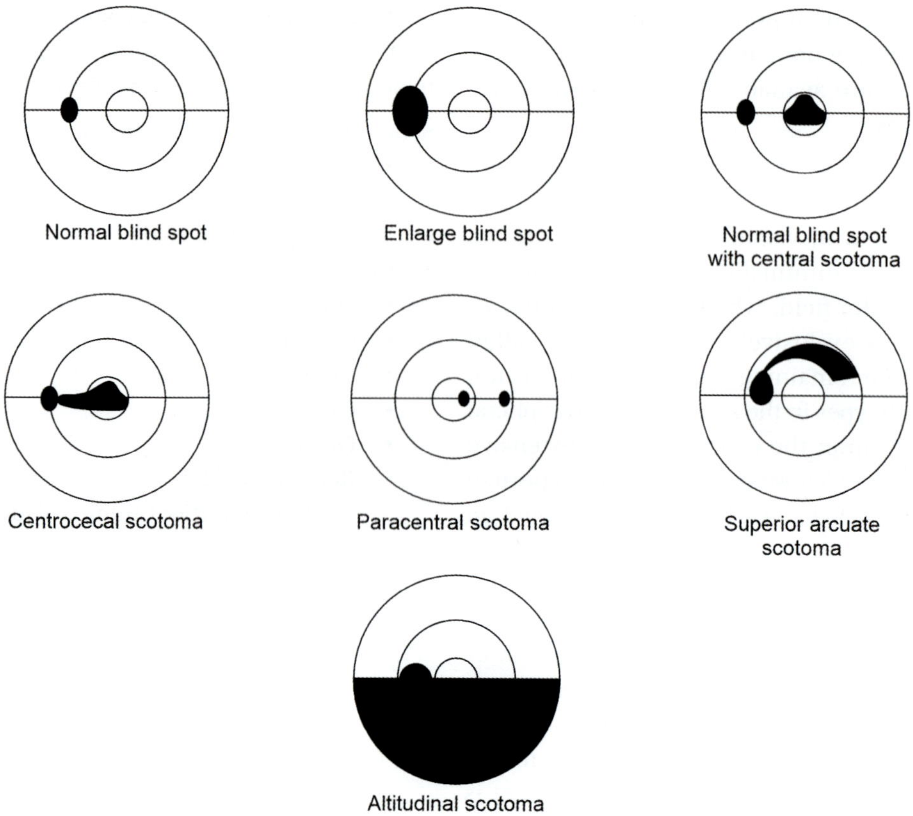

Fig. 29.4: Unilateral field defect.

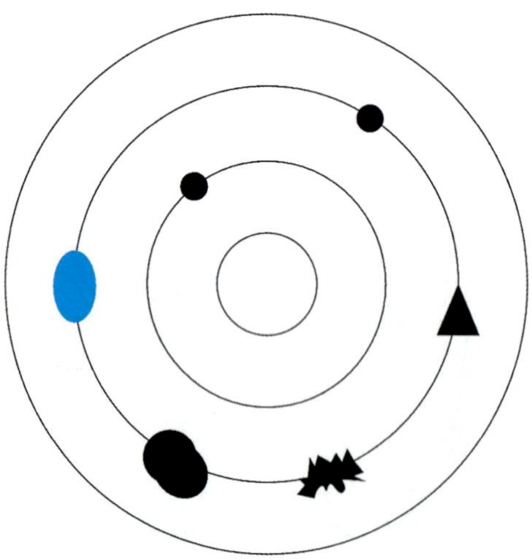

Fig. 29.5: Chorioretinal field defects.

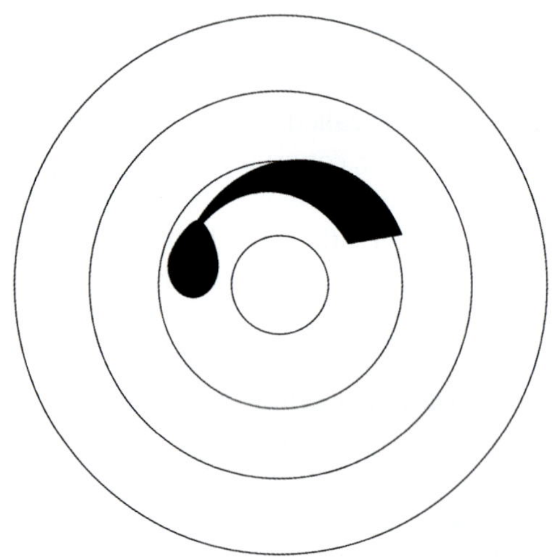

Fig. 29.6: Neuroretinal (nerve fiber layer defect).

Characteristics of Various Scotomas

- *Chorioretinal:* They do not have much diagnostic value. They can be single or multiples of various shapes and sizes. They do not respect the retinal topography, which may be unilateral or bilateral, rarely symmetric.
- *Retinoneural:* They are of diagnostic value. According to topography, they can be central, centrocecal, or paracentral. The retinoneural scotomas are due to the involvement of papillomacular fibers. A scotoma covering points of fixation is called central; if the

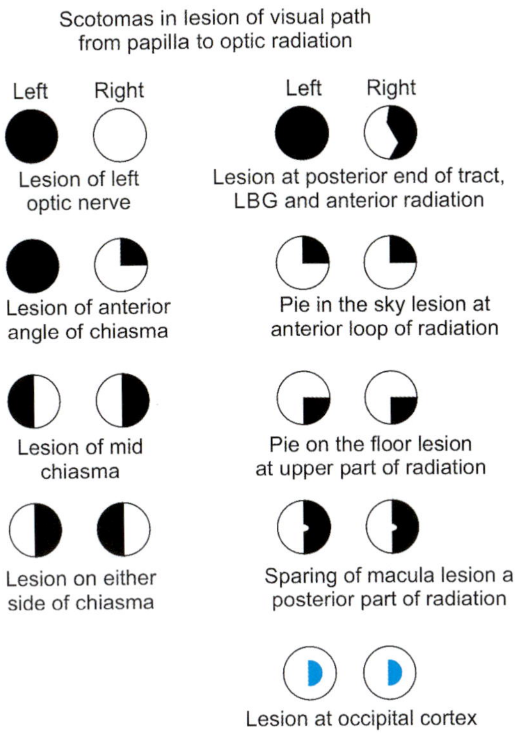

Fig. 29.7: Scotomas due to lesions from the disc to the visual cortex.

central scotoma extends into the blind spot, it is called centrocecal, involvement of fibers other than the macula is called paracentral. Which does not involve either the point of fixation or blind spot. Specific types of scotomas with diagnostic importance; involve the nerve fiber bundle. They are:

- Bjerrum's scotoma (See field changes in glaucoma below)
- Seidel scotoma (See field changes in glaucoma below)
- Roenne's nasal step (See field changes in glaucoma below)

Bjerrum's scotoma may develop superiorly or inferiorly when they meet each other on the horizontal raphe they form an irregular annular scotoma. The ends of meeting Bjerrum's scotomas do not overlap each other; they form a step called the Roenne's nasal step.

The above scotomas can be unilateral or bilateral; when bilateral, they need not be symmetrical. They are independent of each other; they have a bearing in glaucoma.

- *Optic nerve lesion:* Lesions of the optic nerve produce a central scotoma, which may be relative or absolute, mostly unilateral. The central scotomas are symptomatic; they result in diminished vision, color vision, contrast sensitivity, and afferent pupillary change. Extensive lesions reaching the angle of chiasma produce scotomas, which cause ipsilateral diminished vision and central scotomas with contralateral hemianopia.
- *Chiasma lesion*: The scotoma has a specific character due to the peculiar distribution of fibers in the chiasma, i.e., crossed and uncrossed. The scotomas differ from each other due to their location in the chiasma, i.e., anterior, middle, and posterior. The chiasmal lesions may be quadratic, anopic, or hemianopic.

Lesions from Chiasma Produce—Hemi and Quadrantanopia Field Defect

- *Anterior chiasmal* lesions are typically ipsilateral central with contralateral hemianopia.
- *Mid-chiasmal* lesions are the most common field defect due to their association with pituitary tumors, both sellar and suprasellar. The field defect is heteronymous, which produces bitemporal hemianopia. The bitemporal hemianopia does not progress from the temporal to the medial side vertically. They start in one eye in the superior temporal quadrant and gradually spread inferiorly. The defect in the right eye progresses clockwise, while in the left eye it is anticlockwise. Initially, the vertical line is respected, but once the whole of the inferior temporal quadrant has been abolished, the field invades the midline.
- *Posterior chiasmal*: Lesions produce homonymous hemianopia, i.e., temporal loss on one side and nasal on the other side. These defects are incongruous. Lesions of chiasma do not cause an afferent papillary defect.
- *Binasal hemianopia* is caused due to two separate lesions, one on each side of the chiasma. They are rare and, when present, often missed.
- *Optic tract lesion*: The lesions produce homonymous hemianopia split at fixation. The lesions are explained by the following anatomical distribution of visual fibers: the optic tract on each side contains ipsilateral uncrossed temporal fibers along with crossed nasal fibers from the contralateral side. The scotomas are incongruous. The vision is generally good; there may be an afferent pupillary defect.

- *Lesion of the geniculate body:* The lesions at this level are relatively rare; the lesions, when present, mostly involve the macular fibers. The lesions are incongruous homonymous hemianopia, sectorial with apex toward the point of fixation. Generally, good vision is present.
- *Lesions of optic radiation:* The scotomas depend on whether the lesion is in the temporal or parietal lobe.
  - The lesions of the temporal lobe involve the Meyer's loop, a produces typically pie in the sky scotoma with apex toward the point of fixation in the superior quadrant. The scotoma is sectorial, homonymous, respecting the midline. Good vision is possible, and the pupillary reactions are retained.
  - Lesions of the parietal lobe produce pie in the floor; it is a quadra nopic scotoma, which is homonymous and congruous with normal vision and retained pupillary relations.
- *Lesion of visual cortex—lesion of the visual cortex:* The fibers from the optic radiation synapse in the calcarine fissure in the occipital lobe. They are chiefly macular that are found at the top of the occipital cortex. The scotomas are congruous, homonymous, and hemianopic; the macula is not always involved. Thus, a situation of macular spare may result. The scotomas respect the vertical meridian; the probable causes of macular sparing are:
  - Dual blood supply to the occipital cortex.
  - The macular fibers spread over a large area; hence, it is possible that enough macular fibers are spared to retain central vision.
  - It is presumed that there is double innervation of macular area.

Some specific types of field defects are:

- Enlargement of the blind spot is not always diagnostic.
  - Papilledema
  - Glaucoma
  - Opaque nerve fibers
  - Drusen of the optic nerve
  - Coloboma of optic disk
  - Peripapillary edema of the retinal (not seen in children)
  - Juxtapapillary choroiditis (not seen in children)
- *Constriction of peripheral fields:*
  - Onset of optic atrophy—postpapilledematous or postneurotic.
  - Retinitis pigmentosa
  - Advanced glaucoma
  - Hysteria
  - Malingering
- *Altitudinal field defect:*
  - Acute ischemic optic neuropathy (not seen in children)
  - Occlusion of the central retinal artery branch (not seen in children)
  - Trauma to the superior occipital lobe
  - Optic tract syndrome

Specific types of scotoma are:

- Glaucoma
- Pituitary lesion
- Retinitis pigmentosa
- Binasal hemianopia

Scotomas in Chronic Simple Glaucoma

The following are the field defects seen in glaucoma (duration-wise) **(Fig. 29.8)**:

Field defect in pituitary tumor and Field defect in craniopharyngioma.

The pituitary gland is a ductless gland of utmost importance; it indirectly controls other endocrinal glands. Hence, it is called the master gland. It is situated in the pituitary fossa in the body of the sphenoid; it develops from the Rathke's pouch as an ingrowth of neural ectoderm from the developing palate. During its embryogenesis, it gets detached from the palate. It is about 1.00 cm by 1.00 cm under the Sella turcica, through which it is attached to the hypothalamus not by neural tissue but by blood vessels; the connection is called the stalk or infundibulum. The pituitary gland is divided into two unequal parts, a large anterior pituitary and a smaller posterior pituitary. The anterior pituitary secretes many hormones. While the posterior pituitary secretes two hormones, i.e., oxytocin and antidiuretic hormone.

The growths of sella are broadly divided into two groups:

1. Pituitary adenoma
2. Craniopharyngioma

PITUITARY ADENOMA

The pituitary adenomas, also known as pituitary neuroendocrine adenomas, are the most common tumor of the pituitary that produces the most spectacular field-change characteristics of the tumor. The tumor has been put into two groups depending on the hormone it secretes; about one-fourth of the tumors are not secreting. Most pituitary

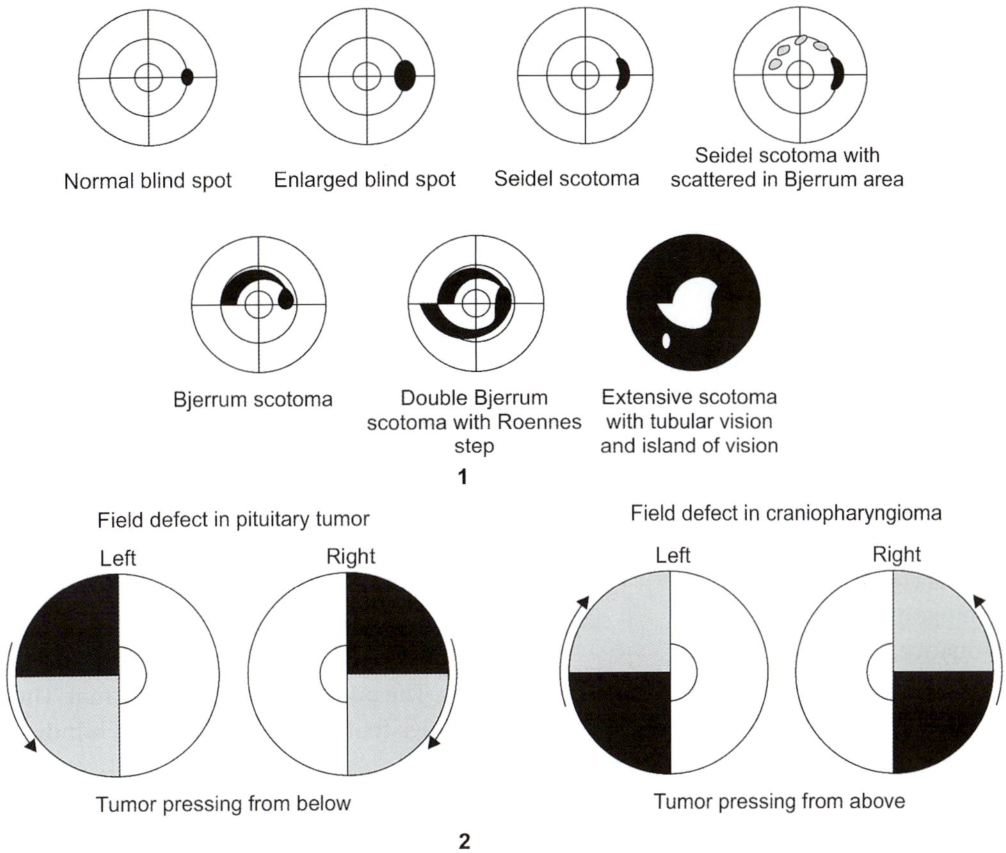

Fig. 29.8: Progress of field changes as per extension of pituitary tumor.

tumors are benign, slow-growing, and do not metastasize. Most of the symptoms are due to its pressure on the visual path that causes specific field changes. The most common age for a patient to present with pituitary adenoma is between 30 and 40 years; however, it can develop at any age in both sexes without any racial preponderance. Pituitary adenoma in children is mostly hormone-secreting; the common hormones produced by pituitary tumors are prolactin, adrenocorticotropic hormone (ACTH), and growth hormone. Nonsecreting tumors are rare; thus, a child with a pituitary tumor may present with surprisingly two different symptoms, i.e., gigantism and dwarfism, hypogonadism, and precocious puberty. The tumors that are nonsecretory are generally large and produce early pressure symptoms. Pituitary adenomas in all ages are slow-growing; a tumor causes symptoms when the tumor is >1.00 cm in size. Pituitary adenomas, to begin with, may be symptomless, but when they present with symptoms, the symptoms are confused with other systemic conditions not related to pituitary tumors.

The symptoms of pituitary adenoma may be broadly divided into two groups: Visual and nonvisual.

The visual symptoms are:

- Fleeting disturbance of visual acuity
- Color desaturation
- *A typical field defect:* The field defects are bitemporal; they generally start in the superior quadrant and spread downward, resulting in bitemporal hemianopia (*see* diagram earlier).
- Symptoms pertaining to the disc, such as optic atrophy and papilledema, are rare and indicate extrasellar extension.

The nonvisual symptoms are:

- Headaches
- Unexplained tiredness
- Mood changes
- Irritability
- Unexplained changes in menstrual cycles
- Erectile dysfunction (in adult)

- Infertility
- Unexpected breast growth or production of breast milk
- Cushing's syndrome, a combination of weight gain, high blood pressure, diabetes, and easy bruising that is caused by overproduction of the adrenocorticotropic hormone.
- Acromegaly is the enlargement of the arms or legs and thickening of the skull and jaw caused by too much growth hormone.

In children, it results in gigantism if the tumor develops before the bone plates have fused and acromegaly after the bone plates have fused.

Diagnosis

Diagnosis is by exclusion; the common investigations ordered are:

- X-ray skull-lateral view
- Computed tomography (CT)
- Magnetic resonance imaging (MRI)

The MRI with gadolinium contrasts is the gold standard of diagnosis. The adenomas are hypointense on T1 and hyperintense on T2 image. CT has been mostly given up in favor of MRI as it demonstrates only enlargement and erosion of the sella. It also shows calcification; the X-ray has mostly been abandoned in favor of CT and MRI.

Treatment

Treatment depends on the size of the tumor and its clinical features. Small tumors detected incidentally are better observed regularly; otherwise, the treatment of choice is neurosurgery and radiation. Adenomas of the pituitary are best managed by a team of ophthalmologists, neurosurgeons, and oncologists.

CRANIOPHARYNGIOMA

Craniopharyngiomas are congenital, non-malignant tumors of childhood and adolescence. They constitute 80–90% of all growths found in the pituitary fossa, and they are responsible for 15% of all brain tumors. The tumors develop from the unabsorbed tissue of the Rathke's pouch; they could be intrasellar or extrasellar. The former contribute only 5% of all cases. Topographically, they can be prechiasmatic or retrochiasmatic. They are generally small tumors that may rarely change into a gigantic form. The sellar tumors are small but large enough to encroach upon the pituitary gland, producing a state of hormonal deficiency.

The prechiasmatic tumors produce field changes and visual loss that may be unilateral or bilateral. The retrochiasmatic tumors invade the third ventricle, producing hydrocephalus with raised intracranial pressure, resulting in papilledema. Generally, they cause visual deficiency and are known to cause hormonal changes. The diagnosis is confirmed by MRI and CT. The MRI gives the exact location. No medical treatment except for hormonal deficiency is available; the two options available are neurosurgery and radiation.

BINASAL HEMIANOPIA

See **Figure 29.9**.

CORTICAL BLINDNESS

Cortical blindness is also known as cerebral blindness or cortical visual impairment.

In these cases, the patient is blind but denies blindness. The pupillary reaction is normal. There are no fundal findings that can be attributed to blindness. The lesion is bilateral.

Other less common visual symptoms are:

- Dyslexia
- Visual aphasia
- Agraphia
- Agnosia
- Visual hallucination

DYSLEXIA

Dyslexia is a more common disorder in children than it is thought to be. In most cases, it goes undetected and unattended. It is a congenital, nontreatable condition that may be managed by a multidisciplinary approach. The other members of the family may have a milder form of the disorder. The genetics involved has not elucidated; the incidence of dyslexia is as high as 4–5% in all school going children in developed countries. It is equally common in boys and girls; the incidence in developing countries is not well documented. It may be as high as in developed countries. Children suffering from dyslexia are first thought to be dim-witted or suffering from diminished vision. This is in contrast to the fact that the children suffering from dyslexia have normal intelligence, with normal intelligence quotient (IQ), with either normal or correctable vision. The color defect, when present,

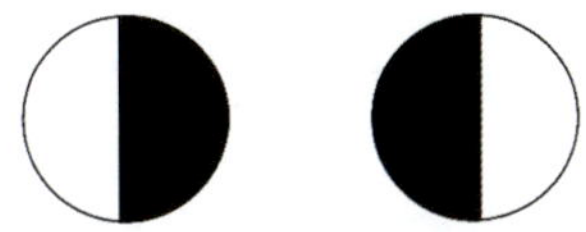

Lesion on either side of the chiasma

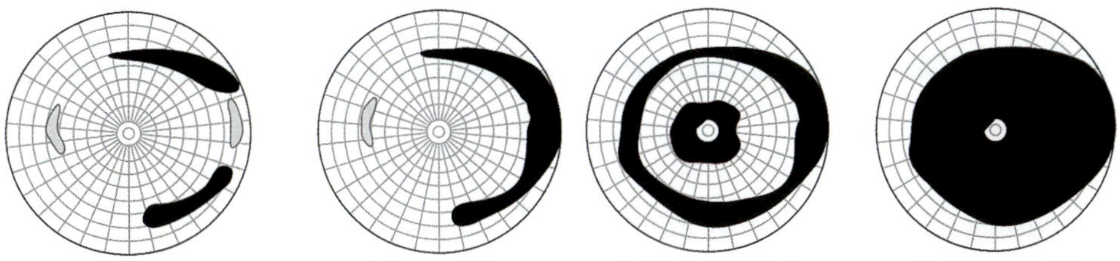

Early Intermediate Fully developed Terminal stage

3

Fig. 29.9: Scotoma in retinitis pigmentosa.

cannot be attributed to dyslexia. The condition is most probably central in origin; the condition is detected when the child goes to school. The child is found to have difficulty relating letters and groups of letters with appropriate sounds. Besides reading and writing difficulties, the child may have any or many of the following symptoms: That may vary with age.

Difficulty with names and sounds of letters; they confuse people with similar appearances by writing "b" when they should write "d." Same is with "p" and "u," which they write as "q" and "n." They also reverse the words, such as stop for "pots" or "was" as "saw." The child may show a tendency to read from right to left. In some cases, there words may be a mirror image of the original words.

- Their abilities to spell are unpredictable and inconsistent.
- They read slowly and wrongly when reading aloud.
- They answer oral questions better than written.
- They take more time copying written text and longer time to complete written text.
- Generally, they have poor handwriting.
- Many of them are left-handed, and some are ambidextrous.

The diagnosis is not simple; it is often missed, and the child is permanently stigmatized as dull. A correct diagnosis depends on the combined efforts of a pediatrician, an ophthalmologist, and a child psychologist. The role of an ophthalmologist does not end with "no visual abnormality found." He should meticulously exclude other causes of reading difficulty, i.e., high errors of refraction, bilateral amblyopia, and muscle imbalance. The above causes should be treated as best as possible, and try to put the child in a normal milieu.

- Visual aphasia (word blindness) is the inability to recognize words, letters, or colors in the presence of normal vision and color sense. The child can write spontaneously but fails to copy written words. This is seen in lesions of optic radiation.
- Alexia has an inability to read.
- *Agraphia* is the inability to express in written language.
- *Agnosia* is a condition where a person cannot recognize an object visually but can recognize it by touch or sound.
- *Color agnosia* is the inability to recognize colors in the absence of color blindness.
- *Amnestic* color aphasia is the inability to name the color.
- *Visual hallucination* is an acquired sensation that makes a person see objects, person, and color patterns that are not present.

SUGGESTED READING

1. Mukherjee PK. Clinical examination in ophthalmology, 2nd edition. New Delhi: Elsevier; 2016.
2. Mukherjee PK. Essentials of neuro-ophthalmology, 1st edition. New Delhi: Jaypee Brothers; 2010.

CHAPTER 30

Ocular Manifestation of Systemic Infection in Pediatric Age Group

The eyes cannot be considered a separate entity from the body. They share all the maladies of the body in some way or another, and infectious diseases are no exception. The eyes may get involved in systemic infection by way of maternal infection or acquire it after birth. The eyes in a systemic infection can be involved in the following ways:

- Direct spread from neighboring structures like skin and the nasopharynx
- Hematogenous
- Fomites

Infections spreading from systemic involvement to the eyes are more common than the reverse.

The infections can be acute or chronic; the former is mostly due to spread from the surrounding structures or bloodborne. An acute systemic infection may release toxins that may be harmful to the body; the involvement of the eyes by such toxins is frequent. Chronic infections are responsible for granulomatous disorders; they are also caused by allergens due to the release of bacterial proteins.

All organisms that cause systemic infection need not involve the eyes. The common organisms that are responsible for ocular involvement in the presence of systemic disease are:

- Bacteria
  - Bacilli
  - Cocci
  - Coccobacilli
    - All of them can be:
      - Gram-negative/positive
      - Motile/nonmotile
      - Aerobic/anaerobic
      - Spore forming/nonspore forming
      - May have an allergic reaction
      - Grown on culture media
      - Maybe opportunistic
      - Some of them are commensals
      - Most of them respond to chemotherapeutic measures
- Viruses
  - Deoxyribonucleic acid (DNA)
  - Ribonucleic acid (RNA)
- Fungi
- Protozoa
- Helminths
- Arthropods
- Myiasis (larva)

The first three are more common than the remaining.

THE BACTERIAL INFECTIONS

The systemic bacterial infections that have ocular involvement are arranged alphabetically in the description that follows. All of them are not equally common.

Acinetobacter (Herellea vaginicola)

Acinetobacter is an opportunistic organism, present widely in water and soil. The organism belongs to the family *Neisseriaceae*. It is aerobic, gram-negative, coccobacilli-pleomorphic, and nonmotile. It infects children with compromised immunity more.

Systemic involvement: Multisystemic infection: Pneumonia, meningitis, urinary tract infection (UTI), and septicemia.

Ocular involvement is less common: They include blepharitis, purulent conjunctivitis, superficial punctate keratitis, sloughing corneal ulcers, and endophthalmitis, mostly following trauma—accidental or surgical.

Management consists of the correct diagnosis by culture. It is sensitive to many antibiotics, both local as well as systemic. Common chemotherapeutics used are trimethoprim, sulfamethoxazole, aminoglycosides, and fluoroquinolones.

Actinomycosis

This was previously thought to be a fungus infection; now it is classified as a nonacid-fast mycobacterium. This is an anaerobic organism. The organism is of low virulence with a chronic course and does not cause impairment of vision.

Systemic involvement can be cutaneous or ocular, the cutaneous involvement is mostly of the skin of face, neck, teeth, and gums.

Ocular involvement is generally unilateral, with canaliculitis of the lower lid leading to epiphora and swelling over the canaliculus. On pressing the inflamed canaliculus, there is regurgitation of yellow, creamy material, which on microscopy contains concretions like sulfur granules. Rarely, there may be chronic dacryoadenitis.

Management consists of systemic tetracycline, cephalosporin, or penicillin. Local antibiotics are tetracycline ointment, or aminoglycoside drops, which are frequently used.

Bacillus cereus

The organism *Bacillus cereus* belongs to the genus *Bacillus,* which also contains *Bacillus anthracis*, or anthrax bacillus, which has acquired notoriety as a tool of biological warfare with lethal effects. *Bacillus cereus* is commonly found in water, soil, air, and dust. It is an aerobic, gram-positive, spore-forming organism that is highly virulent and generally resistant to penicillin and cephalosporins.

Systemic involvement is relatively rare, seen in drug addicts who use infected needles. It reaches the eye as hematogenous spread due to contaminated intravenous injection or more commonly due to penetrating injury, mostly accidental and rarely surgical.

Ocular involvement is a fast-developing endophthalmitis, often leading to panophthalmitis and loss of the eye. As it is a spore-bearing organism, it is resistant to usual autoclaving and requires additional aseptic and antiseptic measures. Otherwise, the wound, whether surgical or accidental, will end in fulminating endophthalmitis, leading to panophthalmitis. The endophthalmitis is hyperacute, developing within 24 hours; the severity depends on the capacity of the organisms to produce exotoxin, which is not neutralized by antibiotics.

Management: It is an ocular emergency that requires anticipation, especially following accidental injuries. The postoperative endophthalmitis presents with unexplained pain that, on examination, is found to have all the signs of hyperacute postoperative endophthalmitis, including a fast fall in vision, corneal edema, a fast-growing hypopyon, and chemosis of the lids and conjunctiva. The condition is confirmed by an anterior chamber (AC) or vitreous tap; the conjunctival swab may not be positive for organisms. In suspected cases of *Bacillus cereus* endophthalmitis, it is better to err on the safer side by starting intravenous ciprofloxacin 400 mg twice a day. Intravitreal vancomycin, gentamycin, and clindamycin give better results. Early vitrectomy may save the eyeball structure but does not guarantee useful vision.

Brucellosis

Brucellosis is a disease that spreads from animals to humans due to consumption of unpasteurized milk or direct contact with affected animals. All animals are known to suffer from the disease. The systemic infection in humans is subacute, presenting with relapsing fever, headache, joint pain, weight loss, lymphadenopathy, and splenomegaly. The ocular findings are milder, in the form of edema of the lids, conjunctivitis, and nummular keratitis. Occasionally, it may cause uveitis ending in endophthalmitis and extraocular palsy. The diagnosis is by exclusion; the organism is sensitive to many antibiotics and sulfa drugs. Complete eradication takes 4–6 weeks.

Clostridium

Clostridium is not a single organism; it consists of many organisms, all of which do not infect the eyes but have far-reaching systemic involvement. Combined ocular and systemic involvements are frequent. The clostridia of ocular importance are:

- *Clostridium perfringens* (gas gangrene and food poisoning)
- *Clostridium tetani* (tetanus)
- *Clostridium botulinum* (botulism)

The organisms are opportunistic, gram-positive bacilli, anaerobic, and sometimes gas-forming and spore-bearing; all of them produce toxins. That is not neutralized by chemotherapy.

Clostridium perfringens (Gangrene and Food Poisoning)

The infections, both systemic and ocular, are hyperacute in onset, starting within a few hours of the onset of the infections.

The systemic manifestations consist of acute food poisoning following consumption of contaminated food, deep tissue infection, skin and soft-tissue infection with accumulation of gas under the skin that gives a bloated appearance, crepitation, foul-smelling exudates, and coloration of the site of entry. The condition may end in shock and renal failure, which may be fatal.

The ocular involvement follows a penetrating, contaminated wound around the eyes that causes changes in the lid and orbit containing gas, resulting in chemosis of the lids and conjunctiva spreading to the cornea. Severe panuveitis with coffee-colored hypopyon endophthalmitis, panophthalmitis, and loss of vision may occur.

Management: The condition is a medical emergency managed by a person specially trained in infectious diseases with the collaboration of a surgeon. The first step is to combat shock, fever, anemia, and pain by standard methods. The specific treatment consists of the administration of 50,000 units of gas gangrene antitoxin every 6 hours for the first 2 days. This will neutralize the toxin but have no effect on the organism, which is sensitive to many broad-spectrum antibiotics. Hyperbaric oxygen seems to usher in early relief.

Ocular management is difficult and should be preceded by systemic management. The ocular management is primarily the management of panophthalmitis and orbital cellulitis.

Clostridium tetani (Tetanus)

The organism causes deadly neuromuscular disorders, which are among the top 10 causes of death in children in underdeveloped countries where proper immunization against the disorder is not available. The condition is fully preventable by the administration of the DPT (diphtheria, pertussis, and tetanus) vaccine under the National Immunization Programme. The disease can occur at any age and is equally common in both sexes; the younger the child, the more fatal the disease is. The organism is found in soil, dust, water, animal, and human stool. It is estimated that about 10% of the population are symptom-free carriers of the disease, harboring the organism in the gastrointestinal (GI) tract. The terminal spores of the organism are responsible for the neurotoxin called tetanospasmin, which is responsible for the clinical picture. The other toxin released is tetanolysin, which causes diminished tissue oxygenation, which in turn encourages the proliferation of the organism. An increased load of organisms releases more toxins that are deleterious to the body.

The disease is caused by the introduction of organisms under the skin or mucus membrane. The incubation period varies from a few hours to many days. The shorter the incubation period, the more serious the disease. Infections near the central nervous system (CNS) are more dangerous than those away. Clinically, there are four forms of the disorders: (1) Neonatal, (2) adult, (3) cephalic, and (4) localized.

Systemic involvement is more frequent and serious than ocular involvement, which consists of a locked jaw (trismus), risus sardonicus, restlessness, irritability, stiffness, cramps, dysphagia, and an arched back. Isolated ocular involvements are not known; when present, they are bilateral blepharospasm, paralysis of all cranial nerves from the 3rd to the 12th, resulting in ptosis, total ophthalmoplegia, facial palsy, supranuclear palsy, corneal exposure, conjunctival congestion, conjunctivitis, and corneal ulcer.

The ocular injuries that predispose to tetanus are corneal and scleral perforations, lacerated wounds of the lids, and periorbital structures. The child with ocular involvement due to tetanus is better treated by a physician trained in infectious diseases. The role of an ophthalmologist is limited to treating anterior segment involvement.

Clostridium botulinum

The disease caused by *Clostridium botulinum* is called botulism, which is a neuroparalytic disease that begins in the CNS. It is fatal if not treated early. The incubation period is short in food-related infections; it may be as short as a few hours or as long as a few days. The condition has a short incubation period. Botulism has been divided into food-related and nonfood-related categories; it could be infantile, childhood, or adult; it may be food- or wound-related. The organism produces the most potent toxin; clinical pictures in all conditions are identical. The systemic involvement begins with ptosis, preceded by diplopia, dysphagia, and dysarthria, which may involve the thorax and neck muscles. The symptoms of food poisoning are nausea, vomiting, abdominal cramps, paralytic ileus, and urinary retention. The ocular involvement may precede, be concurrent with, or follow the acute status. It consists of ptosis, diplopia, iridoplegia, and cycloplegia.

Management: There is no preventive vaccine against botulism. The child should be hospitalized under the care of a physician well versed in the disorder and administered a trivalent antitoxin. Oral antibiotics are given to reduce the number of organisms present in the gut.

Corynebacterium diphtheriae

Infection with *Corynebacterium diphtheria* is acute, more life-threatening than vision-threatening; the ocular involvement when present may involve extraocular structure.

The organism is found in the nasopharynx as a surface saprophyte. Healthy asymptomatic carriers may be the cause of the spread of the disease in nonimmunized children. It affects children more than adults. In adults, it is milder than in children. The organism is a gram-positive, club-shaped, nonmotile organism that produces a strong toxin that involves the heart, CNS, cranial nerves, and eyes.

Systemic involvement in children starts with fever and chills. It soon involves the heart, in the form of myocarditis, and the CNS. The CNS involvement is mostly polyneuritis. Respiratory involvement includes sore throat, rhinorrhea, hoarseness, dysphagia, cough, and pneumonia. The formation of a membrane over the tonsil is diagnostic and may give a positive result on a throat swab. The ocular involvement is mostly extraocular in the form of specific diphtheritic conjunctivitis and superficial corneal ulceration that may perforate.

The cranial nerve involvement results in ptosis, paralysis of extraocular muscles, cycloplegia without mydriasis, internal ophthalmoplegia, convergence, and divergence palsy.

Management: The disease is fully preventable by immunization. The immunization should be repeated after 3 years. Once the disease is confirmed, management is directed toward neutralizing the toxin and reducing the bulk of bacteria with antibiotics. Along with the management of shock and fever. Systemic treatment is best managed by people trained in infectious diseases. The ocular involvement is managed by ophthalmologists with local broad-spectrum antibiotics and cycloplegia. The role of local instillation of antitoxin drops has been questioned.

Escherichia coli

The organism is a gram-negative rod. Systemic infection in children under 5 years may result in fatal hemolytic uremic syndrome. The organism is a commensal found in the GI tract and urinary tract. The systemic involvement consists of recurrent fever, diarrhea, dysentery, and hemorrhagic colitis. UTIs are common. The ocular involvements are rare and mild and may present as bacterial mucopurulent conjunctivitis, pseudomembranous conjunctivitis, keratitis, uveitis, hyphema, and hypopyon; gas in the AC has been reported; unattended uveitis may result in endophthalmitis. The ocular involvement is managed by instilling appropriate antibiotics and cycloplegics. The systemic condition that invariably becomes chronic is best managed by a physician.

Gonococcus

The organism belongs to the family *Neisseria*; the other human pathogen in this group with ocular involvement is *Neisseria meningitidis*, which is less common and less blinding. *Neisseria gonococcus* produces disease only in humans, though it is found in the submucosa of many animals. The organism is intracellular, gram-negative, and diplococci. Found in polymorphonuclear forms, it produces oxidase and catalase; some strains produce beta-lactamase, which is the cause of penicillin resistance, which is becoming more common due to irregular treatment by subtherapeutic dose. The other cause of penicillin resistance is a chromosomal mutation.

The gonococcal infection is a worldwide health problem. Though it is viewed more as a sexually transmitted disease (STD) in adults, it can infect anyone at any age. The prevalence is higher in developing countries than in developed countries, where its incidence in adolescence is increasing; it is seen in both sexes equally. To begin with, it is an acute multisystemic disorder that can be life- and vision-threatening in infants and children.

Systemic involvement in adults begins mostly as purulent urethritis in males and cervicitis in females; men seek medical help earlier than women. Some men do not develop the acute stage and remain asymptomatic; they do not take treatment and remain reservoirs of the disease. The symptomatic adult males always seek medical consultation for dysuria, meatal inflammation, local swelling, pain, fever, epididymitis, and inguinal lymphadenitis. In the females, the infection starts with yellowish discharge due to cervicitis and may result in acute endometritis and salpingitis, which in the long run cause infertility. Urethritis is common and has the most prominent symptoms in both sexes. Patients, irrespective of sex, may develop ocular involvement.

Ocular Infection

In the pre-antibiotic era, gonococcal ocular infections were one of the major causes of bilateral blindness in children. The ocular manifestations in children can be divided into two groups: (1) Neonatal gonococcal infections and (2) pediatric/adolescent gonococcal infections. The neonatal gonococcal infection develops in two ways:

1. Intrauterine infection (rare)
2. Infection in neonates

The most common acquired form is ophthalmia neonatorum; the pediatric and adolescent gonococcal infection does not differ from the adult form. Other ocular involvements in children are bilateral central corneal ulcers and anterior uveitis. Gonococci are one of the organisms that can pass through intact corneal epithelium, making the cornea vulnerable to ulceration and perforation, followed by their train of sequelae. This makes it mandatory to use atropine in an age-related dose in all cases of ophthalmia neonatorum. A small perforation in the center leads to the collapse of the AC, which brings the lens–iris diaphragm into contact with the posterior surface of the cornea. Healing of the perforation results in central leukoma and anterior polar cataracts. Such catastrophic vision loss is generally bilateral, leading to bilateral diminished vision and nystagmus.

Haemophilus influenza and Koch–Weeks *Bacillus*

The two organisms belong to the genus *Haemophilus* and produce similar clinical pictures. The latter is also known as *Haemophilus aegyptius*. All of them are pleomorphic, gram-negative coccobacilli.

The organism is a common infection in children, causing upper respiratory symptoms. The disorder shows seasonal variation, commonly seen in epidemics of seasonal conjunctivitis followed by respiratory infections. The systemic involvement is generally mild, presenting as malaise, fever, upper respiratory tract infection, sinusitis, and bronchitis. In its severe form, it causes pneumonia. Still, severe infections may result in meningitis, bacteremia, and septic arthritis, which is still rare.

Ocular involvements are common and consist of acute mucopurulent conjunctivitis or pseudomembranous conjunctivitis swollen violet-colored lid is almost diagnostic. It is accompanied by keratitis. The conjunctivitis resolves within 10–12 days even without treatment. There is no prophylactic measure against the organism. The mucopurulent conjunctivitis responds well to antibiotic drops given frequently and the same ointment at night. Combined antibiotics are better avoided and corneal involvement should get appropriate cycloplegia.

Leptospirosis

Leptospira is a gram-negative spirochete that stains poorly, is best seen in a dark field examination, and is highly motile. Leptospirosis is seen as an epidemic mostly in the rainy season in tropical and subtropical countries among malnourished populations of all ages. The disease spreads from animals to humans through infected urine or contaminated water. The disease is rarely seen among animals; humans may be asymptomatic carriers. The incubation period is 1–2 weeks. Once the person is infected, organisms can be found in urine, blood, cerebrospinal fluid (CSF), and aqueous solutions within 24 hours. The organism is known to produce toxins. The systemic conditions are divided into two phases. The first is a stage of leptospiremia, and the second is an immune phase. In the first phase, the patient has pain all over the body, a fever with rashes, diarrhea, and an upper respiratory infection. One of the common findings at this stage is conjunctival effusion, which is almost diagnostic in the absence of a craniofacial injury. The conjunctival discharge is invariably positive for organisms. The other ocular features are mild iridocyclitis in 30% of cases that may be self-limiting; however, hypopyon, mutton fat keratic precipitates (KPs), and posterior synechiae may be seen in months to come. The systemic conditions are treated with antibiotics. The most common antibiotics used are doxycycline and penicillin. The ocular features are treated with local antibiotics and cycloplegia when required.

Leprosy (Hansen's Disease)

The disease was one of the conditions recognized centuries ago and is still persisting in many parts of the world, being more common in underdeveloped, tropical, and subtropical countries. It has profound systemic as well as ocular features. The disease is caused by *Mycobacterium leprae*, an acid-fast bacillus. The organism has more affinity for neural tissue than for muscular and bony tissues, both of which are secondarily affected by the neural involvement. The disease is almost unknown in children under the age of 10 years.

It becomes more frequent after 10 years of age; the maximum number of cases is encountered after 30 years of age. Its manifestation when present in children is milder and nonblinding than in adults; however, children exposed to the disease may have ocular involvement in 40–70% of cases.

Leprosy can cause a variety of eye complications, including:

- *Eyelid adnexa:* Madarosis, blepharochalasis, nodules, ectropion, entropion, lagophthalmos, reduced blinking, trichiasis, conjunctivitis, and pterygium
- *Intraocular leprosy:* Iritis, uveitis, low intraocular pressure, corneal anesthesia, corneal ulceration and scarring, episcleritis and scleritis, conjunctival and scleral lepromas, uveal effusion, and retinal pearls and detachment
- *Other manifestations:* Glaucoma, thickened corneal nerves, superficial stromal keratitis, pannus, exposure keratopathy, interstitial keratitis, band-shaped keratopathy, and iris leproma.

The ocular involvements are many, depending on the duration of the disease. The ocular involvement is bilateral. Leprosy has the highest incidence of ocular involvement as compared to other bacterial infections. It is estimated that about 70–75% of patients will develop ocular involvement. The ocular involvements are time-related, never acute, and not seen in children. 10–15% of patients with ocular involvement have clinical features serious enough to cause extensive ocular involvement. The rate of blindness among them is as high as 5–10%. The involvements are mostly extraocular; the intraocular involvements are due to hematogenous spreads of the disease or immune modulated. The sight-threatening conditions are lagophthalmos, exposure keratitis, corneal anesthesia, chronic iridocyclitis, complicated cataracts, and secondary glaucoma. Corneal anesthesia predisposes corneal ulcers. Absence of corneal anesthesia leaves the patients oblivious of the condition. However, other features of corneal ulcers are present that may draw the attention of the patient or caregiver. The unattended corneal ulcer soon develops hypopyon–endophthalmitis–panophthalmitis.

Management of the disease is early detection and initiation of multidrug chemotherapy. The treatment requires months to years to be effective. Early treatment helps in avoiding ocular involvement. The most important part of management of ocular involvement is management of lagophthalmos and corneal anesthesia. The patients without ocular involvement should get their eyes examined every month to avoid serious complications.

Lyme Disease

Lyme disease is a zoonotic disease that may be spread by arthropods. It is a spirochetal disease. The most common arthropod to spread disease is tick *Ixodes*. It is more prevalent in the Western Hemisphere, but its incidence is becoming more frequent in other countries.

The disease is multisystemic and includes skin rashes; cranial nerve palsy, of which facial palsy is the most frequent; meningitis; and peripheral neuritis. The ocular features are mostly due to neurological involvement. Mostly immune-mediated, the common features are sequelae of facial palsy and cranial nerve involvement in the form of optic neuritis and retrobulbar neuritis, optic atrophy, paralytic squint, pseudotumor cerebri, and papilledema. The specific ocular features are conjunctivitis, keratitis, and episcleritis. The condition is confirmed by the enzyme-linked immunosorbent assay (ELISA) test and immunofluorescence assays. The organism is sensitive to many antibiotics, given orally or parenterally.

Moraxella

Moraxella was previously known as Morax–Axenfeld and *Moraxella lacunata*. It is gram-negative bacilli, or diplococci, that are aerobic organisms; due to their bean-shaped appearance, they look similar to *gonococcus*. It is found in half of asymptomatic children; systemic involvement consists of upper respiratory tract infections, pneumonia, and otitis media. In the past, it was one of the common causes of mild-to-moderate conjunctivitis in malnourished children. Besides chronic angular conjunctivitis, it causes dermatitis of the outer canthus, which is almost diagnostic when present in children, and it also causes chronic blepharitis. Corneal ulcers, when present, may result in hypopyon without ciliary congestion. The organism is not only sensitive to many locally instilled antibiotic drops but also to zinc sulfate in 0.25–0.5% drops.

Mycobacterium tuberculosis

Like *Mycobacterium leprae, Mycobacterium tuberculosis* is also an acid-fast organism. The organism is a rod-shaped, nonspore-forming, slender, aerobic bacterium that does not stain with gram stain. The organism causes tuberculosis, which is also a disease of antiquity like leprosy.

The disease has a worldwide distribution and is more common in underdeveloped countries. It directly or indirectly involves many organs at all ages in both sexes and is still a major cause of death in developing countries, with the most common cause of death being pulmonary involvement. The disease has been divided into two broad groups: (1) Pulmonary and (2) extrapulmonary. The systemic conditions include predominantly respiratory systems in the form of pneumonia, consolidation, cavity formation, and pleurisy. Ocular involvement is divided into two groups, i.e., (1) primary and (2) secondary.

The former is less common, mostly seen in the lids, as cutaneous tuberculosis called lupus vulgaris, at the angle of the lids, and is generally associated with lupus of the alae nasi. The second primary involvement is chronic conjunctivitis, which may produce cock's comb-like growths or tuberculomas.

> Children with frank pulmonary tuberculosis rarely develop tuberculosis of the eyes. Conversely, tuberculosis of the eye is rarely associated with frank pulmonary tuberculosis.

The secondary involvement of the eyes can be divided into two groups: (1) Extraocular and (2) intraocular. The extraocular disease involves the conjunctiva, cornea, and sclera. *They are:*

- Phlyctenular conjunctivitis and conjunctival ulcer
- Phlyctenular keratoconjunctivitis, fascicular ulcers, and frank keratitis; the conditions mentioned are rarely caused directly by tubercular bacilli and are rarer than interstitial keratitis; seen from the second decade onward
- Episcleritis is seen in the second decade; it is more common than frank scleritis, and sclerosing keratitis is still rare.
- The above lesions are immune-mediated.

Intraocular involvement

- Intraocular involvement in children under 10 years of age is rare.
- All vascular intraocular structures are involved either by hematogenous spread or due to hypersensitivity, ranging from acute mild iritis to severe posterior uveitis.
- The uveal involvement is granulomatous.
- A granulomatous lesion is generally associated with vitritis.
- Tubercular nodule on the iris surface
- Chronic iridocyclitis
- Choroidal involvement may present either as a solitary nodule or as patches of
- disseminated choroiditis.
- Isolated retinal involvement is rare.
- The retina is involved only in chorioretinitis.
- Optic neuritis is less common than antitubercular drug-induced neuritis.

Management

Prophylaxis: Bacillus Calmette-Guérin (BCG) given at birth does not eliminate the possibility of tuberculosis in later life. It only prevents serious, life-threatening forms of tubercular meningitis and miliary tuberculosis. The best management is early detection and elimination of the disease at the beginning as per national eradication of tuberculosis in children. Prophylactic use of antitubercular chemotherapy has not been found to be effective.

The child with tuberculosis should be treated by a pediatrician with an adequate dose lasting for the prescribed period.

Ocular tuberculosis is managed by:

- Full treatment by antitubercular chemotherapy for an adequate period
- Age-matched cycloplegia
- Local steroid drops in an adequate dose at an adequate frequency and time.
- Local antitubercular drugs do not have any therapeutic value.

Pneumococcal Infection

Pneumococcal infection is common in children; it used to be life-threatening in the pre-chemotherapeutic era. The organism is also known as *Streptococcus pneumoniae* due to its tendency to form chains. The organism is a gram-positive, capsulated diplococcus with a short incubation period, found as a commensal of the human nasopharynx in 10% of the general asymptomatic population. The disease spreads through droplets from infected persons or carriers. The systemic involvement consists of bilateral pneumonia, consolidation, otitis media, sinusitis, meningitis, peritonitis, salpingitis, pericarditis, and osteomyelitis.

Ocular Involvement: The most common ocular involvement by pneumococcus is acute bilateral mucopurulent with or without petechial hemorrhages; more severe cases may develop pseudomembrane. It may be associated with superficial keratitis that may proceed to serpiginous ulcer with prominent hypopyon. Uveal involvement may be due to the spread of pneumococcal ulcer, and due to spread of toxin from the infected lacrimal sac and hematogenic spread from other organs. Uveal involvement may present as a fulminating hypopyon corneal ulcer ending in endophthalmitis.

Chronic dacryocystitis is common. The infected sac may harbor pneumococcal toxin, which is a common cause of early development of fast-growing hypopyons.

Acute orbital cellulitis has been reported in malnourished children.

Management: The systemic involvement that may be more serious than ocular involvement is better treated by a pediatrician with appropriate antibiotics and ancillary treatment. The ocular involvement is treated by ophthalmologist, the conjunctivitis responds well to erythromycin ointment (drops are not available). In the past, it was managed in the same fashion as ophthalmia neonatorum by frequent drops of fresh crystalline penicillin. All cases with corneal involvement should be treated as ophthalmic emergencies and treated with appropriate cycloplegia and frequent instillation of antibiotics along with systemic antibiotics.

Pseudomonas aeruginosa

The organism is one of the most common nosocomial infections all over the world. It is a common infection following injury. The organism is a free-living, ubiquitous, opportunistic organism. It is found in water, plants, animals, humans, and many animals. It involves the skin and mucous membranes that act as reservoirs in asymptomatic carriers.

It is gram-negative, slightly curved or straight, motile bacteria. It produces a blue-green pigment called pyocyanin that imparts green color to pus and exudate. The presence of blue-green pus in a wound is almost diagnostic. The organism produces an enzyme called proteases that causes rapidly growing stromal necrosis in the cornea.

Systemic infections are generally grave that start as respiratory infections associated with cough, fever, chills, dyspnea, and cyanosis/otitis media. Bones and joints may be involved more commonly following injury than as part of a systemic infection. Lacerated wounds are often infected by the organism. The presence of green pus in the wound is a red flag that requires emergent management.

Ocular infections are always devastating that should be treated as an ocular emergency in hospitals. The predisposing factors besides open injury to the eye and its adnexa are contact lenses of all types, contact lens solutions, and contact lens boxes.

Fluorescein drops, which are commonly used as diagnostic tools in ophthalmology, are notorious for being contaminated. If these are used as drops, the drops should be as fresh as possible; if stored for >24 hours, they should be reautoclaved. Presently, drops have given way to single-use sterilized strips impregnated with the die, reducing chances of contamination but not eliminating them. The other sources of contamination are tonometers of all types and gonioscopy.

The *clinical presentation* of ocular involvement is acute with redness, pain, copious discharge that may be tinged green and mucopurulent conjunctivitis. Unexplained pain suggests involvement of the cornea, causing superficial keratitis that is soon converted into a sloughing central corneal ulcer with large green hypopyon. The protease produced by the organism causes necrosis of the stroma, enhancing perforation, and resulting in endophthalmitis that may end in panophthalmitis.

Management: There is no preventive vaccine against the organism. The utmost surgical asepsis is mandatory in all places of surgical intervention. Both systemic and ocular involvement require early diagnosis and prompt treatment. The organism is sensitive to many broad-spectrum antibiotics that should be administered in hospitals.

Staphylococcus

Staphylococcus is one of the most common organisms to inflict human beings all over the world. Infection may be as mild as a boil to devastating nosocomial infection. The organism is ubiquitous and develops on the skin and mucous membrane without being symptomatic. Such colonies are the common causes of its frequent spread; it is found in water, dust, soil, and inanimate objects of clinics and hospitals. People working in hospitals, including doctors, are often asymptomatic carriers. Contaminated bioprosthesis like intraocular lens (IOL) and contact lenses are common sources of infection, so are the irrigating solution and tubes. The organism is small, gram-positive, nonmotile, and nonspore-forming, seen mostly in bunches. It may present in short chains or even scattered singly. The organism has been broadly put into two groups based on its ability to produce an enzyme coagulase. Thus, *Staphylococcus* could be coagulase-positive or negative; out of the two, coagulase-positive is more pathogenic; it produces many enzymes and toxins. There are many species of coagulase-negative *Staphylococcus* by various names, i.e., *S. albus*, *S. aureus*, *S. epidermidis*, *S. haemolyticus*, *S. saprophyticus*, and others. *S. aureus* is the most important human pathogen. It is difficult to treat because of the highly destructive enzyme. The organism is difficult to destroy by usual autoclaving and boiling. It is prone to developing resistance to many antibiotics. In the past, coagulase-negative organisms were thought only to be contamination but have been found to be opportunist organisms that are responsible for many hospital-related infections. There are no vaccines effective against all strains. The organism is sensitive to many chemotherapeutic agents ranging from sulfa, trimethoprim, to broad-spectrum antibiotics. Local administration of drops may suffice for local conditions but require systemic administration in deep-seated infections, sometimes for days together.

Streptococcus

The organism is as common as *Staphylococcus*, with more systemic involvement. The organism is found in the respiratory, gastrointestinal, and urinary tracts of human beings; many of them are silent carriers of various diseases and causes of spread of the disease, and it is as common a nosocomial as Staphylococci. The organism is a main cause of neonatal sepsis; it is a predisposing factor in rheumatic fever and glomerulonephritis. The organism is a commensal, gram-positive, oval, nonmotile, nonspore-bearing, facultative anaerobe. It is mostly seen in chains of various lengths. The organism has been divided into two groups: (1) hemolyticus and (2) nonhemolyticus. The hemolytic strain is again divided into alpha and beta hemolyticus.

Symptomatic involvement consists of acute or chronic infection of many organs in isolation or combination. In the skin, it causes pyoderma, cellulitis, erysipelas, necrotizing fasciitis, boils, and abscesses. In the respiratory system, it causes pharyngitis, tonsillitis, tonsillar abscess, pneumonia, and empyema. More serious conditions include streptococcal shock syndrome, neonatal sepsis, meningitis, and food poisoning. The ocular manifestation may be as mild as simple, self-limiting conjunctivitis to devastating ophthalmia neonatorum, endophthalmitis, and panophthalmitis; it is a common organism to cause postoperative endophthalmitis. The conjunctivitis may cause membranous or pseudomembranous conjunctivitis and keratitis corneal ulcer. It is a common cause of preseptal cellulitis and orbital cellulitis. It is a common cause of preseptal cellulitis in children.

Management: Like *Staphylococcus*, it is also sensitive to an array of chemotherapeutic agents that range from local drops to intravenous administration of broad-spectrum antibiotics. Hospital infections are notorious for being resistant to many antibiotics.

Syphilis

The disease has been known to inflict men and women of all ages for centuries. It is caused by *Treponema pallidum,* a spirochete. The other human pathogens of the same genera are leptospira and borrelia (Lyme disease). It produces chronic infection; it can inflict fetus as well. The organism is spiral in shape, thin, delicate, motile, not staining with gram stain, and not visible on a simple microscope. It is seen only on dark-field examination; it has not been cultured. Humans are the only natural hosts of the organism. The disease is mostly transmitted sexually; it can be transmitted following transfusion of infected blood as well. Congenital syphilis is a trans-placental spread from mother to the growing fetus generally in the 3rd or 4th month of pregnancy. Older children acquire the disease following child abuse. The children with such disease go through all the stages that are found in adults. In adults, it has been divided into the following stages: (1) Primary, (2) secondary, (3) latent, and (4) tertiary.

The systemic involvements are too many to be discussed in short. The disease involves all the organs over years. The congenital form is an extended type of the disease; it can cause multiple disorders, may cause stillbirth, abortion, and may be fatal to the newborn.

Systemic Involvement in Congenital Syphilis

The infection is transmitted from a seropositive mother to the developing fetus via the placenta at any time during pregnancy; the pregnancy in the third and fourth months is the most common period when the disease is transmitted. Early months of pregnancy make the fetus more vulnerable to the disease. Treatment of the mother before 16 weeks is claimed to spare the fetus; abortion and stillbirth are common. It is a common cause of neonatal death, the disease in surviving neonates can be divided into the following stages: (1) Early, (2) Late, and (3) Residual. The early features are seen in the first 2 years; the late manifestations develop after 2 years. The residual effects are seen in still older children, the systemic manifestations in infants differ from those in the older age group. The ocular signs are not seen in neonates. They develop after 2 years without obvious ocular signs. The features in infants are systemic: Hepatosplenomegaly, jaundice, anemia, thrombocytopenia, lymphadenopathy, skin rashes that may be bullae or vesicles, rhinitis, and osteochondritis. Rhinitis is the cause of destruction of the nose bridge, which is considered to be one of the hallmarks of congenital syphilis. In older children, the common systemic features include changes in the bones and joints in the form of periostitis, anterior bowing of the shin, frontal bossing, Clutton's joints, a destroyed nose bridge resulting in a saddle nose, and changes in the mouth consisting of mulberry molars and peg-shaped teeth. Out of all central nervous involvement, the eighth nerve is most commonly involved. The ocular involvements are marked.

The ocular manifestations are delayed changes in congenital syphilis that have remained untreated in earlier stages. The most common and most prominent ocular feature after two years is interstitial keratitis.

Syphilitic Interstitial Keratitis

Syphilitic interstitial keratitis is an acute bilateral feature; it is presumed that the disorder starts in the anterior uvea, and the cornea that shows prominent signs is involved secondary to anterior uveitis. The anterior uveitis presents as endothelial edema, resulting in generalized swelling of the cornea followed by deep vascularization. The deep vascularization is initially located in the stroma, giving rise to a salmon-patch appearance that causes generalized haze of the cornea so much as to obliterate the view of the AC. The stage of deep vascularization lasts for months to years if not treated; the haze is terminated with local treatment with steroids. The deep pink vessels are replaced by white lines that represent obliterated vessels, resulting in a lifelong hazy cornea.

The other ocular features of congenital syphilis are: Bilateral chorioretinitis with typical salt and pepper pigmentation is confused with retinitis pigmentosa. The chorioretinitis of congenital syphilis is differentiated from typical retinitis pigmentosa by the absence of night blindness. Secondary glaucoma is frequent due to changes in the angle.

The differential diagnosis of interstitial keratitis consists of all the causes that present with hazy cornea, i.e., birth injury to the cornea, late acquired corneal injury, corneal endothelial dystrophy, mucopolysaccharidosis, and mucolipidosis. Congenital glaucoma may be primary or secondary to anterior segment changes. The other conditions that give rise to pepper-salt appearance should be differentiated from those caused by congenital syphilis. They are rubella and *Cytomegalovirus* retinitis.

Management: The condition is preventable if the infected mother gets adequate treatment before 16 weeks of pregnancy. The child born to an infected mother should get an adequate dose of antisyphilitic treatment following consultation with a pediatrician.

Ocular involvement consists of a dose of age-related atropine twice a day for 7–10 days. The cornea is initially treated with a strong dose of steroid for the first 10 days, followed by a weaker solution for months in the usual tapering dose. This does not clear corneal haze.

Proteus

In the past, ocular infection by proteus was not thought to be of much importance due to its rarity; with changed environments, more cases of proteus infections are being reported. It is an opportunistic saprophyte found in decaying organic matter, soil, contaminated water, and the GI tract of many animals and human beings. The infection caused by proteus is mild and often neglected; it is a gram-negative motile organism that produces an enzyme urease that makes it a potential cause of UTI infection, which acts as a portal of entry to other organs by hematogenous spread. It may be devastating in immune-compromised persons. It is known to infect wounds, both accidental and surgical. Other infections caused by it are otitis media, mastoiditis, lateral sinus thrombosis, meningitis, and even brain abscess.

Ocular manifestations are mild without any specific sign, mostly following scratches in the extraocular structures in the form of conjunctivitis and keratitis.

Infections of intraocular structures following penetrating accidental or surgical wounds may lead to fulminating endophthalmitis and panophthalmitis. Less-frequent infections by proteus are dacryocystitis and episcleritis. The latter is most probably immune-mediated. Treatment consists of the local and systemic use of many broad-spectrum antibiotics. The ocular treatment is preferably by fortified gentamycin or tobramycin and appropriate cycloplegia.

Salmonella

Salmonellosis, commonly referred to as typhoid (enteric fever), is a common acute febrile condition mostly seen in children. In the past, children under 5 years of age were thought to be immune to the disease. However, it has been reported to inflict children as young as 1 year. Thus, no age is immune to the disease; the older the patient, the milder the disease. The disease is seen worldwide in both sexes, more often in underdeveloped countries where the main source of infection is drinking water and food. The other sources of infection are silent carriers of the disease. The disease is preventable by both oral and intramuscular vaccines; a partially treated child has a higher chance of relapsing than a child who is fully treated. The disease is fatal in untreated children. The organism is gram-negative motile facultative anaerobe, with an incubation period between 3 and 60 days. The systemic involvement is mainly enteritis, due to direct involvement of the small intestine; both diarrhea and constipation are common. Perforation of the small intestine results in fatal peritonitis. The other serious complications are meningitis, encephalitis, paralysis of cranial nerves, pneumonia, bronchitis, myocarditis, cholecystitis, osteomyelitis, and arthritis. The fever is a prominent symptom throughout the disease, ranging from mild to hyperpyrexia. The temperature rises stepwise; pink rashes all over the body are common. Relative bradycardia is a red flag. The untreated case may last for 3–4 weeks or may result in a fatality. The ocular manifestations are few; they may be as mild as mucopurulent conjunctivitis to paralytic squint and ptosis. The other ocular involvements are lid abscesses, dacryoadenitis, and retinal hemorrhage.

Management: The disease is preventable by oral or injectable vaccines; besides vaccines, the incidence can be reduced if the children are given potable water and noncontaminated food. The children should be taught the basic principles of hygiene. The disease is treated by many broad-spectrum antibiotics, and the ocular manifestations are managed by standard methods along with systemic treatment.

Chlamydiasis

Chlamydia is a group of organisms between the smallest bacteria and the largest viruses. In the past, they were thought to be selective ocular pathogens. With the elimination of ocular manifestations by *Chlamydia*, it has been found that it can cause other systemic infections, including a mild form of ophthalmia neonatorum in children and genitourinary infections in adults. *Chlamydia* cell walls are similar to those of bacteria. It possesses both RNA and DNA. It is a gram-negative, obligate intracellular organism. The organism is sensitive to many commonly used antibacterials but not to antiviral drugs.

Based on its antigen, the organism has been put in three broad groups of human pathogens they are *Chlamydia trachomatis*, *Chlamydia pneumoniae*, and *Chlamydia psittaci*. Out of them, *Chlamydia trachomatis* is an exclusively human pathogen, a major cause of a treatable and preventable disease called trachoma.

Lymphogranuloma Venereum

Lymphogranuloma venereum (LGV) is a chronic, chlamydial sexually transmitted disease of the genital tract and inguinal lymph nodes without much systemic or ocular manifestations. It is often missed due to lack of evidence in children who are generally infected following sexual abuse. The infected children may pass it on to other children in schools, hostels, and orphanages. The chlamydia responsible for the disease is *Chlamydia trachomatis* serovars L1, L2, and L3, with an incubation period of <1 week.

The *ocular involvements* consist of granulomatous conjunctivitis with preauricular lymphadenopathy and enlargement of the submandibular, subclavian, and neck glands. Other ocular presentations are generally unilateral, which may be edema of the lids, mucopurulent conjunctivitis, keratitis, interstitial keratitis, episcleritis, uveitis, and retinal hemorrhages. The ocular manifestations are amenable to many broad-spectrum antibiotics, including tetracycline given locally or systemically. Doxycycline 100 mg BD is a convenient mode of treatment. Interstitial keratitis and episcleritis require local steroids drops.

VIRUSES RESPONSIBLE FOR OCULAR AND SYSTEMIC MANIFESTATIONS

The following is a summary of the characteristics of viruses: Viruses are the smallest submicroscopic organisms without a specific staining property. Each virus contains either a DNA or RNA (nucleic acid). The nucleic acid is surrounded by a layer of proteins; the viruses themselves cannot replicate without a host cell, and hence are categorized as obligate intracellular parasites. Some of the viruses have an extra outer cover of protein responsible for their antigenicity. The antigen is responsible for immunity and is used in diagnostic tests. The invading virus gets attached to the host cell membrane at a specific receptor and gets phagocytosed by the host cell. The viruses do not possess enzymes required for multiplication and survival. The enzyme is provided by the host cell. The RNA viruses replicate in the cytoplasm and DNA in the nuclei of the host cell.

The RNA viruses that have ocular involvement are listed in **Table 30.1**.

The DNA viruses that have ocular involvement are given in **Table 30.2**.

TABLE 30.1: Class and name of RNA viruses responsible for ocular involvement.

Class of virus	*Name of virus*
Enterovirus (picornaviruses)	Poliomyelitis virus, Coxsackievirus, and ECHO viruses
Paramyxoviruses	Mumps, togavirus, and measles viruses
Rubivirus *(Matonaviridae)*	Rubella virus
Lentivirus *(Retroviridae)*	Human immunodeficiency virus

(ECHO: enteric cytopathic human orphan; RNA: ribonucleic acid)

TABLE 30.2: Class and name of deoxyribonucleic acid (DNA) viruses responsible for ocular involvement.

Class of virus	*Name of virus*
Pox viruses	Molluscum contagiosum, Smallpox virus (variola), and vaccinia virus
Herpes viruses	Chickenpox (varicella), herpes simplex, herpes zoster, Epstein–Barr virus (EBV), and *Cytomegalovirus*
Other viruses	Human papillomavirus and human adenoviruses and EBV

Coxsackie Virus and ECHO Viruses

The term ECHO virus stands for *enteric cytopathic human orphan virus*.

The virus causes widespread systemic disorders that include myositis of skeletal muscles, spasticity, flaccid paralysis, tremor, encephalomyelitis, and aseptic meningitis. The ocular structures per se are not involved; primarily, they are involved secondary to CNS involvement, which includes extraocular muscle palsy. The most common muscle involved is the lateral rectus. Involvement of seventh nerve is less common. Nystagmus is frequent. Involvement of the third nerve leads to pupillary changes; Horner syndrome too has been reported and involvement of the optic nerve leads to transient blurring of vision. All the neurological changes are self-limiting. The ocular involvements are conjunctivitis, pseudomembranous conjunctivitis, phlycten, keratitis, and superficial vascularization.

Mumps

Mumps is a common, worldwide acute infection in children. Boys and girls are equally infected. The most common presentation is painful, bilaterally symmetrical swelling of the parotids and submandibular glands. The disease spreads by droplet infection. The incubation period is 14–20 days. In the initial stages, the child suffers from fever, body pain, anorexia, and malaise. The disease gives lifelong immunity, which can be acquired by immunization in childhood.

Systemic Involvement

The initial stage lasts for 2–3 days with fast-developing bilateral painful swelling of the parotids, difficulty swallowing, and earache. It is common for the submandibular salivary glands to be enlarged simultaneously; enlargement of the lacrimal gland has also been reported. The involvement of the glands subsides in a week without any scarring. The other organs involved are the testes, pancreas, and ovaries. Orchitis is common in postpubertal age; about 20% of males are affected. The orchitis is unilateral and painful. A late complication of orchitis is testicular atrophy. Oophoritis is less frequent; it presents as pain in the lower abdomen and does not cause sterility. Less common but serious manifestations are aseptic meningitis, encephalitis, transverse myelitis, cerebellar ataxia, and facial palsy.

Ocular involvements are secondary to dacryoadenitis, which is bilateral. The swelling is tense and painful, giving an S-shaped appearance to the pseudoptosis lid with proptosis. Conjunctivitis is generally due to direct invasion by the virus; superficial keratitis is common with conjunctivitis. Scleritis and uveitis are rare and self-limiting. Bilateral optic neuritis, when present, is also self-limiting; involvement of extra- and intraocular muscles has been reported.

Management: The disease is fully preventable by a vaccine that is used as prophylaxis against measles and rubella as well, called MMR (measles, mumps, and rubella), which is administered at the age of 12 months. This gives lifelong immunity; there is no antibiotic or antiviral drug to which the organism is sensitive; hence, the management is symptomatic and includes antipyretics and analgesics orally with bed rest. Ocular involvement is treated as per symptom by standard antibiotics and cycloplegics.

Rubella (German Measles, Three-day Measles)

The organism causes serious systemic infections. It is an RNA paramyxovirus seen worldwide in both sexes; it may affect adults as well in a milder form. Children born to mothers suffering from rubella are at great risk of multiple congenital anomalies. The disease caused by the virus is called measles, which is fully preventable by a single dose of the MMR vaccine given subcutaneously at 12 months of age. This gives lifelong immunity. A nonimmunized mother in her first trimester is in danger of contracting the disease. Mothers infected after 4 months do not cause congenital anomalies in the developing fetus, which are seen only in the first trimester. The disease happens in epidemics among nonimmunized children. The infection spreads by droplets from the infected child who may be in the incubation period. The incubation period ranges between 12 and 24 days; the droplets initially cause respiratory tract infection that spreads to other organs via blood. The disease has been divided into two broad groups; the first is a mild infection seen in school-going children that may go unnoticed. The other is a more serious fatal condition that causes multiple congenital anomalies in a fetus of nonimmunized mother in the first trimester.

Congenital Rubella

Congenital rubella is contracted during the first trimester and is fraught with the danger of multiple congenital anomalies in the fetus, including pronounced bilateral ocular involvement. It remains a major cause of congenital anomalies of the eyes in developing countries; the ocular anomalies may cause permanent subnormal vision. The spread from the mother to the fetus is transplacental; the classical clinical features of congenital rubella result in rubella syndrome that consists of a triad of congenital cataracts, heart disease, and deafness. Other less dangerous systemic involvements are premature birth, abortion, low birth weight, retarded growth, hepatosplenomegaly, pneumonia, and thrombocytopenia. The other anomalies may be microcephaly, cleft palate, and dental anomalies. The less serious ocular features are catarrhal conjunctivitis and superficial keratitis. The graver congenital ocular findings are microphthalmos, central cataract, retinopathy, congenital glaucoma, corneal haze, hypoplasia of the iris, squint, nystagmus, and errors of refraction. Late complications include retinopathy, subretinal neovascularization, and maculopathy.

Rubella Cataract

The following is a summary of rubella cataracts.

Rubella cataracts are typically complete congenital cataracts in the microphthalmic eye; they are generally symmetrical, dense, and nuclear bilateral. The lens is known to harbor a live virus up to 2 years of age; there is no medical treatment for the cataract, and surgery is the only remedy available for the best result. The presence of a live virus in the cataract makes use of strong steroid and cycloplegic from the first postoperative day to the next few months to prevent virus-induced uveitis in postrubella cataract surgery. The surgery should be underway as soon as the child can stand general anesthesia. It is better to operate two eyes with a gap of 6 weeks in between. The results are not as gratifying as in nonrubella congenital cataracts. The role of the IOL is debatable. The child requires frequent changes of glasses for the rest of the life. The child following best surgery may still require low-vision aids for better vision. The congenital glaucoma that is common in Rubella syndrome is a matter of concern; it is independent of the cataract. It is multifactorial; the factors that may cause glaucoma are microphthalmos, anomalies of angle, and spherophakia. The glaucoma is worsened by associated postoperative uveitis, and it prolongs treatment with strong steroids and cycloplegia.

Measles

Measles is a common infectious exanthematous disease of childhood that mostly involves the skin and respiratory tract. It happens in epidemics. A seemingly simple, short-lived disease can be fatal. It has worldwide distribution, affecting boys and girls equally. It is caused by paramyxoviridae viruses belonging to the genus *Morbilli* with one genetic type, seen only in human being. The disease is seen in children between 6 months and 2 years, with an incubation period of 10 days. The disease spreads by droplets. The disease is most contagious between 1 and 2 days before the actual signs and symptoms develop. The disease clinically has been divided into the following stages.

- Prodrome
- Exanthema
- Complications

In the prodromal stage, the child suffers from fever, body ache, rhinitis, cough, and a bluish-white spot in the buccal mucosa called Koplik spots, which is almost diagnostic of the disease. In the next stage, the child develops rashes all over the body lasting for the next 3–4 days and disappears even without treatment; they do not leave any scars common to other exanthematous diseases. In the stage of complication, many organs are involved in the form of respiratory infection, infection of the CNS, and GI infection; more than one system may be involved simultaneously.

The most common ocular involvement is mucopurulent conjunctivitis that develops in the prodromal stage and spills over the next stage. The Koplik spots too have been observed with conjunctivitis. The lids are swollen and covered by rashes; the child suffers from intense photophobia resulting in blepharospasm due to involvement of corneal epithelium. If the conjunctiva is invaded by bacteria, the cornea develops an ulcer. In absence of corneal ulcer, the conjunctivitis and superficial keratitis are self-limiting. The corneal ulcer is worsened in presence of malnutrition with vitamin A deficiency. The other ocular involvements are frequent styes in post-infectious period and dacryocystitis. Complications of measles are more frequent and severe in presence of vitamin A deficiency. The malnourished children are more likely to succumb to the disease. The measles is often accompanied by protein-caloric malnutrition. The cause of vitamin A deficiency is depletion of vitamin A in the liver.

Management: The disease is fully preventable by the MMR vaccine given at 1 year of age; there is no chemotherapy available against the disease. The next important prophylaxis is to provide sufficient additional vitamin A despite the child's vitamin A status. The additional dose of vitamin A is administered as soon as the diagnosis of measles is confirmed. The common recommended dose is 50,000 IU under 6 months, 100,000 IU between 6 months and 1 year, and 200,000 IU above 1 year, in divided doses as per the national program of vitamin supplementation. The child with photophobia should get age-matched cycloplegia and antibiotics for corneal involvement.

Human Immunodeficiency Virus

Human immunodeficiency virus (HIV) virus belongs to the family *Retroviridae* and subfamily *Orthoretrovirinae*; it is an RNA virus. It uses host cellular mechanisms to form DNA for replication, which causes depletion of host cell immunity and nutrition. The virus has been divided into two types, i.e., type 1 and type 2. HIV-1 is found throughout the world; type 2 is localized to West African countries. HIV-1 is more easily transmitted than type 2; the former is more aggressive and causes AIDS. This is a chronic contagious disease of all ages in both sexes. It takes months to years to manifest after contracting the disease, both systemic and ocular. Isolated ocular involvement has not been reported. Two-thirds of patients with the human immunodeficiency virus [acquired immunodeficiency syndrome (AIDS)] will ultimately develop ocular symptoms. The disease, if not treated, will end in death; there is no preventive vaccine against AIDS. The drugs presently available do not change the immunodeficiency but act against the opportunistic organisms that are the cause of its spread in the body and ultimate death. The drugs available are not equally effective against all the invading opportunistic organisms. Thus, multidrug therapy is the rule. The disease spreads by body fluids.

It is the most common mode being sexual transmission. Otherwise, it can be spread through infected blood, infected mother's milk, tears, saliva, and aqueous. The neonates can get the infection from the mother's birth canal. The older children get the disease via infected blood, infected needles in adolescent drug addicts, and sexual assault. It is more common in homosexuals. The virus has affinity for CD4+ lymphocytes, causing a reduction in their number that reduces host immunity.

The ocular infections are early to develop. The ocular lesions are intraocular and extraocular caused by one or more opportunistic organisms.

The intraocular lesions are:

- Retinal microangiopathy
- Progressive outer retinal necrosis (PORN)

- Uveitis
- Uncommon neoplasm
- Neuro-ophthalmic complications

The extraocular lesions are infections of conjunctiva or cornea alone or in combination; the keratitis is superficial, similar to herpes simplex. The opportunistic organisms that worsen immunodeficiency can be viral, bacterial, or protozoal. More than one organism in various combinations and groups can be responsible for the lesions. The common opportunistic organisms are *Mycobacterium tuberculosis*, atypical *Mycobacterium tuberculosis, Pneumocystis carinii*, Cryptococcus, *Toxoplasma, Cytomegalovirus (CMV)*, and *Candida*. Many other organisms are now being added to the ever-growing list.

Out of all intraocular involvements, retinal microvasculopathy, also known as HIV retinopathy, is the most common due to direct invasion of the endothelium, producing cotton wool spots, microaneurysms, and maculopathy. The other retinal involvement is *CMV* retinitis. At least one-third of patients with AIDS are likely to develop CMV retinitis; the lesions develop along the retinal vessels due to invasion by viruses, producing white granular dots, superficial hemorrhages, retinal edema, retinal vasculitis, and retinal necrosis, which is called progressive outer retinal necrosis, caused by opportunistic herpes zoster and simplex viruses; it begins on the retinal periphery, progressing relentlessly toward the center. The condition is not amenable to multidrug therapy, hence a cause of total blindness. The two rare neoplasms encountered with HIV infection are Kaposi's sarcoma and Burkitt's lymphoma. Squamous cell carcinoma of conjunctiva, which is a rare disorder, when found with HIV infection, is pretty aggressive. The neoplasms do not respond to usual anti-HIV chemotherapy; they are best managed by oncologists.

The HIV infection is confirmed by:

- History and clinical examination suggestive of HIV infection
- CD4+ cells <200 cells/mm^3
- Evidence suggesting at least one opportunistic infection
- Evidence of HIV-related neoplasm anywhere in the body

Management: The seemingly fatal disorders, both ocular and systemic, are better treated by people trained in the management of AIDS, with assistance from ophthalmologists and oncologists.

Smallpox (Variola)

The disease is caused by the variola virus; commonly referred to as smallpox. It was a scourge known for centuries, inflicting great loss of life. Those who survived were left with scared bodies and blind eyes. The disease had worldwide distribution, mostly seen in children, till it was eradicated the world over by universal immunization against the disease by a cheap vaccine generally administered either within a few days of birth or within the first 2 years of life. The world was declared smallpox-free in 1980 by the World Health Organization (WHO). The ocular involvements consisted of vesicle on the skin of the lid and conjunctiva; the corneal involvements could be simple corneal opacity, adherent leucoma, or large bilateral total anterior staphyloma with no perception of light or at the most hand movement, with nystagmus. It used to be a very common cause of bilateral blindness in children. The conditions can still be seen in adults born before 1977 when the last case was seen.

Vaccinia

The vaccinia virus is a DNA virus resembling the smallpox virus with some differences. The vaccinia virus is used to prepare a prophylactic vaccine against smallpox. The infection is generally secondary to autoinoculation from the site of vaccination. Primary infection by vaccinia is rare. The lesion following autoinoculation or contact inoculation is generally a single blister, developing 3–4 days after vaccination anywhere on the body; it is more common on the face and lids and less frequent on the conjunctiva. There is diffuse swelling of the lid with preauricular lymphadenopathy. The condition subsides within 10 days without treatment and without scaring. The conjunctiva may develop pustules along with purulent conjunctivitis that may be associated with pseudomembrane formation. The cornea is involved if the lesion is on the lid margin, in the form of superficial punctate keratitis, which heals without treatment. A disciform keratitis may develop after a few days, which is most probably immune-mediated. Involvement of other intraocular structures are rare. Systemic presentation does not require any treatment except counseling of the parents. The ocular involvement is treated by the usual local antibiotic drops and cycloplegic.

Herpesviruses

There are many viruses in this DNA virus group that inflict human beings; they are: herpes simplex type 1 and 2, herpes zoster, varicella, CMV, and Epstein–Barr virus, which has been found to cause Burkitt lymphoma. Other viruses of the group to infect human beings are human herpesviruses 6 and 7.

The conditions mentioned above, i.e., herpes simplex, herpes zoster varicella, and molluscum, have been discussed earlier.

Cytomegalovirus

The infection by CMV can be congenital or acquired. The latter can be in neonatal or adult form. The immunocompromised adults are at a greater risk of being infected. The neonates get infection from the infected birth canal or via the placenta. The congenital CMV infection may be asymptomatic or the neonate may be seriously ill. The common congenital features are underweight children, microcephaly, hepatosplenomegaly, thrombocytopenia, and petechial hemorrhages over the body. The condition is known to cause intracranial calcification and asymptomatic chorioretinitis.

Acquired CMV infection has different presentations in immunocompromised and nonimmunocompetent persons. Later, it presents as infective mononucleosis in sexually active males with fever, chills, body aches, splenomegaly, and rarely pneumonitis. The two common involvements of the eyes are: CMV retinitis and CMV anterior uveitis.

The CMV retinitis is a serious condition that does not respond well to usual anti-HIV treatment; hence, it can cause blindness within 3–4 months of diagnosis. It has been described variously as cheese pizza, pizza pie, and granular forms. The other intraocular involvement is frosted angiitis in patients with HIV. There is a widespread retinal vasculitis with prominent sheathing.

Epstein–Barr Virus

This virus belongs to the herpes group of viruses that cause a mild systemic disease called infectious mononucleosis. The ocular involvement consists of oculoglandular syndrome, conjunctivitis, dry eye, keratitis, uveitis, choroiditis, retinitis, papillitis, and ophthalmoplegia. Recently, it has been found to be a cause of Burkitt lymphoma and nasopharyngeal carcinoma.

Coronavirus

Coronavirus is a severe acute respiratory syndrome coronavirus 2 (SARS-CoV-2) RNA virus; the disease caused is commonly referred to as coronavirus disease (COVID). In recent years, there was a pandemic of the disease, which proved to be fatal to a large population of both sexes in all races worldwide in adults. However, children do not possess immunity to the disease. In children, the symptoms are less serious and less fatal. The disease is spread by droplets in crowded localities. The disease mostly involves the respiratory system, leading to fatal hypoxia and death. Many patients survive the disease because their condition was self-limiting. There are no antivirals or antibiotics against the disease. However, an effective vaccine has been developed, which is administered as two intramuscular injections with a gap of 3–4 weeks to be followed by a booster dose 6 months later. The immunity is short-lived. Aged patients with comorbidities are more likely to develop fatal complications. Persons suffering from COVID are more likely to contract serious fungal infections. The most dangerous and common contaminants is mucormycosis. The COVID is confirmed by a reverse transcription polymerase chain reaction (RT-PCR) test. Ocular involvements by coronavirus are few and mild; they include headaches, pain in the eyeball without tenderness, and mild conjunctivitis; they may have mild keratitis. Both of which are self-limiting.

MYCOTIC (FUNGUS) INFECTION

Fungi are widely distributed microorganisms found worldwide in soil, water, air, and decaying organic matter. Fungi are microorganisms between the largest bacteria and the smallest plant. They belong to the phylum Thallophyta. The fungi do not contain chlorophyll and they do not synthesize carbohydrates. The branched filaments present in many fungi are called hyphae. This divides fungi into two broad groups of fungi with hyphae and those without hyphae. A network of hyphae is called mycelia. The fungi develop on living organisms or on dead organic matter. They are either saprophytes or parasites. The saprophytic fungi can become pathogenic. A change in environment can turn a fungus from saprophyte to parasite if the environment is changed in its favor, that can be brought about by a change in the immunity of the host. An immune-compromised body is more likely to develop a fungal infection than an immunocompetent. AIDS is an example of this change. Prolonged use of antibiotics may eliminate the causative bacteria but encourage relatively benign fungi to become invasive. This is worsened by the use of steroids, both local and systemic. Other situations that work in favor of fungi are general debility, diabetes, drug abuse, chemotherapy, and radiation.

The fungi can reproduce sexually or asexually. The spores are the reproductive bodies. There are about 30–35 species of fungi that cause systemic mycoses in humans. All systemic mycoses have ocular involvement. Occasionally, fungi may get access to the ocular structure following trauma that may be accidental or surgical. The fungi are difficult to grow on culture media; they require special media to thrive and take as much as 3 weeks to give results.

The pathogenic fungi have been put into two broad groups:

1. *Schizomycetes: Nocardia* and Actinomycosis (Actinomycosis is no longer considered a fungus). It has been put between bacteria and higher molds.
2. *Fungi imperfecti* (without spores)

Most of the fungi that have ocular manifestations are:

- Mucormycosis
- Candidiasis
- Aspergillosis
- Blastomycosis
- Coccidioidomycosis
- Histoplasmosis

Mucormycosis

Mucormycosis is a serious blinding and often fatal disease. It belongs to the species *Rhizopus phycomycetes* and order Mucorales. It is found all over the world in soil, water, manure, and the skin of asymptomatic human beings. It is known to contaminate food with high sugar contents. It is a saprophyte that is nonseptate with branching hyphae. The infection spreads most probably by droplet inhalation or ingestion.

The conditions that turn the saprophyte fungi to pathogenic in immune-compromised are diabetic ketosis, postorgan transplant status, lymphomas, and leukemias. Its incidence has shown a sudden peak in COVID patients, resulting in loss of eyes. Ocular involvement generally requires exenteration, which too may not save the life of the patients.

The disease comprises a moderate-to-fast-growing black mass in the sinus that soon invades the surrounding structures like the brain, orbit, nasopharynx, respiratory tract, and GI tract.

The eyes are involved due to the spread from the nasopharynx of a person with mucormycosis. The disease most probably begins in paranasal sinuses, from where it spreads to adjacent structures. The main infected mass is highly vascular with invasive angiopathy, which results in ischemic or hemorrhagic necrosis **(Figs. 30.1 and 30.2)**.

The ocular involvements are mostly in the orbit; involvement of the skin of the lids and conjunctiva is rare. The orbital involvement is secondary to extension from neighboring structures. The orbital involvement in COVID patients is generally overshadowed by systemic symptoms of COVID. By the time its presence is suspected, it is too late. The symptoms start as deep-seated pain in the orbit,

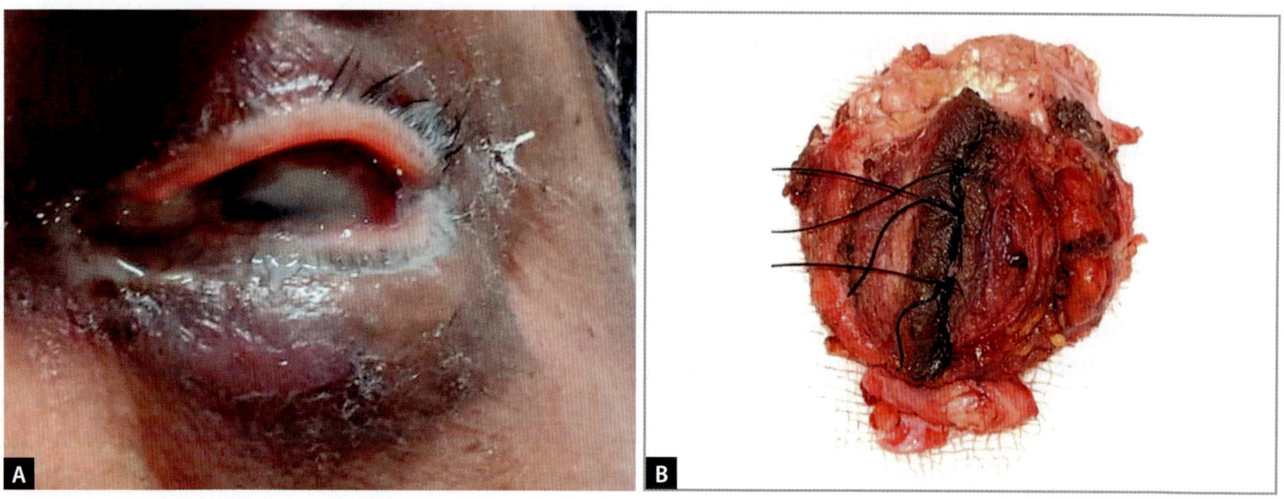

Figs. 30.1A and B: (A) Mucormycosis of orbit and (B) mass removed from orbit in a patient with coronavirus disease (COVID).
Courtesy: Dr Somen Misra.

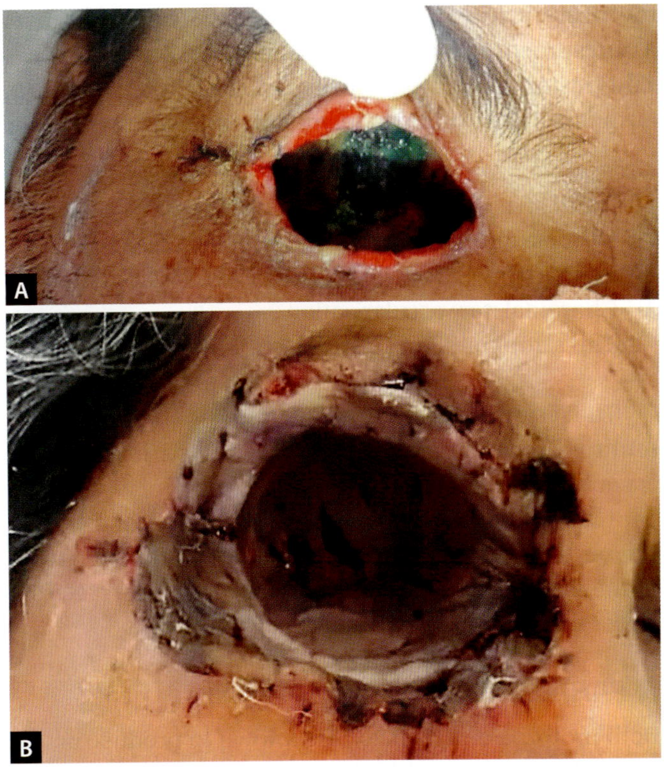

Figs. 30.2A and B: Exenterated orbit following mucormycosis in patients with COVID.
Courtesy: Dr Somen Misra.

headaches, diplopia, and diminished vision with edema of the blackened lids and chemosis of the conjunctiva. A black mass may be present in the conjunctiva. The earliest signs of the disease in orbit are best seen on magnetic resonance imaging (MRI) and computed tomography (CT). Medical treatment with amphotericin B has limited success. Exenteration may save life, leaving an ugly deformity.

Candidiasis

Candidiasis of all exposed mucous membranes is very common in children, especially in the buccal mucosa. It is commonly known as thrush. *Candida albicans* is the most common out of all *Candida* fungi. It is normal flora of all mucous membranes, skin, GI tract, respiratory, and urinary tract. It is occasionally found on the lid margin, from where it gets into the conjunctiva. More common in dry eye and keratitis sicca, it is profusely distributed in soil and water; it may be seen in green vegetables and fruits; and rarely, it may contaminate cooked food. It is a dimorphic fungus with two phases, i.e., yeast and mycelia; the former is more frequent. The infection finds its way into the body through local inoculation or via a contaminated abrasion. It may reach the eye through endogenous primary systemic infection.

Systemic involvement is common in neonates and malnourished children as oral thrush. It may be seen as a chronic mucocutaneous lesion in adults with comorbidities of diabetes, hypoparathyroidism, hypothyroidism, and Addison's disease; it is common in persons suffering from other systemic infections by bacteria. It is common in persons with indwelling catheters. The ocular involvement consists of purulent conjunctivitis, pseudomembranous conjunctivitis, conjunctival ulcer, and rarely phlycten. It is known to produce granulomatous canaliculitis. Intraocular involvement results as frank endophthalmitis, commonly following a penetrating injury either accidental or surgical. Intraocular spread from an infected lesion may cause endogenous endophthalmitis. Free-flowing snowballs in the vitreous heralds on a set of endophthalmitis. The only way to treat endophthalmitis is a timely complete vitrectomy. Intravitreal antifungal drugs too have been advocated with limited success. Keratitis is treated by usual cycloplegia, and locally acting antifungal drops frequently. The results of which are not encouraging; extraocular candidiasis is treated with oral antifungal drugs.

Aspergillosis

Aspergillus is a saprophytic fungus found in soil, decaying vegetable matter with worldwide distribution, more common in humid tropical and temperate countries. The systemic manifestation follows inhalation of spores leading to infection of the paranasal sinuses and respiratory tract. From these primary lesions, the disease may spread to distant organs, including the brain and kidney. Ocular involvement is mainly an orbital mass, less commonly a corneal ulcer. Endophthalmitis in aspergillosis is commonly exogenous following penetrating wound; less common is metastatic endophthalmitis. The first line of treatment is voriconazole, which is administered orally. Intravitreal voriconazole has not been found to be very effective, leaving vitrectomy as an alternate mode of treatment.

Blastomycosis

Blastomycosis is caused by a dimorphic fungus *Blastomyces dermatitidis*, found in two phases, the mycelial phase and the yeast phase. The organism is mostly found in soil. Inhalation of the organism is the most common form of acquiring the disease. The earliest infection is found in the respiratory tract, from where it spreads to many organs. The ocular manifestation consists of granuloma of the skin of the lid, conjunctiva, orbit, and uveitis. The condition is treated with itraconazole under the supervision of an internist.

Coccidioidomycosis

Coccidioidomycosis is caused by a dimorphic fungus *Coccidioides immitis*, that changes its phases with changes in environment. It is a saprophyte that grows like a white fluffy mold on decaying matter and culture media. The organism multiplies by endospores present in spherules. The spherule ruptures, releasing endospores, which again form spherules in a cycle. The systemic involvements are respiratory, which may remain asymptomatic and resolve or may be cause of pulmonary cavity. The organism spreads to other organs by dissemination; immunocompromised patients are at higher risk of pulmonary and extrapulmonary spread. The ocular involvements are few; they are due to hematogenous spread or hypersensitivity. The ocular lesions are progressive chronic granulomatous panuveitis, independent of severity of pulmonary lesion. The cornea may develop keratitis. Granuloma of conjunctiva lid and sac has been reported.

Histoplasmosis

Histoplasmosis is a chronic systemic disease mainly involving the lungs. It is seen in all ages in susceptible races; it is infrequent in dark races. The organism causing the disease is *Histoplasma capsulatum*, with worldwide distribution in soil and water; it is disseminated by the droppings of birds. The organism grows well in Sabouraud's media at room temperature. The fungus is dimorphic; the disease spreads by spores present in the air by inhalation.

The *systemic involvement* is mostly localized to the lungs after the spores have been inhaled. The lungs are involved as multiple granulomas spread all over the lung. The granulomas necrose to get calcified, giving classical round multiple opacities; the granulomas before calcification are confused with tubercular lesions. Immunocompromised patients of all ages are more likely to suffer from the disease that may prove fatal, especially in children. The ocular lesions mostly involve the posterior uvea. The ocular lesions are referred to as presumed ocular histoplasmosis syndrome (POHS). The posterior segment involvement is hematogenous. Surprisingly, the anterior segment is spared in spite of its being vascular.

The triad of ocular involvements consists of:
1. Discrete atrophic choroid scars in the macula
2. Peripapillary atrophic patch
3. Choroidal neovascularization

The atrophic patches in the choroid are called histo spots.

The lesion may disappear without treatment, leaving multiple opacities that may be activated in later life, especially in children.

The systemic condition is treated by itraconazole for 6 months to 1 year, depending on the immunity status of the patients. The ocular lesions may require a steroid under the umbrella of systemic drugs.

PARASITIC INFECTION

Both protozoa and metazoa are known to produce ocular morbidity with or without systemic involvement. The metazoa infections are commonly caused by helminths, both cestodes and nematodes. The organisms other than protozoa or metazoa that inflict eyes are arthropods and insect larvae. The most common protozoa to infect the eye is toxoplasma. The other protozoan of importance is *Trypanosoma*. The arthropods that cause ocular disorders are phthiriasis and demodicosis. Infestation by insect larvae is called ocular myiasis.

Toxoplasmosis

Toxoplasmosis is caused by a universally present protozoan called *Toxoplasma gondii*. About half of the adult populations are asymptomatic carriers of the disease. The ocular infection can either be primary without systemic involvement or secondary to systemic involvement. In children, it can either be congenital or acquired; the former is more common.

Acanthamoeba

The disease caused by protozoan *Acanthamoeba* is called acanthamoebiasis. The organism is found in contaminated water. The most serious systemic involvement is granulomatous acanthamoebic encephalitis. The organism reaches the brain by hematologic spread from sinuses, lungs, and even skin. The most common ocular involvement is kerato-acanthamoeba.

Trypanosomiasis (Sleeping Sickness)

The disease is endemic, localized to certain parts of Africa and South America. The disease has not been reported from places other than endemic areas. The disease is caused by *Trypanosoma gambiense* transmitted by tsetse fly in South America and by the bite of a bug of the genera *Triatoma*. The African and South American trypanosomiasis differ in clinical presentation. The African trypanosomiasis has a more ocular presentation than its counterpart.

African Trypanosomiasis

The disease is seen in both sexes of any age in the endemic area. The disease becomes obvious in 1–2 weeks following the bite of the fly tsetse. The organism has a hematogenous and lymphatic spread, involving lymph glands, CSF, and brain. The first manifestation is seen in the skin as a nodule called *Trypanosoma* chancre. This is followed by fever that may last for weeks and is intermittent; in the meantime, the organism reaches the spleen, resulting in splenomegaly. It takes a few years to develop the sleeping sickness stage with shuffling gate, difficulty to walk, a mask-like face, and mild bilateral ptosis. The patient has a tendency to go to sleep at odd hours; the last stage comprises convulsions, various types of paralysis, and coma that may terminate in death. The ocular manifestations consist of edema of the lids, enlargement of preauricular and submandibular lymph nodes, bilateral interstitial keratitis, and chronic uveitis. In the late stages, there may be paralysis of extraocular muscles and papilledema due to involvement of the brain. The condition becomes worse when associated with onchocerciasis, another blinding disorder of parasitic origin in endemic areas. The South American trypanosomiasis, in contrast to its African counterpart, differs in being spread by the bite of a triatomine bug. The other point of differentiation is that it is devoid of somnolence. The disease is called Chagas disease and the cutaneous lesion is called a chagoma. The Chagas disease is associated with enlargement of lymph nodes, fever, hepatosplenomegaly, endocarditis, and meningoencephalitis. The ocular manifestations are few in the form of unilateral chagoma of the lid. The disease is treated by benznidazole, which is specific for Chagas disease.

Onchocerciasis (River Blindness)

Onchocerciasis is a major cause of preventable and treatable disease commonly known as river blindness. The parasite is a nematode. The two parasites of this group that cause the diseases are *Onchocerca volvulus* and *Onchococesea caecutiens*. The parasite is commonly known as blinding worm and river worm because the larvae of the parasite reproduce in fast-flowing rivers. The disease is mostly seen in remote villages situated on the banks of these rivers. The disease is endemic in 31 tropical and temperate countries of Africa and South America. The disease is not found outside these countries; the vector responsible is female black fly *Simulium*. The fly is an intermediate host. The adult larva develops in the mouth part of the fly. The disease spreads from infected to noninfected persons following a bite of the fly that acts as a host. There may be multiple infections in a single person.

The *systemic involvement* consists predominantly of skin, in the form of intense itching with patches of hypopigmented conglomerated spots called leopard skin. The skin is also wrinkled. Some patients develop multiple subcutaneous palpable nodules. Enlargement of inguinal and femoral lymph nodes and hydroceles are common.

The disease involves all the parts of the eyes. They are:

- Transient edema of the lids may have nodules.
- Mild proptosis
- Conjunctiva is thickened and pigmented.
- Conjunctival snips show living parasites even without stain.
- Parasites are not seen on the surface of the conjunctiva.
- Corneal involvement is the most important cause of blindness. The corneal involvement is bilateral; all the people with onchocerciasis develop corneal morbidity. The corneal involvement is varied that may be in the form of any or many of the following: Longer the history of corneal involvement, more are the corneal signs. All the layers of the cornea are involved. They include various grades of corneal opacities, hazy cornea, superficial and deep vascularization, folds in Descemet's membrane, deposits of calcium, dead microfilaria in the cornea, superficial keratitis, punctate keratitis, sclerosing keratitis, and KPs.
- *AC* shows the number of free-floating microfilaria without any AC reaction. The dead microfilaria accumulates at the bottom of AC, forming a pseudohypopyon.

- *Uvea* shows various grades of chronic uveitis ranging from iritis to chorioretinitis. The pupil is irregular, mostly pear-shaped, spongy iris that is called pumice stone iris.
- *Vitreous* may show free-floating microfilaria.
- Optic neuritis and optic atrophy
- There may be complicated cataracts secondary to chronic uveitis.

Diagnosis: The diagnosis is obvious in endemic areas. Even nonmedical persons can diagnose it due to skin involvement and fast-growing diminished vision in both eyes; many of the persons living in the same village may suffer from the disease, which is nonfatal but blinding. The disease is confirmed by examining a skin snip under a microscope by *hematoxylin and eosin (H&E)*. The subconjunctival living microfilaria are visible without staining.

Management: Prophylaxis consists of wearing long-sleeved shirts and pants and using repellent cream during the day. The fly is active only during the day.

The definitive treatment is oral ivermectin given in doses of 200 micrograms per kg of body weight as a single dose every 6 months for many months. The addition of doxycycline enhances the efficacy of ivermectin. A new drug, moxidectin, which is generally used to deworm animals too, has been tried without equal success. A vaccine has been developed against Onchocerca to immunize children under 5 years of age. The vaccine reduces adult worm number in the body, which results in reduced morbidity of the infestation.

Loiasis

The nematode *Loa-loa*, also known as African eye worm, causes intraocular infections in endemic areas of central and western Africa. The life cycle of the worm is not well established; the disease is vector-borne and caused by a fly called by various names such as deer fly, mango fly, or mangrove fly. The parasitic worm is *Loa-loa*. It is transmitted to humans by way of repeated bites of deer flies of the genus *Chrysops*; only female flies can spread the disease from infected person to noninfected. The worm, which is diurnal in nature, the microfilaria, is seen in the peripheral blood between 12:00 noon and 2:00 PM. The exact incubation period is not known. The disease is caused by adult worms that move under the skin to be picked up by female flies. The cutaneous lesions may form a nodule called Calabar swelling. Systemic involvements are rare. Eosinophilia is a constant feature. The other systemic manifestations are cardiomyopathy, nephropathy, and encephalopathy, which are late manifestations that may prove to be fatal. The ocular manifestations are worms under the conjunctiva and Calabar swelling of the lids.

The organism may be visible on a slit lamp in the AC. The microfilaria may move from anterior to posterior chambers and may cause inflammation of the uvea. The definitive treatment consists of systemic administration of *diethylcarbamazine (DEC)* that eliminates both microfilaria and adult worms. Albendazole needs to be added to the above drug if it does not prove to be curative. The albendazole kills the adult worms. The worms in the anterior chamber and vitreous are removed surgically by standard methods. The associated uveitis is treated by cycloplegia and steroid drops.

Thelaziasis

Thelazia is a small nematode, called an oriental worm, as most of the human cases have been reported from southeast Asia and the Far East, the life cycle of which is not well understood. It commonly lives in the lacrimal glands and lacrimal passages of many mammals, common being dogs and horses. There are two species of thelazia, i.e., *Thelazia callipaeda* and *Thelazia californiensis*. Cockroaches are suspected to be intermediate hosts. It is presumed that the disease is spread by common houseflies.

Systemic infection has not been reported.

It is presumed that the flies deposit the eggs of the nematode in the conjunctiva. The larvae hatch from the eggs and migrate to the lids and lacrimal sac. The larvae may produce conjunctival nodules. The larvae may penetrate the cornea or the sclera to become intraocular, causing uveitis. The dead worm, like most of the nematodes, can cause an allergic reaction. The worm may be seen as a free-floating organism in the AC.

Treatment: The management consists of surgical removal of the worm from AC by slandered method, i.e., constriction of the pupil to prevent the worm from escaping in the posterior chamber; anesthetizing the cornea generally immobilizes the worm, facilitating removal of the worm. Eye drops of ivermectin and diethylcarbamazine drops (when available) kill the worm. Oral ivermectin, diethylcarbamazine, and albendazole eradicate the worm as well. Death of the worm starts an allergic reaction that should be treated with antihistamine tablets.

Trichinosis

Trichinosis is a disease seen in the Western hemisphere, though the parasite has worldwide distribution, caused by larvae of the nematodes *Trichinella spiralis* and *Trichinella pseudospiralis*.

The disease is spread by eating undercooked food, infected pork, or beef. The larva has predilection for striated muscles. The systemic involvement consists of diarrhea, abdominal pain, nausea, and vomiting. The cutaneous involvement includes migration of larvae, allergic reactions, and maculopapular rash. Myocarditis, tachyarrhythmia, and encephalopathy are rare. Muscle involvement is common.

Ocular involvements are edema of periorbital tissue, orbicularis, and extra ocular muscles, palsy, subconjunctival hemorrhages, and retinal hemorrhages.

Treatment of Trichinosis

Metronidazole is the drug of choice to treat trichinosis. The drug is administered as an oral tablet of 500 mg per day for 7 days for adults. Albendazole and ivermectin too are effective against the worm.

Dracunculosis (Guinea Worm)

This parasitic disease is mostly seen in tropical and subtropical, humid areas, caused by a largest thread worm called *Dracunculus medinensis*. The intermediate host is *Cyclops*, a crustacean found in many water bodies and step wells. The larva of the worm lives in the *Cyclops*; the larvae penetrate the walls of the GI tract; the female lives for years after fertilization; the males are short-lived. In humans, the larvae penetrate the gut wall to mature. The female, after fertilization, migrates under the skin to reach the extremities, mostly legs and feet. In fact, they may travel to any part of the body that remains wet for hours, hence, it is not uncommon to see them on the back and head of water carriers. The gravid female migrates under the skin to become superficial, forming a blister. A person may have multiple blisters. The blister ruptures to release the worm in large numbers in stagnant water to be engulfed by Cyclops, which in turn infect human beings following drinking infested water. The cycle is repeated continuously in endemic areas. There is no systemic involvement. The disease has been eradicated in many parts of the world, including India, in 2000. The ocular involvements are local edema of the lids and periorbital skin with blisters that may regularly release the worms. The orbital larvae may cause mild proptosis; the organism gets calcified if it dies in the orbit.

Treatment: There is no medical treatment for dracunculosis; the only way to get the worm out of the body is to remove it mechanically. The most common practice is to wind the worm around a stick about a centimeter each day. Ivermectin has been used with limited success. The best way is to avoid drinking water suspected of being contaminated by *Cyclops*.

Cysticercosis

Cysticercosis is caused by a cestode called *Taenia solium*, commonly referred to as the pork tape worm. Humans are definitive hosts; pigs are intermediate hosts that harbor the larval form of *Taenia solium*. However, sometimes humans can also act as intermediate hosts by ingestion of ova of the cestode. The disease caused by *Taenia solium* is called cysticercosis. The gravid proglottid of the adult worm is passed in the stool of the definitive host, which is picked up by the intermediate host, i.e., a pig or other mammals. In the intestine of the pig, embryos are released from gravid proglottid; the embryos pass the intestinal mucosa to reach the circulation that takes them to other organs. The common tissue to be invaded is the striated muscles of the pig. The embryos get enmeshed in small vessels and are converted to the larval stage called cysticercus. Humans are infected by consuming undercooked pork infested by live cysticercus or consuming food contaminated with ova that makes humans an intermediate host. The ovum thus consumed is converted into cysticercus.

Systemic involvement of cysticercus is manyfold; it may involve all organs, chief being the brain, eyes, muscles, kidney, liver, and spleen. Involvement of the GI tract may remain asymptomatic or may present with vague abdominal pain, diarrhea, or weight loss. Patients pass segments of tapeworm in stool. Out of the conditions mentioned, involvement of the brain is most important. The involvement of the brain is generally in the form of neurocysticercosis. It may be parenchymal, i.e., located in the brain matter; more common is extraparenchymal that may invade meninges, ventricles, cisterna basalis, subarachnoid space, or even the spinal cord. The lesion behaves as a space-occupying lesion. The common symptoms of which are headache, vomiting, focal seizures, convulsions, and raised intracranial pressure reflected as papilledema, best seen on CT and MRI. Ocular involvements are frequent. 50% of persons with systemic cysticercosis develop ocular symptoms that may be intra or extraocular. The left eye is more frequently involved; the cyst has two presentations: (1) It may develop in the orbit, causing proptosis and extraocular muscle palsy and (2) migrate anteriorly along the recti to become subconjunctival. The other mode is the primary subconjunctival cyst without involving the orbit in the conjunctiva; it is more commonly seen on the medial side. The involvement of medial subconjunctiva in the left eye is so frequent that it is almost diagnostic of subconjunctival cysticercosis. There may be more than one cyst in the subconjunctiva space. As the cyst grows, it breaks the conjunctiva and may be expelled. The involvement of the cranial nerve is secondary to growth in the brain. The cyst may be seen in the AC and vitreous. The death of an intraocular organism causes severe endophthalmitis; this happens commonly during medical therapy or surgical intervention.

Management: The worm is killed by systemic administration of many drugs given orally; the most common drug used is albendazole in doses of 15 mg/kg/day in 2 divided doses for 15 days. The other drug used is praziquantel in a dose of 50 mg/kg/day for 15 days. The former is better tolerated; any of the drugs may cause death of the organism, resulting in a local or systemic allergic reaction, which requires a heavy dose of steroids. The ocular lesions are treated by systemic albendazole, local instillation of steroid drops, and cycloplegia. Medical treatment is generally sufficient to eradicate the infection; otherwise, the cyst may be removed surgically. The preventive methods are avoiding raw vegetables, drinking contaminated fluid, and consuming uncooked pork or beef.

Toxocariasis

This is yet another nematode infection caused by *Toxocara*. The disease caused by the nematode is toxocariasis. There are two types of *Toxocara* that infest human beings. They are *Toxocara canis* and *Toxocara cati*; the latter, which was thought to be a major cause of toxocariasis in the past, has been removed from the list, as it has been proved that *Toxocara cati* is not a causative factor. The parasite is seen in dogs of all ages and both sexes; the parasite in puppies is the cause of the disorders. Human children are more likely to develop the disease than adults. The ages of pediatric patients range between 2 and 15 years. It has been observed more commonly in boys; the children with pica are most vulnerable than others. In the puppies, the disease is passed either transplacentally or during suckling and direct ingestion of food infected by the eggs of the worm. Human children acquire the disease following consuming infected food, soil, dust, or water. In children, the ingested eggs hatch to form larva that penetrate the gut wall to reach systemic circulation that carries them to distant organs, including the eyes.

Management: Management is medical, by oral administration of antihelminthics, such as albendazole, mebendazole, and ivermectin. Recurrences are common if the puppies are not treated along with the children.

PROTOZOAN INFECTION

The two protozoa of ocular importance are *Acanthamoeba* and *Toxoplasma*. They have been discussed in detail in previous chapters.

Ocular Myiasis

The term myiasis refers to the invasion of living or dead human (or animal) tissue by fly larvae. That can occur on any exposed part of the body that could be the mucous membrane or an exposed, contaminated wound. The most common invasion is by *Oestrus ovis* (sheep bot fly). The disease is caused mostly by first-stage larvae and is called myiasis external. The second-stage larvae cause myiasis interna. The former is more common than the latter. The condition is seen frequently in people who deal with sheep; however, it can be seen rarely in other persons as well. The ophthalmic myiasis may be caused by the deposition of larvae in the normal conjunctival sac of healthy people as well. Otherwise, it is generally seen in a debilitated, malnourished person with unattended leprosy, diabetes mellitus, open wounds, fungating carcinomas, psychiatric illness, a person on immunosuppressive agents, or suffering from HIV. The exact incubation period is not known. The patient presents with foreign body sensation, redness of the eyelid, edema, acute ocular foreign body sensation, irritation, redness, lacrimation, photophobia, and reduced vision. The condition is worsened following invasion by bacteria. Photophobia indicates corneal involvement. Conjunctival involvement is associated with a pseudomembrane under which live larvae can be seen. Occasionally, the larvae may be seen in the lacrimal sac or canaliculus. The larvae can erode the outer coat of the eyeball to become intraocular to reach AC and vitreous, starting intense endophthalmitis. Sometimes, the larvae can be seen crawling on the conjunctiva sac, both bulbar and tarsal. The ocular myiasis externa does not involve extraocular structures except conjunctiva. The stage 2 larva invades the bony orbit and invades paranasal sinuses and the brain, which may be fatal.

Treatment: The treatment consists of the physical removal of the maggots from the conjunctival surface of healthy persons by sufficient instillation of a local anesthetic agent; this will immobilize the worm that can be picked up by plain forceps. This should be followed by the instillation of broad-spectrum antibiotics in the conjunctival sac. Oral ivermectin has been found to be useful in eradicating the infection.

Ophthalmic myiasis externa is difficult to treat; it is better treated by general surgeons. The principle of management is correction of fluid electrolyte imbalance, correction of diabetes, and management of primary infection and malignancy, along with systemic broad-spectrum antibiotics with anti-inflammatory drugs. The patient requires hospitalization under a mosquito net, isolated from other patients. The infected wound is treated by standard methods.

SUGGESTED READING

1. Latif I, Qamar RR, Attaullah I, Soomro M. Ocular Myiasis. PJO. 2008;24(3).
2. Mukherjee PK, Agrawal S. Subconjunctival twin cysticercosis. Indian J Ophthalmol. 1975;23(3):28-9.
3. Mukherjee PK, Bandyopadhyay P. Infectious Diseases of the Eyes, 1st edition. Gurgaon Haryana: Wolters Kluwer India; 2010.
4. Mukherjee PK, Bandyopadhyay P. Ocular Microbiology, 1st Edition. New Delhi: Jaypee Brothers Medical Publishers (P) Ltd; 2010.
5. Mukherjee PK, Jain PC, Mishra, RK; Exanthemata: A causative factor of chronic dacryocystitis in children. J All India Ophthalmol Soc. 1969;17(1):27-30.
6. Mukherjee PK, Verma S, Agrawal S. Intraocular thelazia. A case report. Indian J Ophthalmol. 1978;25(4):41-2.
7. Mukherjee PK. Thelaziasis. In: Roy FH, Fraunfelder FW, Fraunfelder FT (Eds). Current Ocular Therapy, 5th edition. Philadelphia: WB Saunders Company; 2000. pp. 100-1.
8. Nema HV, Venkatesh P, Sharma YR, Nema N. Eye is Systemic Disorders, 1st edition. New Delhi: Wiley India; 2015.
9. Nene AS, Mishra A, Dhand P. Ocular myiasis caused by Chrysomya bezziana—a case report. Clin Ophthalmology. 2015;9:423-7.
10. Thakur K, Singh G, Chauhan S, Sood A. Vidi, Vini, Vinci: External ophthalmomyiasis infection that occurred, and was diagnosed and treated in a single day: A rare case report: Oman J Ophthalmol. 2009;2(3):130-2.

CHAPTER

31 Examination of Vision in Children

Examination of eyes in children is more time-consuming than in adults. Younger the child, more difficult is the examination, especially recording of vision. It should be remembered that recording vision is the most crucial examination.

Many a time infants are brought by anxious parents to know:

- If the child can see?
- Does the child squint?

> Remembering the dictum that a child is not a compressed adult. This helps in overcoming the predicament.

> The eyes are fully formed at birth, but it takes the next 5 years to develop all the functions. The examination of the eyes can be broadly divided into.

- Physical examination of structures
- Eliciting its function

The latter, which is predominantly recorded of vision, may take as much as 50% of all times spent on examination.

For the purpose of examination, the procedure can be compartmentalized age-wise.

- Examination of neonates and infants
- Examination between 1 and 5 years
- Examination between 5 and 10 years
- Examination above 10 years

A child under 1 year is nonverbal, making it more difficult to examine. The principal of examination, methods, tests, and interpretations of tests in children are similar to adults with little modification.

EXAMINATION OF EYES OF NEONATES AND INFANTS

Before embarking on examination, it is worth noting that the structures of the eyes of a neonate do not differ much from the eyes of infants under 1 year.

> The growth of the eye is maximum in the first 2 years of life.

The eyes of newborns are essentially smaller than adult eyes; hence, it is but natural to assume that as sensory organs, they must be far less efficient than adult eyes. This is far from the truth; the infant's eyes are far more developed as sensory organs when weighed against their size.

The newborn keeps eyes closed almost 15–20 hours a day, making it difficult to elicit many tests.

> To be able to examine well, a neonate should be awake, alert, comfortable, and hungry.

The child's eyes, like adult eyes, are tested under:

- Diffuse light
- Focused light
- Especially adopted optical devices:
    - Hand-held slit lamp
    - Direct ophthalmoscope
    - Indirect ophthalmoscope
    - Operating microscope
    - Non-touch tonometer
    - Gonioscope

The actual examination should be preceded by history.

- *Mother:* History of maternal illness during pregnancy, especially in the first trimester. An inquiry should be made regarding rubella, toxoplasmosis, diabetes, thyroid disorder, myasthenia, eclampsia, difficult past labors, and mode of delivery
- *Child*: Prematurity, low birth weight, oxygenation, difficult labor, fatal distress neonatal apnea, difficulty to suckle, and history of home delivery

The purposes of examination of the eyes of a newborn are twofold, i.e., does the child have vision, if so, how much is the vision, and the next is to identify the conditions that may jeopardize the vision.

> The incidence of absence of vision in newborns is minuscule if detectable causes are excluded.

The causes that may result in bilateral subnormal vision can be ocular or systemic. It is common to have a combination of the two.

The ocular causes are mostly congenital anomalies.

They are:

- Anophthalmos
- Microphthalmos
- Microcornea
- Central congenital cataract
- Buphthalmos
- Aniridia
- Large uveoretinal coloboma
- Persistent corneal haze
- Retinoblastoma and other causes of leukocoria
- Congenital anomalies of disc
- Albinism

The systemic causes are:

- Prematurity
- Low birth weight
- Prolonged administration of oxygen
- Fetal distresses
- Birth trauma to the occipital area
- Cortical blindness (cerebral visual impairment)
- Midline defect

Recording of vision in children:

This is one of the most difficult clinical tasks in ophthalmology. The tests employed to record vision can be divided into two groups:

1. Gross
2. Detailed

1. *Gross examination:* Exclusion of obvious obstruction to the visual path.
    - Congenital ptosis
    - Microphthalmos
    - Microcornea
    - Opacity in media
    - White reflex in pupil
2. *Detailed examination:*
    - Refraction under cycloplegia
    - Examination of fundus:
        - Direct ophthalmoscope
        - Indirect ophthalmoscope
    - Hand-held slit-lamp examination to exclude opacity in media

Points to remember while recording vision in children:

- Recording of vision in a newborn does not give very accurate information, the results are gross.
- Recording of vision between 1 and 3 years gives more definite information than under 1 year.
- After 3 years, the task becomes easier and results in more precise results, barring the fact that the child may be apprehensive, hence noncooperative.
- The child between 1 and 3 years old is nonverbal, hence cannot be tested on usual optotypes.
- The examination in such a situation has to depend on an indirect method.
- The child follows the object by turning the eyes. Turning and tilting the head when the object of interest is moved in the field of vision from side to side or in a vertical plane.
- Changing the size of the target the vision can be roughly estimated and translated Snellen chart.
- The children in this age group have good near vision. The child of 1 year can pick up small particles from the floor generally with the intention to put them in the mouth.
- If the child has very poor vision, the parents are the first to notice it and bring the child with a common question, i.e., does the child see? This is a difficult question to answer. There is nothing worse than assuring the parents that the child is normal, and the latter turns out not to be so. The revere is also possible.
- Straight eyes with good, central, and maintained fixation, a bright cornea, a brisk pupillary reaction, and a normal fundus are indications of fairly good vision.
- Squint, nystagmus, persistent staring, and loss of interest in the object are bad signs they point toward poor to very poor vision.
- Cross fixation is seen in congenital large-angle esotropia, an indication of equal vision in both eyes, which may or may not be age-matched.
- Alternation also denotes good vision.
- The presence of pupillary reaction indicates intact afferent and efferent paths of light. Pupillary reaction is not a measurement of visual acuity.
- In cortical blindness, the pupillary reaction is present.
- A child as young as 1 year resents occluding the eye with better vision.

TABLE 31.1: Various types of examinations and their purpose in recording vision in children.

Types of vision	*Test employed*
1. Acuity detection	i. Catford drum ii. STYACR test (they have been called by two different names, i.e., Snellen's test for young children and retarded and Sheridan test) iii. Boeck candy bead test
2. Acuity recognition	i. Snellen E; ii. Landolt C iii. HOTV test; iv. Sjogren's hand test v. Collins pictures; vi. Allen picture vii. Cardiff cards; viii. Sheridan's letter test
3. Acuity resolution	i. Optokinetic nystagmus test (OKN) ii. *Preferential looking test (PLT):* Teller acuity cards test iii. Visually evoked response (VER)

- The plan followed in recording vision in children above 5 years is similar to recording vision in adults. It consists of:
  - Recording of vision in two eyes separately
  - The right eye is examined first; this is a convention.
  - This is followed by a recording of vision in both eyes.
  - The vision into eyes together should be better than in the individual eye.
  - If vision in two eyes together is not better than vision in a better eye, it should be concluded that vision in eye with poor vision is uncorrectable.
- This routine is changed in children under 5 years.
  - Vision is tested with both eyes open as an initial step, this gives confidence to the child and reduces apprehension.
  - This is followed by examination of the supposed to be better eye.
  - The diseased eye is examined next.
- While recording vision in one eye, the other eye should be occluded completely; otherwise, the child will look over the occluder.
- The vision in children should be recorded in a room with usual illumination.
- One of the attendants may be present at the time of recording vision in the child with instruction, not to prompt.
- Children waiting in the examination room are known to memorize the optotypes and can recite them even without looking at them.
- This can be avoided by asking the child to read the optotypes from right to left instead of the usual practice of left to right.
- A child of any age with searching movement most probably does not have vision in any eye.

One of the formulas used to calculate visual acuity in a nonverbal child is:

$$\text{Visual acuity} = \frac{0.3 \times \text{Distances in meter}}{\text{Size of the object in milimeter}}$$

The above formula gives visual acuity in decimal, i.e., 6/6 on Snellen chart is 1.00 in decimal unit.

A more accurate and detailed examination consists of:

- *Acuity detection:* This is the ability of detect the smallest stimulus without the ability to recognize the stimulus.
- *Acuity recognition:* This estimates the faculty to detect and recognize stimulus and compare to other stimulus that may be an object or optotype. Empirically, the test has been divided into four groups are as follows:
  1. *Direction:* Snellen E, Landolt C, Sjogren's hand
  2. *Identification of optotypes:* Snellen chart, Sheridan letter, HOTV, and its variations, recognizing symbols
  3. *Identifying pictures and toys:* Allen picture cards, Collins picture cards, and Sheridan's miniature toys
  4. *Identifying picture on behavioral pattern:* Cardiff acuity card, Bally–Hall test

  Table 31.1 describes vision and tests performed to elicit them.
- *Acuity resolution*

There are about a hundred of such methods all not suitable for all ages. All the tests listed above are subjective except for visually evoked responses.

VISUAL ACUITY TEST IN INFANCY

- Eliciting of vision should be attempted at every visit.
- Vision should be recorded at every visit.
- Best corrected vision should be noted in each eye.
- Vision in two eyes should be tested separately.

Visual acuity in infants can be tested either directly or indirectly, as depicted in the ***Flowchart 31.1****.*

Common methods used are:

- Preferential looking test
- Optokinetic drum
- Visually evoked response
- Teller cards
- Cardiff acuity card

Vision between birth and 2 months:
At birth, a child can fixate a pattern stimulus.

This faculty has been utilized to evaluate the vision.

- Preferential looking test
- Fixation and following a target
- Pupillary reaction

- *Preferential looking test:* This is a gross subjective test used in children who cannot identify letters or even pictures. This is based on the principle that an infant has a tendency to fixate on a patterned object more often than a monochromatic, dull object of the same brightness at the same distance. To elicit this, infant's eyes are exposed to two stimulus, one with stripes and the other with a uniformly homogeneous gray fields of the same illumination. The child looks at the striped object for as long as the pattern is visible and the eyes can resolve it. The position of the stripes is alternated randomly; the child with vision will look at the stripes rather than at the gray fields. A child without vision will not show preference between the stripes and gray fields. During the test, the child will sit on an adult's lap facing the stimulus, the two stimuli painted on a board side by side with a peep hole between the two fields. The peep hole is meant for the observer to monitor the preference of the child. The observer views the child through the peephole and judges the location of the stripes based on the child's head and eye movements. The narrowest stripes for which the child can fix consistently are considered to be the child's vision.
- *Fixation and following a target:* Fixation is essential for the development of vision and is present at birth. 75% of infants have this faculty at 2 weeks, and all normal children should develop this by 2 months. A newborn has preference for stimuli that are either moving objects or alternating light-patterned figures with contrasting colors. The best fixation is the mother's face.

  Flowchart 31.2 summarizes the fixation pattern with probable vision.
- *Pupillary reaction*: This is a gross indirect method of testing vision in children and infants, less accurate than fixation. Brisk pupillary reaction only denotes intact anterior (afferent) pathway. It does not exclude postgeniculate defect or presence of error of refraction. The ability to fix and follow a target is a better indicator of the presence of gross vision. A central and maintained fixation is the best indication of moderate vision.

Various methods employed to record vision in a child between 1 and 3 years (preschool) are the same as under 1 year with modification. It gives a better and more definite result than under 1 year, but not as accurate as in school going children.

Table 31.2 depicts the age of the child and reaction to stimuli.

Flowchart 31.1: Methods of testing vision in infants.

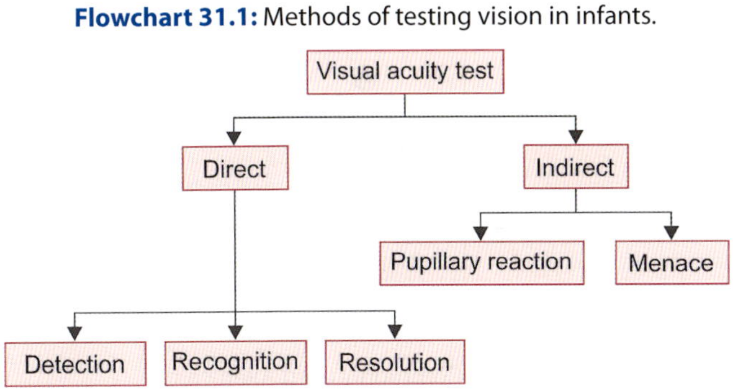

Flowchart 31.2: Importance of fixation in recording vision.

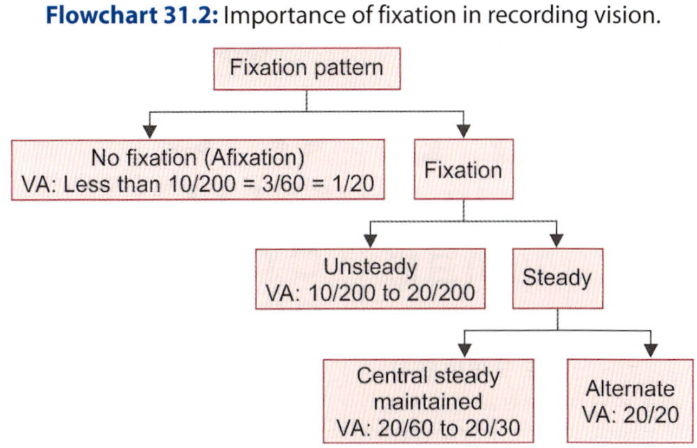

(VA: visual acuity)

TABLE 31.2: Reaction to various photo stimuli at various ages in children.

Age	*Reaction to various stimuli*
6 weeks	Smiles at faces brought near the eye, fixes, light and follows it
3 months	Converges, fixes a nonilluminated target, and follows a slowly moving target
6 months	Can grab small toys in visual field
2 years	Matches pictures (Allen card#, HOTV##)
3 years	Can match single letters in HOTV
5 years	Can read Snellen's chart*, tell various positions of E** and C***. Tumbling E**** is better understood than Landolt C

Snellen's chart* **(Fig. 31.1):

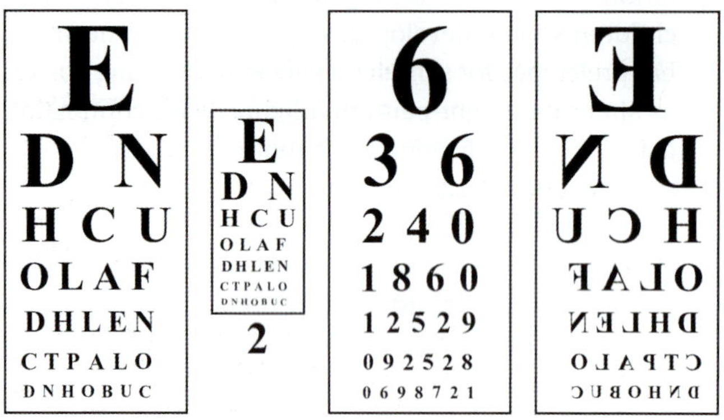

1 2 3 4

Fig. 31.1: Various types of Snellen charts. (1) Snellen's alphabetical chart; (2) Snellen's reduced chart; (3) Snellen's number chart; (4) Snellen's reversible chart.

Snellen alphabetic and number chart can be read at 6 meter or at 3 meter when proportionately reduced it can be in any language or in numbers **(Fig. 31.2)**.

***Snellen's "E" chart*   ****Landolt "C" chart*

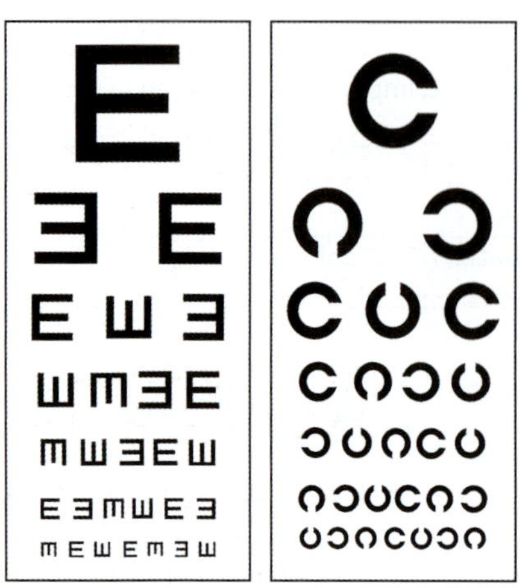

Fig. 31.2: Two types of nonalphabetic optotypes.

*****Tumbling "E"*:

Tumbling "E" chart: The construction of tumbling "E" is similar to that of Snellen's chart. It is used for illiterate/mute children **(Fig. 31.3)**. The child only has to indicate the direction of the E shown to at 3 meters. This is supposed to be as reliable as the Landolt "C" and "E" charts.

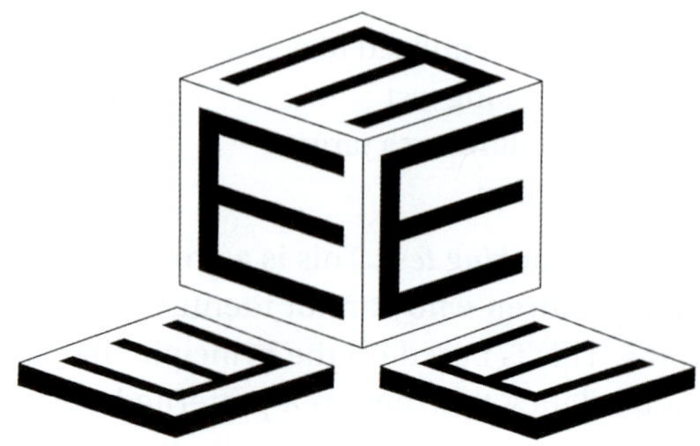

Fig. 31.3: Tumbling E chart.

#Allen card: Allen cards **(Fig. 31.4)** consist of a series of pictures of familial figures arranged in a ratio of 60:36:24:18:12. They can be used at 6 meters like a Snellen's chart or at 3 meters; the child is required to match the picture shown by the examiner in a chart held by the examiner. The chart is less accurate than Snellen's charts.

Fig. 31.4: Commonly used Allen card.

##HOTV:

HOTV chart: This is available in four, five, or seven numbers of letters arranged in a circle; the original test has only four letters, i.e., HOT and V; later, X was added to make it five letters **(Fig. 31.5)**. Still later, A and U were added to make the seven letters. The test is done at 3 meters, and the child either names the letter pointed at or matches on a card held in the hand of the examiner.

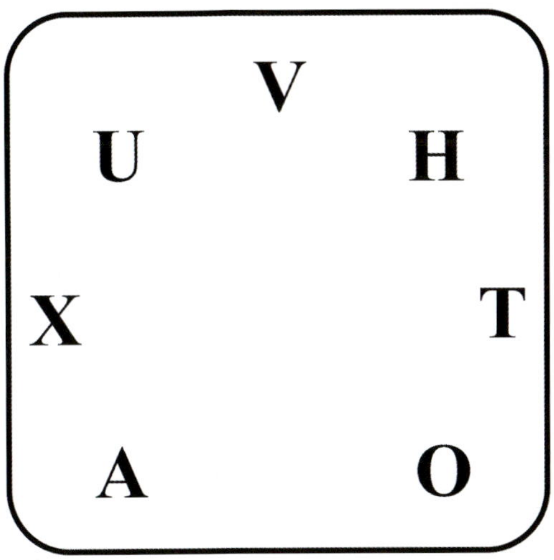

Fig. 31.5: Seven lettered HOTV chart.

LogMAR: LogMAR charts are a recent addition to an array of already existing vision testing charts. It was originally meant for assessment of progress of diabetic retinopathy, hence also known as the Early Treatment Diabetic Retinopathy Study Chart (ETDRS) **(Fig. 31.6)**.

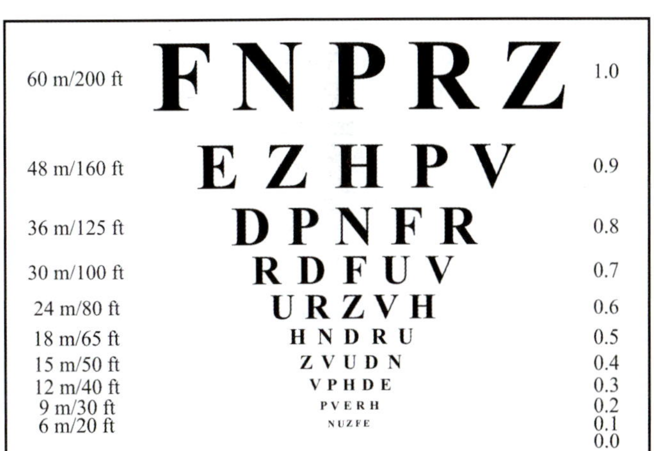

Fig. 31.6: A typical logMAR vision chart.
Note: MAR stands for minimum angle of resolution.

The logMAR chart is more suitable for mathematical calculation than the Snellen's chart. It is based on the logarithm of the minimal angle of resolution in contrast to the geometrical background of the Snellen chart. The logMAR chart was found to be more effective in recording distant vision in low vision, retinal disorders other than diabetic, and errors of refraction in children older than 5 years. It differs from Snellen's chart in many ways.

The differences are:

- The logMAR chart is used at 4 meters.
- It has five letter in each line.
- The number of letter in successive lines gradually becomes smaller.
- The top letters are largest.
- The total number of lines in each chart was 14 originally.
- This is in contrast to Snellen's chart:
  - That generally has seven lines.
  - The seventh line has seven letters.
  - The top line has only one letter that denotes 6/60.
  - The seventh line denotes 6/6.
  - The size of the optotypes in Snellen's chart gradually decreases in ratio of 60:36:24:18:12:9:6.
- The optotypes in logMAR can either be alphabets or Landolt "C" or Snellen's "E".
- The usual recommendation is to have three identical logMAR charts, one each for the right and left eye and the third for error of refraction.
- One of the advantages of a logMAR chart is that there is no crowding phenomenon with five letters in each line and the letters are equally legible.
- The difference between optotypes in the Snellen chart and logMAR is given below.

Table 31.3 describes vision as recorded on the Snellen chart and its equivalent in logMAR.

TABLE 31.3: Relation between optotypes of Snellen chart and logMAR.

Snellen chart	*LogMAR*
6/60	1.0
6/24	0.6
6/12	0.3
6/6	0.0

- If the child habitually fixes with one eye, the other eye has poor vision or uniocular mobility disorder, which can be confirmed by cover test.
- If the child resents occlusion of one eye, the other has poor vision in the uncovered eye* **(Fig. 31.7)**.
- A child with convergent squint, cross fixes**.
- A positive Bruckner test shows unilateral poor vision***.

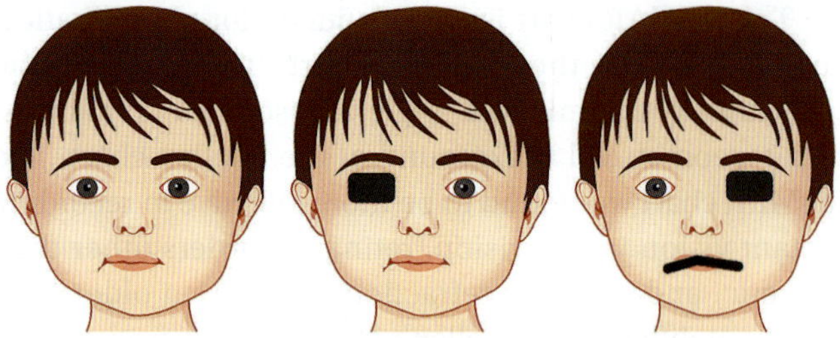

Fig. 31.7: Effects of occlusion of the better eye in a child with diminished vision in the other eye. (1*) Child with grossly diminished vision in right eye; (2*) Child does not resent covering right eye; (3*) Child resents covering normal seeing eye.

- **A child with conversant squint, cross fixes **(Fig. 31.8)**

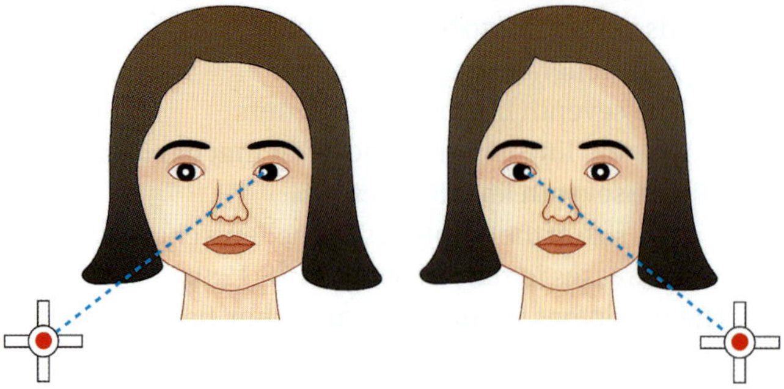

Fig. 31.8: *Cross fixation*: (1) Fixates object of right with left eye; (2) Fixates object of left with right eye.

- ***A positive Bruckner test shows unilateral poor vision

Bruckner test: Both eyes of the patient are simultaneously illuminated from approximately 1 meter distance by a direct ophthalmoscope. First, the position of the corneal light reflex (Hirschberg test) is noted, and then the brightness difference of the fundus reflex in two eyes through the ophthalmoscope is evaluated. When strabismus is present, the fixing eye has a darker reflex in comparison to the deviated eye **(Fig. 31.9)**.

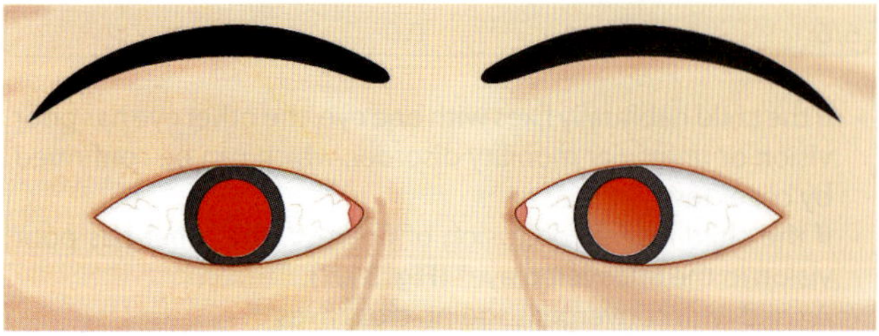

Fig. 31.9: A positive Bruckner test.

TABLE 31.4: Test perform at various ages in years.

Years	*Test*
0–1	Preferential looking test (PLT)
1–2	Cardiff card
2–4	Allen picture
4–8	Snellen's, logMAR
More than 8	As in adult

The gist of tests done to evaluate vision in children is given in ***Table 31.4***.

- Preferential looking test
- Optokinetic drum test of Hare Court
- OKNOVIS
- Catford drum*
- Teller acuity card**
- Cardiff acuity card***
- Boeck candy bead test****
- Visually evoked potential*****

The above test is divided on two principles:

1. Preferential looking
2. Optokinetic nystagmus#

The test based on preferential looking and its modifications are:

- Catford drum test
- OKNOVIS##
- Teller acuity card
- Cardiff acuity card

##*OKNOVIS test:* This is a recently developed test. The procedure has two parts. The first part is to induce optokinetic nystagmus by a especially designed drum. The second part is to introduce optotypes of gradually decreasing size till the nystagmus stops. The optokinetic drum has a fixed rate of 12 rpm. Held at 60 cm. It is an objective test; the vision recorded by this method cannot be converted to Snellen's fraction automatically.

**Catford drum test:* The principle of the test is similar to that of the optokinetic drum of Hare Court, where the usual drum of the optokinetic test is replaced by a circular disc with dots instead of strips of the optokinetic drum. The dots range from 0.5 to 15 mm that evoke a visual response between 6/6 and 2/60. The disc is revolved at a distance of 60 mm that evokes pendular movement and not nystagmus as is seen in OKT. The smallest target that evokes movement resents the vision. It is matched against Snellen's chart. The drawback with the test is that it may overestimate the vision; it is not suitable in amblyopic eyes.

**Teller acuity card:* This is a modification of the preferential looking test. It indicates quantitative grating acuity. The device is made up of 17 cards of 25.5 cm × 51 cm with squares of 12.5 × 12.5 cm in the first 15 cards, which are used for normal vision. The remaining two are low-vision cards. The 17th card is a blank gray card with no grating pattern. The first 15 cards are inscribed with alternate black lines of equal length and width; the size of the grating gradually decreases in steps of half octave.

An octave is having or doubling of spatial frequency.

It is a quantitative measure of grating acuity in infants and nonverbal young children.

The results are expressed in cycles, which are converted to Snellen's equivalent. It does not have a fixed testing distance. The distance varies with the age of the child. The child under 6 months is tested at 36 cm, while the distance is increased to 60 cm between 6 months and 3 years.

***Cardiff acuity card:* The test is a modified preferred-looking test in children between 6 months and 3 years nonverbal children of age and children with mental retardation. The device contains 36 test cards with familiar pictures in gradually decreasing size. To perform the test, the examiner presents the card with the largest picture at a distance of 0.5–1 meter at eye level to observe the eye movement. The smallest picture that stops the movement is roughly the vision.

****Boeck candy bead test:* This is a rough test to fine vision between 1 and 2 years. It is based on the observation that a child, when presented with candy beads of different sizes, picks up only that he can see. It consists of showing the child with an object that acts not only as an object of interest but it has an incentive. To beginning with the child's hand is guided to the candy and then to his mouth. The test is done at 40 cm; it can measure vision equal to 20/200 by this method. The size of the candy picked up regularly represents approximate vision.

*****Visually evoked potential (also known as visually evoked response—VER):* This is an objective test in contrast to the above tests, which are subjective, to record vision in all ages. It indirectly records the action potential of the visual cortex when stimulated by light on the retina. It denotes the integrity of the visual pathway beyond retinal ganglion cells. It is used when the fundus does not show any or very little changes or the media is opaque. It does not give an actual level of visual acuity; it only gives an approximate level of vision. It shows action potential of the visual cortex. The retina is represented in areas 17, 18, and 19 of the visual cortex. The macula occupies a disproportionately large area of the visual cortex; hence, the test results denote the integrity of central vision. The VER is the counterpart of the electroencephalogram; both are seen on an oscillograph and recorded as series of waves. In VER, electrodes are put on the occipital scalp nearest to the visual cortex. The test is evidence of abnormality, shown in amplitude and latency, but not the nature of disorder. Amplitude records the height of electric potential, while latency represents time in milliseconds. Amplitude is measured in μV. The types of stimuli used in VER are flash and patterned stimulus. The flash stimulus is a source of light with good intensity that is flashed on the eyes. The pattern stimulus consists of a flat square board on which alternate black and white squares of equal size are inscribed, resembling chess boards. The colors of the squares are interchangeable. Positive flash tests only denote the presence of light perception. Opacity in media does not affect the results. The pattern reversal result denotes the presence of form sense; hence, it can be taken as a gross estimation of visual acuity. In adults, it is used in—optic neuritis, ischemic optic neuropathy, compressive optic neuropathy, traumatic neuropathy, and evaluation macular disorder in the presence of ocular media. It can also be used to exclude malinger.

STYCAR test: This is used between 1- and 3-year-old children. It is based on the ability to recognize patterns of gradually decreasing optotypes. Called Snellen test for young children and retarded **(Fig. 31.10)**.

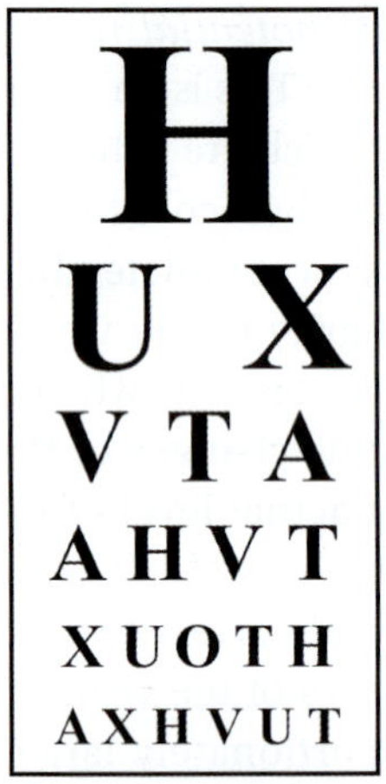

STYCAR

Fig. 31.10: Modify the Snellen test for young children and retarded.

[#]*Optokinetic nystagmus:* Newborns show bizarre ocular movement till fixation develops. This is physiological and should not be confused with nystagmus except in the case of idiopathic congenital nystagmus, which characteristically worsens on fixation. Once the child has developed fixation, he will try to fix bright stimulus in the field of fixation; hence, nystagmus can be elicited by passing successive alternate strips of contrasting colors, i.e., black and white, in front of the eyes as by optokinetic drum. Optokinetic nystagmus is a rhythmic involuntary conjugate ocular movement in response to the movement of full visual field images, either rotation of an image before the subject, such as a drum with vertical black stripes on a white background **(Fig. 31.11)**. The best results one obtained when alternate bands and white strips of the same width under the same illumination are used. Gradually the width of strips is narrowed, the narrowest strip that stops nystagmus is roughly the vision. This does not match the Snellen's test.

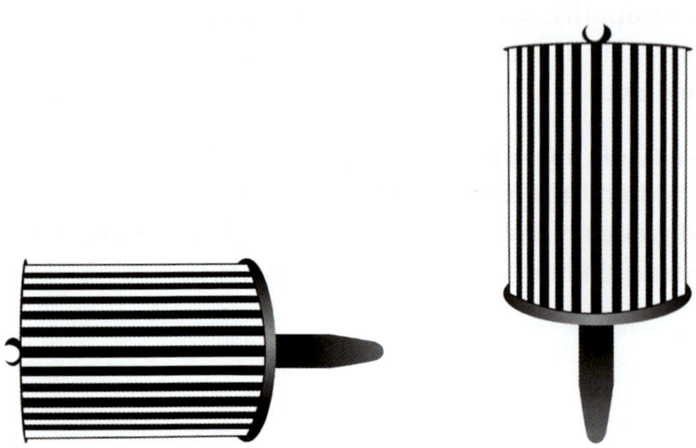

Fig. 31.11: Optokinetic drum.

Point to remember in recording vision infants:

- A newborn can perceive light.
- Will close eyes in the presence of bright light
- By 2 months can follow an object of interest
- May smile at mother's face brought near
- By 4 months, we will reach for an object held in front.
- By 6 months, I will play with the object in hand.
- Children develop good fixation by the age of 2 months.
- If the child under 1 year can pick up small bits of an object of 1 mm size at 35 cm, he has a visual acuity of roughly 6/24, but if the child tries to feel the bits before picking, he has poor vision.
- Vision should be tested at birth (6 months), 3 years, and 5 years.

Recording vision between 2 and 3 years: The vision is well developed by this time.

By this time, the child starts walking and negotiates between obstacles with ease, may reach for things in the field of vision.

Tumbling against obstacles in ambient light is a bad omen. The child most probably has a gross loss of vision.

By 3 years, the child is verbal; hence, the preferential looking test is no more relevant. The only test that can confirm presence of vision is visually evoked potential in such a child. A child may not cooperate on all optotypes. Optotypes suitable to be used at 3 meters are better than one used at 6 meters. Direct-looking optotypes are better than reversed charts. The best chart is the STYCAR test, which is especially made for young and retired children. Basically, it is a Snellen's chart. The HOTV test is the next best option.

Recording vision between 3 and 5 years: Recording vision in this age group is less cumbersome. By 3 years, children even in developing countries start going to primary schools and are acquaint with alphabets and numbers; hence, they can be tested on usual optotypes, i.e.:

- Snellen's chart
- Landolt C chart
- "E" chart
- STYCAR chart
- HOTV chart

The Snellen's charts used are mostly in English but can be in any vernacular language. The advantage of Snellen's E chart is that the letters have straight lines that prevent the child to guess.

Recording vision in a literate child is easy; he can be tested on the usual optotypes, E chart, or C chart at 6 meters or on a chart modified to be used at 3 meters. The testing can be done either directly or through a reversing mirror.

Difficulty arises examining an illiterate of mentally handicapped child; for them, most use full charts (STYCAR and HOTV charts). To examine them, it is essential to explain to the children what they are supposed to express; for this, there should be a smaller version of optotypes that should be shown to them at reading distance and explained how to express them. Thereafter they should be shown the larger optotypes kept at 6 meters or 3 meters defending on the size of optotypes.

Examination of near vision in children:

- Generally, near vision is not tested in children; on the contrary, parents may complain that the child keeps books too close to read; this happens in two situations, i.e., the child can afford to read from such a close quarter due to strong accommodation.
- The child has uncorrected myopia. The children with high uncorrected hypermetropia may complain of asthenopia and the running of letters. A child with albinism also keeps books too close; this gives marginal magnification and to overcome distortion produced by nystagmus, which is common in albinos. If a child complains of diminished near vision, the first is to test his refraction under complete cycloplegia; he may turn out to be a high hypermetropic with or without high estimation.

Other causes diminished near vision in children are:

- Uncorrectable distant vision
- Diminished convergence
- Diminished accommodation due to:
  - Drug induced
  - Internal ophthalmoplegia
- Nystagmus
- Reading disorder
- Malingering

> The most common iatrogenic cause of loss of near vision is use of strong cycloplegic.

SUGGESTED READING

1. All India Ophthalmological Society. (2017). All India Ophthalmological Society Guidelines. National, Expert-Based Consensus Statement Regarding Paediatric Eye Examination, Refraction, and Amblyopia Management. [online] Available from https://boamumbai.com/wp-content/uploads/2023/12/Paedamblopia.pdf. [Last accessed March, 2025].
2. Anstice NS, Thompson B. The measurement of visual acuity in children: an evidence-based update. Clin Exp Optom. 2014;97:3-11.
3. Bhartiya P, Sharma P, Biswas NR, Tendon R, Khokhar SK. Levodopa-carbidopa with occlusion in older children with amblyopia. J AAPOS. 2002;6(6):368-72.
4. Dadeya S, Kaur S. Visual Acuity Assessment in Children. Basic Examination of Strabismus. Delhi: Ophthalmic Society; 2021. pp. 5-13.
5. Diamond GR. "Evaluating vision in preverbal and preliterate infants and children." In: Yanoff M, Duker JS (Eds). Ophthalmology, 3rd edition. St Louis, MO, USA: Mosby (Elsevier Health Sciences); 2009. pp. 1309-12.
6. Duke Elder S, Cook C. Chronology of development in the system of ophthalmology, Volume 3, Part 2. London: Henry Kimpton; 1962.
7. Fern KD, Manny RE. Visual acuity of the preschool children: a review. Am J Optom Physiol Optics. 1986;63:314-45.
8. Flyon JT. Evaluation of visual function in neonates and infants. In: Harley RD (Ed). Paediatric ophthalmology, Volume 1, 2nd edition. Philadelphia: WB Saunders Company; 1983. pp. 1-25.
9. Ghauri AJ, Abbott J, Butler L. Ophthalmic assessment in children. In: Denniston KO, Murray PL (Eds). Oxford Handbook of Ophthalmology, 4th edition. London: Oxford University Press; 2018. pp. 862-7.
10. Gillian GWA, Bates A. Vision Assessment (Paediatric). In: Lackson TL (Ed). Moorfields Manual of Ophthalmology, 2nd edition. New Delhi: Jaypee Brothers Medical Publisher; 2020. pp. 625-6.
11. Hoyt CS, Nickel BL, Billson FA. Ophthalmological examination of the infant serve. Surv Ophthalmol. 1983;26:177-89.
12. Khurana AK. Theory and Practice of Optics and Refraction, 2nd edition. New Delhi: Elsevier; 2008. pp. 42-60.
13. Mukerjee PK. Examination of Eyes in Paediatric Age. In: Mukherjee PK (Ed). Clinical Examination in Ophthalmology, 2nd edition. New Delhi: Elsevier; 2016. pp. 382-4.
14. Mukerjee PK. Recording of Visual Acuity. In: Mukherjee PK (Ed). Ophthalmic Assistant, 1st edition. New Delhi: Jaypee Brothers Medical Publisher; 2013. pp. 108-213.
15. Mukherjee PK. Recording of Vision In: Mukherjee PK (Ed). Manual of Optics & Refraction, 1st edition. New Delhi: Jaypee Brothers Medical Publisher; 2015. pp. 131-40.
16. Prager TC, Zou YL, Jensen CL, Fraley JK, Anderson RE, Heird WC. Evaluation of methods for assessing visual function of infants. J AAPOS. 1999;3:275-82.
17. Saxena R, Sharma P; Paediatric Ophthalmology Expert Group. National consensus statement regarding paediatric

eye examination, refraction, and amblyopia management. Indian J Ophthalmol. 2020;68:325-32.
18. Saxena R, Singh D, Jethani J, Sharma P. AIOS guideline regarding paediatric eye examination. Indian J Ophthalmol. 2020;68(7):1300-5.
19. Sharma P. Visual Acuity Assessment in Strabismus Simplified, 1st edition. New Delhi: Modern Publishers; 1999. pp. 53-62.
20. Singh A, Sharma P, Saxena R. Evaluation of the Role of Monocular Video Game Play as an Adjuvant to Occlusion Therapy in the Management of Anisometropic Amblyopia. J Paediatr Ophthalmol Strabis. 2017;54(4):244-9.
21. Suttle CM. Visual acuity assessment in infants and young children. Clin Exp Optom. 2001;84:337-45.
22. Teller DY, McDonald M, Preston K, Sebris SL, Dobson V. Visual acuity in infants and children: the acuity card procedure. Dev Med Child Neurol. 1986;28:779.
23. Vijayalakshmi P. Paediatric Ophthalmology: A Practitioner's Guide. Maduri, India: Aravind Eye Care System; 2009.
24. Wallace DK, Morse CL, Michele M, Springer DK, Repka MX, Lee KZ, et al. Paediatric Eye Evaluations Preferred Practice Pattern: I. Vision Screening in the Primary Care and Community Setting; II Comprehensive Ophthalmic Examination-Preferred Practice Pattern. Ophthalmology. 2018;125:184-227.
25. Zwan JT. Does this baby see. In: Cibis GW (Ed). Decision Making in Paediatric Ophthalmology. California: Harcourt Brace; 1992. pp. 124-5.

Index

Page numbers followed by *b* refer to box, *f* refer to figure, *fc* refer to flowchart, and *t* refer to table.

A

B

D

E

F

I

J

K

L

N

O

P

Q

R

S

T

U

V